GLOBAL BURDEN OF DISEASE AND INJURY SERIES
VOLUME I

THE GLOBAL BURDEN OF DISEASE

A comprehensive assessment of mortality and disability from diseases, injuries, and risk factors in 1990 and projected to 2020

EDITED BY

CHRISTOPHER J. L. MURRAY
HARVARD UNIVERSITY
BOSTON, MA, USA

ALAN D. LOPEZ
WORLD HEALTH ORGANIZATION
GENEVA, SWITZERLAND

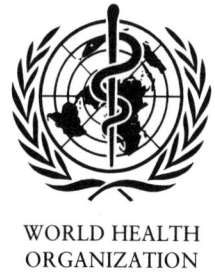

WORLD HEALTH
ORGANIZATION

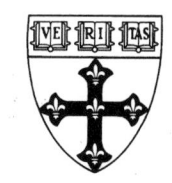

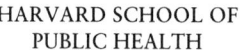

HARVARD SCHOOL OF
PUBLIC HEALTH

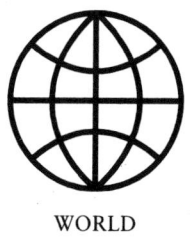

WORLD
BANK

PUBLISHED BY THE HARVARD SCHOOL OF PUBLIC HEALTH ON BEHALF OF
THE WORLD HEALTH ORGANIZATION AND THE WORLD BANK
DISTRIBUTED BY HARVARD UNIVERSITY PRESS

Library of Congress Cataloging-in-Publication (CIP) Data

    The global burden of disease : a comprehensive assessment of
mortality and disability from diseases, injuries, and risk factors in
1990 and projected to 2020 / edited by Christopher J.L. Murray and
Alan D. Lopez.
      p. cm. -- (Global burden of disease and injury series : v. 1)
    Includes bibliographical references and index.
    ISBN 0-674-35448-6
    1. World health-- Statistics. I. Murray, Christopher J. L.
II. Lopez, Alan D. III. Harvard School of Public Health. IV. World
Health Organization. V. World Bank. VI. Series.
    [DNLM: 1. Mortality--trends. 2. Disabled--statistics.
3. Health Status Indicators. 4. Risk Factors. WA 16 G561 1996]
RA441. G56 1996
614.4'2--dc20
DNLM/DLC
for Library of Congress   96-27266
                                                CIP

Printed in the United States of America

The authors alone are responsible for the views expressed in this publication.
    The designations employed and the presentation of the material in this publica-
tion do not imply the expression of any opinion whatsoever on the part of the
World Bank and the Secretariat of the World Health Organization concerning the
legal status of any country, territory, city or area or of its authorities, or concerning
the delimitation of its frontiers or boundaries.

TABLE OF CONTENTS

List of Tables

ANNEX TABLES

LIST OF FIGURES

FOREWORD TO
THE *GLOBAL BURDEN OF DISEASE AND INJURY SERIES*

RALPH H. HENDERSON

The collection and use of timely and reliable health information in support of health policies and programmes have been actively promoted by the World Health Organization since its foundation. Valid health statistics are required at all levels of the health system, ranging from data for health services support at the local community level, through to national statistics and information used to monitor the effectiveness of national health strategies. Equally, regional and global data are required to monitor global epidemics and to continuously assess the effectiveness of global public health approaches to disease and injury prevention and control, as coordinated by WHO technical programmes. Despite the clear need for epidemiological data, reliable and comprehensive health statistics are not available in many Member States of WHO, and, indeed, in many countries the ascertainment of disease levels, patterns and trends is still very uncertain.

In recent years, monitoring systems, community-level research and disease registers have improved in both scope and coverage. Simultaneously, research on the epidemiological transition has increased our understanding of how the cause structure of mortality changes as overall mortality rates decline. As a consequence, estimates and projections of various epidemiological parameters, such as incidence, prevalence and mortality, can now be made at the global and regional level for many diseases and injuries. The Global Burden of Disease Study has now provided the public health community with a set of consistent estimates of disease and injury rates in 1990. The Study has also attempted to provide a comparative index of the burden of each disease or injury, namely the number of Disability-Adjusted Life Years (DALYs) lost as a result of either premature death or years lived with disability.

The findings published in the *Global Burden of Disease and Injury Series* provide a unique and comprehensive assessment of the health of populations as the world enters the third millennium. We also expect that the methods described in the various volumes in the series will stimulate

Member States to improve the functioning and usefulness of their own health information systems. Nonetheless, it must be borne in mind that the results from an undertaking as ambitious as the Global Burden of Disease Study can only be approximate. The reliability of the data for certain diseases, and for some regions, is extremely poor, with only scattered information available in some cases. To extrapolate from these sources to global estimates is clearly very hazardous, and could well result in errors of estimation. The methods that were used for some diseases (e.g. cancer) are not necessarily those applied by other scientists or institutions (e.g. the International Agency for Research on Cancer) and hence the results obtained may differ, sometimes considerably, from theirs. Moreover, the concept of the DALY as used in this Study is still under development, and further work is needed to assess the relevance of the social values that have been incorporated in the calculation of DALYs, as well as their applicability in different sociocultural settings. In this regard, WHO and its various partners are continuing their efforts to investigate burden-of-disease measurements and their use in health policy decision-making.

Dr Ralph H. Henderson is Assistant Director-General of the World Health Organization.

FOREWORD TO
THE *GLOBAL BURDEN OF*
DISEASE AND INJURY SERIES

DEAN T. JAMISON

Rational evaluation of policies for health improvement requires four basic types of information: a detailed, reliable assessment of epidemiological conditions and the burden of disease; an inventory of the availability and disposition of resources for health (i.e. a system of what has become known as national health accounts); an assessment of the institutional and policy environment; and information on the cost-effectiveness of available technologies and strategies for health improvement. The *Global Burden of Disease and Injury Series* provides, on a global and regional level, a detailed and internally consistent approach to meeting the first of these information needs, that concerning epidemiological conditions and disease burden. It fully utilizes what information exists while, at the same time, pointing to great variation—across conditions and across countries—in data quality. In the *Global Burden of Disease and Injury Series*, Christopher Murray, Alan Lopez and literally scores of their collaborators from around the world present us with a *tour de force:* its (initial) 10 volumes summarize epidemiological knowledge about all major conditions and most risk factors; they generate assessments of numbers of deaths by cause that are consistent with the total numbers of deaths by age, sex and region provided by demographers; they provide methodologies for and assessments of aggregate disease burden that combine—into the Disability-Adjusted Life Year or DALY measure— burden from premature mortality with that from living with disability; and they use historical trends in main determinants to project mortality and disease burden forward to 2020. Publication of the *Global Burden of Disease and Injury Series* marks the transition to a new era of health outcome accounting—an era for which these volumes establish vastly higher standards for rigour, comprehensiveness and internal consistency. I firmly predict that by the turn of the century the official reporting of health outcomes in dozens of countries and globally will embody the approach and standards described in this series.

The *Global Burden of Disease and Injury Series* culminates an evolutionary process that began in the late 1980s. Close and effective collaboration between the World Bank and the World Health Organization initiated, supported and contributed substantively to that process.

BACKGROUND

Work leading to the *Global Burden of Disease and Injury Series* proceeded in three distinct phases beginning in 1988. Intellectual antecedents go back much further (see Murray 1996, or Morrow and Bryant 1995); perhaps the most relevant are Ghana's systematic assessment of national health problems (Ghana Health Assessment Project Team 1981) and the introduction of the QALY (quality-adjusted life year)—see, for example Zeckhauser and Shepard (1976). My comments here focus on the three phases leading directly to the *Global Burden of Disease and Injury Series*.

Phase 1 constituted an input to a four-year long "Health Sector Priorities Review" initiated in 1988 by the World Bank; its purpose was to assess "...the significance to public health of individual diseases (or related clusters of diseases)...and what is now known about the cost and effectiveness of relevant interventions for their control" (Jamison et al. 1993, p. 3; that volume provides the results of the review). Dr Christopher Murray of Harvard University introduced the DALY as a common measure of effectiveness for the review to use across interventions dealing with diverse diseases, and Dr Alan Lopez of the World Health Organization prepared estimates of child death by cause that were consistent with death totals provided by demographers at the World Bank (Lopez 1993). At the same time, and in close coordination, a World Bank effort was preparing consistent estimates for adult (ages 15–59) mortality by cause for much of the developing world (Feachem et al. 1992). Ensuring this consistency was a major advance and is a precondition for systematic attempts to measure disease burden. (Estimates of numbers of deaths by cause that are not constrained to sum to a demographically-derived total seem inevitably to result in substantial overestimates of deaths due to each cause.) Phase I of this effort, then, introduced the DALY and established important consistency standards to guide estimation of numbers of deaths by cause.

Phase 2 constituted the first attempt to provide a comprehensive set of estimates not only of numbers of deaths by cause but also of total disease burden including burden from disability. This effort was commissioned as background for the World Bank's *World Development Report 1993: Investing in Health*; it was co-sponsored by the World Bank and the World Health Organization; and it was undertaken under the general guidance of a committee chaired by Dr JP Jardel (then Assistant Director-General of WHO). The actual work was conceptualized, managed and integrated by Drs Murray and Lopez and involved extensive efforts by a large number of individuals, most of whom were on the WHO staff. First publication of the estimates of 1990 disease burden appeared in Appendix B of *Investing in Health* (World Bank 1993); the World Health Organization subsequently published a volume containing a full account of the methods used and a somewhat revised and far more extensive presentation of the results (Murray and Lopez 1994).

Preparation and publication of the *Global Burden of Disease and Injury Series* constitutes Phase 3 of this sequence of efforts. As in the earlier phases, the *Global Burden of Disease and Injury Series* was undertaken to inform a policy analysis—in this case an assessment of priorities for health research and development in developing countries being guided by WHO's Ad Hoc Committee on Health Research Relating to Future Intervention Options. The Committee sought updated estimates of disease burden for 1990, projections to 2020 and an extension of the methods to allow assessment of burden attributable to selected risk factors (volume IX of the *Global Burden of Disease and Injury Series*). The committee's report (Ad Hoc Committee 1996) and the *Global Burden of Disease and Injury Series* appear as companion documents.

Chapters summarizing results from the *Global Burden of Disease and Injury Series* appear in volume I, *The Global Burden of Disease;* underlying epidemiological statistics for over 200 conditions appear in volume II, *Global Health Statistics.* The next six volumes of the *Series* provide, for the first time, chapters detailing the data on each condition or cluster of conditions. These condition-specific chapters were extremely difficult to prepare under the constraints of time, consistency and comprehensiveness imposed by Murray and Lopez. (As co-author of the chapter on intestinal helminthiases I am well aware of the difficulties involved!) Yet the results, individually and collectively, enrich greatly the summaries that were hitherto published. The selection of subjects for the individual volumes—reproductive health, infectious diseases, non-communicable diseases, neurological and psychiatric disorders, injury and malnutrition—will make individual volumes of value to specialist communities. Volume IX reports on the burden due to selected risk factors. The tenth and final volume for the initial series—additional volumes are in the planning stage—reports country-specific analyses (the first of which, for Mexico, had been published previously by Lozano et al. 1994), describes applications of the analyses and introduces alternative methodological approaches.

Will there be a fourth phase? I am sure there will. Reporting of the disease-specific and risk factor analysis in the *Global Burden of Disease and Injury Series* will provoke constructive and perhaps substantial criticism and improvements; country-specific assessments will multiply (over 20 are now under way) and they, too, will modify and enrich current estimates. Country and global estimates for times in the past will most likely be prepared; estimates of years of life lost for the Unites States in 1900 have already been made (Jamison 1995). Methodologies will be criticized and, I would predict, constructively revised. Unfinished elements of the agenda discussed in the next section will be completed. Phase 4, perhaps centred on the estimation of global and regional disease burden for 1995 and including a look at the past, will take us well beyond where we now are.

THE AGENDA

Disease burden (or numbers of deaths by cause) can be partitioned in three separate ways for different age, sex and regional groupings (Murray et al. 1994). One partition is by *risk factor*—genetic, behavioural, environmental and physiological. The second is by *disease*. The third is by consequence—*premature mortality* at different ages and different *types of disability* (e.g. sensory, cognitive functioning, pain, affective state, etc.).

Disaggregation by risk factor helps guide policy concerning primary and secondary prevention, including development of new preventive measures. Disaggregation by disease helps guide policy concerning cure, secondary prevention and palliation; and disaggregation by consequence helps guide policies for rehabilitation.

Work on the disease burden assessment agenda began with assessments of mortality and burden by disease; the *Global Burden of Disease and Injury Series* advances the agenda in that domain by revising and adding great detail on disease burden estimates. Additionally the *Global Burden of Disease and Injury Series* makes a major advance by assessing burden due to selected major risk factors (Volume IX); this extends usefulness of the work to the domain of prevention policy.

There remains, however, an important unfinished agenda. The disease burden associated with different types of disability remains to be assessed; perhaps part of the reason for neglect of rehabilitation in most discussion of health policy is the lack of even approximate information on burden due to disability or on the DALY gains per unit cost of rehabilitative intervention.

A related agenda item—relevant to planning for curative and, particularly, rehabilitative intervention—is to present disease burden estimates from a current prevalence perspective. The dominant perspective of work so far undertaken, including in the *Global Burden of Disease and Injury Series*, is that of adding up over time the burden that will result from all conditions incident in a given year (here 1990); this well serves the development of primary prevention policy and of treatment policy for diseases of short duration. The prevalence perspective complements the incidence one by assessing how much burden is being experienced during a particular year by chronic conditions or by disabilities; those conditions or disabilities will often have been generated some time in the past. From an incidence perspective, disability in this year from, say, an injury occurring a decade ago would generate DALY loss in the year of incidence; but to guide investment in rehabilitation we need to know how much disability exists today, i.e., we need a prevalence perspective. Murray and Lopez in *The Global Burden of Disease* and in *Global Health Statistics* provide the basic estimates of prevalence of different disabilities and first glimpses of the prevalence perspective.

A final major agenda item is to establish for each condition and in the aggregate how much of the potential current burden is in fact being averted by existing interventions and how much of the remaining burden persists because of lack of any intervention, lack of cost-effective interventions, or because of inefficiency of the system.

USES OF DALYS AND DISEASE BURDEN MEASUREMENT

DALYs have six major uses to underpin health policy. Five of these relate to measurement of the burden of disease; the final one concerns judging the relative priority of interventions in terms of cost-effectiveness.

Assessing performance. A country-specific (or regional) assessment of the burden of disease provides a performance indicator that can be used over time to judge progress or across countries or regions to judge relative performance. These comparisons can be either quite aggregated (in terms of DALYs lost per thousand population) or finely disaggregated to allow focused assessment of where relative performance is good and where it is not. The *Global Burden of Disease and Injury Series* with its burden assessments for eight regions in 1990—and with the increasing number of country-specific assessments that it will report—will provide, I predict, the benchmark for all subsequent work. The most natural comparison is to the development of National Income and Product Accounts (NIPAs) by Simon Kuznets and others in the 1930s, which culminated in 1939 with a complete NIPA for the United Kingdom prepared by James Meade and Richard Stone at the request of the UK Treasury. NIPAs have, in the subsequent decades, transformed the empirical underpinnings of economic policy analysis. One of the leading proponents of major changes in NIPAs has put it this way:

> The national income and product accounts for the United States (NIPAs), and kindred accounts in other nations, have been among the major contributions to economic knowledge over the past half century.…Several generations of economists and practitioners have now been able to tie theoretical constructs of income, output, investment, consumption, and savings to the actual numbers of these remarkable accounts with all their fine detail and soundly meshed interrelations. (Eisner 1989)

My own expectation is that this series will, over a decade or two, initiate a transformation of health policy analysis analogous to that initiated for economic policy by the introduction of NIPAs in the late 1930s. Today most health policy work concerns only cost, finance, process and access; burden of disease (and risk factor) assessments should soon allow full incorporation of performance measures in policy analysis.

Generating a forum for informed debate of values and priorities. The assessment of disease burden in a country-specific context in practice involves participation of a broad range of national disease specialists, epidemiologists and, often, policy makers. Debating the appropriate values for, say, disability weights or for years of life lost at different ages helps clarify values and objectives for national health policy. Discussing the inter-relations among diseases and their risk factors in the light of local conditions sharpens consideration of priorities. And the entire process brings technically informed participants to the table where policy is discussed. The preparation of a well-defined product generates a process with much value of its own.

Identifying national control priorities. Many countries now identify a relatively short list of interventions, the full implementation of which becomes an explicit priority for national political and administrative attention. Examples include interventions to control tuberculosis, poliomyelitis, HIV infection, smoking and specific micronutrient deficiencies. Because political attention and administrative capacity are in relatively fixed and short supply, the benefits from using those resources will be maximized if they are directed to interventions that are both cost-effective and aimed at problems associated with a high burden. Thus, national assessments of disease burden are instrumental for establishing this short list of control priorities.

Allocating training time for clinical and public health practitioners. Medical schools offer a fixed number of instructional hours; training programmes for other levels and types of practitioners are likewise limited. A major instrument for implementing policy priorities is to allocate this fixed time resource well—again that means allocation of time to training in interventions where disease burden is high and cost-effective interventions exist.

Allocating research and development resources. Whenever a fixed effort will have a benefit proportional not to the size of the effort but rather to the size of the problem being addressed, estimates of disease burden become essential for formulation of policy. This is the case with political attention and with time in the medical school curriculum; and it is likewise true for the allocation of research and development resources. Developing a vaccine for a broad range of viral pneumonias, for example, would have perhaps hundreds of times the impact of a vaccine against disease from Hanta virus infection. Thus information on disease or risk factor burden is one (of several) vital inputs to inform research and development resource allocation. Indeed, as previously noted, this series—with its disease burden assessments for 1990, its projections to 2020 and its initial assessment of burden due to risk factors—was commissioned to inform a WHO Committee charged with assessing health research and development priorities for developing countries (Ad Hoc Committee 1996).

The Committee sought not only to know the burden by condition, but also to partition the burden remaining for each condition into several distinct parts reflecting the importance of the reasons for the remaining disease burden. This division into four parts was undertaken for several conditions; a major agenda item for future analysis is to undertake such a partitioning systematically for all conditions so that there could be reasonably approximate answers to such questions as "How much of the remaining disease burden cannot be addressed without major biomedical advances?" or, "How much of the remaining disease burden could be averted by utilizing existing interventions more efficiently?" Arguably most of the spectacular gains in human health of the past century have resulted from advances in knowledge (although improvements in income and education have also played a role). If so, improving research and development policy in health may be more important than improving policy in health systems or finance; improved assessments and projections of disease burden will be critical to that undertaking.

Allocating resources across health interventions. Here disease burden assessment often plays a minor role; the task is to shift resources to interventions which, at the margin, will generate the greatest reduction in DALY loss. When there are major fixed costs in mounting an intervention—as is the case with political and managerial attention for national control priorities—burden estimates are indeed required to optimize resource allocation. But, typically, much progress can be made with only an understanding of how the DALYs gained from an intervention vary with the level of expenditure on it; such assessments are the stuff of cost-effectiveness analysis. The DALY as a common measure of effectiveness allows comparison of cost-effectiveness across interventions addressing all conditions; such an initial effort was undertaken for the World Bank's "Health Sector Priorities Review" (Jamison et al. 1993) in the late 1980s using a forerunner to the DALY utilized in this series.

* * *

The *Global Burden of Disease and Injury Series* contains the only available internally consistent, comprehensive and comparable assessments of causes of death, incidence and prevalence of disease and injury, measures and projections of disease burden, and measures of risk factor burden. In that sense the authors' contributions represent a landmark achievement and provide an invaluable resource for policy analysts and scholars. This effort dramatically raises the standard by which future reporting of health conditions will be judged. Yet, the very need for the ad hoc assessments that the volumes in this series report, points to important gaps in the international system for gathering, analysing and distributing policy-relevant data on the health of populations. Without information on how levels and trends in key indicators in their own countries compare with other countries, national decision-makers will lack benchmarks for judging performance. Likewise students of health systems will lack the empirical basis for forming outcome-based judgements on which policies work—and which do not. I hope, then, that one follow-on to the *Global*

Burden of Disease and Injury Series will be the institutionalization of continued efforts to generate and analyse internationally comparable data on health outcomes.

Dean T. Jamison is Professor of Public Health and of Education at the University of California, Los Angeles, and Economic Adviser to the Human Development Department of the World Bank. He recently served as Chairman of the World Health Organization's Ad Hoc Committee on Health Research Relating to Future Intervention Options.

REFERENCES

Ad Hoc Committee on Health Research Relating to Future Intervention Options (1996) *Investing in health research and development.* World Health Organization. Geneva (Document TDR/Gen/96.1).

Eisner R (1989) *The total incomes system of accounts.* Chicago, University of Chicago Press.

Feachem RGA et al., eds. (1992) *The health of adults in the developing world.* New York, Oxford University Press for the World Bank.

Ghana Health Assessment Project Team (1981) A quantitative method of assessing the health impact of different diseases in less developed countries. *International journal of epidemiology,* 10: 73–80.

Goerdt A et al. (1996) Disability: definition and measurement issues. In: Murray CJL and Lopez AD, eds., *The global burden of disease: a comprehensive assessment of mortality and disability from diseases, injuries, and risk factors in 1990 and projected to 2020.* Cambridge, Harvard University Press.

Jamison DT et al., eds. (1993) *Disease control priorities in developing countries.* New York, Oxford University Press for the World Bank.

Jamison JC (1995) The mortal burden: disability adjusted life years lost to premature mortality in the United States in 1900. Economic history paper, MIT Department of Economics.

Lopez AD (1993) Causes of death in industrial and developing countries: estimates for 1985–1990. In: Jamison DT et al., eds. *Disease control priorities in developing countries.* New York, Oxford University Press for the World Bank, 35–50.

Lozano R et al. (1994) *El peso de la enfermedad en México: un doble reto.* [The national burden of disease in México: a double challenge.] Mexico, Mexican Health Foundation, (Documentos para el análisis y la convergencia, No. 3).

Morrow RH, Bryant JH (1995) Health policy approaches to measuring and valuing human life: conceptual and ethical issues. *American journal of public health,* 85(10): 1356–1360.

Murray CJL (1996) Rethinking DALYs. In: Murray CJL and Lopez AD, eds., *The global burden of disease: a comprehensive assessment of mortality and disability from diseases, injuries, and risk factors in 1990 and projected to 2020.* Cambridge, Harvard University Press.

Murray CJL and Lopez AD, eds. (1994) *Global comparative assessments in the health sector: disease burden, expenditures and intervention packages.* Geneva, World Health Organization.

Murray CJL, Lopez AD, Jamison DT (1994) The global burden of disease in 1990: summary results, sensitivity analysis and future directions. *Bulletin of the World Health Organization*, 72(3):495–509.

World Bank (1993) *World development report 1993: investing in health.* New York, Oxford University Press for the World Bank.

World Health Organization. *World health statistics annual*, various years. Geneva, WHO.

Zeckhauser R, Shepard D (1976) Where now for saving lives? *Law and contemporary problems*, 40:5–45.

FOREWORD

WILLIAM H. FOEGE

"You don't have to know where you are to be there, but it is helpful to know where you are if you wish to be someplace else." In public health there has been a great desire to move health to ever higher levels even when we could not measure accurately where we were.

If knowledge is power, the field of public health has remained incredibly weak. Compared with the extensive information on history, physical findings, biochemical tests and x-rays often available to a clinician for a specific patient, collective knowledge about the health conditions of a group, city, country, region or continent is often fragmentary. It is so fragmentary, in fact, that it is remarkable that we have done as well as we have. Our surveillance systems, with few exceptions, have been incomplete, inaccurate and heavily biased towards mortality because of the relative ease of acquiring figures on death compared to those on morbidity.

In the United States, the first nation-wide surveillance system to measure the burden for any disease was not implemented until 1950 when malaria surveillance was developed. It was a surprise to find that malaria had quietly disappeared in the 1940s, and that no one had realized it. Such was the quality of our information. It took five more years until the second surveillance system was initiated, this time for poliomyelitis. It was the crisis of a vaccine problem that prompted the evaluation, but the programme proved so valuable that it was continued. It was not until 1957 that a third surveillance system was inaugurated, that for influenza. The utility of national surveillance in identifying and responding to health problems has led to the institution of comprehensive surveillance on the morbidity and mortality from dozens of conditions.

Many developing countries find it difficult to acquire accurate mortality statistics, let alone morbidity and quality-of-life information. There are exceptions, of course. Smallpox surveillance systems provided all the information required to eliminate the problem. Surveillance for guinea worm and poliomyelitis is rapidly becoming sufficient to eradicate both conditions before the end of the century. Yet many countries face difficulties in accurately determining infant mortality rates, or even AIDS and tuberculosis incidence and prevalence rates, let alone acquiring a comprehensive understanding of the total burden of disease—or its constituent parts—they face. Better information on the burden of disease cannot guarantee appropriate decisions on the use of public health resources, but the probability of good decisions certainly decreases with inferior information.

The *World Development Report 1993*, published by the World Bank, was an exciting revelation for international health workers, but it has also provided a revolution in thinking. Albert Schweitzer reminded us that "Pain is a more terrible lord of mankind than even death itself," prompting the dream of public health workers for a metric that would account for suffering as well as death and provide a way of comparing disease problems in a quantitative way. The report made that dream a possibility. The approach of Disability-Adjusted Life Years (DALYs) reaffirmed and quantified the size of the burden of illness globally, focusing attention on the discrepancies in health between regions of the world (and subsequently as well within countries). In addition, it provided comfort to those challenged to make adequate decisions with inadequate information by showing how good those past choices had been when made in favour of immunization programmes, diarrhoeal disease control programmes, micronutrient supplementation, respiratory infection treatment, etc. But the report also showed that there was better information with which to approach these problems. It gave value to some health care delivery activities that public health practitioners would have ignored.

The *World Development Report 1993* demonstrated that DALYs are to current surveillance systems what Global Positioning Devices are to the guesses made about location by early explorers. They provide a more precise and sophisticated guidance system for our daily activities. Who would want to go back to the guesses on disease burden and the relative importance of different conditions which informed health decisions of even the last decade?

The Global Burden of Disease Study, described in this volume and in subsequent volumes of the *Global Burden of Disease and Injury Series*, takes additional major steps in improving this "Global Positioning Device" and its accuracy and usefulness, by heeding the suggestions and criticisms that have followed the *World Development Report 1993*. In addition it rationalizes the approach and teaches those of us who are practitioners of public health how to use this common international language.

For those still critical of the approach, the challenge is to show a better way. For those of us enthusiastic about one of the great developments in public health, the challenge is to ensure implementation, widespread use, better decisions on resource allocation, and the development of feedback mechanisms to make health information precise, timely, and useful in improving the quality of lives, providing more equitable health within and between countries and ensuring a more rational health future for everyone.

William H. Foege, M.D., M.P.H. is a Fellow for Health Policy at The Carter Center.

Preface

In an era in which the gap between people's expectations for health and health-care resources is widening, prioritization of health actions has become increasingly important. In most decision-making arenas, priorities are determined by many factors such as budgetary inertia (where programmes this year are those funded last year), vocal political constituencies, the effects of past investment decisions in hospitals or other infrastructure, funding agency agendas, perceived public health crises and maximizing health gain for the population given the available resources. While improving the people's health may not be the sole, or even dominant, basis on which priorities are established, information on the magnitude of different health problems (diseases, injuries or risk factors) and an understanding of the cost-effectiveness of different options for intervention can have a powerful influence on health sector priorities. Quantification sets boundaries on the claims made in health policy debates and, in some cases, can put new problems and intervention options on the agenda.

To inform health policy debates, epidemiological information may be required at all levels of health systems. Compilations of mortality and morbidity statistics at the national and sub-national levels have been published by many countries, in some cases for more than 100 years. However, to our knowledge, there does not exist a publication giving comparable regional and global estimates and projections of disease and injury burden based on a common set of methods and denominated in a common metric, despite the clear need for it. This book is an attempt to meet that need.

In describing and documenting the methods and main findings of the Global Burden of Disease Study (GBD), we have tried to address the interests and needs of two audiences. Those readers who wish to use this book as a reference on the global and regional patterns of ill-health are directed to the introductory comments, results and discussion sections of each chapter herein. For those readers interested in technical discussions of the analytical bases of the GBD, the more detailed and, at times, lengthy methods sections will be of interest.

The book is divided into two parts. In the first part, seven chapters provide the conceptual underpinnings, methods and results of the GBD. A series of detailed Annex tables are provided in the second part of the book. These tables give the reader access to complete detail of the study results by age, sex, region and cause.

The first two chapters—by Murray and by Goerdt and colleagues, respectively—outline the concepts and methods used to develop a single measure of health outcome, namely the Disability-Adjusted Life Year (DALY). Chapter 1 by Murray describes in considerable detail the conceptual framework from which DALYs have been developed. Most of the chapter is devoted to an analysis of social preferences which are incorporated into measures of population health status: the duration of life lost due to a death at each age, the valuation of time lived with various disabilities compared to time lost due to premature mortality, discounting future health, the relative importance of years of life lived at different ages, and the distributions within populations of years of life lost or years lived with disability. After reviewing the extensive literature on each of these topics, the particular and at times arbitrary approach taken in formulating DALYs is outlined and justified. The chapter ends with a series of general formulae for calculating the two classes of DALYs: Years of Life Lost due to premature mortality (YLLs); and Years Lived with Disability adjusted for the severity of disability (YLDs). These formulae will facilitate testing the sensitivity of any DALY-based analysis to the various social preferences incorporated into the analysis. Chapter 2, by Goerdt, Koplan, Robine, Thuriaux and van Ginneken, provides an alternative perspective on the various conceptual frameworks used in the measurement of disability, including that of the International Classification of Impairments, Disabilities and Handicaps (ICIDH), health-related quality of life, and the welfare economics framework emerging from the work by health economists on quality-adjusted life years (QALYs).

The burden of any condition can be divided into two components: the years of life lost due to premature mortality and the years of life lived with disability. In the absence of reliable vital registration systems for much of the developing world, various methods have been employed to estimate mortality by age, sex, cause and region, as described in Chapter 3 by Murray and Lopez. Plausible estimates of mortality by cause have been constructed based on compilations of nearly 14 million death certificates, epidemiological estimates of the importance of each cause (described in the disease-specific chapters in other volumes of the *Global Burden of Disease and Injury Series*), and several indirect methods developed for this study. The methods section of Chapter 3 reports on several sub-studies in which we and other colleagues, most importantly Rafael Lozano, have developed new methods for cause-of-death analysis and estimation. These sub-studies include analyses of probable cardiovascular disease miscoding, the inequalities in death distributions across geographic sub-units, cause-of-death models, methods for quantifying deviations of actual cause-of-death patterns from expected patterns, and estimates of neonatal mortality by region. The results and discussion sections of this chapter highlight the major patterns in cause-specific mortality that emerged from the GBD. Estimates of deaths and YLLs by age, sex, region and cause are provided in the Annex.

In Chapter 4, Murray and Lopez present the methods and results of the estimation of years of life lived with disability, adjusted for the severity of disability (YLDs) in 1990. The methods section emphasizes the use of internal consistency checks on estimates from disease experts in order to develop plausible evaluations of the incidence, prevalence, and average duration of some 483 sequelae of the 107 diseases and injuries included in the GBD. The sources of the data used to estimate these epidemiological parameters for each sequela from each disease or injury are discussed in detail in the respective disease and injury specific chapters in Volumes III-VIII of the *Global Burden of Disease and Injury Series*. In addition to the quantification of non-fatal health outcomes required for the calculation of DALYs, the chapter provides, for the first time, global and regional estimates of the prevalence of disabilities, by severity class. Additionally, the chapter provides global and regional estimates for a variety of measures of health expectancy including disability-free life expectancy and Disability-Adjusted Life Expectancy (DALE).

The main findings of the Global Burden of Disease Study for 1990, where the burden of premature mortality and non-fatal health outcomes are combined, are described by Murray and Lopez in Chapter 5. The sensitivity of the main findings of the GBD to changes in the underlying social values incorporated into DALYs is analysed—i.e. the discount rate, the age-weighting function, and disability weights. The effect of changing the epidemiological perspective incorporated in DALYs—from the incidence perspective to the prevalence perspective—is also explored. An important conclusion to emerge from this analysis is that the uncertainty associated with selected epidemiological parameters, such as incidence or duration, is much more significant than the effect of changing any of the social preferences incorporated into DALYs.

In Chapter 6, Murray and Lopez summarize the application of the DALY approach to the quantification of the impact of selected risk factors in 1990. Analyses of ten risk factors have been undertaken by experts in the field. Chapter 6 provides a summary of the results presented in full detail in Volume IX of the *Global Burden of Disease and Injury Series*: *Quantifying Global Health Risks*. The ten risk factors analysed include the major addictive substances (tobacco, alcohol, and other drugs), environmental exposures and other individual behaviours. Methods used to assess attributable fractions for each risk factor are briefly reviewed but the major emphasis in the chapter is on the results and their implications.

Although the assessments of burden attributable to various risk factors are crude, such information is a critical input to global health policy debate.

Projections of causes of death and DALYs to the year 2020 are provided by Murray and Lopez in Chapter 7. A simple model for nine major clusters of causes relating age-specific death rates to a limited set of socio-economic variables is developed in the chapter. Three alternative scenarios are projected based on pessimistic, baseline and optimistic forecasts for changes in the socio-economic independent variables. The chapter distinguishes between changes in the burden of disease that are likely due to demographic change and the effects of other changes, such as the epidemic of smoking-related mortality, that are expected as a result of changes in the *risk* of disease or injury arising from epidemiological factors.

By bringing together the extensive detail on the methods and findings of the Global Burden of Disease Study into one summary volume, we hope to provide policy-makers, scientists, public health specialists and the public with a convenient reference book describing global health status in 1990, with projections of some indicators into the 21st century. Certainly, an undertaking as ambitious as that described in the following pages must contain errors and inconsistencies which, despite all efforts to identify and correct them, have escaped detection. Undoubtedly, some methodological aspects of the GBD could be improved, and, as our understanding of the science of the epidemiological transition and the determinants of disease improves, they will be. It is our hope that if the estimates and methods are made widely available, they will be used, scrutinized and improved. For in this way, the question of whether the estimates are right or wrong will become secondary to the more fundamental issue of whether or not they prove useful for promoting public health.

CJLM
ADL

Acknowledgements

An undertaking such as this book is simply not possible without the support and contribution of many individuals and institutions throughout the world. A large number of scientists, both within the World Health Organization and elsewhere, provided epidemiological data, research reports, and other information on specific diseases and injuries, which greatly facilitated the preparation of regional estimates published in this book. Many, but not all, of those involved have authored chapters on their particular disease that appear in other volumes of the *Global Burden of Disease and Injury Series*. The cooperation of several scientific organizations, government research institutes and non-governmental organizations in providing datasets and advice on their reliability is also gratefully acknowledged.

We wish to acknowledge particularly the dedication, long days and long nights, and truly extraordinary contribution made by Steven Goodreau, Caroline Cook, Emmanuela Gakidou, Joshua Salomon, Robert Ashley, William Whang, Arnab Acharya, Xinjian Qiao, Rafael Lozano, Bonifasiyo Ssenyamantono, Catherine Michaud, Prasanta Mahapatra, Kenji Shibuya, and Andrina Ngo at the Burden of Disease Unit, Harvard Center for Population and Development Studies. Input from the large number of collaborators based in the United Kingdom was coordinated by Jonathan Broomberg, Julian Lob-Levyt and Sharon Huttly. Their time and committment to reviewing the material were invaluable to the success of this project. Helpful comments and suggestions were provided by several WHO staff. Theo Vos provided valuable suggestions on measuring disability from injuries and on other aspects on disability.

A special acknowledgement is due to Dean Jamison who inspired all of this.

This work would not have been possible without the financial support of the Edna McConnell Clark Foundation, the Rockefeller Foundation, and the World Bank. We wish to specifically acknowledge the collegial environment and financial support provided by the WHO Ad Hoc Committee on Health Research Relating to Future Intervention

Options. Although the preparation of the *Global Burden of Disease and Injury Series* began prior to the Committee's establishment, these books describe in some detail the analytical basis of the Committee's Report, and are thus complementary to it.

The secretarial support of Marie-Claude von Rulach is gratefully acknowledged. Many other individuals have provided critical comments and suggestions on various aspects of this study. We particularly wish to acknowledge Seth Berkley, Jose Luis Bobadilla, Sissela Bok, Patricia Butler, Lincoln Chen, Tim Evans, Richard Feachem, Julio Frenk, Tore Godal, Ralph Henderson, Jean-Paul Jardel, Jeff Koplan, Juan Luis Londoño, Richard Peto, and Jim Tulloch.

While these individuals and institutions played a substantial role in the preparation of this book, they are not responsible for the estimates reported herein. Rather, these numbers represent the outcome of a long series of discussions with scientists, and we alone assume responsibility for their accuracy and plausibility.

We wish to particularly thank our wives, Agnes and Lene, and our families for their understanding, encouragement, and support throughout the nearly five years of this undertaking.

CJLM
ADL

Chapter 1

RETHINKING DALYs

CHRISTOPHER J. L. MURRAY

The Global Burden of Disease Study (GBD) began in 1992 with the objective of quantifying the burden of disease and injury on human populations. Quantification requires a unit of measure and this chapter is devoted to exploring the rationale for such health-outcome measures. Building on three decades of work on time-based measures of health status that incorporate non-fatal health outcomes, Disability-Adjusted Life Years (DALYs) were developed as the measurement unit for the Global Burden of Disease Study (Murray 1994). The publication, wide dissemination and subsequent use of DALYs has prompted considerable discussion in the literature and in various international forums (see for example Anand and Hanson 1995, Arellano 1996, Barker and Green 1996, Berman 1995, Desjarlais et al. 1995, Fernandez et al. 1995, Finlay et al. 1995, Foege 1993, Karkal 1995, Kleinman and Kleinman 1996, Laurell and Lopez 1996, Lozano et al. 1995, Martens et al. 1995, Morrow and Bryant 1995, Politi et al. 1995, Schwuebel 1994, Shepard 1994, Ugalde and Jackson 1995, Werner 1994).[1,2] The publication in this volume of the final results of the GBD for 1990 provides an opportunity to rethink the basis and design of DALYs. In this chapter, the logical thread, which at times is tortuous, that ties together DALYs is outlined, some important modifications are proposed, and some future directions that may usefully be pursued are suggested.

To understand the rationale for DALYs, the overall goals of this five-year exercise in quantifying the burden of disease must be kept in mind. The study had three major objectives. The first objective was to facilitate the inclusion of non-fatal health outcomes in debates on international health policy, which were all too often focused on mortality in children under 5 years of age. Second, we wanted to decouple epidemiological assessment from advocacy so that estimates of the mortality or disability from a condition are developed as objectively as possible. Decision-makers at the national and international level are frequently presented with evaluations of the burden of a disease or injury that have been produced by groups advocating a particular policy change. What they require are independent objective evaluations. Third, we wanted to quantify the burden of disease using a measure that could also be used for cost-effectiveness analysis. The power of using a common metric for burden assessment and economic appraisal of intervention options warranted the difficulties of crafting a measure for both purposes. While recognizing this third objective, the primary focus of this chapter will be on the development of an appropriate measure of the burden of disease and injury.

LAYING THE GROUNDWORK

Five key social choices are explicitly or implicitly incorporated in any burden measure. Before embarking on a detailed analysis of these five choices, two issues need to be addressed. Should DALYs be designed as a positive or normative measure? And what is the parent intellectual tradition for DALYs—welfare, human rights, capabilities, or "justice as fairness"? To forewarn the reader, a fully worked out maximalist view of human worth is not proposed; rather, a less satisfying but more pragmatic approach somewhere between the various major traditions is used.[3]

NORMATIVE OR POSITIVE MEASURES OF HEALTH

Economists like to draw a sharp distinction between positive analysis, in which no value choices are incorporated, and normative analysis, in which value choices are included.[4] Is a measure of the burden of disease—the gap between a population's health status and some reference standard—a positive or normative measure? One could reasonably argue that quantifying units of time lost due to premature death and time "lost" due to non-fatal health outcomes is a purely positive exercise. Going on to use such an indicator to influence how health problems are prioritized and ultimately how resources for health improvement are allocated would, of course, be a normative exercise. While theoretically correct, the distinction between the positive nature of a health indicator and the normative use of a health indicator to influence resource allocation may be difficult to maintain. Two recent examples will illustrate the difficulty of sustaining a sharp distinction between the positive design of a health or development indicator and its normative use.

The infant mortality rate (IMR), the proportion of live newborns who die before their first birthday, would, at first glance, appear to be a purely positive measure. It is routinely published, although not so routinely measured, in various international compendiums each year (UNICEF 1995, World Bank 1995).[5] The infant mortality rate is often advocated as a "sensitive" measure of population health status, supposedly a type of early warning indicator of general health conditions. The World Health Organization encourages governments to set explicit targets for a decrease in the infant mortality rate as a primary objective of public policy (World Health Organization 1981). Perhaps initially a "sensitive" indicator of general health status, the IMR over the past two decades has become an object of public policy. Many governments, with urging from UNICEF and the World Health Organization, have set explicit goals for the health sector in terms of reductions in the IMR and improvements in their position in league tables of the IMR. At the margin, decision-makers have therefore become more interested in policies that specifically target infants and reduce the IMR than policies which benefit other groups. What may have been initially a purely positive indicator has become a normative measure because it is widely used and influences policy choice.

Another case-study of the normative uses of new indicators is the Human Development Index (United Nations Development Programme 1991). Published annually in the *Human Development Report* (United Nations Development Programme 1995), the Human Development Index (HDI) is approximately the average of life expectancy, literacy and income per capita.[6] Already, the United Nations Development Programme and some governments are articulating goals for public policy in terms of the HDI and trying to measure achievements towards these goals by the change in the HDI. At some point in the policy debate, the HDI shifts from being an indicator of development to an object of development policy. These normative uses bring into sharp focus the equal weights assigned to life expectancy, literacy and income in the calculation of the HDI. Perhaps, people care much more about life expectancy or income than literacy. If this is the case, maximizing the HDI may not be as desirable to some groups as maximizing some alternatively weighted combination of life expectancy, income and literacy.

Paradoxically, if a measure is used, it will influence policy debate, permeate the thinking of decision-makers and become part of the culture of the subject. In other words, an indicator that is widely used will soon become normative through its use. The infant mortality rate, life expectancy and, to the extent they are adopted, DALYs, are used normatively and thus become normative measures. The normative aspects of indicators should be recognized clearly in the design of an indicator. This is not to suggest that the proponent of a new indicator bears responsibility for all intended or unintended uses of the measure *in perpetuo*. Rather, it is prudent to recognize the normative shadow that health measures cast and to try to reason carefully about their likely normative uses and the implications of such uses for the design of health indicators.

A FRAMEWORK FOR THINKING ABOUT THE NORMATIVE ASPECTS OF DALYs

An intellectually satisfying and academically secure approach to developing a measure of the burden of disease would be to start with a given conception of "goodness"[7] and proceed to develop an indicator. A welfarist might choose to design an indicator of burden based on assigning a value to each health event according to its contribution to welfare loss. An advocate of human rights might believe that the right to life has lexicographic dominance over a right to a better quality of life and propose the crude death rate as the best measure of burden. Perhaps, someone inspired by Rawls would argue for a measure that emphasizes the health conditions of those who have the worst health.[8] A soldier for the one true conception of the good (that he or she believed in) would march to battle for the indicator founded on his or her maximalist system of beliefs.

The advantages of such soldiering are clear: internal consistency, intellectual elegance and the appeal of the proselytizing missionary. The disadvantages, however, are great. The resulting measure of health may well be unappealing to those who disagree with the starting maximalist position. If the purpose of studying the burden of disease is to enhance debate over the appropriate objects of health policy and to create a common mode of communication about the magnitude of different health problems and the costs versus benefits of alternative efforts to improve health, the maximalist approach may well be self-defeating. It was not and is not my intention to argue through the design of DALYs for any particular conception of the good life. Rather, I have sought an approach which a large proportion of society might accept as reasonable even if it cannot wholly endorse it.

The work on common values (Bok 1995) provides a useful parallel.[9] Bok argues that a minimalist common value set is needed for societies "to have some common ground for cross-cultural dialogue and for debate about how best to cope with military, environmental, and other hazards that, themselves, do not stop at such boundaries." (Bok 1995, p.13). Common values are not simply the values of the majority (whether tyrannical or benevolent). Rather, they are a set of minimal values that nearly everyone in a society recognizes as legitimate for their own but that have not been universally applied in society.

Another way of thinking about developing an acceptable set of values that generally reflects a consensus of society but goes beyond is exposed by Goodin (1986). He argues for "laundering of preferences":

> Want regarding moralities are continually embarrassed by the fact that some preferences are so awfully perverse as to forfeit any right to our respect....We want to bring 'non-utility information' to bear on the social choice, most especially in the form of vested rights guarantees protecting people from the meddlesome (or, indeed, sadistic) preferences of others....Recourse to non-utility information seems necessary merely because we work with such an impoverished conception of individual preferences in the first place. For the most part, they are just taken to be an individual's rankings of various social states. Whatever underlies this ordering ordinarily goes undiscussed. But, in truth, there is much more to individual utilities than is captured by simple numbers and rank-orderings. 'Utility information' can and should be seen to include information about why individuals want what they want, about the other things they also want, about the interconnections between and implications of their various desires, etc....The ultimate goal of

> enriching our utility information in this way is to use it to launder
> people's preferences. (Goodin 1986, p.75–77)

The common values approach and Goodin's laundering of preferences
share an uneasy position. In both, a clear set of internally consistent first
principles is not defined. Goodin provides five arguments why individuals' revealed preferences should be laundered for reasons still consistent
with individual wants, but he recognizes that "Ultimately, we may want
to launder preferences more thoroughly than we can find internal justifications for doing, and will be forced to fall back on ideal-regarding principles to do so."(p.86)[10] One might ask why we do not construct an
approach with reference to these ideal regarding principles in the first
place. Common values projects can likewise be challenged. But Bok (1995)
defends them:

> A constructivist basis for morality thus interpreted calls for no
> extrahuman or superhuman guarantees of objectivity or absolute-
> ness. To the extent that it is a minimalist basis, it offers, rather, a
> common groundwork or footing upon which to undertake dia-
> logue, debate, and negotiations within and between otherwise
> disparate traditions: a set of values that can be agreed upon as a
> starting point for negotiation or action. However, differently par-
> ticipants may view this set of values as itself founded or justified…it
> represents the 'chief or most stable component' of what they can
> hold in common. (p.76)

A mixed conception is promoted in a large part driven by the need to
find a functional common ground or set of operating principles. Such a
mixed view probably lies closer to the view of an individual who has
deliberated on these issues without pressing limits of time.

For the construction of DALYs, I propose a principle of "filtered consensus" which borrows from the common values and "laundering preferences" approaches. If many individuals after deliberation hold a
preference or value then this value should be considered seriously. We
should investigate, and if need be, speculate on, the likely reasons why
many individuals hold such a view. If these reasons appear to be persuasive and do not contravene important "ideal-regarding principles," these
preferences should be incorporated into the construction of DALYs. There
will be cases (see the discussion on discounting), however, where cogent
arguments can be marshalled to modify or reject a common view, even if
it has emerged from appropriate deliberation. The final filtered consensus that arises from this reflective process will be used to select the social
preferences incorporated in DALYs.

Certain issues emerge several times in the discussion of social preferences for different key choices in the design of DALYs. To facilitate the
argument and to make the filtering process more transparent, let me make
two propositions that I will use for filtering on several occasions. Both of

these propositions will have an important influence on the arguments for different social values and on the final form of DALYs.

Proposition 1. The burden calculated for like health outcomes should be the same.

The "like as like" proposition appeals to the most elementary notion of fairness. The interpretation of this statement, however, depends critically on the information set used to define like health outcomes. Every health outcome, such as the premature death of a 45 year-old man from a heart attack or permanent disability from blindness in a 19 year-old woman due to a road traffic accident, can be characterized by a set of variables. Some of these variables define the specific health outcome itself, such as the etiology, type, severity or duration of disability. Others are properties of the individual, such as sex, age, income, educational attainment, religion, ethnicity, occupation and even individual preferences. At the limit, if all possible information is used, every health outcome is unique and thus the "like as like" principle has no meaning. The importance of this proposition in the formulation of DALYs arises when it is combined with the following proposition for a very restricted information set.

Proposition 2. The non-health characteristics of the individual affected by a health outcome that should be considered in calculating the associated burden of disease should be restricted to age and sex.

Such a restricted information set combined with the "like as like" proposition has profound implications for the design of DALYs. I shall first address the part of the proposition excluding certain information from the calculation method for DALYs; later on in this chapter, I will make arguments for the part of the proposition that the age and sex of the individual should be considered. I will assume that few disagree with excluding information on race, religion, beauty, and other individual characteristics. (Although I claim no further argument is needed, it is sobering to recognize that some groups have invoked repugnant reasons to attach greater importance to the same health outcome in different races or religions— the former apartheid government of South Africa implicitly put a higher relative weight on the same health outcomes in whites compared with other races.)

When it comes to certain socio-economic characteristics of individuals, however, there are strong objections to these Propositions from some quarters. Many economists might argue that the health of higher income earners or the well-educated should be accorded greater weight than the same health outcome in lower-income or less educated groups (Rice and Hodgson 1982):[11] the higher-income earners contribute more to the economy, to the accumulation of capital and to future growth and hence to the well-being of the entire society. The net welfare contribution argument could extend beyond income groups to many other socio-economic categories to the extent that average income differs between socio-economic groups. Others (e.g. Anand and Hanson 1995) have argued that we should accord greater importance to the same health outcome in the *disadvantaged* as compared to the advantaged. The death of a poor 40 year-old, according to them, is worse that the death of a rich 40 year-old. They justify this discriminatory viewpoint with reference to "Rawls' Difference Principle in the space of capabilities."[12]

The proposition that we should exclude information on the income, education or other aspects of the social status of an individual in estimating the burden due to a health outcome is clearly a middle-ground between these two points of view. Imagine a situation where two patients arrive at an emergency room both in a coma from meningitis, but there is only enough antibiotic to treat one of them. The two patients are totally identical in every respect except that one is rich and the other is poor. The welfare maximizers might choose to treat the rich patient, while others, such as Anand and Hanson, would choose to treat the poor patient. I argue through the restricted information proposition that we should be completely indifferent to treating one over the other.[13] The income of the patients has no bearing on who should receive the life saving intervention. As survival and, to a large extent, good health are required for all other forms of well-being, few individuals are willing, after deliberation, to discriminate by socio-economic status. For example, there are no formalized rules for the allocation of organs for transplantation that give preference based on income or educational attainment (see for example Starzl et al. 1987 on rules for kidney allocation).[14]

A more troublesome objection to the restricted information proposition is that the consequences of a health outcome on an individual will depend on many individual characteristics. Some individuals may be better able to cope with adversity than others. The adversity faced because of a given outcome, such as infertility, may differ greatly among people based on their cultures and social responses. The consequences of any health outcome are ultimately unique to the individual. Nevertheless, the notion that we should count a given health outcome, for example blindness due to onchocerciasis, as more important in an individual who has a lower capacity to adapt psychologically than in an individual who has a higher capacity to adapt psychologically would appear to be manifestly unfair. This argument will be taken up again later in the sections on disability and handicap as well as in the section discussing de Tocqueville's "happy slave."

The combination of Propositions 1 and 2 give DALYs a strongly egalitarian flavor. This may be unappealing for those who are welfare maximizers or those who believe in maximizing the conditions of the worst off. While more involved justifications for restricting the information set for calculating DALYs could be constructed with reference to concepts of opportunity, fairness or preferences on preferences,[15] these justifications are not pursued further. In keeping with the notions of common values and laundering preferences, I argue that these propositions are acceptable to many and can form the basis of a dialogue for the construction of DA-LYs and, hopefully, for the patterns of the burden of disease denominated in DALYs.

SOME GENERAL ISSUES IN THE DESIGN OF A BURDEN OF DISEASE INDICATOR

The specific objective of the Global Burden of Disease Study was to quantify the burden of premature mortality and non-fatal health outcomes. The term "burden" is not used in the vernacular sense, where it conjures up a very individual phenomenon. As has already been noted, the impact of blindness on the individual depends on a host of personal, social and economic factors. However, from a population viewpoint, the interest is in quantifying the burden from a condition given average conditions of individuals and social responses. In the section on measuring preferences for health states, the exact meaning of average individual and social conditions will be discussed.

It is also necessary to explain the meaning of the qualifiers "disease" and "injury." Ultimately all deaths and non-fatal health outcomes have a proximal biological causes in the form of disease or injury. Distal socio-economic causes, however, also act through diseases and injuries to affect health—for example, Mosley and Chen (1984) have developed a framework of distal and proximal causes of child mortality. The term "the burden of disease and injury" does not suggest in any way that the policies and priorities for reducing the burden of mortality and non-fatal health outcomes are solely narrow medical interventions targeted to specific diseases and injuries. Educating young girls, for example, may well be one of the most effective means of reducing the burden of disease. In fact, DALYs can be and have been used to evaluate the cost-effectiveness of interventions far beyond a narrowly defined biomedical focus (Jamison et al. 1993).

Developing a composite measure of premature death and non-fatal health outcomes requires a common dimension in which both can be measured. Most health measures are event rates per unit time and/or per unit population, such as the crude death rate or the smear-positive tuberculosis incidence rate. For a composite health indicator, a more general unit of measure is required. The best candidate for a general unit of measure is time itself, denominated in years or days. Nearly 50 years ago, Dempsey (1947) proposed that premature mortality should be measured in units of time lost. Her fundamental insight opened up the possibility of developing combined measures of premature mortality and non-fatal health outcomes which were proposed two decades later (Berg 1973, Chiang 1965, Fanshel and Bush 1970, Patrick et al. 1973, Piot and Sundaresan 1967). The remainder of this chapter is based on the premise that the best approach for measuring the burden of disease is to use units of time.[16]

Having chosen units of time as the unit of measure, the burden of disease can still be calculated using incidences or prevalences. Time lost due to premature mortality is a function of death rates and the duration of life lost due to a death at each age. Because death rates are incidence rates, there is no obvious alternative for mortality to using an incidence perspective—there are no calculated measures of the prevalence of the dead. By contrast, for non-fatal health outcomes both incidence and prevalence measures have been routinely used. In the calculation of disability-free life expectancy, for example, both prevalence (Sullivan 1971) and incidence based methods have been proposed (Bebbington 1991, Crimmins et al. 1993, Robine and Ritchie 1991). Using the prevalence perspective, time lived with non-fatal health outcomes is estimated using point prevalences, adjusting for seasonal variation if present, multiplied by one year. The alternative is to measure the incidence and the expected duration of non-fatal health outcomes. Expected durations require information on remission rates and case-fatality rates. If the incidence of disability is constant over time and the population age-structure is also constant, then the prevalence and incidence approaches yield exactly the same total amount of time lived with a non-fatal health outcome. For nearly all populations the age structure is not constant and for many diseases such as lung cancer, cervical cancer, stomach cancer, HIV disease and leprosy, the incidence is changing over time.

For measuring the global burden of disease and injury, an incidence perspective has been chosen for three reasons. First, the method of calculating time lived with disability is more consistent with the method for calculating time lost due to premature mortality. Second, an incidence perspective is more sensitive to current epidemiological trends. Third, measuring incidence or deriving it from prevalence data and information on case-fatality and remission rates imposes a level of internal consistency and discipline that would be missing if prevalence data were used uncritically.[17] To demonstrate the effect on changing from an incidence to a prevalence perspective, the results of the Global Burden of Disease Study have also been calculated using the prevalences of non-fatal health outcomes and are presented in Chapter 5 in this volume (Murray and Lopez 1996b). The best measure for the assessment of the benefits of an intervention is the volume of life-years added, appropriately adjusted for time lived with a non-fatal health outcome, irrespective of the perspective adopted for measuring the burden of disease.[18]

In the following sections, the options, and the moral and technical arguments for or against these options, are described in detail for five important social choices: estimating the duration of life lost due to a death at each age, comparing time lived with a non-fatal health outcome with time lost due to premature mortality, discounting future health, age-weighting, and incorporating considerations of equity.

THE DURATION OF LIFE LOST DUE TO A DEATH AT EACH AGE

Since Dempsey (1947) first proposed time based measures of premature mortality, a wide array of alternatives has been suggested (Centers for Disease Control 1986, Dickinson and Welker 1948, Feachem et al. 1992, Greville 1948, Haenszel 1950, Kohn 1951, Murray 1987, Perloff et al. 1984, Robinson 1948, Romeder and McWhinnie 1977). For the purposes of measuring burden, or the gap between current mortality levels and some idealized goal, there are advantages and disadvantages of each of the methods. To help clarify the range of approaches, methods have been clustered into four families: potential years of life lost, period expected years of life lost, cohort expected years of life lost, and standard expected years of life lost. Each measure is defined and its advantages and disadvantages are reviewed.

In the earliest literature on measuring years of life lost, there was also considerable debate about the "zero mortality assumption" (Dickinson and Welker 1948, Greville 1948, Haenszel 1950). Using the zero mortality assumption in calculating years of life lost due to a particular disease requires recalculating a life table in the absence of mortality from that cause at any age. Each death from a cause is weighted by the life expectancy of the population in the absence of that cause. As a result, the number of years of life lost due to a tuberculosis death at age 40 would be different from those lost due to a road traffic accident at age 40. These methods are inconsistent with the "like as like" proposition and are not discussed further here.

To help illustrate measures of the duration of life lost, a graphical display of a survivorship function (Figure 1.1) is useful. A survivorship function shows the probability of survival to each age for a newborn who

Figure 1.1   Survivorship function for a population with a life expectancy at birth of 50 years

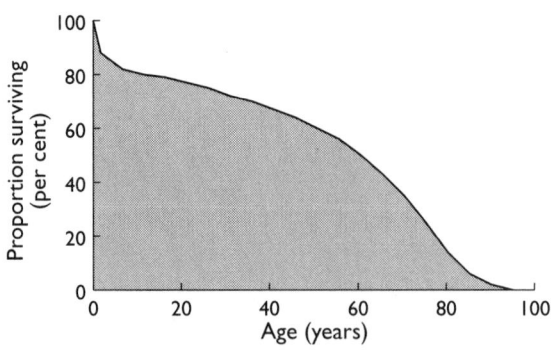

experiences a set of age-specific mortality rates. The y-axis shows the probability that a newborn will be alive at each age and the x-axis indicates age. One-hundred per cent of newborns are alive at age zero; thereafter the survivorship function steadily drops as individuals are exposed to risks of death For example, in Figure 1.1, sixty per cent of newborns are still alive at age fifty. A convenient characteristic of a survivorship curve is that the shaded area under the curve equals life expectancy at birth. In a population where there is no growth and mortality rates are constant, the survivorship function also represents the distribution of population by age. This latter property is useful for illustrating the meaning of different measures of time lost due to premature mortality on a two-dimensional graph. Survivorship graphs are used below to illustrate what each type of indicator measures in such a stable population with no growth.

POTENTIAL YEARS OF LIFE LOST

Potential years of life lost (PYLL) is the simplest measure of time lost due to premature death. A potential limit to life is chosen arbitrarily and the duration of life lost due to a death is simply the potential limit to life minus the age at death. Formally, PYLL for a population is:

$$PYLL = \sum_{x=0}^{L} d_x (L - x)$$

where L is the arbitrary limit to life, x is the age at death, and d_x is the number of deaths in the population at each age. A wide range of potential limits to life have been used, ranging from 60 to 85 (Centers for Disease Control 1986, Feachem et al. 1992, Ghana Health Assessment Project Team 1981, Haenszel 1950, Romeder and McWhinnie 1977). The choice of the upper limit is arbitrary, often justified on the basis of limited statistical arguments. Dempsey (1947) proposed that the limit to life should be set equal to life expectancy at birth for a given population. Others have selected arbitrary limits slightly in excess of period life expectancy (e.g. Feachem et al. 1992) or substantially below period life expectancy as in the United States (Centers for Disease Control 1986). For clarity, the convention of putting the potential limit to life used in calculating PYLL in brackets after the initialism is followed here.

Using the survivorship function in Figure 1.2, PYLL(70) can be represented as the triangle at the top right formed by the survivorship curve and the vertical line at the potential limit to life. For a population with zero growth and constant death rates, the area of the triangle equals the number of PYLL(70).[19] PYLL(70) for a population with a life expectancy at birth of 50 years is shown on the left and for a population with a life expectancy of 65 years on the right.

What is the sum of life expectancy at birth, which is the area under the survivorship curve, and PYLL(70), the area between the survivorship curve and the vertical line drawn at the potential limit to life? In theory, the combination of these two areas would be the life expectancy at birth of a cohort

Figure 1.2   Various measures of years of life lost in a stable population
with zero population growth

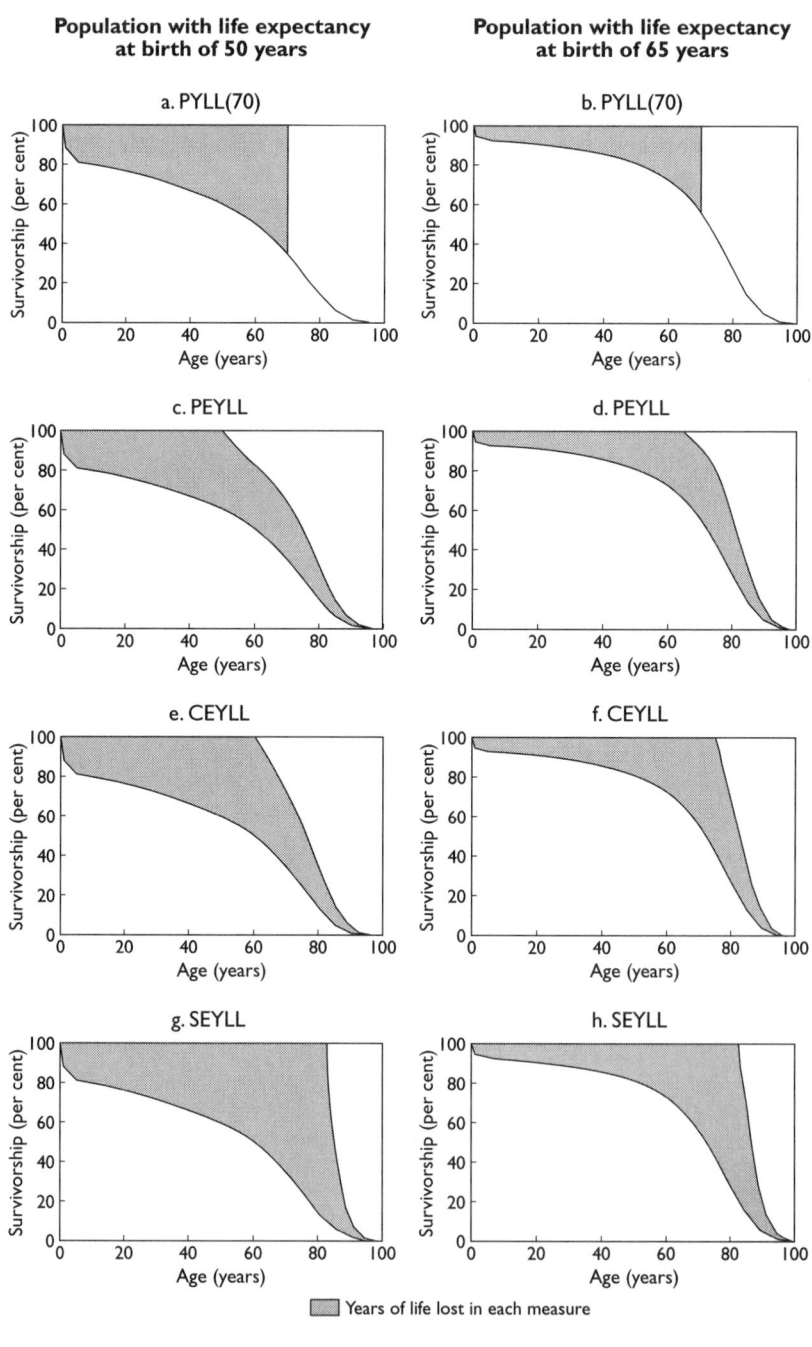

Years of life lost in each measure

in which the burden of premature death measured by PYLL was completely averted. In Figure 1.2a, the sum of these two areas equals 73.2 years; and in Figure 1.2b the sum equals 75.9 years. Perhaps surprisingly, the sum of life expectancy and PYLL(70) exceeds 70 years. Moreover, this excess increases as life expectancy increases. As life expectancy increases, there are more years lived by the population over the potential limit to life, in this case 70 years, as illustrated in Figure 1.2a and 1.2b. The sum of life expectancy at birth and PYLL, therefore, must also grow.

The main advantages of PYLL as a measure of the burden of premature mortality are the ease of its calculation and the egalitarian treatment of all deaths at a given age. There are, however, several major disadvantages. Deaths beyond the arbitrarily selected potential limit to life do not contribute to burden. If PYLL is used to measure burden, and change in PYLL is used to assess the benefits of a health intervention, any programme which reduces mortality after the potential limit to life would have zero benefits. In the United States, where 65 is used as the limit to life by the Centers for Disease Control and Prevention in these calculations, health interventions reducing mortality at age 66 would have no benefit according to this method. Attaching a value of zero to health gains over some arbitrary limit is at odds with the revealed preferences of nearly every society in which substantial resources are devoted to extending life even at ages over 70, 75 or 80. When a very high potential limit to life is used such as 85, 90 or 100, the magnitude of this age discrimination problem is diminished, but the problem still exists in principle.

PERIOD EXPECTED YEARS OF LIFE LOST

A popular alternative to PYLL is to calculate period expected years of life lost (PEYLL), where the duration of life lost is the local period life expectancy at each age. Formally,

$$PEYLL = \sum_{x=0}^{l} d_x e_x$$

where e_x is the period life expectancy at each age, l is the last age to which people survive and d_x is the number of deaths at age x. In this measure, deaths at all ages contribute to the estimated burden of premature death. There is no arbitrary age after which deaths are ignored in burden calculations.

As a measure of burden for the same community over time or across communities, PEYLL can yield perverse results. Such results stem from the fact that in PEYLL a population's current mortality level is being used as the "ideal" against which it is compared in order to calculate the burden of disease. Over time and across communities, local life expectancies vary and thus the reference standards vary, creating, at times, peculiar findings.

Figures 1.2c and 1.2d illustrate, using survivorship curves, PEYLL in two stable populations with zero growth—one with a life expectancy at birth of 50 years and one with a life expectancy at birth of 65 years. As with PYLL, the figures show a hypothetical survivorship curve as a second line. The area between the survivorship curve and the second line in each figure is PEYLL. When we measure the burden of premature mortality, we are measuring the gap between current mortality conditions and some ideal reference value. For PEYLL, the implicit ideal reference is the sum of the area under the survivorship curve, life expectancy at birth, and the shaded area. For the population with a life expectancy at birth of 50 years in Figure 1.2c, the shaded area divided by the size of the birth cohort is 22.9 years. The implicit ideal reference life expectancy for this population is thus 72.9 years (50+22.9). For the population with a life expectancy at birth of 65 in Figure 1.2d, the shaded area divided by the size of the birth cohort is 16.5 and the ideal reference life expectancy is 81.5 years. The change from a reference life expectancy of 72.9 to 81.5 years shows how dramatically the goal posts are moving as mortality declines when PEYLL is used as a measure of burden. As life expectancy increases by 15 years from 50 to 65, the reference life expectancy increases by 8.6 years. Less than half the gain in life expectancy at birth is being translated into a reduction in PEYLL for a given birth cohort.

Because the expectation of life does not fall to zero at an arbitrary age, PEYLL has the advantage of providing a more appealing estimate of the streams of life lost to deaths in the older age groups. However, application of the period expectation method would lead us to conclude that the death of a 40 year-old woman in Kigali contributes less to the global burden of disease than the death of a 40 year-old woman in Paris because the expectation of life at age 40 is lower in Rwanda than in France. Equivalent health outcomes would be a greater burden in richer communities than in poorer communities. As this runs counter to the "like as like" proposition, this method has not been used for calculating the duration of life lost due to a death at each age in Disability-Adjusted Life Years.

Cohort Expected Years of Life Lost

Period life expectancies are calculated based on the assumption that a child born today will be exposed in the future to currently observed age-specific mortality rates at every age. Twentieth-century mortality history demonstrates that this is a fallacious assumption, particularly in populations with moderate or high mortality. Mortality has been declining at a steady pace throughout the last decades so that the life expectancy of a birth cohort is much higher than the period life expectancy based on currently observed rates. Figure 1.3 shows that the cohort life expectancy at birth for females in the United States has been 10–15 years higher than period life expectancy calculated from death rates observed in each year from 1900 to 1950.[20]

Cohort expected years of life lost (CEYLL) can be calculated using cohort expectations of life at each age rather than period expectations:

$$CEYLL = \sum_{x=0}^{l} d_x e_x^c$$

Figure 1.3   Period and cohort life expectancies at birth, United States, females, 1900-1950

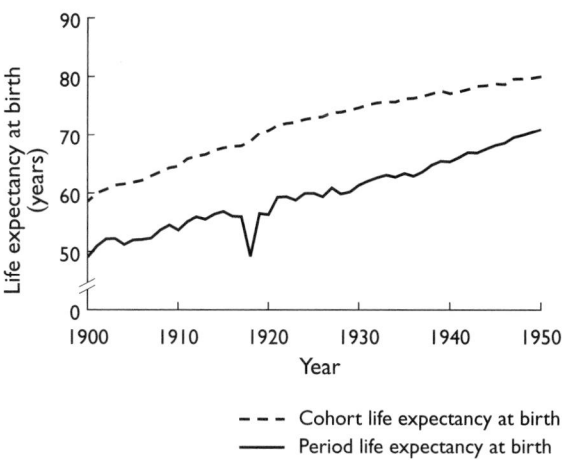

where e_x^c is the cohort expectation of life at each age, l is the last age to which people survive, and dx is the number of deaths at age x. Cohort life expectancies for a population alive today must be estimated since we obviously do not know today what the mortality experience of a cohort will be in the future. Estimates of cohort life expectancy based on various projection models are more likely to be unbiased estimates of the true expectation of life of a cohort than estimates based on period life expectancy. The difference between period and cohort life expectancies will, in general, be greatest for high mortality populations where substantial declines in mortality can be expected over the next few decades.

Figures 1.2e and 1.2f illustrate that CEYLL has the same properties as PEYLL. The reference life expectancy shifts as mortality declines. Using the CEYLL approach, like outcomes would not be treated as like since cohortlife expectancy at age 40 is still much higher in Kalamazoo than in Kinshasa.

STANDARD EXPECTED YEARS OF LIFE LOST

The advantages of the expectation approach in the treatment of deaths at older ages and the egalitarian nature of the potential years of life lost method can be combined using "standard" expected years of life lost. Standard expected years of life lost can be defined as:

$$SEYLL = \sum_{x=0}^{l} d_x e_x^*$$

where e_x^* is the expectation of life at each age x based on some ideal standard. As a measure of the burden of premature mortality, SEYLL has several advantages. As for PEYLL and CEYLL, in SEYLL deaths at all ages contribute to the burden of disease. In SEYLL, deaths at the same age in all communities contribute equally to the burden of disease so that like outcomes are treated as like. Figures 1.2g and 1.2h illustrate values of SEYLL for a population with constant mortality rates and zero growth. The standard used for the figures is a life expectancy of 82.5 years at birth. As with the other measures of the burden of premature mortality, we can determine the sum of life expectancy at birth and SEYLL. For two populations, one with a life expectancy at birth of 50 years and another with a life expectancy at birth of 65 years, the sum equals 85.7 and 87.5, respectively. That is for a 15 year increase in life expectancy, SEYLL for a birth cohort decreases by 13.2 years. In other words, compared with PEYLL, changes in the real number of life years lived is much closer to changes in SEYLL.[21]

For measuring the global burden of disease due to premature mortality, the SEYLL method has been adopted. To define the standard, the highest national life expectancy observed was taken; Japanese females have already achieved a period life expectancy at birth higher than 82 years. The standard expectations that were used are, therefore, based on a model life table, namely Coale and Demeny West Level 26 which has a life expectancy at birth for females of 82.5 years (Coale and Guo 1989). These standard expectancies are shown in Table 1.1. Using a model life table ensures that the standard expectations at each age are easily available through publications and software distributed by the United Nations Population Division and eliminates some peculiarities of Japanese age-specific mortality. Choosing one family of model life tables over any other makes little or no difference to the results at such low mortality levels. In this indicator, deaths at all ages contribute to the total estimated burden of disease while all deaths at the same age will contribute equally to the total estimated burden of disease.

Male and Female Standard Life Tables

Should the same standard expectation of life at each age be used for males as well as for females? The average sex difference in life expectancy at birth in more developed regions according to the United Nations (1995) is 7.4 years. The observed differences in survival for males and females, even in low mortality populations, are complex functions of genetic potential, exposures, occupation, social role, command over resources, etc. While the proximal cause of every male or female death is a disease or injury, one of the distal causes of death for males and females may be genetic survival potential. Even if some of the differences between male and female survival are not due to risk factors such as smoking, alcohol, or occupational exposures, narrowing this "biological" difference in survival potential may become technologically possible in the future and thus a focus of public policy.

Table 1.1   Standard life expectancies at each age and YLLs due to a
death at each age used in the GBD

Age (years)	Life expectancy (years)		YLLs due to a death at each age	
	Females	Males	Females	Males
0	82.50	80.00	33.12	33.01
1	81.84	79.36	34.07	33.95
5	77.95	75.38	36.59	36.46
10	72.99	70.40	37.62	37.47
15	68.02	65.41	36.99	36.80
20	63.08	60.44	35.24	35.02
25	58.17	55.47	32.78	32.53
30	53.27	50.51	29.92	29.62
35	48.38	45.57	26.86	26.50
40	43.53	40.64	23.74	23.32
45	38.72	35.77	20.66	20.17
50	33.99	30.99	17.69	17.12
55	29.37	26.32	14.87	14.21
60	24.83	21.81	12.22	11.48
65	20.44	17.50	9.75	8.95
70	16.20	13.58	7.48	6.69
75	12.28	10.17	5.46	4.77
80	8.90	7.45	3.76	3.27
85	6.22	5.24	2.45	2.12
90	4.25	3.54	1.53	1.30
95	2.89	2.31	0.94	0.76
100	2.00	1.46	0.57	0.42

Note: Years of Life Lost used in the GBD are calculated from the standard life expectancies shown, but are subject to age-weighting and discounting.

One could argue on grounds of equity that a male death at age 40 should count as the same duration of life lost as a female death at age 40. Nevertheless, I have chosen to incorporate into the calculation of standard expected years of life lost a biological difference in survival potential for males and females. Clearly, this is a controversial issue and a strong case could be made for including the component of burden due to biological differences between males and females in the estimation of burden. Perhaps, in future iterations of the burden of disease and revisions of DALYs, this discrimination against males should be removed.

Having chosen to exclude the biological difference in survival between males and females from the calculation of burden, the evidence for the magnitude of such a difference must be examined. Clearly, the average difference in life expectancy at birth in industrialized countries is far greater than the biological differences in survival potential. Males smoke more, drink more, engage in risky behaviors more often and are exposed to more occupational hazards. Unless we are to ascribe all of these male behaviors to genetic determinism, we must attempt to estimate the biological differences in survival potential correcting for these hazards. A number of authors (see for example Fries 1980, Manton 1986, Pressat 1973, Ryder 1975) have attempted to estimate the maximum lifespan for males and females. Using a range of modeling methods, estimates of the difference between male and female maximum lifespan range from 1.9 to 3.2 years, with females having greater lifespans than males. The results of these modeling exercises are consistent with the observation that in rich low-mortality populations male life expectancy approximates female life expectancy more closely. This is well illustrated in Figure 1.4 which shows the male-female gender differences in life expectancy by geographical regions ranked by average income per capita in Canada (Wilkins et al. 1989). A further example of reduced gender differences in life expectancy in low mortality populations is the case of Asians living in the United States; Hahn and Eberhardt (1995) report that Asian/Pacific Islander life expectancy at birth for males and females is 82.0 and 85.8 years, respectively. For whites, they report a life expectancy of 72.9 and 79.4 years for males and females, respectively, and for blacks 65.5 and 73.3 for males and females respectively. A biological difference in life expectancy at birth of 2.5 years has been chosen for the measurement of the burden of disease. The standard life expectancy at birth for males of 80 years has been based on the female schedule for Coale and Demeny Model life table West level 25, as there is no male schedule with a life expectancy of 80.[22] For the GBD, Years of Life

Figure 1.4   Differences in life expectancy at birth for males and females, by income quintile, in urban Canada, 1986

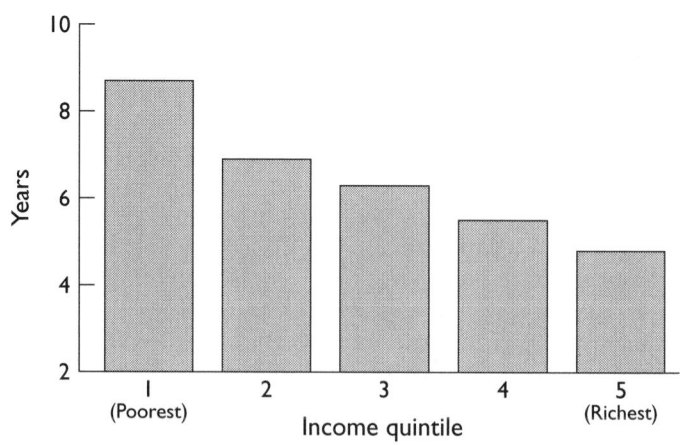

Lost (YLLs) are used to refer to standard expected years of life lost with age-weighting and discounting applied—these are discussed below.

MEASURING CHANGES IN THE BURDEN OF PREMATURE MORTALITY CAUSED BY INTERVENTIONS

In the discussions that have followed the publication of the *World Development Report 1993* (World Bank 1993) and *Global Comparative Assessments in the Health Sector* (Murray and Lopez 1994), there has been considerable confusion over how to estimate the gains achieved through the application of an intervention. It is critical to draw a sharp distinction between the previous discussion of how to measure the burden of premature mortality in terms of years of life lost and a discussion of how to measure changes in burden due to the application of an intervention. While this discussion of how to measure changes in life years is not central to the discussion of YLLs and DALYs, it is important enough to warrant a digression.

Logically, if we choose to measure burden in a given manner, we should measure the benefits of an intervention as the change in that measure. For example, if we choose to measure the burden of premature death by PYLL, then the benefits of an intervention should be:

$$B_i = \sum_{t=0}^{\infty} PYLL_{t,NO} - \sum_{t=0}^{\infty} PYLL_{t,i}$$

where B_i is the benefits of intervention i, $PYLL_{t,NO}$ is the PYLL in the population without the intervention at time t, and $PYLL_{t,i}$ is the PYLL in the population with intervention i at time t. A similar equation could be written for evaluating the benefits of an intervention using PEYLL, CEYLL or SEYLL.[23]

To explore the relationships between the number of extra life-years added and the change in various indicators such as PYLL, PEYLL and SEYLL, a model has been constructed for a population in which each single-year age group is followed for 100 years. Initially, the population has a stable age-structure, a life expectancy at birth of 50 years, and the birth rate set so that the population growth rate is zero. The number of life-years added by an intervention that prevents exactly 1 death at a given age has been analysed first. The individual saved is subsequently exposed to the currently observed mortality rates at all subsequent ages. Figure 1.5 shows how various indicators of the burden of premature mortality change, given the prevention of a single death at each age. The x-axis is the age at which the death is prevented and the y-axis shows the ratio of the change in burden for a given indicator to the change in the actual number of life-years lived. If the indicator of the burden of premature mortality decreases by exactly the quantity of extra life-years lived, this ratio would be one to one. Up to age 50, the ratio of change in burden to change in life-years lived due to the intervention is close to one for PYLL(75) and SEYLL. Even for deaths below age 50, the change in PEYLL is much less than the number

Figure 1.5   Ratio of changes in SEYLL, PEYLL or PYLL to changes in the
number of life-years lived by the population due to the
application of an intervention that prevents a single death
at a given age

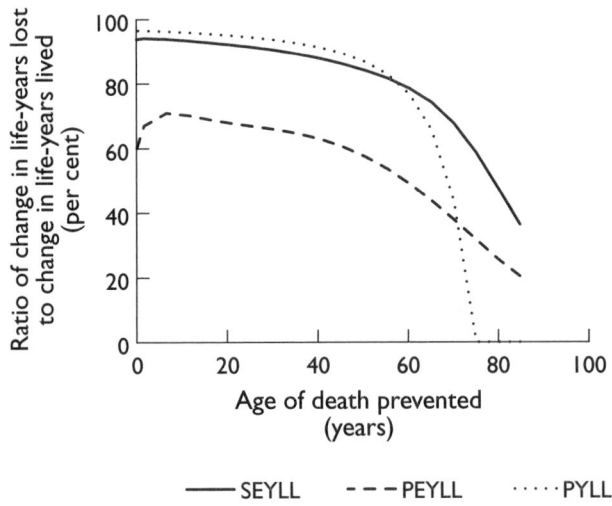

of extra life-years lived. For deaths over 50, the change in all three indicators is substantially less than the change in life-years lived. Preventing
deaths over age 75 does not change PYLL(75) and the ratio falls to zero.
Of all three indicators evaluated, the change in SEYLL is closest to the
change in life-years lived. Strictly measuring the benefits of an intervention using the change in SEYLL or PYLL may underestimate the number
of life-years added through an intervention and thus worsen the estimated
cost-effectiveness ratio.

    In most cost-effectiveness studies, it is often not possible to estimate
burden with and without an intervention over several decades after the
intervention is implemented. Life-years added through an intervention
must be approximated. Local life expectancy is a good first-order approximation of the change in burden for simple single-year interventions. Preston (1993) has analysed the number of life years added to a population
through different types of interventions and has shown that life expectancy at each age is a good estimate of the number of extra-life years lived
by the population. Where mortality is changing over time, we would need
to revise his statement to say that *cohort* life expectancy is a good estima-
tor of life-years added through an intervention. Figure 1.6 shows that using discounted measures of the burden of premature mortality—see the
section below on discounting—does not alter the basic patterns. As an
indicator of burden, changes in SEYLL are closest to the increment in life-
years lived because of an intervention that prevents one death at a given age.

Figure 1.6   Ratio of changes in discounted SEYLL, PEYLL or PYLL to
changes in the number of discounted life-years lived by the
population due to the application of an intervention that
prevents a single death at a given age

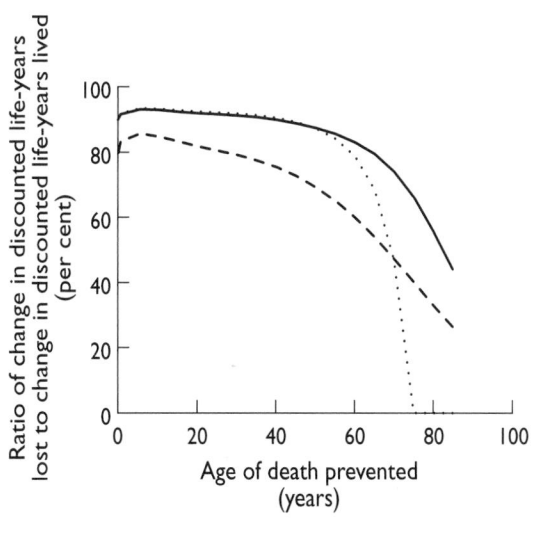

——Discounted SEYLL - - -Discounted PEYLL · · · · ·Discounted PYLL

Analysing the benefits of an intervention that changes age-specific
mortality rates for a sustained period is more challenging. Consider a ten-
year intervention, which, while it operates, reduces the mortality rate for
a given age group by ten per cent. What would the number of extra life-
years lived by the population be and how does this compare to the change
in PYLL(75), PEYLL and SEYLL? As Preston (1993) has noted, evaluating long-term changes in mortality is more complicated because the period life expectancy is changing. Figure 1.7 dramatically demonstrates how
the change in PEYLL deviates from the change in the number of life-years
lived by the population. In fact, programmes that reduce mortality rates
over age 55, in this example, increase PEYLL because the increase in life
expectancy at these ages outweighs the decrease in the number of deaths.
Using PEYLL, the benefits of an intervention which reduces mortality by
10 per cent at age 60 would be negative. Of the three measures, the change
in SEYLL correlates most closely with the volume of extra life-years lived.
Even for SEYLL, however, there is a substantial difference at older ages.

On a more practical level, life-years added through simple single year
interventions that do not substantially change age-specific mortality rates
estimated using cohort life expectancy is a good first-order approximation of the expected change in SEYLL. To estimate life-years added or the

Figure 1.7   Ratio of changes in SEYLL, PEYLL or PYLL to changes in the
                   number of life-years lived by the population due to the
                   application of an intervention that reduces mortality at a
                   given age by 10 per cent for 10 years

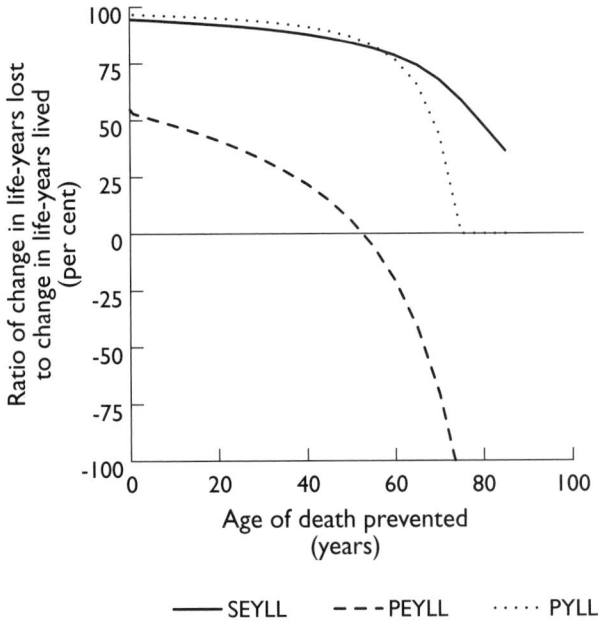

change in burden from more complex multi-year programmes, a population projection model should be used, as suggested by Preston (1993).

COMPARING TIME LOST DUE TO PREMATURE DEATH AND TIME LIVED WITH A NON-FATAL HEALTH OUTCOME

Despite lip service paid to morbidity and disability, too often health policy
debates are focused on mortality. One reason for this is the lack of comparable information on non-fatal health outcomes that can be juxtaposed
with information on the burden of premature mortality. A key objective
of the GBD has been to promote awareness of the magnitude, cost-effectiveness of prevention, and cost-effectiveness in health policy debates of
rehabilitation of non-fatal health outcomes. The definition of death is clear
and its measurement, even in the absence of an established vital registration system, well developed. This is not the case with non-fatal health
outcomes, for which many aspects of the definition, measurement and
valuation are controversial.

Each non-fatal health outcome is unique, characterized by the initial
pathological process, by its antecedent biological, social and economic

causes, by the characteristics of the individual affected and the characteristics of the social milieu and by society's response to the individual with the condition. In order to quantify time lived with non-fatal health outcomes in a manner comparable to time lost due to premature mortality which is standardized across communities and over time, a great degree of simplification is required. Not all the information defining each unique non-fatal health outcome can be incorporated; in the interest of capturing the major patterns, a certain level of reductionism must be accepted. This must be based on a careful consideration of what information is relevant to defining, measuring and valuing non-fatal health outcomes for this study, what information is acceptable given the propositions set out at the beginning of this chapter and what approaches are feasible at the global and regional levels.

In the following section, some conceptualizations of non-fatal health outcomes are given, alternative methods for the measurement of incidence and prevalence of non-fatal health outcomes are presented, and the challenge of linking or apportioning outcomes to diseases and injuries and the methods available to measure preferences for health states are described, with some judgments on their strengths and weaknesses. This review will be used to discuss the original formulation of non-fatal health outcomes used for calculating Years Lived with Disability (YLDs), the non-fatal health outcome part of DALYs, as well as criticisms of this approach that have emerged since 1993. The latter part of this section is devoted to the revision of the approach undertaken for this study including the development and application of a new protocol for measuring preferences for 22 indicator conditions. The results of this protocol have been used to generate weights for several hundred conditions in the untreated and treated state. The section concludes with a discussion of future directions for the global study and strategies for country adaptation.

CONCEPTUALIZING NON-FATAL HEALTH OUTCOMES

Since the first proposals for synthetic indicators of health status appeared in the 1960s, a substantial literature on measuring the health-related quality of life has developed (see Lohr 1989, 1992, Lohr and Ware 1987 for proceedings of three general conferences). Conceptualizations of various health-related quality of life (HRQL) approaches differ but certain facets are common (Patrick and Erickson 1993, Ware et al. 1981).[24] A number of different "concepts" of health-related quality of life have been identified: opportunity, health perceptions, functional states, and impairments. Within these concepts, Patrick and Erickson (1993) identify 17 domains which include: social or cultural disadvantage, resilience, general health perceptions, limitations in usual roles, integration, contact, intimacy and sexual function, affective psychological function, cognitive psychological function, activity restrictions, fitness, symptoms/subjective complaints, signs, self-reported disease, physiological measures, tissue alterations and diagnoses. Initial work on HRQL began with a more limited focus on domains of physical function, such as measures of the activities of daily living. During the 1970s and 1980s, the domains included in HRQL measurements were expanded to include psychological and social function as well as broader concepts such as opportunity. While much of the HRQL work has been undertaken in North America, there is increasing international experience with some HRQL instruments (Anderson et al. 1995). Despite the common themes in various HRQL measures, Ziebland et al. (1993) point out that there are different conceptual models operating within the field. They identify the functional model, subjective distress model, comparative model and the dependence model. The conceptualization of non-fatal health outcomes and their significance remains controversial (Verbrugge and Jette 1994).

An alternative conceptualization of non-fatal health outcomes, one with much more structure, is embedded in the *International Classification of Impairments, Disabilities and Handicaps* (ICIDH) (World Health Organization 1980). A World Health Organization initiative, in collaboration with the WHO Centre for the Classification of Diseases in Paris and various non-governmental organizations, led to the publication of a draft classification of impairments, disabilities and handicaps in 1975 (Wood 1975) and the *International Classification of Impairments, Disabilities and Handicaps* in 1980 (World Health Organization 1980). The conceptual framework that emerged from this process is substantially different from the health-related quality of life approach. In the manual of the ICIDH, a linear progression from disease to pathology to manifestation to impairment to disability to handicap is proposed. Impairment is defined at the level of the organ system, disability in terms of the impact on the performance of the individual and handicap in the context of the overall consequences which depend on the social environment. For example, a loss of a finger or an eye is an impairment. The consequent disability may be the loss of fine motor function or seeing. Depending on the individual's need in particular environments, the loss of function could lead to a handicap. The loss of fine motor function may be a greater handicap, following this terminology, for a concert violinist than for a bank teller. There is a major difference between this approach, which views handicap on a completely different axis, and much of the health-related quality of life literature which treats social function as one of many variables.

MEASUREMENT OF NON-FATAL HEALTH OUTCOMES

Given the diffuse nature of the conceptualization of non-fatal health outcomes in the HRQL field, it is not surprising that there are over 300 instruments reported in the literature (Spilker et al. 1996). Few individuals have read the vast literature on these instruments, let alone been in a position to describe their relative merits and limitations. Only some general observations on this collection are possible (and these with trepidation). At one level, one can distinguish between generic measures capturing a range of domains and those instruments more tailored to a specific disease. Well known examples of generic measures include the Nottingham Health Profile (Hunt et al. 1981), the Sickness Impact Profile (Bergner et al. 1981), Medical Outcomes Study 36-Item Short Form Health Survey (Ware and Sherbourne 1992), EuroQol (EuroQol Group 1990), and the Quality of Well-Being Scale (Kaplan and Anderson 1988). A large number of instruments have been developed that are tailored to capture the effects of specific types of problems on various domains such as musculo-skeletal conditions on activities of daily living. The large and expanding set of disease or condition-specific instruments is brought about by the need in clinical trials, and perhaps clinical practice, for instruments that are sensitive to slight improvements or decrements in health status. There appears to be a trade-off between the simplicity of an instrument and its responsiveness to subtle change. Second, in recent years, there has been increasing emphasis on the international comparability of these measures but there has been little experience with them in developing countries (Shumaker and Berzon 1995). Third, nearly all instruments with the exception of a few condition-specific instruments are based on self-reports.

Much of the literature is devoted to investigating the reliability and validity of the various instruments (Hays et al. 1993). Reliability is most often measured using internal consistency of an individual's responses to repeated questions or by looking at their test-retest reliability by comparing an individuals response to the same instrument at different times. Measuring the validity of HRQL instruments is much more problematic. Because there is no agreed upon gold standard measure of health-related quality of life, traditional measures of validity, called "criterion validity" in the psychometric literature, are absent. Much weaker forms of validity, such as content or construct validity, are often used to support HRQL instruments.[25] The lack of criterion validity remains as a concern in cross-national and inter-temporal comparisons using most HRQL instruments.

The difficulties of interpreting self-reported health status become clearer when inter-community and inter-temporal comparisons are attempted. Figure 1.8 illustrates how in the Living Standards Measurement Survey of Ghana, rich households reported more episodes of illness than poor households. Murray and Chen (1992) suggest that individuals in the United States report more episodes of illness than do individuals in India and that within India, individuals in the poorest and highest mortality states, namely Assam and Bihar, report lower rates of illness than in Kerala state which has the lowest mortality rates. Counter-intuitive patterns such as these are common.[26] These results are not at all surprising (Murray 1995, Johansson 1991). Different individuals have different perceptions and expectations of health. These perceptions and expectations are likely to be complex functions of socio-demographic variables including education, household income, contact with health services and cultural conceptions of health. As societies change in terms of their socio-economic composition and cultural beliefs, we might expect that perceptions and expectations of health would change as well (Mackenbach et al. 1990).

Defenders of self-reported measures point to several studies (Idler and Angel 1990, Idler et al. 1990, Kaplan and Kotler 1985, McCallum et al. 1994, Mossey and Shapiro 1982) showing that those who rate their health as poor experience higher mortality than those who rate their health as excellent. There are two reasons why this finding does not validate self-reported illness for inter-temporal or cross-community assessments. First, if those individuals who have been given a diagnosis of disease that carries with it a substantially increased risk of death are likely to report their health status as poor then, of course, those who report poor health status will have a higher death rate. The proportion given such diagnoses, however, will vary over time and across communities as a function of access to health care. Second, in both Kerala State, India and in the United States, those who rate their health as poor may have a higher death rate than those who rate their health as excellent, but the proportion that report their health as poor may not explain any of the difference in mortality between Kerala and the United States. For example, the aboriginal population in Australia has substantially higher mortality rates than the rest of the Australian population, but 2 per cent report their health as poor and 10 per cent report their health as fair, as compared to 4.5 per cent in the rest of the Australian population reporting poor health and 16 per cent reporting fair health (Australian Institute of Health and Welfare 1996).

Given these difficulties, we have endeavoured to use observations on non-fatal health outcomes wherever possible in the Global Burden of Disease Study. There is a category of health outcomes which cannot be

Figure 1.8   Percentage of adults aged 15–39 years reporting illness during one month

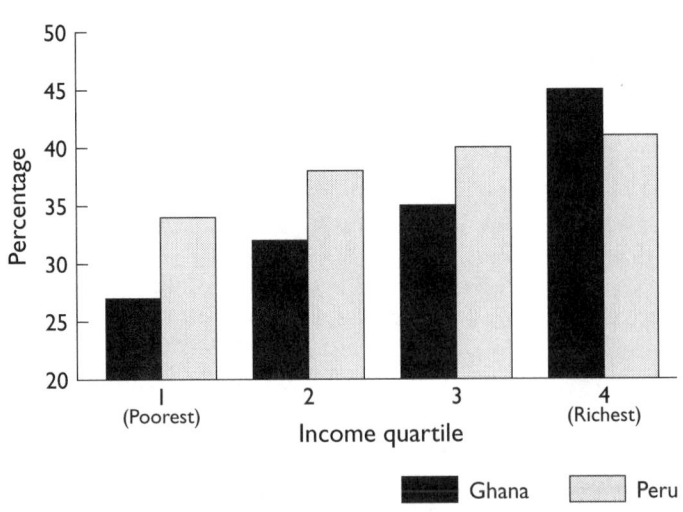

observed, namely pain and suffering (Murray and Chen 1992). For such conditions, the only option is to use self-reported measures, bearing in mind the substantial potential for confounding by socio-economic and cultural factors when making cross-community comparisons.

APPORTIONING NON-FATAL HEALTH OUTCOMES TO SPECIFIC ETIOLOGIES

If measurements of non-fatal health outcomes are to be useful in discussions about the allocation of scarce resources for promotive, preventive, curative or rehabilitative interventions, some attempt must be made to apportion the burden by etiology. Ascribing outcomes to proximal pathological causes does not imply that there are not important distal socio-economic determinants of an individual's non-fatal health outcome. One of the greatest limitations of the available literature on non-fatal health outcomes is that it does not apportion burden by proximal cause. There are two ways to approach the issue; tracing the individual back to a set of proximal causes or projecting forward from a pathological event to the probable non-fatal health outcome. Many factors will determine the probability of transition from a pathological event through to an impairment, disability or handicap. These transition probabilities depend on access to treatment, social, economic and cultural factors and contexts. Linking disease specific epidemiology with non-fatal health outcomes through some probabilistic causal web will be a critical step in developing useful measures of non-fatal health outcomes. Such measures can then inform debates on health policy and intervention choice. As we shall see later in this chapter and in other chapters of this book, a substantial effort was made in the Global Burden of Disease Study to develop a mapping of these transition probabilities for a large number of conditions.

VALUING TIME LIVED WITH VARIOUS HEALTH OUTCOMES

In order to compare time lived in various health states with years of life lost due to premature mortality, one needs to develop a set of weights for time spent in different health states. An important issue is to define what exactly we are intending to value. For example, we could value time spent being blind, time spent with a reading disability or time spent unable to work because of blindness. In this section, methods available to measure preferences or values are discussed, as well as the appropriate place in the causal web where it is most feasible to undertake these valuations.

There are five main methods that have been proposed to measure health state preferences: rating scales or visual analogue, magnitude estimation, standard gamble, time trade-off and person trade-off (Nord 1992, Richardson 1994, Torrance 1986). [27] A second important issue in measuring preferences for time lived with different non-fatal health outcomes is the choice of respondents, or in other words, whose values should be measured. At least four groups are often distinguished: those living in a given health state, families of individuals in a health state, the general public and health care providers. Because health state preference measurement is a rapidly changing field, it may be useful to review briefly the strengths and weaknesses of various approaches before returning to the approach that has been taken for Years Lived with Disability (YLDs), the component of DALYs pertaining to non-fatal health outcomes.

Opinions on which preference measurement method is best and which respondents are most appropriate vary widely (Froberg and Kane 1989, Hornberger et al. 1992, Kaplan and Ernst 1983, Mehrez and Gafni 1987, Mulley 1989, Nord 1991, 1992, 1995, Nord et al. 1993, Revicki and Kaplan 1995, Richardson 1994, Rosser and Kind 1978, Torrance and Feeny 1989). The best method depends on the ultimate use to be made of the preference measurements. In burden of disease analyses and sectoral cost-effectiveness analyses, comparisons between different groups of individuals are inevitable. Such comparisons introduce additional considerations that are not strictly present in individual choices. For burden and cost-effectiveness analyses, health state preferences need to have at least interval scale properties so that a change in health state weight from 0.1 to 0.2 is equivalent to a change from 0.7 to 0.8.[28] Richardson (1994) and Nord (1991) have challenged whether individual's preferences measured using ratings scales or visual analogues report preferences that have interval scale properties. Eddy (1991) and Nord (1993) have argued that rating scale measures like the Quality of Well-Being Scale (QWB) yield utility values for mild conditions that are too low. In such measures, utilities are scaled such that 0 is equivalent to death and 1 to perfect health. For example, in the Oregon health prioritization exercise using QWB, 50 dental pulp extractions were considered equivalent to saving a life. Likewise, magnitude estimation methods have yielded results that are different than rating scales and that are not likely to have interval scale properties (Kaplan et al. 1979, Richardson 1994).

Torrance and colleagues (Torrance 1986, Torrance and Feeny 1989) argue that the standard gamble is the gold standard measure of health state preference because it is based directly on the von Neumann-Morgenstern formulation of expected utility.[29] Yet the standard gamble is one of the most difficult approaches to incorporate in the measurement of health state preferences (Mulley 1989, Nord 1992). For mild health states, the standard gamble depends on an individual's ability to discriminate between probabilities close to one; however, there is a considerable literature suggesting that individuals have biased perceptions of risks at low and high probabilities (Fischhoff et al. 1981, Viscusi 1993). The difficulty in evaluating probabilities would tend to bias health state preferences for very mild or very severe states towards either pole. Based on theoretical and empirical evidence, individuals confound standard gamble health state preferences with their like or dislike of gambling (Nord 1992, Richardson 1994, Wolfson et al. 1982).[30]

The time trade-off was originally proposed by Torrance (1976) and justified because the health state preferences measured using this method correlated with measurements based on the standard gamble. In fact, it measures the individual's preference for the two health states. Richardson (1994) notes that it has the interval scale properties desired because the respondent is asked to make a direct equivalence between two outcomes in the dimension of life-years. A major disadvantage is that preference measurements are confounded by time preference. Johannesson et al. (1994) argue that depending on the risk aversion of individuals for QALYs, health state preferences can be estimated that are not confounded by time preference; although this approach has not been applied in practice.

The person trade-off method (PTO) was first proposed by Patrick et al. (1973) and more recently has been advocated by Nord and others (Nord 1991, 1992, 1993, 1995, Nord et al. 1995, Olsen 1993). Because individuals are forced in the PTO method to undertake interpersonal comparisons of utility for different groups of individuals, Nord (1995) argues that the content validity of the resulting weights is greater if the weights are to influence the allocation of resources between groups.[31] As with time preference—see discussion below—individuals may have different preferences for trade-offs between quantity of life for one set of individuals and quality of life for another set of individuals and trade-offs between quantity and quality of life for themselves. Nord (1995) has pointed out that the PTO may be confounded by respondent's preferences for the distribution of health benefits. For example, individuals may prefer to save one life-year for 1000 individuals as opposed to saving ten life-years for 100 individuals or vice-versa. Opposite results can also be obtained depending on the magnitude of the benefits being compared—see the discussion below under equity. While the exact distributional preferences of different populations have not yet been fully defined (Nord et al. 1995), by its construction the PTO methods appears to include some element of distributional preference in the estimated magnitude of health state preference.

RESPONDENTS, COPING, ADAPTATION AND DE TOCQUEVILLE'S "HAPPY SLAVE"

Whatever method is used to elicit preferences for health states, the results appear to depend on the type of respondent used (Carter et al. 1976, Froberg and Kane 1989b, Kane et al. 1986, Mulley 1989, Nord 1992, Sackett and Torrance 1978). In general, health-care providers and families of persons in a specific health state rate health states as worse than the general public does, and the general public in turn rates the same health states worse than those living in the health state do. As responses vary, considerable debate has emerged on whose values should be used. Torrance (1986) argues that for decisions about the allocation of scarce societal resources among different groups of recipients, valuations of the general public should be used. For the choice among different interventions for the same individual, many advocate using the evaluations of individuals in a particular health state (Drummond 1987, Hornberger et al. 1992, Kaplan and Bush 1982). Advocates of the rights of the disabled feel strongly that only the preferences of those living in a given health state should be used (Nagler 1993). The debate on respondent types can be interpreted in terms of knowledge and adaptation.

It is my own experience in undertaking preference measurement exercises that knowledge of a health state has a profound effect on preference evaluations. Various respondent types can be re-categorized into two groups: those with no knowledge of a health state, such as much of the general public, and those with knowledge. The latter group can be subdivided into those living in a health state, those whose life has been affected (usually adversely) by someone they know in a health state, and those with knowledge but without a direct personal effect (usually health care providers). In one exercise, a group representative of the general public were asked to evaluate their preferences for active delusional psychosis. Despite verbal descriptions of the state, the participants were uncomfortable undertaking the evaluation. Moreover, if someone was present with knowledge of the state, individual assessments would gravitate to the assessment of the individual with knowledge, if respondents are allowed to change their preferences after group discussion. Re-interpreting the variation in preference values for health states, knowledge leads to lower utility weights (death is zero) but knowledge derived from experiencing a health state may lead to a higher utility weight.

Fortunately for the human condition, man adapts. Coping with adversity and readjusting expectations have important effects on measuring preferences. Adaptation can be seen to have both negative and positive aspects. One manifestation of readjusting expectations is the "hedonic treadmill" where an individual's satisfaction or well-being appears not to improve despite substantial increases in material well-being overtime (Diener 1984, Kahneman and Varey 1991, van de Stadt et al. 1985). Subjective well-being could worsen despite improvements in material well-being particularly if neighbours have improved more. A more positive example of adaptation can be seen in those who live permanently in a health state worse than perfect health. Figure 1.9 shows a hypothetical individual who suffers a spinal cord transection. Immediately after the injury the individual might assign a very low preference weight for his health state. With time the individual will adapt to his paraplegia, and serial assessments of his preference weight for his health state might steadily rise, perhaps reaching a plateau a few years after the injury. At the limit, there may be individuals who adapt so perfectly that their preference weight returns to one. Which preference should be used for burden of disease or cost-effectiveness analyses, the adapted or the pre-adapted weight? The coping/adaptation phenomenon has profound resource implications: using pre-adapted weights will make prevention and rehabilitation look more cost-effective, but life extension for those with paraplegia will appear to be less cost-effective. Using the adapted weights will make prevention and rehabilitation much less attractive in cost-effectiveness terms, but it will make life extension more cost-effective.

Figure 1.9   Health state utility over time of an individual who experiences a spinal cord transection at age 30 and becomes a paraplegic

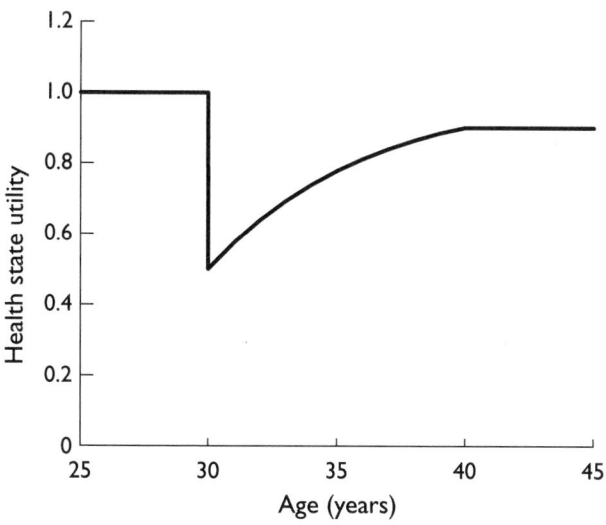

Note: With time after the accident, this hypothetical individual adapts to his condition and assigns a higher health state utility to being paraplegic.

The adaptation phenomenon has long plagued social theorists (Helson 1964, Ittleson et al. 1974, Elster and Roemer 1991). Indeed, as De Tocqueville (1839) noted in a now-classic passage:

> Should I call it a blessing of God, or a last malediction of his anger, this disposition of the soul that makes men insensible to extreme misery? Plunged in this abyss of wretchedness, the slave hardly notices his ill fortune; he was reduced to slavery by violence, and the habit of servitude has given him the thoughts and ambitions of a slave.

The fact that some slaves may have been happy does not in any way make the reality of slavery more acceptable. By analogy, the adaptive powers of man should not make the prevention or rehabilitation of those with a non-fatal health outcome less valuable. It would be exceedingly perverse to argue that we should not prevent deafness simply because those who are deaf are able to adapt so well to their loss of hearing. It would be equally perverse to argue against preventing cognitive impairment due to micronutrient deficiencies because the cognitively impaired are happy.

An opposing viewpoint is that using non-adaptive weights devalues the importance of interventions that extend the life of those living in a health state worse than perfect health. I find this attribute of cost-effectiveness, as currently practiced, a vexing moral problem. Instinctively, I would like to use the adapted weights for evaluating life-extending interventions and the pre-adapted weights for evaluating preventive or rehabilitative interventions. Yet, giving up internal consistency, which requires a single weight for a time lived in a given health state, would come with a high price. The potential for confusing or conflicting results in burden and cost-effectiveness analyses would be too great. In reality, few interventions are specifically tailored to extend the life of individuals in a given health state; thus there are few cost-effectiveness analyses of such interventions. In fact, in the normal practice of a cost-effectiveness analysis, studies of the cost-effectiveness of the same intervention in different population sub-groups of recipients are rarely elaborated. While we may avoid this problem in the near future, ultimately, the dilemma posed by pre-adapted and adapted preference weights for cost-effectiveness must be addressed.

THE IMPORTANCE OF DELIBERATION

Characteristics which have not yet been discussed are the duration, intensity and degree of reflection built into the preference measurement process. Nord (1992, 1995) has proposed that one method to validate preference measurements is through a "reflective equilibrium" where individuals are faced with the policy consequences of their value choices. His call for more reflection in the elicitation of preferences is an example of a more general subject in political theory: the importance of deliberation. In the Federalist Papers, Madison argued that a representative democracy would be preferable to a direct democracy because some judgments require deliberation: reflection on the implications of a choice and sufficient time to arrive at an informed judgment (Rossiter 1961). Since the general public would not have adequate time and opportunity for such deliberation, Madison argued, indirect representative democracy would be preferable to direct democracy. Fishkin (1991) has argued that the United States Presidential primary system needs to be revised to include a deliberative process at the beginning, so that polls of opinions based on little or no deliberation do not determine the outcome of the primary process. There is a similarity between arriving at valuations for different health states and making difficult policy choices in democratic societies. The choice of health state weights may have profound implications for many members of society. Such weighty choices are difficult and benefit from considered deliberation. I believe that it can only enhance the value of preference judgments if the individuals are confronted with the direct implications of their choices and allowed to discuss the bases for their viewpoints with their peers.

There is clearly a trade-off between the number of individuals whose preferences are measured and the degree of deliberation. A deliberative approach to preference measurement requires much time and should probably be undertaken in groups. A deliberative approach could not, for example, be integrated into a large-scale household survey. Contrast the deliberative approach with that of the Oregon Health Plan's telephone survey used to elicit, through brief conversations, valuations using the Quality of Well-Being Scale (Eddy 1991). Perhaps it is not surprising that in community consultations, the policy implication of the valuations in the telephone survey were rejected by the community. I believe that preference measurements for health states which are intended to inform social choices must be based on a deliberative process, but empirical evidence on the difference between deliberative and rapid judgments has yet to be collected.

YEARS LIVED WITH DISABILITY

Given the diverse approaches to conceptualizing, measuring and valuing non-fatal health outcomes, many possible strategies could have been used for measuring the burden of non-fatal health outcomes. Prior to the Global Burden of Disease Study, the only effort to evaluate the burden of disease due to disability and premature mortality by cause for an entire population was the Ghana Health Assessment Project (1981). While this study was path breaking, the methods and rationale used for defining, measuring and weighting disability were never published.[32] Building on this and other experiences, a practical approach that could be applied to over 100 diseases and their sequelae was developed for this version of the GBD. With this opportunity to rethink DALYs, the approach to non-fatal health outcomes has been substantially revised. The conceptual approach is outlined below, after which the original application is presented, followed by the substantive revisions.

In the terminology of the *International Classification of Impairments, Disabilities and Handicaps*, I have chosen to measure disability, not handicap. The principle of treating "like as like" requires using disability instead of handicap. Handicap is an attractive concept because it focuses on the impact given the particular social context of the individual. In some cases, similar disabilities may lead to a greater handicap for an already disadvantaged person than for the more fortunate. In many cases, however, allocating resources to avert handicap as opposed to disability could exacerbate inequalities. The manual of the ICIDH itself gives the following example:

> A subnormality of intelligence is an impairment, but it may not lead to appreciable activity restriction; factors other than the impairment may determine the handicap because the disadvantage may be minimal if the individual lives in a remote rural community, whereas it could be severe in the child of university graduates living in a large city, of whom more might be expected. (p.31)

Pursuing handicap could, and probably would, lead us to invest in avoiding mental retardation in the rich and well educated but not in the poor. To avoid the obvious problems with such an approach, one must focus on disability rather than handicap.

Having stated this, the actual approach implemented in the Global Burden of Disease Study has been to use a construct somewhere between disability and handicap. More precisely, given the method used to elicit preferences for health states in this revision of DALYs, perhaps the concept is best described as an average level of handicap.[33] Since the construct used lies somewhere between disability and handicap and in order to maintain consistency with the earlier versions of the GBD, time lived with non-fatal health outcomes weighted as outlined below is labelled Years Lived with Disability (YLDs).

THE ORIGINAL APPROACH TO YLDS

In 1992, four domains of disability were defined for the original version of DALYs: procreation, occupation, education and recreation. Six classes of disability severity were arbitrarily defined using word definitions related to activities of daily living, instrumental activities of daily living and the four domains. Based on available literature and expert panels, the probabilities of transition from the onset of major disease or injury through to disabling sequelae were estimated. Finally, a panel of public health practitioners used a rating scale method to choose the severity weight for each of the six classes. At the time that the severity weights were chosen, the panel was aware of the set of disabling sequelae included in each class. Subsequently, in country applications and scientific meetings,[34] a number of important criticisms of this approach have been raised, four of which are worth considering here. First, the word definitions of the six disability classes were developed based on the literature on adult disability; they are clearly not appropriate for defining disability in children. Strictly speaking, young children would automatically be in a disability class because they are dependent on care-givers for many activities of daily living (Murray 1994). Second, for those analysts undertaking a national burden of disease study, the process of selecting disability weights is not easily reproduced as there was no formalized protocol available for reproducing the disability weights selection process. Third, the first class of disability already carried a disability weight of 0.096 which is very severe for many mild conditions—remember that in YLDs the disability scale is inverted compared with QALYs so that 0 is perfect health and 1 is equivalent to death. As a consequence, the scale is insensitive to changes in the severity of mild disabilities. Finally, the panel of public health practitioners who selected the class weights used a rating scale approach and was not challenged with the policy implications of their valuations. In other words, the exercise was not a deliberative process.

Based on these criticisms and the expanding literature and debate on alternative methods for preference measurement discussed above, the approach used to define, measure and value disabilities for YLDs—the component of DALYs due to non-fatal health outcomes—was revised for the present estimates of the GBD. The major change resulting from this revision has been to shift away from defining disability classes in terms of the four domains of recreation, education, procreation and occupation and to move to a deliberative process for choosing weights for any given disabling sequela based on several variants of the person-trade-off method. The approach has been designed so that it can be replicated at the national or sub-national level without too much difficulty. As the ultimate goal is a set of weights for the treated and untreated forms of several hundred outcomes included in the Global Burden of Disease Study, it is perforce a complicated process. The following discussion is divided into several sections for clarity: the PTO protocol and its development, the consensus meeting on disability weights convened at the World Health Organization, the definition of seven classes of disability, estimation of disability distributions for several hundred conditions (treated and untreated) and some comments on future challenges and opportunities in this area.

PERSON TRADE-OFF (PTO) PROTOCOL

Based on the discussions in the previous sections, a protocol has been developed for preference measurement. The details on the protocol are provided in Appendix 1 of this chapter. A few aspects of the design and development of the protocol are worth noting.

- The process has been designed to be deliberative. Participants are challenged with the implications of their valuations, pushed to make valuations from different perspectives and forced to reconcile the differences that emerge from different framings. As the ultimate purpose is to achieve a consensus, the process is a group exercise which allows for substantial exchange and revision.

- At a maximum, a group exercise can last one day, or more specifically eight to ten hours. Even a process of this length will severely restrict the number of group exercises that can realistically be undertaken. In eight to ten hours, deliberative valuations of approximately twenty conditions are feasible.

- The final version of the protocol includes 22 indicator conditions. The set of conditions has been chosen to reflect the different dimensions of non-fatal health outcomes. Conditions with largely physical manifestations include blindness, deafness and a below-the-knee amputation; neuro-psychiatric conditions include unipolar major depression, active psychosis, Down Syndrome, and mild mental retardation; one condition has exclusively social or group interaction consequences, namely vitiligo, and several conditions represent varying degrees of pain: severe migraine, angina and sore throat. Finally, three conditions that affect sexual/reproductive function have been included in the list: impotence, infertility and recto-vaginal fistula. For the remainder of the conditions included in the GBD, short-cut methods have been used to estimate the disability weight, as described later in this chapter.

- Two forms of the PTO are used. In the first form, participants are asked to trade-off life extension of healthy individuals and life extension of individuals in a given health state—herein labeled PTO1. For example, would you as decision-maker prefer to purchase, through a health intervention, one year of life for 1000 perfectly healthy individuals or 2000 blind individuals? In a second form of the PTO, participants trade-off between raising the quality of life of those in health state *i* to perfect health for 1 year versus extending life for healthy individuals for one year—labelled PTO2. Both forms of the PTO yield preference weights for the health state under consideration.

In general, however, most individuals will give a low disability weight based on PTO1 and a high disability weight based on PTO2, on a scale where 0 is perfect health and 1 is equivalent to death.[35] Using a set of tables that show the equivalence between PTO1 and PTO2 judgments, participants are instructed to resolve the inconsistency in their valuations. There are three possible explanations for the common inconsistency between the PTO1 and PTO2 assessments: framing effects, individuals may be giving adapted weights for PTO1 and pre-adapted weights for PTO2, or the differential effect of distributional considerations in the two judgments. Based on the group discussions built into this protocol, the most important explanation appears to be the difference between adapted and pre-adapted weights.

- For each condition, five assessments of PTO1 and PTO2 are undertaken. After learning the PTO1 and PTO2 method, each participant first makes an assessment of PTO1 and PTO2 in private. Then using the PTO1–PTO2 equivalence tables, participants must reconcile differences in the disability weight implied by the two judgments. Participants in a group then share their internally consistent PTO1 and PTO2 assessments for a given indicator condition and discuss the reasons for their valuations. After discussion, participants can, and often do, revise their PTO1 and PTO2 assessments. This cycle is repeated for each of the 22 indicator conditions. In a second phase, each participant ranks by severity each of the 22 indicator conditions. The individual then compares his or her ordinal ranking with the ranking implied by his or her PTO assessments. After reflecting on why the two rankings may differ, each person is asked to reconcile differences which may include changing the PTO1 and PTO2 assessments. These revised PTO assessments are shared amongst group members and may be revised for a final time, after discussion.

- The protocol was tested on students and fellows from a number of countries at the Harvard School of Public Health. Based on this experience, the definitions of the 22 conditions were revised, facilitator instructions were developed and operational aspects, such as the use of marker boards and flashcards, were finalized. Details of these aspects are provided in Appendix 1 of this chapter.

- To speed up the already demanding process, the protocol has been designed to be used with health-care providers so that less time needs to be invested to describe each of the conditions. Health care providers are selected because of their knowledge, not because they have "better" judgment. Non health-care providers could be used but much more time would be required to educate them about each indicator condition.

The protocol has been applied to nine groups: an international consensus meeting on disability weights convened at the World Health Organization in Geneva, 14–19 August 1995, a meeting of members of the Japan national burden of disease team, a meeting of public health and quality of life experts at Rotterdam University, a joint meeting of the national burden of disease teams of Algeria, Tunisia and Morocco and five groups of international participants at a conference on burden of disease and cost-effectiveness methods. For the purposes of this study, I have used the results of the meeting convened at the World Health Organization and sponsored by the World Bank expressly to choose revised weights for the fifth version Global Burden of Disease Study.[36] The limited experience in other settings raises some interesting but not definitive hypotheses that are relevant to this discussion. Table 1.2 shows the Spearman's and Pearson's correlation coefficients for the median disability weight from eight other exercises compared with each of the others. Both the ordinal ranks and the cardinal values are highly correlated across all settings. Compared to the results of the Geneva meeting, the lowest correlation coefficient among the other eight exercises was 0.873, six of the eight exercises had a Pearson's correlation coefficient greater than 0.9, and seven of the eight had a Spearman's rank order correlation coefficient greater than 0.9. Putting it very bluntly, nearly everyone in all cultures appears to agree that blindness is worse than watery diarrhoea.

While the experience with this protocol is limited, the results to date raise an important issue. Many participants substantially revise their PTO1 and PTO2 assessments after the ordinal ranking phase of the exercise. In addition, the ordinal rankings of conditions appears to be highly preserved across groups. Rankings of conditions based on isolated judgments of the same individual (and presumably of different individuals to an even greater extent) are often inconsistent with deliberative judgments. If subsequent research confirms this finding, then ad hoc preference measurements undertaken for a limited number of health states should be compared with preference valuations from other studies with great caution. Likewise, comparisons of the cost-effectiveness of different interventions based on the preferences measured in different groups may be biased. In the near future, this protocol will hopefully be used on a much larger pool of respondents which will provide a more rigorous test of this phenomenon.

GENEVA MEETING ON DISABILITY WEIGHTS FOR THE GLOBAL BURDEN
OF DISEASE STUDY, VERSION 5

In the absence of a large volume of deliberative PTO health state preference
measurements, for the Global Burden of Disease Study, a consultative process has been followed. A meeting to which individuals from each region of
the world were invited—the sex ratio of those that were able to attend was
60 per cent male and 40 per cent female—sponsored by the World Bank
was convened at the World Health Organization in August 1995.[36] In the
first phase of this meeting, the invitees participated in the 22 indicator condition PTO protocol. When making their assessments, they were asked to
evaluate the average individual with the condition described taking into
account the average social response or milieu. The resulting valuations prob-

Table 1.2   Pearson's correlation coefficients and Spearman's rank
order correlation coefficients for the Geneva meeting on
disability weights and eight other exercises using the PTO
protocol (numbers I–VIII)

		Pearson's correlation coefficients							
Exercise	Geneva	I	II	III	IV	V	VI	VII	VIII
Geneva	1.00								
I	0.97	1.00							
II	0.87	0.87	1.00						
III	0.95	0.96	0.84	1.00					
IV	0.92	0.89	0.93	0.93	1.00				
V	0.92	0.89	0.87	0.95	0.96	1.00			
VI	0.94	0.89	0.81	0.94	0.91	0.93	1.00		
VII	0.90	0.95	0.77	0.90	0.83	0.81	0.84	1.00	
VIII	0.89	0.85	0.84	0.87	0.89	0.85	0.88	0.75	1.00

		Spearman's rank order correlation coefficients							
Exercise	Geneva	I	II	III	IV	V	VI	VII	VIII
Geneva	1.00								
I	0.99	1.00							
II	0.91	0.90	1.00						
III	0.94	0.95	0.90	1.00					
IV	0.94	0.92	0.94	0.93	1.00				
V	0.89	0.87	0.86	0.90	0.92	1.00			
VI	0.92	0.92	0.84	0.95	0.91	0.90	1.00		
VII	0.96	0.97	0.86	0.93	0.91	0.84	0.92	1.00	
VIII	0.93	0.92	0.92	0.92	0.91	0.84	0.84	0.88	1.00

Note: Pearson's correlation coefficient indicates the correlation of the cardinal values. Spearman's correlation
coefficient indicates the correlation of the ordinal rank.

Table 1.3 Preference weights for 22 indicator conditions based on the PTO protocol used at the Geneva meeting on disability weights

	Average disability weight	Median disability weight	Disability weight based on average PTO1	Disability weight based on median PTO1	Standard deviation of disability weight	Coefficient of variation of disability weight
Vitiligo on face	0.020	0.005	0.022	0.005	0.038	1.86
2 SD weight/height	0.024	0.020	0.024	0.020	0.019	0.80
Watery diarrhoea	0.066	0.045	0.068	0.045	0.046	0.70
Severe sore throat	0.077	0.082	0.081	0.083	0.054	0.70
Severe anaemia	0.111	0.099	0.117	0.099	0.066	0.59
Fractured radius in a stiff cast	0.136	0.107	0.140	0.107	0.058	0.43
Infertility	0.191	0.177	0.204	0.177	0.095	0.50
Erectile dysfunction	0.195	0.201	0.199	0.202	0.054	0.28
Rheumatoid arthritis	0.209	0.200	0.216	0.200	0.071	0.34
Angina	0.223	0.231	0.228	0.231	0.057	0.26
Below-the-knee amputation	0.281	0.272	0.286	0.273	0.059	0.21
Deafness	0.333	0.333	0.349	0.333	0.099	0.30
Mild mental retardation	0.361	0.410	0.394	0.412	0.148	0.41
Recto-vaginal fistula	0.373	0.333	0.392	0.333	0.102	0.27
Down syndrome without cardiac malformation	0.407	0.373	0.440	0.375	0.126	0.31
Unipolar major depression	0.619	0.633	0.636	0.636	0.079	0.13
Blindness	0.624	0.641	0.634	0.643	0.060	0.10
Paraplegia	0.671	0.672	0.691	0.672	0.080	0.12
Active psychosis	0.722	0.714	0.737	0.714	0.062	0.09
Severe migraine	0.738	0.753	0.831	0.762	0.146	0.20
Dementia	0.762	0.770	0.784	0.770	0.071	0.09
Quadriplegia	0.895	0.894	0.903	0.895	0.027	0.03

ably reflect average handicap stemming from each condition. Table 1.3 shows the average, median and standard deviation of the disability weights emerging from the exercise.[37] Spearman's rank order correlation coefficients between participants were all high—in excess of 0.86. The results show that despite diverse cultural backgrounds, the international group meeting at WHO achieved a high degree of consensus. It is also comforting to note that the results of this Geneva meeting closely match the pooled results of all nine exercises using the same protocol (see Figure 1.10).

Based on the PTO protocol results, with the Geneva meeting participants, we arbitrarily divided the spectrum from health to death into seven disability classes, shown in Table 1.4. The classes are exclusively defined by a range of disability weights; there are no longer any word definitions

Figure 1.10 Disability weights for the 22 indicator conditions based on the combined results of nine exercises using the PTO protocol compared with the results of the Geneva meeting on disability weights

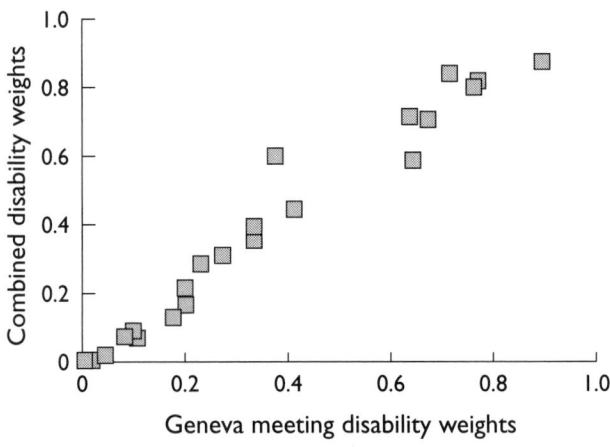

Table 1.4 Revised disability classes for the Global Burden of Disease Study based on the results of the PTO protocol used at the Geneva meeting on disability weights

Disability class	Severity weights	Indicator conditions
1	0.00–0.02	Vitiligo on face, weight-for-height less than 2 SDs
2	0.02–0.12	Watery diarrhoea, severe sore throat, severe anemia
3	0.12–0.24	Radius fracture in a stiff cast, infertility, erectile dysfunction, rheumatoid arthritis, angina
4	0.24–0.36	Below-the-knee amputation, deafness
5	0.36–0.50	Rectovaginal fistula, mild mental retardation, Down syndrome
6	0.50–0.70	Unipolar major depression, blindness, paraplegia
7	0.70–1.00	Active psychosis, dementia, severe migraine, quadriplegia

Note: For a complete description of the indicator conditions see Appendix 1 of this chapter.

for each class. Based on the Geneva meeting, each class includes 2–3 indicator conditions. The number of disability classes and the range of disability weights used to define these classes are entirely arbitrary. The classes and the benchmark conditions in each class are needed to facilitate a short-cut approach to estimating disability weights for the several hundred other conditions included in the study.

For the GBD, disability weights for treated and untreated forms of several hundred different outcomes were required. A number of these outcomes are fundamentally the same, for example blindness from retinopathy, trachoma or trauma. The participants at the Geneva meeting were asked to use a rating scale approach to decide the distribution of each condition in the treated and untreated form across the seven disability classes. The process used was deliberative; each participant chose a distribution across the seven classes in private, shared their results with the group, discussed discrepancies, and made revised distributions based on the discussion. Where treatment was judged to change the distribution of severity by class, and not simply the incidence, duration or case-fatality rate of a condition, the group developed a separate distribution for the treated form of a condition—for example, angina pectoris.

Ideally, any group convened to choose disability weights should be asked to render exclusively preference judgments for various health states. Unfortunately, at the Geneva meeting the group were presented with a mixed task, both epidemiological estimation and preference assessment. For example, when asked to choose a distribution by severity class of asthma, ideally the group would value each type of asthma as defined by frequency and intensity of episodes. Epidemiologists would provide information on the population distribution of asthma cases by severity group. In reality, our understanding of the descriptive epidemiology of many, if not most, conditions is not advanced. The participants at the Geneva meeting were therefore called upon at times to make a composite judgment of the distribution of different forms of a condition and the valuation of time spent with each form of the condition. As the epidemiology of non-fatal health outcomes by cause advances, future iterations of this process should result in a much sharper distinction between epidemiology and valuation of health state preferences.

Annex Table 3 provides the disability weights by age for treated and untreated forms of various conditions included in the Global Burden of Disease Study. Distributions of a condition across the seven disability classes were converted into a single disability weight for each condition by multiplying the per cent in each class by the mid-point severity weight for the range defining that class. For ease of reference, the weights are provided in the same format as Annex Table 2. As a consequence, the same outcome may appear several times in the table. Since access to treatment varies by region, the composite disability weight for a condition where the treated and untreated weights are different is a function of the proportion of incidence cases that receive treatment.

CO-DISABILITY

With few exceptions, there is no explicit recognition of co-disability in the development of the disability weights for this study. In other words, if an individual simultaneously has more than one condition each of which has a disability weight, the composite disability weight for the combination of two conditions is simply the sum of their disability weights. This crude assumption could lead to nonsensical situations where the individual disability weight is greater than one.[38] One way forward would be to explicitly develop disability weights for a selected number of common co-morbid conditions using the methods described above. The current version of the Global Burden of Disease Study includes a few such composites, including Down syndrome with mental retardation and mental retardation with cerebral palsy.

It is important in this regard to distinguish dependent and independent co-disabilities. Some combinations occur more frequently than at random, such as neuropathy, retinopathy and ischaemic heart disease—three pathologies related to diabetes mellitus. For such dependent co-disabilities, future iterations of this study will need to move towards direct preference valuations for the combination itself.

For co-disability due solely to chance, there is the suggestion that the disability weights for such co-disability should remain the sum of the individual disability weights. One of the initial propositions in this chapter is the principle of treating like health outcomes as like. The same non-fatal health outcome such as cognitive impairment should contribute the same amount to the burden of disease regardless of location. If we "correct" disability weights for co-disability—reduce them such that the disability weight for the combination of two conditions is less than the sum of the disability weights for each condition separately—becoming blind in a population with a high prevalence of disability would lead to a smaller incremental increase in burden than becoming blind in a population with low disability prevalence. Correcting for independent co-disability would introduce a bias in favor of saying the same event caused more burden in the better off than in the worse off. As a result, adjustments have not been made for co-disability except for a few major examples of dependent co-disability.

ALTERNATIVE INDICATORS OF TIME LIVED WITH DISABILITY

Where information on the incidence, prevalence, duration and severity of non-fatal health outcomes is available, a variety of other population indicators of non-fatal health outcomes can be calculated. These alternative population indicators are not designed to facilitate disaggregating the burden of premature mortality and non-fatal health outcomes into component causes. Rather, they are health expectancies that summarize incidence or prevalence data in terms of the average length of life lived in various health states.

REVES is an independent network of academics and government agencies that are concerned with quantifying healthy life (Robine et al. 1993a). In line with the ICIDH, REVES has proposed three such expectancies: impairment-free life expectancy, disability-free life expectancy and handicap-free life expectancy (Robine et al. 1993b). Proponents of these measures sometimes argue that disability-free life expectancy avoids the vexing problem of preference weights for disabilities. Barendregt (personal communication, 1995) has pointed out that these measures actually incorporate extreme preference weights of zero and one, a position now accepted by some members of REVES (Robine et al. 1993b). In disability-free life expectancy, all time spent with a moderate or severe disability is considered equivalent to time lost due to premature mortality, a weight of one. Mild disability is given a weight of zero. Unfortunately, because the threshold below which disability is weighted as zero is inconsistently defined between studies, estimates of disability-free life expectancy cannot reliably be compared between populations (REVES 1993).

If time lived with non-fatal health outcomes is weighted by a health state preference weight, a health-adjusted life expectancy can be calculated. For example, Wolfson (1994) has advocated using a health-adjusted life expectancy, namely, the population health index, as the summary health status measure for Canada. Murray and Lopez (1996a) in Chapter 4 in this volume use the data generated through the burden of disease study on the prevalence of various disabilities and the severity weights reported here to calculate Disability-Adjusted Life Expectancy (DALE), an indicator closely related to DALYs in which period life expectancy is corrected for the number of years lived with disability, adjusted for the severity of disability.[39] Such an indicator is a useful alternative summary measure of the global burden of disease. When disaggregating burden into specific causes or risk factors, however, DALYs are a preferable measure.

FUTURE DIRECTIONS FOR DISABILITY PREFERENCE MEASUREMENT

For those groups that wish to replicate the Global Burden of Disease Study at the national or sub-national level, the following steps are recommended. It is probably worthwhile to apply the PTO protocol to at least one but preferably several groups. If the results are similar and most of the 22 indicator conditions fall into the same classes as defined at the Geneva meeting then it would seem reasonable to adopt the entire set of disability weights in Annex Table 3. If the results are markedly different, the task is much more difficult. Options would include replicating the entire exercise, revising those conditions closely linked to the indicator conditions that changed classes, or simply rescaling the ranges for each class and the median disability weight for each class.

The GBD and the calculation of DALYs linked with it must be viewed as an ongoing process with methods, data and results in steady evolution. For the next revision of the GBD, substantially more data on the PTO protocol and alternative approaches will, hopefully, have been collected. Regardless of how the methods are developed, there needs to be an institutionalized process whereby a representative group is periodically convened by the World Health Organization and/or other international health bodies. This representative group is needed to choose a new set of disability weights for global and comparative analyses. The weights presented in this chapter should be viewed as indicative of the current state of knowledge with revisions expected in the future.

Discounting Future Health

At the simplest level, discounting is the economic concept which reflects the fact that most individuals prefer benefits now rather than in the future. If offered the choice between $100 from a completely reliable source today or $100 in one year, most will prefer their money today. If offered $110 in one year versus $100 today, some may choose the $110. The interest rate on a savings account is the rate at which individuals must be compensated to forgo consumption today for consumption in the future. The market rate of interest is the aggregate rate at which individuals in society as a whole discount future consumption. It is standard practice in economic appraisal of projects to use the discount rate to discount benefits in the future (Das Gupta 1972, Layard and Glaister 1994). The process of discounting future benefits converts them into present value terms; they can then be compared with project costs to determine cost-effectiveness.

Despite widespread use of discounting in the evaluation of health projects (Evans and Hurley 1995, Sloan 1995), the practice has recently come under scrutiny and challenge (Anonymous 1992, Cairns 1992, Cropper et al. 1994, Fuchs 1986, Fuchs and Zeckhauser 1987, Ganiats 1992, Hammit 1993, Johannesson 1992, Krahn and Gafni 1993, Martens and Doorslover 1990, Olsen 1993, Parsonage and Neuberger 1992, Redelmeier and Heller 1993, Viscusi and Moore 1989). The issues involved are complex and the range and types of arguments for and against discounting health benefits are extensive. It is beyond the scope of this chapter to present an exhaustive review of the practice, or an original set of arguments for and against discounting future health. Discounting as a practice, however, can have a profound effect on the results of cost-effectiveness analysis and, to a lesser extent, alter the importance attached to deaths in children compared with adults in burden of disease analyses. In this section, the major arguments for discounting dollars and health benefits from both the individual and the societal perspectives will be reviewed, leading towards a justification for the arbitrary three per cent discount rate used in YLLs, YLDs and their sum, DALYs.

Although they are often used interchangeably, discounting and time preference are not synonymous. Discounting refers to the practice of valuing the same thing in the future as less (or more) valuable than the present. There may be many reasons to discount the future, such as uncertainty that increases with time or the likelihood that we will be better off in the future. Time preference refers to a preference for utility or well-being sooner rather than later, chosen simply because it is sooner and not because of other changes that might be correlated with time. The term "time preference" is used here only when referring to the latter concept.

This section begins by examining individuals' discount rates for dollars and proceeds to examine individuals discounting of prospects for their own future health. Next, the extent to which discount rates for social decisions deviate from individual discount rates both for dollars and for health benefits are discussed. This is followed by a brief review of a series of consequentialist arguments for discounting future health, concluding with arguments for discounting future health in the calculation of DALYs.

INDIVIDUAL DISCOUNT RATES

Individual behaviour in the marketplace consistently shows that individuals discount future dollars compared to present dollars. Why do individuals prefer money today rather than tomorrow? Individuals may not intrinsically prefer dollars today over tomorrow. They may simply prefer to receive a dollar today because that dollar can be invested and yield more than one dollar in the future. This opportunity cost argument for discounting by individuals, however, is circular. If all individuals were indifferent between consumption today versus tomorrow, the interest rate would approach zero because as long as the interest rate was non-zero some individuals would choose to invest. At the limit, there would be no opportunity cost to consuming a dollar today and individuals would not discount future consumption. In reality, it is individuals' preference for consumption today rather than later that creates a positive interest rate and thus an opportunity cost of money. We must return then to reasons why individuals might prefer to consume a dollar today over consuming a dollar in the future.

An individual's probability of being alive at any point in the future is steadily declining—see the earlier discussion of survivorship functions. The average risk of dying for the entire world's population is approximately one per cent per year. It would be rational for individuals to discount a dollar in the future according to the likelihood of being alive next year to use it. As the risk of death rises with age, we expect the discount rate to rise *ceteris paribus* with age, a proposition supported in part by some surveys.[40] Likewise, we might predict *ceteris paribus* higher discount rates in the poor than in the rich because mortality rates are higher among the poor (Strotz 1956).

Figure 1.11 shows the hypothetical relationship between utility and an individual's level of consumption. The curve is concave[41] so that as an individual's level of consumption rises, the increment in utility derived from each dollar is smaller. This phenomenon of declining marginal utility of increased consumption appears to be a common human trait. If individuals expect to be richer in the future and marginal utility decreases as consumption increases, individuals would derive less utility from $1 in the future than the present. Of course, if individuals expect to be poorer in the future then a future dollar may be more valued than a present dollar. As most economies are growing, most individuals will tend to discount future dollars.

In addition to discounting for a risk of death and declining marginal utility of future consumption, combined with an expectation of growing income, individuals may simply prefer utility now over equivalent amounts of utility in the future. Undoubtedly many individuals do have

Figure 1.11   Utility as a function of consumption

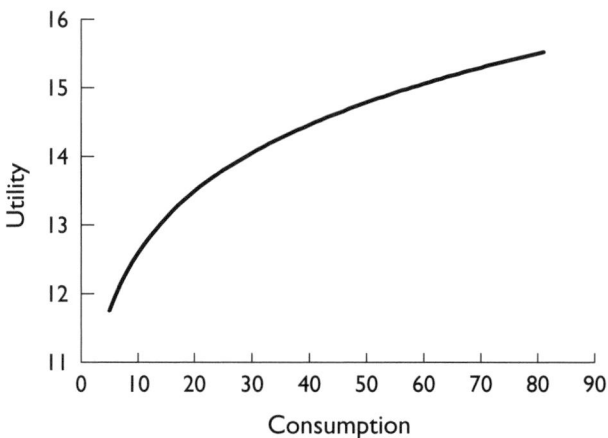

Note: The curve is concave so that equal increases in consumption lead to smaller increments in utility at higher levels of consumption.

a positive rate of time preference and many economists of the revealed preference school would accept these preferences as expressed in market behavior. Other philosophers and economists view pure time preference as a form of myopia, a simple defect in human judgment (Pigou 1932, Ramsey 1928, Sidgewick 1907). Pure time preference is an emotive issue; one for which there is unlikely to ever be a consensus (Anand and Hanson 1995).

Individual Discount Rates for Future Health

Even if individuals choose to discount future dollars, do they or should they discount their own future health? The evidence based on market behaviour and surveys is mixed: Viscusi and Moore (1989) find rates of 2–3 per cent or 11 per cent depending on the method used to impute the discount rate from market behaviour. Redelmeier and Heller (1993) surveyed individuals and found a mean discount rate of 3.3 per cent, but 10 per cent of those surveyed had a negative discount rate, 62.1 per cent had a zero discount rate and 15.7 per cent has a discount rate greater than 10 per cent. As with dollars, we can speculate on the reasons why an individual might discount his or her own future health. The probability of death is already captured in the estimation of future life-years or health status so that this component of an individual's discount rate for dollars is clearly not relevant to discounting future health. Is there a declining marginal utility of an extra life-year in the future? Life-years provide the capacity to derive utility from consumption and are not just another good or service. There is simply no reason to presume that there is a declining marginal utility of extra life-years. In fact, if an individual expects to be better off in the future, a future life-year may confer a larger increase in lifetime expected utility than a proximal life-year because the average level of utility will be higher.[42]

If individuals have a positive rate of pure time preference for utility, we might expect that it would also apply to future health. Acharya and Murray (1996) have shown that an individual will discount expected increments in life expectancy at a rate that is a function of many factors: the growth rate of consumption, pure time preference, the concavity of utility as a function of consumption and the size of the increase in life expectancy.[43] Individual discount rates for life-years need not be positive and could be negative. In the formulation of Acharya and Murray, for example, negative discounting will occur if the growth rate of consumption exceeds the individual's rate of pure time preference. Redelmeier and Heller (1993) found, moreover, that some individuals do have a negative discount rate for life-years. The relevance for social choices of these individual discount rates for future health is discussed in the next section.

THE SOCIAL DISCOUNT RATE

In the literature on economic analysis, there is an extensive debate on the choice of a discount rate for decisions taken by society (see Lind et al. 1984). Social discount rates may differ from individual discount rates for dollars and health because individuals view social choices differently and because of the way in which individual preferences are aggregated. Part of an individual's discount rate is the risk of death, which is on average one per cent per year. When considering choices affecting society, individuals may exclude from consideration their risk of death and consider instead the much smaller risks of extinction for society. The risk of environmental or geological cataclysmic events that would destroy societies is clearly very small, but non-zero; other risks for the survival of societies include war and natural disasters. The combined risk of extinction due to all possible causes is, nevertheless, likely to be far less than one per cent per year in most societies.

Sen (1961, 1972) and Marglin (1963) have pointed out that an individual may have different rates of pure time preferences for decisions affecting society as compared to decisions exclusively affecting himself or herself. Sen (1984) gives two reasons for this: (1) the dual argument, namely that members of the present generation in their political or public role may be more concerned about the welfare of future generations than they are in their day to day market activities; and (2) the isolation argument, whereby even with a given set of preferences, members of the present generation may be willing to join in a collective contract of more savings by all, though unwilling to save more in isolation.

Recognizing that individuals may have different discount rates for social decisions, the issue of whose preferences are relevant to choosing a social discount rate is equally important. Many economists would argue that only the preferences of those individuals that are currently alive or, even more narrowly, active in the marketplace should be taken into consideration in choosing the social discount rate. Other writers such as Parfit (1984) and Goodin (1982) have questioned why the preferences of future generations should not be taken into consideration. Parfit argues that pure time preference for society is as reasonable as a rate of pure spatial preference, where we would prefer utility gained by individuals living closer to us to utility gained by those that live farther away.[44] Even among those economists who argue for considering only the preferences of the currently living, some such as Feldstein (1964) have argued that an alternative to the market, such as the ballot box, may be needed to aggregate individual preferences for social discount rates.

Cropper and colleagues (Cropper and Portney 1992, Cropper et al. 1994) have studied individual's preferences for saving lives from a societal perspective. They found that individuals have a positive social discount rate for life years ranging on average from 16.8 per cent in the next 5 years to 3.8 per cent over the next 100 years. Few other studies have explicitly investigated individual's discount rates for saving social lives. The dominant reasons explaining a social discount rate for future health are similar to the reasons for individuals discounting future health. Negative social discount rates for future health are possible if the expected growth in future consumption, and thus utility, are high enough.

CONSEQUENTIALIST ARGUMENTS

It is both theoretically and empirically unclear whether or not individuals would always discount their own future health. The arguments reviewed so far that society should discount future health are even less convincing. Other types of arguments for discounting future health, however, have been very persuasive to some, but are peculiar in nature. They are not arguments that future life-years are intrinsically less important. Rather, it is suggested that we are induced to discount future life-years because of the consequences of not discounting. The two major consequentialist arguments for this position are outlined below. I propose a third which may be the most difficult to deal with.

The Opportunity Cost Argument

Weinstein (1981, 1990) makes an argument for "induced" discounting of life-years as follows:

> A choice has to be made between Program A that costs $10 million today and saves 500 QALYs today and Program B that also costs $10 million today but saves 500 QALYs 30 years in the future. If Program B were not adopted, the $10 million *not* spent could have been invested (say, at a real interest rate of 5%) to yield approximately $40 million in 30 years' time, after correcting for inflation. This $40 million, which would have been available in 30 years, is the true opportunity cost of the $10 million present cost of Program B. Thus, Program B is equivalent to a hypothetical

Program B that costs $40 million 30 years from now and saves 500
QALYs at that same point in time. To summarize, Program A costs
$20,000 per QALY *at the time the resources are spent* and Program
B is equivalent to a program that costs $80,000 per QALY saved
at the time the resources are spent. As long as society's marginal
willingness to pay for QALYs is constant with time (in real terms),
Program A should be preferred to Program B. (1990, p. 97)

There are two reasons why this apparently persuasive argument may
not hold. First, Weinstein is arguing that because of the opportunity cost
for dollars, we are "induced" to discount future life-years. This need not
be the case.

Imagine a decision-maker with three options: spend dollars now on
curative interventions and save life-years now, spend dollars now on preventive interventions and save life-years in 30 years, or invest dollars now
and after 30 years purchase curative interventions to save life-years in that
same year. The beneficiaries of the different types of interventions will most
likely not be the same individuals. Within each type of intervention there
is a wide range of interventions with different cost-effectiveness ratios.
Table 1.5 illustrates that there are five types of interventions within each
class ranging from $10 to $100 000 per year of life saved. The number of
life-years that can be purchased through each intervention is also limited
to 10 life-years per intervention.

Next, imagine that you are a decision-maker who is indifferent to the
time period when life-years are gained, but you recognize a real opportunity cost for dollars and you have $50 000 to spend on saving life-years.

Table 1.5 Costs and benefits of three types of interventions: curative
interventions where costs and benefits are experienced
now, preventive interventions where costs are incurred
now and benefits accrued in 30 years, and curative
interventions where costs and benefits occur in 30 years

	Real cost per life-year			Present value per life-year		
Intervention	Cost now, benefits now	Cost now, benefits in 30 years	Cost is 30 years, benefits in 30 years	Cost now, benefits now	Cost now, benefits in 30 years	Cost in 30 years, benefits in 30 years
I	$100 000.00	$100 000.00	$100 000.00	$100 000.00	$100 000.00	$23 137.74
II	$10 000.00	$10 000.00	$10 000.00	$10 000.00	$10 000.00	*$2 313.77*
III	$1 000.00	$1 000.00	$1 000.00	*$1 000.00*	*$1 000.00*	*$231.38*
IV	$100.00	$100.00	$100.00	*$100.00*	*$100.00*	*$23.14*
V	$10.00	$10.00	$10.00	*$10.00*	*$10.00*	*$2.31*
VI	$1.00	$1.00	$1.00	*$1.00*	*$1.00*	*$0.23*

Note: For each type of intervention six different interventions in descending order of cost per year of life saved
are shown. The cost per year of life saved and the present value of the cost per year of life saved are shown.

You want to allocate your budget in this year so as to purchase the maximum number of life-years, irrespective of the time period in which they will occur. You can calculate the cost-effectiveness ratios of the various options by converting costs into present value terms and dividing by life-years gained—for this illustration, let us assume that the real discount rate is five per cent. The curative interventions to be used in 30 years appear to be very attractive because, in present value terms, their cost is low but the benefits are high. With a budget of $50 000 one could purchase all the interventions listed in italics in Table 1.5. Fifty-one per cent of the budget would be set aside for investment to purchase curative interventions in the future, 24 per cent for prevention now and 24 per cent for curative interventions now. In other words, because there is a real opportunity cost to money, investing dollars today to purchase curative interventions in 30 years is attractive for a number of interventions but that realization does not "induce" us to discount future life-years. The cost-effectiveness ratio of the invest-now-buy-curative-in-30-years option reflects the opportunity cost of money without any need to discount life-years.[45] In reality, if the budget is not fixed, decision-makers with a zero discount rate for life-years will buy all interventions up to the point that the cost of a life-year equals the social value of a life-year, irrespective of the year in which the life-year is gained.

The Time Paradox

Keeler and Cretin (1983) formalized an old argument called the time paradox. Olsen (1993) notes that some health economists view this argument as the "grand argument" for discounting health benefits. Imagine a decision-maker with a fixed budget for health improvement but with the flexibility to put the budget into private investments yielding a return. Furthermore, imagine that this decision-maker is secure in the knowledge that the return from these investments will be reserved for purchasing health interventions in the future—a rather unrealistic scenario from the start. Imagine that the set of health interventions, their cost-effectiveness and the volume of the intervention that can be delivered at that cost-effectiveness ratio are all constant over time. If we choose not to discount future life-years, the decision-maker will always get more health gain by deferring a programme into the future, when the budget through investment will be larger but the present value of the benefits would remain the same.

This argument is an artifact of the contrived nature of the choice. Parsonage and Neuberger (1992) have pointed out that most health sector decision-makers do not have the option of investing resources for health and reaping greater gains in the future. Investments made in productive sectors would not necessarily be returned to the Ministry of Health; rather they would accrue in nearly every government to the treasury or its equivalent. If health dollars can only be spent this year, there is no longer any time paradox or a necessity to discount future health benefits.

The assumption that the opportunity set for intervention and the cost-effectiveness of interventions is constant over time is inconsistent with the experience of the last 50 years. In countries with good information systems, it is clear that mortality rates have been steadily declining, with few exceptions, and that the cost of most health interventions rises faster than the general price level. With either assumption relaxed, the time paradox will no longer hold.

Based on more realistic assumptions about a decision-maker such as the government itself, the time paradox can be shown not to hold. Imagine a government that, on the basis of some unspecified but quantitative and replicable method, has decided on a threshold cost it is willing to spend to save a life-year. This government chooses to discount future life-years in the evaluation of prevention projects at the same rate as the social opportunity cost of capital. With these decision criteria and the marginal cost-effectiveness functions for health interventions, x per cent of the budget is spent on health interventions. According to Keeler and Cretin, if a discount rate slightly lower than the social opportunity cost of capital is used, the government would immediately cease to invest in any health interventions this year. Of course, if future life-years are discounted at a rate lower than the social opportunity cost of capital, all curative and preventive projects that the government chose to fund when life-years were discounted by the social opportunity cost of capital will still be attractive according to the government's decision criteria. Such projects remain attractive since costs are the same but benefits are at least as large or larger. In addition, however, some preventive project previously considered cost-ineffective will now be cost-effective, as the present value of benefits will now be greater and costs unchanged. The health sector budget would necessarily increase from x to $x+n$ per cent, where n is a positive number. As the discount rate is reduced, rather than spending less on health interventions as suggested by Keeler and Cretin, we would be induced to spend more on health interventions.

The Disease Eradication and Health Research Paradoxes

There is an even more difficult consequentialist argument to confront which might be called the "disease eradication paradox." Imagine a disease for which the incidence rate is stable so that the sum of all future burden of the disease (without discounting) is infinite. If there are programmes with a finite probability of eradicating a disease then the benefits of such programmes evaluated without discounting are infinite. Society would necessarily redirect all its resources to disease eradication programmes and reduce all other investments in all curative and preventive programmes to zero. A similar counter-intuitive conclusion would be reached when evaluating the benefits of some types of health research. Even if the benefits of a disease eradication or research project are not infinite, if they are very large they will lead to unacceptable redistributions of health dollars from the current generation to future generations. If future health benefits are discounted, the magnitude of benefits from research are finite. If the discount rate is high enough, we may not call upon the current generation to undertake excessive sacrifices.

In fact, the eradication and research paradoxes are not arguments for valuing future life-years as less important. Rather, they suggest that without some means of discounting future life-years in aggregate, the current generation will be asked to make excessive sacrifices. Anand and Hanson (1995) attempt to argue that this problem can be solved by using an inter-temporal welfare function. But even with such a function, the current generation may well be called upon to make an excessive sacrifice. [46] Some form of discounting the future appears to be required to avoid this paradox. As noted by Parfit (1984), an excessive sacrifice argument may lead to a different form of discounting the future than a classical exponential decay discounting function, where more distal generations are discounted more than proximal generations. Based purely on the argument of excessive sacrifice, life-years for generation $n+k$ are no more or less important than life-years for generation n. We simply cannot call upon the current generation to sacrifice so much of currently available health resources to improve the health of future generations. Each future generation, however, would have an equal claim on current resources. Of course, the small but non-zero probability of global disaster and the extinction of society means that we would slightly discount the claims of generation $n+k$ compared with generation n.

Figure 1.12 demonstrates a hypothetical discount function based on an argument of excessive sacrifice. Life-years for distant generations would all be discounted by a constant multiplier. However, a declining discount

Figure 1.12   Hypothetical discounting function for life-years based on an argument of excessive sacrifice

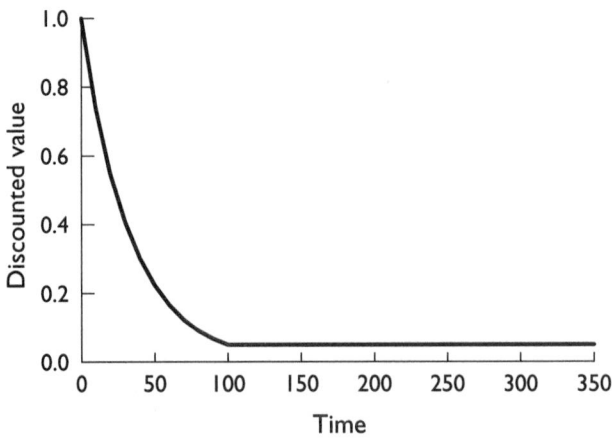

rate perhaps similar to an exponential decay may be used for proximal generations for two reasons. First, there is substantial but steadily decreasing generation overlap for the next 2–4 generations. Beneficiaries of an intervention purchased today which prevents burden in 50 years would be a mix of currently living and future generations. Second, the current generations may have some legitimate special concern for specific members of the next generation such as their children and grand-children beyond their concern for all future generations. We could, therefore, conclude that a discount function which approximates the classical exponential decay function for 100–150 years and is thereafter flat may adequately reflect concerns over excessive sacrifice brought about by the eradication and research paradoxes. The empirical findings of Cropper and Portney (1992) are consistent with the notion that individuals may have a much lower marginal discount rate for distant events than proximal events.[47] Of course, apart from the democratic process itself, there is no way to measure or objectively define the form and level of this type of discount function.

DISCOUNTING DALYS

A wide array of arguments for and against discounting future health have been reviewed here. These are summarized below.[48]

- Discounting life-years is different than discounting future dollars. Life is the capacity to generate utility. One representation of this concept is the multiplicative form of the QALY utility function. In this formulation, there is no declining marginal utility of extra life-years. Individuals and society could, under certain circumstances, have a negative discount rate for life-years, if the expected growth in income exceeds the effects of pure time preference.

- There is a small uncertainty of survival for a society that monotonically increases over time. While few would disagree with discounting future life-years for this uncertainty, the appropriate rate may be very small.

- The disease eradication and health research paradoxes are powerful arguments for a doctrine of legitimate sacrifice. Legitimate sacrifice arguments can justify discounting but the form of such discounting may differ from a continuous exponential decay.

In the construction of DALYs, I have struggled with two options: to use a low positive discount rate to capture uncertainty that increases with time and, more importantly, to reduce the problems of excessive sacrifice; or to use a zero discount rate, ignoring the cumulative small effects of uncertainty, and to capture the problems of excessive sacrifice through other means, such as an arbitrary division of the health resources into separate budgets for the health of the current generations and the health of future generations. Since the issue of discounting is not easily resolved, in this book we have published DALYs calculated with and without discounting.

As with previous versions of this study, the baseline DALY measure incorporates a three per cent discount rate. The choice of three per cent is entirely arbitrary. Three per cent is a low positive rate that is probably at the lower limit of acceptability for those economists who are persuaded by opportunity cost arguments and is at the upper limit for public health practitioners who are willing to accept a positive discount rate for the reasons already reviewed.

Discounting the Benefits of Health Interventions

For cost-effectiveness analyses, another important issue must be addressed which does not often enter into the discussion of discounting. As there has been a century of steady progress in reducing the burden of disease, the benefits of a preventive intervention may be significantly smaller than estimated. If we immunize a child today for hepatitis B, we expect to reduce mortality from cirrhosis and liver cancer approximately 40 years from now. Technological progress may be such that in 40 years the case-fatality rate or the rate at which patients with chronic hepatitis B develop cancer or cirrhosis may be much lower. The expected benefits of hepatitis B intervention are thus uncertain and, given past trends, likely to be smaller than estimated based on current epidemiological patterns. Uncertainty over the magnitude of benefits from preventive interventions may vary by type of condition so that the discount rate may vary by condition. For example, the annual decline in communicable disease mortality rates has been much faster than the annual decline in non-communicable disease mortality rates. Perhaps we should discount the expected benefits from preventive interventions for communicable conditions more than the benefits from those interventions that prevent burden from non-communicable conditions. Whether or not to introduce different discount rates for different types of interventions, where the mortality or disability reductions will be observed in the future, remains an issue for further debate.

Age-Weighting

Recall the scenario mentioned earlier in this chapter where there is only one course of antibiotics available and two individuals with meningitis arrive simultaneously at the emergency room. The only difference between the two that you know about is their age: one is two years old and one is twenty-two. Their prognosis is identical. Which patient would you choose to treat? Such a stark case forces consideration of a difficult choice. According to the principle of reducing the duration of life lost, we should always prefer to save the younger patient who has the prospect of more years of life to be saved. Several studies, however, including some population surveys have found that individuals prefer to save the lives of young adults over young children (Institute of Medicine 1986, Johannesson and Johansson 1996, Lewis and Charny 1989, Nord et al. 1995).

Figure 1.13 Relative value of preventing a death at different ages in four group valuation exercises

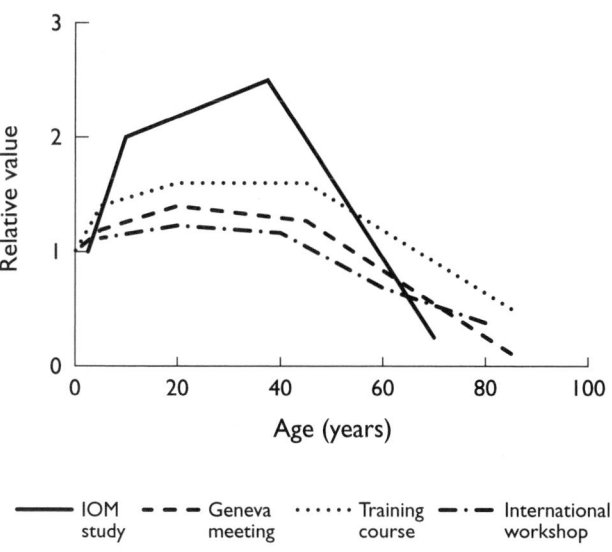

For the Institute of Medicine's 1986 vaccine priority study, a panel of public health experts selected relative valuations of a death at each age, shown in Figure 1.13.[49] Over a five year period, I have undertaken a similar valuation exercise with 116 participants from developing countries in a tuberculosis training course; their average relative valuation of the importance of preventing a death at each age is also shown in Figure 1.13. The figure also shows for comparison the values given for the trade-offs of saving lives at different ages by responses of the participants at the Geneva meeting and at an international workshop. All three of these group consultations show a preference, of varying intensity, for saving lives of young adults over young children and for young adults over older adults. As part of the Cardiff Health Survey, 721 adults were interviewed about age preferences (Lewis and Charny 1989). Ninety-four per cent of the population preferred saving a 5-year-old over a 70 year-old, 80 per cent preferred saving a 35 year-old over a 60 year-old and 34 per cent preferred saving an 8 year-old over a 2 year-old—although for the latter choice, 46 per cent were unable to choose and 21 per cent chose the 2 year-old. Nord et al. (1995) found in a survey of 551 individuals that given the choice of saving a young child or a newborn, 55 per cent were unable to choose but 44 per cent preferred the young child. At least in these populations studied, many individuals appear to assign greater importance to preventing the deaths of young adults and adolescents than of very young children or older adults.[50]

Should this apparently widely held preference be reflected in DALYs? The answer depends on two questions. Why do individuals hold this preference? And, once these reasons are identified, do they justify using these preferences in calculating the burden of disease? A preference for preventing a young adult death over a newborn death cannot be explained by the duration of expected life lost, even when these durations are discounted. Such preferences imply some other age-dependent preference whereby life-years lived at different ages are valued differentially. These age-dependent preferences that explain the difference between preferences for saving lives at different ages and those predicted on the basis of duration of expected life lost with or without discounting are defined as age-weights.[51] Johannesson and Johansson (1996) surveyed population preferences for saving life-years at different ages and found strong non-uniform age-weighting, such that one QALY for a 30 year-old was equivalent to three QALYs at age 50 and nine QALYs at age 70.

While age-weighting may be nearly ubiquitous, the reasons for age-weighting may well vary. At least three types of arguments have been advanced to explain preferences for years of life lived at different ages. Individuals may value their own health at various ages differently. Wright (1986) found that individuals in the population assigned greater importance to being healthy during "infancy" and the "period of raising children." Bussbach et al. (1993) used a form of trade-off to investigate preferences of student and elderly respondents for healthy time lived at different ages. Both groups attached the greatest importance to years of life lived at age 10 and lower weights to ages 5 followed in descending order by 35, 60 and 70.

Even if every year of life has the same intrinsic value to the individual, we may be "induced" to attach greater importance to years of productive adult life. All consumers in society depend on producers for food and other items of consumption. Net producers, therefore, have a magnified role in contributing to social welfare. This type of argument is often labeled the human capital approach—man as a productive machine inspires the name.

To illustrate human capital arguments, we can make use of a simple model of a growing economy. Imagine a population where only young and middle-aged adults produce, and where their product is divided according to some social contract into three shares: investment in capital, investment in educating the next generation of producers, and consumption. In this egalitarian society, the consumption share is divided equally amongst all those living. We further assume that everyone has the same utility function so that the utility value of every life-year is identical. The economy grows as a function of capital, healthy labour and the average level of education of the labour force.[52]

The individual and social willingness-to-pay to prevent a death at each age for six variants of this model are shown in Figure 1.14. Willingness-to-pay is shown in terms of multiples of income per capita. Individuals, who in this model are not interested in the role of net producers contrib-

Figure 1.14   Willingness-to-pay to prevent a death at each age—
six variants of the human capital model

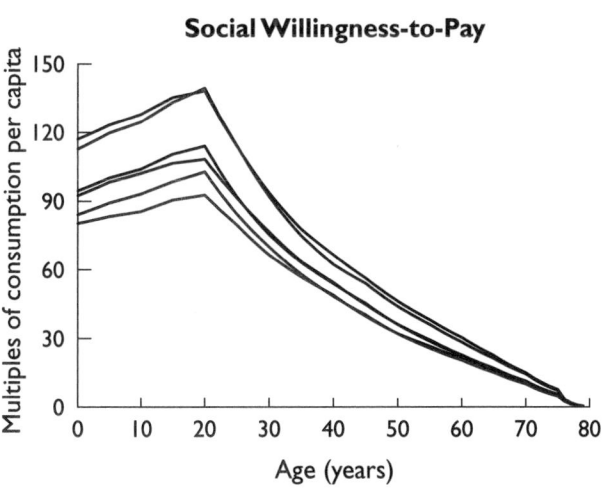

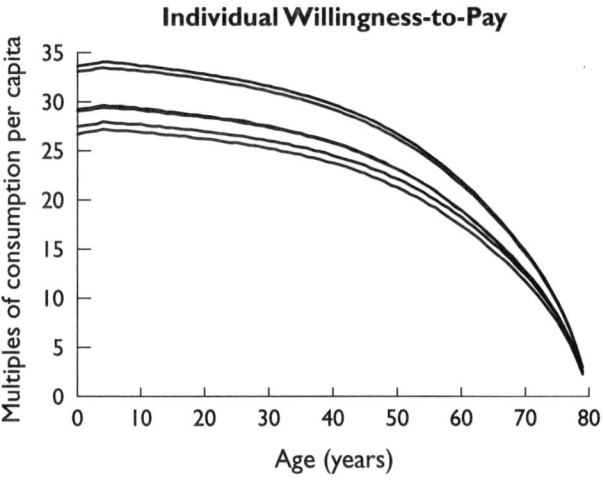

uting to the well-being of the rest of society, value preventing a death at younger ages as more important because more life has been lost. Society, on the other hand, is willing to pay relatively more to prevent a young adult death than a death at any other age. This is because young adults have already been educated and are about to contribute to overall production for society. Their deaths are a loss of individual utility and of the invest-ment in their education. Preventing deaths of individuals over age 60 low-

Figure 1.15   Willingness-to-pay to add a single year of life at different ages

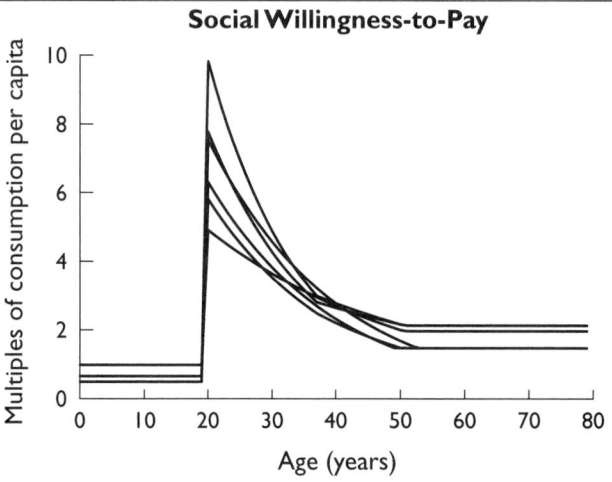

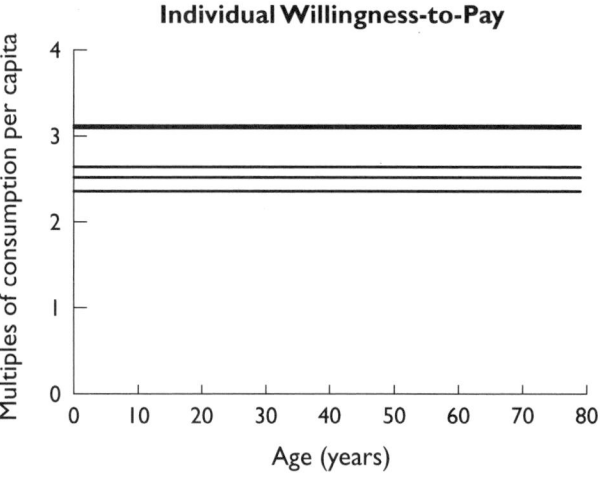

ers the average level of consumption for everyone in society and, thus, is less attractive than preventing deaths at an earlier age.

Figure 1.15 shows the individual and social willingness-to-pay (WTP) for adding a single year of life at each age. Adding a year of life to the producing population has two effects in a growing economy: it immediately raises the total volume of production and thus the average level of consumption of every individual, and it increases investment in capital and education of children and thus improves future growth. Increased growth rates will raise the welfare level of the population for several generations into the future. The addition of one child life-year without increasing the future number of adult life-years will decrease utility in the current and future time periods. The immediate effect is due to the fact that the same level of total production is being divided between more individuals thus lowering everyone's average level of consumption. The long-term effects of adding a child life-year will be the expenditure of money on the child's education which is lost because that child will not live to be a producer; therefore, long-term growth will also be adversely affected. In some variants of the model, the social WTP for a child life-year is negative while for others it is positive but still much lower than for productive adults. These simulations suggest that those individuals that assign a much higher value to preventing an adult death (2–4 times higher) are, in fact, assigning a negative value to single years of life added during childhood.

If we decide to treat all life-years as the same irrespective of the age at which they are lived, we are de facto saying that the value of an adult life year *per se* is less than a child or elderly life-year *per se*. Otherwise, how can the welfare bonus of saving a productive adult life-year be ignored? The human capital logic can be extended; why stop with age? Shouldn't more educated and higher income groups who contribute more to total economic product be accorded a higher weight for exactly the same reasons as put forward for age? In fact, the standard practice in cost of illness studies (Cooper and Rice 1976, Rice 1994, Rice and Hodgson 1982) is to calculate income-weighted years of life lost—although for obvious political reasons these cost of illness calculations are not explicitly labelled as income-weighted years of life lost.[53] The fully elaborated human capital approach would not be consistent with the propositions on restricted information proposed for the formulation of DALYs at the beginning of this chapter.

While there is an unavoidable element of truth in the human capital calculus, however distasteful the logical extension of the argument may be, it fails to capture non-monetary transfers between individuals such as care-giving. Welfare interdependence clearly exists as some individuals play a critical role in providing for the well-being of others—consider parents and their young children. A more general notion of welfare interdependence would also generate age-weights of some form. In such a framework, the greatest contributors to the welfare of others would not necessarily be those who earn the most. Some net contributors to the welfare of others may earn no dollars but may work within the household. *A priori*, we would not expect rich individuals or more educated individuals to contribute more to the welfare of others than poor or less educated individuals. This broader concept of flows between individuals contributing to welfare provides a much more convincing argument for age weights if these flows are a function of age. The empirical evidence reviewed above on population preferences for age-weighting suggests that these flows are a function of age with years of life lived as a young or middle-aged adult being valued more.

As with net dollar transfers between individuals, age does not explain all of the variation in net flows contributing to the welfare of others. There must be individuals who contribute more to the well-being of others than their peers of the same age. Should the life-years of these individuals be assigned a greater relative value? If such individuals could reliably be identified, some may sympathize with this argument. The appeal of age-weighting, however, is that it is a variable which does not discriminate between the lives of different individuals but simply differentiates between periods of the life cycle for a cohort. Taking into consideration altruism, or some other factor that predicted net flows to the well-being of others, would lead to discrimination between different peoples' lives. Based on the proposition to restrict the information used to establish relative values to age, it seems reasonable to consider age-weighting because of different roles and contributions of different age groups but to reject proposals to pursue this logic to identify other variables predicting net flows.

Given the widespread preference for age-weighting and a reasonable justification for this view, I have included in the formulation of DALYs age weights that assign a greater value to a year of young or middle-aged adult life as compared to a year of life lived by young children or the elderly. To operationalize age-weighting, we must choose between establishing a set of discrete weights for each age or defining a continuous mathematical function for the weights at each age. Discrete weighting schemes, where a numerical weight is chosen for each specific age group, have been used (Barnum 1987, Prost and Prescott 1984). They allow for great flexibility in the pattern chosen but require time consuming iterative computations in their application.

Figure 1.16   Relative value of a year of life lived at different ages incorporated into DALYs

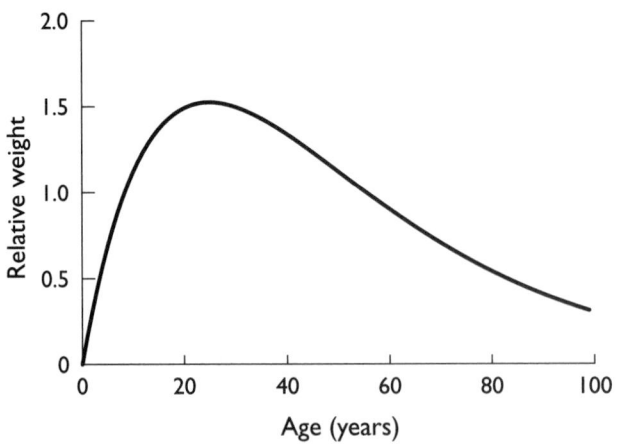

For reasons of convenience, it is far more preferable to define a continuous age-weighting function which can be mathematically manipulated to provide a summary formula for YLLs or YLDs. Functions of the form:

$$Cxe^{-\beta x}$$

where β and C are constants and have the general form shown in Figure 1.16. This conforms to the basic age-weighting pattern desired. Only a narrow range of β and C approximately between 0.03 and 0.05, provides age-patterns consistent with the various surveys and group exercises reviewed above.[54] Based on consultations with the advisory board for this study, a β of 0.04 was chosen. Concern raised by the arbitrary nature of the choice of this age-weighting function is offset to some extent by the findings reported by Murray and Lopez (1996b), Chapter 5 in this volume. They find that the results of the GBD are basically insensitive to the choice of β. The important issue is not the exact form of an age-weighting function but the presence of non-uniform age-weights. Murray and Lopez (1996b), Chapter 5 in this volume have demonstrated that the qualitative effect of age-weighting on the relative rank assigned to different conditions is quite small.

The constant C in the equation has been included so that the introduction of unequal age weights will not change the global estimated burden of disease. Its value thus depends on the results of the Global Burden of Disease Study, as described in Murray and Lopez (1996b). For the final version of the Global Burden of Disease Study for 1990 published in this volume, C equals 0.1658. If the age-weighting function were changed, for example by altering β, the constant would necessarily change as well.

EQUITY AND DALYs

Should the basic measurement unit, a DALY, a QALY or, more generally, a health adjusted life-year, be considered as the same in all settings? If the burden of disease and cost-effectiveness of interventions are measured using such units, the question arises as to whether the goal of the health sector should be maximizing health denominated in these units? Several authors have been concerned with the distributional aspects of QALY maximization as a social goal (Broome 1988, Harris 1995, Lockwood 1988, Nord et al. 1995, Olsen 1994, Rawles 1989, Singer et al. 1995, Smith 1987, Wagstaff 1991). The discussion has centered on three types of distributional issues: the distribution of benefits across individuals, distribution across age groups (already discussed), and the distribution across socio-economic groups. In this section, the first and the last of these are addressed.

DISTRIBUTION OF BENEFITS ACROSS INDIVIDUALS

Nord et al. (1995) and Olsen (1994) have found in surveys that individuals appear to have preferences over programmes with the same cost and

same volume of life-years gained but with different numbers of beneficiaries. For example, Olsen found that survey respondents preferred 10 years
of life gained by 100 people to 20 years of life gained by 80 people (1000
total life-years). Williams (1981) describes a common viewpoint that it is
"better for many people to get a little than for a few people to get a lot
(i.e. contradicting the notion that one person getting ten years additional
life expenditure is the same as ten people getting one each)" (p.277). Is this
a universally held preference? If it is, should some form of distributional
concern be incorporated into the calculation of DALYs?

The experience from the Oregon Health Service's Commission is in-
structive (Eddy 1991). Preference weights based on the Quality of Well-
Being Scale elicited through a telephone survey were used in a study of the
cost-effectiveness of over 700 health interventions. Given the budget available to the state government, it was proposed that the most cost-effective
interventions be funded, in descending order until the budget was ex-
hausted. In town meetings, the results of the cost-effectiveness rankings
were challenged. The public felt that interventions for relatively minor conditions were given too much importance as compared to interventions for
more life threatening conditions. Nord (1993) and Eddy (1991) have
suggested that this was due to the effects of visual analog scales; alternatively, there may have been a preference in Oregon for large benefits for
a few as compared to minor benefits for many. In a group of students from
many countries at the Harvard School of Public Health, I found a preference for large benefits for a few over small benefits for many. Given the
choice of saving one day of health-adjusted life for 36 500 individuals and
one year for 100 individuals, 57 of out of 69 preferred one year for 100
individuals. Given the choice between 10 years of life for 100 individuals
and one year of life for 1 000 individuals, 47 of our of 69 preferred 10
years of life for 100 individuals. Previous group consultations have yielded
similar results. It would seem that individuals assign more importance to
large benefits for a few than small benefits to many when the difference
in duration is great, such as an order of magnitude. In these choices, minor or even trivial gains do not add up to large gains to the individual.
However, when large substantive gains such as 10 years or 20 years are
compared, then individuals may have a preference for a larger number of
beneficiaries.

For burden of disease analyses, none of the preference measurement
exercises are directly relevant, since they are all framed as questions about
alternative intervention options. Even if individuals may have preferences
over the distribution of benefits from interventions, it would be extremely
difficult to incorporate these values into the calculation of burden by cause
without altering the total burden and losing the tremendous advantages
of a completely additive measure. For cost-effectiveness analysis, as Nord
(1995) has pointed out, health state preferences based on the person trade-
off approach already incorporate some distributional preferences. Of
course, distributional preferences for interventions that reduce YLLs alone

are not incorporated. At this juncture, given the conflicting nature of the evidence on distributional concerns and the contentious basis for these concerns, it would seem more reasonable not to explicitly incorporate distributional preferences into cost-effectiveness calculations.

DISTRIBUTION BY SOCIO-ECONOMIC STATUS

Anand and Hanson (1995) argue that a QALY or a DALY for a disadvantaged person should be given more importance than a QALY or a DALY for an advantaged person. Disadvantage apparently means lower health status or socio-economic status. The premise that life-years for poor individuals or other disadvantaged socio-economic groups should count more than life-years for rich individuals runs counter to most of the literature on medical ethics. As noted in the example provided at the beginning of this chapter, many would find it unacceptable to discriminate in the allocation of a scarce medical therapy such as organ transplantation between two individuals solely on the basis of their income or wealth. On the other hand, the notion that there may be settings in which we may prefer to avert fewer DALYs, so that the DALYs averted are more equally distributed, has some appeal—for example, immunizing children in remote rural areas may be more costly and thus less cost-effective than immunizing poor children in urban slums, nevertheless we may prefer to spend some scarce resources on the remote community at the cost of lowering the total number of immunizations delivered. Unfortunately, we must recognize that the latter type of group equity consideration ultimately maps into the former individual discrimination. We would be preferring poor life-years over rich life-years.

Many people are concerned with the situation common to most countries where the rich receive highly expensive cost-ineffective interventions while many effective simple and cheap interventions are not delivered to the poor. Clearly, a goal of health maximization in the face of such allocative inefficiencies will lead to a substantial reallocation of resources to the health problems of the poor. The question addressed here is different. Few can challenge the conclusion that pursuing a goal of health maximization would improve the health of the poor dramatically in so far as resources are reallocated from cost-ineffective interventions to cost-effective interventions that will primarily benefit the poor. Do we need an extra value assigned to poor life-years? For DALYs, given the restricted information proposition at the beginning of this chapter, the answer is clearly no. The premise that we should value a life-year as more or less important based on the income or wealth of an individual is difficult to accept as an ethical premise. On the other hand, studying and reporting patterns of burden in different socio-economic groups as a contribution to describing the extent of inequity is important and should be pursued. This descriptive task, however, does not require any elaboration in the method of calculation of burden.

Formulae and Nomenclature for YLLs, YLDs and DALYs

As defined, YLLs and YLDs are two types of DALYs. Thus, DALYs from any given condition are simply the sum of YLLs and YLDs from the condition such that:

$$DALY_i = YLL_i + YLD_i$$

where i is a condition. Following the reasoning developed in this chapter, Years of Life Lost (YLLs) are calculated using standard expected years of life lost. Coale and Demeny model life table West with an expectation of life at birth for females of 82.5 years and males 80 years has been chosen as the standard. Time lived at different ages has been valued using an exponential function of the form $cxe^{-\beta x}$. Time lost due to premature mortality has been discounted at three per cent. A continuous discounting function of the form e^{-rt} has been used where r is the discount rate, and t is time.[55]

The formula for YLLs has been generalized from a single death at age a to include a parameter K which can be used in sensitivity analysis to remove non-uniform age-weights. The general formula for calculating YLLs is thus:

Figure 1.17   Years of Life Lost (YLLs) due to deaths at each age, males and females

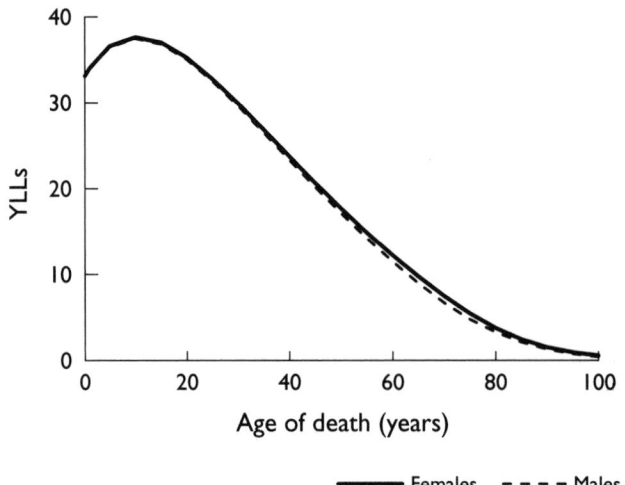

$$YLLs = \frac{KCe^{ra}}{(r+\beta)^2}\left[e^{-(r+\beta)(L+a)}\left[-(r+\beta)(L+a)-1\right]-\right.$$
$$\left. e^{-(r+\beta)a}\left[-(r+\beta)a-1\right]\right]+\frac{1-K}{r}\left(1-e^{-rL}\right)$$

where r is the discount rate, β is the parameter from the age weighting function, K is the age-weighting modulation factor, C is a constant, a is the age at death and L is the standard expectation of life at age a. For standard YYLs used in the GBD, r is 0.03, β is 0.04, K is 1, and C is 0.1658. If K is set to 0 then YLLs are calculated with uniform age-weights. Figure 1.17 presents the number of YLLs due to a death at each age for a male and a female. The curve incorporates the duration of time lost due to premature mortality, age-weighting and discounting. To calculate the number of YLLs lost to a condition, the number of YLLs lost per death at each age must be multiplied by the number of deaths at each age and then summed across all ages.

Without further notation, YLLs are calculated using a three per cent discount rate and age-weights. When YLLs are calculated with different discount rates or age-weights, we recommend reporting such valuations as YLLs [r,K]. For example, YLLs calculated with a zero discount rate and no age-weights would be denoted by YLLs [0,0]. Similar notation is recommended for YLDs and DALYs.

When the discount rate is set equal to zero, the formula can be simplified to:

$$YLLs\,[0, K] = \frac{KCe^{-\beta a}}{\beta^2}\left[e^{-\beta L}\left(-\beta(L+a)-1\right)-\left(-\beta a-1\right)\right]+\left[(1-K)(L)\right]$$

where each of the parameters is defined as above. When the discount rate is zero and K is set equal to zero so that there is uniform age-weighting, the length of life lost due to a death at age a is simply:

$$YLLs\,[0,0] = L$$

where L is the standard life expectancy at age a.

Years Lived with Disability (YLDs) is time lived in health states worse than perfect health, weighted by a preference weight for each health state. Preference weights for 22 indicator conditions have been developed using a person trade-off method. Seven classes of disability have been defined based on these 22 indicator conditions and distributions of disabling severity generated for several hundred treated and untreated disabling sequelae. Time lived with disability is also age-weighted and discounted in the same manner as YLLs.

The formula for YLDs differs from the formula for YLLs because of the addition of a disability weight and slightly different interpretations of a and L. The general formula for YLDs from a single disabling event is:

$$YLDs = D\{ \frac{KCe^{ra}}{(r+\beta)^2}[e^{-(r+\beta)(L+a)}[-(r+\beta)(L+a)-1] - e^{-(r+\beta)a}[-(r+\beta)a-1]]+\frac{1-K}{r}(1-e^{-rL}) \}$$

where a is the age of onset of the disability, L is the duration of disability, r is the discount rate ($r=0.03$), is the age-weighting parameter ($\beta=0.04$), K is the age-weighting modulation factor ($K=1$), C is the adjustment constant necessary because of unequal age-weights ($C=0.1658$) and D is the disability weight. To calculate the number of YLDs lost due to a condition, the number of YLDs lost per incident case must be multiplied by the number of incident cases.

When the discount rate is set equal to zero, the formula for YLDs becomes:

$$YLDs[0,K] = D\{ \frac{KCe^{-\beta a}}{\beta^2}[e^{-\beta L}(-\beta(L+a)-1) - (-\beta a-1)]+[(1-K)(L)] \}$$

where each of the parameters is defined as above. When the discount rate is set equal to zero and uniform age-weighting is used, the formula for a disabling event at age a simplifies to:

$$YLDs[0,0] = DL$$

where D is the disability weight and L is the duration of disability.

CONCLUSIONS

In this chapter, I have attempted to explain the origin and arguments for the construction of Disability-Adjusted Life Years (DALYs) which are the sum of Years of Life Lost (YLLs) and Years Lived with Disability, adjusted for the severity of disability (YLDs). As presented in this chapter, DALYs can be viewed as a special variant of a more general type of time-based measure that incorporates judgments about the value of time spent in different health states. Such time-based measures are often categorized as Quality Adjusted Life Years or QALYs. The term QALY, however, does not imply any specific set of value choices or methods used to elicit preferences for particular values choices. DALYs, therefore, are a form of QALYs in which the value choices have been standardized and have been increasingly used in international analyses. As with all efforts at standardization, many choices made in the standardization process are ultimately arbitrary and various individuals will hold well-reasoned but differing views. Inter-community comparisons and intertemporal comparisons for the same community, nevertheless, require standardized measures. The present variant of DALYs is a contribution towards such standardization.

Estimates of the burden of disease denominated in DALYs can readily be used in conjunction with the literature on cost-effectiveness of health interventions. The largest compendium of international health interventions to date has reported results in terms of cost per DALY averted (Jamison et al. 1993). This facilitates using estimates of the burden of disease in determining health resource allocations (Bobadilla et al. 1994, Murray et al. 1994).

As the chapters in this volume demonstrate, using a time-based measure that incorporates non-fatal health outcomes such as DALYs does not imply any particular model of causation. The fact that DALYs can be, and have been, used to measure the burden of disease due to certain diseases and injuries, does not mean that the only determinants of burden are biomedical. Murray and Lopez (1996c), Chapter 6 in this volume summarize the results of different approaches to estimating the burden of disease denominated in DALYs due to certain risk factors such as poor water supply, air pollution, unsafe sex or tobacco use. DALYs due to socio-economic determinants could be estimated as well, if the data and investigations were available to do so.

Any new method or approach will evolve over time and DALYs are no exception. In this book, the first round of substantial revisions of DALYs has been presented. As we learn more through national and specific applications of the burden of disease approach, DALYs will inevitably evolve further. In their present state DALYs are intended to be a transparent tool to enhance dialogue on the major health challenges facing humanity.

NOTES

1   To this short list of published documents should be added the large number of reports from country studies which have been undertaken or are ongoing, including: Mauritius, Mexico, Colombia, Chile, Uruguay, Andhra Pradesh State, Japan and others. In addition, the World Bank has undertaken a number of "short-cut" exercises in other countries in which regional results of the Global Burden of Disease have been modified to local demographic parameters—Bobadilla (1996) provides a summary of this experience in a large number of countries.

2   DALYs, and the social preferences incorporated into DALYs, and all other health measures are literally matters of life and death, evoking extraordinary passion on the part of some authors. Werner (1994, p.9), for example, writes "The DALY prioritization method which authoritatively deprecates disability

has the stench of eugenics. Disabled activists need to join with health rights activists to protest this potentially neo-fascist policy." Much of this passion appears to be misdirected as the authors (such as Werner 1994 or Ugalde and Jackson 1995) are clearly unfamiliar with the technical basis and ethical debates underlying the construction of DALYs as discussed in Murray (1994). It is my contention that a careful and deliberative review of the major debates will help clarify the issues and engender a common framework for discussion.

3   The term maximalist is used, as by Sissela Bok, to mean a fully worked out system of ethics (Bok 1995)

4   The MIT dictionary of economics (Pearce 1992) describes positive economics as "that part of economic science which concerns itself with statements that are capable of verification with reference to the facts," and normative economics as "economic analysis which provides prescriptions or statements about what 'should be' rather than what 'is'."

5   For readers interested in the difficulties of measuring the infant mortality rate in many developing countries with poor vital registration systems and the consequent use of models to generate yearly estimates of the infant mortality rate, see Murray (1987).

6   The exact specification of the Human Development Index (HDI) is slightly more complicated: "The HDI is constructed in three steps. The first step was to defined a country's measure of deprivation for each of the three basic variables—life expectancy (X1), literacy (X2) and (the log of) per capita GDP (X3). A maximum and a minimum value was identified for the actual values of each of the three variables. The deprivation measure then placed the country in the 0–1 range defined by the difference between the maximum and the minimum. ... The second step was to define an average deprivation indicator by taking a simple average of the three indicators. ... The third step was to measure the human development index (HDI) as one minus the average deprivation index." (United Nations Development Programme 1991, p88).

7   The *Cambridge Dictionary of Philosophy* (Audi 1995) provides a useful definition of "goodness." "Philosophers have typically treated the question of the ends we sought to pursue in one of two ways: whether as a question about the components of a good life or as a question about what sorts of things are good in themselves. On the first way of treating the question, it is assumed that we naturally seek a good life; hence, determining its components amounts to determining, relative to our desire for such a life, what ends we sought to pursue. On the second way, no such assumption about human nature is made; rather it is assumed that whatever is good in itself is worth choosing or pursuing. The first way of treating the question leads directly to the theory of human well-being. The second way leads directly to the theory of intrinsic value." (p.245).

8   Rawls published *A Theory of Justice* in 1971; one aspect of his theory is the notion that individuals ignorant of their position in society, behind a "veil of ignorance" would choose to maximize the position of the worst off. A number of authors have tried to use an original position to speculate on appropriate health measures (Harris 1995, Singer et al. 1995).

9   Bok (1995) cites a substantial recent literature on common values, including Hampshire (1989), Jones (1991), Maxwell (1990), Pogge (1989), and Walzer (1992).

10 The five internal reasons to launder the preferences revealed by individuals according to Goodin are: (1) a person's choices do not always perfectly reflect their preferences because of incomplete information, ignorance of their own future desires or the absence of awareness of all alternatives; (2) reciprocal forbearances such that individuals agree to forego their own meddlesome preferences; (3) explicit preferences for sets of preferences where individuals explicitly recognize they would rather operate with a different set of preferences; (4) implicit preferences for sets of preferences and (5) the internal logic of preference aggregation.

11 Although many may not publicly acknowledge this position, it is widely held in many governments and development organizations.

12 The *Oxford Companion to Philosophy* (Honderich 1995) explains the difference principle of Rawls as: "The principle, proposed by John Rawls, that economic and social advantages for the better-off members of a society are justified only if they benefit the worst-off."(p.201) Sugden (1993) explains Sen's concept of capability: "Sen starts from the idea that 'living may be seen as consisting of a set of interrelated "functionings," consisting of beings and doings.' 'Being adequately nourished,' 'avoiding premature mortality,' and 'being happy,' are all examples of functionings....A person's state of being is understood as a vector of functionings. In choosing what kind of life to live, a person chooses among such vectors. The set of feasible vectors for any person is that person's capability set. A capability set represents a person's opportunities to achieve well-being."(p. 1951)

13 This example does not depend on it being a comparison of two individuals. One can construct a somewhat fanciful but, nevertheless, possible choice where there are two groups of individuals, all members of each group have a deadly contagious disease. The two groups are exactly identical in every way except one group is richer than the other. While the symptoms and death rates for the two groups are identical they suffer from different diseases. To receive treatment they must be put in an isolation ward and a vaccine must be developed based on sera from the affected individuals. There is capacity only for one group. The two groups cannot be mixed because they will then co-infect each other, all will die and technologically a vaccine cannot be developed for both. I would argue that in such a case, we would not prefer to save either the rich or the poor group; and if forced to choose, we would be indifferent.

14 It has been pointed out that this restricted information proposition accords well with traditional physician's professional ethics where only information about the health state and perhaps age of the individual is considered relevant for the choice of treatment. While this is clearly the case, I am proposing that this restricted information proposition has a broader appeal.

15 There is a concept that individuals may have preferences over different sets of preferences. For example, someone who is a sadist may prefer to have a set of non-sadistic preferences.

16 The use of time-based measures of health status to influence resource allocation has been criticized on ethical grounds (Harris 1987, 1995, Rawles 1989). Their objection is that the length of life that an individual loses does not determine an individual's interest in continued life. Rather, two individuals with equal

interest in continued life should have equal command on resources to extend life.

17 One could subject epidemiological information to rigorous internal consistency checks and subsequently use the prevalence estimates to calculate burden using a prevalence perspective. In practice, however, it is likely that less effort would be invested in developing internally consistent epidemiological profiles of conditions if the prevalence perspective were used.

18 For example, if one uses an incidence perspective for measuring the burden of disease and a rehabilitation intervention is implemented so that the expected duration of a non-fatal health outcome is decreased, estimates of incidence-based burden would decrease for past years but not for the year that the intervention is deployed. By measuring the volume of life-years adjusted for non-fatal health outcomes actually added through an intervention, the evaluation of the benefits of an intervention would not be confounded by perspective.

19 The area is exactly the number of PYLL lost for a population with a birth cohort of magnitude 1 each year. The number of PYLL for a population with a larger birth cohort each year would simply be the area in the figure, multiplied by the size of the birth cohort.

20 The dramatic drop in period life expectancy for US females in 1918 was due to the effects of the influenza pandemic. The effect of such a mortality "shock" is spread over all cohorts living in 1918 and as a result does not show up on the cohort life expectancy curve.

21 Many readers may find the discussion of SEYLL confusing. Another perspective on the meaning of these indicators can be gained by asking how many standard expected years of life are lost in a population with exactly the mortality rates of the reference population. The answer is not zero. With reflection, the nature of these indicators (PEYLL, CEYLL and SEYLL) implies that unless everyone lives to an extraordinarily old age (beyond 100), there will always be years of life lost calculated using these methods.

22 In Coale and Guo (1989), the latest revision of the Coale and Demeny (1966) model life tables, two new levels were added, Level 26 and Level 27. In Level 27, model life table West male life expectancy at birth is 78.98. I have therefore used the female life table for Level 25 with a life expectancy at birth of 80 as the standard for males. For the convenience of readers, I have used the Second Edition of West Level 25 available in the United Nations Population Division software package MORTPAK (Coale et al. 1983). Note that the life table for females Level 25 has changed from the second version of the Coale and Demeny model life tables and the Coale and Guo revisions.

23 If the method of estimating burden includes discounting, the formula for calculating the benefits for an intervention would have to be modified to calculate the present value of burden with and without the intervention at each time t.

24 The discussion of the concepts and domains of health-related quality of life follows closely from the typology presented by Patrick and Erickson (1993).

25 Content validity is a subjective judgment on the part of the investigator, or of a panel of experts, of the extent to which the instrument asks about the aspect

of HRQL under study. Construct validity is the extent to which an instrument behaves in a manner consistent with some theoretical construct. In practice, much of the literature is devoted to a form of construct validity called convergent validity where a new instrument is "validated" if it correlates with previously used instruments measuring a similar trait. Alternatively, discriminant validity can be measured where an instrument is shown to discriminate between different traits.

26 Many of these socio-economic reversals within communities and across communities are not reported in the literature. Investigators often assume that if the results of their survey do not accord with their prior hypotheses then there must be a problem in the application of the survey. Given the widespread nature of this finding, an alternative and equally plausible hypothesis is that self-reports of illness are confounded by different conceptions and expectations of health for different socio-economic groups and different communities. For example, in an unpublished manuscript, Maggi and colleagues investigated the relationship between self-reported activities of daily living and performance tests measuring similar traits. They used the same approach for Italians aged 71–84 years and Americans aged 71–84. On every measure, Italians reported lower rates of inability to perform a given task than Americans. Conversely, on the performance tests, Americans had lower rates of inability to perform each task than Italians.

27 The following explanation of the five methods is adapted from Richardson (1994), Nord (1992) and Torrance (1986):

Rating Scale/Visual Analogue—A typical rating scale consists of a line with clearly defined end points. The most preferred health state is placed at one end of the line and the least preferred at the other. The remaining states are placed between these two so that the intervals between the placements correspond to the differences in preferences as perceived by the subject.

Magnitude Estimation—Subjects are asked to provide the ratio of undesirability of pairs of health states. For instance, State A is two or three times worse than State B. A series of questions allows all states to be located on a scale of undesirability.

Standard Gamble—A subject is offered two alternatives. Alternative 1 is a treatment with two possible outcomes: probability p of being restored to normal health and living t years or probability $(1-p)$ of dying immediately. Alternative 2 is the certain outcome of living in a given health state i for t years. The probability p is varied until the respondent is indifferent to the choice of the two alternatives. The probability p at the point of indifference is the preference weight for health state i.

Time Trade-Off—A subject is offered two alternatives. Alternative 1 is health state i for t years followed by death and alternative 2 is normal health for x years. x is varied until the respondent is indifferent to the choice between the two alternatives at which point the preference weight for state i is x/t.

Person Trade-Off—A subject is offered two alternatives. Alternative 1 is to extend life for x individuals in normal health and alternative 2 is to extend life for y individuals in health state i. y is varied until the respondent is indifferent to the choice between the two alternatives, at which point the preference for state *i* is x/y. Other forms of person trade-offs can be structured where subjects are asked to trade-off restoring health to x individuals in health state *i* versus restoring health to y individuals in health state *j*.

28 In the literature on preference measurement, various types of scales are discussed. For readers unfamiliar with the terminology of ordinal and cardinal scales, some simple definitions are given. An ordinal scale is one in which a variety of items can be ranked relative to each other. For example, A is worse than B and B is worse than C. An interval scale resembles a temperature scale where the differences in values have meaning. If A is one unit greater than B and B is one unit greater than C then these differences are equivalent. An even more exacting scale is a ratio scale where the ratio of values can also be interpreted. Length measured in inches has ratio scale properties: 10 inches is twice as long as 5 inches. Temperature has interval scale, but not ratio scale, properties.

The consensus in the cost-effectiveness literature is that interval scale properties are required. Jamison (personal communication), however, has argued that ratio scale properties are required. Preferences derived from a von Neumann-Morgenstern (1944) expected utility framework do not have ratio scale properties.

29 von Neumann and Morgenstern (1944) developed a representation theorem such that the preferences of individuals for various uncertain outcomes (called lotteries) can be represented by an index of expected utility which is the sum of the probabilities of each outcome multiplied by the utility under uncertainty of each outcome.

30 Even among economists there is considerable confusion over the meaning and interpretation of risk aversion. As Schoemaker (1982) points out there is a critical distinction in expected utility theory between the utility of an outcome under certainty $v(x)$ and the utility of an outcome under uncertainty $u(x)$. A standard gamble equates the utility of an outcome under certainty, such as living in health state i, with the a gamble with probability p of health state j and probability $(1-p)$ of another state k (usually death). The equivalence is such that:

$$v(x_1) \equiv pu(x_2) + (1-p)u(x_3)$$

where $v(x_1)$ is the utility under certainty of health state 1, $u(x_2)$ is the utility under uncertainty of health state 2 (usually perfect health) and $u(x_3)$ is the utility under uncertainty of health state 3. There is no reason to assume that utility of $v(x_1)$ will equal $u(x_1)$ although under certain circumstances it may be reasonable to assume that they are monotone transformations of each other. Therefore a functional relationship is postulated between u and v:

$$u(x) = f(v(x))$$

We may expect that under certainty the utility of death is negative infinity but under uncertainty human behaviour suggests that it has a finite, but negative value. In fact, the distinction between the utility of death under certainty and uncertainty may underlie several criticisms of QALYs (Broome 1988) and raises serious doubts about von Neumann-Morgenstern representations of choices involving death, which are far beyond the scope of this chapter. In addition, $u(x)$ may well be a function of variables other than simply $v(x)$, such as the probabilities in the gamble itself. Unfortunately, there is little empirical evidence on the difference between individual's utility for health state x under certainty and uncertainty and its determinants.

As Richardson (1994) has pointed out (using other notation) the result of a standard gamble is identical to the preference valuation under certainty when $u(x) = v(x)$. When $u(x)$ is not a linear transformation of $v(x)$ then the result of a standard gamble will be confounded. If $u(x)$ is a function of the gamble itself, then the confounding may be even more problematic.

31 Since Robbins (1932), many economists loath to make interpersonal comparisons of well-being. As almost all social choices involve comparing gains to some with losses to others, a variety of methods (Kaldor 1939, Hicks 1939) have been developed to avoid explicit interpersonal comparisons of utility but still to permit statements about alternative social choices. All of these approaches ultimately require a judgment about whether the gains to the winners outweigh the losses to the losers (Sugden 1993). Recently, there has been increased recognition and discussion among some economists about the need for interpersonal comparisons of well-being (Elster and Roemer 1991).

32 The original paper on the Ghana exercise provides per cent disablement figures for 29 conditions—for 11 of these conditions, the per cent disablement was 25. The method used to derive these per cent disablements was not specified: "A document detailing the basis on which the estimates in Table 1 were made is available on request from the authors." (Ghana Health Assessment Report 1981, p.76).

33 I am indebted to Tim Evans who pointed this out at a seminar at the Harvard Center for Population and Development Studies in September 1994.

34 A major review meeting of the Global Burden of Disease Study was held at the Royal Society, in London, December 1993. A variety of smaller conferences and workshops on various aspects of DALYs and the Global Burden of Disease Study have been held at, or sponsored by, the Harvard Center for Population and Development Studies.

35 There is a minority of respondents who assign a lower disability weight based on PTO2 than on PTO1. This sub-group of respondents usually state that the right to extra life of the 1000 healthy individuals in the PTO2 choice must take precedence over the right to improved quality of life for the individuals in a given health state. My experience is that these individuals often have the same ordinal ranking of the 22 conditions but tend to scale the disability weights for all 22 conditions lower, reflecting their belief in the relative dominance of a right to life over a right to life of a given quality.

36 This meeting on disability weights at the World Health Organization was kindly funded by the Rockefeller Foundation.

37 Various methods could be used to estimate the group disability weights from the results of the person-trade-off protocol. Because PTO1 and PTO2 values are not bounded by zero and one as are disability weights, a single outlying response can substantially alter the average PTO1 or PTO2 values. To avoid this problem, the group composite disability weight has been calculated using the median PTO value for each condition.

38 There is a literature on health states considered by some individuals to be worse than death; for recent examples see Patrick et al. (1994) and Pearlman et al.

(1993). From the perspective of measuring the global burden of disease, health states worse than death can be treated as equivalent to death without substantively affecting the results by disease problem. For individual clinical decision-making, health states worse than death are important, but from the standpoint of a social decision-maker choosing between competing health interventions, health states worse than death could lead to some perverse conclusions such as the cost-effectiveness of encouraging premature death.

39 Barendregt et al. (1995) were the first to propose using the disability weights from DALYs to calculate a health-adjusted life expectancy and suggested the name Disability-Adjusted Life Expectancy (DALE).

40 The relationship between the probability of death at each age and individual discount rates at each age is confounded by the desire of some individuals to leave some wealth to their family or others.

41 A function is concave towards the origin if the second derivative of the function is negative. A circle is concave with respect to the center of the circle.

42 Underlying much of the QALY literature is a special form of an expected utility function, apparently first formalized in discrete time by Garber and Phelphs (1992). Acharya and Murray (1996) explore various implications of this multiplicative form of a utility function, a continuous form of which is:

$$EU(t) = \int_0^\infty p(t)k(t)U(C(t))e^{rt}dt$$

where $p(t)$ is the probability of surviving to time t, $k(t)$ is a variable representing the quality of life of the individual's health state, $U(C(t))$ is the utility from consumption in time period t, and r is the rate of pure time preference.

43 Acharya and Murray (1996) derive an expression for the willingness-to-pay for a fixed increase in survivorship in a given year. If an individual is willing to pay more for a distal life-year than a proximal life-year then the individual must have a negative discount rate for life-years, whereas if the willingness to pay for a distal life-year is less than the willingness-to-pay for a proximal life-year, the individual must have a positive discount rate for life-years. Individual's discount rates for future life-years are assumed to equal the willingness-to-pay for a future life-year divided by the WTP for a proximal life year. A three-period model is constructed using a discrete form of the expected utility expression in the previous note. To solve a three-period model, a specific form of a utility function was used, namely:

$$U(C) = \frac{C^{1-\alpha}}{1-\alpha}$$

In addition, $C(t)$ is assumed to grow at a constant rate such that:

$$C(t) = C_0(1+\tau)^t$$

where τ is the annual growth rate in consumption for the individual. If $(1+\tau)$ is greater than $(1+r)$ where r is the individual's rate of pure time preference then the individual will have a negative discount rate for future life-years; if $(1+\tau)$ is less than $(1+r)$ then the discount rate is positive. If τ equals r then the individual will value distal life-years as equal to proximal life-years.

This result is based on an assumption that the consumption level is exogenous to the model. In other words, the individual does not smooth consumption over different time periods. Empirical evidence strongly suggests that individuals do not smooth consumption over time periods so as to maximize expected utility (Lowenstein and Thaler 1989).

44 Temkin (1995) discusses the literature on justice and equality including those views that assert that the extent to which inequality is objectionable depends on whether it is between individuals of the same society and/or the same time period. Such views could imply a form of spatial or social distance discounting.

45 Weinstein (1983) makes an important argument that if the "cost of health" which I interpret as the dollar value of health to the society, is expected to increase over time then society might discount life-years at a lower rate than dollars or consumption. This is not an argument for induced discounting. Rather, it is an argument that is based on a model of why the individual or society may discount. Theoretically, we expect society and an individual to value future life-years more if consumption per capita is expected to rise. The growth in consumption per capita and the average level of utility derived from a life-year may exceed the marginal opportunity cost of money thus leading to negative discounting.

46 Anand and Hanson suggest that an inter-temporal welfare function for DALYs of the following form would solve the research and eradication paradoxes:

$$\sum_i \sum_t D_{it}^{\alpha} \text{ where } \alpha > 1$$

D is the DALYs lost to individual i at time t.

However, imagine that in every year burden is expected to be identical. The benefits of a health research project that permanently reduces the burden in each year will be infinite. The current generation will still be called upon to make excessive sacrifices. Although, Anand and Hanson do not add any other conditions to their inter-temporal welfare function, they might argue that by adding bliss points (Ramsey 1928) or certain boundedness conditions to the objective function (for a basic discussion see Takayama 1985), the infinite magnitude of benefits is solved. However, neither of these restrictions to their analysis appear to be justified for DALYs.

47 Using the results reported by Cropper and Portney (1992) we can calculate the marginal discount rate for lives saved as follows: 0–5 years 13.9 per cent, 5–10 years 8.1 per cent, 10–25 years 4.6 per cent, 25–50 years 2.4 per cent and 50–100 years 2.8 per cent.

48 One argument that I have not discussed in the text is Scanlon's (1975) argument for urgency. D. Little in a seminar at the Harvard Center for Population and Development Studies in March 1996 argued for discounting future well-being on the basis of the urgent needs of the poor today. In the context of the arguments presented, the urgent concerns of the current generation suggest that only a small degree of sacrifice for the health of future generations is reasonable.

49 In the IOM study, the relative valuations are reported as infant death equiva-
lents so that the scale is inverted. For example, 0.5 deaths at 5–14 years is
equivalent to an infant death.

50 While most group consultations and population surveys find a consistent
pattern of age-preference, Anand and Hanson (1995) express their personal
view that "we can see no reason for valuing time lived at different ages
differently." Of course, in all populations there must surely be individuals who,
like these authors, hold different preferences. They provide, however, no
supporting documentation that many others share their view.

51 Two functional forms of age-weighting would meet this definition. One would
simply be a multiplier that would be the ratio of the value of preventing a death
at each age divided by the relative value expected on the basis of discounted
duration. An intuitive interpretation of such age-weights, however, is hard to
find. Alternatively, we can define the relative value of each year of life lived at
each age. There are a number of reasons discussed in the text why the value of
each year of life lived may differ. Because this functional form has a more direct
interpretation, I have exclusively examined age-weights of the form that attach
a value to each year of life lived at each age.

52 I have constructed a simple model of an economy to explore the relationships
between individual and social willingness-to-pay to add lives or years of life.
This model has been constructed to explore other questions as well, but only
the key aspects of the model are summarized below.

• In the absence of any health expenditure, life expectancy at birth is 55 years.

• Only the population between the ages of twenty and sixty produce. The total
production of the economy is determined by the following modified Cobb-
Douglas production function:

$$P = \gamma K_t^{\alpha} \left(\sum_{a=20}^{59} E_{a,t} L_{a,t} \right)^{\beta}$$

where γ and α are user-defined parameters, β is equal to $(1-\alpha)$, $E_{a,t}$ is the
cumulative expenditure on education of individuals aged a at time t, $L_{a,t}$ is
the number of individuals aged α that are healthy and working at time t and
K_t is the capital stock of the economy.

• The total product of this economy is divided according to an arbitrary social
contract among three categories: education of children, capital investment
and consumption. In this egalitarian society, the share of total production
assigned to consumption is divided equally amongst all those living.

• A specific form of the utility function has been assumed for all individuals:

$$U_t(C_t) = \omega Ln(C_t)$$

where ω is a constant and C_t is consumption in time period t.

• Social welfare is assumed to simply be the aggregation of individual utilties.
As everyone in this simple form of the model is assumed to have the same
level of consumption and the same utility function, alternative forms of a
welfare function would not substantially alter the results. However, if the

levels of consumption between consumers differ then alternative formulations of a welfare function would have important effects on the results.

• We assume that there is a health intervention that can increase survivorship at given ages. There are two forms of these health interventions. In one form, a death is averted at a given age and the individual that survives is subject to the same conditional probabilities of survival at each age thereafter as the rest of the population. In the second type of intervention, a single year of life is added so that the individual saved will die in one year. For both types of intervention, we can calculate the individual willingness-to-pay and the social willingness-to-pay, by calculating the amount an individual is willing to forego in consumption this time period and the amount society is willing to forego such that the expected utility for the individual and the expected welfare for society is equivalent to the situation where the health intervention is not purchased. The individual discount rate is assumed to be 10 per cent and the social discount rate is assumed to be three per cent.

• This variant of the model has six parameters. Credible ranges for each of these parameters were selected. Latin Hypercube Sampling has been used to sample this six-dimensional parameter space 7000 times. Combinations of parameters that yield a growth rate per annum for the economy between two and ten per cent have been used for subsequent analyses.

• The extent to which social WTP for deaths in adults was greater than the social WTP for deaths in children was a function of income per capita and the growth rate. Low income and a high growth rate predicted a strong degree of age-weighting. In high income populations with a low growth rate, the social WTP for years of life was nearly equal to individual WTP and was largely a function of life expectancy at each age. The figures in the text, provide results of six variants selected arbitrarily from among the low to moderate income variants with growth rates in excess of 5 per cent.

53 Rice and Hodgson (1982) write "We no longer argue about whether we should attach a value to human life for cost-benefit analyses of health programmes. The debate now is on the method to be used..."(p536). Despite their claims, human capital calculations of the value of human life remain highly controversial and there is no consensus on the desirability of using cost-benefit analysis as opposed to cost-effectiveness analysis in which a dollar value is not assigned to a year of life.

54 Johannesson and Johansson (1996) report on much more extreme age-weights from a survey 1000 Swedes. They found that 9 QALYs gained for 70 year-olds was equivalent to 3 QALYs gained for 50 year-olds and one QALY gained for a 30 year-old. The age-weighting function used in DALYs, the equivalence numbers would be 2.1 and 1.3 for 70 year-olds and 50 year-olds, respectively, compared to 30 year-olds.

55 Note that in a continuous discount function r is not precisely the same as r in the discrete form. The formula for the discrete form is simply

$$\frac{1}{(1+r)^t}$$

If the discount rate in the discrete formula is r then the equivalent result is achieved with a continuous discount rate of $\ln(1+r)$.

BIBLIOGRAPHY

Acharya AK, Murray CJL (1996) *Do individuals discount future health?* Harvard Center for Population and Development Studies, Working Paper.

Anand S, Hanson K (1995) *Disability-adjusted life years: a critical review.* Harvard Center for Population and Development Studies, Working Paper #95.06.

Anderson RT, Aaronson NK, Wilkin D (1995) Critical review of the international assessments of health-related quality of life: generic instruments. In: Schumaker SA, Berzon R, eds. *The international assessment of health-related quality of life: theory, translation, measurement and analysis.* Oxford, Rapid Communications.

Anonymous (1992) Discounting health care: only a matter of timing? *Lancet,* 340:148–149.

Audi R (1995) *The Cambridge dictionary of philosophy.* Cambridge, Cambridge University Press.

Australian Institute of Health and Welfare (1996) Australia's health 1996: the fifth biennial report of the Australian Institute of Health and Welfare. Canberra, AGPS.

Barendregt JJ, Bonneux L, van der Maas PJ (1995) Health expectancy: froma population health indicator to a tool for policy making. Paper presented at REVES 8, October 5–7 1995.

Barker C, Green A (1996) Opening the debate on DALYs. *Health Policy and Planning,* 11(2):179–183.

Barnum H (1987) Evaluating healthy days of life gained from health projects. *Social science and medicine,* 24(10):833–841.

Bebbington AC (1991) The expectation of life without disability in England and Wales: 1976–88. *Population trends,* 66:26–29.

Berg RL (1973) Weighted life expectancy as a health status index. *Health services research,* 8:153–156.

Bergner M et al. (1981) The Sickness Impact Profile: development and final revision of a health status measure. *Medical care,* 19:787–805.

Berman S (1995) Otitis media in developing countries. *Pediatrics,* 96(1):126–131

Bobadilla JL et al. (1994) Design, content and financing of an essential national package of health services. *Bulletin of the World Health Organization,* 72(4):653–662.

Bobadilla JL (1996) *Searching for essential health services in low- and middle-income countries. A review of recent studies on health priorities.* Washington DC, Human Development Department Report.

Bok S (1995) *Common values.* Colombia, MO, University of Missouri Press.

Brickman P, Coates D, Janoff-Bulman R (1978) Lottery winners and accident victims: is happiness relative? *Journal of personality and social psychology,* 36(8):917–927.

Bussbach JJV, Jessing DJ, de Charro FT (1993) The utility of health at different stages of life: a quantitative approach. *Social science and medicine,* 37(2):153–158.

Cairns J (1992) Discounting and health benefits: another perspective. *Health economics,* 1:76–79.

Carter et al. (1976) Validation of and interval scaling: the sickness impact profile. *Health services research,* Winter:516–528.

Centers for Disease Control (1986) Premature mortality in the United States: public health issues in the use of years of potential life lost. *Morbidity and mortality weekly report,* 35(Suppl 2):15–115.

Chiang CL (1965) *An index of health: mathematical models. Public Health Services Publications 1000 Series 2. No. 5.* Washington DC, National Center for Health Statistics.

Coale A, Guo G (1989) Revised regional model life tables at very low levels of mortality. *Population index,* 55(4):613–643.

Coale A, Demeny P, Vaughan B (1983) *Regional model life tables and stable populations. Second edition.* New York, Academic Press.

Coale A, Demeny P (1966) *Regional model life tables and stable populations.* Princeton, Princeton University Press.

Cooper BS, Rice DP (1976) The economic costs of illness revisited. *Social security bulletin,* 39(2):21–36.

Crimmins EM, Saito Y, Hayward MD (1993) Sullivan and multistate methods of estimating active life expectancy: two methods, two answers. In: Robine JM et al., eds. *Calculation of health expectancies: harmonization, consensus achieved and future perspectives.* London, John Libbey Eurotext.

Cropper ML, Portney PR (1992) Discounting human lives. *Resources for the future,* 108:1–4.

Cropper ML, Aydede SK, Portney PR (1994) Preferences for life saving programs: how the public discounts time and age. *Journal of risk and uncertainty,* 8:243–265.

Dasbach EJ et al. (1994) Self-rated health and mortality in people with diabetes. *American Journal of Public Health,* 84(11): 1775–1779

Dasgupta P, Sen A, Marglin S (1972) *Guidelines for project evaluation.* New York, United Nations.

de Tocqueville A (1839) *Democracy in America.* New York, Anchor Books.

Dempsey M. (1947) Decline in tuberculosis. The death rate fails to tell the entire story. *American review of tuberculosis,* 56:157–164.

Desjarlais R et al. (1995) *World mental health: problems and priorities in low-income countries.* New York, Oxford University Press.

Dickinson FG, Welker EL (1948) What is the leading cause of death? Two new measures. *American Medical Association Bureau of Medical Economic Research bulletin,* 64.

Diener E (1984) Subjective well-being. *Psychological bulletin,* 95(3):542–575.

Drummond MF (1987) Resource allocation decisions in health care: a role for quality of life assessments. *Journal of chronic disease,* 40:605–619.

Eddy DM. (1991) Oregon's methods: did cost-effectiveness analysis fail? *Journal of the American Medical Association,* 266:2135–2141.

Elster J, Roemer JE, eds. (1991) *Interpersonal comparisons of well-being.* Cambridge, Cambridge University Press.

EuroQol Group (1990) EuroQol—a new facility for the measurement of health-related quality of life. *Health policy,* 16:199–208.

Evans DB, Hurley SF (1995) The application of economic evaluation techniques in the health sector: the state of the art. *Journal of international development,* 7(3):503–524.

Fanshel S, Bush JW (1970) A health-status index and its application to health services outcomes. *Operations research,* 18(6):1021–1066.

Feachem RGA et al., eds. (1992) *The health of adults in the developing world.* New York, Oxford University Press for the World Bank.

Feldstein, MS (1964) The social time preference discount rate in cost benefit analysis. *Economic journal,* 74:360–379.

Fernandez JM, Pereira JC, Torres AC (1995) Una agenda a debate: el informe del banco mundial "Invertir en Salud." *Rev Esp salud publica,* 69:385–391.

Finlay JF et al. (1995) A new Canadian health care initiative in Tanzania. *Canadian Medical Association journal,* 153(8):1081–1085.

Fischhoff B et al. (1981) *Acceptable risk.* Cambridge, Cambridge University Press.

Fishkin JS (1991) *Democracy and deliberation: new directions for democratic reform.* New Haven, Yale University Press.

Foege W (1994) Preventive medicine and public health. *Journal of the American Medical Association,* 271(21):1704–5.

Fries JF (1980) Aging, natural death and the compression of morbidity. *New England journal of medicine,* 303:130–135.

Froberg DG, Kane RL (1989a) Methodology for measuring health-state preferences—II: scaling methods. *Journal of clinical epidemiology,* 42(5):459–471.

Froberg DG, Kane RL (1989b) Methodology for measuring health-state preferences — III: population and context effects. *Journal of clinical epidemiology,* 42(6):585–592.

Fuchs VR (1986) *The health economy.* Cambridge, MA, Harvard University Press.

Fuchs V, Zeckhauser R (1987) Valuing health—a priceless commodity? *American economic review,* 77:263–268.

Gafni A, Torrance GW (1984) Risk attitude and time preference for health. *Management science,* 30(4):440–451.

Garber AM, Phelphs CE (1992) *Economic foundations of cost-effectiveness analysis.* Cambridge, MA, National Bureau of Economic Research Working paper no. 4164.

Ganiats TG (1992) On sale: future health care. The paradox of discounting. *Western journal of medicine,* 156(5):550–553.

Ghana Health Assessment Project Team (1981) A quantitative method of assessing the health impact of different diseases in less developed countries. *International journal of epidemiology,* 10(1):73–80.

Goodin RE (1982) Discounting discounting. *Journal of public policy*, 2(1):53–72.

Goodin RE (1986) Laundering preferences. In: Elster J, Hylland A, eds. *Foundations of social choice theory*. Cambridge, Cambridge University Press.

Grant MD, Piotrowski ZH, Chappell R (1995) Self-reported health and survival in the Longitudinal Study of Aging, 1984-1986. *Journal of Clinical Epidemiology*, 48(3): 375-387.

Greville TNE (1948) Comments on Mary Dempsey's articles on "decline in tuberculosis: the death rate fails to tell the entire story." *American review of tuberculosis*, 57:417–419.

Haenszel W (1950) A standardized rate for mortality defined in units of lost years of life. *American journal of public health*, 40:17–26.

Hahn RA, Eberhardt S (1995) Life expectancy in four US racial/ethnic populations: 1990. *Epidemiology*, 6:350–355.

Hammit JK (1993) Discounting health increments: editorial. *Journal of health economics*, 12:117–120.

Hampshire, S (1989) *Innocence and experience*. Cambridge, MA, Harvard University Press.

Harris J (1987) QALYfying the value of life. *Journal of medical ethics*, 13(3):117–123.

Harris J (1995) Double jeopardy and the veil of ignorance—a reply. *Journal of medical ethics*, 21:151–157.

Hays RD, Anderson R, Revicki D (1993) Psychometric considerations in evaluating health-related quality of life measures. *Quality of life research*, 2:441–449.

Helson J (1964) *Adaptation-level theory*. New York, Harper and Row.

Hicks J (1939) The foundations of welfare economics. *Economic journal*, 49(146):696–712.

Honderich T (1995) *The Oxford Companion to Philosophy*. New York, Oxford University Press.

Hornberger JC, Redelmeier DA, Petersen J (1992) Variability among methods to assess patients' well-being and consequent effect on a cost-effectiveness analysis. *Journal of clinical epidemiology*, 45(5):505–512.

Hunt SM, Mckenna SP, Williams J (1981) Reliability of a population survey tool for measuring perceived health problems: a study of patients with osteoarthrosis. *Journal of epidemiology and community health*, 35:297–300.

Idler EL, Angel RJ (1990) Self-rated health and mortality in the NHANES-I Epidemiologic Follow-up Study. *American Journal of Public Health*, 80(4):446–452.

Idler EL, Kasl SV, Lemke JH (1990) Self-evaluated health and mortality among the elderly in New Haven, Connecticut, and Iowa and Washington counties, Iowa, 1982–1986. *American Journal of Epidemiology*, 131(1):91–103.

Institute of Medicine (1986) *New vaccine development. Establishing priorities. Volume II. Disease of importance in developing countries*. Washington DC, National Academy Press.

Ittleson WH et al. (1974) *An introduction to environmental psychology*. New York, Hold, Rinehart and Winston.

Jamison DT et al., eds. (1993) *Disease control priorities in developing countries.* New York, Oxford University Press for the World Bank.

Johannesson M, Johansson PO (1996) *Is the valuation of a QALY gained independent of age? Some empirical evidence.* Mimeo

Johannesson M, Pliskin JS, Weinstein MC (1994) A note on QALYs, time tradeoff, and discounting. *Medical decision making,* 14:188–193.

Johannesson M. (1992) On the discounting of gained life-years in cost-effectiveness analysis. *International journal of technology assessment in health care,* 8(2):359–364.

Johansson SR. (1991) The health transition: the cultural inflation of morbidity during the decline of mortality. *Health transition review,* 1:39–68.

Jones, DV (1991) *Code of peace: ethics and security in the world of the warlord states.* Chicago, U of Chicago Press.

Kahneman D, Varey C (1991) Notes on the psychology of utility. In: Elster J, Roemer J, eds. *Interpersonal comparisons of well-being.* Cambridge, Cambridge University Press

Kaldor N (1939) Welfare propositions of economics and interpersonal comparisons of utility. *Economic journal,* 49(145): 549–552.

Kane RL, Bell RM, Riegler SZ (1986) Value preferences for nursing home outcomes. *Gerontologist,* 26:303–308.

Kaplan GA, Kotler PL (1985) Self-reorts predictive of mortality from ischemic heart disease: a nine year follow-up of the human population laboratory cohort. Journal of Chronic Diseases, 38(2):195-201.

Kaplan RM, Anderson JP (1988) A general health model: update and applications. *Health services research,* 23:203–35.

Kaplan RM, Ernst JA. (1983) Do category rating scales produce biased preference weights for a health index. *Medical care* 21:193–207.

Kaplan RM, Bush JW (1982) Health related quality of life measurement for evaluation of research and policy analysis. *Health psychology,* 1:62–???.

Kaplan RM, Bush JW, Berry CC (1979) Category rating versus magnitude estimation for measuring levels of well being. *Medical care,* 17:501–525.

Karkal M (1995) *Our lives, our health.* New Delhi, Co-ordination Unit, World Conference on Women—Beijing '95.

Keeler EB, Cretin S (1983) Discounting of life-savings and other non-monetary effects. *Management science,* 29:300–6.

Kleinman A, Kleinman J (1996) The appeal of experience; the dismay of images: cultural appropriations of suffering in our times. *Daedalus,* 125(1):1–23.

Kohn R (1951) An objective mortality indicator. *Canadian journal of public health,* 42:375–379.

Krahn M, Gafni A (1993) Discounting in the economic evaluation of health care interventions. *Medical care,* 31:403–418.

Laurell AC, Lopez Arellano O (1996) Market commodities and poor relief: the World Bank proposal for health. *International journal of health services* 26(1):1–18.

Layard R, Glaister S, eds. (1994) *Cost-benefit analysis*. Cambridge, Cambridge University Press.

Lewis PA, Charny M (1989) Which of two individuals do you treat when only their ages are different and you can't treat both? *Journal of medical ethics*, 15:28–34.

Lind RC et al. (1982) *Discounting for time and risk in energy policy*. Baltimore, Johns Hopkins University Press.

Lindsted KD, Tonstod S, Kuzma JW (1991) Self-report of physical activity and patterns of mortality in Seventh-Day Adventist men. *Journal of clinical epidemiology*, 44(4–5):355–64.

Lockwood M (1988) Quality of life and resource allocation. In: Bell M, Mendus S, eds. *Philosophy and medical welfare*. Cambridge, Cambridge University Press.

Lohr KN (1992) Advances in health status assessment: fostering the application of health status measures in clinical settings. Proceedings of a conference. *Medical care*, 30(Suppl 5): MS1–293.

Lohr KN, ed. (1989) Advances in health status assessment: overview of the conference proceedings. *Medical care*, 27(Suppl 3):S1–11.

Lohr KN, Ware JE Jr., eds. (1987) Proceedings of the advances in health assessment conference. *Journal of chronic disease*, 40(Suppl 1):S1–191.

Lowenstein G, Thaler RH (1989) Anomalies. Intertemporal choice. *Journal of economic perspectives*, 3(4):181–193.

Lozano R et al. (1995) Burden of disease assessment and health system. Reform results of a study in Mexico. *Journal of international development*, 7(3):555–563.

Mackenbach J, Looman C, van de Meer J (1996) Differences in the misreporting of chronic conditions by level of education: the effect on inequalities in prevelance rates. *American Journal of Public Health*, 86(5):706-711

Manton KG (1986) Past and future life expectancy increases at later ages: their implications for the linkage of chronic morbidity, disability and mortality. *Journal of gerontology*, 41(5):672–681

Marglin SA (1963) The opportunity costs of public investment. *Quarterly journal of economics*, 77:274–289.

Martens WJ et al. (1995) Potential impact of global climate change on malaria risk. *Environmental health perspectives*, 103(5):458–464.

Martens L, van Doorslaer E (1990) Dealing with discounting. *International journal of technology assessment of health care*, 6:139–145.

Max W, Rice DP, Mackenzie EJ (1990) The lifetime cost of injury. *Inquiry*, 27(4):332–343.

Maxwell M (1990) *Morality among nations: an evolutionary view*. Albany, State University of New York Press.

McCallum J, Shadbolt B, Wang D (1994) Self-rated health and survival: a 7-year follow-up study of Australian elderly. *American journal of public health,* 84(7):1100–1105.

Mehrez A, Gafni A (1987) An empirical evaluation of two assessment methods for utility measurement for life years. *Socio-economic planning sciences,* 21(6):371–375.

Morrow RH, Bryant JH (1995) Health policy approaches to measuring and valuing human life: conceptual and ethical issues. *American journal of public health,* 85(10):1356–1360.

Mosley WH, Chen LC (1984) An analytical framework for studying child survival in developing countries. *Population and development review,* 10(Suppl):25–45.

Mossey IM, Shapiro E (1982) Self-rated health: a predictor of mortality among the elderly. *American Journal of Public Health,* 72(8):800–808.

Mulley AG (1989) Assessing patients' utilities. Can the ends justify the means? *Medical care,* 27(Suppl 3):S269–281.

Murray CJL (1987) A critical review of international mortality data. *Social science and medicine,* 25(7):773–781.

Murray CJL (1988) The infant mortality rate, life expectancy at birth and a Linear Index of Mortality as measures of general health status. *International journal of epidemiology,* 17(1):122–128.

Murray CJL (1994) Quantifying the burden of disease: the technical basis for DALYs. *Bulletin of the World Health Organization,* 72(3):429–445.

Murray CJL (1995) Epidemiologic and morbidity transitions in India. In: Dasgupta P, ed. *Health, poverty and development in India.* Oxford, Oxford University Press.

Murray CJL, Chen LC (1992) Understanding morbidity change. *Population and development review,* 18(3):481–503.

Murray CJL, Kreuser J, Whang W (1994) Cost-effectiveness analysis and policy choices: investing in health systems. *Bulletin of the World Health Organization* 72(4):663–674.

Murray CJL, Lopez AD, eds. (1994) *Global comparative assesments in the health sector.* Geneva, World Health Organization.

Murray CJL, Lopez AD (1996a) Global and regional descriptive epidemiology of disability: incidence, prevalence, health expectancies and years lived with disability. In: Murray CJL, Lopez AD, eds. *The Global Burden of Disease: a comprehensive assessment of mortality and disability from diseases, injuries, and risk factors in 1990 and projected to 2020.* Cambridge, Harvard University Press.

Murray CJL, Lopez AD (1996b) The global burden of disease in 1990: final results and their sensitivity to alternative epidemiologic perspectives, discount rates, age-weights and disability weights. In: Murray CJL, Lopez AD, eds. *The Global Burden of Disease: a comprehensive assessment of mortality and disability from diseases, injuries, and risk factors in 1990 and projected to 2020.* Cambridge, Harvard University Press.

Murray CJL, Lopez AD (1996c) Quantifying the burden of disease and injury attributable to ten major risk factors. In: Murray CJL, Lopez AD, eds. *The Global Burden of Disease: a comprehensive assessment of mortality and disability from diseases, injuries, and risk factors in 1990 and projected to 2020.* Cambridge, Harvard University Press.

Nagler M, ed. (1993) *Perspectives on disability. Second edition.* Palo Alto (CA), Health Market Research.

Nord E (1991) The validity of a visual analogue scale in determining social utility weights for health states. *International journal of health planning and management,* 6:234–242.

Nord E (1992) Methods for quality adjustment of life years. *Social science and medicine,* 34(5):559–569.

Nord E (1993) Unjustified use of the Quality of well-being scale in priority setting in Oregon. *Health policy,* 24:45–53.

Nord E (1995) The person-trade-off approach to valuing health care programs. *Medical decision making,* 15(3):201–208.

Nord E et al. (1995) Maximizing health benefits vs. egalitarianism: an Australian survey of health issues. *Social science and medicine,* 41(10):1429–1437.

Nord E, Richardson J, Macarounas-Kirchmann K (1993) Social evaluation of health care versus personal evaluation of health states. Evidence on the validity of four health-state scaling instruments using Norwegian and Australian Surveys. *International journal of technology assessment in health care,* 9(4):463–478.

Olsen J (1993) On what basis should health be discounted? *Journal of health economics,* 12:39–53.

Olsen JA (1994) Persons vs. years: two ways of eliciting implicit weights. *Health economics,* 3:39–46.

Parfit D (1984) *Reasons and persons.* Oxford, Oxford University Press.

Parsonage M, Neuburger H (1992) Discounting and health benefits. *Health economics,* 1:71–76.

Patrick DL, Erickson P (1993) *Health status and health policy: quality of life in health care evaluation and resource allocation.* New York, Oxford University Press.

Patrick DL, Bush JW, Chen MM (1973) Methods for measuring levels of well-being for a health-status index. *Health services research,* 8(3):228–245.

Patrick DL et al. (1994) Measuring preferences for health states worse than death. *Medical Decision Making,* 14(1):9–18.

Pearce DW, ed. (1992) *The MIT dictionary of modern economics.* Cambridge, MIT Press.

Pearlman RA et al. (1993) Insights pertaining to patient assesments of states worth than death. *Journal of clinical ethics,* 4(1):33–41.

Perloff JD et al. (1984) Premature death in the United States: Years of life lost and health priorities. *Journal of public health policy,* 5:167–184.

Pigou AC (1932) *The economics of welfare. Fourth edition.* London, Macmillan.

Piot M, Sundaresan TK (1967) A linear programme decision model for tuberculosis control. Progress report on the first test-runs. Geneva: World Health Organization, WHO/TB/Techn.Information/67.55.

Pogge TWM (1989) *Realizing rawls.* Ithaca, Cornell University Press.

Politi C et al. (1995) Cost-effectiveness analysis of alternative treatments of African gambiense trypanosomiasis in Uganda. *Health economics,* 4(4):273–287.

Pressat R (1973) Surmortalite biologique et surmortalite sociale. *Revue Francaise de sociologie,* 14:103–110.

Preston SH (1993) Health indices as a guide to health sector planning: a demographic critique. In: Gribble JN, Preston SH, eds. *The epidemiological transition. policy and planning implications for developing countries.* Washington DC, National Academy Press.

Prost A, Prescott N (1984) Cost-effectiveness of blindness prevention by the Onchocerciasis Control Programme in Upper Volta. *Bulletin of the World Health Organization,* 62:795–802.

Ramsey FP (1928) A mathematical theory of savings. *Economic journal,* 38:543–559.

Rawles J (1989) Castigating QALYs. *Journal of medical ethics,* 15:143–147.

Rawls J (1971) *A theory of justice.* Cambridge, Harvard University Press.

Redelmeier DA, Heller DN (1993) Time preference in medical decision making and cost-effectiveness analysis. *Medical decision making,* 13(3):212–217.

Reseau Esperance de Vie en Sante (1993) *Statistical world yearbook. Retrospective 1993 Issue.* Montpellier, INSERM.

Revicki DA, Kaplan RM (1995) Relationship between psychomoetric and utility-based approaches to the measurement of health-related quality of life. In: Shumaker SA, Berzon RA, eds. *The international assessment of health-related quality of life: theory translation, measurement and analysis.* Oxford, Rapid Communications.

Rice DP, Kelman S, Miller LS (1991) Estimates of economic costs of alcohol and drug abuse and mental illness, 1985 and 1988. *Public health reports,* 106(3):280–292.

Rice DP, Hodgson TA (1982) The value of human life revisited. *American journal of public health,* 72(6):536–538.

Rice DP (1994) Cost-of-illness studies: fact or fiction? *Lancet,* 344:1519–1520.

Richardson J (1994) Cost utility analysis: what should be measure? *Social science and medicine,* 39(1):7–21.

Robbins L (1932) *An essay on the nature and significance of economic science.* London, Macmillan.

Robine JM et al., eds. (1993a) *Calculation of health expectancies: harmonization, consensus achieved and future perspectives.* London, John Libbey Eurotext.

Robine JM, Mathers CD, Bucquet D (1993b) Distinguishing health expectancies and health-adjusted life expectancies from quality-adjusted life years. *American journal of public health,* 83(6):797–798.

Robine JM, Ritchie K (1991) Healthy life expectancy: evaluation of a global indicator for change in population health. *British medical journal,* 302:457–460.

Robinson HL (1948) Mortality trends and public health in Canada. *Canadian journal of public health*, 39(2):60–70.

Romeder JM, McWhinnie JR (1977) Potential years of life lost between ages 1 and 70: an indicator of premature mortality for health planning. *International journal of epidemiology*, 6:143–151.

Rosser R, Kind P (1978) A scale of valuations of states of illness: is there a social consensus? *International journal of epidemiology*, 7(4):347–358.

Rossiter C, ed. (1961) *The Federalist papers*. New York, New American Library.

Ryder NB (1975) Notes on stationary populations. *Population index*, 41:3–28.

Sackett DL, Torrance GW (1978) The utility of different health states as perceived by the general public. *Journal of chronic disease*, 31:697–704.

Scanlon TM (1975) Preference and urgency. *Journal of philosophy*, 72:655–669.

Schoemaker PJH (1982) The expected utility model: its variants, purposes, evidence and limitations. *Journal of economic literature*, 20:529–563.

Schwuebel V (1994) [The DALY: an indicator for measuring disease burden]. *Revue d'epidemiologie et de sante publique*, 42(2):183–4.

Sen AK (1961) On optimizing the rate of savings. *Economic journal*.

Sen AK (1972) *Choice of techniques*. Oxford: Blackwell.

Sen AK (1984) Approaches to the choice of discount rates for social benefit-cost analysis. In: Lind RC, ed. *Discounting for time and risk in energy policy*. Baltimore, Johns Hopkins University Press.

Shepard DS (1994) Economic analysis of investment priorities for measles control. *Journal of infectious diseases*, 170(Suppl 1):S56–62

Shumaker SA, Berzon R, eds. (1995) *The international assessment of health-related quality of life: theory translation, measurement and analysis*. Oxford, Rapid Communications.

Sidgwick H (1922) *The methods of ethics. Seventh edition*. London, Macmillan and Company.

Singer P et al. (1995) Double jeopardy and the use of QALYs in health care allocation. *Journal of medical ethics*, 21:144–150.

Sloan FA, ed. (1995) *Valuing health care: costs, benefits, and effectiveness of pharmaceuticals and other medical technologies*. Cambridge, Cambridge University Press.

Smith A (1987) Qualms about QALYs. *Lancet*, 1 (8542):1134–1136.

Spilker B et al. (1996) Quality of life bibliography and indexes. *Medical care*, 28(12 Suppl):D51–77.

Starzl TE et al. (1987) A multifactorial system for equitable selection of cadaver kidney recipients. *Journal of the American Medical Association*, 257:3073–75.

Strotz RH (1956) Myopia and inconsistency in dynamic utility maximization. *Review of economic studies*, 23:165–180.

Sullivan DF (1966) *Conceptual problems in developing an index of health. US Public Health Service Publication Series No. 1000. Vital and Health Statistics Series 2. No. 17.* National Center for Health Statistics.

Sullivan DF (1971) A single index of mortality and morbidity. *HSMHA health reports,* 86:347–354.

Sugden R (1993) A review of *Inequality reexamined* by Amartya Sen. *Journal of economic literature,* 31(4):1947–1986.

Takayama A (1985) *Mathematical economics. Second edition.* Cambridge, Cambridge University Press.

Temkin LS (1995) Justice and equality: some questions about scope. *Social philosophy and policy,* 12(2):72–104.

Torrance GW (1976) Social preferences for health states: an empirical evaluation of three measurement techniques. *Socio-economic planning sciences,* 10:129–136.

Torrance GW (1986) Measurement of health-state utilities for economic appraisal: a review. *Journal of health economics,* 5:1–30.

Torrance GW, Feeny D (1989) Utilities and quality adjusted life years. *International journal of technology assessment of health care,* 5:559–575.

Ugalde A, Jackson JT (1995) The World Bank and international health policy: a critical review. *Journal of international development,* 7(3):525–541.

UNICEF (1995) *State of the world's children.* Oxford, Oxford University Press.

United Nations (1995) World population prospects: 1994 assessment. New York, United Nations.

United Nations Development Programme (1991). *Human Development Report 1991,* New York, Oxford University Press.

United Nations Development Programme (1995). *Human Development Report 1995,* New York, Oxford University Press.

van de Stadt H, Kapteyn A, van de Geer S (1985) The relativity of utility: evidence from panel data. *Review of economics and statistics,* 67(2):179–187.

Verbrugge LM, Jette AM (1994) The disablement process. *Social science and medicine,* 38(1):1–14.

Viscusi WK (1993) The value of risks to life and health. *Journal of economic literature,* 31:1912–1946.

Viscusi WK, Moore M (1989) Rates of time preference and valuations of the durations of life. *Journal of public economics,* 38:297–317.

von Neumann J, Morgenstern O (1994) *Theory of games and economic behavior,* Princeton University Press.

Wagstaff A (1991) QALYs and the equity-efficiency trade-off. *Journal of health economics,* 10:21–41.

Walzer M (1992) Moral minimalism. In: Shea WR, Spadafora A, eds. *From the twilight of probability: ethics and politics.* Canton, MA, Science History Publications.

Ware JE et al. (1981) Choosing measures of health status for individuals in general populations. *American journal of public health,* 71:620–625.

Ware JE, Sherbourne CD (1992) The MOS 36-item Short-Form Health Survey (SF-36): conceptual framework and item selection. *Medical care*, 30:473–483.

Weinstein MC (1981) Economic assessments of medical practices and technologies. *Medical decision making*, 1:309–330.

Weinstein MC (1990) Principles of cost-effective resource allocation in health care organizations. *International journal of technology assessment in health care*, 6:93–103.

Werner D (1994) *Turning health into an investment: the latest high-power assaults on third world health care.* Keynote address, Seminar of Health Communications, Xavier Institute of Communications, 25th Anniversary 17 November 1994, Mimeo.

Wilkins R, Adams O, Brancker A (1989) Changes in mortality by income in urban Canada from 1971 to 1986. *Health reports*, 1(2):137–174.

Williams A (1981) Welfare economics and health status measurement. In: van der Gaag J, Perlman M, eds. *Health, economics and health economics.* Amsterdam, North-Holland.

Wolfson AD, et al. (1982) Preference measurements for functional status in stroke patients: interrater and intertechnique comparisons. In: Kane RL, Kane RA, eds. *Values and long term care.* Lexington, MA, Lexington Books.

Wolfson MC (1994) Social proprioception: measurement, data, and information from a population health perspective. In: Evans RG, Barer ML, Marmor TR, eds. *Why are some people healthy and others not?: the determinants of health of populations,* New York.

Wood PHN (1975) *Classification of impairments and handicaps.* Geneva, World Health Organization, WHO/ICD9/REV.CONF/75.15.

World Bank (1995) *World development report 1995.* New York, Oxford University Press.

World Health Organization (1980) *International classification of impairments, disability and handicap.* Geneva, World Health Organization.

World Health Organization (1981) *Development of indicators for monitoring progress towards health for all by the year 2000.* Geneva, World Health Organization.

Ziebland S, Fitzpatrick R, Jenkinson C (1993) Tacit models of disability underlying health status instruments. *Social science and medicine*, 37(1):69–75.

APPENDIX I

PROTOCOL FOR MEASURING DISABILITY SEVERITY
WEIGHTS USING THE PERSON-TRADE-OFF METHOD

For Version 5 of the Global Burden of Disease Study, the method for deriving the disability weights and the distribution of different sequelae across the various disability classes has been elaborated. The changes have been designed to facilitate local validation of the disability weights for National Burden of Disease Studies. Disability weights for each of the hundreds of sequelae in the burden of disease study are developed in a two-step process. First, for 22 indicator conditions, a formal assessment using the person-trade-off method is undertaken. The process is designed to emphasize simultaneously consistent ordinal rankings and ratio scale valuations for each individual and group consensus. Disability weights for each of the 22 indicator conditions generated through this exercise are then used to define seven classes of disability spanning the spectrum from perfect health to death. Each class contains several of the indicator conditions, thus providing an intuitive and easily conveyed operational definition of the severity of each class. For the remaining conditions and sequelae, magnitude estimation and group consensus are used to estimate the distribution across the seven classes of disability using the conditions in each class as pegs on the scale from perfect health to near death. In this protocol, the process used to elicit preference weights for the 22 indicator conditions is described.

DESIGN OF THE 22 INDICATOR CONDITION EXERCISE

The objective of the exercise is to develop, in a short period of time, (approximately 8 hours), a set of disability weights for 22 indicator conditions that has a high degree of internal consistency and group consensus. The protocol has been developed to ensure that individuals are giving internally consistent valuations, to minimize framing effects, and to promote group consensus. Several design issues are worth emphasizing: the selection of the 22 conditions, the variant of the person-trade-off method used, distinctions between disability and handicap, and the importance of not factoring in extraneous epidemiological information.

The 22 indicator conditions have been chosen to incorporate a diverse set of conditions that capture many of the dimensions of health status including physical, mental, and social function as well as pain. The definitions of the conditions have been elaborated to minimize the variation between individual respondents in their images of the person with the condition. Examples of conditions that capture major physical disabilities include blindness, deafness, paraplegia, quadriplegia, and below-the-knee amputation. Conditions with a significant cognitive function component include mild mental retardation, Down syndrome, and dementia. Mental health problems include major depression, and active psychosis. Some conditions are included that are physical or mental disabilities with complex social overtones such as recto-vaginal fistula, infertility in those desiring a child, and erectile dysfunction. Several conditions have been included to represent the spectrum of pain including continuous pain that does not impede major functions but can be very annoying, such as severe sore throat; pain related to exertion, such as angina; intermittent pain, such as rheumatoid arthritis; and the extreme form of totally debilitating pain, represented by a continuous severe migraine headache.

A specific variant of the person-trade-off method is used. Each trade-off is framed in two ways. In the first, the participants are given a choice of trading quantity of life for healthy individuals and disabled individuals. In the second, they are asked to trade-off quantity of life for healthy individuals versus improved quality of life for a group of disabled individuals. By approaching the valuation of disability in both ways, we are able to reveal to the individual their own inconsistencies (often referred to as the framing effects).

1. Each member of the group is asked to undertake the following thought experiment. You are a decision maker that has only enough money to buy one of two mutually exclusive health interventions. If you purchase intervention A, you will extend the life of 1000 healthy individuals for exactly one year, at which point they will all die. If you do not purchase intervention A, they will all die today. The alternative use of your scarce resources is intervention B, with which you can extend the life of n individuals with a particular disabling condition for one year. If you do not buy intervention B, they will all die today; if you do purchase intervention B, they will all die at the end of exactly one year. For example, you may be faced with a choice between extending the life of (A) 1000 healthy individuals for one year, or (B) 2000 blind individuals for one year. If you prefer intervention B, the number of individuals with the disabling condition in intervention B is reduced. This process of choosing between the alternatives is continued until you reach the number of disabled individuals at which point you cannot choose between the two alternatives; at this point you are indifferent between the choices. This trade-off exercise is hereafter referred to as PTO1.

2. Each member of the group is asked to undertake a second thought experiment. You are a decision maker that has only enough money to buy one of two mutually exclusive health interventions. If you purchase intervention A, you will extend the life of 1000 healthy individuals for exactly one year, at which point they will all die. If you do not purchase intervention A, they will all die today. The alternative use of your scarce resources is intervention B, with which you can cure the disability of n individuals who will live exactly one year with or without the intervention. With the intervention they will be in perfect health; without the intervention they will continue with

the given disabling condition. For example, you may be faced with a choice between extending the life of (A) 1000 healthy individuals for one year, or (B) giving perfect vision back to 2000 blind individuals who will live for one year. If you prefer intervention B, the number of individuals with the disabling condition in intervention B is reduced. This process of choosing between the alternatives is continued until you reach the point at which you are indifferent between the choices. This exercise is hereafter referred to as PTO2.

Invariably, the individual's two assessments of the severity of disability from PTO1 and PTO2 are inconsistent with each other. To use health state preferences or disability weights in the calculation of burden or cost-effectiveness, a single disability weight for each health state is required. An important part of this protocol is to require that the individual reflect on why the two methods have generated different assessments of the severity of the same condition. The difference may reflect in part using adapted weights for PTO1 and pre-adapted weights for PTO2. Each individual is provided with a conversion table that shows the internally consistent PTO2 for a given PTO1 and vice-versa.

The protocol is a group process intended for approximately 8-12 individuals. It is designed as a group process to encourage individuals to reflect on their own reasoning for making various trade-offs and to encourage the development of group consensus. These ends are achieved by asking each individual to share with each other their PTO1 and PTO2 results after they have arrived at an internally consistent evaluations. Those with the highest and lowest evaluations are asked to explain their reasoning to the group, and an open discussion follows. Individuals are then given the opportunity to revise their assessments of PTO1 or PTO2 in private, based on the discussion.

Assessments of the severities of a given set of conditions, undertaken on a condition-by-condition basis, may not be consistent with an individual's notion of the ordinal ranking of the severity of each of the 22 conditions. To force further reflection of the PTO1 and PTO2 valuations, the protocol includes an exercise to ensure ordinal rank consistency after each of the 22 conditions has been evaluated. Each individual is asked to rank in order, from least to most severe, the 22 indicator conditions. The individual then compares this ranking with the ordering implied by his assessments of PTO1 and PTO2. If the two orderings are inconsistent, individuals are asked to revise both the ordinal rankings and their PTO1 and PTO2 estimates to produce a final ordinal and ratio scale evaluation that they are comfortable with. As a final step, these final rankings are shared with the group, and after open discussion, revisions in private are allowed.

In this exercise, the distinction between disability and handicap is somewhat blurred. In the person-trade-off valuations, individuals will factor in any considerations that they consciously or unconsciously consider important. Nevertheless, for the calculation of Disability-Adjusted Life

Years, we do not want to factor in very specific circumstances where a disability may or may not lead to handicap because of a particular social milieu. Rather, assessments should be based on average social conditions. At the global level, this tends to make the assessment closer to disability, while at the national level, the assessment will be a step closer to handicap, assuming that the variation within social conditions in a country is less than between countries in the world. Thus, vitiligo is included in the list of 22 indicator conditions. Some might argue that there is little or no disability associated with vitiligo. Yet in nearly all societies, there would be some social dysfunction associated with vitiligo on the face, albeit mild.

IMPLEMENTING THE PROTOCOL

The following series of specific steps for the basis for implementing this protocol with a group of 8-12 respondents who have knowledge of the 22 indicator conditions but do not suffer from them. We believe that it is important to have approximately equal numbers of men and women in the group. In this exercise, the role of the facilitator is critical. The activity is long and requires constant encouragement from the facilitator. With all such exercises in valuation using hypothetical scenarios, there is a very real danger that some will not take it seriously or will try to cut corners and make rapid assessments without going through the process of personal reflection required to arrive at reliable and valid assessments. It is the role of the facilitator and the group discussions to challenge individuals to search for their own valuations based on careful reflection.

1. Teaching the PTO1 and PTO2 methods. The process starts with the facilitator using blindness as the initial condition to evaluate. In public, on a marker board or equivalent, the facilitator will lead one volunteer through the exercise of finding their PTO1 for blindness. Immediately, the facilitator will lead the same individual in public through the PTO2 question for blindness. Once the two assessments have been elicited, the facilitator will lead the group through using the PTO1 and PTO2 conversion table to determine whether the two valuations are internally consistent. Invariably, they will not be consistent. The individual will then be asked to revise his or her PTO1 and PTO2 to yield an internally consistent valuation. The facilitator will then repeat the exact same sequence of events with every member of the group. This is time consuming but necessary to ensure that every member fully understands the nature of the two methods and also understands the requirement to arrive at internally consistent assessments. Once each member has generated an internally consistent estimate of PTO1 and PTO2, the results are shared with the group by writing on small marker boards their PTO1 and PTO2 results— both must be written down to discourage individuals from fixing on one or the other method in making his or her assessment. The individual with the highest PTO1 is asked to comment, followed by the

individual with the lowest PTO1. This is followed by a general group discussion. Individuals are then asked to write on their forms a revised set of PTO1 and PTO2 values.

2. For the remaining 21 conditions, each individual is asked to make their first assessments of PTO1 and PTO2 on their own. They should then use the PTO1-PTO2 conversion table to identify internal inconsistency and then choose internally consistent values for PTO1 and PTO2. These are shared with the group on the marker boards. The individual with the highest PTO1 is asked to comment, followed by the individual with the lowest PTO1. This is followed by a general group discussion. Individuals are then asked to write on their forms a revised set of PTO1 and PTO2 values.

3. On the summary sheets provided, each individual is then asked to rank each of the 22 conditions from least severe to most severe without looking back at the PTO1 and PTO2 assessments. To facilitate the ordinal ranking, a series of cards with the name of each condition should be used so that individuals can more easily change rankings. Once each individual is comfortable with his or her ordinal ranking, they are asked to go back to each of their sheets for each disease and transcribe onto the summary sheet both their PTO1 and PTO2 assessments. Based on these assessments, each individual is asked to record the ranking of the 22 indicator conditions from least to most severe. In most cases, the ordinal ranking based solely at looking at the 22 conditions and that implied by the PTO1 and PTO2 results will not be identical. The participants are then asked to revise their ordinal rankings and PTO1 and PTO2 assessments to produce an internally consistent set with which they are comfortable. As a final step, these rankings are shared with the group, followed by group discussion. At this point, the facilitator will want to draw attention to major differences between participants and prompt discussion of the reasons for varying evaluations. After discussion, individuals are given a final opportunity to revise their ordinal ranks and PTO1 and PTO2 results.

DESCRIPTIONS OF INDICATOR CONDITIONS

1. *Blindness*—maximum visual acuity with the best possible correction is less than 3/60. (A person is unable to distinguish the fingers of a hand at the distance of 3 metres, or, has less than 5 per cent of remaining vision as compared to a normally sighted individual.).

2. *Severe sore throat*—while artificial for this exercise, one must imagine an individual having a continuous severe sore throat for one year.

3. *Active psychosis*—an individual with paranoid delusions, auditory hallucinations and disorganized speech.

4. *Infertility*—in someone who desires a child. Given that the PTO1 and PTO2 questions use a single year as the period of life extension or disability cure, you must try and imagine that the infertile individual would in fact have the opportunity to conceive and deliver in the time period.

5. *Paraplegia*—with a rudimentary wheelchair. Associated complications may be factored in, for example, decubitus ulcers and frequent urinary tract infections.

6. *Fracture of radius in a stiff cast*—the cast extends above the elbow, the finger tips are free and the arm affected is the writing arm.

7. *Mild mental retardation* (IQ level between 55 and 70)—people with this level of mental retardation typically develop social and communication skills during the pre-school years (ages 0–5), have minimal impairment in sensorimotor areas, and often are not distinguishable from children without mental retardation until a later age. By their late teens, they can acquire academic skills up to approximately the sixth-grade level. During their adult years, they usually achieve social and vocational skills adequate for minimum self-support, but may need supervision, guidance, and assistance, especially when under unusual social or economic stress.

8. *Down syndrome without cardiac malformation*—Down syndrome has a spectrum of severity, so for the purpose of this evaluation consider the average individual with Down syndrome.

9. *Dementia*—an individual with multiple cognitive deficits that include memory impairment and aphasia (difficulty producing the names of individuals and objects) and apraxia (impaired ability to execute motor activities despite intact motor abilities, sensory function, and comprehension of the required task).

10. *Below-the-knee amputation*—in an individual without a prosthesis but with the basic aids, such as crude crutches, that are available in all societies.

11. *Severe anaemia*—for this assessment imagine an individual exactly at the cutoff of severe anaemia which for pregnant women and children is a haemoglobin equal to 7mmol/l, for adult women a haemoglobin equal to 8mmol/l, and for adult men a haemoglobin equal to 9mmol/l.

12. *Quadriplegia*—with a rudimentary wheelchair. Associated complications may be factored in, for example, decubitus ulcers and frequent urinary tract infections.

13. *Unipolar major depression*—the loss of interest or pleasure in nearly all activities. The depressed individual has change in appetite or weight, sleep, and psychomotor activity; decreased energy; feeling of

worthlessness or guilt; difficulty thinking, concentrating, or making decisions.

14. *Severe migraine*—imagine a person with a continuous severe migraine for one year. This individual would effectively be bed-ridden and unable to undertake any organized physical or mental activity. This condition is intended to be the proxy indicator condition for severe pain.

15. *Deafness*—an adult whose average hearing threshold level for pure tone stimuli of 500, 1000, and 2000 hertz with reference to ISO is less than 70 dB. Shouting at a close distance can be heard as sound but the words cannot be distinguished. The individual acquired deafness as an adult.

16. *Recto-vaginal fistula*—part of the assessment includes the social dysfunction brought about because of the women leaking faeces through her vagina and the associated odour which is difficult to mask.

17. *Watery diarrhoea*—five episodes a day without major pain or cramps.

18. *2 standard deviation below weight/height*—for your assessment assume the individual has a weight for height exactly 2 standard deviations below the US National Center for Health Statistics reference population mean weight for height.

19. *Rheumatoid arthritis*—the individual has rheumatoid arthritis afflicting the interphalangeal, metacarpophalangeal and wrist joints. The individual has morning stiffness and pain, which largely subsides by the afternoon, and has deformity of the metocarpophalangeal joints.

20. *Vitiligo on face*—the individual has 10 percent of the face afflicted, and this condition is evident at a distance.

21. *Erectile dysfunction*—the individual is unable to have an erection but is not infertile.

22. *Angina*—the individual has reproducible chest pain when walking 50 metres or more. On a subjective scale from 0 to 10, where 10 is the worst pain they have ever experienced, they would rate the pain as a 5. When assessing the severity of this exertional pain, *do not* take into consideration your clinical judgment that someone with this degree of angina may have an increased risk of death.

Appendix Table 1 Conversion table between PTO1 and PTO2

PTO1	PTO2	PTO1	PTO2	PTO1	PTO2
1 001	1 001 000	1 180	6 556	3 300	1 435
1 002	501 000	1 190	6 263	3 400	1 417
1 003	334 333	1 200	6 000	3 500	1 400
1 004	251 000	1 210	5 762	3 600	1 385
1 005	201 000	1 220	5 545	3 700	1 370
1 006	167 667	1 230	5 348	3 800	1 357
1 007	143 857	1 240	5 167	3 900	1 345
1 008	126 000	1 250	5 000	4 000	1 333
1 009	112 111	1 300	4 333	4 100	1 323
1 010	101 000	1 350	3 857	4 200	1 313
1 011	91 909	1 400	3 500	4 300	1 303
1 012	84 333	1 450	3 222	4 400	1 294
1 013	77 923	1 500	3 000	4 500	1 286
1 014	72 429	1 550	2 818	4 600	1 278
1 015	67 667	1 600	2 667	4 700	1 270
1 016	63 500	1 650	2 538	4 800	1 263
1 017	59 824	1 700	2 429	4 900	1 256
1 018	56 556	1 750	2 333	5 000	1 250
1 019	53 632	1 800	2 250	5 500	1 222
1 020	51 000	1 850	2 176	6 000	1 200
1 021	48 619	1 900	2 111	6 500	1 182
1 022	46 455	1 950	2 053	7 000	1 167
1 023	44 478	2 000	2 000	7 500	1 154
1 024	42 667	2 050	1 952	8 000	1 143
1 025	41 000	2 100	1 909	8 500	1 133
1 030	34 333	2 150	1 870	9 000	1 125
1 040	26 000	2 200	1 833	9 500	1 118
1 050	21 000	2 250	1 800	10 000	1 111
1 060	17 667	2 300	1 769	11 000	1 100
1 070	15 286	2 350	1 741	12 000	1 091
1 080	13 500	2 400	1 714	13 000	1 083
1 090	12 111	2 450	1 690	14 000	1 077
1 100	11 000	2 500	1 667	15 000	1 071
1 110	10 091	2 600	1 625	16 000	1 067
1 120	9 333	2 700	1 588	17 000	1 063
1 130	8 692	2 800	1 556	18 000	1 059
1 140	8 143	2 900	1 526	19 000	1 056
1 150	7 667	3 000	1 500	20 000	1 053
1 160	7 250	3 100	1 476	21 000	1 050
1 170	6 882	3 200	1 455	22 000	1 048

Appendix Table 1 (continued)

PTO1	PTO2	PTO1	PTO2	PTO1	PTO2
23 000	1 045	60 000	1 017	150 000	1 007
24 000	1 043	65 000	1 016	200 000	1 005
25 000	1 042	70 000	1 014	250 000	1 004
30 000	1 034	75 000	1 014	300 000	1 003
35 000	1 029	80 000	1 013	350 000	1 003
40 000	1 026	85 000	1 012	400 000	1 003
45 000	1 023	90 000	1 011	450 000	1 002
50 000	1 020	95 000	1 011	500 000	1 002
55 000	1 019	100 000	1 010	1 000 000	1 001

Note: the value of PT02 should be consistent with the value of PT01 on the same row, so that, for example, if PT02 is 5000 one would be indifferent between intervention A and an intervention B through which the life of 1250 disabled individuals could be extended for exactly one year.

Mathematical formulations: $$PTO2 = \frac{1000}{1 - \dfrac{1000}{PTO1}}$$

CHAPTER 2

NON-FATAL HEALTH OUTCOMES: CONCEPTS, INSTRUMENTS AND INDICATORS

A. GOERDT, J. P. KOPLAN, J. M. ROBINE,
M. C. THURIAUX, J. K. VAN GINNEKEN

Concern with the human and financial consequences of disease has increased over the past three decades as the ageing of populations has led to a greater prevalence of disability in developed countries and spiralling health care costs have made it difficult to meet the increasing needs for services. Traditional analyses based on mortality and morbidity are inadequate to assess the situation in which people who are not ill are limited in their abilities to function in a manner considered to be normal. The definition of health according to the World Health Organization, i.e. "a state of complete physical, mental and social well-being and not merely the absence of disease or infirmity" (World Health Organization 1996), provides a basis for the broad perspective needed to analyse the situation. Other definitions, concepts and methods have been developed to assess the health status of individuals, communities and nations. This work has been carried out by individuals from a variety of disciplines, including health care professionals, social scientists and economists. During the past two decades in particular, new health indicators have been developed for the analysis of the consequences of disease.

The development of Disability-Adjusted Life Years (DALYs) as an indicator for the consequences of specific diseases on a global and national level is the latest addition to a process of developing concepts and methodologies for the assessment of health status. This new measure has been applied to the estimation of both disability and mortality from over 100 diseases in all regions of the world. As a perspective on DALYs, this chapter provides an overview of several major themes that have dominated the extensive literature on the measurement of non-fatal health outcomes. While important issues are reviewed, no attempt is made to provide a consensus framework. Rather, this chapter highlights the diversity of available conceptual approaches, measurement methods, indicator designs and applications.

The chapter is divided into three sections. First, the main conceptual frameworks used by various investigators are reviewed. Second, issues in the measurement of the incidence and prevalence of different health states, and the preferences individuals have for spending time in these states, are discussed. Third, the evolution and computation of various indicators are reviewed with a focus on Disability-Free Life Expectancy (DFLE) and Quality-Adjusted Life Years (QALYs). Research and policy uses of these indicators are also explored.

CONCEPTUAL FRAMEWORKS AND CLASSIFICATION SYSTEMS

Most measures of non-fatal health outcomes can be traced to a particular conceptualization of health. While the WHO definition of health is broad and all encompassing, there has been considerable effort to conceptualize the notion of non-fatal health outcomes over the last two decades. In the following sub-sections, three important conceptual frameworks are discussed: the *International Classification of Impairments, Disabilities and Handicaps,* the health-related quality-of-life approach, and the utilitarian framework underlying most work on health economics.

International Classification of Impairments, Disabilities and Handicaps (ICIDH)

The ICIDH (World Health Organization 1980) was developed in response to the need for a framework to describe the consequences of disease. It classifies three dimensions of the consequences of disease: impairment, disability and handicap.

- An *impairment* is any loss or abnormality of psychological, physiological or anatomical structure or function.

- A *disability* is any restriction or lack (resulting from an impairment) of ability to perform an activity in the manner or within the range considered normal for a human being.

- A *handicap* is a disadvantage for a given individual resulting from an impairment or a disability that limits or prevents the fulfilment of a role that is normal (depending on age, sex and social and cultural factors) for that individual.

The sequence, which is not necessarily unidirectional, is defined as follows (see Figure 2.1):

- exteriorization of symptoms and signs through awareness of these manifestations (**impairments**)—at the organ level;

- objective alteration of behaviour or performance (**disabilities**)—at the level of the individual;

- interaction with society, resulting in disadvantages (**handicaps**)—at the level of environmental and social interaction.

The ICIDH already exists in fourteen languages while other translations are in preparation. It has been used in developed and developing countries

Figure 2.1   Schema for assessing non-fatal health outcomes

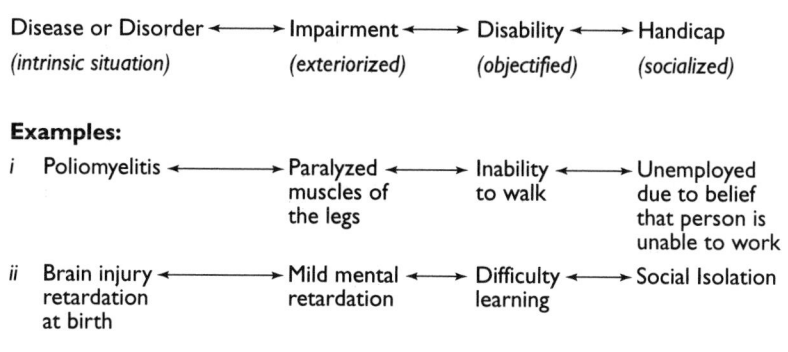

Disease or Disorder ←——→ Impairment ←——→ Disability ←——→ Handicap

(intrinsic situation)   *(exteriorized)*   *(objectified)*   *(socialized)*

Examples:

i   Poliomyelitis ←————→ Paralyzed ←——→ Inability ←——→ Unemployed
                          muscles of   to walk   due to belief
                          the legs   that person is
                                                              unable to work

ii Brain injury ←————→ Mild mental ←——→ Difficulty ←——→ Social Isolation
    retardation   retardation   learning
    at birth

as a conceptual framework (Minaire 1992) applicable to personal health care, the mitigation of environmental and societal barriers (Minaire et al. 1989), and the study of health care systems in terms of evaluation and policy formulation (Fougeyrollas 1990). Applications cover activities in social security (*Nomenclature des déficiences, incapacités, et désavantages* 1988), the design of population surveys at local, national and international levels (Bezzaoucha and Dekkar 1990, Chamie 1989, Gomez-Rodriguez 1989), and areas such as the assessment of working capacities (Schian 1991), demography (Robine 1989), and community needs assessment (Minaire et al. 1989). Although the ICIDH is primarily a health-related classification, it reflects a broad spectrum of applications and uses.

The ICIDH belongs to the "family of classifications" developed by WHO and centred around the *International Classification of Diseases* (ICD) (World Health Organization 1993a). The tenth revision of the ICD, published in 1992, includes changes which will be taken into account in the revised version of the ICIDH (ICIDH-2), scheduled for publication in 1999.

The ICIDH concept of *impairment* is used in the assessment of the health status of individuals for purposes of prevention and treatment in health care services, and in screening, as well as in survey and census questions. *Disability* is used in rehabilitation services as well as by policy makers and planners in both the rehabilitation and the social integration of people with disabilities. There is also an interest in focusing census and survey questions on disability-based rather than impairment-based data (Chamie 1989). It is regarding the need for a better clarification by the ICIDH of the role of the social and physical environment in the development of *handicap* that discussion has been most active.

The ICIDH has served as a guide for assessment, planning and policy formulation related to community; it has underpinned national-level policies and practices which affect equal opportunities and social integration of people with disabilities. The combination of the three concepts has, in general, raised awareness about issues which have been of concern to people with disabilities, service providers, community leaders and policy makers.

The current model of the consequences of disease is effective in distinguishing between impairments, disabilities and handicaps as separate concepts, but does not always provide adequate information on the relationship between these concepts. In particular, the arrows linking disease or disorder, impairment, disability and handicap have occasionally been interpreted as representing a causal model and unidirectional change over time. The original text of the ICIDH states that the situation is more complex than a simple linear progression; this statement needs to be made more strongly—the arrows in Figure 2.1 must be understood as meaning no more than "may lead to." Graphic representations of the ICIDH framework must also better reflect the role of the social and physical environment in the handicap process.

Classifications of environmental factors may prove useful in the analysis of situations and in the development of solutions at the national level, but it is unlikely that a universally acceptable classification of these determinant factors is achievable at present. This is because, even though they are major components of the handicap process, environmental factors are also strongly culture-bound; thus they should not be developed as an additional classification scheme within ICIDH.

Health-Related Quality of Life

The second major conceptual framework for non-fatal health outcomes falls under the rubric health-related quality of life. Following the description of Patrick and Erickson (1993), health-related quality of life (HRQL) includes at least four broad concepts: opportunity, health perceptions, functional status, and impairment. Unfortunately, the same vocabulary as in the ICIDH is used in different ways in the HRQL field. Within each of these concepts various domains have been identified. For example, the domains of social or cultural disadvantage and resilience are within opportunity. Within health perceptions, some authors include general health perceptions and satisfaction with health. Functional status can include the domains of social function, psychological function and physical function. Each of these three domains can in turn be sub-divided into domains such as affect, integration, contact, intimacy and fitness. Impairment includes domains such as symptoms, signs, tissue alterations or diagnoses.

There is some conceptual confusion, which arises from the fact that different investigators started to develop instruments independently of each other and without coordination. The first instruments were developed by clinicians and clinical psychologists and focused on the measurement of quality of life after various therapies. Later, several of these instruments were adapted by epidemiologists, psychologists and sociologists for use in cross-sectional surveys of the general population.

While an entire chapter could be devoted to distinctions among the various concepts and domains and to differentiating the conceptual approach of HRQL from that in the ICIDH, we will focus on some general differences. There is no one overreaching conceptualization of HRQL. Instruments used to measure HRQL have a multidimensional approach. At a minimum, most would agree that the domains of physical functioning, psychological well-being, social and role functioning, and health perceptions should be included (Ware 1987). Some conceptions of HRQL (Patrick and Bergner 1990) include the additional domains of opportunities and resources to pursue and achieve life goals, which have particular relevance to persons with disabilities. Because HRQL contains a phenomenological component, that is, individual values and expectations regarding health, it is recognized as including both objective and subjective measures of functional status and well-being (Kaplan and Anderson 1990). Finally, HRQL may also be defined at the level of the community, to include factors such as public policy and health resources (Flynn 1992).

Unlike the ICIDH, where the distinction between disability and handicap lies in the consequences for the individual given the environmental conditions and social response, the HRQL approach does not draw such a sharp distinction. Rather the impact on the individual is one out of many domains making up HRQL. Furthermore, a clear distinction is not made between living in a particular health state and the valuation of time spent in the health state. Some domains, such as satisfaction with health, are obviously a mixture of perceived health status and the valuation of that health status by the individual. Notably, no overarching conceptual framework that provides an ordered relationship between concepts and domains is available in the HRQL literature.

Utilitarian Perspective

Most health economics research on non-fatal health outcomes has as its conceptual basis a utilitarian model. In this theory, non-fatal health outcomes matter only in as much as they alter the individual's utility. In the most widely used form, utility in modern economics is taken to be synonymous with the satisfaction of individual preferences. One can then use the terminology of utilities or preferences for different health states somewhat interchangeably.

Some authors such as Torrance et al. (1972) have developed an approach in which health states between perfect health and death are weighted by the utility to the individual of time spent in each of these states. Such a concept was formulated in order to select health interventions; those that maximized utility-weighted time lived by individuals for a given expense were the most desirable. Zeckhauser and Shephard (1976) were the first to label such a measure of utility or preference-weighted time as Quality-Adjusted Life Years. The Quality-Adjusted Life Year (QALY) measures the equivalent number of years of full health that a series of years lived in some state other than health represent, according to individual's expressed preferences. Because individual preferences are measured directly, the definition and measurement of particular health states is seen as less critical. As long as the individual evaluating the utility of each health state has sufficient information to predict his or her preference for time spent in that state, the approach should in theory work. Not surprisingly, the focus of research in this area is on the measurement of preferences rather than on the conceptualization or measurement of the characteristics of health that individuals value. As such, the utilitarian approach lies closest to the ICIDH concept of handicap.

MEASURING HEALTH STATES AND PREFERENCES FOR HEALTH STATES

For the purposes of organizing the wide array of material on the measurement of non-fatal health outcomes, we have somewhat arbitrarily divided this into two components: measurement of incidence and prevalence of different health states and measurement of preferences for time spent in different health states. Some measures in the HRQL field, such as level of satisfaction with health, are a mixture of both, but for the majority of instruments this distinction is useful. We also note the work that has been done to determine the prevalence of disability within a population.

MEASURING HEALTH STATES
Observed Versus Self-Reported Measures

Instruments to measure the incidence or prevalence of different health states can be divided into self-reported measures and observed measures. Murray and Chen (1992) divide health states into three types: those that can be only be perceived by the individual, such as pain, those that can be only perceived by an observer, such as many cognitive or affective disorders, and those that can be perceived by both the individual and an observer, such as blindness or loss of a limb. Clearly, the first and second categories imply that to measure all health states one must use a combination of self-reports and observations.

For those states that can be observed and self-perceived, one can study the divergence between observations and self-reports of self-perceptions. In many cases, investigators have found dramatic differences between self-reports and observations of diseases, impairments and disabilities (Murray and Chen 1992, Murray et al. 1992). In Ghana, for example, in a study of self-reported morbidity versus clinical diagnosis, only six per cent of the individuals with missing extremities reported their condition (Belcher et al. 1976). In Cote d'Ivoire, the rich reported more episodes of illness and more days of disability than the poor (Murray et al. 1992).

The explanations for the divergence between self-reports and observations are complex (Murray and Chen 1992, Johannesson 1992). One might expect an individual's perceptions of health status to be made with respect to some norm or expectation of health. The disadvantaged in a community with poor health status may well have such diminished expectations of health, that health states other than perfect health go unrecognized. Increasing income, education, exposure to health services and changing social expectations of health may all play an important role in altering health perceptions. Such factors may explain why the better educated report more illness and more days of incapacity in developing countries than the poor do.

Considerable research will need to be undertaken to fully understand the determinants of the difference between self-reported and observed measures of health status. When discussing this distinction, however, it is critical to recognize that the individual's valuations of time spent in different health states when fully informed about the range of possible health states for their age and sex can only be reported, never observed.

Instruments to Measure the Incidence or Prevalence of Health States

To date, the richest source of instruments for measuring the incidence or prevalence of health states in the community has come from the HRQL field. Most of the research on HRQL has been conducted in conjunction with clinical trials focused on measuring the impact of medical interventions on patient well-being. Instrumentation for HRQL assessment for specific diseases has been developed, particularly in the areas of cancer, cardiovascular, rheumatic, and chronic pulmonary diseases (Nissinen and Wahl 1992). Such instruments typically include symptom-related items, for example, on pain and fatigue, in addition to questions on functional status, psychological state, and performance of normal activities.

Several generic instruments have been designed to provide a profile of health status relevant to quality of life (QOL). These instruments comprehensively measure function, disability and distress, and some compile item scores into a summary index (Guyatt and Jaeschke 1990). Among such tools are the Sickness Impact Profile (SIP), the Nottingham Health Profile, the McMaster Health Index Questionnaire, and the Rand Medical Outcomes Study (MOS) Health Survey. The Sickness Impact Profile, for example, is comprised of 136 items within five independent categories and two dimensions (physical and psychosocial functioning). These domains include items covering twelve areas of behaviour, such as work, home management, mobility, body care and movement, and communication, for which separate sub-scores may be obtained. One of the best known of the disability scales in this category is the Activities of Daily Living (ADL) Index developed by Katz and colleagues (Katz et al. 1963). Although originally developed for clinical purposes, it is frequently adapted and applied in cross-sectional surveys in the general population, particularly among the elderly. Some of these instruments have been tested for reliability and validity.

Another type of instrument consists of a series of questions on various aspects of health which provide the opportunity to rank individuals above or below an average score. This has been called the "thermometer" approach as described by Dohrenwend and Dohrenwend (1982). These instruments have had little or no testing for reliability and validity. One other instrument which may be used consists of a single question concerning the individual's overall quality of life.

The majority of existing QOL instruments has been developed within the Anglo-American context (Bullinger and Hasford 1991), and, although a number of QOL instruments, including the Sickness Impact Profile and the Nottingham Health Profile, have been translated from English into other languages, their validity for other cultures remains to be established.

The World Health Organization has developed a generic Quality of Life measure, the WHOQOL (World Health Organization 1993). This provides an assessment in six broad domains: physical, psychological, environmental, spiritual, level of independence, and social relationships. These have been developed by simultaneous work in fifteen centres around the world, involving twelve languages. Although English was the working language of the group, the questions were developed in all twelve languages and pooled together for extensive pilot and field testing, resulting in a 100 item instrument, which is under field testing.

Regional and local surveillance of QOL is conducted in the Netherlands, for example, as part of the Healthy Cities Project, and in Canada through the Ontario Health Survey (Garretsen et al. 1991). In the United States, data on self-perceived health, recent limitations in physical and/or mental health, and recent disability days, are now collected annually by 48 States through the Behavioral Risk Factor Surveillance System (BRFSS) (Hennessy et al. 1993). The BRFSS uses telephone surveys of the adult population to provide state-level prevalence information that can direct public health programme priorities, including interventions related to disabilities.

In less developed countries (LDCs), few cross-sectional sample surveys dealing with aspects of self-perceived health in the general population or in major age groups have been carried out. With respect to children under the age of 5, the Demographic and Health Surveys can be mentioned; they are limited to certain diseases only (but have information on nutritional status). The evidence with respect to adults has been summarized by Murray et al. (1992). In so far as data are available, they are limited to the approach dealing with illness, conditions and symptoms. Surveys dealing with consequences of diseases in general and with health-related quality of life in particular have rarely been done. It will not be easy to conduct such surveys in LDCs because a considerable amount of illness takes place in children below the age of 5 and instruments which adequately measure the consequences of diseases in this population group do not exist. In addition, the existing instruments for adult populations can only be applied in LDCs after adjustments have been made and after validation.

At present, routine surveillance of QOL among persons with physical and mental impairments is limited, despite the increasing importance of disability data for health resource allocation and intervention planning and evaluation (Centers for Disease Control 1991). In the United States, for example, some QOL data are collected annually through the National Health Interview Survey (NHIS) conducted by the National Center for Health Statistics, Centers for Disease Control and Prevention. The NHIS includes items on physical health impairments, activity limitations, and self-perceived health. However, the survey does not currently provide information on other major disabling conditions such as mental health impairments.

Measures of health resources and opportunities have been relatively peripheral in QOL research, but these domains assume heightened importance for persons with disabilities, and instruments should elaborate on these disadvantage risk factors, such as unmet needs for rehabilitation or support services. Community-level measures of QOL, moreover, would permit an assessment of the extent to which community environments are supportive of the needs of persons with disabilities.

The value of assessing QOL as an indicator of needs and outcomes related to the burden of disease enjoys a broad consensus. A growing body of instrumentation for measuring QOL has developed, primarily in the area of chronic diseases. To date, however, no single one of these tools has emerged as a "gold standard." Thus, researchers and clinicians using existing instruments to evaluate QOL for persons with disabilities need to select tools to match their particular purposes. These choices should be guided by an awareness of the desired features and limitations of these measurement systems as discussed above. In addition, work needs to be done to further refine and elaborate existing instruments to capture important QOL consequences of disability, such as self-perception of autonomy.

Measuring Preferences for Time Spent in Different Health States

Because there is no market for health, and individuals cannot buy and sell health states like cars or televisions, indirect methods have been developed by health economists to elicit from individuals their valuation of different health states. These indirect methods are largely based on asking individuals a series of questions. Five types of methods have been used: rating scales, standard gambles, time trade-offs, person trade-offs and magnitude estimation techniques (Nord 1992, Froberg and Kane 1989). In all of these methods, individuals are asked to compare a given health state with another, usually either perfect health or death. In the trade-off methods, the comparison is repeatedly changed until individuals are indifferent *vis-à-vis* two options.

At least four different groups can be asked these five types of preference questions. One gets different responses if the general public, health care providers, individuals living in particular health states or these individuals' family members are surveyed. While only few such studies have been conducted, the general pattern is that health-care providers rate health states as worse than the general public, who in turn rate them worse than those living in the particular health states. It remains quite controversial who is the most appropriate group to derive utility weights to be used in the construction of indicators such as quality-adjusted life years. For example, some members of the disabled community believe that normative values assigned to health states by persons without disabilities may lack validity for those whose health and functioning is not likely to improve significantly. On the other hand, using utilities derived from surveying those living in a particular state of ill-health may underrate the importance of preventing these conditions.

This consistent difference in *ex ante* and *ex post* valuation may be a reflection of the process of adaptation so that with time an individual's utility from living in a health state other than perfect health improves as the individual copes with the new situation. The impact of coping on health state utilities is a priority for future research in this area.

Measurement of Disability Prevalence

In addition to measuring the prevalence of health states, there has been a growing interest in determining the prevalence of disability through censuses and surveys to obtain data for policy formulation and programme planning. The Statistical Division of the United Nations Department of Social and Economic Development (UNSTAT) has established a Disability Statistics Data Base (DISTAT), which has documented data on the prevalence of impairments and disabilities in over 90 countries. The *Disability Statistics Compendium* (United Nations 1990) presents these data from 55 countries, some of which include information on causes of disabilities; social, economic and environmental characteristics; and on the availability and use of support services.

DISTAT uses the ICIDH as a framework for the presentation of data from countries, so that data submitted are categorized as impairment, disability or handicap. In the *Compendium*, this revealed that survey or census questions which identify impairments will lead to lower reported rates than questions which identify disabilities. Among the 55 countries, impairment rates varied from 0.2 per cent to approximately 6 per cent, while disability rates varied from approximately 7 per cent to 20.9 per cent. The use of the ICIDH in DISTAT has raised awareness in countries about the importance of using the concepts and definitions of impairment and disability and also about the advantages of identifying disability rather than impairments.

Member States of the World Health Organization have included information on the prevalence of disability in their monitoring and evaluation of progress towards Health for All (World Health Organization 1985, 1993b), at both regional and global levels. At the global level, only a few Member States in each Region provided answers according to the proposed format, which asked for data on disabilities. A similar format was also developed jointly by UNICEF, UNSTAT, and WHO for the monitoring of Child Summit goals and objectives.

Screening strategies in censuses and surveys influence the results in a number of ways. Estimates vary widely, primarily because they are sensitive to specific survey conditions, but also because of variations in chronic and infectious disease patterns, in life expectancy, in the age-structure of populations, in nutritional status, in rates of exposure to environmental, occupational and traffic hazards, and in public health practices. When comparing disability rates within national data sets according to age or to residence, for example, the relationships between disability and other demographic and socio-economic variables are reasonably consistent, even though the magnitude of the relationships may vary from one survey to another. Presentations may be used to highlight the relationship between disability and related characteristics (age, geographical residence, educational attainment, school attendance, labour force participation and employment opportunities, marital status and family formation, living arrangements). In addition, surveys have made it possible to identify causes of impairment or reasons for disability and special aids used.

There is a great need for improved measurement of the prevalence of disability, but it is also necessary to go beyond the counting of disabilities towards the development of indicators that can be used for an assessment of changes in disability at community and national levels.

CONSTRUCTION OF INDICATORS OF NON-FATAL HEALTH OUTCOMES

Given information on the incidence or prevalence of different health states and valuations of time spent in these health states, a wide variety of indicators could be constructed. These indicators can be distinguished by three important aspects: the level of analysis, their intended use, and the use of information on preferences for different health states (see Table 2.1).

First, indicators of non-fatal health outcomes can be used at the individual level or the population level. Measures such as quality-adjusted life years have primarily been used at the individual level. Other indicators

Table 2.1   Indicators of non-fatal health outcomes

Indicator	Level of analysis	Intended use	Use of information on preference for different health states
QALY	Individual	Assessment, planning for interventions; Research	Weights selected by individuals
DFLE*, IFLE*, HFLE*	Population	Comparisons, research; Regional and national planning	Assigned weights implied
DALY	Individual and Population	Comparisons, research; Regional and national planning	Assigned weights stated

* Disability, impairment and handicap-free life expectancy, respectively.

such as disability-free life expectancy can only be used at the population level. Disability-adjusted life years as discussed in Chapter 1 in this volume (Murray 1996), are unusual in that the measure has been used both at the individual level in cost-effectiveness studies and at the population level as an indicator of the burden of disease.

Second, indicators can be used for many purposes. In specific health care settings, indicators of individual performance can be useful for choosing interventions such as rehabilitation strategies or for evaluating progress towards certain treatment goals. Population indicators such as disability-free life expectancy or impairment-free life expectancy may be used primarily for purposes of comparison or research. Frequently, comparisons between communities or within a community over time are required, and such population indicators may be extremely useful. Another critical use of such indicators lies in the identification of priorities for public health action. Such applications require indicators that can be used at the individual level for cost-effectiveness analysis of interventions, and at the population level to evaluate the importance of different problems in contributing to non-fatal health outcomes.

Third, various indicators differ in their use of information on the valuation of health states by individuals. Quality-adjusted life years, health-adjusted life expectancies and disability-adjusted life years all make use of weights to reflect the utility of time spent in different health states. Other indicators such as impairment-free life expectancy, disability-free life expectancy and handicap-free life expectancy claim to not incorporate information on the utility of time spent in different health states (Robine et al. 1992, Robine and Mathers 1993). However, it can be argued that these indicators implicitly incorporate weights. The normal practice in calculating disability-free life expectancy is to count only moderate to severe disabilities and to ignore mild disabilities. This is equivalent to using a weight of zero for the mild disabilities and a weight of one for moderate and severe disabilities. Thus, these indicators incorporate weights which are not based on the values expressed by the individuals themselves but are arbitrary and constrained to be zero or one.

Because disability-free life expectancy is now in wide use, it is useful to briefly review the history of this indicator and its calculation since it is now being applied by a number of countries. In the mid-1970s, the growth in life expectancy at birth in the more developed countries was felt to have virtually ended, according to the mortality hypotheses used for population projections. The sustained and continuous increase in life expectancy over the last two decades was totally unexpected. The decline in mortality among the very old in Western countries was particularly surprising. As a result, there was concern about whether people who survive heart disease, for example, do so only to live in poor health.

The principle of the calculation of disability-free life expectancy was postulated as early as 1964 (Sanders 1964) and a first method of calculation was proposed in 1971 (Sullivan 1971). Sullivan's method is very simple and has been reviewed by many authors (e.g. Robine 1989). The years lived at various ages by the population of a life table are qualified on the basis of the institutionalization rate (generally from a recent census) and the prevalence of permanent and temporary limitation of activity (from national health or disability surveys). Once the table is modified, the period life expectancy is calculated in the traditional manner, according to various states of functional disability, yielding the value of *disability-free life expectancy*. In 1973, it was proposed that a weight be introduced in the calculation in order to obtain a single value, the weighted life expectancy (Berg 1973) or the value-adjusted life expectancy (Bush et al. 1973), which should make it possible to measure the social value of future gains in life expectancy (Robine 1992).

There exist essentially three different methods of calculation of health expectancies: (i) Sullivan's method; (ii) the double decrement life table method; and (iii) the multi-state life table method.

The main advantage of Sullivan's method lies in the separate treatment of mortality and disability data and in the availability of the data necessary for the calculation. Basic cross-sectional surveys are sufficient to collect the observed prevalence of disability within the population. However the indicator obtained is not really a period indicator. The problem with this method is that it approximates the period prevalence by the observed prevalence of disability.

The double decrement life table method is based on the observation, during the study period, of the occurrence of two events corresponding to the two possible outcomes: mortality and disability. The simplified method used by Katz et al. (1983) results from using the probabilities of survival without disability, directly observed at the end of the study period. This implies that the two studied outcomes are irreversible. The advantage of this method is that it provides a *period indicator* based on data that are not too difficult to collect. The main drawback of the method lies, as for the following method, in the joint collection of mortality and disability data; the accuracy of mortality data depends on the size and representativeness of the study sample.

The multi-state life table method has been proposed by Rogers et al. (1989) in order to take into account *the recovery of lost functions* and the return to a state of good health. The advantage of this method is that it provides a period indicator that takes into account the *reversibility of disability*. The specific drawback of the multi-state life table method arises from the scarceness of adequate data. Data requirements for multi-state methods are considerable and there are very few countries where national data are available or likely to be available for some time (Robine et al. 1992).

As of the early 1990s, a first calculation of health expectancy has been carried out for more than 30 countries (REVES 1993), mainly using Sullivan's method. The limits of this method are increasingly well understood. Simulations provide a better means of assessing its imprecision

(Robine and Mathers 1993). In order to improve data collection to facilitate the application of the method, REVES (the International Network on Health Expectancy and Disability) has proposed the inclusion of a retrospective question on health status into cross-sectional health surveys, one or two years prior to the survey, in order to obtain information about flows into and out of health states (Robine et al. 1992). This would allow one to combine the advantages of Sullivan's method with those of the multi-state method.

Summary

This chapter has reviewed the concepts, methods and indicators which have been developed to analyse health states and non-fatal outcomes at the individual and population levels. The review highlights the diversity of approaches, but does not lead to a conclusion regarding the likelihood of reaching a universally applicable approach to assessing health outcomes.

Clinicians in medical, psychiatric and rehabilitation services, as well as social scientists have used the concepts of the ICIDH and HRQL to assess individuals and to determine the health status of populations, as a basis for programme planning and for policy formulation. Although the ICIDH and HRQL both address health states with reference to different levels, i.e. the organ, the person and the society, the categories and definitions of the two approaches are different. Health economists have applied a utilitarian approach to assess the cost-effectiveness of interventions relevant to survival time and quality of life. The utilitarian approach considers the health states that are preferred, whether by the individual, the family, the health care provider or the general public. The preference rather than the health state itself is measured.

The number and type of instruments used to measure health states vary a great deal depending on the concept applied and the domains addressed. The instruments may vary from a single question focused on quality of life, or functional limitations, to a lengthy questionnaire ranging from specific personal limitations to societal barriers. The instruments used to measure preferences also vary although they can be categorized as rating scales, standard gambles, time trade-offs and person trade-offs. Census and survey questions are used to determine disability rates at community and national levels.

The QALY, and particularly the DFLE, are the indicators which are the focus of this chapter. Both attempt to determine the period of time people may live with limited functions. QALYs can measure health gained from a health intervention and are based on the combination of survival time and the health-related quality of life for that period. QALYs are used at the individual level. DFLE, which is used for populations, is a measure based on a combination of mortality and disability data. The empirical applicaton of both indicators lacks precision because of inadequate data.

Chapter 1 in this volume (Murray 1996) introduces the concept of disability-adjusted life years (DALYs), an indicator which is another step in the development of measures of non-fatal health outcomes and premature mortality. DALYs are an indicator for assessing the consequences of specific diseases at national and global levels, though they can be applied at the individual level as well. The differences with previous indicators include different value choices for the duration of life lost, the value of life lived at different ages, comparison of time lived with a disability with the time lost due to mortality, and time preference. In addition, DALYs include the time lived with a disability, so that disability which does not cause premature death is considered. Like other indicators, the data available for calculating DALYs are not yet adequate, particularly with regard to the disabling sequelae of diseases and injuries.

REFERENCES

Belcher DW et al. (1976) Comparison of morbidity interviews with a health examination survey in rural Africa. *American journal of tropical medicine and hygiene*, 25: 751–758.

Berg RL (1973) Weighted life expectancy as a health status index. *Health services research*, 8:153–156.

Bezzaoucha A, Dekkar N (1990) Handicaps in Algiers according to a household survey. *International journal of epidemiology*, 19(2):466–471.

Bullinger M, Hasford J (1991) Evaluating Quality-of-Life Measures for Clinical Trials in Germany. *Controlled clinical trials*, 12:91S–105S.

Bush JW, Chen MM, Patrick DL (1973) Health status index in cost effectiveness: analysis of PKU program. In: Berg RL, ed. *Health status indexes*. Chicago, Hospital Research and Educational Trust, pp. 172–208.

Centers for Disease Control (1991) *Draft working papers on the prevention of primary and secondary disabilities*. National Conference on the Prevention of Primary and Secondary Disabilities, Atlanta, GA.

Chamie M (1989) Survey design strategies for the study of disability. *World health statistics quarterly*, 42(3):122–146.

Dohrenwend BP, Dohrenwend BS (1982) Perspectives on the past and future of psychiatric epidemiology. *American journal of public health*, 72:1271–1279.

Flynn P (1992) Measuring Health in Cities. In: Ashton J, ed. *Healthy cities*. Milton Keynes, England, Open University Press, pp. 30–40.

Fougeyrollas P (1990) Les implications de la diffusion de la Classification internationale des Handicaps sur les politiques concernant les personnes handicapées [Implications of the diffusion of the International Classification of Impairments, Disabilities, and Handicaps on policies concerning disabled persons]. *World health statistics quarterly*, 43(4):281–285.

Froberg DG, Kane RL (1989) Methodology for measuring health-state preference. *Journal of clinical epidemiology* I: Measurement strategies, 42(4): 345–54. II: Scaling methods, 42(5): 459–71. III: Population and context effects, 42(6):585–92.

Garretsen HFL, Gilst ECH, Van Oers HAM (1991) Collecting health information at a local level. *Health promotion international,* 6:121–133.

Gomez-Rodriguez P (1989) Using the International Classification of Impairments, Disabilities, and Handicaps in surveys: the case of Spain. *World health statistics quarterly,* 42(3):161–166.

Guyatt GH, Jaeschke R (1990) Measurement in Clinical Trials. In: Spilker B, ed. *Quality of life assessments in clinical trials.* New York, Raven Press, pp. 37–46.

Hennessy et al. (1993) *Measuring quality of life for public health surveillance.* Unpublished manuscript. Atlanta, GA, National Center for Chronic Disease Prevention and Health Promotion, Centers for Disease Control and Prevention.

Johannesson M (1992) On discounting of gained life-years in cost-effectiveness analysis. *International journal of technology assessment in health care,* 8(2): 359–364.

Kaplan RM, Anderson JP (1990) The General Health Policy Model: An Integrated Approach. In: Spilker B, ed. *Quality of life assessments in clinical trials.* New York, Raven Press, pp. 131–149.

Katz S et al. (1983) Active life expectancy. *New England Journal of Medicine,* 309:1218–1224.

Katz S et al. (1963) Studies of illness in the aged. The Index of ADL: a standardized measure of biological and psychosocial function. *Journal of the American Medical Association,* 216:185–194.

McMaster University Health Priorities Analysis Unit (1991) 1989 Hamilton-Wentworth Health Survey. *Infowatch,* 3:4.

Minaire P et al. (1989) La mesure du handicap dans la communauté: une micro-enquête dans un village français [Measurement of handicap in the community: a micro survey in a French village]. *World health statistics quarterly,* 42(3):167–176.

Minaire P (1992) Disease, illness and health: theoretical models of the disablement process. *Bulletin of the World Health Organization,* 70(3):373–379.

Murray CJL, Chen LC (1992) Understanding morbidity change. *Population and development review,* 18(3):481–503, 593, 595.

Murray CJL (1996) Rethinking DALYs. In: Murray CJL, Lopez AD, eds. *The Global Burden of Disease: a comprehensive assessment of mortality and disability from diseases, injuries and risk factors in 1990 and projected to 2020.* Cambridge, Harvard University Press.

Murray CJL et al. (1992) Adult morbidity: limited data and methodological uncertainty. In Feachem, RC et al. (eds.), *The health of adults in the developing world.* New York, Oxford University Press, pp. 113–160.

Nissinen A, Wahl M (1992) health promotion and quality of life. *Hygie: International journal of health education,* 11:90.

Nomenclature des déficiences, incapacités, et désavantages (1988) Journal Officiel de la République Française, document spécial 88/13bis, 54.

Nord E (1992) Methods for quality adjustment of life years. *Social science and medicine,* 34:559–569.

Patrick DL, Erickson P (1993) Concepts of health-related quality of life and types of health-related quality of life assessments. In: Patrick DL, Erickson P *Health status and policy: allocating resources to health care.* New York, Oxford University Press, Chapters 4 and 5.

Patrick DL, Bergner M (1990) Measurement of health status in the 1990s. *Annual review of public health,* 11:165–83.

REVES (1993) *Statistical World Yearbook "Health expectancy".* Paris, Les Editions INSERM.

Robine JM, Mathers C (1993) Measuring the compression or expansion of morbidity through changes in health expectancy. In: *Calculation of health expectancies: harmonization, consensus achieved and future perspectives,* John Libbey Eurotext.

Robine JM, Romieu I, Mathers C (1992) *Multiplication of health expectancy calculations and problems of international comparison.* WHO/Netherlands CBS Consultation to develop common methods and instruments for health interview surveys: Third consultation, September 1992.

Robine JM (1992) Disability-free life expectancy. In: *Health expectancy.* London, HMSO.

Robine JM (1989) Estimation de la valeur de l'espérance de vie sans incapacité (EVSI) pour les pays occidentaux au cours de la dernière décennie. Quelle peut être l'utilité de ce nouvel indicateur de l'état de santé ? [Estimating the value of disability-free life expectancy for western countries in the last decade. How can this new health status indicator be used? (published erratum *World health statistics quarterly,* 1989, 42(4): following Table of Contents)]. *World health statistics quarterly,* 42(3):141–150.

Rogers A, Rogers RG, Branch LG (1989) A multistate analysis of active life expectancy. *Public health reports,* 104:222–225.

Sanders BS (1964) Measuring community health levels. *American journal of public health,* 54:1063–1070.

Schian HM (1991) Erhebung der beruflichen Fahigkeiten Behinderter unter Verwendung der WHO-Klassifikation ICIDH—Bericht über die internationale Sachverstandigensitzung vom 20.–21.3.1991 in Siegen [Assessment of the vocational capabilities of the handicapped using the WHO classification ICIDH—report of the International Expert meeting, Siegen FRG, March 20–21, 1991]. *Rehabilitation (Stuttgart),* 30(3):159–160.

Sullivan DF (1971) A single index of mortality and morbidity. HSMHA *Health reports,* 86:347–354.

Torrance G, Thomas WH, Sackett DL (1972) A utility maximization model for evaluation of health care programmes. *Health services research,* 7:118–133.

United Nations (1990) *Disability Statistics Compendium.* New York, United Nations Statistical Office, Statistics on Special Population Groups, Series Y, No 4.

Ware JE (1987) Standards for validating health measures: definition and content. *Journal of chronic diseases.* 40:473–480.

World Health Organization (1980) *International classification of impairments, disabilities, and handicaps: A manual of classification relating to the consequences of disease*, WHO, Geneva.

World Health Organization (1985) *Targets for Health for All*. Copenhagen, WHO Regional Office for Europe.

World Health Organization (1993a) *International statistical classification of diseases, injuries and causes of death*—Tenth Revision (1993) WHO, Geneva.

World Health Organization (1993b) *Implementation of strategies for Health for All by the year 2000. Third monitoring of progress. Common framework.* WHO, WHO/HST/GSP/93.3, Geneva.

World Health Organization (1993c) *Measuring quality of life. The development of the World Health Organization Quality of Life Instrument (WHOQOL).* Geneva, WHO, Division of Mental Health, MNH/PSF/93.1.

World Health Organization (1996) *Constitution, Basic documents*, 40th edition, WHO, Geneva.

Zeckhauser R, Shephard, D (1976) Where now for saving lives? *Law and contemporary problems,* 40(b):5–45.

Chapter 3

ESTIMATING CAUSES OF DEATH: NEW METHODS AND GLOBAL AND REGIONAL APPLICATIONS FOR 1990

CHRISTOPHER J. L. MURRAY
ALAN D. LOPEZ

Reliable information on deaths by cause is an essential input for planning, managing and evaluating the performance of the health sector in all countries. In an earlier attempt to address this need, Murray and Lopez (1994) published detailed estimates of global and regional mortality patterns for 1990, disaggregated by age and sex for over 100 specific causes of death. Because of the limitations of space, only a broad overview of the methods used to derive the global and regional estimates of mortality by cause were presented. In this chapter, much more extensive detail on the materials and methods used to develop global and regional estimates of causes of death are given. With the recent availability of new data sets for large populations in the developing world, and upon a critical appraisal of data sources and methods, a new revised set of estimates of mortality by cause are presented here. The number of deaths assigned to different causes has, in some cases, changed significantly from the previous analysis (Murray and Lopez 1994).

The estimates presented in this chapter use a combination of data sources and approaches, exploiting vital registration data where available, using models of the epidemiological transition to estimate broad causes, and supplementing these with a distillation of disease-specific data sources. The chapter is organized into sections concerning: the classification of causes of death used for the Global Burden of Disease Study (GBD); quality of cause-of-death attribution; sources of data for estimating causes of death; methods; results; and discussion. In each section, we have attempted to provide as much detail as is necessary for the reader to in sequence follow each step of the analysis that has been undertaken.

ASSIGNING A CAUSE TO A DEATH

To estimate global and regional patterns of causes of death, it is important first to delineate the steps involved in assigning a cause to a death. While there is an extensive literature on cause-of-death attribution, we will limit our focus here to several key issues. Perhaps the most important factor is the information available at the time of a death. Such information may include the clinical course of the disease prior to death as described in medical records or provided directly by the health care provider who cared for the individual prior to death, or, alternatively, the clinical course as perceived by relatives or associates and provided *post mortem* for the purposes of certification. Clinical histories can be supplemented with information from medical diagnostics and imaging studies (where these facilities are available) completed before death and with pathological studies undertaken after death. Second, even given the same information about a death, the final diagnosis will be affected by the training of the individual assigning a cause, his or her experience in diagnosis, and the level of detail sought in assigning a cause of death. For example, depending on the training of an individual, the same death may be recorded as tuberculosis, pulmonary tuberculosis, smear-positive pulmonary tuberculosis, or smear-positive pulmonary tuberculosis affecting particular segments of the lung. The third critical dimension is the coding of medical diagnoses according to a specific set of rules and to a set of rubrics such as those specified in the International Classification of Diseases (ICD).

In practice, most populations are characterized by one of two situations. In one scenario there is extensive information including clinical history, diagnostics and imaging tests available, and medical diagnosis is assigned by a physician according to the procedures of the International Classification of Diseases (or a near-equivalent). The other typical situation is one where most deaths are not recorded and those that are reported tend to have only a post-mortem clinical history obtained from relatives or associates, with no diagnostics or imaging studies, and the cause of death is assigned in accordance with a rudimentary classification scheme including a very limited number of major causes. In the following sections we address a series of issues relevant to the first type of community, where most deaths are registered, namely: the classification system, the International Classification of Diseases, the use of ill-defined or "garbage" codes, cardiovascular coding, and validation studies. We shall also briefly review some experiences in the second type of community, that with much more rudimentary information.

CAUSE-OF-DEATH CLASSIFICATION

In the transformation of data and estimates of mortality from different causes into information that is useful for health policy debate, a critical decision is the selection of a classification scheme to represent mortality by cause. At the simplest end of the spectrum, causes of death can be aggregated into just two categories: infectious and parasitic diseases, and chronic diseases. While providing useful insights into the overall pattern of mortality, such aggregate data are not useful for identifying specific health priorities or the potential for improving survival through specific intervention strategies. Even somewhat more disaggregated clusters of causes—such as infectious and parasitic diseases, maternal causes, cancer, cardiovascular diseases and so on (see, for example, Preston 1976)—are not sufficiently detailed to adequately inform health policy choices. On the other hand, overly detailed lists make cross-national and inter-temporal comparisons difficult to interpret because of the mass of detail and the likelihood of spurious patterns arising from differences in diagnostic practices.

For the Global Burden of Disease Study, we have proposed a tree structure of causes of death (Murray et al. 1992). The structure and content of the list of causes of death is shown in Table 3.1. At the first level of disaggregation, overall mortality is divided into three broad groups of causes: Group I, consisting of communicable diseases, maternal causes, conditions arising in the perinatal period, and nutritional deficiencies;[1] Group II, encompassing the noncommunicable diseases; and Group III, comprising all injuries, whether intentional or unintentional.

Group I causes of death consist of the cluster of conditions that typically decline at a faster pace than all-cause mortality during the process of the epidemiological transition. As a result, in low mortality populations, these causes account for only a small proportion of deaths (and, conversely, in high mortality populations they dominate the cause-of-death pattern). The noncommunicable diseases listed together in Group II are the most important health problems in populations that have undergone the epidemiological transition. (While it is true that mortality rates from some noncommunicable conditions, such as stomach cancer, may decline faster than all-cause mortality, these conditions have been maintained in Group II along with other cancers, since death rates from cancer as a whole appear to be relatively constant throughout the epidemiological transition.) Finally, injuries are classified into Group III, in part because their etiology is very different from that of most diseases, but also because there is no generalized pattern of change in injury mortality that accompanies the epidemiological transition.

Each Group has been divided into several major sub-categories of disease and injury that are mutually exclusive and exhaustive. These sub-categories are identified with capital letters in Table 3.1. Specifically, Group I has been divided into infectious and parasitic causes, respiratory infections, maternal causes, conditions arising during the perinatal period, and nutritional deficiencies. Noncommunicable causes (Group II) have been divided into 14 categories (see Table 3.1). Group III (Injuries) has been divided into two major sub-categories, unintentional injuries and intentional injuries.

A third level of disaggregation is used to identify more specific causes of death within each of these second-level categories. For example, within the category of infectious and parasitic diseases (IA), specific causes such as tuberculosis (IA1), HIV (IA3) and diarrhoeal diseases (IA4) have been identified. Finally, for some diseases, such as sexually transmitted diseases (IA2), a fourth level of disaggregation is provided, in this case syphilis

Table 3.1 Global Burden of Disease Study (GBD) classification system for diseases and injuries

Title of GBD cause	ICD-9 Code	ICD-9 BTL Code	ICD-10 Code
I. Communicable, maternal, perinatal and nutritional conditions	001-139, 243, 260-269, 280-285,320-322, 381-382, 614-616, 460-465, 466, 480-487, 614-616, 630-676, 760-779	01-07, 19, 200, 220, 240, 310-312, 320-322, 371-373, 38-41, 45	A00-B99, G00, N70-N73, J00-J06, J10-J18, J20-J22, H65-H66, O00-O99, P00-P06, E00-E02, E40-E46, E50, D50
A. Infectious and parasitic diseases	001-139,320-322,614-616	01-07, 220, 371-373	A00-B99, G00, N70-N73
1. Tuberculosis	010-018, 137	02, 077	A15-A19, B90
2. Sexually transmitted diseases excluding HIV	090-099, 614-616	06, 371-373	A50-A64, N70-N73
a. Syphilis	090-097	060	A50-A53
b. Chlamydia	i	ii	A55-A56
c. Gonorrhoea	098	061	A54
3. HIV	i	ii	B20-B24
4. Diarrhoeal diseases	001, 002, 004, 006-009	01 minus 013	A01-A04, A06-A09
5. Childhood-cluster diseases	032, 033, 037, 045, 050, 055, 056, 138	033, 034, 037, 040-043, 078	A33-37, A80, B05, B91
a. Pertussis	033	034	A37
b. Poliomyelitis	045, 138	040, 078	A80, B91
c. Diphtheria	032	033	A36
d. Measles	055	042	B05
e. Tetanus	037, 771.3	037[iii]	A33-A35
6. Bacterial meningitis and meningococcaemia	036, 320-322	036, 220[iv]	A39, G00
7. Hepatitis B and hepatitis C	070.2-070.9	046[v]	B16-B19
8. Malaria	084	052	B50-B54
9. Tropical-cluster diseases	085, 086, 120, 125	053, 054, 072, 074	B55-B57, B65, B73-B74
a. Trypanosomiasis	086.3, 086.4, 086.5, 086.9[vi]	054[ii]	B56
b. Chagas disease	086.0, 086.1, 086.2, 086.9[vi]	054[vii]	B57
c. Schistosomiasis	120	072	B65
d. Leishmaniasis	085	053	B55
e. Lymphatic filariasis	125.0, 125.1	ii	B74.0-B74.2
f. Onchocerciasis	125.3	ii	B73
10. Leprosy	030	032	A30
11. Dengue	061	ii	A90-A91
12. Japanese encephalitis	062.0	ii	A83.0
13. Trachoma	076	048	A71
14. Intestinal nematode infections	126-129	ii	
a. Ascariasis	127.0	ii	B77
b. Trichuriasis	127.3	ii	B79
c. Ancylostomiasis and necatoriasis	126	ii	B76
B. Respiratory infections	460-466, 480-487, 381-382	310-312, 320-322, 240	J00-J06, J10-J18, J20-J22, H65-H66
1. Lower respiratory infections	466, 480-487	320-322	J10-J18, J20-J22
2. Upper respiratory infections	460-465	310-312	J00-J06
3. Otitis media	381-382	240	H65-H66
C. Maternal conditions	630-676	38-41	O00-O99
1. Maternal haemorrhage	640, 641, 666	390	O44-O46, 067, 072
2. Maternal sepsis	670	ii	O85-O86
3. Hypertensive disorders of pregnancy	642	ii	O10-O16
4. Obstructed labour	660	393	O64-O66
5. Abortion	630-639	38	O00-O08
D. Conditions arising during the perinatal period	760-779	45	P00-P06
1. Low birth weight	764-765	452	P05-P07
2. Birth asphyxia and birth trauma	767-770	453-454	P03, P10-P15, P20-P29

Table 3.1   (continued)

Title of GBD cause	ICD-9 Code	ICD-9 BTL Code	ICD-10 Code
E. Nutritional deficiencies	243, 260-269, 280-285	19, 200[viii]	E00-E02, E40-E46, E50, D50
1. Protein-energy malnutrition	260-263	190-192	E40-E46
2. Iodine deficiency	243	ii	E00-E02
3. Vitamin A deficiency	264	ii	E50
4. Iron-deficiency anaemia	280	200[viii]	D50
II. Noncommunicable diseases	140-242, 244-259, 270-279, 286-319, 323-380, 383-459, 467-479, 488-613, 617-629, 680-759	08-18, 20-37, 42-44. [minus 200, 220, 240, 310-312, 320-322, 371-373]	C00-C97, D00-D48, D55-D80, E03-E07, E10-E16, E20-E34, E51-E89, F00-F99, G03-G99, H00-H61, H68-H95, I00-I99, J30-J99, K20-K99, N00-N64, N75-N99, L00-L99, M00-M99, Q00-Q99, K00-K99
A. Malignant neoplasms	140-209	08-14	C00-C97
1. Mouth and oropharynx cancers	140-149	08	C00-C14
2. Oesophagus cancer	150	090	C15
3. Stomach cancer	151	091	C16
4. Colon and rectum cancers	153, 154	093, 094	C18-C21
5. Liver cancer	155	095	C22
6. Pancreas cancer	157	096	C25
7. Trachea, bronchus and lung cancers	162	101	C33-C34
8. Melanoma and other skin cancers	172-173	111, 112	C43-C44
9. Breast cancer	174	113	C50
10. Cervix uteri cancer	180	120	C53
11. Corpus uteri cancer	179, 182	122	C54-C55
12. Ovary cancer	183	123	C56
13. Prostate cancer	185	124	C61
14. Bladder cancer	188	126	C67
15. Lymphomas and multiple myeloma	200-202	14 [minus 141]	C81-C90, C96
16. Leukaemia	204-208	141	C91-C95
B. Other neoplasms	210-239	15, 16, 17	D00-D48
C. Diabetes mellitus	250	181	E10-E14
D. Endocrine disorders	240-242, 244-249, 251-259, 270-279, 281-289	18, 20 [minus 200[ix]]	D55-D80, E03-E07, E15-E16, E20-E34, E51-E89
E. Neuro-psychiatric conditions	290-319, 323-359	21-22 [minus 220]	F00-F99, G03-G99
1. Unipolar major depression	i	ii	F32-F33
2. Bipolar disorder	296	212	F30-F31
3. Schizophrenia	295	211	F20-F29
4. Epilepsy	345	225	G40-G41
5. Alcohol use	291, 303, 305.0	215[x]	F10
6. Dementia and other degenerative and hereditary CNS disorders	330, 331, 290	222, 210[xi]	F01, F03, G30-G31
7. Parkinson disease	332	221	G20-G21
8. Multiple sclerosis	340	223	G35
9. Drug use	304, 305.2-305.9	216[xii]	F11-F16, F18-F19
10. Post-traumatic stress disorder	i	ii	xvii
11. Obsessive-compulsive disorders	300.3	ii	F42
12. Panic disorder	300.2	ii	F40.0, F41.0
F. Sense organ diseases	360-380, 383-389	23, 24 [minus 240]	H00-H61, H68-H95
1. Glaucoma	365	230	H40
2. Cataracts	366	231	H25-H26
G. Cardiovascular diseases	390-459	25-30	I00-I99
1. Rheumatic heart disease	390-398	25	I01-I09
2. Ischaemic heart disease	410-414, Proportion of: 428, 427.1, 427.4, 427.5, 440.9, 429.0-429.2, 429.9[xiii]	27 xiv	I20-I25 xv
3. Cerebrovascular disease	430-438	29	I60-I69
4. Inflammatory heart diseases	420, 421, 422, 425, Proportion of 428[xvi]	ii	I30-I33, I38, I40, I42

Table 3.1   (continued)

Title of GBD cause	ICD-9 Code	ICD-9 BTL Code	ICD-10 Code
H. Respiratory diseases	470-478, 490-519	31-32 [minus 310-312, 320-322]	J30-J99
1. Chronic obstructive pulmonary disease	490-492, 495-496	ii	J40-J44
2. Asthma	493	ii	J45-J46
I. Digestive diseases	530-579	34	K20-K99
1. Peptic ulcer disease	531-533	341	K25-K27
2. Cirrhosis of the liver	571	347	K70, K74
3. Appendicitis	540-543	342	K35-K37
J. Genito-urinary diseases	580-611, 617-629	35-37 [minus 371-373]	N00-N64, N75-N99
1. Nephritis and nephrosis	580-589	350	N00-N19
2. Benign prostatic hypertrophy	600	360	N40
K. Skin diseases	680-709	42	L00-L99
L. Musculo-skeletal diseases	740-759	43	M00-M99
1. Rheumatoid arthritis	714	430	M05-M06
2. Osteoarthritis	715	ii	M15-M19
M. Congenital anomalies	740-759	44	Q00-Q99
1. Abdominal wall defect	i	ii	xvii
2. Anencephaly	740.0	ii	Q00
3. Anorectal atresia	751.2	ii	Q42
4. Cleft lip	749.1	ii	Q36
5. Cleft palate	749.0	ii	Q35,Q37
6. Oesophageal atresia	750.3	ii	Q39.0-Q39.1
7. Renal agenesis	753.0	ii	Q60
8. Down syndrome	758.0	ii	Q90
9. Congenital heart disease	745-747	442	Q20-Q28
10. Spina bifida	741	ii	Q05
N. Oral conditions	520-529	33	K00-K14
1. Dental caries	521.0	ii	K02
2. Periodontal disease	523	ii	K05
3. Edentulism	i	ii	xvii
III. Injuries	E800-999	E47-E56	V01-Y98
A. Unintentional injuries	E800-921, 923-949	E47-E51, E520-E523, E53	V01-X59, Y40-Y98
1. Road traffic accidents	E810-819, 826-829, 928-929	E471,E472	V01-V89
2. Poisonings	E850-869	E48	X40-X49
3. Falls	E880-888	E50	W00-W19
4. Fires	E890-899	E51	X00-X09
5. Drownings	E910	E521	W65-W74
6. Other unintentional injuries	E800-E807, E820-825, E830-E848, E870-E879, E900-E909, E911-E921, E923-E949	E470, E473-E474, E49, E520, E522-E523, E53	V90-V99, W20-W64, W75-W99, X10-X39, X50-X59
B. Intentional injuries	E922, 950-979, 990-999	E524, E54-E55, E561	X60-Y09,Y35-Y36
1. Self-inflicted injuries	E950-959	E54	X60-X84
2. Violence	E922, 960-969	E55	X85-Y09
3. War	E990-999	E561	Y35-Y36

Notes

- "Symptoms, signs, and ill-defined conditions" (Chapter XVI in ICD-9 and R00-R99 in ICD-10) are included in Group I for persons aged under 5 years and in Group II for persons aged 5 years and over, and distributed proportionally to all causes below the Group level.

- Cause E560 of ICD-9 BTL code (E980-E989 of ICD-9, Y10-Y34 in ICD-10) is distributed proportionally among all injury causes below the Group level.

[i] No ICD-9 code is available.
[ii] No ICD-9 BTL code is available.
[iii] There is no BTL code for neonatal tetanus.
[iv] BTL 220 includes unspecified causes of meningitis which can be excluded when 4-digit ICD-9 data are available.
[v] BTL 046 includes hepatitis A which should not be part of this category.
[vi] 086.9 in SSA is African trypanosomiasis and 086.9 in LAC is Chagas disease.
[vii] 054 in SSA is African trypanosomiasis and 054 in LAC is Chagas disease.

Table 3.1   (continued)

---

viii BTL 200 includes anaemias other than iron-deficiency anaemia that should be classified in IID, "Endocrine disorders."
ix Some of BTL 200, anaemias other than from iron deficiency, should be included here.
x BTL 215 does not include deaths from ICD-9 detailed codes 303 and 305.0.
xi BTL 210 includes ICD-9 detailed codes 330-336 which should not be part of this category.
xii BTL 216 does not include ICD-9 detailed codes 305.2-305.9 which should be included here.
xiii The proportion of these ill-defined cardiovascular codes that should be included with ischaemic heart disease depends on the proportion of cardiovascular deaths that were originally coded to 410-414. See p. 128 for a detailed analysis and recommended correction methods.
xiv See p. 133 for an equation to approximate ischaemic heart disease mortality using BTL data.
xv No correction algorithm has been developed yet for ICD-10 data to correct for miscoding of ischaemic heart disease deaths.
xvi 2.5 per cent of deaths at ages 30–44, 5 per cent of deaths at ages 45–59, and 10 per cent of deaths at ages 60+.
xvii No ICD-10 code is available.

(IA2a), chlamydia (IA2b), and gonorrhoea (IA2c). The set of disaggregated causes was selected on the basis of three criteria: the probable magnitude of the disease or injury as a cause of death or disability as evaluated at the beginning of the study (e.g. ischaemic heart disease; malaria); the level of health services provided for the cause (e.g. appendicitis); and the attention attracted by the cause in current health policy debate (e.g. leprosy, HIV). The aggregations used, such as childhood cluster, sexually transmitted diseases and tropical cluster, are somewhat arbitrary and have been maintained for consistency with prior analyses.

The category, "Symptoms, signs and ill-defined conditions"—Chapter XVI of the Ninth Revision of the ICD (Chapter XVIII in ICD-10)—is not listed as one of the major causes in our classification system. Deaths assigned to this category, as well as some other codes used for ill-defined conditions, have been reassigned to specific causes of death in the GBD classification scheme. From the perspective of generating useful information to inform the choice of alternative health policies, the assignment of a death to a category for deaths of ill-defined causes can be misleading. Each person who dies does so from some specific underlying cause and the best possible estimate of the magnitude of each cause is required for policy formulation. The advantages and disadvantages of reassigning deaths due to ill-defined causes are further discussed below.

For reference, Table 3.1 provides the four-digit ICD-9 codes used to define each cause of death in the GBD classification tree. International collections of cause-of-death data, such as that maintained by the World Health Organization, are often compiled according to a condensed list of causes (for example, the Basic Tabulation List (BTL) has been used to store data coded according to ICD-9). Much important detail, however, is lost when the full ICD-9 four-digit codes are collapsed into the Basic Tabulation List. For example, there is no BTL code for asthma, nor for a number of parasitic diseases, nor for appendicitis. In order to estimate mortality due to causes for which there is no BTL code, either four-digit ICD-9 cause-of-death data must be obtained or causes must be estimated based on the BTL codes that best approximate the cause. Table 3.1 provides those BTL codes that map (some more precisely than others) to each cause in the GBD list. Countries are now in the process of adopting the Tenth Revision of the ICD. While no ICD-10 data have been included in this study, we have provided our equivalent ICD-10 codes for each cause. In the section on cause-of-death models, we have made use of data coded according to previous revisions of the ICD for Groups I, II and III. Table3.2 provides the equivalent Short List codes (the A-List) for the Sixth, Seventh and Eighth Revisions of the ICD.

ICD CODING RULES

The rules of the ICD specify that, while several causes of death can be listed on a death certificate, each death must be attributed to one cause in the primary tabulations. Rather than the immediate cause of death, the underlying cause of death is to be specified. "For this purpose, the underlying cause has been defined as (a) the disease or injury which initiated the train of morbid events leading directly to death, or (b) the circumstances of the accident or violence which produced the fatal injury"(World Health Organization 1993). In reality, there may often be multiple conditions present at or around the time of death. For example, a person with diabetes and hypertension could have a myocardial infarction complicated by congestive heart failure and might ultimately die of pneumonia in the intensive care unit. What is the underlying cause of death? By convention, this death would not be coded to the immediate pulmonary demise but rather to ischaemic heart disease with diabetes and hypertension perhaps listed as associated causes. The various conventions that have been agreed upon are, in fact, an arbitrary method to deal with the multi-causal nature of mortality. For example, deaths from liver cancer even in an individual known to have hepatitis B are still coded to liver cancer. In contrast,

Table 3.2   ICD-6, ICD-7 and ICD-8 A-List codes for the Global Burden of Disease Study classification Groups I, II and III

Title of GBD disease or injury category	ICD-6 A-List	ICD-7 A-List	ICD-8 A-List
I. Communicable, maternal, perinatal and nutritional conditions	A1-A43, A64-A65, A71, A77, A87-A92, A104, A115-A120, A130-A135	A1-A43, A64-A65, A71, A77, A87-A92, A104, A115-A120, A130-A135	A1-A44, A65, A67, A72, A78, A89-A92, A112-A18, A131-A135
II. Noncommunicable diseases	A44-A63, A66-A70, A72-A76, A78-A86, A93-A103, A105-A115, A121-A129	A44-A63, A66-A70, A72-A76, A78-A86, A93-A103, A105-A115, A121-A129	A45-A64, A66, A68-A71, A73-A77, A79-A88, A93-A111, A119-A130
III. Injuries	AE138-AE150	AE138-AE150	AE138-AE150

Notes

• "Symptoms, signs, and ill-defined conditions" (A135-A136 in ICD-6 and ICD-7 and A136-A137 in ICD-8) are included in Group I for persons aged under 5 years and in Group II for persons aged 5 years and over.

• No A-List codes are available in ICD-6, ICD-7 and ICD-8 for pelvic inflammatory disease which should be included in Group I.

in ICD-10, deaths from lymphoma among persons with HIV are coded to HIV and not to lymphoma.

For the purposes of this study, we have followed the principles of the ICD and have therefore insisted that there can only be a single cause of death in the primary tabulations. In Chapter 5 in this volume, which includes information on diseases as risk factors for death from other diseases, we have estimated the fraction of deaths associated with a given cause. In some cases, however, the ICD-9 rules and conventions are ambiguous. Table 3.3 summarizes a few important combinations of causes that may be frequently encountered in different populations, and the arbitrary conventions that we have adopted or modified to estimate the underlying causes of death for the primary tabulations.

VALIDITY OF MEDICALLY CERTIFIED CAUSES OF DEATH

Even in those regions of the world where deaths are registered and causes are assigned by medically qualified staff with the aid of substantial diagnostic information, the quality of cause-of-death attribution is still of concern. Many physicians are skeptical of the reliability of cause-of-death attribution and coding. In such populations, the quality of the cause-of-death data depends strongly on two considerations: do physicians make the correct diagnosis of the cause of death in the absence of an autopsy, and does a trained coder assign an appropriate ICD code to the physician's diagnosis? In most countries with complete vital registration, well over 90 per cent of causes are assigned by a physician. There are exceptions, such as

Table 3.3 GBD conventions for primary tabulation of major cause combinations

Cause combination			Primary tabulation cause selected
HIV	&	Tuberculosis	HIV
HIV	&	Lymphoma	HIV
Hepatitis B	&	Liver Cancer	Liver Cancer
Hepatitis B	&	Cirrhosis	Cirrhosis
STDs	&	Ectopic pregnancy	Ectopic pregnancy
Diarrhoea	&	Lower respiratory infection	Lower respiratory infection
Meningitis	&	Lower respiratory infection	Meningitis
Measles	&	Lower respiratory infection	Measles
Pertussis	&	Lower respiratory infection	Pertussis
Measles	&	Diarrhoea	Measles
Tuberculosis	&	Protein-energy malnutrition	Tuberculosis
Malaria	&	Protein-energy malnutrition	Malaria
Measles	&	Protein-energy malnutrition	Measles
Meningitis	&	Otitis media	Meningitis

Sri Lanka, where "lay-coders" assign causes to a substantial proportion of deaths. Persons who are not medically qualified tend to assign a larger proportion of deaths to "Symptoms, signs and ill-defined conditions" and other "garbage" codes. For example, the code for epilepsy is often used by lay-reporters as a code of convenience. In Morocco in 1992, 47 per cent of all deaths were coded by non-physicians whereas 85 per cent of all epilepsy deaths were coded by non-physicians; in Colombia between 1989 and 1991, nine per cent of all deaths were coded by non-physicians while 21 per cent of all epilepsy deaths were coded by non-physicians.

A variety of autopsy studies have examined the accuracy of physician-assigned causes of death (e.g. Battle et al. 1987, Britton 1974, Carvalho et al. 1991, Gough 1985, Middleton et al. 1989, Stehbens 1987, Veress and Alafuzoff 1994). In general, clinical attribution of causes of death can be quite inaccurate when evaluated at the individual level. Britton (1974) summarized 11 studies from 1950 to 1971 reporting diagnostic error rates from 6 to 55 per cent. Battle et al. (1987) found that in one-third of 2067 autopsies there was a major diagnostic discrepancy between the clinical and post-mortem diagnosis. Carvalho et al. (1991) found a similar rate of diagnostic discrepancy (31 per cent) in 910 autopsies performed in Brazil. Veress and Alafuzoff (1994) reported similar findings for Sweden. Often in these studies, however, the difference in diagnoses is only minor and even for major errors, false positives often tend to balance false negatives. From a public health perspective, diagnostic error only matters if it changes the measured rates of a particular cause. Unfortunately, many of the studies only report diagnostic discrepancy rates for each individual diagnosis and do not show if the false positives balance the false negatives. The few studies that do provide such information, in general, suggest that the numbers of deaths assigned to a cause are quite reliable even if the particular cause assigned to any individual death is less so. Not surprisingly, this tendency for false positives to balance false negatives is observed more in broad cause groupings, such as all cardiovascular deaths, than in more detailed sub-causes, such as hypertensive heart disease or aortic aneurysms.

ICD-9 Chapter XVI and Other Codes for Ill-defined Conditions

While vital registration data are generally a reliable source of information on the broad cause-of-death pattern in a community, the use of some ICD-9 codes can affect their usefulness. Some codes present problems that affect the interpretation of data from nearly all communities. Chapter XVI in ICD-9 ("Symptoms, signs and ill-defined conditions") is the most important of these. Less than three per cent of deaths are assigned to this category in most high-income countries. Unfortunately, in a number of developing countries, this category can account for a large share of deaths, particularly those at older ages. In Egypt in 1987, for example, 21 per cent of deaths overall and 49 per cent of deaths in the age groups 75 years and over were assigned to this category (World Health Organization 1991).

With development, the proportion of deaths assigned to "Symptoms, signs and ill-defined conditions" or its equivalent has steadily declined. In 1960, twelve per cent of deaths were assigned to the equivalent category in Mexico, declining to two per cent in 1994. The most important public health implication of the steady decline in this category is that it can create spurious increases in the reported age-specific death rates from specific causes (e.g. heart diseases).

There is considerable evidence to suggest that in adults, deaths coded to ill-defined causes (ICD-9 Chapter XVI) are in fact most likely miscoded deaths from noncommunicable diseases. Preston (1976) investigated how specific cause-of-death patterns changed with the reduction in all-cause mortality using a pooled time series cross-sectional dataset. He found that age-standardized mortality rates for cardiovascular diseases tended to increase as all-cause mortality rates declined. However, he found a strong relationship between residual cardiovascular disease mortality and the mortality from other and unknown causes; age-standardized cardiovascular disease mortality *declined* with all-cause mortality, after adjusting for miscoding of deaths to ill-defined conditions (ICD-9 Chapter XVI or its equivalent). Murray et al. (1992), analysing cause-specific mortality in adults aged 15–59, also concluded that deaths assigned to ill-defined conditions were miscoded noncommunicable disease deaths, a large portion of which are deaths from cardiovascular disease.

Only a detailed validation study of deaths coded to ill-defined conditions in each population could fully resolve the uncertainty surrounding the true causes of these deaths. In the absence of such information and in the light of the research mentioned above, we have established an arbitrary algorithm for redistributing these ill-defined deaths based on three hypotheses. First, we have assumed that deaths due to injuries are much less likely to be assigned to "Symptoms, signs and ill-defined conditions" than are deaths from diseases in Group I (communicable, maternal, perinatal or nutritional) or Group II (noncommunicable). Second, we have assumed that among adults, ICD-9 Chapter XVI deaths are likely to be miscoded noncommunicable diseases. Third, in children, these deaths could well be miscoded Group I deaths because of the greater difficulty in obtaining a clear clinical history in this population group. For this study, we have redistributed ICD-9 Chapter XVI deaths in the age group 0–4 years proportionately across all (known) Group I causes within that age and sex group. For each age group above 5, we redistributed deaths proportionately across (known) Group II causes. Given the relative importance of Group I below age 5 and Group II above age 5, this algorithm gives similar results to simple proportionate redistribution of ICD-9 Chapter XVI deaths across both Groups I and II at all ages.

Within Group III (Injuries), there are also two widely used groups of codes in ICD-9 for assigning unspecified causes: E980–E989 and E928. E980–E989, *Injury undetermined whether accidentally or purposefully inflicted*, varies from less than two per cent of all injury deaths in the

United States to 42.9 per cent in Chile in 1993. (High proportions of in-juries assigned to this set of codes can be an unintended consequence of medico-legal practice [Taucher 1989].) In some countries further infor-mation on injuries can be obtained from dual E and N coding—E codes represent external causes of injuries such as a road traffic accidents, falls or fires, and N codes represent the nature of injuries, such as skull frac-tures, spinal cord transections or burns. E980–989 deaths in these coun-tries can be redistributed according to the distribution of each N code across the remaining E codes. In most countries, however, such dual cod-ing is either unavailable or incomplete and we have therefore chosen to redistribute E980–E989 deaths proportionately across all other (known) E codes. In some National Burden of Disease studies a third method has been used (Lozano et al. 1994) whereby a panel of experts has developed an arbitrary redistribution algorithm to allocate these ill-defined injury deaths to specific external causes.

For a number of countries, E928 *Other and unspecified environmen-tal and accidental causes*—which includes E928.9 *Unspecified accidents* (stated as accidentally inflicted but not otherwise specified)—is an im-portant code for unspecified injury deaths. In Mexico in 1991, E928 ac-counted for twenty per cent of all unintentional injury deaths. As there is no Basic Tabulation List code in ICD-9 for this cause, it is not possible to identify deaths assigned to this code using the WHO collection of inter-national cause-of-death data. In countries where three or four digit ICD-9 data are available, we have redistributed E928 deaths proportionately across all unintentional injury causes. Alternatively where dual E and N coding is available, the E/N matrix can be used to redistribute these E928 deaths to other external causes within Group IIIA (unintentional injuries).

Coding of Cardiovascular Diseases

Cardiovascular deaths account for a significant proportion of adult deaths in all countries. Even for such an important cause of death, coding prac-tices across communities and within the same community over time have been notoriously variable (Campbell 1963, Robb-Smith 1967, Stehbens 1987). For example, Figure 3.1 shows death rates from two cardiovascu-lar diseases in Mexico for males aged 60 years and over for the period 1986–1991, namely ventricular dysrhythmias and ischaemic heart dis-ease. During this period, ventricular dysrhythmias declined and ischaemic heart disease increased in nearly inverse proportion. It appears likely that in the early 1980s, many ischaemic heart disease deaths were coded as ventricular dysryhthmias and that over the decade coding improved, cre-ating false trends in both causes. This is but one example of a common phenomenon. To enhance the comparability of our cardiovascular dis-ease mortality estimates in countries with complete medical certification of causes of death, we have undertaken a sub-study of cardiovascular disease coding, which is reported more fully elsewhere (Lozano et al. 1996).

Figure 3.1   Probable effects of changing coding practices on reported death rates for two cardiovascular diseases in males, Mexico, 1986–1991

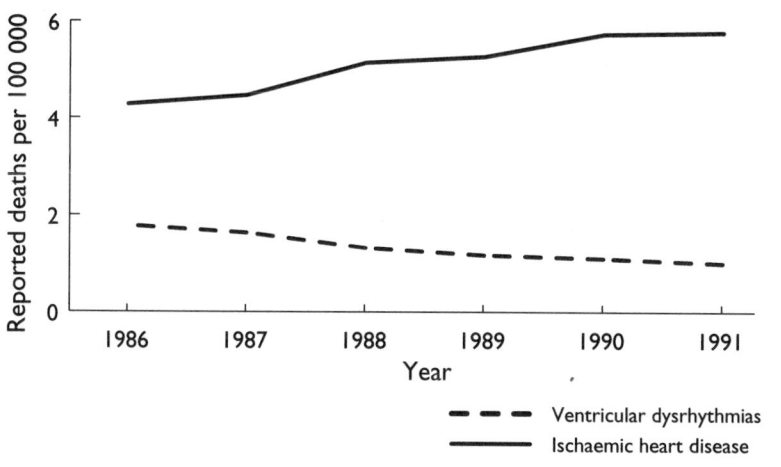

The two most important causes of cardiovascular mortality are cerebrovascular accidents (or stroke) and ischaemic heart disease; each is discussed here in turn. Because the diagnosis of stroke is often clearer than for ischaemic heart disease, we suspect that the coding of deaths due to cerebrovascular accidents is, in general, better than for ischaemic heart disease. At the very least, stroke death rates are not under-estimated but may actually be over-estimated by vital registration systems. Stroke incidence registries indicate that vital registration systems tend to overcode cerebrovascular mortality (Bonita et al. 1996, Kojima et al. 1990). Bonita et al. (1996) suggest that over the age of 75 years, stroke mortality may be over-estimated by a factor of two. While we suspect that vital registration systems do indeed overcode stroke mortality, we have decided for the purposes of the Global Burden of Disease Study not to reassign some of the stroke deaths to other causes since we do not yet have sufficient information on which to base a reallocation algorithm. Further research may yield a rational basis for revising downward estimated stroke mortality in high income countries.

Figure 3.2 shows the age-standardized death rates at ages 30 years and over for cardiovascular diseases, excluding stroke, and the age-standardized death rates for ischaemic heart disease (ICD-9 codes 410–414) for those countries for which three-digit ICD-9 data are available. There is wide variation in the gap between ischaemic heart disease mortality rates and cardiovascular disease (excluding stroke) mortality rates. Much of this variation may be due to differential attribution of ischaemic heart disease deaths to selected codes for ill-defined cardiovascular deaths,

Figure 3.2   Age-standardized mortality rates from cardiovascular diseases
(excluding stroke) and from ischaemic heart disease for
selected countries, both sexes combined, ages 30 and over,
circa 1990

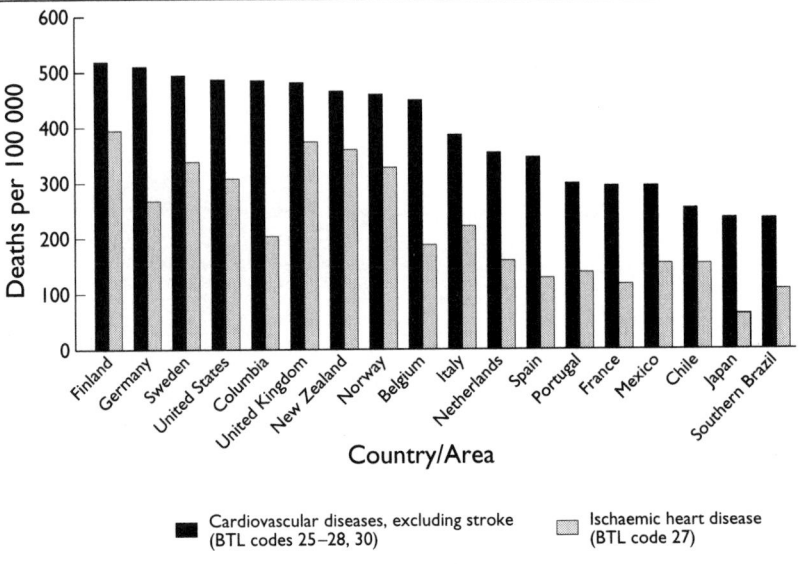

Cardiovascular diseases, excluding stroke
(BTL codes 25–28, 30)

Ischaemic heart disease
(BTL code 27)

particularly heart failure (ICD-9 code 428), ventricular dysrhythmias
(ICD-9 codes 427.1, 427.4, 427.5), general atherosclerosis (ICD-9 code
440.9), and ill-defined descriptions and complications of heart disease
(ICD-9 codes 429.0, 429.1, 429.2 and 429.9).

In Figure 3.3, the vertical axis shows the percentage of cardiovascular
disease (CVD) deaths (excluding stroke) assigned to these codes for ill-
defined cardiovascular conditions. The horizontal axis shows the proportion of cardiovascular deaths assigned to ischaemic heart disease
(410–414). At one extreme, coders in Canada, Finland, Norway, New
Zealand, the United Kingdom and Sweden assign, on average, a small
proportion of deaths to these "garbage" codes—8.3 per cent at ages 30–44
years, 4.0 per cent at ages 45–59 and 11.7 per cent at ages 60 years and
above. At the other extreme, coders in Japan, Germany, Spain, Belgium
and Portugal assign more than 40 per cent of cardiovascular disease deaths
(excluding stroke) to these four groups of codes at ages 10 years and over.
This analysis would suggest that many of the deaths assigned to the CVD
"garbage" codes are in fact miscoded ischaemic heart disease deaths, given
the strong inverse relation shown in Figure 3.3.

In order to correct for the likely undercoding of ischaemic heart disease in countries such as Japan, France and Spain, we have developed the
following algorithm. We assume that the cluster of countries comprising
Canada, Finland, Norway, New Zealand, the United Kingdom and Swe-

Figure 3.3   Proportions of cardiovascular disease deaths (excluding stroke) assigned to selected codes for ill-defined causes and directly to ischaemic heart disease, for selected countries, circa 1990

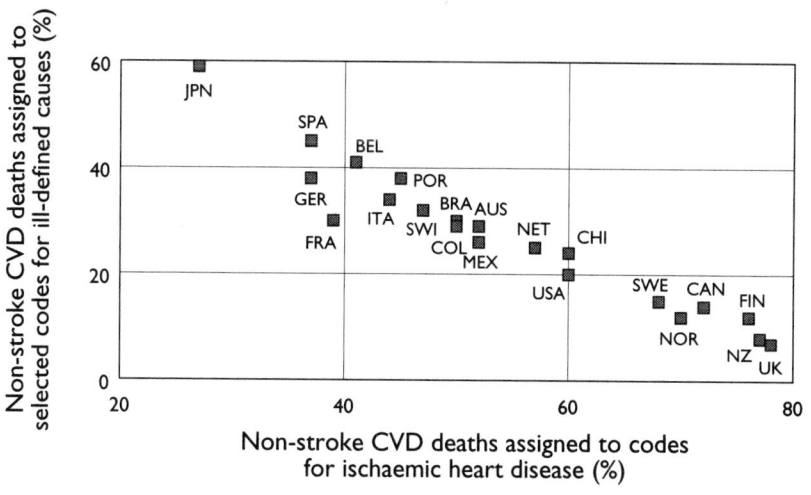

den define the "standard" coding practice and that the percentage of cardiovascular deaths (excluding stroke) assigned to these ill-defined codes (in aggregate) is acceptable. The percentage of cardiovascular deaths (excluding stroke) assigned to these codes in excess of this percentage is then assumed to be largely miscoded ischaemic heart disease. However, to take into account possible real variations in the proportion of deaths that should be assigned to these ill-defined codes, we followed a two-step procedure. First, an ordinary least squares (OLS) regression equation has been estimated for each age group predicting the proportion of cardiovascular deaths (excluding stroke) assigned to these ill-defined codes as a function of the proportion of deaths assigned to ischaemic heart disease, as follows:

$$G_{30-44} = 0.46 - 0.56\, I_{30-44} \qquad R^2 = 0.59$$

$$G_{45-59} = 0.48 - 0.55\, I_{45-59} \qquad R^2 = 0.82$$

$$G_{60+} = 0.71 - 0.80\, I_{60+} \qquad R^2 = 0.93$$

where G is the percentage of cardiovascular deaths (excluding stroke) assigned to the ill-defined codes, and I is the percentage of CVD deaths (excluding stroke) that are directly coded to ischaemic heart disease (410-414). To estimate the regression parameters we have excluded Japan, as it has a profound effect on the fitted slope and intercept. Note that the R^2 increases with increasing age, providing further indirect evidence that the ill-defined codes are indeed being used for ischaemic heart disease which is more common at older ages.

Next, we have estimated a corrected proportion for CVD ill-defined codes and the corrected ischaemic heart disease proportion for each country, with the constraint that the percentage of CVD deaths with ill-defined codes does not exceed the average of Canada, Finland, Norway, New Zealand, the United Kingdom and Sweden, using the following formula:

$$I_n^* = I_n + G_n \left(1 - \frac{G_n^{ref}}{G_n^{pred}}\right)$$

where I_n^* is the adjusted percentage of cardiovascular deaths (excluding stroke) attributed to ischaemic heart disease for age group n, I_n is the measured percentage of cardiovascular deaths (excluding stroke) coded to 410–414, G_n is the measured percentage of cardiovascular deaths (excluding stroke) assigned to the four ill-defined codes, G_n^{ref} is the average percentage of cardiovascular deaths (excluding stroke) assigned to the ill-defined codes in the reference group of countries (Canada, Finland, Norway, New Zealand, United Kingdom and Sweden), and G_n^{pred} is the percentage of cardiovascular deaths (excluding stroke) assigned to the ill-defined codes predicted from the regression equation on the basis of I_n.

Figure 3.4   Adjusted and unadjusted ischaemic heart disease (IHD) mortality rates for selected countries: age-standardized mortality rates at ages 30 and over, both sexes, circa 1990

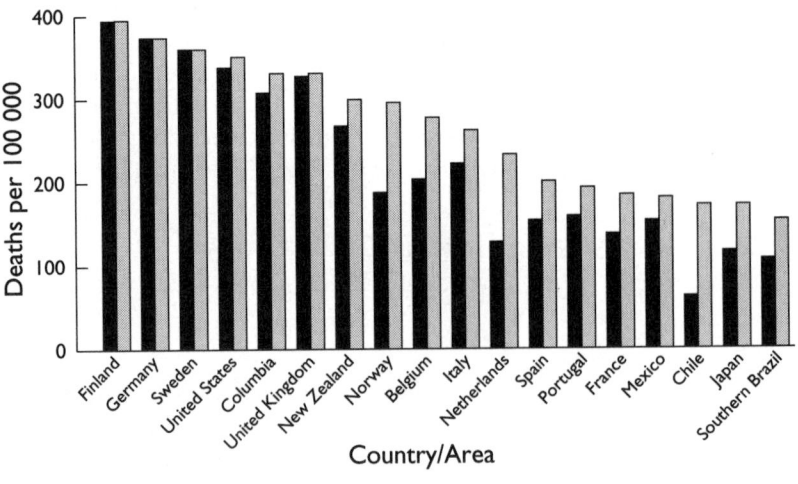

IHD death rates before correction   IHD death rates after correction

The adjusted and directly reported ischaemic heart disease death rates are compared in Figure 3.4. Prior to correction, the ratio of the highest ischaemic heart disease mortality rate at ages 30 years and over (Finland) to the lowest (Japan) was 6.3. After correcting for possible miscoding, this ratio of rates was reduced to 2.3. The coefficient of variation for age-standardized ischaemic heart disease mortality rates at ages 30 and over decreased from 0.44 to 0.28 as a result of the adjustments. It is interesting to note that while France (and some other Mediterranean countries) still had lower IHD rates than other industrialized countries, even after correcting in this fashion, it would appear that at least some part of the "French Paradox" (Burr 1995, Criqui and Ringel 1994) might be due to differential coding of ischaemic heart disease.

The correction algorithm described above is only applicable for countries where four-digit ICD-9 codes or equivalent data are available. Where only ICD-9 BTL codes (or the equivalent) can be used, the proportion of deaths assigned to these ill-defined codes cannot be directly estimated. For these situations, an approximate correction algorithm can be derived based solely on the proportion of non-stroke cardiovascular mortality assigned to ischaemic heart disease (410–414). In this case, the estimated regression equations are as follows:

$$I^*_{30-44} = 0.38 + 0.44 I_{30-44}$$

$$I^*_{45-59} = 0.44 + 0.45 I_{45-59}$$

$$I^*_{60+} = 0.60 + 0.2 I_{60+}$$

where I^* is the adjusted proportion of cardiovascular deaths (excluding stroke) due to ischaemic heart disease for the specific age group, and I is the observed proportion of cardiovascular deaths (excluding stroke) coded to 410–414.

We also suspect that some of the deaths coded to the cluster of cardiovascular "garbage" codes are misclassified inflammatory heart disease deaths—pericarditis, endocarditis, myocarditis and cardiomyopathy. In younger age groups, this cluster of inflammatory heart conditions, especially cardiomyopathies, form a substantial percentage of cardiovascular deaths in countries such as the United States or the United Kingdom. We have not been able to develop any statistical method to suggest what proportion of deaths assigned to "garbage" codes should be reassigned to inflammatory heart diseases. Nevertheless, based on consultations with several cardiologists and cardiovascular epidemiologists, we have chosen to assign an arbitrary percentage of ill-defined CVD deaths to this category—2.5 per cent at ages 30–44, 5 per cent at ages 45–59 and 10 per cent at ages 60 and over.

LOCAL CODING PRACTICES

In addition to the general problems with ICD-9 Chapter XVI, E980–989, E928 and cardiovascular disease coding, there are local peculiarities of cause-of-death coding in countries despite the fact that they use the ICD. When using BTL datasets, many of these local preferences codes are hidden in larger residual categories and cannot be identified, analysed or reassigned. When three- or four-digit ICD-9 data are available however, a careful analysis of each code can help identify local peculiarities. In the National Burden of Disease studies in Mexico, Chile, Mauritius, Colombia and Uruguay, a number of these local preferred codes were identified (Gareeboo et al. 1995, Londoño et al. 1994, Lozano et al. 1994, 1995). In each of these studies, algorithms for redistributing some of the deaths assigned to these codes based on local expert consultation have been formulated. We strongly recommend this type of detailed local analysis when applying burden of disease methods to a national or sub-national population. Likewise, it would be extremely useful if international collections of cause-of-death data based on ICD-10 (such as that to be maintained by WHO) make available more detail on cause of death, so that more careful assessments of local coding practices can be undertaken before international comparisons are made.

CAUSE-OF-DEATH ATTRIBUTION WITH LIMITED INFORMATION

For the majority of countries in the world, deaths are not fully registered and sentinel surveillance systems to ascertain causes of death are often based on limited information about the clinical course of disease ascertained *post-mortem* from relatives or associates. Methods to assign causes of death in these circumstances are commonly referred to as "verbal autopsy" procedures. A number of studies have investigated the effect on data reliability of classification systems, questionnaire design, interviewer background and training, respondent's relationship to the deceased, and the algorithms for assigning a diagnosis from the information obtained (Bang et al. 1992, Chandramohan et al. 1994, Gray 1991, Kalter et al. 1990, Snow et al. 1992, Snow et al. 1993). These verbal autopsy methods are based on two assumptions: (a) family members can recall the symptoms of a dead family member accurately, and (b) the symptom cluster is specific to one cause of death. These restrictive conditions are met for some causes but not for others. The results of verbal autopsy methods have been compared with hospital diagnoses for several child death instruments (Bang et al. 1992, Snow et al. 1992). For example, Snow et al. (1992) found that the sensitivity and specificity of the verbal autopsy method applied in Kenya were both over 80 per cent for malnutrition, measles and tetanus. Predictive value positive was 50 per cent or below for acute respiratory infections, gastroenteritis, anaemia and meningitis. Similar results have been found in other validation studies (World Health Organization 1993). Sensitivity, specificity and predictive value positive tend to exaggerate the weakness of the verbal autopsy methods for public health applications. False positives will be balanced to some extent by false negatives; therefore, the error in the measured proportion assigned to a particular cause is not likely to be as great. Verbal autopsy methods to identify the causes of adult deaths are not as well developed. Validation studies for one adult instrument are only now being conducted (Chandramohan et al. 1994). As discussed in the following section on sources, verbal autopsy data have therefore been used only sparingly and for a limited set of causes in this analysis.

SOURCES FOR ESTIMATING MORTALITY BY CAUSE

For the Global Burden of Disease Study, there were four types of sources of information on mortality by cause available to us: vital registration systems, sample registration systems, epidemiological assessments and cause-of-death models. In this section, we review the availability of data derived from these four types of sources. The ways in which each of these types of data were used is outlined in the methods section.

VITAL REGISTRATION

Vital registration data on causes of death are available for a large number of countries from national governments, WHO and other inter-governmental organizations. Table 3.4 summarizes the countries, years and ICD revisions for which vital registration data were available to us for this study.[2] In a number of these countries, however, the coverage of the vital registration system is considered to be less than 90 per cent complete. In addition, in some of these countries such as Sri Lanka, less than 90 per cent of deaths are medically certified. Three- and four-digit ICD-9 cause-of-death data were also obtained for some 22 countries. Vital registration cause-of-death data obtained for the newly independent states of Central and Eastern Europe listed in Table 3.4 were coded according to the cause-of-death classification in use in the former USSR at the time. This coding system was mapped to the GBD cause list based exclusively on content validity criteria and not on any death certificate bridge-coding exercise (which, to our knowledge, has never been done).[3]

SAMPLE REGISTRATION SYSTEMS

Sample registration systems provide cause-of-death information for China and India (and for other countries as well). The routine vital registration system in China is far from complete. Several sources provide information on patterns of mortality by cause for China, which contains one-fifth of the world's population. In 1976 a retrospective survey of nearly one million deaths which occurred during the period 1973–1975 was undertaken, primarily to investigate mortality rates from different cancers (Chen et al. 1990, Li et al. 1981). Unfortunately, full details from this large survey have not yet been published; hence, it was not extensively used for this study. In cooperation with the World Bank, the Chinese Academy of

Table 3.4   Countries and years for which vital registration data are
available by ICD revision

Region and	Years of available data			
country/territory[1]	ICD-6	ICD-7	ICD-8	ICD-9[2]
Established Market Economies				
Australia	50-57	58-67	68-78	79-93
Austria	55-57	58-68	69-79	80-94
Belgium	54-57	58-67	68-78	79-89
Canada	50-57	58-68	69-78	79-92
Denmark	51-57	58-68	69-93	
Finland	52-57	58-68	69-86	
France	50-57	58-67	68-78	79-92
Former Federal Republic of Germany	52-57	58-67	68-78	79-94
Germany				90-94
Greece	56-57	58-67	68-78	79-93
Iceland	51-57	58-70	71-80	81-90
Ireland	50-57	58-67	68-78	79-92
Italy	51-57	58-67	68-78	79-92
Japan	50-57	58-67	68-78	79-93
Luxembourg	55-57	58-62, 65-70	71-78	79-90
Malta	55-57	58-67	68-78	79-90
Monaco				86-87
Netherlands	50-57	58-68	69-78	79-93
New Zealand	50-57	58-67	68-78	79-92
Norway	51-57	58-68	69-85	86-92
Portugal	55-57	58-70	71-79	80-93
Spain	51-57	58-67	68-79	80-92
Sweden	51-57	58-68	69-86	87-92
Switzerland	51-57	58-68	69-93	
United Kingdom	50-57	58-67	68-78	79-92
USA	50-57	58-67	68-78	79-91
Formerly Socialist Economies of Europe				
Albania				87-89, 92
Belarus				85-90, 92-93
Bulgaria		64-67	68-79	80-93
Former Czechoslovakia	53-57	58-67	68-78	79-91
Czech Republic				86-93
Estonia				90-93
Former German Democratic Republic			69-78	80-94
Georgia				89
Hungary		55-68	69-78	79-94
Latvia				88-93
Lithuania				88-94
Moldova				89
Poland		59-68	69-79	80-93
Romania		59-68	69-78	80-93
Russian Federation				88-93
Slovenia				85-94
Ukraine				85-92
Former USSR				85-90
Former Yugoslavia		60-67	68-78	79-90

Table 3.4   (continued)

Region and country/territory	ICD-6	ICD-7	ICD-8	ICD-9
Other Asia and Islands				
Hong Kong	55-57	58-68	69-78	79-89
Malaysia (Peninsular)			77-79	
Mauritius		57-68	69-80	81-94
Philippines		63-72	73-78, 81	
Republic of Korea				85-87
Sao Tome & Principe				85, 87
Seychelles				85-87
Singapore	55-57	58-68	69-78	79-89
Sri Lanka	50-57	58-68	77	80-86
Thailand	55-57	58-68	69-78	79-87
Sub-Saharan Africa				
South Africa				89-91
Latin America and the Carribean				
Anguilla			73, 75-76	
Antigua & Barbuda		61-64, 66	69-78	83
Argentina		66-68	69-70, 77-78	79-91
Bahamas			69, 71-72, 73-77, 79	80-81, 83-85, 87
Barbados	55-57	58-67	68-78	79-84, 85-88
Belize		64-67	68-79	80-84, 86
Bermuda		64-65, 67	68-78	
Brazil—Southern Region[3]				84-86
Brazil—Northern Region				86
British Virgin Islands			68-70, 75-78	81-82
Cayman Islands			73-74, 78-79	
Chile	54-57	58-67	68-79	80-89
Colombia	53-57	58-67	68-70, 72, 74-77	86, 91
Costa Rica	56-57	58-67	68-79	80-88
Cuba		59, 64-65	68-78	79-90
Dominica		61-62, 67-68	69-78	79-82, 84-85
Dominican Republic	56-57	58-63, 65-67	68-79	80-85
Ecuador		61.63-67	68-75, 77-78	79-80, 82, 84-88
El Salvador	50-57	58-67	68-74	81-84
French Guiana			68-78	79
Guadeloupe			74	81
Guyana			77	79, 84
Haiti				81
Honduras		66	68-78	79-82
Jamaica		60-61, 64-65, 67	77	84
Martinique			70-71, 73-75	81-82, 85
Mexico		55-67	68-78	79-90
Montserrat			79	
Netherland Antilles				81
Nicaragua		59, 61-65	68-69, 73-78	
Panama	54-57	58-67	68-79	79-87
Paraguay		61-63, 65-67	68-78	79-86

Table 3.4   (continued)

Region and country/territory	Years of available data			
	ICD-6	ICD-7	ICD-8	ICD-9
Peru		66-67	68-78	79-86
Puerto Rico	55-57	58-66	69-77	79-89
St. Kitts & Nevis		61-63, 65-67	69-78	79-85
St. Lucia			68, 72-73, 75-77	79-81, 83, 86-88
St. Vincent & Grenadines			70-72, 74, 77-79	82-83, 85-86
Suriname		63-66	71-73, 75-78	79-82, 84-85
Trinidad and Tobago	51-57	58-68	69-78	79-91
Turks & Caicos Islands			79	80, 87
Uruguay	55-57	58-60, 63-67	68-78	80-90
Venezuela	55-57	58-67	68-78	79-83, 85-89
Middle Eastern Crescent				
Armenia				88-92
Azerbaijan				89
Bahrain				85, 87-88
Egypt	54-57	58-67	70-79	80, 87
Israel			75-78	79-92
Iran (Cities)			74-75, 78-85, 87	
Kazakhstan		59-60, 62-66, 68	70-75, 78-79	88-93
Kuwait			72, 75-78	79-87
Kyrgyzstan				81-82, 85-90
Syria			73-78	80-81, 84-85
Tajikistan				91
Turkey			78-79, 81-84, 87	
Turkmenistan				89
Uzbekistan				91-92

Notes:

1   The GBD analysis was carried out for the geographical regions developed specifically by the World Bank for the *World Development Report 1993* (World Bank 1993).

2   The sixth revision of the ICD (ICD-6) was adopted in 1948, the seventh (ICD-7) in 1955, the eighth (ICD-8) in 1965, and the ninth (ICD-9) in 1975.

3   The Southern Region of Brazil includes those states for which vital registration data are reasonably complete and reliable.

Preventive Medicine established a sample monitoring system of causes of death in the early 1980s in a representative sample of counties called the Disease Surveillance Points (DSPs). By 1986 there were 69 DSPs, but an analysis in 1989 revealed that the points were biased towards richer counties, with poor rural counties being particularly under-represented. The system was subsequently expanded to 145 DSPs to provide a fully representative sample of counties (Yang et al. 1991). Overall, 10 million people living in urban and rural areas are covered by the system. At each surveillance point, a team that includes a physician investigates each death using medical records and interviews with family members to assign a cause of death. Deaths coded in the DSP system are assigned to a limited set of ICD-9 codes that approximates the Basic Tabulation List with some minor differences. Yang et al. (1991) have attempted to provide a correspondence mapping from the DSP codes to equivalent ICD BTL codes. In addition, China provides WHO with cause-of-death data collected from those counties that report ICD-coded vital registration data to the Ministry of Public Health. This system provides data on a large number of deaths; about 392 900 deaths in 1989 (World health Organization 1991). However, compared to the DSP system, the vital registration data are not adequately representative of poor urban or rural counties.

Another valuable source of data on causes of death in China are large-scale prospective or case-control studies being carried out to assess and monitor the effects of certain exposures, particularly cigarette smoking. One such study has investigated the causes of over 1.1 million deaths using medical records, interviews with families and health workers, and physician's diagnoses (R. Peto, personal communication). Only very limited results from this large undertaking were available at the time of writing this chapter.

India, like China, does not have complete vital registration and cause-of-death attribution. Two systems, however, provide information that can be used to assess causes of death. In urban areas, medically certified deaths which occur in hospitals are collated each year by the Office of the Registrar-General. In most states, however, the coverage of this system is low and the sample of deaths reported suffers from severe selection bias. In Maharashtra State, however, coverage of medical certification of causes of death is estimated to be at least 80 per cent (Government of India, Registrar-General 1992a). Manipur state also appears to have a high level of coverage. The Registrar-General collects and publishes the results for a subset of ICD-9 codes that approximates the BTL list. For this study, we were able to obtain these vital registration data for 1986–1990 through the kind collaboration of the Andhra Pradesh Burden of Disease Study (APBD) Team.

Because there is virtually no medical certification of causes of death in rural areas of India, in 1965 the Registrar-General initiated the Model Registration Scheme, a verbal autopsy sample registration system centred on Primary Health Centre (PHC) villages. The system was renamed the "Survey of Causes of Death (Rural)" (SCD(R)) in 1982 and by the 1990s covered over 1300 PHCs (Government of India, Registrar-General 1992b). The survey includes 21 000–23 000 deaths each year. Trained para-medical staff at selected Primary Health Centres contact local residents at regular intervals to ascertain whether there have been any births or deaths. The field workers use a standard protocol to collect information on symptoms prior to death in order to assign a cause of death to a limited set of categories. The assignment of causes of death for a sample of the diagnoses is reviewed by the Medical Officer of the Primary Health Centre. The protocol used to elicit symptoms, and the guidelines for assigning a cause to the rudimentary cause list, have not been independently validated. Moreover, the cause list in use does not correspond to ICD codes. To enhance the utility of the information from the SCD(R), the APBD undertook a follow-up study of 440 deaths coded to "Symptoms, signs and ill-defined conditions" in the SCD(R) in Andhra Pradesh State. Through their analysis, they were able to reassign 99 per cent of these ill-defined deaths to more specific categories. (P. Mahapatra and G.N.V. Ramana, personal communication)

POPULATION LABORATORIES

In parts of sub-Saharan Africa, Bangladesh, Pakistan and a few other countries, small populations have been intensively monitored in the context of so-called population laboratories, such as in Niakhar (Senegal) (Garenne et al. 1991), Farafenni (The Gambia) (deFrancisco et al. 1994), Navrongo (Ghana) (Ghana VAST Study Team 1993), Machakos (Kenya) (Omondi-Odhiambo et al. 1990), Morogoro, Hai and Dar es Salaam (AMMP 1993) and Matlab (Bangladesh) (D'Souza 1986). These population laboratories provide some information on causes of death based on a variety of verbal-autopsy methods. While providing some useful information on local patterns of causes of death, their usefulness for estimating regional patterns of causes of death is limited. In most cases, the cause-of-death list includes very general categories, with many deaths assigned to causes such as fevers, epilepsy or dropsy. Because the total population monitored is comparatively small, the number of deaths registered each year is small. Even after pooling data for many years, the information is rarely sufficient to estimate age-specific mortality, even for the three broad cause-of-death Groups; at best, child deaths can be distinguished from adult deaths. Because verbal-autopsy methods are probably more reliable for injury deaths, the population laboratories do provide some rough indication of the extent of injury deaths and their causes. Table 3.5 provides illustrative data from the registration areas in Hai, Morogoro and Dar es Salaam in Tanzania. Based on the description of the cause-of-death categories, we have grouped the deaths into approximations of Groups I, II and III. These data illustrate the type of broad observations for large aggregated age groups that are possible from such studies.

EPIDEMIOLOGICAL ESTIMATES

For a number of causes in several regions, epidemiologists have developed estimates of cause-specific mortality based on the natural history of a given disease. Incidence and/or prevalence estimates from surveys are combined with information on case-fatality rates for treated and untreated cases to yield approximate death rates. For some causes of death, such as lower respiratory infections, diarrhoea and malaria, surveys have been undertaken to measure more directly (with limited success) cause-specific mortality—see the relevant chapters in other volumes in this series.

Table 3.5 Distribution of deaths by broad cause Group in three population laboratories in Tanzania based on a verbal-autopsy system

Region	Age group (years)	Male deaths				Female deaths			
		Total	% Group I	% Group II	% Group III	Total	% Group I	% Group II	% Group III
Dar es Salaam	0–4	135	62.1	37.1	0.7	95	71.7	28.5	0.0
	5–14	33	60.6	36.4	3.0	22	63.4	22.5	13.6
	15–59	179	60.3	27.6	12.3	165	69.2	30.2	0.6
	60+	77	40.3	54.6	5.2	46	30.3	67.3	2.2
Morogoro rural	0–4	361	77.7	22.2	0.3	313	78.1	20.4	1.6
	5–14	82	73.1	28.1	6.1	76	73.5	19.6	6.6
	15–59	468	61.5	27.4	11.0	414	72.0	26.3	1.7
	60+	308	57.4	36.8	5.5	254	52.4	46.5	1.2
Hai	0–4	200	44.5	53.0	2.5	184	48.4	47.7	3.8
	5–14	46	26.1	54.4	19.6	35	48.7	43.1	8.6
	15–59	318	42.2	36.4	21.1	228	58.4	36.8	4.9
	60+	304	29.0	66.9	1.3	243	29.1	66.9	3.7
All three regions	0–4	696	65.1	33.9	1.0	592	67.8	30.2	2.0
	5–14	161	57.1	37.3	9.3	133	65.3	26.3	8.3
	15–59	965	54.9	30.4	14.6	807	67.6	30.1	2.4
	60+	689	43.0	52.1	3.6	543	40.1	57.4	2.4

Notes

• Percentages may not always sum to 100 due to rounding.

• Group I includes communicable, maternal, perinatal and nutritional conditions; Group II includes noncommunicable diseases; and Group III includes injuries.

The major limitation of epidemiological estimates is that they tend to over-estimate the amount of mortality from of a particular disease or condition. Thus, when epidemiological estimates for major causes of death are summed, the total number of deaths claimed often exceeds the plausible number of deaths from all causes based on demographic analyses. The tendency of epidemiological estimates to be over-estimates can be traced to several sources of bias. First, because many deaths are multi-causal, they are often fully attributed to more than one cause in epidemiological assessments. Second, when there is uncertainty as to incidence, prevalence, or case-fatality rates, analysts tend to err on the side of higher rates despite frequent claims to the contrary. Third, because epidemiological assessments are usually undertaken without consideration of other causes of death, authors of epidemiological assessments are often unaware of the comparative magnitude of their claims of mortality. Epidemiological assessments of the magnitude of health problems can be very informative but, when considered independently of other causes of death and disability, they can be misleading. In the methods section, we describe the efforts undertaken in this study to use constructively the information from epidemiological assessments.

CAUSE-OF-DEATH MODELS

Where no vital registration, sample registration or epidemiological estimates are available, cause-of-death models may be helpful to estimate patterns. Indirect techniques to estimate cause-of-death structure were first developed by Preston (1976) who modelled the relationship between total mortality and cause-specific mortality for twelve broad groups of causes, based on an analysis of historical vital registration data for industrialized countries and a few developing countries. In particular, cause-specific mortality was postulated to be a linear function of total mortality. Preston's work has formed the basis of nearly all subsequent approaches to estimating cause-of-death patterns in regions without vital registration. Typically, these refinements have involved estimating equations for specific age groups, incorporating more recent data or examining more detailed causes (Bulutao 1993, Hakulinen et al. 1986, Hull et al. 1981, Lopez and Hull 1983, Murray et al. 1992).

These previous attempts to use models to estimate cause-of-death patterns in regions or countries without reliable data have been hampered by a number of concerns, including the diversity of cause-of-death patterns by age and sex, the limited range of reliable observations on cause-of-death structure at high mortality levels, the analytical complications created by the use of Chapter XVI of the ICD-9 ("Symptoms, signs and ill-defined conditions"), and the true functional form of the relationship between cause-specific mortality and all-cause mortality. We have endeavoured to address each of these limitations in the models developed for this study and these approaches are outlined below. In view of the requirements of the GBD to estimate cause-of-death patterns by age and sex for

GLOBAL BURDEN OF DISEASE AND INJURY SERIES

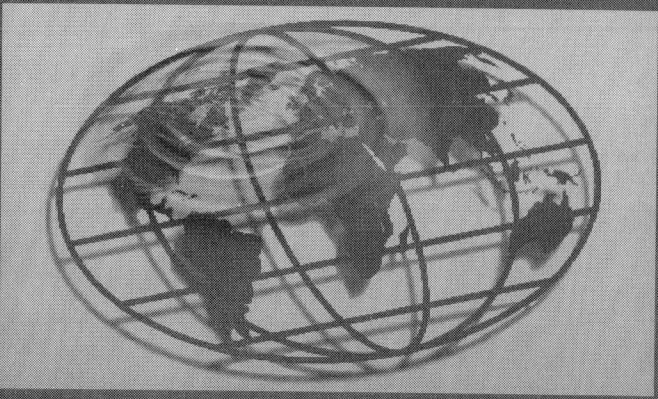

THE GLOBAL
BURDEN OF DISEASE

EDITED BY

CHRISTOPHER J. L. MURRAY
ALAN D. LOPEZ

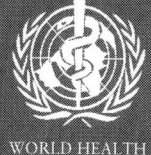

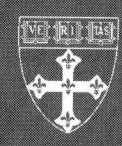

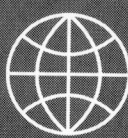

WORLD HEALTH
ORGANIZATION

HARVARD SCHOOL OF
PUBLIC HEALTH

WORLD
BANK

Annex Table 2, continued.

GBD Classification Code	Cause group, disease, injury, or sequela
IA5	Childhood-cluster diseases
IA5a	Pertussis
IA5a-1	Episodes
IA5a-2	Mental retardation
IA5b	Poliomyelitis
IA5b-1	Lameness
IA5c	Diphtheria
IA5c-1	Episodes
IA5c-2	Neurological complications
IA5c-3	Myocarditis
IA5d	Measles
IA5d-1	Episodes
IA5e	Tetanus
IA5e-1	Episodes
IA6	Bacterial meningitis and meningococcaemia
IA6-1	All forms – episodes
IA6-2	Streptococcus pneumoniae – episodes
IA6-3	Haemophilus influenzae – episodes
IA6-4	Neisseria meningitidis – episodes
IA6-5	Meningococcaemia without meningitis – episodes
IA6-6	Deafness
IA6-7	Seizure disorder
IA6-8	Motor deficit
IA6-9	Mental retardation
IA7	Hepatitis B and hepatitis C
IA7-1	Episodes
IA7-2	Cirrhosis of the liver – symptomatic cases
IA7-3	Hepatoma
IA8	Malaria
IA8-1	Episodes
IA8-2	Anaemia
IA8-3	Neurological sequelae
IA9	Tropical-cluster diseases
IA9a	Trypanosomiasis
IA9a-1	Episodes
IA9b	Chagas disease
IA9b-1	Infection
IA9b-2	Cardiomyopathy without congestive heart failure
IA9b-3	Cardiomyopathy with congestive heart failure
IA9b-4	Megaviscera
IA9c	Schistosomiasis
IA9c-1	Infection
IA9d	Leishmaniasis
IA9d-1	Visceral
IA9d-2	Cutaneous
IA9e	Lymphatic filariasis
IA9e-1	Hydrocele > 15 cm0
IA9e-2	Bancroftian lymphoedema
IA9e-3	Brugian lymphoedema
IA9f	Onchocerciasis
IA9f-1	Blindness

Annex Table 2. **Cause groups, diseases and injuries, and sequelae included in the Global Burden of Disease Study**

GBD Classification Code	Cause group, disease, injury, or sequela
I	Communicable, maternal, perinatal, and nutritional conditions
IA	Infectious and parasitic diseases
IA1	Tuberculosis
IA1-1	HIV sero-negative cases
IA1-2	HIV sero-positive cases
IA2	Sexually transmitted diseases excluding HIV
IA2a	Syphilis
IA2a-1	Congenital syphilis
IA2a-2	Low birth weight
IA2a-3	Primary
IA2a-4	Secondary
IA2a-5	Tertiary – cardiovascular
IA2a-6	Tertiary – gummas
IA2a-7	Tertiary – neurologic
IA2b	Chlamydia
IA2b-1	Ophthalmia neonatorum
IA2b-2	Low birth weight
IA2b-3	Corneal scar – blindness
IA2b-4	Corneal scar – low vision
IA2b-5	Cervicitis
IA2b-6	Neonatal pneumonia
IA2b-7	Pelvic inflammatory disease
IA2b-8	Ectopic pregnancy
IA2b-9	Tubo-ovarian abscess
IA2b-10	Chronic pelvic pain
IA2b-11	Infertility
IA2b-12	Symptomatic urethritis
IA2b-13	Epididymitis
IA2b-14	Stricture
IA2c	Gonorrhoea
IA2c-1	Ophthalmia neonatorum
IA2c-2	Low birth weight
IA2c-3	Corneal scar – blindness
IA2c-4	Corneal scar – low vision
IA2c-5	Cervicitis
IA2c-6	Pelvic inflammatory disease
IA2c-7	Ectopic pregnancy
IA2c-8	Tubo-ovarian abscess
IA2c-9	Chronic pelvic pain
IA2c-10	Infertility
IA2c-11	Symptomatic urethritis
IA2c-12	Epididymitis
IA2c-13	Stricture
IA3	HIV
IA3-1	Cases
IA3-2	AIDS
IA4	Diarrhoeal diseases
IA4-1	Episodes

several broad age groups, cause-of-death models were developed separately for males and females for each of the seven age groups: 0–4 years, 5–14, 15–29, 30–44, 45–59, 60–69, and 70 and over.[4] One of the most important problems with cause-of-death models is that there are few recent reliable observations of cause-of-death structure for populations with moderate to high mortality levels. Not coincidentally, those countries with complete vital registration coverage and medical certification are usually countries with low mortality; yet, the need to use models to approximate cause-of-death structure is greatest in high mortality populations. Studies, such as those by Hakulinen et al. (1986) and Bulutao (1993), have estimated cause-of-death models based only on observations from Established Market Economies and a small number of countries from Latin America and the Caribbean in the 1980s. These models are then used to make predictions for countries or regions with all-cause mortality rates far outside the range of those for the countries included in the dataset. Not surprisingly, the estimates for diseases such as tuberculosis and malaria based on these models are implausibly low (Bulutao 1993). The range of mortality rates represented in the dataset can be expanded by using historical data. For example, Preston (1976) used cause-of-death data from 1861–1964 to estimate relationships for 12 broad causes. Using older data, however, raises other issues; the quality of diagnosis and coding, and the the structure of International Classification of Diseases have changed considerably over the past century. In addition, the advent of major new health technologies may have altered the cause-of-death structures at some levels of total mortality. The focus of the last decade and a half on enhancing child survival through mass immunization and the application of a limited number of effective health interventions may have substantially altered the mixture of causes at some levels of all-cause mortality.

For this study, we selected two different datasets: one for the estimation of models for Groups I, II and III as a function of all-cause mortality in a given age-sex group, and another for estimating models for more detailed causes, e.g. cardiovascular disease, as a function of mortality for the respective Group. To estimate the relationships between the three large cause Groups and all-cause mortality, we have chosen to use the subset of countries given in Table 3.4 for which we are confident that vital registration coverage is 90 per cent or better. To expand the range of all-cause mortality rates included in the analysis, we have used recent observations from 67 countries and supplemented this information with the oldest data sets available for the 36 countries for which reliable data were available before 1965. Data prior to 1965 have been coded according to ICD-6 or ICD-7. We suspect that bridge coding between these older revisions of the ICD and ICD-9 for Group I, Group II and Group III is reasonable—a conversion system is provided in Table 3.2.

Differences between populations or within a population over time in the proportion of deaths assigned to ICD-9 Chapter XVI ("Symptoms, signs and ill-defined conditions") or its equivalent in previous revisions of the ICD can create spurious relationships between cause-specific mortality and total mortality. For example, Preston (1976) reported a negative coefficient for the regression between cardiovascular disease and total mortality in adult age groups—he chose to correct for this finding by analysing the trend in the other and ill-defined category. As noted above, we have chosen to redistribute deaths coded to ICD-9 Chapter XVI at ages over 5 years proportionately across all known Group II causes and in the age group 0–4 proportionately across Group I causes. These poorly coded deaths were thus redistributed *before* estimating the regression equations.

Figure 3.5 shows the mortality rate for Group I plotted against total mortality rate for males aged 30–44 years using a log-log scale. The relationship is well represented by a straight line. As all-cause mortality increases, Group I mortality rate increases at a faster rate—a 10 per cent increase in all-cause mortality is accompanied by a 17 per cent increase in Group I mortality. Ordinary least squares regression of Group I mortality rates on total mortality rates are likely to give biased predictions, particularly at higher mortality. We have, therefore, estimated equations of the form similar to that shown in Figure 3.5, namely:

Figure 3.5   Group I and all-cause mortality rates in males aged 30–44 for 103 national populations with reliable cause-of-death registration

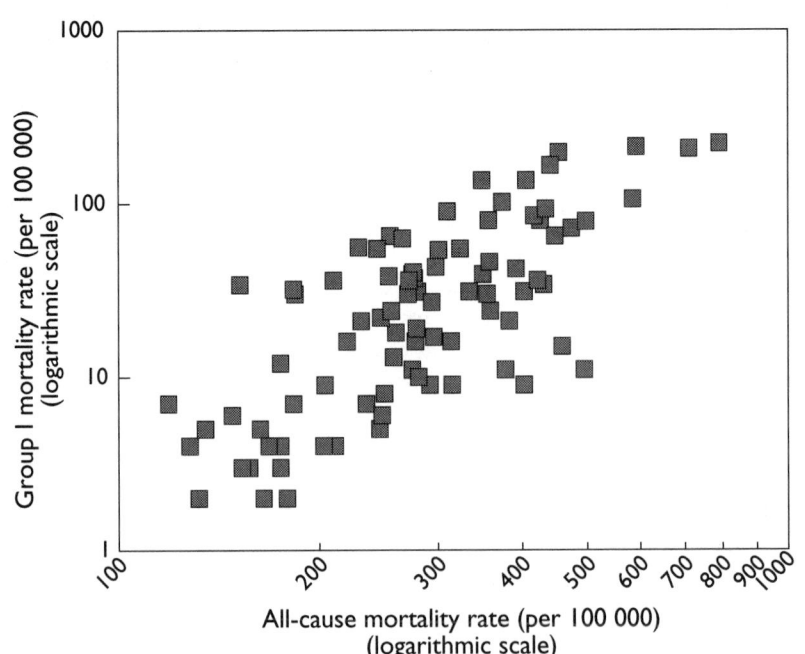

All-cause mortality rate (per 100 000)
(logarithmic scale)

$$\ln M_{a,k,i} = \beta_{a,k,i} \ln M_{a,k,t} + C_{a,k,i}$$

where $M_{a,k,i}$ is mortality in age group a, sex k and cause Group i, $M_{a,k,t}$ is all-cause mortality in age group a and sex k, $\beta_{a,k,i}$ is the age, sex and cause-specific regression coefficient and $C_{a,k,i}$ is an age, sex and cause-specific constant. The equations have been estimated for seven age groups: 0–4 years, 5–14, 15–29, 30–44, 45–59, 60–69, and 70 and over.

Table 3.6 shows the coefficients and slopes (with standard errors) and the proportion of variation explained for Groups I, II and III for each age and sex group. For 10 of the 14 age-sex groups, the R^2 for Group I exceeds 40 per cent, for all age-sex groups the R^2 for Group II exceeds 40 per cent, and for 4 of the 14 age-sex groups, the R^2 for Group III exceeds 40 per cent. It is clear that for all but a few age groups, only a small proportion of the variation in Group III causes is related to the level of all-cause mortality. In the age group 70 years and over, the relationships for Group I and Group III are particularly weak. These weak relationships are perhaps not surprising, because in this age group the basic cause-of-death data for Group II are the least reliable and Group II dominates mortality in that age group in nearly every population. The regression coefficients indicate the percentage change in death rates for a Group which might be expected for a unit percentage change in all-cause mortality. The highest coefficient, for Group I causes in females aged 30–44 is 2.54, implying that a 10 per cent increase in all-cause mortality in females aged 30–44 would be accompanied by a 25.4 per cent increase in Group I mortality. Interestingly, there are no negative coefficients. In other words, at the Group level, mortality rates all rise as all-cause mortality rises (and fall as all-cause mortality falls). This finding is in sharp contrast to the notion that, with the epidemiological transition, death *rates* from non-communicable diseases *rise* as all-cause mortality declines. In fact, among the adult age groups, the lowest slope for Group II was estimated for males aged 15–29 where a 1 per cent decline in all-cause mortality is associated with a 0.8 per cent decline in Group II mortality.

Preston (1976) earlier observed the convenient property that if total mortality is split into three causes (say A, B and C), then in linear regressions of A, B and C on total mortality, the sum of the slopes will always be 1. Put another way, the sum of predicted mortality for causes A, B and C will be equal to total mortality. Unfortunately, the sum of predicted mortality for Groups I, II and III based on the logarithmic forms of the equations does not equal total mortality. When using these equations to predict Group mortality from total mortality we have, therefore, adjusted the predictions so that they sum to total mortality using the following equation:

$$M_{a,k,i}^* = \frac{M_{a,k,i}}{M_{a,k,I} + M_{a,k,II} + M_{a,k,III}} M_{a,k,t}$$

Table 3.6   Results of regression analysis of cause Group mortality on
all-cause mortality by age and sex based on 103
observations from 67 countries, 1950–1991

Cause Group	Sex	Age group (years)	R² (%)	Intercept	Standard error of intercept	X-coefficient	Standard error of X-coefficient
Group I	Female	0–4	97	-2.352	0.061	1.308	0.010
Group I	Female	5–14	73	-4.809	0.169	1.802	0.050
Group I	Female	15–29	73	-6.481	0.226	2.027	0.056
Group I	Female	30–44	70	-9.877	0.350	2.454	0.072
Group I	Female	45–59	49	-10.148	0.591	2.103	0.096
Group I	Female	60–69	44	-7.213	0.557	1.526	0.076
Group I	Female	70+	13	-3.335	0.929	1.010	0.115
Group II	Female	0–4	53	2.059	0.111	0.453	0.019
Group II	Female	5–14	83	-0.162	0.059	0.858	0.017
Group II	Female	15–29	82	-0.563	0.081	0.960	0.020
Group II	Female	30–44	93	0.161	0.054	0.907	0.011
Group II	Female	45–59	97	-0.020	0.047	0.984	0.008
Group II	Female	60–69	99	-0.025	0.034	0.993	0.005
Group II	Female	70+	97	-0.190	0.061	1.014	0.008
Group III	Female	0–4	24	0.276	0.218	0.466	0.037
Group III	Female	5–14	41	0.323	0.099	0.547	0.029
Group III	Female	15–29	28	0.611	0.169	0.589	0.042
Group III	Female	30–44	19	0.348	0.248	0.544	0.051
Group III	Female	45–59	7	0.588	0.441	0.444	0.072
Group III	Female	60–69	5	1.207	0.509	0.347	0.070
Group III	Female	70+	11	-0.819	0.674	0.632	0.084
Group I	Male	0–4	96	-2.253	0.072	1.287	0.012
Group I	Male	5–14	67	-5.712	0.227	1.903	0.061
Group I	Male	15–29	28	-5.275	0.501	1.421	0.103
Group I	Male	30–44	56	-6.854	0.368	1.680	0.067
Group I	Male	45–59	32	-7.689	0.727	1.645	0.107
Group I	Male	60–69	21	-4.931	0.809	1.205	0.102
Group I	Male	70+	2	1.378	1.145	0.469	0.134
Group II	Male	0–4	54	2.007	0.116	0.469	0.019
Group II	Male	5–14	80	-0.487	0.074	0.904	0.020
Group II	Male	15–29	46	-0.124	0.178	0.773	0.037
Group II	Male	30–44	87	-0.060	0.086	0.911	0.016
Group II	Male	45–59	93	-0.096	0.084	0.987	0.012
Group II	Male	60–69	97	-0.246	0.063	1.018	0.008
Group II	Male	70+	95	-0.618	0.093	1.062	0.011
Group III	Male	0–4	26	0.205	0.232	0.509	0.038
Group III	Male	5–14	50	0.337	0.111	0.675	0.030
Group III	Male	15–29	64	-0.536	0.162	1.012	0.033
Group III	Male	30–44	68	-1.269	0.171	1.035	0.031
Group III	Male	45–59	30	-1.803	0.426	0.938	0.063
Group III	Male	60–69	9	0.858	0.541	0.493	0.069
Group III	Male	70+	9	-0.685	0.797	0.667	0.093

where $M^*_{a,k,i}$ is the adjusted mortality rate for age group a, sex k and cause Group i, and $M_{a,k,i}$ is the predicted mortality rate for age group a, sex k and cause Group i, and where I, II, III and t represent cause Groups I, II and III, and all causes, respectively.

As discussed below in the methods section, there are a number of situations where we would like to be able to compare an observed pattern of Group-specific mortality rates with those predicted by these models and also to measure the extent to which the two differ. To investigate the probability distribution of predicted values for each Group, we have used Monte Carlo simulation.[5] For each mortality level for each age and sex group, we defined a probability distribution for the coefficients and constants for Groups I, II and III, using a normal distribution with the mean equal to the estimated X-coefficient from the regression and the standard deviation equal to the standard error from the regression. Eight thousand simulations were run where a coefficient and constant for each Group was chosen from the probability distribution and these values were used to predict the sizes of Groups I, II and III, respectively. Each set of predictions was then adjusted so that the sum of Groups I, II and III was equal to the total mortality using the equation above. This procedure yielded 8,000 predicted values for each age, sex and cause Group at each mortality level. For this large set of predicted values we then calculated the standard deviation and confidence interval for predictions. As an example, Figure 3.6 shows the expected value for Group I for males aged 5–14 and the -2 and +2 standard deviation predictions. The width of the interval between plus and minus 2 standard deviations increases dramatically as

Figure 3.6 Predicted per cent of mortality due to Group I causes as a function of the all-cause mortality rate in males aged 5–14.

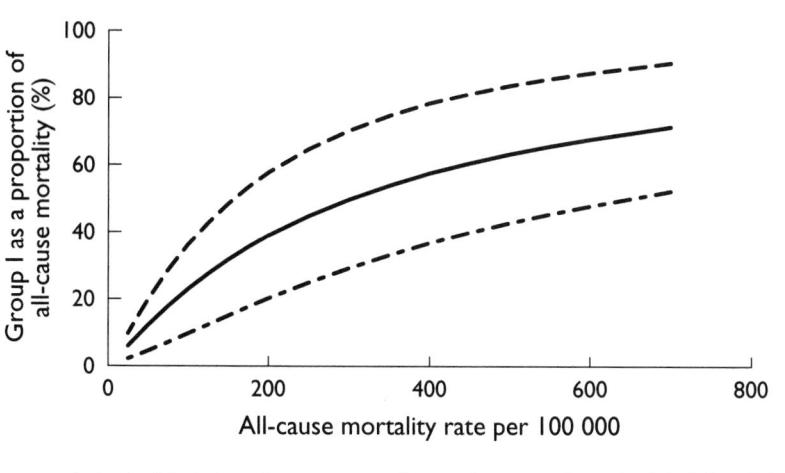

Group I as a proportion of all-cause mortality (%)

All-cause mortality rate per 100 000

- - - 2 standard deviations above ——— Expected - - - 2 standard deviations below

all-cause mortality increases from 25 per 100 000 to 200 per 100 000 and then is relatively constant at higher mortality rates.

A new family of cause-of-death models can be defined by choosing a particular number of standard deviations from the expected value that will be used for prediction. For example, if there are some data to suggest that Group I in SSA is likely to be 2.5 standard deviations higher than predicted by the models at a given mortality level, a value 2.5 standard deviations above the expected value can be used as an SSA model at all mortality levels. Annex Table 5 provides the reader with the predicted proportion of total mortality for Groups I, II and III and predictions for 3, 2, 1, -1, -2, and -3 standard deviations. This Annex table can be used to determine how deviant an observed population is compared with the aggregate experience of the set of countries embodied in the cause-of-death models.

In addition to models predicting Group-specific mortality from all-cause age-specific mortality, in rare situations we have also used models to predict the age-specific mortality rates for more detailed causes. Because of variations in coding practices among countries, we suspect that models for more detailed causes of death are less reliable than for the major Groups. Given the uncertainties in reliably mapping between the various revisions of the ICD for detailed causes, we have only used ICD-9 coded mortality data for estimating these detailed cause regressions. For each detailed cause in Table 3.1, we have estimated the following equation relating cause-specific mortality to the corresponding Group mortality:

$$\ln M_{a,k,j} = \beta_{a,k,j} \ln M_{a,k,i} + C_{a,k,j}$$

where $M_{a,k,j}$ is the mortality rate for age group a, sex k and detailed cause j, $M_{a,k,i}$ is the mortality rate for age group a, sex k and Group i, $\beta_{a,k,j}$ is an age, sex and cause-specific regression coefficient and $C_{a,k,j}$ is an age, sex and cause-specific constant. We have chosen to use a log-log form of the equation so that, as mortality declines, we do not arrive at predictions of zero or negative mortality from certain causes (such predictions might emerge using linear forms of the relationship).[6] As noted in the methods section, these small cause regressions are not used for the global or regional estimates presented here.

METHODS

The sequential procedure for estimating age, sex, region and cause-specific mortality can be divided into four steps: (1) generating preliminary estimates largely from vital registration and sample registration data; (2) correcting selected cause-groups using specific methods; (3) adjusting cause-specific mortality for selected causes based on epidemiological analyses; and (4) carrying out final adjustments as required so that the sum of cause-specific mortality rates equals total age-specific mortality. Each of

Table 3.7 Sources used to estimate mortality by cause for each region in 1990

| | Vital registration (% coverage) | | | Sample registration[1] | |
	Under 5 years	5 years and over	TOTAL	Urban	Rural
EME	99	99	99		
FSE	99	99	99		
IND				ICD	SCD(R)
CHN				DSP	DSP
OAI	2.1	13.6	10.2		
SSA	0.4	1.7	1.1		
LAC	27.6	47.2	42.6		
MEC	12.3	27.1	21.8		

[1] *Abbreviations:*	ICD	=	ICD-9 coded medically certified hospital deaths in Maharashtra state
	SCD(R)	=	Survey of Causes of Death (Rural)
	DSP	=	Disease Surveillance Point System

these steps is explained on a region by region basis in the following sections since the approaches used often differed by region. Table 3.7 summarizes the information used to generate the final estimates.

PRELIMINARY ESTIMATES

For EME and FSE, preliminary estimates were derived solely from vital registration data. Cause-specific deaths have been adjusted proportionately to equal regional total deaths in each age group because some countries with comparatively small populations, such as Iceland, Luxembourg and Albania, had not been included in the cause-of-death data, and in order to adjust for changes in total death numbers due to population changes between the last year of data available and 1990 (the base year for the estimates).

For China, preliminary estimates were calculated using 1991 Disease Surveillance Points data. Unfortunately, prior to 1991 the new DSPs which were added to make the system more representative of poorer areas were not fully functional. Detailed returns for later years have not yet become available. In total, detailed information was available for 52 734 deaths out of a population of 10 million. These included 10 906 deaths in urban DSPs and 41 828 deaths in rural DSPs. Follow-up studies undertaken by the Chinese Academy of Preventive Medicine suggest an under-registration of about 10 per cent in urban areas and 15 per cent in rural areas. To estimate the number of deaths due to each cause in each age-sex group for the entire population of China, taking into account the relative rates of under-registration and the population distribution between urban and rural areas, we have used the following equation:

$$D_{a,k,j}^{China} = D_{a,k,t}^{China} \left(\frac{1.10 \, D_{a,k,j}^{DSPURBAN} + 1.15 \, D_{a,k,j}^{DSPRURAL}}{1.10 \, D_{a,k,t}^{DSPURBAN} + 1.15 \, D_{a,k,t}^{DSPRURAL}} \right)$$

where $D_{a,k,j}^{China}$ is the estimated number of deaths from cause j in age group a and sex k in China, $D_{a,k,t}^{China}$ is the number of deaths from all causes in China in age group a and sex k, $D_{a,k,j}^{DSPURBAN}$ is the number of deaths registered in the urban DSPs for cause j in age group a and sex k, $D_{a,k,j}^{DSPRURAL}$ is the number of deaths registered in the rural DSPs for cause j in age group a and sex k, $D_{a,k,t}^{DSPURBAN}$ and $D_{a,k,t}^{DSPRURAL}$ are the number of deaths from all causes in urban and rural DSPs, respectively. For some causes in specific age-sex groups, there were fewer than five deaths. When inflated to national estimates for China, a single death in the DSPs may appear as several hundred deaths. Due to a small-numbers effect, the age-specific rates for some of the these causes are not reliable. We have attempted to correct for this effect as described below.

For India, preliminary estimates for urban areas were derived from the Maharashtra ICD-9 Medical Certification of Causes of Death database (described earlier) inflated to the estimated urban deaths in each age and sex group based on the Sample Registration Scheme.[7] Estimates of mortality by cause in rural areas were based on the Survey of Causes of Death (Rural) results for 1991–1993, corrected on the basis of the Andhra Pradesh SCD(R) validation study and on the epidemiological adjustments made to the SCD(R) results by the Andhra Pradesh Burden of Disease Study (APBD). The resulting estimated structure of mortality by cause for each age group was then inflated to equal the estimated number of rural deaths in India based on the Sample Registration Scheme. All India estimates were then obtained as the sum of the urban and rural estimates of mortality by cause.

In the four remaining regions, LAC, OAI, MEC and SSA, some vital registration data are available but many deaths are not captured by existing systems (see Table 3.7). Those deaths that are registered cannot be considered as representative of mortality for the entire region. The major challenge for these regions was then to estimate the cause-of-death structure in the residual areas not covered by vital registration systems. Cause-of-death models could be used to help estimate the division of total mortality into the three broad Groups if the overall death rate in the residual areas could be estimated. The regional demographic estimates provide an assessment of total deaths in each age group. Subtracting registered deaths from this total gives the absolute number of deaths expected in the residual area in each region, but the denominator, i.e. the population of the residual areas, is not known. To address this problem, we have developed a two-stage procedure: first we estimated the total mortality rate in the residual areas, and then we used the probability models of cause-of-death structure and the deviation pattern in the registered areas to estimate the Group I, II and III distribution of causes for each age-sex group.

LORENZ CURVE METHOD

To estimate the mortality rate in the residual areas of a region, we have developed an approach based on two hypotheses. First, deaths are assumed to be unevenly distributed across geographic subunits of a population. Second, those geographic subunits that have functioning vital registration systems are likely to have a higher socio-economic status and to have lower mortality rates than those areas without vital registration systems. One way of representing an unequal distribution of a quantity such as income across groups or individuals, often used by economists, is a Lorenz curve. Figure 3.7 shows the relationship between the proportion of the population covered on the x-axis as one moves from geographic units with the lowest mortality rate to the highest mortality rate. On the y-axis, the cumulative proportion of deaths covered, as each geographic subunit is added, is shown. If the death rates in all geographic subunits were identical, the curve would be a straight line from the origin to 100 per cent coverage of deaths and population. The more unequal the distribution of mortality is across geographic subunits, the more the curve will bow towards the bottom right of the Figure. In practice such a curve is constructed by ranking geographic subunits (regions or states) from the lowest to highest mortality rates. As the next lowest mortality region is considered, the percentage of all deaths occurring in that region is added to the cumulative total of deaths on the y-axis and the percentage of total population living in that region is added to the cumulative proportion of population shown on the x-axis. In this

Figure 3.7   Hypothetical set of geographic Lorenz curves for mortality

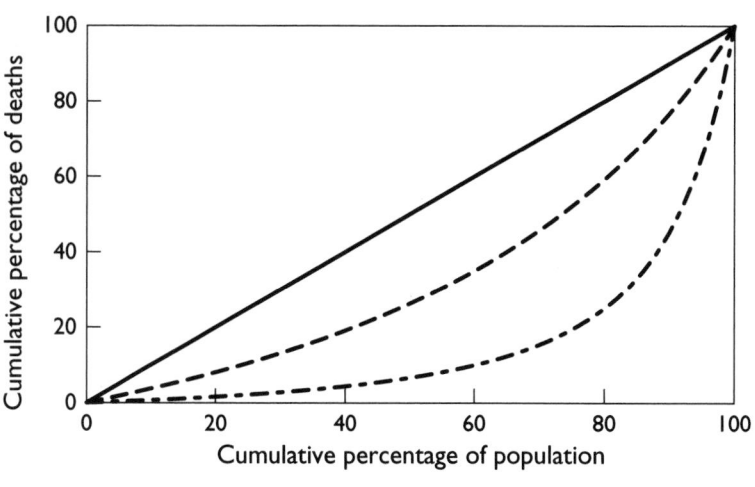

manner, the populations and deaths in each subunit are progressively added until all populations and deaths have been included.

Using mortality and population data for the 50 states of the USA in 1988 (NCHS 1990), 28 major provinces of China based on the 1982 Census,[8] the 16 largest states of India based on data from the Sample Registration System for 1991 (Registrar-General 1992), and 32 states of Mexico in 1990,[9] we have constructed Lorenz curves for mortality for six age groups (0–4, 5–14, 15–29, 30–44, 45–59, 60 years and over) and for both sexes. Figure 3.8 illustrates the curves for each of these groups. A number of interesting findings from the graphs deserve comment. In children, there are considerable differences between India, Mexico, China and the United States in the inequality of death distribution by geographic subunits. For both boys and girls, inequalities in child mortality appear greatest in China, followed by India then Mexico and finally the United States. Inequality is approximately the same for male and female children, despite the fact that in most places male mortality at ages 0–4 is greater than female mortality at these ages. Beginning with the age group 5–14 years, and becoming more pronounced at older ages, two major patterns emerge. First, after age 15, there is remarkably little inequality by geographic subunit and the inequality that is present is nearly identical in countries as different as the United States and India. Second, at all ages, the inequality of death distribution across geographic subunits is greater in females than in males of the same age. In females, for all age groups, the most unequal distribution of mortality by geographic subunit is found in China.

The finding that adult males in the United States, India, China and Mexico have nearly identical Lorenz curves of death distribution by geographic subunit is difficult to explain. The scale of the geographic subdivision in each country is different; in India the average state size is close to 50 million while in the United States the average state size is five million. One suspects that if the data were available for counties in China, we might find the exact same Lorenz curve constructed with county-level mortality data for any province in China. While we must await an adequate theory explaining this finding, the similarity of Lorenz curves across countries for each of the adult age groups is convenient for our purposes, as we use this relationship to estimate mortality rates in the residual areas of each of the regions with vital registration data.

These empirical Lorenz curves can be well represented by a function of the form:

$$y = c_2(e^{\frac{x}{c_1 - x}} - 1) \quad \text{where} \quad c_2 = \frac{1}{e^{\frac{1}{(c_1-1)}} - 1}$$

where y is the cumulative proportion of deaths, x is the cumulative proportion of population, c_1 is a constant, and c_2 is used in the equation to simplify the notation and is a simple transformation of c_1. The degree of convexity of the curve is determined solely by the value of c_1. The lower

Figure 3.8   Geographic Lorenz curves for mortality in the United
States, Mexico, China and India

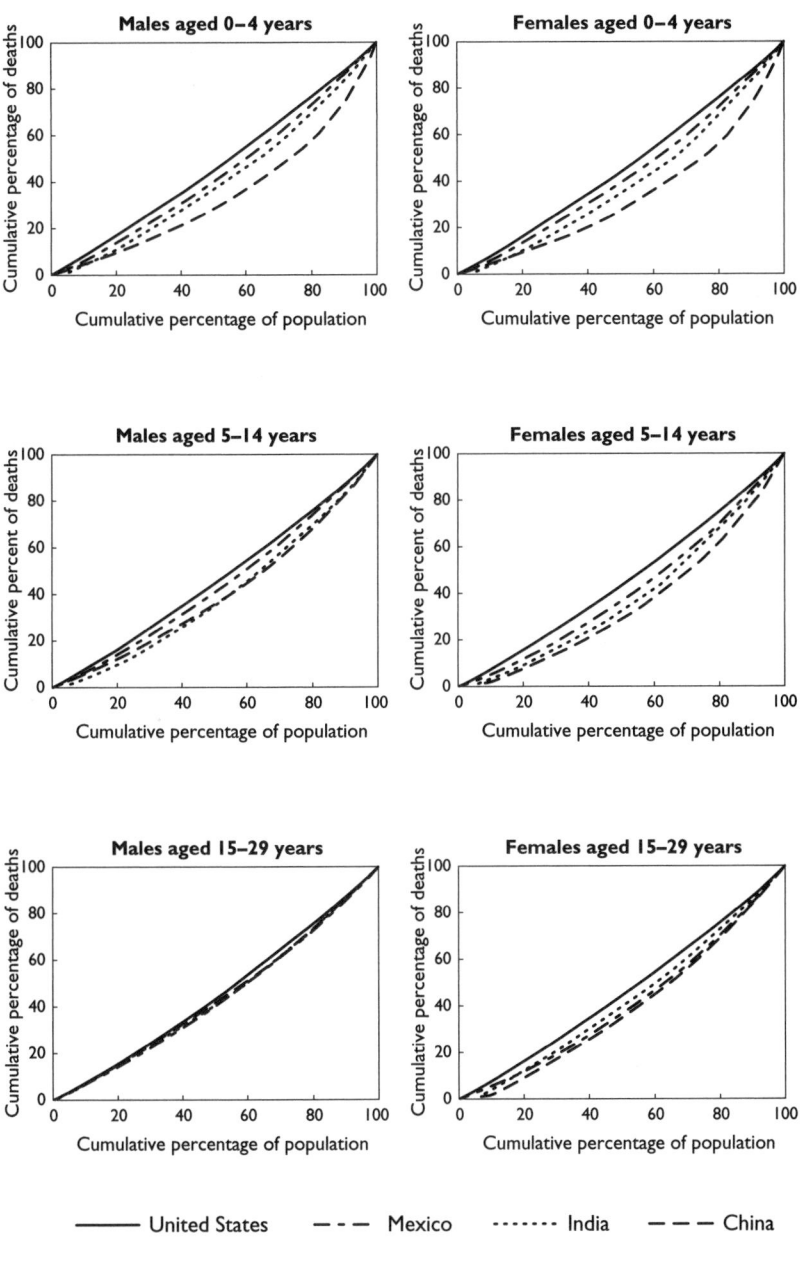

Figure 3.8   (continued)

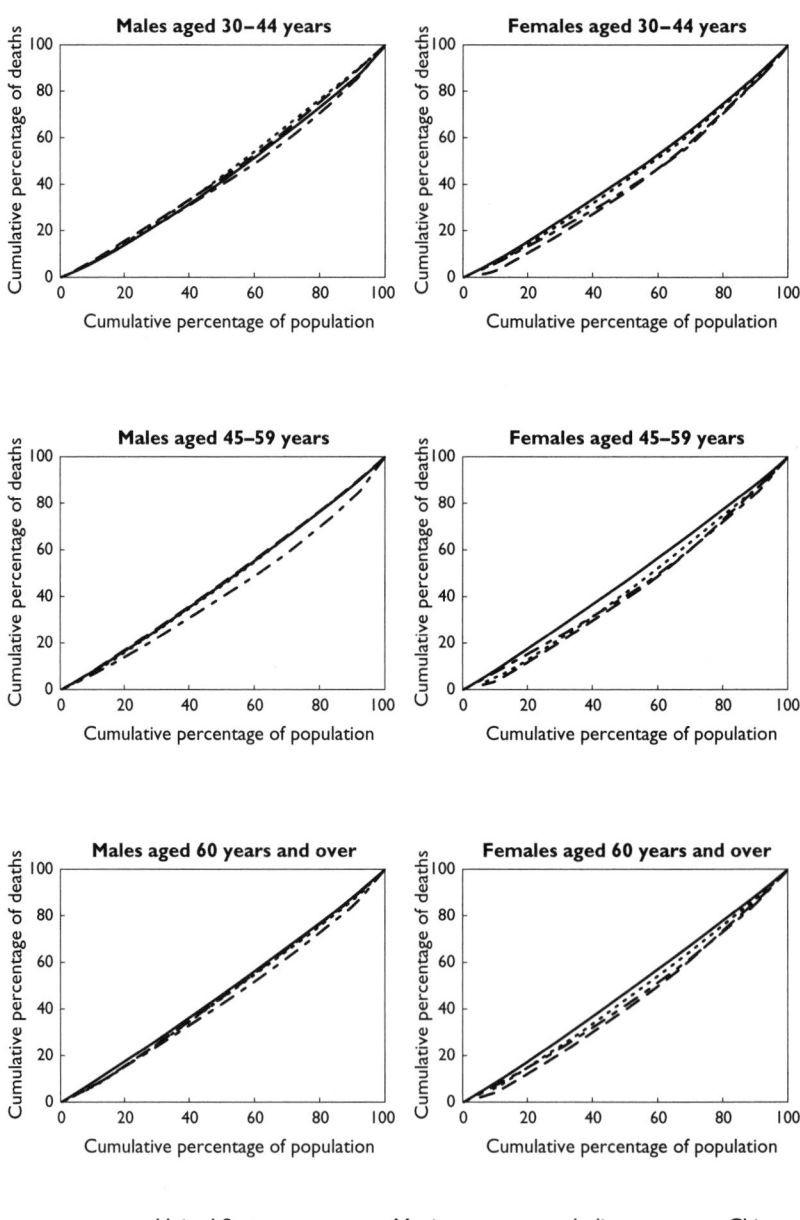

Table 3.8   Least squares estimates for c_1 and c_2 based on data for India, China and Mexico

Age group (years)	c_1	c_2
Males		
0–4	2.96	1.50
5–14	3.53	2.06
15–29	4.65	3.17
30–44	5.00	3.52
45–59	5.52	4.04
60–69	5.89	4.41
70+	5.89	4.41
Females		
0–4	2.81	1.36
5–14	2.80	1.35
15–29	3.34	1.88
30–44	3.68	2.21
45–59	4.25	2.78
60–69	4.76	3.28
70+	4.76	3.28

the value of c_1 the greater the inequality of death distribution by geographic subunits. As we intended to apply this method in developing regions only, we have estimated values of c_1 using the data from India, China and Mexico, excluding the United States. Table 3.8 shows the estimates of c_1 (and, by inference, c_2) based on minimum least squares methods. Excluding the United States makes a significant difference to the estimate of c_1 for males and females at ages 0–4, and for females aged 5–14 and 15–29 as well.

For LAC, MEC, OAI and SSA, we have used the Lorenz curve method to estimate total mortality in the residual areas for each age and sex group. Knowing the percentage of regional deaths recorded in the registration areas, we use the Lorenz curve for the appropriate age group to estimate the population covered in the registration area. The above equation can be rearranged so that the cumulative proportion of population (x) is a function of the cumulative proportion of deaths (y), as follows:

$$x = \frac{c_1 \ln \left(\dfrac{y + c_2}{c_2} \right)}{1 + \ln \left(\dfrac{y + c_2}{c_2} \right)}$$

The death rate in each residual area is easily calculated by subtracting the deaths and population, respectively for the registration area (estimated from the above equation) from the regional totals for deaths and popula-

Figure 3.9   Number of standard deviations by which recorded cause-
Group mortality rates for LAC registration areas deviate
from predictions of cause-of-death models

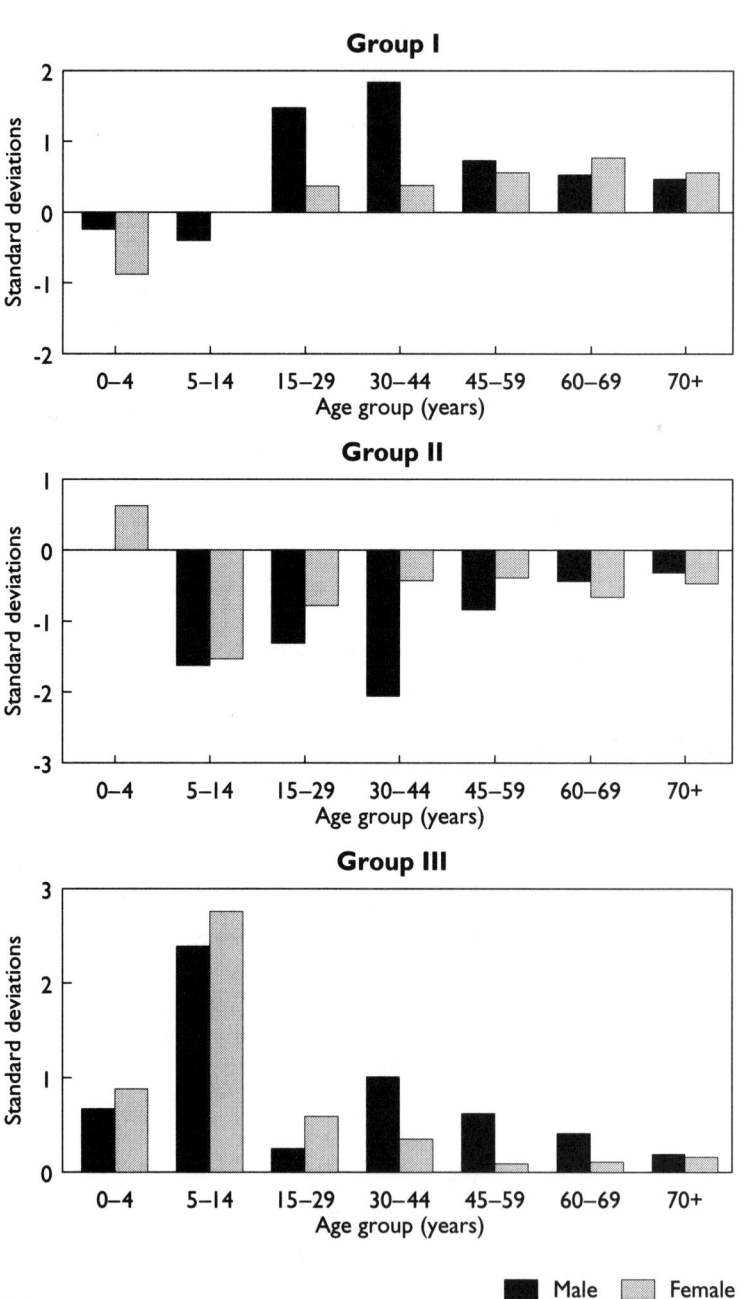

tion. Estimates of deaths and population in the residual areas of each region were then used to calculate the all-cause mortality rate for each age and sex group.

For the registration areas, we have compared the recorded percentage of deaths in each age group coded to Groups I, II and III with the percentages predicted by the cause-of-death models. The number of standard deviations above or below the predicted value for each Group is a measure of how the registration areas in the region deviate from the cause-of-death patterns specified by the models. Figure 3.9 illustrates the pattern of deviation from the models for Groups I, II and III for LAC males. To estimate the division of all-cause mortality into Groups I, II and III in the residual areas, we have assumed that, where all-cause mortality for a given age group is higher, the pattern of deviation of the cause-of-death structure as compared to the cause-of-death models is similar to those for the registration areas. In other words, if the registration areas in LAC have a percentage of all-cause mortality due to Group I that is 2.3 standard deviations higher than expected, then we have assumed that the residual areas also have a percentage of all-cause mortality due to Group I that is 2.3 standard deviations higher than predicted. While this is only a hypothesis, we believe that it is a preferable hypothesis to the alternative, which is to assume that the residual

Figure 3.10   Confidence bands for estimating the proportion of Group II deaths in females aged 30–44 in the residual areas of LAC using the cause-of-death models

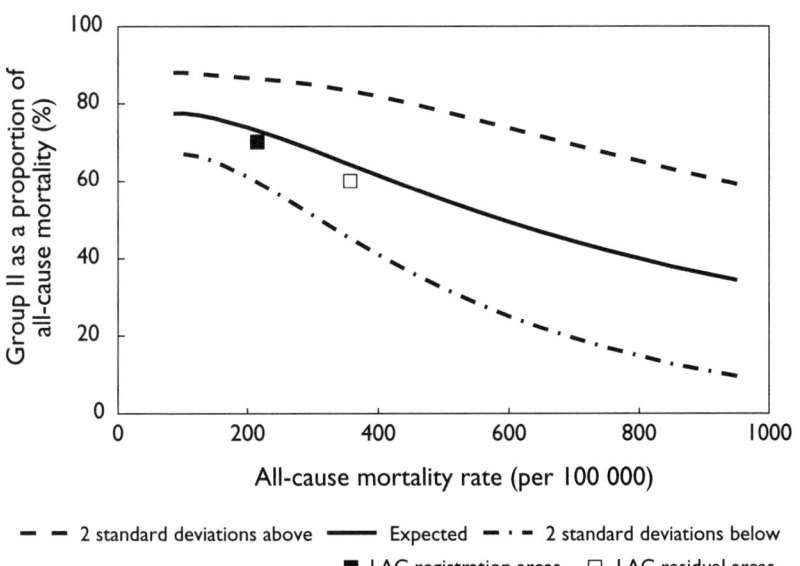

areas have the same cause-of-death pattern as Europe did at a similar mortality level—the assumption implicit in the simple prediction from the regression models. The estimation of Group II for males aged 30–44 in the residual areas of LAC is illustrated in Figure 3.10.

In SSA, a slightly different method was used because registration data were available only for South Africa.[10] The region was divided into two components: Southern Africa (South Africa, Botswana, Namibia, Mozambique, Zimbabwe, Swaziland, Zambia and Malawi) and the remainder of the region (Northern SSA). Sub-regional estimates of mortality and population were based on work commissioned by the World Bank for the 1993 World Development Report (World Bank 1993).[11] The Lorenz curve method was then used to estimate the pattern for these areas. For the northern SSA, the mortality pattern was based on the difference between the regional estimates and the estimates for the Southern African subregion. The distribution of registered deaths across Groups I, II and III in South Africa was within 1 standard deviation of that predicted by the models. For the Northern SSA sub-region, we have therefore chosen to use the same pattern of deviations as in the registration areas of South Africa.

For more detailed causes in the residual areas of LAC, MEC, SSA and OAI, we have assumed that the proportionate distribution of deaths for a given age-sex group within each Group is the same as in the registration areas. The alternative would have been to use the small-cause regressions discussed above. We felt, however, that it is preferable to base the preliminary distribution of more detailed causes on local data rather than on the patterns implied by vital registration data from industrialized countries.

SPECIFIC CORRECTIONS

For the FSE region and for some major cause groups—such as for malignant neoplasms, cardiovascular diseases, neuro-psychiatric conditions and chronic respiratory conditions—additional corrections were made to the estimates as described below.

FSE

At ages 70 years and over, there is evidence to suggest that a number of causes are substantially undercoded in this region. For neuro-psychiatric disorders, for example, there is a characteristic age-pattern of mortality that is observed in all other regions which is not apparent in the vital registration data for FSE. Similarly unusual deviations from characteristic age-patterns of mortality were found for respiratory infections, nutritional deficiencies, and other infectious and parasitic diseases, particularly at ages 70 years and over. For both males and females at older ages in FSE, we have therefore modified the redistribution algorithm for ICD-9 Chapter XVI deaths to preferentially distribute them to these causes in FSE, so that the age-pattern of mortality is consistent with that observed in other regions. The expected mortality rates at ages 70 years and over for various conditions were estimated based on the average ratio of rates for those aged 70 and over to those aged 60–69 for corresponding cause Groups in other regions with good registration data, such as EME, parts of LAC and China. Once these corrections had been made, the remainder of deaths coded to ICD-9 Chapter XVI were then proportionately redistributed across Group II causes in the same manner as was done for other regions.

Malignant Neoplasms

More is known about the descriptive epidemiology of malignant neoplasms than most other chronic diseases since there is an extensive network of population-based cancer registries in a number of countries, coordinated by the International Agency for Research on Cancer (IARC) (Parkin et al. 1992). The most recently published compendium of data by the IARC contains data from 163 registries in 50 countries. Results from cancer registries are published by IARC only if they satisfy certain validity criteria, as assessed by the percentage of cases with age not known, relative frequency of different sites of cancer, crude rates, age-standardized rates, average annual percentage change in the age-standardized rate, percentage of cases verified histologically, percentage of cases notified on the basis of a death certificate only, and the mortality to incidence ratio. For many populations, cancer registry incidence rates are likely to be the best source of information on the occurence of cancer. However, even a cursory examination of the reported death rates by site from registries in the developing world suggests that they are less useful as a source of information on cancer mortality. Death to incidence ratios in many of these developing country registries are lower than in the United States SEER[12] registry and other industrialized country registries. As access to treatment is likely to be much higher in industrialized countries, it seems likely that the lower death to incidence ratios reported from registries in developing countries are due to differential under-reporting of deaths as compared with incidence.

Parkin et al. (1992) have used the IARC network of registries to develop global and regional estimates of mortality from various sites. For those parts of the developing world where either there are no cancer registries or the number of cancer deaths reported by registries is considered too low, they used the site-specific distribution of incidence and a plausible set of death-to-incidence ratios based on industrialized country experience, combined with estimates of total cancer deaths in each region from Bulutao (1993). While this basic approach is reasonable, the final estimates which were obtained are highly dependent on the estimates of cancer death rates from Bulutao (1993) which we believe consistently underestimate cancer mortality in developing regions.[13]

To estimate total cancer death rates for each age-sex group, we first applied the methods described earlier in the section to generate preliminary estimates. In EME, FSE, China and in the registration areas of LAC, vital registration data were used to estimate the distribution of total cancer deaths by site. In India, the urban site distribution is based on the vital registration data from Maharashtra and for rural areas the distribution by site has been based on the APBD. The estimates for India prepared by Parkin et al. (1994) were based on the incidence of cancers recorded in the cancer registries of Ahmedabad, Bangalore, Bombay, and Madras, and on plausible death to incidence ratios based on the SEER cancer registry data adjusted on the basis of expert opinions from India. For other regions, and for the residual population in LAC, a recent set of published estimates of site-specific mortality for 1985 based on the IARC network of registries was used to estimate site-specific distributions (Parkin et al. 1994). However, in these estimates, the proportion of total cancer deaths which were attributed to other and unknown primary sites was very small in comparison to areas with better vital registration, such as EME and FSE. We therefore corrected the site distribution of cancer deaths in these estimates on the assumption that the low proportion of cancer deaths estimated for other and unknown cancers by Parkin et al. (1994) is due to misdiagnosis of metastatic cancers or other coding problems. The site-specific distribution of death has, therefore, been adjusted so that the proportion of other and unknown cancers is equal to (or not lower than) the proportion observed in the vital registration data from EME.[14]

Cardiovascular Diseases

As described in detail in the section dealing with the coding of cardiovascular disease deaths, we have corrected for under-registration of ischaemic heart disease mortality in every region. While there is good evidence for an over-registration of stroke deaths, we have chosen not to reduce the registered number of stroke deaths, as it is not clear to which cause these should be reassigned. Using BTL codes, it is not possible to identify deaths due to the group of conditions labelled as inflammatory heart diseases, i.e. pericarditis, endocarditis, myocarditis and cardiomyopathies. As the proportions are relatively consistent across regions, we used the average age-sex-specific percentages of deaths due to inflammatory heart diseases in countries for which three digit ICD-9 data were available to estimate inflammatory heart disease deaths in each region.

Neuro-Psychiatric Disorders

The coding of neuro-psychiatric disorders appears to be less precise than for most other diseases in many countries. The estimation of mortality from neuro-psychiatric conditions is problematic for at least three reasons. First, in some countries, such as Thailand, a very large number of deaths are assigned to the neuro-psychiatric category but not to a particular BTL code. The category of residual neuro-psychiatric disorders appears to function as a depository for ill-defined conditions, similar to ICD-9 Chapter XVI. Second, in other countries, such as South Africa and countries where lay coders are used, epilepsy is often used as a code for classifying ill-defined conditions. Third, there appears to be substantial variation between countries in the diagnostic practices of physicians in assigning a neuro-psychiatric code as the cause of death. For example, in some regions, almost no deaths are assigned to dementia despite epidemiological evidence that the prevalence of dementia is relatively constant across regions.

In India total neuro-psychiatric death numbers were based on the preliminary estimates with only minor modifications. However, epidemiological estimates were made for psychoses, dementia, Parkinson disease, multiple sclerosis, and drug dependence. For bipolar disorder, the average proportion of neuro-psychiatric conditions (excluding alcohol dependence) by age and sex in EME, FSE and LAC was used to estimate the number of deaths. Alcohol dependence deaths were estimated in a similar fashion using the OAI proportions of neuro-psychiatric deaths due to alcohol dependence.

In China, deaths from the cluster of neuro-psychiatric conditions were based on the DSPs as described in the section on preliminary estimates. Amongst the detailed neuro-psychiatric causes, the DSPs provide data only on deaths due to psychoses. Epidemiological estimates have been used for several causes not reported with unique codes in the DSPs, namely dementia, Parkinson disease, multiple sclerosis, and drug dependence. The number of deaths due to alcohol dependence was estimated by taking the percentage of neuro-psychiatric deaths in the OAI registration areas attributed to alcohol dependence and applying this to the total number of neuro-psychiatric deaths in China for each age-sex group. Bipolar disorder and epilepsy death numbers were estimated in a different way. Firstly, the percentage of remaining neuro-psychiatric deaths in each age-sex group which were attributed to these two causes in regions with good vital registration (EME, FSE and LAC registration areas) was calculated. The average of the EME, FSE and LAC percentage distributions was then applied to China.

In the OAI registration areas, the neuro-psychiatric category appears to be substantially inflated by the use of a code in the neuro-psychiatric residual category for coding ill-defined causes of death. We therefore calculated a revised OAI total for neuro-psychiatric deaths by taking the average of the age-sex specific total neuro-psychiatric death rates in EME, LAC and India. Alcohol-dependence deaths were based on the OAI vital registration data. Epidemiological estimates were used for psychoses, dementia, Parkinson disease, multiple sclerosis, and drug dependence. Bipolar disorder and epilepsy estimates were calculated using the same method as for China. The residual category of other neuro-psychiatric disorders was based on the average of EME and LAC rates.

In SSA, total neuro-psychiatric mortality rates were based on the preliminary estimates except that the residual category of other neuro-psychiatric disorders was corrected for probable use as a depository for ill-defined deaths and set equal to the average of EME and LAC rates. In LAC, total neuro-psychiatric deaths were taken from the preliminary estimates. Epidemiological estimates were then used for psychoses,

Parkinson disease, multiple sclerosis and drug dependence. The percentage distribution of the remaining neuro-psychiatric causes within the neuro-psychiatric total was based on the average percentage distribution for EME, FSE and LAC registration areas. In MEC, total neuro-psychiatric conditions from the preliminary estimates were used. Epidemiological estimates were then used for psychoses, dementias, Parkinson disease, multiple sclerosis, and drug dependence. Bipolar disorder and epilepsy estimates were calculated by applying the average percentage distribution from EME, FSE and LAC registration areas. Deaths due to the residual category of other neuro-psychiatric disorders were based on the average of EME and LAC rates.

Chronic Obstructive Pulmonary Disease (COPD) and Asthma

Unfortunately, using BTL codes one cannot distinguish asthma from other chronic respiratory diseases. This distinction is only possible when three-digit ICD-9 data are available. To obtain preliminary estimates of mortality from COPD and asthma, we first examined the distribution of COPD and asthma deaths within the category of chronic respiratory diseases for those countries where three-digit ICD-9 data were available. For these countries, we then estimated the proportion of deaths due to asthma and to COPD by age and sex. The percentages of chronic respiratory mortality by age-sex group from the 22 countries with detailed data due to COPD were used for all regions except FSE, where data from the Russian Federation on the proportion of chronic respiratory mortality due to COPD were used. In China, a large number of deaths are coded to pulmonary heart disease. Based on what is known about coding preferences in China, we transferred most of these deaths to COPD. For asthma, we used the percentage of chronic respiratory deaths assigned in the 17 EME countries with detailed ICD-9 data to estimate asthma deaths in EME. In FSE, we used detailed data from the Russian Federation. For all other regions, epidemiological estimates have been used to estimate asthma deaths by age and sex.

Oral Conditions

In SSA, MEC, and China, baseline estimates resulted in a considerable number of deaths being assigned to oral health conditions. Other than noma, which is uncommon in MEC, China and South Africa, and which is the only major disease causing death among these conditions, we suspect that these deaths were due to local coding differences. In these three regions, we have modified the oral health deaths so that age-specific rates are similar to all other regions.

Protein-Energy Malnutrition

In OAI and SSA, the number of deaths directly coded to protein-energy malnutrition (PEM) was estimated by using the average proportion of PEM deaths among Group I deaths in EME and China, by age and sex, applied to the regional Group I total. Alternative methods such as esti-mating a case-fatality rate for wasted or stunted children based on vital registration data in EME, LAC or China gave much lower figures which did not seem plausible. Using a fixed proportion of all Group I causes implies that nutritional status improves as Group I mortality declines. Given the postulated close relationship between infectious disease mor-tality and nutritional status, this hypothesis is not unreasonable.

EPIDEMIOLOGICAL CORRECTIONS

Table 3.9 identifies those diseases and regions for which estimates of mortality by cause for at least one age-sex group in a region have been generated from a disease-specific epidemiological approach. Because of the greater concentration on infectious disease epidemiology in most developing countries, epidemiologically-based estimates of mortality are available for many more Group I diseases than for Group II. As epide-miological assessments tend to be higher than those based on vital reg-istration, this tends to bias the final results towards Group I diseases and away from Group II diseases. For the detailed basis of each epidemio-logical assessment, the reader is referred to the relevant chapters in the respective volumes of the *Global Burden of Disease and Injury Series*.

Because of the sporadic but intense effect of war on mortality, the epi-demiological estimates of war deaths were incorporated in a slightly dif-ferent manner. In brief, we chose to consider war deaths as additional to the number of deaths estimated from the basic demographic analyses used to determine the number of deaths in each age-sex group in each region. Thus, the epidemiological estimates of war deaths have not been subject to the final adjustment algorithm described below.

FINAL ADJUSTMENTS

One of the characteristics of the approach taken in this study to estimat-ing causes of death is the requirement that each death be assigned to a single cause in the primary tabulations. After correcting estimates for a number of causes based on epidemiological assessments, the sum of cause-specific mortality exceeded the total mortality in a number of age groups in several regions. In other cases, the sum of Group-specific causes of death exceeds the total Group mortality in a given age group—a common prob-lem for Group I in the adult age groups. To ensure that the sum of cause-specific deaths was the same as the number of deaths from all causes in any given age-sex group, two final adjustment algorithms were used, one for neonatal causes and one for all other age groups.

Neonatal Death Adjustment Algorithm[15]

In most regions, 85 per cent of neonatal deaths are due to a limited number of causes namely: congenital syphilis, neonatal tetanus, conditions arising during the perinatal period, and congenital anomalies. To obtain estimates of deaths from these causes, we first estimated the number of neonatal

Table 3.9   Diseases and injuries for which disease-specific corrections were made to adjust mortality estimates for at least one age group

	Region							
Cause	EME	FSE	IND	CHN	OAI	SSA	LAC	MEC
I. Communicable, maternal, perinatal and nutritional conditions								
A. Infectious and parasitic diseases								
1. Tuberculosis			•	•	•	•	•	•
2. Sexually transmitted diseases excluding HIV			•		•	•	•	•
a. Syphilis			•		•	•	•	•
b. Chlamydia			•	•	•	•	•	•
c. Gonorrhoea			•	•	•	•	•	•
3. HIV	•	•	•	•	•	•	•	•
4. Diarrhoeal diseases			•		•	•	•	•
2. Childhood-cluster diseases			•	•	•	•	•	•
a. Pertussis			•	•	•	•	•	•
b. Poliomyelitis			•	•	•	•	•	•
c. Diphtheria			•		•	•		•
d. Measles			•	•	•	•	•	•
e. Tetanus			•		•	•	•	•
6. Bacterial meningitis and meningococcaemia			•	•	•	•	•	•
7. Hepatitis B and hepatitis C			•		•	•		•
8. Malaria				•	•	•	•	•
9. Tropical-cluster diseases			•	•	•	•	•	•
a. Trypanosomiasis						•		
b. Chagas disease							•	
c. Schistosomiasis				•	•	•		•
d. Leishmaniasis			•	•	•	•	•	•
e. Lymphatic filariasis								
f. Onchocerciasis								
10. Leprosy				•		•		
11. Dengue			•	•	•	•	•	
12. Japanese encephalitis			•	•	•			
13. Trachoma								
14. Intestinal nematode infections			•	•	•	•	•	•
a. Ascariasis			•	•	•	•	•	•
b. Trichuriasis			•	•	•	•	•	•
c. Ancylostomiasis and necatoriasis			•	•	•	•	•	•
15. Other infectious and parasitic diseases								
B. Respiratory infections			•	•	•	•		•
1. Lower respiratory infections			•	•	•	•		•
2. Upper respiratory infections			•	•	•	•		•

Table 3.9   (continued)

Cause	EME	FSE	IND	CHN	OAI	SSA	LAC	MEC
3. Otitis media			•	•	•	•	•	•
C. Maternal conditions	•	•	•	•	•	•	•	•
1. Maternal haemorrhage	•	•	•	•	•	•	•	•
2. Maternal sepsis	•	•	•	•	•	•	•	•
3. Hypertensive disorders of pregnancy	•	•	•	•	•	•	•	•
4. Obstructed labour	•	•	•	•	•	•	•	•
5. Abortion	•	•	•	•	•	•	•	•
D. Conditions arising during the perinatal period	•		•	•	•	•	•	•
1. Low birth weight	•	•	•	•	•	•	•	•
2. Birth asphyxia and birth trauma	•	•	•	•	•	•	•	•
E. Nutritional deficiencies					•	•	•	•
1. Protein-energy malnutrition								
2. Iodine deficiency	•	•	•	•	•	•	•	•
3. Vitamin A deficiency	•	•	•	•	•	•	•	•
4. Iron-deficiency anaemia	•				•	•		•
II. Noncommunicable diseases								
A. Malignant neoplasms								
1. Mouth and oropharynx cancer								
2. Oesophagus cancer								
3. Stomach cancer								
4. Colon and rectum cancers								
5. Liver cancer								
6. Pancreas cancer								
7. Trachea, bronchus and lung cancers								
8. Melanoma and other skin cancers								
9. Breast cancer								
10. Cervix uteri cancer								
11. Corpus uteri cancer								
12. Ovary cancer								
13. Prostate cancer								
14. Bladder cancer								
15. Lymphomas and multiple myeloma								
16. Leukaemia								
B. Other neoplasms								
C. Diabetes mellitus	•	•	•	•	•	•	•	•
D. Endocrine disorders								
E. Neuro-psychiatric conditions								
1. Unipolar major depression								
2. Bipolar disorder								
3. Schizophrenia	•				•	•	•	•
4. Epilepsy								

Table 3.9   (continued)

Cause	EME	FSE	IND	CHN	OAI	SSA	LAC	MEC
5. Alcohol use						•		
6. Dementia and other degenerative and hereditary CNS disorders			•	•	•	•		•
7. Parkinson disease			•	•	•	•	•	•
8. Multiple sclerosis			•	•	•	•	•	•
9. Drug use			•	•	•	•	•	•
10. Post-traumatic stress disorder			•	•	•	•	•	•
11. Obsessive-compulsive disorders			•	•	•	•	•	•
12. Panic disorder			•	•	•	•	•	•
F. Sense organ diseases								
1. Glaucoma								
2. Cataracts								
G. Cardiovascular diseases								
1. Rheumatic heart disease			•		•	•		•
2. Ischaemic heart disease								
3. Cerebrovascular disease								
4. Inflammatory heart diseases								
H. Respiratory diseases								
1. Chronic obstructive pulmonary disease								
2. Asthma	•	•	•	•	•	•	•	•
I. Digestive diseases								
1. Peptic ulcer								
2. Cirrhosis of the liver								
3. Appendicitis			•	•	•	•	•	•
J. Genito-urinary diseases								
1. Nephritis and nephrosis								
2. Benign prostatic hypertrophy								
K. Skin diseases								
L. Musculo-skeletal diseases								
1. Rheumatoid arthritis								
2. Osteoarthritis								
M. Congenital anomalies			•		•	•		•
1. Abdominal wall defect			•	•	•	•	•	•
2. Anencephaly			•	•	•	•	•	•
3. Anorectal atresia			•	•	•	•	•	•
4. Cleft lip			•	•	•	•	•	•
5. Cleft palate			•	•	•	•	•	•
6. Oesophageal atresia			•	•	•	•	•	•
7. Renal agenesis			•	•	•	•	•	•
8. Down syndrome			•	•	•	•	•	•
9. Congenital heart anomalies			•	•	•	•	•	•

Table 3.9   (continued)

Cause	EME	FSE	IND	CHN	OAI	SSA	LAC	MEC
			Region					
10. Spina bifida			•	•	•	•	•	•
N. Oral conditions								
1. Dental caries								
2. Periodontal disease								
3. Edentulism								
III. Injuries								
A. Unintentional injuries								
1. Road traffic accidents								
2. Poisonings								
3. Falls								
4. Fires								
5. Drownings								
6. Other unintentional injuries								
B. Intentional injuries								
1. Self-inflicted injuries								
2. Violence								
3. War	•	•	•	•	•	•	•	•

deaths in each region and then required that the sum of deaths from congenital syphilis, neonatal tetanus, conditions arising during the perinatal period, and congenital anomalies during the neonatal period must equal 85 per cent of estimated neonatal deaths.

The demographic analyses undertaken by the World Bank for the 1993 World Development Report (WDR) provided estimates of deaths at ages 0–4 years and the probability of death between birth and age 5, for each of the eight WDR regions. Estimates of mortality at ages 0–4 years for more detailed age groups, such as for neonatal deaths, infant deaths and childhood deaths were not undertaken. In all regions, neonatal deaths are an important fraction of all infant deaths and can easily be under-estimated unless reliable bounds on the neonatal mortality rate are derived. We therefore estimated neonatal deaths based on the extensive recent survey data collected through the Demographic and Health Surveys (Sullivan et al. 1994). For 28 of these national surveys in developing countries, estimates of the probability of death between birth and one month, birth and one year, and birth and five years have been calculated for males and females. Figure 3.11 shows the relationship between the ratio of the probability of neonatal death to the probability of childhood death ($_5q_0$), and the overall probability of childhood death. Using ordinary least squares regression, the following equation was estimated:

Figure 3.11 Relationship between the ratio of the probability of neonatal death to $_5q_0$ and $_5q_0$ in 28 demographic and health surveys in developing countries

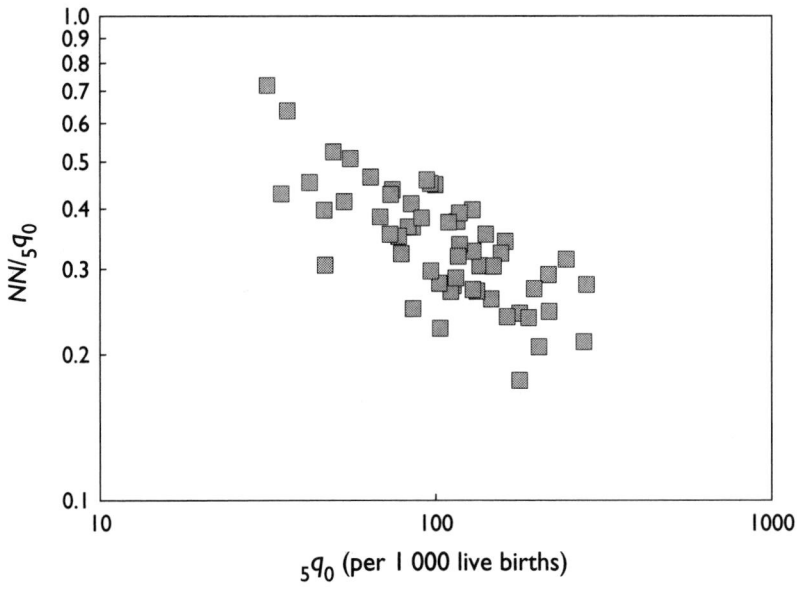

$_5q_0$ (per 1 000 live births)

Source: Sullivan et al. (1994)

Notes:

• NN = probability of neonatal death; $_5q_0$ = probability of death between birth and age 5.

• Rate ratios and rates in males and females are shown as separate observations.

$$\ln(\frac{NN}{_5q_0}) = -0.394 \ln(_5q_0) + 0.749$$

where NN is the ratio of the probability of neonatal to child death, and $_5q_0$ is the probability of death between birth and age 5. In conjunction with World Bank estimates of mortality at ages 0–4, this equation was then used to estimate the neonatal death rate for each region and the absolute number of neonatal deaths. Not all deaths from conditions arising during the perinatal period or from congenital anomalies occur within the first month of life. Based on data from countries with detailed vital registration information on the timing of deaths from these two causes, it was estimated that 95 per cent of deaths under age 5 due to conditions arising during the perinatal period occur in the neonatal period, and that 65 per cent of congenital deaths in children under age 5 occur within one month of birth. We then summed deaths from conditions arising during the perinatal period and congenital anomalies expected in the first month, neonatal tetanus deaths and congenital syphilis deaths. The estimates of deaths from each of these conditions were then proportionately adjusted so that their total was equal to 85 per cent of the estimated number of neonatal deaths in a given region.

Final Adjustment Algorithm

The extent of overestimation of mortality in each of the fourteen age-sex groups and in each region can be evaluated by comparing the number of standard deviations above or below the proportionate mortality for each cause Group predicted by the cause-of-death models with the number of standard deviations above or below in the preliminary estimates. Figure 3.12 illustrates this comparison for Group I diseases in SSA. The preliminary estimates suggest much higher than predicted levels of Group I mortality for males aged 5 and over and for females aged 45 and over. Despite the higher than expected Group I estimates based on the available registration data, epidemiological assessments would increase Group I mortality in all age groups except at ages 5–14 for both males and females, and 70 and over in males. In the adult age groups, the increases range from 1.2 to 2.1 standard deviations for males and from 1.6 to 2.5 standard deviations for females. We have assumed that the magnitude of Group III mortality is correct in the baseline estimates because we suspect that injury patterns are highly region-specific but are not strongly related to the level of mortality, unlike Group I or Group II. Higher levels of Group I mortality therefore imply lower and thus more deviant levels of Group II mortality. Figure 3.13 illustrates the profound increase in standard deviations below the mean this would imply for Group II in SSA— in the age group under five, -5.9 standard deviations for males and -11.9 standard deviations for females. Epidemiological assessments for other regions imply similarly large increases in the model-derived deviation from the cause-of-death patterns—Table 3.10 summarizes the differences between preliminary and epidemiological estimates for OAI, SSA, LAC and MEC.

Accepting the epidemiological assessments for Group I causes and directly reducing Group II mortality in proportion to Group I would very likely result in a significant underestimate of Group II mortality. In effect, this would mean biasing the GBD study results towards diseases that are better studied and underestimating those conditions whose epidemiology in developing countries is currently neglected. If as much epidemiological work had been done on Group II diseases as for Group I, epidemiological assessments might be much larger than the levels suggested by the preliminary estimates. Historical time series of cause-of-death data for EME and some LAC countries also provide a strong basis for rejecting the option of reducing Group II mortality so drastically. This body of data suggests that Group II age-specific mortality rates have in fact been *declining* for many decades (Murray et al. 1992, Preston 1976). This marked secular trend in Group II mortality implies that Group II age-specific death rates in poor regions should be *higher* than in wealthier regions. The results of the cause-of-death models presented earlier also support this hypothesis.

Figure 3.12   Number of standard deviations by which *prelimary* estimates
of mortality by cause for SSA deviate from the level
predicted by cause-of-death models

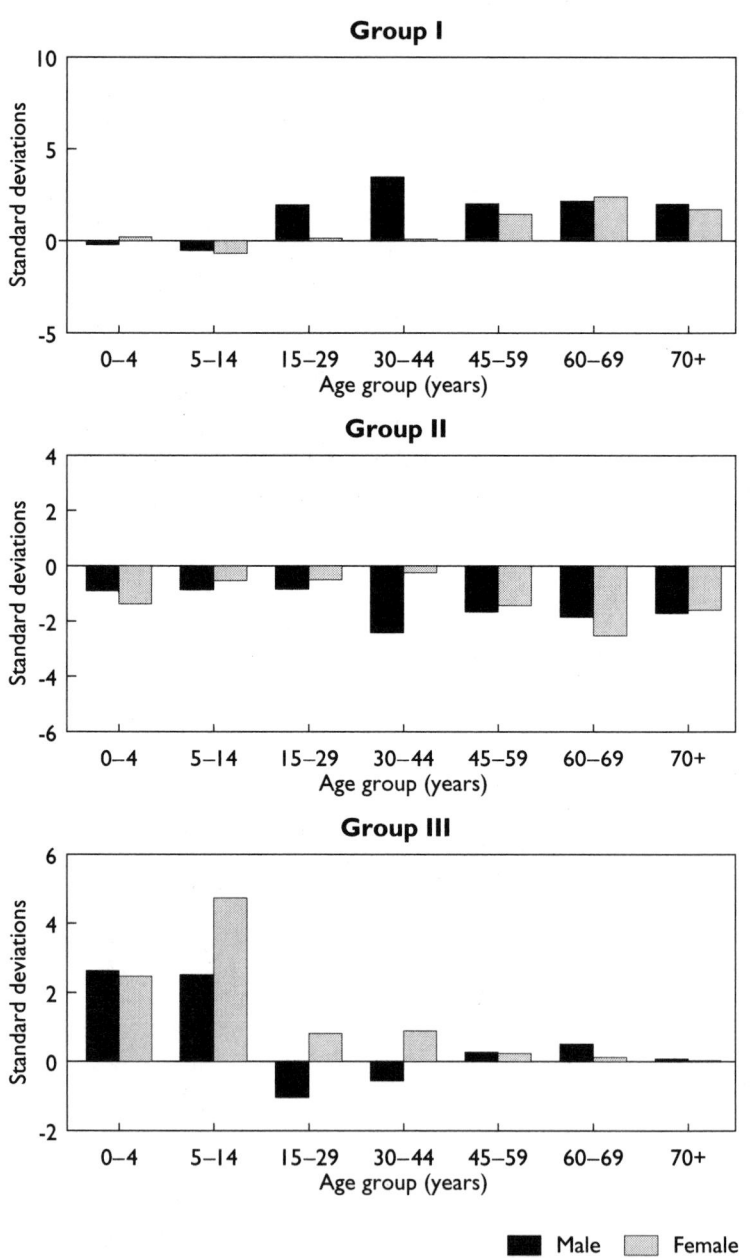

Figure 3.13 Number of standard deviations by which *epidemiological* estimates of mortality by cause for SSA deviate from the level predicted by cause-of-death models

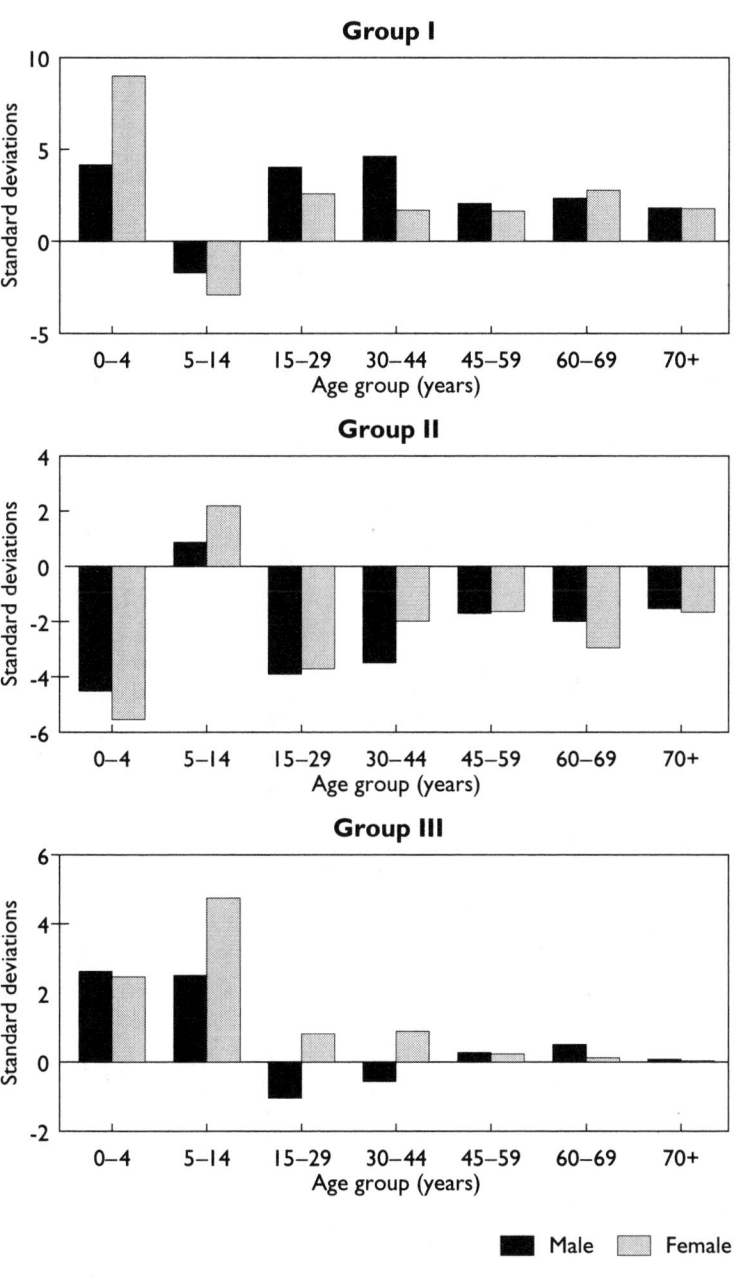

Table 3.10 Difference (in number of standard deviations) of estimates of mortality patterns from cause-of-death models, by region, cause Group, sex and age group predicted

Region and cause Group	Males							Females						
	0–4	5–9	14–29	30–44	45–59	60–69	70+	0–4	5–9	14–29	30–44	45–59	60–69	70+
Preliminary Estimates														
OAI														
Group I	-2.92	-1.01	0.99	1.29	0.92	0.56	0.12	-3.28	-1.48	-0.50	0.26	0.97	0.60	0.04
Group II	1.92	1.20	0.79	-0.10	-0.54	-0.29	0.10	1.86	1.11	0.03	-0.49	-0.88	-0.58	0.13
Group III	3.06	0.44	-1.24	-0.56	0.04	0.01	-0.05	3.89	2.05	0.85	0.73	0.25	0.22	-0.14
SSA														
Group I	-0.22	-0.53	1.97	3.48	2.03	2.17	2.01	0.20	-0.69	0.14	0.09	1.44	2.40	1.70
Group II	-0.90	-0.87	-0.85	-2.43	-1.66	-1.85	-1.71	-1.38	-0.54	-0.50	-0.24	-1.43	-2.53	-1.59
Group III	2.63	2.51	-1.04	-0.56	0.27	0.51	0.08	2.47	4.74	0.82	0.89	0.23	0.12	0.03
LAC														
Group I	-0.24	-0.40	1.48	1.84	0.73	0.53	0.47	-0.88	-0.00	0.37	0.38	0.56	0.77	0.56
Group II	0.00	-1.63	-1.31	-2.06	-0.84	-0.44	-0.32	0.63	-1.53	-0.78	-0.43	-0.39	-0.66	-0.47
Group III	0.67	2.39	0.25	1.01	0.62	0.41	0.19	0.88	2.76	0.59	0.35	0.09	0.11	0.16
MEC														
Group I	-1.63	-0.71	1.07	1.02	0.11	-0.37	-0.10	-2.57	-1.69	-0.66	0.59	-0.04	-0.31	-0.22
Group II	1.60	1.22	1.93	0.17	0.54	0.82	0.35	2.19	2.15	2.05	-0.22	0.27	0.55	0.40
Group III	0.65	-0.16	-2.38	-0.63	-0.50	-0.58	-0.17	1.33	0.22	-1.36	-0.44	-0.14	-0.17	-0.17
Epidemiological Estimates														
OAI														
Group I	-0.91	-1.44	3.19	3.36	1.65	1.91	1.01	1.01	-1.45	3.75	3.01	2.70	3.88	1.15
Group II	-0.34	1.84	-0.81	-1.39	-1.09	-1.37	-0.73	-3.02	1.06	-4.95	-3.41	-2.53	-4.04	-0.99
Group III	3.06	0.44	-1.24	-0.56	0.04	0.01	-0.05	3.89	2.05	0.85	0.73	0.25	0.22	-0.14
SSA														
Group I	4.17	-1.71	4.04	4.63	2.07	2.36	1.81	8.98	-2.91	2.59	1.67	1.63	2.78	1.76
Group II	-4.51	0.87	-3.90	-3.49	-1.70	-2.00	-1.52	-5.54	2.18	-3.71	-1.99	-1.63	-2.96	-1.66
Group III	2.63	2.51	-1.04	-0.56	0.27	0.51	0.08	2.47	4.74	0.82	0.89	0.23	0.12	0.03
LAC														
Group I	1.15	0.77	2.77	3.60	1.26	1.10	0.54	3.25	1.86	1.96	1.43	1.20	1.50	0.64
Group II	-1.53	-3.24	-2.41	-3.17	-1.23	-0.85	-0.39	-3.99	-3.84	-2.62	-1.52	-0.99	-1.40	-0.55
Group III	0.67	2.39	0.25	1.01	0.62	0.41	0.19	0.88	2.76	0.59	0.35	0.09	0.11	0.10
MEC														
Group I	-0.97	-1.25	4.53	3.61	0.85	1.46	0.51	-1.69	-2.68	2.79	4.25	1.03	2.00	0.46
Group II	0.85	2.02	-0.26	-1.27	-0.20	-0.83	-0.22	1.29	3.39	-2.03	-3.99	-0.74	-1.87	-0.28
Group III	0.65	-0.16	-2.38	-0.63	-0.50	-0.58	-0.17	1.33	0.22	-1.36	-0.44	-0.14	-0.17	-0.17

Table 3.10 (continued)

Region and cause Group	Males							Females						
	0–4	5–9	14–29	30–44	45–59	60–69	70+	0–4	5–9	14–29	30–44	45–59	60–69	70+
Final Estimates														
EME Group I	0.29	-0.73	0.67	3.61	0.15	-0.29	0.25	0.68	-0.37	-0.03	1.05	-0.02	0.00	0.26
Group II	-0.54	-0.34	-1.13	-1.48	0.15	0.61	-0.07	-0.74	-0.52	-1.87	-1.08	0.08	0.20	-0.19
Group III	0.55	0.65	0.89	0.04	-0.04	-0.21	0.06	0.30	0.76	1.94	0.79	0.16	-0.02	0.26
FSE Group I	-1.64	-1.98	-0.89	-0.51	-0.57	-0.49	0.17	-1.47	-2.03	-1.32	-0.54	-0.52	-0.33	0.11
Group II	-0.32	-3.02	-1.16	-1.74	-0.22	0.21	-0.02	-0.75	-3.71	-2.44	-1.91	-0.23	0.20	-0.02
Group III	**4.04**	**4.67**	1.61	2.17	0.83	0.43	0.10	**4.47**	**5.98**	3.60	2.85	1.40	0.50	0.17
India Group I	0.10	0.53	**6.07**	**8.56**	2.98	2.78	1.81	-0.32	-0.52	0.31	2.44	2.29	2.40	1.52
Group II	-1.23	-2.15	-0.78	-3.87	-2.18	-2.07	-1.52	-0.73	-1.71	-2.24	-3.62	-2.79	-2.85	-1.47
Group III	2.56	1.75	-3.14	-1.55	-0.05	-0.24	0.06	2.51	**6.78**	3.10	2.79	1.78	1.06	0.24
China Group I	-1.79	-0.42	0.55	1.62	0.78	0.42	0.47	-2.44	0.11	-1.22	0.49	0.37	0.48	0.29
Group II	-1.11	-1.95	1.05	-0.26	-0.40	-0.33	-0.38	-0.40	**-4.39**	-2.25	-2.11	-1.11	-0.99	-0.41
Group III	**6.35**	2.42	-1.20	-0.46	0.01	0.33	0.32	**6.91**	**6.01**	**4.21**	2.72	1.81	1.44	0.90
OAI Group I	-1.02	-1.13	2.41	2.66	1.72	2.03	1.09	-1.42	-1.44	1.24	2.22	2.77	2.55	1.24
Group II	-0.29	0.98	-0.32	-1.04	-1.15	-1.47	-0.81	-0.15	1.00	-2.21	-2.65	-2.61	-2.66	-1.08
Group III	3.21	0.94	-1.16	-0.49	0.05	0.02	-0.05	**4.10**	2.18	1.09	0.88	0.28	0.26	-0.14
SSA Group I	0.44	-1.28	1.83	2.76	2.04	2.38	1.91	0.10	-1.84	0.45	1.10	1.65	2.97	1.87
Group II	-2.50	-0.87	-1.80	-2.75	-1.90	-2.20	-1.66	-2.50	-0.07	-2.41	-1.90	-1.84	-3.49	-1.80
Group III	**4.46**	**4.22**	-0.44	0.31	0.59	0.92	0.18	**4.89**	**7.98**	**4.09**	3.66	0.97	1.09	0.17
LAC Group I	1.01	-0.49	2.36	2.41	1.26	1.09	0.54	0.71	0.65	1.59	1.33	1.19	1.50	0.64
Group II	-1.54	-1.67	-2.21	-2.54	-1.25	-0.86	-0.40	-1.38	-2.53	-2.57	-1.57	-1.01	-1.43	-0.55
Group III	1.00	2.57	0.36	1.11	0.65	0.44	0.19	1.33	3.11	1.04	0.64	0.15	0.17	0.16
MEC Group I	-1.68	-1.49	1.30	1.66	0.80	1.43	0.51	-2.53	-2.75	-0.58	1.42	0.95	1.55	0.46
Group II	0.83	1.35	0.10	-1.60	-0.36	-0.92	-0.23	1.26	2.62	-0.93	-2.49	-0.95	-1.66	-0.30
Group III	2.44	1.09	-0.80	0.71	-0.11	-0.13	-0.13	3.57	2.31	2.43	2.34	0.44	0.40	-0.11

Note: Age-sex groups that differ from model predictions by more than four standard deviations are shown in bold.

Unqualified reductions of Group II death rates would, in our view, produce implausible regional patterns.

For these reasons, we have chosen to limit the changes to the preliminary estimates of the cause Group structure of mortality suggested on the basis of epidemiological assessments. We have arbitrarily chosen the following algorithm. If preliminary estimates for Group I or Group II are already more than 2.5 standard deviations above or below the expected value, we did not allow epidemiological assessments to increase the degree of deviation. If the baseline assessment for Group I is less than 2.5 standard deviations above that expected or Group II is more than 2.5 standard deviations below predicted, then epidemiological assessments were allowed to change the proportion in either group by 2 standard deviations. If a change of 2 standard deviations would increase Group I to be above 2.5 standard deviations or decrease Group II to be below -2.5 standard deviations, Group I was set to 2.5 standard deviations and Group II to -2.5, respectively.

The vital registration data on which the cause-of-death models are based do not include many observations from country-years where war was a prominent cause of death. Therefore, we have analysed the deviation pattern for preliminary estimates and epidemiological estimates prior to adding estimated war-related deaths to Group III and all-cause mortality. Table 3.10 shows the deviation pattern for each region after all corrections have been undertaken. In some regions, war-related mortality raises the all-cause mortality rate enough to alter the deviation pattern for all three Groups. In Table 3.10, the age-sex groups with more than 4 standard deviations above or below the rate expected for a cause Group are shown in bold. In FSE, Group III deaths in children aged 0–14 are 4–6 standard deviations higher than expected on the basis of the cause-of-death models. Indian males aged 15–44 have extraordinarily high levels of Group I mortality, as do Indian females aged 5–14. Other examples of higher levels of mortality include Group III in China for children and females aged 5–29. The high rates of war-related deaths in SSA give very high rates of deviation for Group III in males aged 0–14 and females aged 0–29.

RESULTS

Figure 3.14 illustrates the estimated distribution of all deaths in the world by age and region. Because of a much younger age-distribution of population and higher mortality rates in children, 98 per cent of deaths under age 5 and indeed under age 15 are in the developing world (for this analysis, we have defined the developing world as comprising the regions of India, China, OAI, SSA, LAC and MEC). Not surprisingly, 32 per cent of all deaths in the developing world occur among children less than 5 years old, and 63 per cent occur before age 60. Within the developing regions, the age-structure of death varies widely; 53 per cent of all deaths in SSA occur at ages 0–4 years compared with 11 per cent in China. Interestingly, 83 per cent of all adult deaths at ages 15–59 years occur in developing countries. By any standard, these must be considered premature deaths. Even at ages 70 and above, 59 per cent of deaths globally are in the developing world. In EME, 4.6 million deaths occur each year over age 70, as do 3.6 million in China alone. What this emphasizes is that the epidemiological transition in developing regions is sufficiently advanced so that there are only a handful of causes for which there are more deaths in EME and FSE than in the developing world—the list is restricted to several sites of cancer (e.g. colon, lung and pancreas), dementias, Parkinson disease and a few others.

Table 3.11 summarizes the estimated number and percentage distribution of deaths in each region from Groups I, II and III. Globally, one death out of every three arises from one of the diseases in Group I (communicable, maternal, perinatal and nutritional conditions). One death in ten is from an injury, and just slightly more than one death in two is from Group II, the noncommunicable diseases. Because of differences in population age-structure, mortality rates and epidemiological patterns, there is a dramatic difference between EME and FSE and the developing regions in the distribution of deaths. For the developing regions as a whole, Group I conditions account for four out of every ten deaths, Group II one death in two, and injuries one death in ten. For countries in EME and FSE, only 1 death in 16 is due to Group I diseases, while Group II accounts for over 85 per cent of all deaths.

The variation in the extent of the demographic and epidemiological transitions in the developing regions is evident from Table 3.11 as well.

Figure 3.14   Distribution of deaths by age in developing and developed regions, 1990

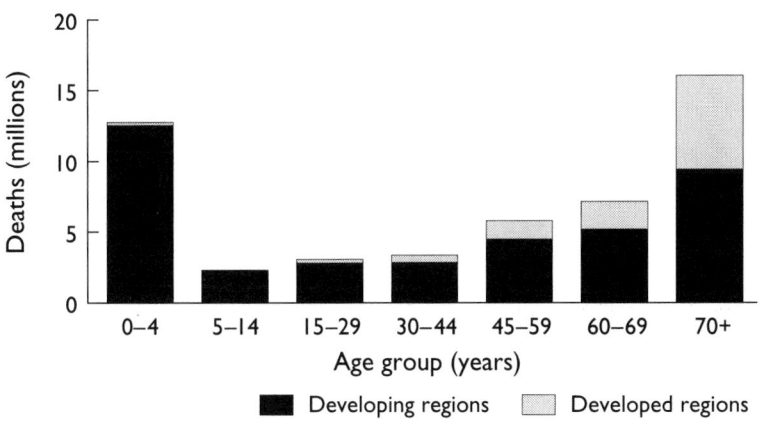

Table 3.11   Distribution of deaths by broad cause Group and region, 1990

	Group I	Group II	Group III	Total	Group II/ Group I Ratio
		Deaths (thousands)			
EME	453	6 223	445	7 121	13.7
FSE	214	3 188	389	3 791	14.9
IND	4 775	3 788	808	9 371	0.8
CHN	1 405	6 460	1 020	8 885	4.6
OAI	2 190	2 785	559	5 534	1.3
SSA	5 316	1 864	1 022	8 202	0.4
LAC	943	1 676	389	3 009	1.8
MEC	1 945	2 156	452	4 553	1.1
World	17 241	28 141	5 084	50 467	1.6
Developed	667	9 411	834	10 912	14.1
Developing	16 573	18 730	4 251	39 554	1.1
		Deaths (as percentage of regional total)			
EME	6.4	87.4	6.3	100.0	
FSE	5.6	84.1	10.3	100.0	
IND	50.9	40.4	8.6	100.0	
CHN	15.8	72.7	11.5	100.0	
OAI	39.6	50.3	10.1	100.0	
SSA	64.8	22.7	12.5	100.0	
LAC	31.3	55.7	12.9	100.0	
MEC	42.7	47.4	9.9	100.0	
World	34.2	55.8	10.1	100.0	
Developed	6.1	86.2	7.6	100.0	
Developing	41.9	47.4	10.7	100.0	

Notes:

Group I: Communicable, maternal, perinatal and nutritional conditions
Group II: Noncommunicable diseases
Group III: Injuries

In SSA, Group I diseases account for 65 per cent of all deaths while in China these diseases account for only 16 per cent of deaths. The ratio of Group II deaths to Group I deaths has been proposed as a crude but useful indicator of the epidemiological transition (Frenk et al. 1989). In fact, this ratio is a function of both population age-structure as well as the epidemiological transition. These ratios (shown in Table 3.11) range from more than 13 in EME and FSE to 0.4 in SSA. According to this criterion, China, followed distantly by LAC and OAI, is the developing region farthest along on the path of the combined demographic and epidemiological transitions. One surprising finding is that for the develop-

Figure 3.15 Regional probabilities of death by age, sex and broad cause Group, 1990

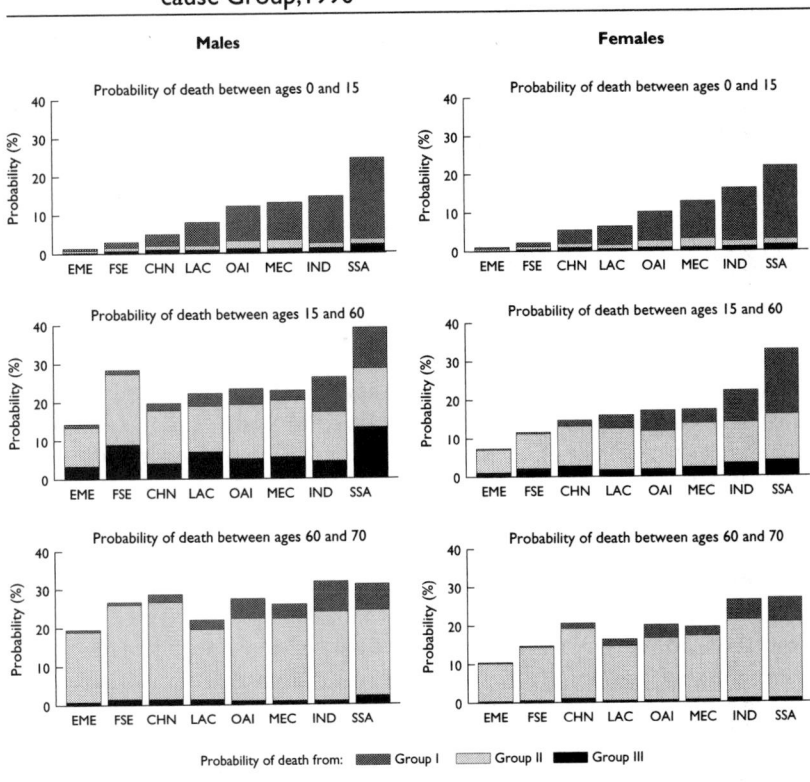

ing world as a whole, and more specifically in China, OAI, LAC and MEC, more people die from noncommunicable diseases than Group I causes. From the perspective of the potential demand for health services in developing countries, the epidemiological transition would thus appear to be much further advanced than is generally appreciated.

A useful way of summarizing the results of this study of global and regional patterns of mortality by cause is in terms of probabilities of death. Figure 3.15 is comprised of six histograms showing probabilities of death for males and females during different periods of life. The top histograms show the probability of dying between birth and age 15 for newborns in each of the 8 regions. Each probability is divided into the probabilities of death from Group I, Group II or Group III causes. As expected, for females the probability of death between birth and age 15 is highest in SSA, (22.0 per cent) and the lowest is EME (1.1 per cent). At these ages, most of the difference between regions is due to differences in the probability of a Group I death. The middle histograms show the probability of death between ages 15 and 60, by region, divided into probabilities of Group I, Group II and Group III death. The regional rankings for females are the same as those for the probabilities of child and adolescent death. For adult women a large part of the difference between regions is the higher probability of Group I death, but the probability of a noncommunicable disease death (Group II) is also higher in developing regions (such as SSA) than in EME or FSE. For many public health specialists, the higher probability of dying from a noncommunicable disease in high-mortality developing regions contradicts the conventional wisdom that the epidemic of chronic diseases is limited to industrialized countries. The results of this study, however, clearly suggest that mortality rates from noncommunicable diseases are higher in low income, high mortality populations than in EME. The middle histogram in Figure 3.15 also demonstrates the unusually high probability of injury death among adult women in China, due mainly to high suicide rates in rural China. The bottom histograms show the probability of death between ages 60 and 70 years, according to the risk of death from Group I, II and III conditions. Again, most of the differences between high and low mortality regions are due to differences in the probability of death from noncommunicable diseases.

The regional rankings and prominence of Group I in explaining regional differences in the probability of death between birth and age 15 are the same for males as for females. Regional differences in the probability of death for adult males between ages 15 and 60 are surprisingly different than those for children, and for adult females. Most notably males in FSE have a higher probability of death (28.4 per cent) than any other region except SSA (39.1 per cent). Differences in adult risks of death are due to a substantial variation in the probability of death from all three Groups. SSA and India have higher risks of adult male death largely because of Group I causes, such as tuberculosis and HIV. The remarkable excess mortality in FSE males is due to much higher risks of Group II death and higher probabilities of Group III death compared with EME. The probability of death from Group III (Injuries) at ages 15–59 varies widely among regions from a low of 3.4 per cent to a high of 13.3 per cent. The bottom histogram shows the probability of male death between ages 60 and 70. Much of the differences across regions is attributable to the risk of death from Group II.

Leading Causes of Death in 1990

Just over 50 million people are estimated to have died in the world in 1990, 53 per cent of whom were males. Ischaemic heart disease (IHD) was the leading cause of death worldwide, accounting for just under 6.3 million deaths (2.7 million in EME and FSE; 3.6 million in the developing regions) (see Table 3.12). Cerebrovascular disease was the next most common cause of death (4.4 million deaths, almost 3 million of which occurred in developing countries), closely followed by lower respiratory infections (4.3 million total, 3.9 million in developing countries). Other leading causes include diarrhoeal diseases (2.9 million deaths, virtually all in developing countries), chronic obstructive pulmonary disease (2.2

Table 3.12   Leading causes of death, world, developed and developing regions, by sex, 1990

Rank	Both Sexes — Cause	Deaths (thousands)	Cumulative %	Males — Cause	Deaths (thousands)	Cumulative %	Females — Cause	Deaths (thousands)	Cumulative %
World									
	All Causes	50 467		All Causes	26 692		All Causes	23 775	
1	Ischaemic heart disease	6 260	12.4	Ischaemic heart disease	3 126	11.7	Ischaemic heart disease	3 134	13.2
2	Cerebrovascular disease	4 381	21.1	Lower respiratory infections	2 196	19.9	Cerebrovascular disease	2 359	23.1
3	Lower respiratory infections	4 299	29.6	Cerebrovascular disease	2 022	27.5	Lower respiratory infections	2 103	32.0
4	Diarrhoeal diseases	2 946	35.4	Diarrhoeal diseases	1 533	33.3	Diarrhoeal diseases	1 414	37.9
5	Conditions arising during the perinatal period	2 443	39.8	Conditions arising during the perinatal period	1 266	37.8	Conditions arising during the perinatal period	1 177	42.1
6	Chronic obstructive pulmonary disease	2 211	43.7	Chronic obstructive pulmonary disease	1 214	42.2	Chronic obstructive pulmonary disease	997	45.4
7	Tuberculosis	1 960	45.8	Tuberculosis	1 166	44.9	Tuberculosis	794	47.6
8	Measles	1 058	47.9	Road traffic accidents	730	47.6	Measles	512	49.7
9	Road traffic accidents	999	49.8	Trachea, bronchus and lung cancers	708	49.6	Malaria	400	51.6
10	Trachea, bronchus and lung cancers	945	51.7	Measles	547	51.6	Self-inflicted injuries	330	53.3
Developed Regions									
	All Causes	10 912		All Causes	5 567		All Causes	5 345	
1	Ischaemic heart disease	2 695	24.7	Ischaemic heart disease	1 297	23.3	Ischaemic heart disease	1 398	26.1
2	Cerebrovascular disease	1 427	37.8	Cerebrovascular disease	561	33.4	Cerebrovascular disease	867	42.4
3	Trachea, bronchus and lung cancers	523	42.6	Trachea, bronchus and lung cancers	399	40.5	Lower respiratory infections	205	46.2
4	Lower respiratory infections	385	46.1	Chronic obstructive pulmonary disease	205	44.2	Breast cancer	174	49.4
5	Chronic obstructive pulmonary disease	324	49.1	Lower respiratory infections	180	47.5	Colon and rectum cancers	142	52.1

Table 3.12 (continued)

	Both Sexes		Males			Females		
Rank	Cause	Deaths (thousands)	Cumula-tive %	Cause	Deaths (thousands)	Cumula-tive %	Cause	Deaths (thousands)	Cumula-tive %

Developed Regions (continued)

Rank	Cause	Deaths (thousands)	Cumula-tive %	Cause	Deaths (thousands)	Cumula-tive %	Cause	Deaths (thousands)	Cumula-tive %
6	Colon and rectum cancers	277	51.6	Road traffic accidents	165	50.4	Trachea, bronchus and lung cancers	124	54.4
7	Stomach cancer	241	53.8	Self-inflicted injuries	143	53.0	Chronic obstructive pulmonary disease	119	56.6
8	Road traffic accidents	222	55.8	Stomach cancer	142	55.5	Diabetes mellitus	107	58.6
9	Self-inflicted injuries	193	57.6	Colon and rectum cancers	135	58.0	Stomach cancer	99	60.5
10	Diabetes mellitus	176	59.2	Cirrhosis of the liver	110	59.9	Dementia and other degenerative and hereditary CNS disorders	70	61.8

Developing Regions

Rank	Cause	Deaths (thousands)	Cumula-tive %	Cause	Deaths (thousands)	Cumula-tive %	Cause	Deaths (thousands)	Cumula-tive %
	All Causes	39 554		All Causes	21 124		All Causes	18 430	
1	Lower respiratory infections	3 915	9.9	Lower respiratory infections	2 016	9.5	Lower respiratory infections	1 899	10.3
2	Ischaemic heart disease	3 565	18.9	Ischaemic heart disease	1 829	18.2	Ischaemic heart disease	1 736	19.7
3	Cerebrovascular disease	2 954	26.4	Diarrhoeal diseases	1 529	25.4	Cerebrovascular disease	1 492	27.8
4	Diarrhoeal diseases	2 940	33.8	Cerebrovascular disease	1 461	32.4	Diarrhoeal diseases	1 410	35.5
5	Conditions arising during the perinatal period	2 361	38.7	Conditions arising during the perinatal period	1 217	37.7	Conditions arising during the perinatal period	1 144	40.2
6	Tuberculosis	1 922	43.4	Tuberculosis	1 137	42.5	Chronic obstructive pulmonary disease	878	44.5
7	Chronic obstructive pulmonary disease	1 887	46.1	Chronic obstructive pulmonary disease	1 009	45.2	Tuberculosis	785	47.3
8	Measles	1 058	48.7	Road traffic accidents	565	47.8	Measles	512	50.0
9	Malaria	856	50.9	Measles	546	50.3	Malaria	399	52.4
10	Road traffic accidents	777	52.8	Malaria	457	52.4	Self-inflicted injuries	280	54.6

million), tuberculosis (2 million), measles (just over 1 million), low birth weight and road traffic accidents (each causing about 1 million deaths) and lung cancer (950 thousand). At the global level, the ten leading causes explain just over fifty per cent of all deaths.

Not only do virtually all deaths from causes such as tuberculosis, measles and low birth weight occur in developing countries, but, interestingly, three-quarters of all road traffic accident deaths occur in developing countries. In terms of absolute numbers of deaths in the developing world as a whole (39.6 million), chronic diseases were already a major public health problem in 1990, with IHD, stroke and chronic lung diseases collectively accounting for over 8.4 million deaths (ranking 2nd, 3rd and 7th respectively in the list of leading causes in developing countries). In developed regions, three other cancers (lung, colon/rectum and stomach) are among the ten leading causes of death, as are suicide and diabetes mellitus. In developed regions, the top ten causes account for nearly sixty per cent of deaths.

Table 3.12 shows the top ten causes of death in men and women for the world, developed and developing regions. In men, the set of top ten causes is the same as for both sexes combined, although the ranks change slightly—road traffic accidents and lung cancer are more important causes of male death. However, in women, road traffic accidents and lung cancer are replaced by malaria and suicide as the 9th and 10th most important causes of death, respectively.

Because of the strong international interest in the health of women during the reproductive ages, defined here as ages 15–44, Table 3.13 lists the top ten causes of death for women (and men, for contrast) in these age groups. In 1990, an estimated 2.7 million women died at these ages. Tuberculosis was the leading cause of these deaths, accounting for about 258 thousand deaths (19.4 per cent of all deaths in this age group). Suicide remains a major cause of death among women in this age group, causing an estimated 7 per cent of deaths. War (4.4 per cent of deaths), maternal haemorrhage (3.9 per cent), road traffic accidents (3.7 per cent), HIV (3.3. per cent), and stroke (2.7 per cent) are also significant causes of death among young women.

COMMUNICABLE, MATERNAL, PERINATAL, AND NUTRITIONAL CONDITIONS

Worldwide, this group of causes is estimated to have accounted for about 17.25 million deaths in 1990, with very few of these (666 thousand) occurring in the two developed regions (EME and FSE). The reduction of mortality from these conditions in developing regions remains, therefore, a priority for global public health action. Of these more than 17 million deaths, 4.3 million (25 per cent) are estimated to have arisen from lower respiratory infections, and another 2.95 million from diarrhoeal diseases (17 per cent of all Group I deaths). In other words, 4 out of 10 deaths from Group I diseases are attributable to these two categories of infec-

Table 3.13   Leading causes of death at ages 15–44, by sex, world, 1990

Rank	Cause	Deaths (thousands)	% of all deaths	Cumulative %
Male				
	All Causes	3 691		
1	Road traffic accidents	403	10.9	10.9
2	Tuberculosis	333	9.0	19.9
3	Violence	325	8.8	28.7
4	Self-inflicted injuries	243	6.6	35.3
5	War	185	5.0	40.3
6	Ischaemic heart disease	136	3.7	44.0
7	HIV	108	2.9	47.0
8	Cirrhosis of the liver	107	2.9	49.9
9	Drownings	103	2.8	52.7
10	Cerebrovascular disease	102	2.8	55.4
Female				
	All Causes	2 734		
1	Tuberculosis	258	9.4	9.4
2	Self-inflicted injuries	195	7.1	16.6
3	War	121	4.4	21.0
4	Maternal haemorrhage	108	4.0	24.9
5	Road traffic accidents	100	3.7	28.6
6	HIV	92	3.4	31.9
7	Cerebrovascular disease	74	2.7	34.6
8	Ischaemic heart disease	73	2.7	37.3
9	Fires	70	2.5	39.8
10	Lower respiratory infections	66	2.4	42.3

tious diseases. Perinatal causes were the third leading cause among Group I causes, claiming over 2.4 million lives in 1990, followed by tuberculosis (1.96 million deaths, or about 11 per cent of Group I causes). No other condition in this Group is estimated to have caused more than 10 per cent of all deaths in Group I, with only measles (6 per cent of Group I deaths), and malaria (5 per cent) causing more than 5 per cent of deaths in this pre-transition category. HIV infection is estimated to have caused only about 2 per cent of all Group I deaths in 1990, but this proportion is expected to rise rapidly as the impact of widespread infection during the 1980s becomes evident over the next two decades.

CARDIOVASCULAR DISEASES

Of the various cardiovascular disease pathologies listed in Table 3.14, ischaemic heart disease and stroke predominate in the developed regions accounting for 75–80 per cent of all CVD deaths; stroke is proportion-

Table 3.14   Cause distribution of cardiovascular diseases (CVD) deaths, by region, 1990

	Region								
Cause	EME	FSE	IND	CHI	OAI	SSA	LAC	MEC	World
All CVD deaths (000s)	3 175	2 071	2 266	2 568	1 349	815	789	1 295	14 327
Percentage of CVD deaths attributable to:									
Rheumatic heart disease	0.6	1.2	3.1	6.3	0.8	2.4	1.0	1.9	2.4
Ischaemic heart disease	52.5	49.6	51.9	29.7	34.2	25.6	44.1	47.1	43.7
Cerebrovascular disease	24.8	30.9	19.8	49.5	28.9	47.0	31.5	16.3	30.6
Inflammatory heart diseases	2.1	1.9	3.7	2.6	6.1	7.8	3.1	5.5	3.5
Other CVD	19.9	16.5	21.6	11.9	30.1	17.1	20.3	29.1	19.9

ately more important as a cause of cardiovascular disease death in FSE (31 per cent) than in EME (25 per cent). Rheumatic heart disease is estimated to cause from 1 per cent to 6 per cent of all CVD deaths in the developing regions (and about 2.4 per cent globally). The category labelled as inflammatory heart diseases (pericarditis, endocarditis, myocarditis and cardiomyopathies) accounts for similar proportions of CVD deaths, being highest in sub-Saharan Africa (7.8 per cent). It is also worth noting the very substantial contribution of ischaemic heart disease in all developing regions, ranging from 52 per cent of cardiovascular deaths in India to 26 per cent in SSA. Stroke, on the other hand, is by far the leading cause of cardiovascular deaths in China and SSA, causing roughly half of all cardiovascular disease deaths in 1990.

CANCER

Cancer caused about 6 million deaths in 1990, 3.4 million of which occurred in men. Of this total of 6 million deaths, about 2.4 million occurred in EME and FSE. By 1990, therefore, there were already 50 per cent more cancer deaths in less developed countries compared with developed countries. Globally, lung cancer (trachea, bronchus and lung) is the leading site of cancer deaths, claiming an estimated 945 thousand victims each year. Stomach cancer is the next most important site of cancer mortality (752 thousand deaths), followed by liver (500 thousand), colon/ rectum (472 thousand), oesophagus (358 thousand) and breast (322 thousand). Most lung cancer deaths in 1990 still occurred among males (708 thousand). Indeed, lung cancer caused 1.5 times as many male deaths in 1990 than the next most important site for males (stomach cancer, with 469 thousand deaths). Other leading sites of cancer mortality for males worldwide include the liver (357 thousand deaths), oesophagus (240 thousand), colon/rectum (237 thousand), prostate (193 thousand) and mouth and oropharynx (186 thousand). Breast cancer was the leading site of cancer deaths for females in 1990, claiming about 50 thousand more victims than the next most important site for cancer mortality (stomach, with 282 thousand deaths). Interestingly, lung cancer was already the third leading site of mortality from cancer in women in 1990, accounting for an estimated 237 thousand deaths, slightly more than cervical cancer (200 thousand). More than half of these female lung cancer deaths (124 thousand) occurred among women in developed countries.

As mortality declines, two major cancer transitions occur. One is that lung cancer rises and stomach cancer declines, while the other is that breast cancer rises and cervical cancer declines. The ratios of lung to stomach cancer deaths in males and breast to cervix cancer in females are useful indicators of the evolution of this transition (Figure 3.16). These two cancer transitions follow a similar pattern for most regions. In EME, there are 8.6 times more breast cancer deaths than cervical cancer deaths and 3.4 times more lung cancer deaths compared with stomach cancer. FSE, the next closest region in epidemiological profile, has a breast cancer to cervix cancer mortality ratio of 2.6 and a lung cancer to stomach cancer ratio of 2. In contrast, SSA has a breast cancer to cervix cancer ratio of 0.5 and a lung cancer to stomach cancer mortality ratio of 0.8. Of note, the breast cancer to cervix cancer ratio in China is about 1.2, similar to that for LAC and MEC, whereas the lung cancer to stomach cancer mortality ratio is much lower in China than in these two regions.

INTENTIONAL AND UNINTENTIONAL INJURIES

Injuries, whether intentional or unintentional, are a major cause of death worldwide. In 1990, 5 million people are estimated to have died from Group III causes (injuries and poisonings), representing 10 per cent of

Figure 3.16   Indicators of the cancer transition, by region, 1990

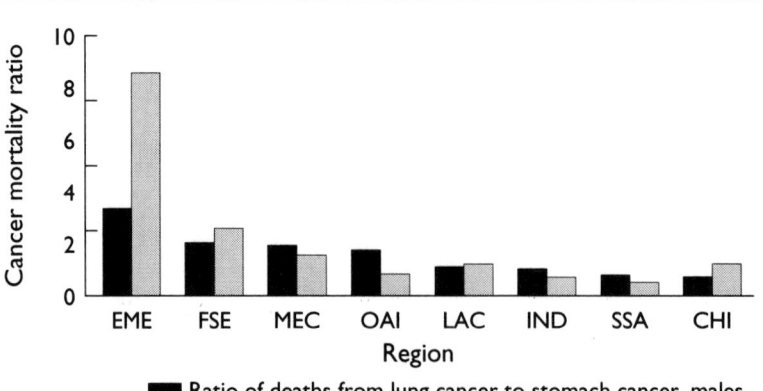

deaths that year. The risk of injury death varies strongly by region, age and sex. Globally, there are about 2 male deaths from violence for every female death (3.3 million compared with 1.7 million). Injuries account for about 12.5 per cent of all male deaths, compared with 7.4 per cent among females. Equally striking is the marked regional variation in mortality from violent causes. In EME, for example, injuries caused about 6 per cent of all deaths in 1990, compared with 9–11 per cent in other regions, rising to 12–13 per cent in sub-Saharan Africa and Latin America. Indeed, violence is a major cause of male deaths in these two regions, accounting for 16–17 per cent of all male deaths.

Worth noting also are the marked regional differences in the causes of injury deaths. Thus, in EME and FSE, road traffic accidents were the leading cause of Group III deaths in 1990 accounting for 30 per cent and 23 per cent, respectively, of all injury deaths in these two regions. Suicide is also a leading cause of injury death in both regions (25 per cent and 21 per cent of Group III deaths, respectively). Fires are not a major cause of injury death in EME (2.4 per cent of Group III deaths), but are much more significant in India where they cause about 15 per cent of Group III deaths, second only to road traffic accidents (21.6 per cent). More importantly, fires are estimated to be by far the leading cause of Group III deaths among Indian females, accounting for one out of every four injury deaths. Suicide is a major cause of injury death in China, causing over 40 per cent of female injury deaths and one in four male injury deaths. Drownings and road traffic accidents are the next most important causes of injury death in both males and females in China. War, on the other hand, is estimated to be the leading cause of injury death in sub-Saharan Africa, particularly among females (causing almost 40 per cent of all female deaths from injuries). Taken together, war and violence are estimated to be responsible for almost half (46 per cent) of all injury deaths in sub-Saharan Africa. Violence is also a major cause of male mortality in Latin America and the Caribbean, causing an estimated 30 per cent of all male deaths from external causes. Road traffic accidents in LAC rank second for males (27 per cent of male injury deaths) and first for females (30 per cent of all Group III deaths).

What makes injury deaths particularly important for public health is their very skewed age distribution, with the majority of those killed by these causes being comparatively young. Globally, 30 per cent of male injury deaths occur at ages 15–29 years, as do one-quarter of female injury deaths.

MALE-FEMALE DIFFERENTIALS IN MORTALITY

The estimated age-patterns of mortality for males and females vary by region, age and cause Group. The ratio of male to female crude mortality rates for Groups I and II are close to 1 (Table 3.15)—ranging from 0.95 for Group I in China to 1.19 for Group I in LAC. The sex mortality ratio of crude death rates from Group III (Injuries), however, ranges from 1.21

in India to 3.13 in FSE. Moreover, the male-female ratio of Group mortality rates for the world (Figure 3.17) shows a markedly different age-pattern for each Group. Group I mortality rates are slightly higher in males under age 5 than in females, but from age 5 through to age 44, female Group I death rates for the world are higher than male. This reflects the fact that, in these age groups, the increased risk of death from reproductive causes exceeds the slight excess death rate from tuberculosis in males. As shown in Table 3.15, as mortality declines, the excess Group I death rate in females at these ages shifts to an excess male mortality. The ratio at ages 30–44 for EME is 4.33, reflecting the substantial impact of the HIV epidemic in this age group among males.

Globally, Group II mortality rates are higher in males than females in all age groups, but the excess begins to rise substantially after age 30. (Table 3.15 indicates that in a few regions male Group II mortality rates are lower than female for selected age groups between 0 and 29). The largest excess Group II male mortality rates are in SSA at ages 30–44 and in FSE ages 45–59. Clearly, the most dramatic differences in mortality risk between the two sexes are for Group III (Injuries). In all age groups in all regions with only one exception, males die at a higher rate from injuries than do females. (The exception is Indian women aged 15–29.) Globally, excess male mortality rises from childhood (a rate ratio of 1.16) to a peak at ages 30–44 (rate ratio of 2.73). The same age-pattern of male-female mortality ratios is observed in all eight regions. FSE and LAC have the highest male-female ratios — more than three times as many men die from injuries as do women.

Figure 3.17   Male-female ratio of mortality rates by age, world, 1990

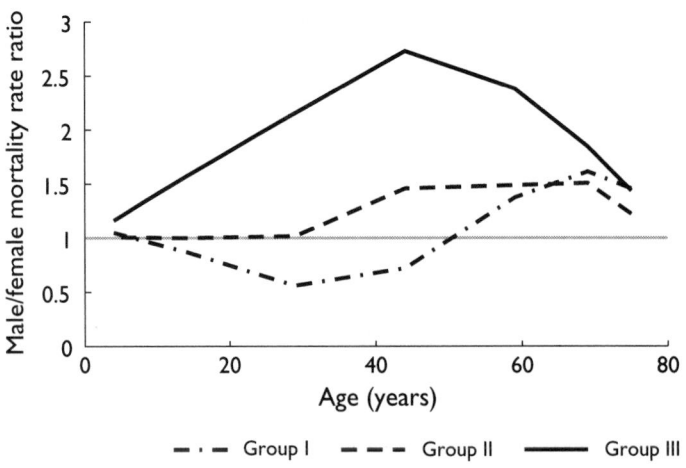

Table 3.15 Ratio of male to female death rates by age and region, for all causes and for broad cause Groups

Region	All ages	Age group (years)						
		0–4	5–14	15–29	30–44	45–59	60–69	70+
All Causes								
EME	1.10	1.26	1.48	2.79	2.11	1.97	1.97	1.34
FSE	1.11	1.31	1.70	2.97	3.00	2.60	1.95	1.37
IND	1.01	0.92	0.82	0.75	1.20	1.34	1.25	1.07
CHI	1.12	0.86	1.27	1.13	1.37	1.43	1.46	1.22
OAI	1.21	1.21	1.28	1.30	1.34	1.47	1.43	1.16
SSA	1.14	1.15	1.08	1.25	1.18	1.28	1.19	1.09
LAC	1.23	1.27	1.30	1.54	1.51	1.40	1.39	1.20
MEC	1.07	1.02	1.07	1.15	1.27	1.46	1.38	1.17
World	1.11	1.05	1.06	1.20	1.39	1.54	1.53	1.25
Group 1								
EME	1.14	1.31	0.98	2.44	4.33	3.08	1.94	1.34
FSE	1.14	1.37	1.14	1.02	2.58	4.56	2.31	1.34
IND	0.96	0.90	0.70	0.62	0.99	1.45	1.62	1.33
CHI	0.95	0.82	0.85	0.49	0.90	1.72	1.50	1.49
OAI	1.12	1.22	1.09	0.62	0.57	1.03	1.55	1.13
SSA	1.03	1.16	0.94	0.49	0.50	1.17	1.13	1.17
LAC	1.19	1.30	0.84	0.74	0.85	1.36	1.45	1.19
MEC	0.98	1.01	0.95	0.50	0.48	1.21	1.62	1.23
World	1.03	1.05	0.87	0.56	0.72	1.37	1.61	1.46

Table 3.15 (continued)

Region	All ages	0–4	5–14	15–29	30–44	45–59	60–69	70+
Group II								
EME	1.05	1.18	1.21	1.59	1.52	1.86	1.95	1.34
FSE	0.99	1.23	1.27	1.54	2.06	2.36	1.91	1.36
IND	1.04	0.95	0.84	0.72	1.30	1.26	1.17	1.00
CHI	1.13	0.89	1.40	1.23	1.31	1.40	1.46	1.21
OAI	1.15	1.13	1.20	1.02	1.48	1.51	1.39	1.16
SSA	1.03	0.96	0.85	1.33	2.39	1.16	1.15	1.05
LAC	1.03	1.06	1.23	0.60	1.07	1.22	1.32	1.19
MEC	1.05	1.03	0.90	0.84	1.26	1.42	1.34	1.15
World	1.06	1.01	1.00	1.02	1.46	1.49	1.51	1.22
Group III								
EME	2.12	1.40	1.94	3.76	3.41	2.90	2.40	1.43
FSE	3.13	1.25	2.14	4.25	5.24	4.27	2.80	1.78
IND	1.21	1.27	1.07	0.97	1.59	1.55	1.03	1.27
CHI	1.29	1.02	1.45	1.26	1.80	1.44	1.45	1.15
OAI	2.17	1.16	1.95	2.53	3.17	3.12	2.04	2.01
SSA	2.42	1.28	1.77	3.42	3.40	3.31	2.31	1.76
LAC	3.04	1.25	2.07	3.64	4.82	4.40	3.03	1.92
MEC	1.82	1.03	1.82	2.11	2.58	2.55	1.64	1.51
World	1.86	1.16	1.57	2.15	2.73	2.38	1.85	1.44

The patterns of male-female mortality ratios presented here do not address the question of how much of the difference in male and female mortality experience is biological and how much is amenable to intervention. Clearly, in developing countries, as the risks of reproduction are reduced, higher rates of Group I mortality in women would be expected to disappear. On the other hand, the relatively higher rates of Group II and Group III mortality in men do not seem to have declined with the reduction in all-cause mortality except in high-income groups with low mortality populations. If exposure to critical risk factors that explain much of the excess Group II mortality in males—i.e. tobacco, occupational hazards and hazardous alcohol use—are reduced through concerted public action, we might expect the future gap in Group II mortality rates between males and females to decline. Likewise, if the massive excess of male mortality from Group III at all ages could be reduced, in the future, male survival might much more closely approximate female survival, at least in the young adult age groups.

YEARS OF LIFE LOST

To adequately describe and monitor health status on the basis of mortality rates (or numbers) requires a vast array of age-specific indicators, simply because mortality rates are strongly age (and sex) dependent. Thus while the actual number of deaths from two (or more) diseases or injuries may be similar, their public health importance may be quite different depending on the age at which death typically occurs (and other considerations, such as the cost-effectiveness of interventions). Injuries and cancers (each causing around 5–6 million deaths a year) are a good example, with injuries concentrated in the middle age groups and cancers concentrated in the elderly. One method of capturing this age-pattern of mortality is to weight each death by the number of years of life lost due to premature death, this weight being higher for deaths at younger ages than at older ages. There are many methods in use for calculating the length of life lost due to premature mortality; for this study, however, we have calculated Years of Life Lost (YLLs) using the methods fully explained in Chapter 1 in this volume (Murray 1996).

Globally, it is estimated that there were about 898 million years of life lost in 1990 due to premature death, of which more than half (54 per cent) arose from Group I causes, and a further 15 per cent from injuries (Group III)—see Table 3.16. Noncommunicable diseases, on the other hand, accounted for 31 per cent of YLLs, considerably less than their proportionate share of mortality (56 per cent), reflecting the fact that these diseases claim lives among older adults. This predominant influence of Group I conditions on YLLs calculations is also reflected in the pattern of regional contributions to the global total. Thus, one-quarter of all YLLs in 1990 is estimated to have occurred in sub-Saharan Africa, and, of these, 74 per cent arose from Group I causes. Premature death in India contrib-

Table 3.16   Years of Life Lost (YLLs) by broad cause Group, 1990

	Group I	Group II	Group III	Total
YLLs (in millions)				
EME	4.4	37.4	7.9	49.7
FSE	3.4	24.3	8.3	35.9
IND	132.9	45.2	22.0	200.1
CHN	33.3	60.7	23.8	117.9
OAI	61.4	37.4	15.9	114.6
SSA	167.7	28.2	31.0	226.9
LAC	26.7	19.1	10.4	56.2
MEC	60.8	31.2	13.2	105.2
World	**490.6**	**283.4**	**132.5**	**906.5**
Percentage of regional YLLs				
EME	8.8	75.3	15.9	100.0
FSE	9.4	67.6	23.0	100.0
IND	66.4	22.6	11.0	100.0
CHN	28.3	51.5	20.2	100.0
OAI	53.6	32.6	13.8	100.0
SSA	73.9	12.4	13.7	100.0
LAC	47.5	34.0	18.5	100.0
MEC	57.8	29.7	12.6	100.0
World	**54.1**	**31.3**	**14.6**	**100.0**

Notes:

Group I: Communicable, maternal, perinatal and nutritional conditions
Group II: Noncommunicable diseases
Group III: Injuries

uted about 22 per cent to this global total. China, OAI, and MEC each contributed 12–13 per cent to this total.

Not only is there a substantial difference in the contributions of different regions to the global total of YLLs, but the composition of leading causes of YLLs varies dramatically from region to region. Thus in EME and FSE, ischaemic heart disease is by far the largest public health problem, as assessed by this metric, accounting for 16–17 per cent of all YLLs. Road traffic accidents (for males) and stroke (for females) rank second, followed by suicide and lung cancer. Lower respiratory infections, diarrhoeal diseases, low birth weight, tuberculosis and measles are the most important causes of YLLs in the developing regions (Table 3.17), although there is considerable regional variation. For example, in China, stroke is the second leading cause, accounting for about 8 per cent of YLLs, about the same as perinatal conditions, and only marginally more than chronic lung diseases and suicide. Malaria is an important cause of YLLs in sub-

Saharan Africa (11 per cent of YLLs), as is measles (9 per cent). In LAC, low birth weight is estimated to be the second most important cause of YLLs (after perinatal conditions), with important contributions from violence and road traffic accidents as well.

ANNEX TABLES[16]

Annex Table 6 provides detailed estimates of mortality for seven age groups, two sexes, eight regions and the world for over 100 causes using the methods described in this chapter. The table also provides the populations for each age-sex group so that the interested reader can calculate age-specific death rates for each cause. Annex Table 7 provides in the same detail Years of Life Lost for each cause.

DISCUSSION

Few of those entrusted with improving the public health would doubt the importance of having reliable data on the cause structure of mortality. Death, unlike morbidity, is an unambiguous event which is clearly defined and thus is, in principle at least, more reliably assessed and monitored at the population level. Death registration and medical certification become progressively more complete and reliable with overall health and socio-economic development. It remains, however, extremely uncommon for developing countries to possess good cause-of-death data for their entire population, although very useful data can be obtained from sentinel surveillance systems covering fractions of the population, as seen in China. The overwhelming conclusion to emerge from this attempt at global and regional mortality estimation is that, as we enter the third millennium, still very little is reliably known about causes of death in much of the developing world.

We have attempted to generate what we believe are the most credible estimates of mortality by cause for each region, but substantial uncertainty will remain for many years about the precise distribution of mortality by cause for most of the developing world. Within developing regions, some estimates are more uncertain than others. In general, the estimates with largest confidence intervals are those for SSA. As noted in the text, there is considerable uncertainty about the levels of adult mortality in much of the developing world. While we are reasonably confident about the estimates of the magnitudes of Groups I, II and III, the exact distributions of mortality within each of these Groups must be considered as much less reliable.

What are the implications of these data lacunae for monitoring progress with global health promotion strategies and specific disease prevention activities? Firstly, much more research is required on the application and adaptation of promising methods for epidemiological surveillance in poorer populations. The Disease Surveillance Points system operating throughout China would seem to be the most useful alternative to complete vital

Table 3.17   Leading causes of Years of Life Lost (YLLs), world, developed and developing regions, by sex, 1990

Rank	Both Sexes Cause	YLLs (thousands)	Cumula-tive %	Males Cause	YLLs (thousands)	Cumula-tive %	Females Cause	YLLs (thousands)	Cumula-tive %
World									
	All Causes	906 501		All Causes	486 937		All Causes	419 565	
1	Lower respiratory infections	108 601	12.0	Lower respiratory infections	55 547	11.4	Lower respiratory infections	53 054	12.6
2	Diarrhoeal diseases	94 434	22.4	Diarrhoeal diseases	49 016	21.5	Diarrhoeal diseases	45 418	23.5
3	Conditions arising during the perinatal period	82 681	31.5	Conditions arising during the perinatal period	42 626	30.2	Conditions arising during the perinatal period	40 055	33.0
4	Ischaemic heart disease	41 595	36.1	Ischaemic heart disease	23 093	35.0	Ischaemic heart disease	18 501	37.4
5	Measles	36 450	40.1	Tuberculosis	19 334	38.9	Measles	17 713	41.6
6	Tuberculosis	34 304	43.9	Road traffic accidents	19 184	42.9	Cerebrovascular disease	16 017	45.5
7	Cerebrovascular disease	32 115	47.5	Measles	18 737	46.7	Tuberculosis	14 971	49.0
8	Malaria	28 038	50.5	Cerebrovascular disease	16 098	50.0	Malaria	13 081	52.2
9	Road traffic accidents	26 162	53.4	Malaria	14 957	53.1	Congenital anomalies	9 582	54.4
10	Congenital anomalies	19 414	55.6	Violence	12 174	55.6	Tetanus	8 718	56.5
Developed Regions									
	All Causes	85 605		All Causes	52 137		All Causes	33 468	
1	Ischaemic heart disease	14 478	16.9	Ischaemic heart disease	8 675	16.6	Ischaemic heart disease	5 803	17.3
2	Cerebrovascular disease	7 081	25.2	Road traffic accidents	3 906	24.1	Cerebrovascular disease	3 740	28.5
3	Road traffic accidents	5 050	31.1	Cerebrovascular disease	3 341	30.5	Breast cancer	1 684	33.5
4	Trachea bronchus and lung cancers	4 269	36.1	Trachea bronchus and lung cancers	3 311	36.9	Road traffic accidents	1 143	37.0
5	Self-inflicted injuries	3 495	40.2	Self-inflicted injuries	2 722	42.1	Conditions arising during the	1 126	40.3

Table 3.17 (continued)

	Both Sexes			Males			Females		
Rank	Cause	YLLs (thousands)	Cumulative %	Cause	YLLs (thousands)	Cumulative %	Cause	YLLs (thousands)	Cumulative %
Developed Regions (continued)									
							perinatal period		
6	Conditions arising during the perinatal period	2 751	43.4	Conditions arising during the perinatal period	1 625	45.2	Lower respiratory infections	1 031	43.4
7	Lower respiratory infections	2 290	46.0	Cirrhosis of the liver	1 272	47.7	Trachea bronchus and lung cancers	958	46.3
8	Congenital anomalies	2 044	48.4	Lower respiratory infections	1 259	50.1	Congenital anomalies	915	49.0
9	Colon and rectum cancers	1 866	50.6	Stomach cancer	1 164	52.3	Colon and rectum cancers	896	51.7
10	Stomach cancer	1 856	52.8	Violence	1 131	54.5	Self-inflicted injuries	773	54.0
Developing Regions									
	All Causes	820 897		All Causes	434 800		All Causes	386 097	
1	Lower respiratory infections	106 311	13.0	Lower respiratory infections	54 288	12.5	Lower respiratory infections	52 023	13.5
2	Diarrhoeal diseases	94 283	24.4	Diarrhoeal diseases	48 933	23.7	Diarrhoeal diseases	45 350	25.2
3	Conditions arising during the perinatal period	79 930	34.2	Conditions arising during the perinatal period	41 001	33.2	Conditions arising during the perinatal period	38 929	35.3
4	Measles	36 437	38.6	Tuberculosis	18 952	37.5	Measles	17 707	39.9
5	Tuberculosis	33 846	42.7	Measles	18 730	41.8	Tuberculosis	14 894	43.7
6	Malaria	28 036	46.1	Road traffic accidents	15 278	45.3	Malaria	13 080	47.1
7	Ischaemic heart disease	27 117	49.5	Malaria	14 956	48.8	Ischaemic heart disease	12 698	50.4
8	Cerebrovascular disease	25 034	52.5	Ischaemic heart disease	14 418	52.1	Cerebrovascular disease	12 277	53.6
9	Road traffic accidents	21 113	55.1	Cerebrovascular disease	12 757	55.0	Tetanus	8 716	55.9
10	Tetanus	17 504	57.2	Violence	11 043	57.6	Congenital anomalies	8 668	58.1

registration but much more research is required on how adaptable this approach might prove to be in different socio-political environments. Applied research on the cost-effectiveness of different systems for data collection is also urgently required. The system of collecting cause-of-death data via "verbal autopsies" needs to be evaluated and improved in order to provide reliable data on broad causes-of-death categories at low cost. What is also clear from this attempt at global estimation of mortality patterns is that even the levels of mortality rates among adults are not well known in many parts of the developing world. As more and more regions move through the epidemiological transition, death, and particularly premature death among adults, will increasingly become a major public health concern. Surveillance systems and research methods to measure and monitor adult mortality must anticipate this trend.

Indeed, the results of this estimation exercise would suggest that the epidemiological transition in developing regions is considerably more advanced than is generally thought. Noncommunicable diseases already cause more deaths in the developing world than communicable diseases and, in some regions, notably China and to a lesser extent LAC, noncommunicable diseases are the most important causes of death. Without detracting from the appropriate focus of global public health activities on reducing infant and child mortality, health promotion and disease prevention programmes in developing countries will need to increasingly adapt to this emerging public health reality. Equally, the global importance of injuries (Group III causes) as a major cause of death and YLLs in all regions (although the composition of leading causes may vary) suggests that much more attention will need to be given by all countries to reducing premature death from unintentional and intentional injuries of all forms.

The fundamental question which must be asked at the conclusion of any attempt at global and regional estimation is whether or not the estimates are useful. Estimates can indeed be counterproductive as an information support for policies and programmes if they are substantially wrong. On the basis of currently available data and research, we do not believe that these estimates are substantially wrong, but they may very well differ from other, independently derived estimates, and they will certainly change as more reliable data and information appear. Part of the difference between these estimates and those developed by disease experts lies in the estimation process we have used, whereby dozens of causes are competing for deaths, as it were. Disease-specific estimates, on the other hand, are generally derived in isolation from other competing causes and may well include co-morbidities which, following the procedures outlined in this chapter, have been allocated to other causes. Differences may also arise from genuine differences in methods of estimation and the extent to which epidemiological models are thought to be applicable.

We do not know how reliable these estimates are. This can only be known once more reliable data become available, by which time the need for estimates will be obviated. Until then, however, we believe that a comprehensive, uniformly-derived set of mortality estimates such as that presented here is required, and will prove useful for public health programmes and policies. Surely, whether or not a disease or injury kills one, two or even three million people a year is not the issue. What matters is that the disease or injury is a major (or minor) cause of death and that, while much more reliable assessment is required, enough is already known about the magnitude of the hazard to take appropriate public health measures. That, after all, is the purpose of mortality statistics and, where these are not available, mortality estimates.

NOTES

1   In earlier versions of the Global Burden of Disease Study, the nutritional deficiencies—namely protein-energy malnutrition, vitamin A deficiency, iodine deficiency disorders, and anaemias—were included in Group II. These conditions clearly meet the criterion defining the pre-transitional cluster of diseases belonging to Group I. However, they were not included in Group I in earlier versions of this study because of the difficulty in distinguishing some of these deaths from other nutritional and endocrine causes using the data available at that time. Considerably more effort has gone into the analysis of these conditions in this fifth version of the study, permitting the appropriate transfer of these causes to Group I.

2   On request, WHO can provide data for a number of countries coded according to the Basic Tabulation List. Not all data for countries listed in Table 3.4 are currently available from WHO since special tabulations of mortality statistics for some populations were provided specifically for this study.

3   Mesle et al. (1992) have reconstructed mortality trends by cause for the USSR for the period 1970–1987. Their analysis was also based on content validity criteria and not on a formal bridge-coding excercise.

4   The cause-of-death models used in earlier versions of the Global Burden of Disease Study are not exactly the same as presented here. Although the functional forms of the two sets of models are similar, the specific results differ because of the addition of more recent information and refinements of the estimation procedures as described in this chapter.

5   In fact, we have used "Latin hypercube sampling" which is a more efficient means of sampling than traditional Monte Carlo simulation (Blower et al. 1991).

6   Results of these detailed-cause regressions are presented in Chapter 7 in this volume (Murray and Lopez 1996).

7   The Sample Registration Scheme is a nationally-representative system for estimating birth and death rates in the various states and territories of India.

8   We are grateful to Judith Bannister for making available the US Bureau of the Census life tables for 28 provinces based on an analysis of data from the 12-month recall of deaths in the household as assessed in the 1982 Census.

9   We are grateful to Rafael Lozano for providing data on population and deaths by age, sex and state.

10 We are grateful to Stephen Hendrix for providing us with preliminary results from his research on causes of death in South Africa. Our analysis of vital registration data from South Africa is based largely on his findings.

11 Timeus IM. *Estimation of age-specific mortality in sub-Saharan Africa for use in modelling the world burden of disease.* Report to PHR-HN, The World Bank, July 1992.

12 The US National Cancer Institute maintains the Surveillance, Epidemiology and End Results (SEER) Program, which is considered to be the most reliable of all cancer registration systems. The SEER system is based on registration data from Connecticut, Hawaii, Iowa, New Mexico and Utah, and Detroit, Atlanta, San Francisco-Oakland, and Seattle-Puget Sound (Ries et al. 1994).

13 Bulutao (1993) found a negative coefficient between age-specific cancer mortality rates and all-cause mortality rates. When he used these models to estimate mortality by cause in high mortality populations, he predicted very low age-specific cancer mortality rates. We believe this result is a direct consequence of not correcting for temporal and cross-sectional patterns in the death rate from "Symptoms, signs and ill-defined conditions" (ICD-9 Chapter XVI).

14 Parkin and colleagues have more recently generated a revised set of estimates of incidence and mortality by site based on new data and a revision of their estimation methods. These estimates were kindly made available to the authors for comparison with the estimates based on the methods described above, but, since this information is not yet in the public domain, it could not be used directly for preparing the estimates for the GBD. As before, the most important difference between the two sets of estimates is not in the site-specific distribution of deaths, but in the total cancer death rate for each age-sex group and region.

15 Neonatal death is defined as a death which occurs in the first 28 days of life.

16 We have compared the detailed results of this revised set of cause-of-death estimates with those that we have previously published (Murray and Lopez 1994). The six changes of more than 100 thousand deaths are as follows: an increase in ischaemic heart disease mortality of 1.1 million deaths globally due to improved corrections of cardiovascular coding; a decrease of 870 thousand deaths assigned to inflammatory heart diseases because much more detailed data on cardiovascular coding was available for this excercise; a decrease of 250 thousand deaths assigned to stroke, most of which is due to reassignment to ischaemic heart disease; an increase of 144 thousand deaths from road traffic accidents and an increase of 139 thousand deaths from COPD; and an increase of 120 thousand deaths from drownings.

BIBLIOGRAPHY

Adult Mortality and Morbidity Project Team (1993) *Policy implications of adult morbidity and mortality: a preliminary report of the adult morbidity and mortality project, Tanzania.* Dar es Salaam, AMMP.

Bang AT, Bang RA, SEARCH team (1992) Diagnosis of causes of childhood deaths in developing countries by verbal autopsy: suggested criteria. *Bulletin of the World Health Organization,* 70(4):499–507.

Battle RM et al. (1987) Factors influencing discrepancies between premortem and postmortem diagnoses. *Journal of the American Medical Association*, 258(3):339–344.

Blower SM et al. (1991) Drugs, sex and HIV: a mathematical model for New York City. *Philosophical transactions of the Royal Society series B*, 331:171–187.

Bonita R et al. (1995) Approaches to the problems of measuring the incidence of stroke: the Auckland Stroke Study. *International journal of epidemiology*, 24(3):535–542.

Bonita R et al. (1996) Stroke. In: Murray CJL, Lopez AD, eds *Global perspectives on non-communicable diseases: the epidemiology of cancers, cardiovascular diseases, diabetes mellitus, respiratory disorders and other major conditions.* Cambridge, Harvard University.

Britton M (1974) Diagnostic errors discovered at autopsy. *Acta Medica Scandinavia* 196:203–210.

Bulutao R (1993) Mortality by cause, 1970 to 2015. In: Gribble JN, Preston SH, eds. *The epidemiological transition. Policy and planning implications for developing countries. Workshop proceedings.* Washington, DC, National Academy Press.

Burr ML (1995) Explaining the French paradox. *Journal of the Royal Society of Health*, 115(4):217–9.

Campbell M (1963) Death rate from diseases of the heart: 1876–1959. *British medical journal*, ii:528–35.

Carvalho F et al. (1991) Clinical diagnosis versus autopsy. *Bulletin of the Pan-American Health Organization*, 25(1):41–46.

Chandramohan D et al. (1994) Verbal autopsies for adult deaths: issues in their deveolpment and validation. *International Journal of Epidemiology*, 23(2): 213–222.

Chen Junshi et al. (1990) *Diet, life-style, and mortality in China. A study of the characteristics of 65 Chinese counties.* Oxford, Oxford University Press.

Chinese Academy of Preventive Medicine (1992) *1992 Annual report on Chinese disease surveillance.* Beijing, Hua Zia Publishing House.

Criqui MH, Ringel BL (1994) Does diet or alcohol explain the French paradox? *Lancet* 344(8939–8940):1719–23.

de Francisco A et al. (1994) Comparison of mortality between villages with and without primary health care workers in Upper River Division, The Gambia. *Journal of tropical medicine and hygiene*, 97:69–74.

Desjarlais R et al. (1995) *World mental health. Problems and priorities in low-income countries.* New York, Oxford University Press.

D'Souza S (1986) Mortality structure in Matlab (Bangladesh) and the effect of selected health interventions. In: United Nations *Determinants of mortality change and differentials in developing countries. The five-country case study project.* New York, United Nations.

Foege W (1994) Preventive medicine and public health. *Journal of the American medical association*, 271(21):1704–1705.

Frenk J (1989) Health transition in middle-income countries: new challenges for health care. *Health policy and planning*, 4(1):29–39.

Garenne M et al. (1991) Child mortality after high-titre measles vaccines: prospective study in Senegal. *Lancet*, 338(8772):903–907.

Gareeboo H et al. (1995) *The national burden of disease of Mauritius.* Report to the Government of Mauritius.

Ghana VAST Study Team (1993) Vitamin A supplementation in northern Ghana: effects on clinic attendances, hospital admissions and child mortality. *Lancet*, 342:7–12.

Gough J (1985) Correlation between clinical and autopsy diagnoses in a community hospital. *Canadian medical association journal*, 133:420–422.

Gray RH (1991) *Verbal autopsy: using interviews to determine causes of death in children.* Johns Hopkins University Institute for International Programs Occasional Paper Series No. 14, Baltimore.

Hakulinen T et al. (1986) Global and regional mortality patterns by cause of death in 1980. *International journal of epidemiology*, 15:226–233.

Hull TH et al. (1981) A framework for estimating causes of death in Indonesia. *Majalah demografi Indonesia*, 15:77–125.

Kalter H et al. (1990) Validation of postmortem interviews to ascertain selected causes of childhood death in children. *International journal of epidemiology*, 19:380–386.

Kojima S et al. (1990) Prognosis and disability of stroke patients after 5 years in Akita, Japan. *Stroke*, 21(1):72–77.

Lopez AD, Hull TH (1983) A note on estimating the cause of death structure in high mortality populations. *Population bulletin of the United Nations*, 14:66–70.

Li J et al. (1981) Atlas of cancer mortality in the Peoples' Republic of China. An aid for cancer control and research. *International journal of epidemiology*, 10:127–33.

Londoño JL et al. (1994) La carga de la enfermedad en Colombia. Ministerio de Salud, Bogota, Colombia. [The burden of disease in Colombia. Ministry of Health, Bogota, Colombia.]

Lozano R et al. (1995) Burden of disease assessment and health system reform: results of a study in Mexico. *Journal of international development*, 7(3):555–563.

Lozano R et al. (1994) El peso de la enfermedad en Mexico: un doble reto. [The burden of disease in Mexico: a double burden] *Documentos de analisis y convergencia*, 3. Mexico, FUNSALUD.

Lozano R, Murray CJL, Lopez AD (1996) *The French Paradox revisited: undercoding of ischemic heart disease mortality.* Harvard Center for Population and Development Studies Working Papers.

Mesle F, Shkolnikov V, Vallin J (1992) Mortality by cause in the USSR in 1970–1987: reconstruction of time series. *Revue Europeene de demographie* 8:281–308.

Middleton K et al. (1989) An autopsy-based study of diagnostic errors in geriatric and nongeriatric adult patients. *Archives of internal medicine*, 149:1809–1812.

Murray CJL (1996) Rethinking DALYs. In: Murray CJL, Lopez AD, eds. *The Global Burden of Disease: a comprehensive assessment of mortality and disability from diseases, injuries, and risk factors in 1990 and projected to 2020.* Cambridge, Harvard University Press.

Murray CJL, Lopez AD (1994) Global and regional cause-of-death patterns in 1990. *Bulletin of the World Health Organization,* 72(3):447–480.

Murray CJL, Lopez AD (1996) Alternative visions of the future: projecting mortality and disability, 1990–2020. In: Murray CJL, Lopez AD, eds. *The Global Burden of Disease: a comprehensive assessment of mortality and disability from diseases, injuries, and risk factors in 1990 and projected to 2020.* Cambridge, Harvard University Press.

Murray CJL, Yang G, Qiao X (1992) Adult mortality: levels, patterns and causes. In: Feachem, RGS et al., eds. *The health of adults in the developing world.* Oxford, Oxford University Press, pp. 23–111.

Government of India, Registrar-General (1992a) *Medical certification of causes of death. Annual report 1991.* New Delhi, Ministry of Home Affairs.

Government of India, Registrar-General (1992b) *Survey of causes of death (rural). Annual report 1991.* New Delhi, Ministry of Home Affairs.

Omondi-Odhiambo, van Ginneken JK, Voorhoeve AM (1990) Mortality by cause of death in a rural area of Machakos district, Kenya in 1975–78. *Journal of biosocial science,* 22:63–75.

Parkin DM et al. (1992) *Cancer incidence in five continents. Volume VI.* Lyon, International Agency for Research on Cancer.

Preston SH (1976) *Mortality patterns in national populations.* New York, Academic Press.

Preston SH, Keyfitz N, Schoen R (1972) Causes of death. In: *Life tables for national populations.* New York, Seminar Press.

Ries LAG et al., eds. (1994) *SEER cancer statistics review, 1973–1991: tables and graphs, National Cancer Institute.* Betheseda, National Institutes of Health, No. 94–2789.

Robb-Smith AHT (1967) *The enigma of coronary heart disease.* Chicago, Year Book Medical Publishers.

Snow RW et al. (1992) Childhood deaths in Africa: uses and limitations of verbal autopsies. *Lancet,* 340:351–355.

Snow RW et al. (1993) Maternal recall of symptoms associated with childhood deaths in rural East Africa. *International journal of epidemiology,* 22(4): 677–683.

Stehbens UE (1987) An appraisal of the epidemic rise of CHD and its decline. *Lancet,* 1(8533):606–611.

Sullivan JM, Rutstein SO, Bicego GT (1994) Infant and child mortality. In: *Demographic and health surveys comparative study No. 15.* Calverton, MD, Macro International Incorporated.

Taucher E, Perez P (1989) Mortalidad del adulto en Chile: 1975 a 1987. [Mortality in adults in Chile, 1975–1987] *Cuadernos medico sociales* 30(2).

Veress B, Alafuzoff I (1994) A retrospective analysis of clinical diagnoses and autopsy findings in 3,042 cases during two different time periods. *Human pathology*, 25:140–145.

Vital and Health Statistics, Series 10. Data from the national health survey. (1990) National Center for Health Statistics, Washington, D.C.

World Bank (1993) *World Development Report 1993: investing in health* New York, Oxford University Press for the World Bank.

World Health Organization (1993) The measurement of overall and cause-specific mortality in infants and children. In: *Report of a joint WHO/UNICEF consultation 15–17 December 1992*. Geneva, WHO.

World Health Organization (1993) *International classification of diseases and related health problems. Tenth revision. Volume 2 Instruction manual*. Geneva, WHO.

World Health Organization (1991) *World health statitstics annual 1990*. Geneva, WHO.

Yang G, Murray CJL Zheng X (1991) Exploring adult mortality in China: levels, patterns and causes. Beijing, Hua Xia Press.

Chapter 4

GLOBAL AND REGIONAL DESCRIPTIVE EPIDEMIOLOGY OF DISABILITY: INCIDENCE, PREVALENCE, HEALTH EXPECTANCIES AND YEARS LIVED WITH DISABILITY

CHRISTOPHER J. L. MURRAY
ALAN D. LOPEZ

One of the primary objectives of the Global Burden of Disease Study (GBD) has been to focus attention on non-fatal health outcomes and, more specifically, on disability. In this chapter, we provide a broad overview of the strategy used to quantify disability by cause and, using a variety of indicators, summarize a large body of information on regional patterns of disability. Details of the epidemiological estimates for each condition are provided in the specific chapters for each disease and injury published in other volumes of this series. The development of the primary indicator of the burden of non-fatal health outcomes, namely Years Lived with Disability (YLDs), is presented in more detail in Chapter 1 in this volume (Murray 1996).

Compared to the challenges of estimating the patterns of mortality by cause, the difficulties of quantifying non-fatal health outcomes by cause are much greater. In all respects, the definition and measurement of non-fatal health outcomes are less precise than for mortality. Even the general magnitude of the problem is much better known for mortality than for non-fatal health outcomes since decades of research and development of demographic estimation methods have led to reasonably robust estimates of the total number of deaths by age and sex in various regions.[1] Unfortunately, similarly reliable estimates of the total burden of disease and injury due to non-fatal health outcomes disaggregated by age, sex and geographic region are not available. As explained in Chapter 1 (Murray 1996), we have chosen to focus on disability in measuring the burden of non-fatal health outcomes. Our basic strategy used to estimate the burden of disability has been to construct robust estimates of the epidemiology of individual conditions. Total incidence and prevalence of disability, therefore, are based on these condition-specific estimates.

For some regions, data on the epidemiology of important non-fatal health conditions are extremely limited. Few community studies, for example, are available on heart disease in sub-Saharan Africa. Knowledge of the disabling sequelae of even well-studied diseases is lacking for large parts of the developing and, perhaps surprisingly, the developed world as well. Nevertheless, choices between competing health priorities are made every day by decision-makers in the public and private sectors. These choices reflect each decision-maker's implicit understanding of a population's epidemiological profile, as well as opportunities for intervention. We believe that it is preferable to make an informed estimate of disability due to a particular condition than to have no estimate at all. The absence of an estimate often fosters the tacit assumption that there is no problem. For example, it may well be that the continued neglect of primary and secondary prevention and rehabilitation of disability is related to the lack of data on its magnitude, especially when compared to the information available about life lost due to premature mortality. When estimates are made, however, it is imperative that the assumptions and empirical observations that are used are made explicit so that the estimation methods can be debated and modified in the future. *Ex cathedra* statements without supporting empirical evidence do not contribute constructively to informed policy debate and should be avoided.

METHODS

For each disease and injury included in the GBD (see Table 3.1), a limited set of disabling sequelae have been selected to be evaluated in depth. For example, for diabetes mellitus we have restricted our analysis to five sequelae: diabetes *per se*, retinopathy, neuropathy, diabetic foot and amputation. Clearly, there are other sequelae for diabetes, just as there are many sequelae for other conditions in the study that have not been directly evaluated. Such an exhaustive analysis of all sequelae for each condition is well beyond the scope of this study. Therefore, in consultation with the disease experts who have collaborated on the GBD, a set of disabling sequelae (see Annex Table 2) have been selected for direct evaluation. In total, 483 disabling sequelae have been separately evaluated including 132 Group I (communicable diseases) sequelae, 68 Group II (noncommunicable diseases) sequelae and 283 Group III (injuries) sequelae. A larger number of Group III sequelae were evaluated since a standard approach was used for seven of the injuries, including 40 sequelae per injury. This standardized approach to injuries is discussed in more detail below.

In order to calculate Years Lived with a Disability (YLDs) from each sequela, it is necessary to know its incidence, average age of onset, duration and disability severity weight. Disability severity weights have been developed for all sequelae included in the study through an independent process described in Chapter 1 in this volume (Murray 1996). In addition to the basic epidemiological parameters of incidence, average age of onset and duration, considerations of internal consistency led to the estimation of prevalence, case-fatality, remission and death rates. These epidemiological parameters have been estimated for five broad age groups, both sexes and eight geographical regions. While it would have been preferable to estimate these parameters for the same seven age groups that were used for the mortality estimates in this study, the lack of data on many disabling sequelae restricted the estimation of epidemiological parameters to five age groups: 0–4 years, 5–14, 15–44, 45–59 and 60 and over. For certain conditions that are much more common at older ages, such as dementia or stroke, lumping all individuals over age 60 into one age group is extremely crude and highly unsatisfactory. In chapters on these conditions in other volumes in this series, more detailed age groups are used to report some epidemiological parameters. For consistency, YLDs have been calculated for all conditions using the five standard age groups.

In most regions, valid community-based epidemiological studies do not exist for several of these epidemiological parameters. In order to identify all useful sources of data and information, and to supplement empirical data with informed judgment, estimates of disabling sequelae were developed in close collaboration with a large number of experts familiar with specific diseases or injuries. The final estimates reported here are the result of an iterative process spanning four and one-half years. The following steps describe the process which was used to develop the disability estimates.

- In 1992, disease experts, or groups of experts in some cases, were identified for each of the more than 100 diseases or injuries included in the GBD. These experts were drawn from the World Health Organization, the International Agency for Research on Cancer, the World Bank, the United States Centers for Disease Control and Prevention, and academic institutions in many countries, including the United States, the United Kingdom, France, Mexico, New Zealand, Japan, India, Sri Lanka, China and South Africa.

- First-round estimates of the duration of the disease and of incidence, remission, case-fatality, prevalence and death rates were made by experts on the basis of published and unpublished studies. Where no data for a region were available, experts were encouraged to make informed estimates. Frequently, age-patterns of incidence or remission rates were based on the assumption that some regions have similar epidemiological patterns but may differ in the level of incidence or prevalence of a condition. In the worst cases, where no information was available at all, the preliminary estimates were based exclusively on data or information from other regions.

- The first-round estimates were critically reviewed and the internal consistency of the estimates of incidence, remission, case-fatality, duration and prevalence was ascertained using DISMOD, a model of the disease/injury process (a more complete discussion of DISMOD is given later in this chapter). This process identified major inconsistencies for many estimates. Disease experts were subsequently invited to revise their estimates, in order to make them internally consistent.

- Revised estimates were used to produce the first version of the GBD estimates of YLDs. These estimates were extensively reviewed by a group of international health experts at a meeting hosted by the World Health Organization in Geneva, 8–11 December 1992.

- A second version of the estimates was generated incorporating the critical comments provided at the WHO meeting; these revised estimates were again subjected to internal consistency validation and consultation with experts.

- Version 3 of the study was generated using the finalized set of disability severity weights developed for the GBD and these modified estimates formed the basis of the YLDs and DALYs published in the *World Development Report 1993: Investing in health* (World Bank 1993).

- Some computational errors were corrected and a limited number of changes to the epidemiological estimates were made based on various reviews of the Version 3 estimates. This fourth version of the GBD was presented in the *Bulletin of the World Health Organization* in 1994 and separately, in greater detail, in *Global Comparative Assessments in the Health Sector* published by the World Health Organization (Murray and Lopez 1994a, 1994b, 1994c; Murray et al. 1994).

- As part of the follow-up to the *World Development Report 1993*, disease experts were asked to write detailed chapters for inclusion in this series of volumes on the data and methods used to generate the estimates of incidence, prevalence, duration and average age of onset. This process provided authors with the opportunity to incorporate new datasets, revise estimates and synthesis methods, and consult colleagues more widely. These modified estimates of duration and of incidence, prevalence, remission, case-fatality, and mortality rates were in turn subjected to internal consistency checks using DisMod. In consultation with these authors, their modified estimates were revised and returned to them for further review. This process of re-estimation, internal consistency checking and revision has gone through three iterations since July 1993. For certain clusters of conditions such as the neuro-psychiatric disorders, international seminars have been convened to review the final sets of estimates. These final estimates are published in full detail in *Global Health Statistics*, the second volume of this series.

TESTING FOR INTERNAL CONSISTENCY

Throughout the course of the GBD, we have strongly emphasized the need to achieve internal consistency of epidemiological profiles for each disease and its associated disabling sequelae. In other words, estimated prevalence must be consistent with estimated incidence and vice-versa. We have also required similar relationships for other epidemiological parameters, such as death and case-fatality rates. In fact, of the more than 40 person-years invested in the preparation of this study, the largest share has been devoted to the development of internally consistent estimates for the epidemiological parameters of each disease in each region. This emphasis was decided upon very early in the GBD when we realized that estimates from experts based on the published and unpublished literature were often not internally consistent.

To assist in identifying inconsistent estimates and modifying them to be consistent, a simple model formalizing the relationship between incidence, remission, case-fatality and prevalence was developed. Figure 4.1 illustrates the basic relationships. Susceptibles in the population are assumed to be at risk of incurring a disease or disability at rate i and can die at a general mortality rate m.[2] Cases of disease can remit at rate r, die from general causes at the same rate as the susceptibles m, or die from cause-specific mortality from the condition at rate f. If these rates can be assumed to be constant over a short time interval such as one year, we can define a set of ordinary differential equations that characterize movement between the four states as follows:

$$\frac{dS(t)}{dt} = -(i+m)S(t)$$

$$\frac{dC(t)}{dt} = iS(t) - (r+f+m)C(t)$$

$$\frac{dM(t)}{dt} = m(S(t)+C(t))$$

$$\frac{dD(t)}{dt} = fC(t)$$

Figure 4.1   Basic relationships between susceptibles, cases and deaths used in developing DISMOD

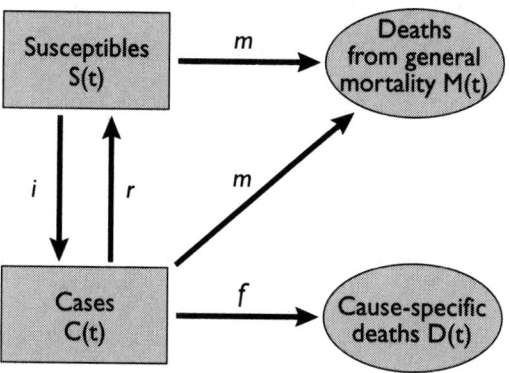

where *S(t)* is the number of susceptibles at time *t*, *C(t)* is the number of cases (of disease or injury) at time *t*, *M(t)* is the number of individuals who have died from general causes of mortality at time *t*, and *D(t)* is the number of individuals who have died from the condition at time *t*; *i*, *m*, *r* and *f* are as described above.

With colleagues at the Burden of Disease Unit, Harvard Center for Population and Development Studies, we have developed a software programme called DisMod, that can solve this system of equations using the finite difference method. DisMod runs in the Microsoft Windows 3.1 environment and was coded in the C++ programming language. In DisMod, the user specifies a set of age-specific incidence, remission and case-fatality rates for a specific disease, region and sex. The program then solves the set of differential equations for a hypothetical birth cohort exposed to the set of region-specific general mortality rates and the disease-specific incidence, remission and case-fatality rates specified by the user. DisMod then outputs the age-specific prevalence implied by these incidence, remission and death rates. In addition, the program provides estimates of incident cases by age as well as the average duration of incident cases within an age group.

Table 4.1 provides an illustrative example of the operation of DisMod. The user specifies the general mortality pattern equal to one of the eight GBD regions, in this case SSA, or a user-determined mortality pattern. A set of input age groups and output age groups are selected by the user; in this example, nine age groups are used for the input and the five standard GBD age groups have been used for the output. Incidence rises steadily with age, beginning with 1 per 1000 individuals per year in the youngest age group reaching 9 per 1000 per year in the oldest age group; the remission rate is 0.1 per individual per year in all age groups and the case-fatality rate is 0.05 per individual per year. The output provides the implied population prevalence, incidence, and cause-specific mortality rates, durations by age, and the prevalence, incidence and death numbers which would be observed if these rates had applied to the population age-structure of SSA.

DisMod has been used extensively in the development of the epidemiological estimates for the GBD. At least four common uses are worth describing in some detail.

1. *Estimating Durations*—To calculate the number of YLDs, an estimate of the average duration for each disabling sequela, by age, is required. The commonly cited relationship:

$$P = ID$$

where *P* is prevalence, *I* is incidence and *D* is duration, is an oversimplification of the true relationship. When age-specific prevalence and incidence rates are used to estimate average duration for an age group, the result is not even a good first-order approximation. For example, consider any chronic disease where the population prevalence rises

Table 4.1   Inputs and outputs from DISMOD: a hypothetical example for sub-Saharan African males

Inputs to model

| Age groups (years) | Instantaneous rates | | | Relative risk minus one coefficient |
	Incidence rate	Remission rate	Case fatality rate	
0–4	0.001	0.100	0.050	0.000
5–14	0.002	0.100	0.050	0.000
15–24	0.003	0.100	0.050	0.000
25–34	0.004	0.100	0.050	0.000
35–44	0.005	0.100	0.050	0.000
45–54	0.006	0.100	0.050	0.000
55–64	0.007	0.100	0.050	0.000
65–74	0.008	0.100	0.050	0.000
75–89	0.009	0.100	0.050	0.000

Output from model

Age groups (years)	Expected duration (years)	Average age of onset (years)	Prevalence rate (per 1000)	Annual incidence rate (per 1000)	Annual cause-specific mortality rate (per 1000)
0–4	5.86	2.4	1.92	1.00	0.09
5–14	6.41	10.0	8.20	1.98	0.41
15–44	6.21	30.9	21.41	3.85	1.07
45–59	5.63	52.4	36.17	6.07	1.81
60–89	4.19	69.7	46.82	7.50	2.35

Age groups (years)	Population (thousands)	Prevalence	Annual incidence	Annual cause-specific deaths
0–4	47 484	91 019	47 430	4 472
5–14	70 258	576 044	139 379	28 680
15–44	103 764	2 222 000	399 404	110 978
45–59	20 308	734 494	123 308	36 721
60–89	10 481	490 677	78 623	24 603

Crude incidence rate (per 1000):   3.12
Crude prevalence rate (per 1000):   16.31

steadily with age but incidence is constant or even declining with age. Duration, if estimated by dividing prevalence by incidence, rises steadily with age. However, the real duration of disease or disability must *decline* with age since the risk of general mortality is greater at older ages. Even for all ages combined, prevalence will not equal the product of incidence and duration when the population size or age-structure is changing, or where there is a trend in the incidence rate over time. DISMOD has been used to estimate the average duration of nearly every disabling sequelae by age, sex and geographical region, except those where the duration is less than a few days.

2. *Estimating incidence from prevalence*—For some disabling sequelae, the primary sources of information are cross-sectional population prevalence surveys. Examples include blindness, deafness or lameness. Incidence rates need to be estimated based on these observed prevalence rates. For some conditions where there is essentially no remission, DisMod can be used iteratively to specify a set of age-specific incidence rates that can explain the observed prevalence rates. For conditions where there is re-mission, case-fatality or an increased risk of death from all causes, such as blindness, more than one combination of age-specific incidence, re-mission and case-fatality rates are consistent with, or can explain, an ob-served set of prevalence rates. Other sources of information such as small-scale studies, case-series, clinical experience, and studies of aver-age duration may be useful in suggesting a credible range of incidence, remission or case-fatality rates. Information on the relative age-pattern of incidence, remission or case-fatality can also be used to narrow the range of possible solutions or more specifically, to estimate incidence rates by age that are consistent with an observed prevalence. In some cases, information on prevalence and mortality may be available which will further restrict the possible set of solutions to the problem. DisMod can also be used to compute incidence from prevalence when trends in inci-dence rates over time are known. Shibuya and Murray (1996) provide an illustration of how lameness surveys of older children as well as trends in incidence rates due to the wider use of polio vaccination have been used in DisMod to estimate 1990 incidence rates of disabling polio.

3. *Estimating prevalence from incidence*—For a number of conditions including many injuries, cancers, myocardial infarction and infertility, information is much easier to obtain on incidence than for prevalence. Where incidence is known and some information is available to guide the selection of remission and/or case-fatality rates, it is a simple task to use DisMod to estimate the implied prevalence. For certain outcomes this provides an excellent basis on which to review estimated incidence. The following example illustrates the importance of examining all es-timates of incidence in terms of prevalence as well: earlier in this study, claims about the incidence of cognitive impairment due to certain Group I conditions suggested that the prevalence of cognitive impairment in some regions was in excess of one-hundred per cent. Critical appraisal of the evidence on the incidence rates of these Group I conditions, and the likelihood of developing cognitive impairment, have resulted in more plausible incidence and prevalence estimates.

4. *Other applications*—As this study has unfolded, other uses of DisMod have emerged. Two in particular are worth noting here. Some studies report their results using different age groupings which can be very unusual, such as 18–32 years or 26–57 years. When incidence and prevalence are age-dependent, results from such studies are difficult to compare with results from studies using other age groups. By manipu-

lating the input and output age groups in DISMOD, a set of incidence rates for a standard set of age groups can be estimated according to prevalence in a series of non-standard age groups. In turn, these incidence rates can be used to estimate prevalence in a standard set of age groups, thus facilitating a more useful comparison between studies with different age groupings. Another important use of DISMOD is the estimation of deaths attributable to a condition, such as blindness or diabetes, for which there is an associated increased risk of death due to other causes. By using the relative risk option included in DISMOD, the number of deaths associated with the cause can be estimated.

DISABLING SEQUELAE FROM INJURIES

For all of the injuries except poisonings and drownings, the definition of an incident case and the approach to estimating disabling sequelae are different from those used for other diseases. An incident episode of an injury has been defined as an episode which is severe enough for the person to be hospitalized or which requires emergency room care, if such care is accessible. In most regions of the world, incidence rates have been estimated for these injuries on the basis of estimated deaths, using the ratio of age and sex-specific deaths to incidence. Where these have been studied, death-to-incidence ratios by age and sex for a number of injuries are quite consistent; Figure 2 shows death-to-incidence ratios for fires in New Zealand, the United States, and Mauritius. Using data from New Zealand, the United States, Sweden and Mauritius, death-to-incidence ratios have been estimated for each injury and modified by region to reflect the expected differences in access to and quality of care, as well as known differences in the nature of a given injury. More details about these methods are available in the chapters on specific injuries included in *The Global burden of injuries: mortality and disability from suicide, violence, war and unintentional injuries* (Volume VIII in the *Global Burden of Disease and Injury Series*). Incidence estimated using this approach has been reviewed in the light of other sources, including police records and other indirect estimation methods.

The literature on the disabling sequelae of injuries is very limited.[3] Follow-up studies of injury cohorts should, in principle, be relatively easy to undertake but to date few have been completed. Because of the dearth of literature on the long-term disabling sequelae of different types of injuries, an alternative approach was developed for this study.[4] Details of this method are reported by Lozano et al. (1996) in *The Global Burden of Injuries*, volume VII in this series. A brief overview of the approach is given below. Following the rules of the Ninth Revision of the International Classification of Diseases (ICD-9), injuries can be coded in two ways: according to the external cause of the injury, such as a fire or a road traffic accident, or according to the nature of the injury such as spinal cord transection or cranial trauma. We believe that the disabling sequelae of an injury can be estimated more easily on the basis of the nature of the

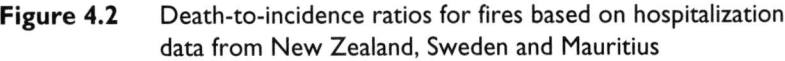

Figure 4.2   Death-to-incidence ratios for fires based on hospitalization
data from New Zealand, Sweden and Mauritius

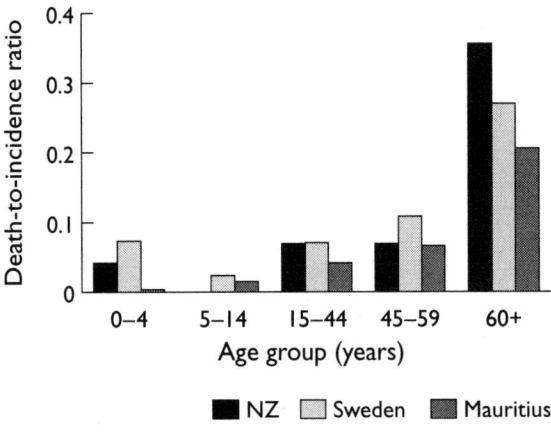

injury than on the external cause of the injury. The relationship between
the external causes of injury and the nature of injury was defined first, and
this information was then used to estimate the likely short-term and long-
term disabling sequelae from injuries assigned to each nature of injury code.

To define the average relationship in each region between the external
cause of injury and the associated natures of injury, countries which meet
the following three criteria were identified: routine use of dual coding for
all injury deaths and hospitalizations using the external codes (E-codes)
and nature of injury codes (N-codes); complete national coverage of all
hospitalizations; and nearly complete access to hospitals for emergency
injury care. We were able to identify three countries that met these criteria and that could provide the relevant data, namely Mauritius, Sweden
and Chile.

In the ICD-9 and in the datasets for these three countries, a large number
of detailed N-codes are used. To facilitate our analysis, we first developed
a list of thirty-three N-codes (see Table 4.2) that combined similar categories of outcome from the perspective of this study. For the three countries,
a matrix of our nine detailed causes of injury, including other unintentional
injuries, and the thirty-three N-codes, was generated. Table 4.3 illustrates
the matrix for road traffic accidents. The distribution of the nature of
injury for a given external cause such as road traffic accidents was similar across the three countries. On the other hand, the distribution of N-
codes for a given E-code differed by age. To estimate the distribution of
incident episodes according to the nature of injury for each region, composite E-code/N-code matrices for each age group 0–14, 15–59 and 60
and older were developed separately. In all three countries, there were

virtually no hospitalizations coded to war. We have, therefore, constructed a matrix for war, starting with the N-code distribution for violence and modifying it on the basis of small-scale studies reviewed by Zwi (1996).

Next, estimates were required for both short-term and long-term disabilities and their severities, stemming from each nature of injury. In the absence of cohort studies on the outcomes of various natures of injury, more indirect and imprecise methods were used. For the thirty-three categories of the nature of injury, participants at the Geneva meeting on disability weights (see Murray 1996, Chapter 1 in this volume for a description of the objectives and outcomes of this meeting) were asked to estimate the average duration of treated and untreated forms of each nature of injury, as well as their distribution across the seven classes of disability, based on information provided by the authors of the various injury chapters in Volume VII of this series. The results of this phase of the exercise are summarized in Table 4.4.

ESTIMATING DISABILITY FROM RESIDUAL CATEGORIES

A large number of diseases and their sequelae have been evaluated in this study. Nevertheless, there remain many that have not been explicitly evaluated. Because YLLs have been calculated for all deaths, they are as complete as the data allow. Some of these YLLs, however, have been assigned to residual categories within each sub-category in the GBD cause list, such as chronic respiratory diseases or other malignant neoplasms. If no attempt had been made to estimate the residual categories of YLDs, the results of the study would have been biased towards YLLs. An attempt was made, therefore, to approximate the YLDs expected for the residual diseases for which YLLs have been estimated. For each age-sex group in each region, the ratio of YLDs–YLLs was calculated. On average, for all ages combined, this ratio varied from 0.3 in SSA to 1.0 in EME. Because the ratio of YLDs–YLLs is likely to vary by cause cluster, we have chosen to estimate separate ratios for Group I conditions, malignant neoplasms, cardiovascular diseases and other Group II conditions. This method was not used for Group III (Injuries) since the E/N code matrix was used to estimate the YLDs more directly for the residual category "other unintentional injuries." Of total YLDs for each region, the proportion estimated to have arisen from the residual categories was, on average, 11.5 per cent for males and 13.9 per cent for females. Much of this residual has been attributed to respiratory diseases, digestive diseases and genito-urinary diseases because of the relatively large number of deaths attributed to the residuals of these categories. The per cent of all YLDs attributed to the residual categories ranges from 8.1 per cent in India to 21.4 per cent in MEC. In addition to the YLDs estimated using this crude approach, there may also be YLDs due to conditions for which there are no deaths. Given the extensive list of sequelae included in this study, however, it is unlikely that there are many conditions which are not at least partially reflected in the analysis.

Table 4.2   GBD classification system for ICD-9 nature-of-injury codes

	Nature of injury	ICD-9 N code
I	Fractured skull	800–801
2	Fractured face bones	802
3	Fractured vertebral column	805
4	Injured spinal cord	806 and 952
5	Fractured rib or sternum	807
6	Fractured pelvis	808
7	Fractured clavicle, scapula, or humerus	810–812
8	Fractured radius or ulna	813
9	Fractured hand bones	814–817
10	Fractured femur	820–821
11	Fractured patella, tibia, or fibula	822–823
12	Fractured ankle	824
13	Fractured foot bones	825–826
14	Other dislocation	830, 833–834, 836–839
15	Dislocated shoulder, elbow, or hip	831, 832, 835
16	Sprains	840–848
17	Intracranial injury	850–854
18	Internal injuries	860–869
19	Open wound	870, 872–884, 890–894
20	Injury to eyes	871, 950
21	Amputated thumb	885
22	Amputated finger	886
23	Amputated arm	887
24	Amputated toe	895
25	Amputated foot	896, 897.0–897.1
26	Amputated leg	897.2–897.3
27	Crushing	925–929
28	Burns < 20%	940–947, 948.0–948.1
29	Burns > 20% and < 60%	948.2–948.5
30	Burns > 60%	948.6–948.9
31	Injured nerves	951, 953–957
32	Poisoning	960–979, 980–989
33	Residual	900–924, 930–939

Notes:

A number of other N codes for ill-defined or minor categories have been distributed across these 33 categories according to the following rules:

- The N codes 803 and 804 were proportionately redistributed across N codes 801 and 802.
- The N code 809 was proportionately redistributed across N codes 807 and 808.
- The N codes 818 and 819 were proportionately redistributed across N codes 810–817.
- The N codes 827 and 828 were proportionately redistributed across N codes 822–826.
- The N codes 897.4–897.7 were proportionately redistributed across N codes 895, 896 and 897.0–897.3.
- The N code 949 was proportionately redistributed across N codes 940–948.
- The N codes 958–959 and 909–999 were proportionately redistributed across all 33 categories after the previous steps.

Table 4.3   Percentage distribution of road traffic accident hospitalizations and emergency ward visits across the 33 GBD nature-of-injury categories, by age, for both sexes combined

	Nature of injury	Age group (years)				
		0–4	5–14	15–44	45–59	60+
1	Fractured skull	2.36	2.36	1.52	1.52	1.71
2	Fratured face	1.86	1.86	4.04	4.04	2.37
3	Fractured vertebral column	0.58	0.58	4.12	4.12	4.62
4	Injured spinal cord	0.31	0.31	2.49	2.49	1.43
5	Fractured rib or sternum	0.24	0.24	2.66	2.66	8.07
6	Fractured pelvis	0.68	0.68	2.31	2.31	3.90
7	Fractured clavicle, scapula, or humerus	5.55	5.55	3.87	3.87	4.44
8	Fractured radius or ulna	7.70	7.70	3.61	3.61	4.00
9	Fractured hand bones	0.79	0.79	1.40	1.40	0.79
10	Fractured femur	5.79	5.79	5.16	5.16	13.43
11	Fractured patella, tibia, or fibula	7.51	7.51	8.39	8.39	11.41
12	Fractured ankle	1.42	1.42	3.70	3.70	4.25
13	Fractured bones in foot	0.49	0.49	1.31	1.31	0.63
14	Other dislocation	0.03	0.03	0.01	0.01	0.01
15	Dislocated shoulder, elbow, or hip	0.77	0.77	2.03	2.03	1.26
16	Sprains	1.02	1.02	3.93	3.93	1.51
17	Intracranial injury	43.75	43.75	30.51	30.51	23.50
18	Internal injuries	2.65	2.65	2.33	2.33	2.30
19	Open wound	5.99	5.99	4.96	4.96	2.85
20	Injury to eyes	0.05	0.05	0.18	0.18	0.06
21	Amputated thumb	0.06	0.06	0.02	0.02	0.02
22	Amputated finger	0.08	0.08	0.07	0.07	0.03
23	Amputated arm	0.00	0.00	0.05	0.05	0.01
24	Amputated toe	0.05	0.05	0.03	0.03	0.00
25	Amputated foot	0.00	0.00	0.07	0.07	0.11
26	Amputated leg	0.00	0.00	0.14	0.14	0.02
27	Crushing	1.11	1.11	0.47	0.47	0.49
28	Burns <20%	0.13	0.13	0.18	0.18	0.02
29	Burns >20% and <60%	0.00	0.00	0.01	0.01	0.00
30	Burns >60%	0.00	0.00	0.09	0.09	0.00
31	Injured nerves	0.07	0.07	0.37	0.37	0.05
32	Poisoning	0.04	0.04	1.02	1.02	0.76
33	Residual	8.92	8.92	8.96	8.96	5.96
	Total	100.00	100.00	100.00	100.00	100.00

Table 4.4   Disability severity weights and durations for treated and untreated natures of injury

Code	Nature of injury	Age group	Disability weight		Duration	
			Untreated	Treated	Untreated	Treated
1a	Fractured skull:	0–4	0.431	0.431	0.107	0.107
	short term	5–14	0.431	0.431	0.107	0.107
		15–44	0.431	0.431	0.107	0.107
		45–59	0.431	0.431	0.107	0.107
		60+	0.431	0.431	0.107	0.107
1b	Fractured skull:	0–4	0.410	0.350	LL*	LL
	life long	5–14	0.410	0.350	LL	LL
	(15% of incident cases)	15–44	0.410	0.350	LL	LL
		45–59	0.419	0.350	LL	LL
		60+	0.471	0.404	LL	LL
2	Fratured face	0–4	0.223	0.223	0.118	0.118
		5–14	0.223	0.223	0.118	0.118
		15–44	0.223	0.223	0.118	0.118
		45–59	0.223	0.223	0.118	0.118
		60+	0.223	0.223	0.118	0.118
3	Fractured vertebral column:	0–4	0.266	0.266	0.140	0.140
	short term	5–14	0.266	0.266	0.140	0.140
		15–44	0.266	0.266	0.140	0.140
		45–59	0.266	0.266	0.140	0.140
		60+	0.266	0.266	0.140	0.140
4	Injured spinal cord:	0–4	0.725	0.725	LL	LL
	life long	5–14	0.725	0.725	LL	LL
		15–44	0.725	0.725	LL	LL
		45–59	0.725	0.725	LL	LL
		60+	0.725	0.725	LL	LL
5	Fractured rib or sternum:	0–4	0.199	0.199	0.115	0.115
	short term	5–14	0.199	0.199	0.115	0.115
		15–44	0.199	0.199	0.115	0.115
		45–59	0.199	0.199	0.115	0.115
		60+	0.199	0.199	0.115	0.115
6	Fractured pelvis:	0–4	0.247	0.247	0.126	0.126
	short term	5–14	0.247	0.247	0.126	0.126
		15–44	0.247	0.247	0.126	0.126
		45–59	0.247	0.247	0.126	0.126
		60+	0.247	0.247	0.126	0.126
7	Fractured clavicle, scapula,	0–4	0.153	0.153	0.112	0.112
	or humerus:	5–14	0.153	0.153	0.112	0.112
	short term	15–44	0.136	0.136	0.112	0.112
		45–59	0.136	0.136	0.112	0.112
		60+	0.136	0.136	0.112	0.112
8	Fractured radius or ulna:	0–4	0.180	0.180	0.112	0.112
	short term	5–14	0.180	0.180	0.112	0.112
		15–44	0.180	0.180	0.112	0.112
		45–59	0.180	0.180	0.112	0.112
		60+	0.180	0.180	0.112	0.112
9	Fractured hand bones	0–4	0.100	0.100	0.070	0.070
		5–14	0.100	0.100	0.070	0.070
		15–44	0.100	0.100	0.070	0.070
		45–59	0.100	0.100	0.070	0.070
		60+	0.100	0.100	0.070	0.070

Table 4.4   (continued)

Code	Nature of injury	Age group	Disability weight Untreated	Disability weight Treated	Duration Untreated	Duration Treated
10a	Fractured femur:	0–4	0.372	0.372	0.241	0.139
	short term	5–14	0.372	0.372	0.241	0.139
		15–44	0.372	0.372	0.241	0.139
		45–59	0.372	0.372	0.241	0.139
		60+	0.372	0.372	0.241	0.139
10b	Fractured femur:	0–4	0.272	0.272	LL	LL
	life long	5–14	0.272	0.272	LL	LL
	(5% of treated)	15–44	0.272	0.272	LL	LL
	(50% untreated)	45–59	0.272	0.272	LL	LL
		60+	0.272	0.272	LL	LL
11	Fractured patella, tibia,	0–4	0.271	0.271	0.179	0.090
	or fibula:	5–14	0.271	0.271	0.179	0.090
	short term	15–44	0.271	0.271	0.179	0.090
		45–59	0.271	0.271	0.179	0.090
		60+	0.271	0.271	0.179	0.090
12	Fractured ankle:	0–4	0.196	0.196	0.146	0.096
	short term	5–14	0.196	0.196	0.146	0.096
		15–44	0.196	0.196	0.146	0.096
		45–59	0.196	0.196	0.146	0.096
		60+	0.196	0.196	0.146	0.096
13	Fractured bones in foot:	0–4	0.077	0.077	0.073	0.073
	short term	5–14	0.077	0.077	0.073	0.073
		15–44	0.077	0.077	0.073	0.073
		45–59	0.077	0.077	0.073	0.073
		60+	0.077	0.077	0.073	0.073
14	Other dislocation	0–4	0.000	0.000		
		5–14	0.000	0.000		
		15–44	0.000	0.000		
		45–59	0.000	0.000		
		60+	0.000	0.000		
15	Dislocated shoulder, elbow,	0–4	0.074	0.074	0.035	0.035
	or hip:	5–14	0.074	0.074	0.035	0.035
	short term	15–44	0.074	0.074	0.035	0.035
		45–59	0.074	0.074	0.035	0.035
		60+	0.074	0.074	0.035	0.035
16	Sprains	0–4	0.064	0.064	0.038	0.038
		5–14	0.064	0.064	0.038	0.038
		15–44	0.064	0.064	0.038	0.038
		45–59	0.064	0.064	0.038	0.038
		60+	0.064	0.064	0.038	0.038
17a	Intracranial injury:	0–4	0.359	0.359	0.067	0.067
	short term	5–14	0.359	0.359	0.067	0.067
		15–44	0.359	0.359	0.067	0.067
		45–59	0.359	0.359	0.067	0.067
		60+	0.359	0.359	0.067	0.067
17b	Intracranial injury:	0–4	0.410	0.350	LL	LL
	life long	5–14	0.410	0.350	LL	LL
	(5% of incident cases)	15–44	0.410	0.350	LL	LL
		45–59	0.419	0.350	LL	LL
		60+	0.471	0.404	LL	LL

Table 4.4   (continued)

Code	Nature of injury	Age group	Disability weight		Duration	
			Untreated	Treated	Untreated	Treated
18	Internal injuries:	0–4	0.000	0.208	0.000	0.042
	short term	5–14	0.000	0.208	0.000	0.042
		15–44	0.000	0.208	0.000	0.042
		45–59	0.000	0.208	0.000	0.042
		60+	0.000	0.208	0.000	0.042
19	Open wound	0–4	0.108	0.108	0.052	0.024
		5–14	0.108	0.108	0.052	0.024
		15–44	0.108	0.108	0.052	0.024
		45–59	0.108	0.108	0.052	0.024
		60+	0.108	0.108	0.052	0.024
20	Injury to eyes:	0–4	0.354	0.301	LL	LL
	life long	5–14	0.354	0.300	LL	LL
		15–44	0.354	0.298	LL	LL
		45–59	0.354	0.298	LL	LL
		60+	0.354	0.298	LL	LL
21	Amputated thumb:	0–4	0.165	0.165	LL	LL
	life long	5–14	0.165	0.165	LL	LL
		15–44	0.165	0.165	LL	LL
		45–59	0.165	0.165	LL	LL
		60+	0.165	0.165	LL	LL
22	Amputated finger:	0–4	0.102	0.102	LL	LL
	life long	5–14	0.102	0.102	LL	LL
		15–44	0.102	0.102	LL	LL
		45–59	0.102	0.102	LL	LL
		60+	0.102	0.102	LL	LL
23	Amputated arm:	0–4	0.308	0.257	LL	LL
	life long	5–14	0.308	0.257	LL	LL
		15–44	0.308	0.257	LL	LL
		45–59	0.308	0.257	LL	LL
		60+	0.308	0.257	LL	LL
24	Amputated toe:	0–4	0.102	0.102	LL	LL
	life long	5–14	0.102	0.102	LL	LL
		15–44	0.102	0.102	LL	LL
		45–59	0.102	0.102	LL	LL
		60+	0.102	0.102	LL	LL
25	Amputated foot:	0–4	0.300	0.300	LL	LL
	life long	5–14	0.300	0.300	LL	LL
		15–44	0.300	0.300	LL	LL
		45–59	0.300	0.300	LL	LL
		60+	0.300	0.300	LL	LL
26	Amputated leg:	0–4	0.300	0.300	LL	LL
	life long	5–14	0.300	0.300	LL	LL
		15–44	0.300	0.300	LL	LL
		45–59	0.300	0.300	LL	LL
		60+	0.300	0.300	LL	LL
27	Crushing:	0–4	0.218	0.218	0.094	0.094
	short term	5–14	0.218	0.218	0.094	0.094
		15–44	0.218	0.218	0.094	0.094
		45–59	0.218	0.218	0.094	0.094
		60+	0.218	0.218	0.094	0.094

Table 4.4   (continued)

Code	Nature of injury	Age group	Disability weight Untreated	Disability weight Treated	Duration Untreated	Duration Treated
28a	Burns <20%:	0–4	0.186	0.158	0.124	0.083
	short term	5–14	0.186	0.158	0.124	0.083
		15–44	0.186	0.158	0.124	0.083
		45–59	0.186	0.158	0.124	0.083
		60+	0.186	0.158	0.124	0.083
28b	Burns <20%:	0–4	0.002	0.001	LL	LL
	life long	5–14	0.002	0.001	LL	LL
	(100% incident cases)	15–44	0.002	0.001	LL	LL
		45–59	0.002	0.001	LL	LL
		60+	0.002	0.001	LL	LL
29a	Burns >20% and <60%:	0–4	0.469	0.441	0.360	0.279
	short term	5–14	0.469	0.441	0.360	0.279
		15–44	0.469	0.441	0.360	0.279
		45–59	0.469	0.441	0.360	0.279
		60+	0.469	0.441	0.360	0.279
29b	Burns >20% and <60%:	0–4	0.255	0.255	LL	LL
	life long	5–14	0.255	0.255	LL	LL
	(100% incident cases)	15–44	0.255	0.255	LL	LL
		45–59	0.255	0.255	LL	LL
		60+	0.255	0.255	LL	LL
30a	Burns >60%:	0–4	0.469	0.441	0.360	0.279
	short term	5–14	0.469	0.441	0.360	0.279
		15–44	0.469	0.441	0.360	0.279
		45–59	0.469	0.441	0.360	0.279
		60+	0.469	0.441	0.360	0.279
30b	Burns >60%:	0–4	0.255	0.255	LL	LL
	life long	5–14	0.255	0.255	LL	LL
	(100% incident cases)	15–44	0.255	0.255	LL	LL
		45–59	0.255	0.255	LL	LL
		60+	0.255	0.255	LL	LL
31	Injured nerves:	0–4	0.078	0.064	LL	LL
	life long	5–14	0.078	0.064	LL	LL
	(100% incident cases)	15–44	0.078	0.064	LL	LL
		45–59	0.078	0.064	LL	LL
		60+	0.078	0.064	LL	LL
32	Poisoning:	0–4	0.611	0.611	0.008	0.008
	short-term	5–14	0.611	0.611	0.008	0.008
		15–44	0.608	0.608	0.008	0.008
		45–59	0.608	0.608	0.008	0.008
		60+	0.608	0.608	0.008	0.008

*   LL: Life long. Duration depends on age, sex and region. In some cases individuals have a heightened average risk of death which has been included in the calculation of average duration used in the final calculation of Years Lived with Disability from these conditions.

Note: In many cases, the duration and severity of disability from a nature of injury category is the same for treated and untreated individuals that survive, although in those cases, the initial case-fatality rate may be different.

ESTIMATING HEALTH EXPECTANCIES

To facilitate comparison of the results of the Global Burden of Disease Study with the results of other studies that have used different indicators of non-fatal health outcomes, we have recalculated the GBD disability component using indicators other than YLDs. Van Ginneken (1994) has proposed that the results of the GBD be used to calculate health-adjusted expectancies for each region and attempted some sample calculations for EME and SSA using the results of the earlier versions of this study (Murray and Lopez 1994). Barendregt et al. (1995) have proposed that the health-adjusted expectancy, which can be calculated using the disability weights from the GBD, be termed Disability-Adjusted Life Expectancy or DALE. In other words, DALE would be the expectation of the equivalent number of healthy years of life at birth. In order to calculate DALE for each region, estimates of the prevalence of disability are required. For this version of the study, we have estimated the prevalence of each disabling sequelae. These figures are reported in *Global Health Statistics* (Murray and Lopez 1996b). With this information on prevalence, and the disability weights for each disabling sequelae by age, sex and region, we have calculated DALE using the Sullivan method (1971). Very briefly, the steps in the method are as follows. The L_x column from a life table is modified so that

$$HL_x = L_x (1 - \sum_j P_{jx} D_{jx})$$

where HL_x is the number of years of healthy life lived at age x, L_x is the number of years of life lived at age x from a life table, P_{jx} is the prevalence of disabling sequela j at age x, and D_{jx} is the disability weight for disabling sequela j at age x. DALE is calculated in the same manner as life expectancy at birth, except that instead of the L_x column being used, the HL_x column is used. The prevalence estimates for each disabling sequela have been estimated only for five standard age groups: 0–4 years, 5–14, 15–44, 45–59 and 60 and over. For the calculation of DALE, we have assumed that the prevalence of a disabling sequelae is constant within each of the five age groups. While this simplifying assumption is clearly not true, it is unlikely that the estimate of DALE will be strongly biased because of it.

Prevalence has been estimated for each of the disabling sequelae included in the GBD but not for the residual categories of YLDs mentioned above. For the residual categories, prevalence multiplied by the disability severity weight has been estimated, using a two-step procedure. First, the ratios of YLDs[0,0] for each residual category to YLDs[0,0] for the disabling sequelae that have been explicitly evaluated were calculated by sex for each region.[5] We then multiplied the $P_{jx} D_{jx}$ values for each age group by one plus this ratio. HL_x was then re-estimated using these adjusted severity-weighted prevalences to calculate DALE for both sexes in each region.

In addition to calculating DALE, the results of this study were used to calculate various forms of Disability-Free Life Expectancy (DFLE) using the Sullivan method. For each disabling sequela, we have back calculated the prevalence of each of the seven classes of disability by using the distribution of each disabling sequela across the seven classes—see Murray 1996, Chapter 1 in this volume, for a description of the seven classes of disability. Because the epidemiological estimates in this study have been constructed for each condition, individuals may have more than one disabling sequelae. Given that class I and class II disabilities are common, the sum of the prevalences of all classes of disability exceeds one-hundred per cent in a number of age groups in various regions. While, on average, individuals may have more than one disabling sequelae in these groups, there will still be individuals who do not have any disability at all.

Co-disability can occur for a variety of reasons. First, simply due to chance, individuals may have more than one disabling sequelae. This form of co-disability can be labeled independent co-disability when the probability of having one disabling sequela does not alter the probability of having other disabling sequelae. Independent co-disability could occur within a class, or between classes. An individual could have two class III disabling sequelae or, for example, an individual might have a class I and class IV disability. Individuals with one disability may also be at higher risk of having other disabilities that are related to the disease process causing their disability or at a lower risk, if having one disease protects against others. This form of co-disability is called dependent co-disability and would occur more or less often than at random. It is easy to estimate independent co-disability between different classes of disability and somewhat harder to estimate independent co-disability within a class but quite difficult to estimate dependent co-disability.

Co-disability may introduce a bias into the estimation of DALE. As described above, DALE is calculated by multiplying the prevalence of each class of disability by the severity weight for that class. *De facto*, we have assumed that the severity weight for an individual with more than one disability is simply the sum of the disability weights for each sequela. This assumption of additivity may bias the estimates of DALE up or down. Clearly, the sum of class VI and class VII disability weights would exceed 1; however, this combination would occur by chance only rarely—even in the age group 60 years and over in the region with the highest prevalences of both classes (EME), less than 0.5 per cent of those alive at these ages would be expected to have both classes of disability. For other combinations of sequela from the same or different classes, the true preference weight for the combined entity might be higher or lower than the sum of the disability weights. Disability weights for the combination of sequelae might depend on the nature of the condition and not simply on the sequela. For example, the severity of blindness and a below-the-knee amputation might be different than major depression and deafness, but both represent class IV and class VI combinations. While recognizing that DALE may be biased by this approach of dealing with the severity of co-disabilities, it was the only practical method that could be applied in this study. Further methodological research is required to reduce the bias due to co-disabilities in such calculations.

For DFLE, the sum of the expectations of life lived in each class, obtained by multiplying the L_x column from the regional life table by the age-specific prevalence of each disability class, exceeds life expectancy in some regions. While there is no method currently available to correct for dependent co-disability, we can correct for independent co-disability between classes in the calculation of DFLE. To do this, seven forms of DFLE were first defined: life expectancy free of class I (or worse) disability (DFLE-I), life expectancy free of class II (or worse) disability (DFLE-II)..., life expectancy free of class VII disability (DFLE-VII). DFLE-I is calculated by first estimating the proportion of each age group without any disability as follows:

$$H_{1x} = (1 - P_{1x})(1 - P_{2x})(1 - P_{3x})(1 - P_{4x})(1 - P_{5x})(1 - P_{6x})(1 - P_{7x})$$

where P_{ix} is the prevalence of class i disability for age group x and H_{1x} is the prevalence of individuals without a class I (or worse) disability. DFLE-I is calculated by multiplying the L_x column in a life table by H_{1x} and calculating the expectation of life free of disability at each age using standard life table methods. DFLE-II, the expectation of life at birth free of class II (or worse) disability is calculated in a similar fashion, the only difference being that H_{2x} in this case is calculated as:

$$H_{2x} = (1 - P_{2x})(1 - P_{3x})(1 - P_{4x})(1 - P_{5x})(1 - P_{6x})(1 - P_{7x})$$

where P_{ix} are defined as before. In the same way, other values of H_{ix} can be calculated and applied, as described above, to produce other variants of DFLE.

RESULTS

The GBD provides estimates of the incidence, prevalence and durations of a large number of disabling sequelae, many of which are presented in detail in the second volume of this series, *Global Health Statistics* (Murray and Lopez 1996b). In the following section some of the more important results obtained by applying various summary measures are described in order to provide an overview of the estimated burden of non-fatal health outcomes and its public health significance. Interested readers are referred to the Annex Table 8 for more detail on disability from specific conditions.

PREVALENCE OF DISABILITY BY CLASS

Although the primary focus of the GBD has been on estimating the incidence of disability in view of the incidence perspective used for calculating YLDs, we begin this section by summarizing the prevalence of different classes of disability by age, sex and region (see Table 4.5). For nearly every class of disability and every region, prevalence rises with age. The notable exception is class III disability among females, for which prevalence reaches a peak in the age group 15–44 years in the six developing regions. This is largely due to infertility caused by sexually transmitted diseases and maternal conditions, which are concentrated in this age group. For class I disability, the rise in prevalence with age is much less marked than for other classes of disability.

For most disability classes, prevalence is highest in SSA and lowest in EME, although there is considerable variation in the rank order of the regions depending on age and on the class of disability under consideration. A notable exception to this general pattern is the high prevalence of class V disability in Chinese men and women, which is largely due to high rates of chronic obstructive pulmonary disease (COPD). Prevalence of class VII disabilities is highest in China, EME and FSE. This is due to higher crude prevalences of dementia in these three regions compared with other regions. Crude prevalence is lower in the other five regions because the population over 75 is a smaller fraction of the population aged 60 years and over.

As expected, class I and class II disabilities are substantially more prevalent than higher-order classes of disability in all regions. More specifically, among the elderly (i.e. those aged 60 and over), class II disabilities tend to be the most common, with typically 40–50 per cent of the elderly population affected in EME and FSE, and 70–80 per cent in the developing world. At younger ages, class I disabilities are the most common, ranging from 7–14 per cent in males aged 0–44 years in EME and FSE, to 30–40 per cent of males at these ages in developing regions. These patterns can be largely explained by the different epidemiological environment of developed and developing regions, with the cumulative incidence and effects of disease and injury being more common in poorer countries.

PREVALENCE OF DISABILITY WEIGHTED BY SEVERITY

By multiplying the prevalence of each class of disability by the severity weight of that class, we have calculated severity-weighted prevalences of disability. This measure can be interpreted as the equivalent prevalence of total disability or the proportion of each year of life lost due to disability. One minus severity-weighted disability prevalence is then equivalent to the percentage of time lived in complete health. Figure 4.3 shows severity-weighted disability prevalences by age and sex for all causes combined and for conditions in Groups I, II and III. In all age groups and regions, severity-weighted disability prevalence due to Group I conditions is higher for females than for males. The severity-weighted disability prevalence from Group I conditions is relatively even across the life cycle but has a notable peak among young adult women aged 15–44. Conversely severity-weighted prevalence of Group II conditions rises steadily with age, reflecting the older age of onset for most of these conditions. In most regions and in most age groups, severity-weighted disability prevalence of Group II conditions is higher for males than for females, except in some

Table 4.5   Prevalence (per 1000) of seven classes of disability, by age, sex and region

Age group (years)	EME	FSE	IND	CHN	OAI	SSA	LAC	MEC
Males								
Class I								
0–4	65.1	137.3	451.9	224.8	357.5	403.6	224.6	365.9
5–14	63.6	110.6	329.2	282.5	297.5	467.4	208.1	293.8
15–44	87.1	140.6	337.8	278.3	338.3	463.4	221.4	287.8
45–59	163.9	261.1	401.3	311.5	411.3	550.9	327.4	392.5
60+	341.4	414.8	556.6	394.1	562.5	656.3	482.6	553.4
Class II								
0–4	71.2	118.5	237.0	196.5	203.2	248.9	179.3	260.2
5–14	59.3	79.3	213.0	158.6	164.2	258.7	176.7	181.9
15–44	90.3	144.4	258.2	182.2	242.9	441.2	210.5	205.9
45–59	172.8	301.1	386.7	267.9	404.2	668.9	344.8	395.8
60+	378.8	490.2	643.6	465.0	749.8	927.6	629.7	705.4
Class III								
0–4	21.2	33.1	64.6	47.0	55.9	69.9	48.9	60.4
5–14	17.9	21.2	43.0	28.7	33.2	45.9	43.5	33.5
15–44	59.9	78.4	77.5	47.6	78.6	139.9	111.3	57.6
45–59	81.2	136.2	126.9	89.2	122.1	203.1	161.7	106.7
60+	169.0	215.8	225.0	200.4	230.3	300.4	282.2	203.1
Class IV								
0–4	8.5	13.2	28.6	17.1	25.1	33.9	20.8	24.7
5–14	8.4	10.4	24.3	13.1	17.1	21.6	16.0	17.4
15–44	35.2	44.8	38.2	24.7	40.6	63.6	57.5	37.8
45–59	43.7	72.6	65.7	53.5	62.3	99.4	78.1	63.8
60+	90.7	111.5	119.9	137.3	122.6	153.0	132.5	121.3
Class V								
0–4	4.8	8.0	16.5	11.4	14.1	16.2	11.3	13.4
5–14	4.7	5.9	15.2	7.2	9.8	11.5	9.0	10.4
15–44	17.6	20.7	22.6	14.9	21.2	26.3	27.2	20.6
45–59	21.9	32.5	37.7	34.3	32.0	39.0	35.8	29.0
60+	55.0	57.5	70.5	99.1	64.3	64.5	68.4	61.1
Class VI								
0–4	1.9	4.7	8.1	6.6	7.2	10.2	5.3	6.5
5–14	2.0	3.0	10.4	4.4	6.3	10.4	4.9	5.9
15–44	25.6	32.1	38.2	32.0	36.0	46.0	35.6	37.6
45–59	30.1	42.0	65.1	47.0	55.9	90.8	46.7	55.9
60+	54.9	58.7	118.6	100.3	98.6	193.7	86.9	103.0
Class VII								
0–4	1.1	3.3	4.3	4.6	3.7	2.7	2.7	3.7
5–14	1.2	1.7	5.7	2.6	3.4	2.3	2.6	3.4
15–44	7.3	10.3	12.1	8.3	11.8	11.1	10.8	11.0
45–59	13.4	21.1	18.1	17.8	19.2	19.3	18.3	15.8
60+	46.0	46.9	36.3	52.0	41.1	34.7	42.9	29.9

Table 4.5   (continued)

Age group (years)	EME	FSE	IND	CHN	OAI	SSA	LAC	MEC
Females								
Class I								
0–4	60.2	139.8	455.2	226.2	365.4	393.6	237.5	364.5
5–14	57.1	105.3	333.6	281.8	297.0	417.9	215.2	284.6
15–44	111.3	156.4	494.0	267.9	450.8	538.9	321.4	503.2
45–59	195.7	268.8	615.5	360.5	535.7	689.0	407.4	622.4
60+	337.6	400.3	679.7	405.3	621.4	728.7	527.5	706.3
Class II								
0–4	71.4	123.4	237.8	200.3	207.9	248.3	189.9	260.2
5–14	58.6	82.1	216.7	159.4	161.0	243.2	182.0	175.5
15–44	88.4	125.3	326.8	172.9	263.0	379.8	214.1	284.4
45–59	180.6	263.4	463.7	284.4	400.8	521.2	327.9	451.8
60+	389.2	483.3	705.6	469.5	725.0	800.3	649.5	781.7
Class III								
0–4	21.3	34.2	65.0	48.6	56.1	70.9	50.7	60.0
5–14	17.2	20.9	38.2	28.8	31.1	44.2	40.6	30.1
15–44	47.9	88.3	160.9	52.1	129.2	251.6	122.5	106.5
45–59	65.9	96.1	97.2	81.7	86.6	122.1	110.1	78.4
60+	145.0	183.7	173.4	171.3	164.2	213.9	229.8	157.2
Class IV								
0–4	8.8	13.7	28.7	17.7	25.0	34.5	21.9	24.4
5–14	7.4	9.1	20.3	13.3	14.8	20.1	15.8	14.8
15–44	20.5	25.7	31.0	21.2	25.3	40.2	31.8	28.0
45–59	31.8	44.5	50.0	46.1	42.4	65.7	51.5	49.0
60+	72.8	87.7	90.9	115.2	84.0	114.3	104.6	93.9
Class V								
0–4	4.7	7.9	16.2	11.0	13.8	16.3	11.5	13.0
5–14	4.2	5.1	12.9	7.4	8.5	10.6	8.9	8.9
15–44	11.8	13.5	19.9	13.4	15.4	20.8	18.2	16.3
45–59	17.5	21.9	30.8	31.2	24.1	29.0	26.7	27.1
60+	49.8	50.5	59.0	90.6	53.0	53.0	60.3	53.3
Class VI								
0–4	1.9	4.5	8.5	6.2	7.2	10.7	5.6	6.5
5–14	1.8	2.5	8.5	4.7	5.3	9.9	4.5	5.0
15–44	34.6	41.0	47.5	45.7	45.9	53.2	45.8	49.4
45–59	35.1	41.7	68.4	60.6	64.6	88.2	50.5	66.8
60+	56.9	56.5	126.8	112.7	110.7	199.3	90.3	113.7
Class VII								
0–4	1.1	3.1	4.3	3.8	3.7	2.8	2.8	3.7
5–14	1.1	1.6	4.9	2.9	3.0	2.1	2.4	3.1
15–44	5.4	6.5	9.8	7.1	8.7	6.9	7.7	8.3
45–59	10.4	12.6	16.0	15.2	14.2	11.4	13.0	12.6
60+	47.5	44.5	33.3	46.9	37.5	25.0	40.0	25.0

Figure 4.3   Severity-weighted prevalence of disability for Groups I, II
                   and III and from all causes, by age, sex and region, 1990

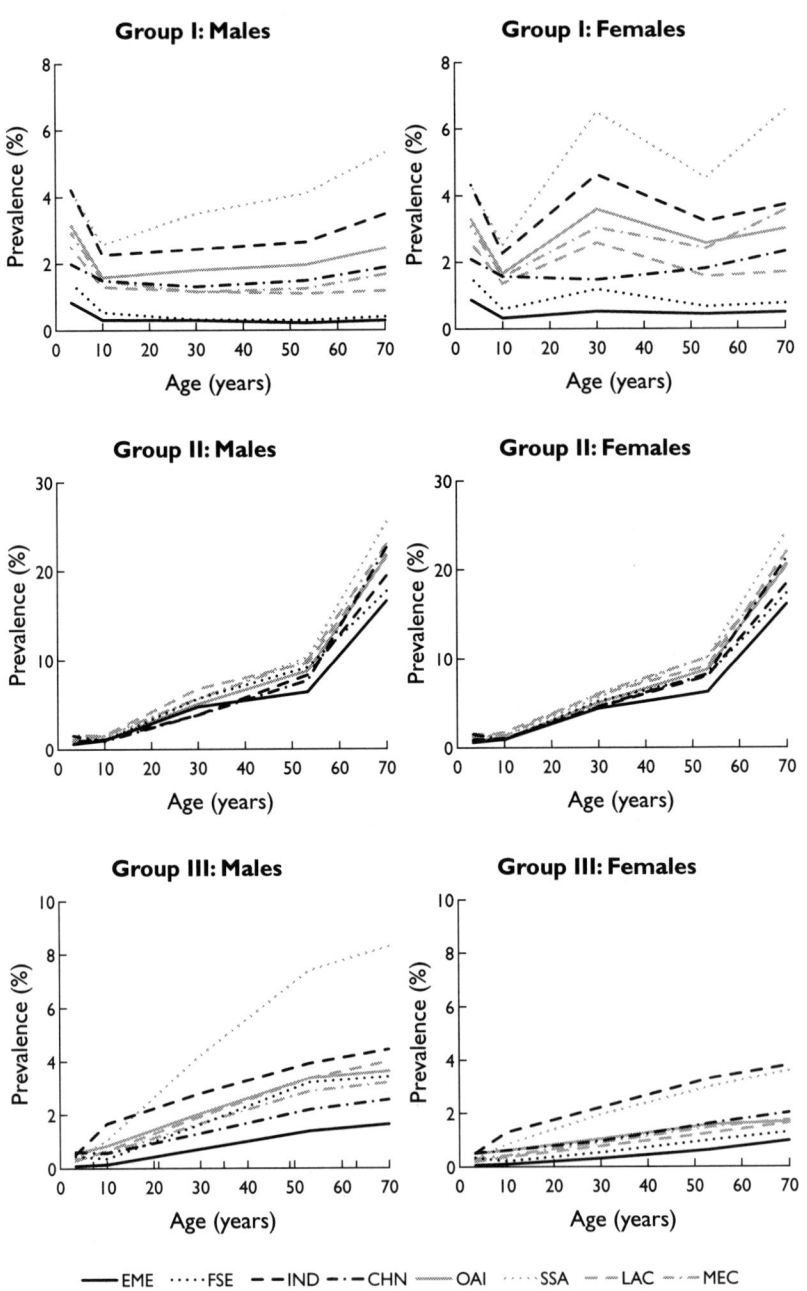

Figure 4.3   (continued)

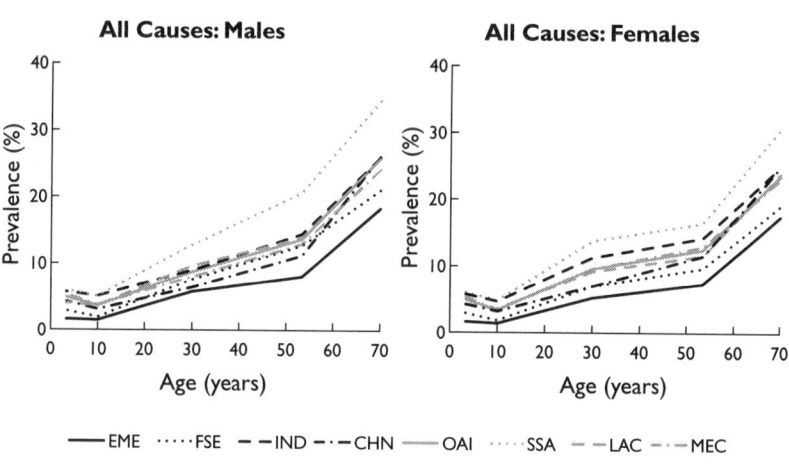

age groups in India, China and MEC. For Group III conditions, severity-weighted disability prevalence rises with age although not as steeply as for Group II conditions, and is substantially higher among males than females in every age group and every region.

Comparative regional patterns of severity-weighted disability are similar to the more familiar regional patterns of mortality. Thus the severity-weighted prevalence of disability is greater in SSA than in EME, for example, for all cause-groups and at all ages; however, this difference is much less obvious than that for mortality. For noncommunicable diseases, regional patterns and levels of severity-weighted disability are remarkably similar across regions, with a noticeable difference in levels apparent only at the older ages (60 years and over). These patterns of severity-weighted disability prevalence are influenced in some cases by the regional differences in mortality; nevertheless, the finding that regions with high mortality tend to have high levels of severity-weighted prevalence, and vice versa, is likely to be generally applicable.

HEALTH-ADJUSTED EXPECTANCIES

Another perspective on age and regional differences in disability is provided in Table 4.6, which shows the average number of disabling sequelae per individual with at least one condition. These co-disability rates have been calculated assuming independence between classes of disability and have not been corrected for dependent co-disability or independent co-disability within a class. Calculated in this manner, co-disability is more common at older ages in all regions, especially in high mortality populations. The average number of disabilities per individual ranges from 1.05 in EME among males and females aged 5–14 years, to 2.36 in SSA among males 60 years and over. If attention is limited to moderate to severe disabilities (classes IV and higher), the highest rate of co-disability is 1.16 conditions per individual estimated for SSA males aged over 60 years. These summary figures indicated that much of the co-disability that arises is due to individuals having more than one mild disability.

Table 4.7 provides estimates of various types of Disability-Free Life Expectancy (DFLE-I,...,DFLE-VII) for males and females in each region. The same information can also be represented in terms of the expectation at birth of the number of years to be lived in each class of disability (see Table 4.8 and Figure 4.4)—in cases of co-disability individuals are assigned to the disability class of the highest order, i.e. an individual with a class III and a class I disability is assigned to class III. The regional rankings of DFLE-I at birth for females exactly parallels the rankings of the expectation of life at birth. In males, the only difference in the regional rankings of DFLE-I at birth and life expectancy at birth is the reversal of MEC and OAI. The rank order for other types of DFLE, however, varies by region. These estimates would suggest that there is considerable heterogeneity across regions in the distribution of disability by class for the two sexes. The expectation at birth of class I disability (6.5–14.7 years) and class II disability (8.5–18.4 years) is large compared to the other classes. Indeed the sum of these two classes exceeds the sum of the other five classes in all regions. Group I conditions account for a large share of the common mild disabilities in these two classes.

Even excluding common mild conditions, i.e. class I and class II disabilities, DFLE varies significantly among regions. The difference between DFLE-VII and DFLE-III varies from 10.9 years (MEC) to 15.4 years (LAC) in males and from 10.6 to 14.8 years in females. Clearly, changing the threshold definition of disability for the calculation of DFLE can have a

Table 4.6   Average number of disabling sequelae per individual with at least one disabling sequela

	EME	FSE	IND	CHN	OAI	SSA	LAC	MEC
Males								
0–4	1.06	1.11	1.29	1.18	1.23	1.29	1.18	1.27
5–14	1.05	1.08	1.23	1.16	1.17	1.28	1.16	1.18
15–44	1.14	1.20	1.32	1.22	1.31	1.53	1.29	1.26
45–59	1.22	1.39	1.50	1.35	1.49	1.84	1.46	1.47
60+	1.54	1.69	1.94	1.75	1.99	2.36	1.91	1.92
Females								
0–4	1.06	1.12	1.29	1.18	1.24	1.29	1.19	1.27
5–14	1.05	1.08	1.22	1.16	1.17	1.26	1.16	1.17
15–44	1.13	1.19	1.47	1.22	1.38	1.60	1.32	1.40
45–59	1.22	1.32	1.61	1.37	1.50	1.74	1.43	1.56
60+	1.51	1.63	2.01	1.72	1.93	2.23	1.88	2.01

Table 4.7 Disability-Free Life Expectancy (DFLE) at birth and
Disability-Adjusted Life Expectancy (DALE) at birth by sex
and region

	I	II	III	IV	V	VI	VII	DALE
				DFLE				
Males								
EME	45.2	51.8	60.7	65.7	68.6	70.2	72.2	67.4
FSE	34.6	41.9	52.3	57.8	60.9	62.5	64.6	59.4
CHN	29.5	41.5	53.7	57.8	60.5	62.4	65.1	59.5
LAC	26.1	34.9	48.6	56.1	60.0	62.0	64.7	57.6
OAI	21.0	32.4	47.5	52.7	55.6	57.2	59.8	53.7
MEC	22.5	33.4	48.0	52.4	55.2	56.7	59.4	53.6
IND	19.4	30.8	44.9	49.8	52.5	54.2	57.0	51.0
SSA	10.1	18.8	34.6	40.4	43.4	44.7	47.8	41.0
Females								
EME	47.7	56.1	67.3	72.3	74.8	76.4	79.1	73.9
FSE	38.3	47.6	60.2	66.6	69.3	70.9	73.6	67.8
CHN	30.0	42.7	56.0	60.4	63.0	65.0	68.7	62.2
LAC	25.0	37.1	53.4	61.0	64.0	65.8	69.2	61.9
OAI	18.5	33.0	50.4	56.5	58.8	60.2	63.6	56.9
MEC	16.4	31.1	50.0	55.2	57.7	59.1	62.6	55.8
IND	14.0	27.5	44.7	51.1	53.4	54.9	58.2	51.5
SSA	9.9	20.7	35.7	43.3	45.6	46.8	50.5	43.4

Note:

Seven forms of DFLE are shown. DFLE-I is the expectation of life free of disability of Class I or higher severity, DFLE-II is the expectation of life free of disability of Class II or higher severity, etc.

dramatic effect on the results. This suggests that national-level estimates of DFLE should only be compared when detailed information is available about the severity of disabilities included in the calculations and provided there is a standardized threshold for defining disability.

The sex ratios of the expectations of disability in each class suggests that on average, the expectation of class I disability is nearly 25 per cent higher in females than in males. In India and MEC, similarly high sex ratios of expectations of disability are apparent for classes II and III as well.

By using the disability severity weights for each class, one can collapse the information on life expectancy and on the prevalence of each class of disability into a composite measure, namely Disability-Adjusted Life Expectancy (DALE). Table 4.9 provides comparative regional estimates of the expectation of life at birth, the Disability-Adjusted Life Expectancy at birth (DALE(0)), the expectation at birth of life with disability, and the proportion of the expected lifespan lived with disability. The expectation of life with disability is defined as the difference between life expectancy and DALE. Expectation of life at birth is 2–14 per cent higher for females than for males, depending on the region; the lowest female to male life-expectancy ratio is observed in India and the highest in FSE. Even after adjusting for time lived with disability, DALE(0), this comparative gap in favour of females remains essentially unchanged. Moreover, the male-female difference in life expectancy is not much larger than the male-female difference in DALE(0), which suggests that the female advantage in Disability-Adjusted Life Expectancy is largely due to lower rates of mortality, not disability.

Figure 4.5 shows the proportion of the expected lifespan lived with disability. This ranges for males from 8.1 per cent in EME to 15.3 per cent in SSA, and for females from 8.3 per cent in EME to 14.9 per cent in SSA. The proportion of the expected lifespan lived with a disability is marginally higher for males than females in EME, FSE, LAC and SSA, whereas the reverse is true in China, OAI, MEC and India. The differences between the sexes, however, are not substantial. Since women live longer than men at older ages where the prevalence of disability is more common, the expectation at birth of years lived with disability is greater for females than for males in all regions, with the differences varying from 0.3 years in LAC to 0.9 years in MEC.

Table 4.10 summarizes the estimates of DFLE and DALE at age 60. As might be expected, there is less variation in the expectation of life at age 60 among regions compared with life expectancy at birth. Nevertheless, life expectancy at age 60 for males is still 20 per cent higher in EME than

Table 4.8   Expectation at birth of time spent in different classes of disability by sex and region

	Class of Disability								
	0	I	II	III	IV	V	VI	VII	E(0)
Males									
EME	45.2	6.5	9.0	4.9	2.9	1.6	2.0	1.1	73.4
FSE	34.6	7.3	10.4	5.5	3.2	1.6	2.1	1.1	65.7
CHN	29.5	12.0	12.2	4.2	2.7	1.9	2.6	1.1	66.2
LAC	26.1	8.9	13.7	7.4	3.9	2.0	2.7	1.1	65.8
OAI	21.0	11.4	15.0	5.2	2.9	1.6	2.6	1.0	60.8
MEC	22.5	10.9	14.6	4.4	2.9	1.5	2.7	0.8	60.3
IND	19.4	11.4	14.1	4.9	2.7	1.7	2.8	0.9	57.9
SSA	10.1	8.8	15.8	5.7	3.0	1.3	3.1	0.7	48.4
Females									
EME	47.7	8.4	11.2	5.0	2.5	1.6	2.7	1.4	80.5
FSE	38.3	9.3	12.7	6.4	2.7	1.5	2.7	1.2	74.8
CHN	30.0	12.7	13.3	4.4	2.6	2.0	3.7	1.1	69.8
LAC	25.0	12.1	16.3	7.6	3.1	1.8	3.4	1.1	70.3
OAI	18.5	14.5	17.5	6.1	2.2	1.4	3.5	1.0	64.6
MEC	16.4	14.7	18.9	5.3	2.4	1.4	3.5	0.7	63.4
IND	14.0	13.5	17.2	6.4	2.3	1.5	3.4	0.8	59.1
SSA	9.9	10.8	15.0	7.6	2.3	1.2	3.7	0.5	51.0

Note: Expectation of time spent with Class X – time classified by worst disability

Figure 4.4   Expectations at birth of time spent in the seven different classes of disability, by sex and region, 1990

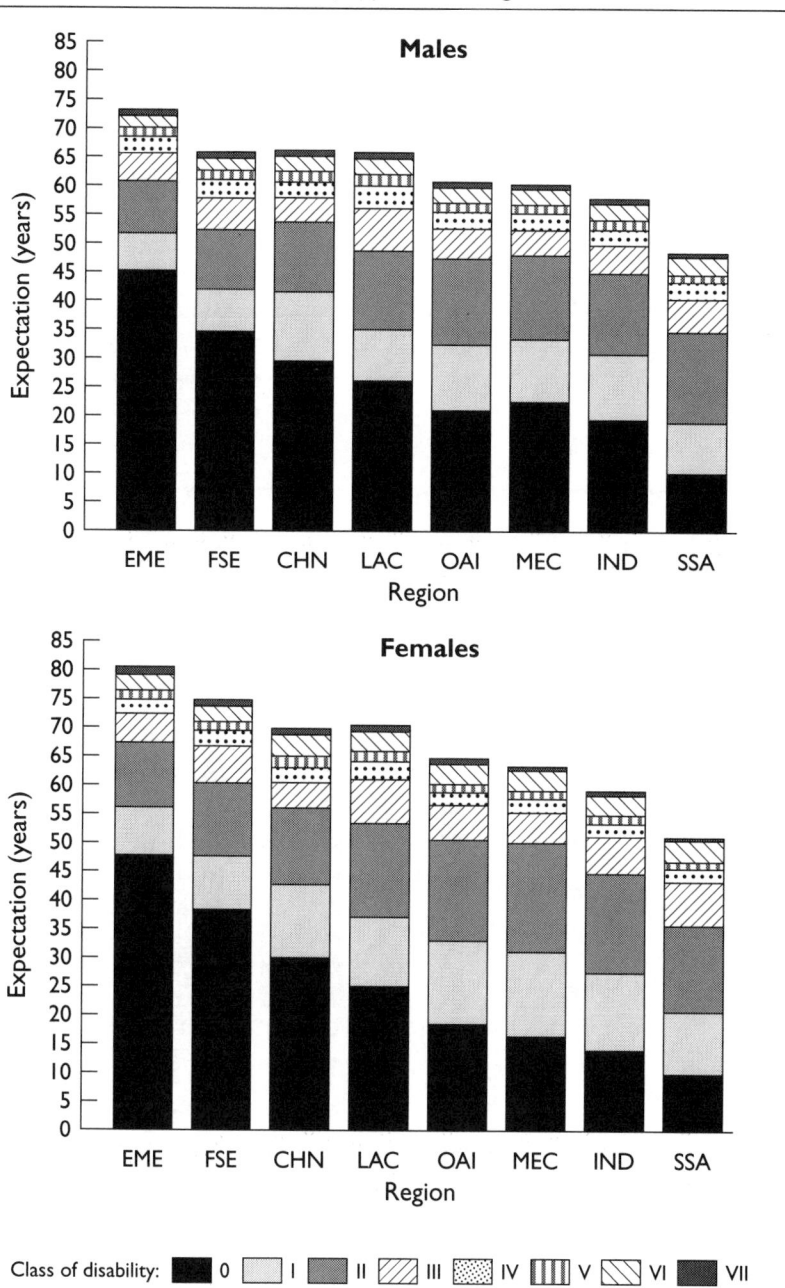

Note: Time with disability is classified by the worst disability in cases of co-disability.

Table 4.9   Life expectancy at birth, Disability-Adjusted Life Expectancy at birth, the expectation of disability at birth, and the proportion of the expected lifespan at birth lost due to disability

	E(0)		DALE(0)		Expectation of disability		Per cent of lifespan lost due to disability	
	Male	**Female**	**Male**	**Female**	**Male**	**Female**	**Male**	**Female**
EME	73.4	80.5	67.4	73.9	5.9	6.6	8.1	8.3
FSE	65.7	74.8	59.4	67.8	6.3	7.0	9.6	9.4
CHN	66.2	69.8	59.5	62.2	6.7	7.6	10.1	10.9
LAC	65.8	70.3	57.6	61.9	8.1	8.4	12.4	12.0
OAI	60.8	64.6	53.7	56.9	7.1	7.6	11.6	11.8
MEC	60.3	63.4	53.6	55.8	6.6	7.5	11.0	11.9
IND	57.9	59.1	51.0	51.5	6.9	7.6	11.9	12.9
SSA	48.4	51.0	41.0	43.4	7.4	7.6	15.3	14.9

Figure 4.5   Proportion of the expected lifespan at birth lost due to disability, by sex and region, 1990

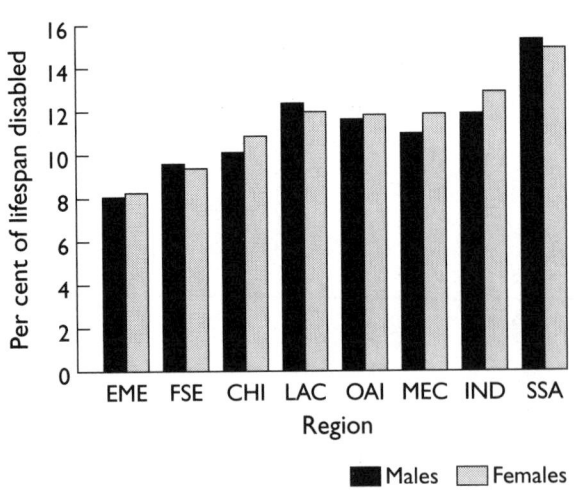

in SSA and 29 per cent higher for females. Figure 4.6 shows that at these older ages, the proportion of the expected lifespan lost due to disability ranges from approximately 20 per cent in EME to nearly 50 per cent in SSA. Even at these ages, the differential in disability between rich and poor regions remains. Reduction of disability, along with reduction of mortal-

Table 4.10   Life expectancy at 60, Disability-Adjusted Life Expectancy at 60, the expectation of disability at 60, and the proportion of the expected lifespan at 60 lost due to disability

	E(60) Male	E(60) Female	DALE(60) Male	DALE(60) Female	Expectation of disability at 60 Male	Expectation of disability at 60 Female	Per cent of lifespan lost due to disability Male	Per cent of lifespan lost due to disability Female
EME	19.0	24.1	15.5	19.9	3.5	4.2	22.4	21.1
FSE	15.8	20.4	12.5	16.5	3.3	3.9	26.7	23.6
CHN	15.2	18.0	11.3	13.5	4.0	4.5	35.3	33.2
LAC	18.5	21.3	13.7	16.2	4.8	5.1	34.7	31.3
OAI	16.2	18.6	12.0	14.2	4.2	4.4	34.8	30.7
MEC	16.3	18.6	12.4	14.3	3.9	4.3	31.8	30.0
IND	15.1	16.3	11.2	12.2	3.9	4.1	35.0	33.2
SSA	14.7	15.9	9.6	11.1	5.1	4.9	52.7	44.2

ity, must therefore be common goals for health development in sub-Saharan Africa and other developing regions into the 21st century.

YEARS LIVED WITH DISABILITY

The primary indicator used in this study to analyse the burden of disease and injury by cause is DALYs, with the component of DALYs due to time lived with disability, labelled as Years Lived with Disability (YLDs). The percentage distribution of YLDs by age and region and by Groups I, II and III is given in Table 4.11. YLDs are calculated based on the incidence of each sequela, assigning the stream of disability from each incident case to the age of onset. Globally, nearly half of all disability due to disease or injury occurs in young adults (15–44 years) and almost one-fifth (18 per cent) is attributable to conditions arising in early childhood (0–4 years). Even though the prevalence of disability rises steadily with age and is highest in those aged over 60, less than 10 per cent of the global burden of disability is due to incidence of disease and injury in these older individuals. This striking age-pattern, which is consistent across all regions, strongly emphasizes the need for disease and injury prevention among young adults if disability is to be reduced, irrespective of region.

The proportions of YLDs from Group I, II and III vary markedly across regions (Figure 4.7), in a fashion similar to that for mortality. Globally, 24 per cent of YLDs is due to Group I conditions, 60 per cent is due to Group II diseases and 16 per cent arises from injuries (Group III). Because of differences in the distribution of population by age and lower rates of Group I sequelae as mortality declines, Group I conditions account for only six per cent of YLDs in developed regions; Groups II and III explain 84 and 10 per cent, respectively. In developing regions, YLDs due to Group I conditions are proportionately much more important (28 per cent), as

Figure 4.6 Proportion of expected lifespan at age 60 lost to disability, by sex and region, 1990

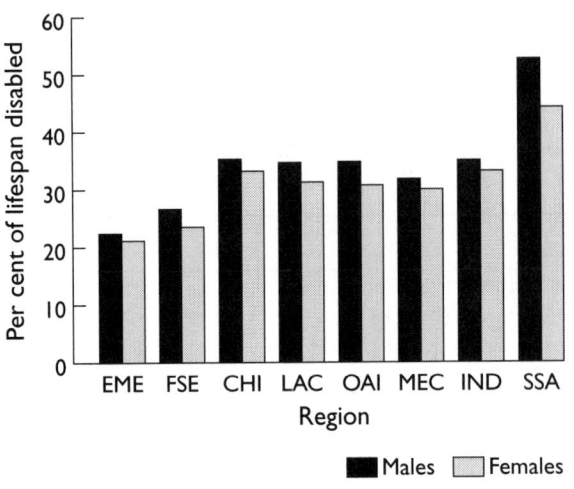

Table 4.11 Percentage distribution of YLDs according to region, by broad cause Group and age group, 1990

Region	Cause Group			All causes	Age group (years)					All ages
	I	II	III		0–4	5–14	15–44	45–59	60+	
EME	0.6	9.0	0.8	10.4	0.5	0.4	5.5	1.9	2.1	10.4
FSE	0.4	4.4	0.7	5.6	0.3	0.2	3.0	1.1	0.8	5.6
CHN	3.6	12.8	2.7	19.1	3.2	1.2	9.8	2.7	2.3	19.1
LAC	1.7	6.0	1.2	8.9	1.3	1.1	4.9	1.0	0.6	8.9
OAI	3.8	7.5	2.1	13.3	2.5	1.4	7.0	1.6	0.9	13.3
MEC	2.4	5.9	1.3	9.6	2.7	0.9	4.5	1.0	0.6	9.6
IND	6.2	8.1	4.2	18.5	4.2	3.2	7.8	2.0	1.3	18.5
SSA	5.7	5.8	3.0	14.5	3.7	2.0	6.9	1.3	0.7	14.5
World	24.4	59.5	16.1	100.0	18.3	10.5	49.4	12.6	9.3	100.0
Developed	1.0	13.4	1.5	15.9	0.8	0.6	8.5	3.0	3.0	15.9
Developing	23.4	46.1	14.6	84.1	17.5	9.9	40.8	9.6	6.3	84.1

are YLDs from Group III (17 per cent). Figure 4.7 also illustrates that there is considerable variation even among developing regions. In SSA, nearly equal shares of YLDs are due to Groups I and II, while injuries (Group III) account for over one-fifth of all YLDs. By contrast, in EME, nearly 9 out of 10 YLDs are due to noncommunicable diseases (Group II).

Figure 4.7   Distribution of YLDs for both sexes combined and all age groups, by cause Group and region

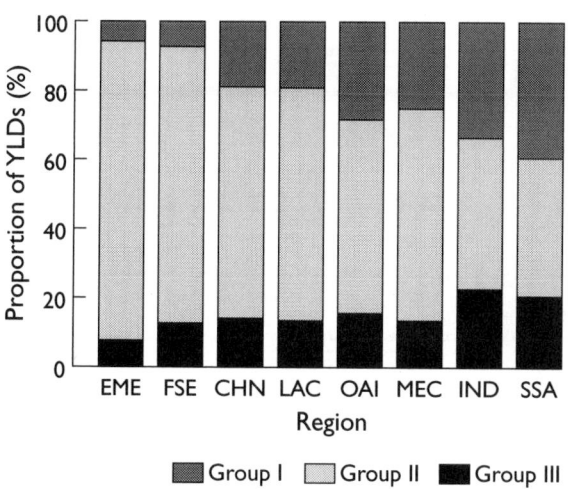

Note:

Group I: Communicable, maternal, perinatal and nutritional conditions

Group II: Noncommunicable diseases

Group III: Injuries

The contribution of major disease or injury categories within Groups I, II and III to YLDs is shown in Table 4.12. Interestingly, the most important contributor to YLDs in all regions (except SSA) are the neuro-psychiatric conditions, ranging from 16 per cent in SSA to 47 per cent in EME. Globally, neuro-psychiatric conditions are estimated to account for almost 30 per cent of all YLDs, far in excess of any other specific category. Infectious and parasitic diseases contribute approximately 11 per cent of YLDs globally, relatively little (3 per cent) in EME, but rather more (22 per cent) in SSA. Other leading causes of YLDs globally include nutritional deficiencies and chronic respiratory diseases, both of which account for more than seven per cent of global YLDs. About one in six YLDs arise from injuries, almost all of which are unintentional injuries. Even for this group of causes, there is marked variation among regions with the proportionate contribution to YLDs ranging from seven per cent in EME to 23 per cent in India.

Finally, it is of some interest to examine the leading specific causes of YLDs for the world, and for developing and developed regions. These are listed in Table 4.13 for males and females separately. The ten leading causes of global YLDs together account for 40 per cent of all YLDs and include five neuro-psychiatric conditions (unipolar major depression, alcohol use, bipolar disorder, schizophrenia and obsessive-compulsive dis-

Table 4.12   Percentage distribution of YLDs for specific causes (level two categories), 1990

Condition group	Region										
	EME	FSE	IND	CHN	OAI	SSA	LAC	MEC	Developed	Developing	World
All Causes	100.0	100.0	100.0	100.0	100.0	100.0	100.0	100.0	100.0	100.0	100.0
I. Communicable, maternal, perinatal and nutritional conditions	5.5	7.8	33.6	18.9	28.5	39.3	19.0	24.6	6.3	27.8	24.4
A. Infectious and parasitic diseases	2.6	3.0	14.3	6.4	12.6	22.4	9.7	6.4	2.7	12.3	10.7
B. Respiratory infections	0.3	0.4	1.4	1.4	1.4	1.3	1.0	1.8	0.4	1.4	1.2
C. Maternal conditions	0.6	1.9	4.7	1.9	4.0	5.8	2.7	5.0	1.1	4.0	3.5
D. Conditions arising during the perinatal period	0.5	0.5	3.5	1.1	1.7	3.2	1.6	2.9	0.5	2.3	2.0
E. Nutritional deficiencies	1.5	2.0	9.8	8.2	8.7	6.6	4.1	8.6	1.7	7.9	6.9
II. Noncommunicable diseases	86.7	79.5	43.7	66.9	56.1	39.8	67.3	61.5	84.2	54.8	59.5
A. Malignant neoplasms	3.8	2.5	0.6	1.2	0.9	0.5	0.8	0.5	3.3	0.8	1.2
B. Other neoplasms	1.2	1.1	0.2	0.6	0.4	0.4	0.8	0.4	1.2	0.4	0.5
C. Diabetes mellitus	3.2	1.5	1.0	0.5	1.0	0.3	1.3	1.5	2.6	0.9	1.1
D. Endocrine disorders	1.7	0.7	0.1	0.4	0.4	0.9	2.1	1.2	1.4	0.7	0.8
E. Neuro-psychiatric conditions	47.2	37.6	20.9	30.7	28.5	16.3	34.6	25.4	43.9	25.5	28.5
F. Sense organ diseases	0.2	0.2	3.4	2.0	2.7	2.9	1.4	2.0	0.2	2.5	2.1
G. Cardiovascular diseases	6.2	7.1	3.6	3.5	2.9	1.6	2.4	3.8	6.5	3.0	3.6
H. Respiratory diseases	6.1	7.1	5.0	14.0	4.7	6.6	6.1	7.8	6.5	7.7	7.5
I. Digestive diseases	4.1	5.5	2.4	5.1	5.8	3.6	4.3	7.1	4.6	4.5	4.5
J. Genito-urinary diseases	1.1	2.0	0.5	0.8	0.8	0.9	1.3	3.4	1.4	1.1	1.2
K. Musculo-skeletal diseases	8.0	10.2	1.6	3.6	3.1	1.5	6.9	1.8	8.8	2.9	3.8
L. Congenital anomalies	2.0	1.8	3.2	3.0	2.6	3.1	2.8	3.6	1.9	3.0	2.9
M. Oral conditions	1.8	1.8	1.2	1.1	2.0	0.6	2.4	3.0	1.8	1.5	1.6
III. Injuries	7.9	12.7	22.8	14.2	15.4	20.9	13.6	13.9	9.5	17.4	16.1
A. Unintentional injuries	7.1	10.7	22.4	12.9	14.6	16.3	12.3	10.0	8.3	15.4	14.3
B. Intentional injuries	0.8	2.0	0.4	1.3	0.8	4.6	1.4	3.9	1.2	1.9	1.8

order). Unipolar major depression alone accounts for 11 per cent of global YLDs. Other important causes of YLDs include anaemia, disabilities stemming from falls, and maternal conditions. COPD and osteoarthritis are also major contributors to the global burden of disability.

Some important differences between males and females, and between developed and developing regions are apparent from the table. Alcohol use, road traffic accidents and asthma are among the ten leading causes of YLDs for males globally, but not for females, among whom maternal conditions (2nd) and chlamydia (8th) cause substantial YLDs. In rich countries, alcohol use (1st) and drug use (5th) are estimated to be major causes of YLDs among males, but not females (although alcohol use ranks 10th for females, accounting for 2.5 per cent of all YLDs in developed countries). Alcohol use is similarly a major cause of YLDs among males in developing regions, causing about twice as much disability as either road traffic accidents or asthma. Dementia, stroke (cerebrovascular disease) and diabetes mellitus also rank in the ten leading causes of YLDs in developed regions, as does protein-energy malnutrition (for both sexes) in developing countries.

DISCUSSION

Trends in the duration of life lived with disability that accompany the epidemiological transition have been subject to extensive debate (Crimmins 1990, Murray and Chen 1992, Robine et al. 1987). There are three types of theories or postulates put forward to explain the changes in disability that accompany mortality decline. Fries (1980,1989) and colleagues (Fries et al. 1989, Leigh and Fries 1994) argue that with improvements in survival, the prevalence of disability will decline and therefore the proportion of the lifespan lived in a disabled state will decrease. This theory is often called the "compression of morbidity" hypothesis. Conversely, a variety of theories have been proposed predicting that the proportion of the lifespan lived with disability will increase as mortality declines. Gruenberg (1977) and Kramer (1980) suggest that as the survival of individuals with chronic conditions such as Down syndrome improves, the prevalence of these conditions must rise. Other authors (Alter and Riley 1989, Feldman 1983, Shephard and Zeckhauser 1980) forecast an increase in the prevalence of disability. According to them, medical intervention will improve survival for more frail individuals who will subsequently experience higher incidence rates of disability. More recently, Olshansky et al. (1991) further refined the expansion of the morbidity hypothesis. A third theory (Manton 1982), which shares elements of both of these viewpoints, predicts that the progression of chronic diseases to severe disability will be slowed leading to a decline in the prevalence of severe disability but a rise in the prevalence of mild disability; the latter would occur because of the decline in mortality.

International comparisons of Disability-Free Life Expectancy, health-adjusted life expectancy and other health expectancies have been severely

Table 4.13   Ten leading causes of YLDs, by sex, 1990

	Both Sexes			Males			Females		
Rank	Disease or Injury	YLDs	Cumula-tive %	Disease or Injury	YLDs	Cumula-tive %	Disease or Injury	YLDs	Cumula-tive %
World									
	All Causes	472 736		All Causes	235 096		All Causes	237 641	
1	Unipolar major depression	50 810	10.7	Unipolar major depression	18 070	7.7	Unipolar major depression	32 740	13.8
2	Iron-deficiency anaemia	21 987	15.4	Alcohol use	13 935	13.6	Iron-deficiency anaemia	12 239	18.9
3	Falls	21 949	20.0	Falls	13 474	19.3	Falls	8 475	22.5
4	Alcohol use	15 770	23.4	Iron-deficiency anaemia	9 748	23.5	Osteoarthritis	7 934	25.8
5	Chronic obstructive pulmonary disease	14 692	26.5	Chronic obstructive pulmonary disease	8 357	27.0	Bipolar disorder	6 938	28.8
6	Bipolar disorder	14 141	29.5	Bipolar disorder	7 203	30.1	Congenital anomalies	6 767	31.6
7	Congenital anomalies	13 507	32.3	Congenital anomalies	6 740	33.0	Chronic obstructive pulmonary disease	6 335	34.3
8	Osteoarthritis	13 275	35.1	Schizophrenia	6 397	35.7	Chlamydia	5 834	36.7
9	Schizophrenia	12 183	37.7	Road traffic accidents	5 834	38.2	Schizophrenia	5 786	39.2
10	Obsessive-compulsive disorders	10 213	39.9	Osteoarthritis	5 341	40.5	Obsessive-compulsive disorders	5 778	41.6
Developed Regions									
	All Causes	75 389		All Causes	38 242		All Causes	37 147	
1	Unipolar major depression	9780	13.0	Alcohol use	5 231	13.7	Unipolar major depression	6 392	17.2
2	Alcohol use	6 112	21.1	Unipolar major depression	3 388	22.5	Osteoarthritis	2 811	24.8
3	Osteoarthritis	4 681	27.3	Osteoarthritis	1 870	27.4	Dementia and other degenerative and hereditary CNS disorders	2 054	30.3
4	Dementia and other degenerative and hereditary CNS disorders	3 264	31.6	Schizophrenia	1 557	31.5	Schizophrenia	1 443	34.2
5	Schizophrenia	2 999	35.6	Drug use	1 484	35.4	Bipolar disorder	1 248	37.5

Table 4.13 (continued)

	Both Sexes			Males			Females		
Rank	Disease or Injury	YLDs	Cumulative %	Disease or Injury	YLDs	Cumulative %	Disease or Injury	YLDs	Cumulative %
Developed Regions (continued)									
6	Bipolar disorder	2 505	38.9	Road traffic accidents	1 446	39.2	Cerebrovascular disease	1 216	40.8
7	Cerebrovascular disease	2 343	42.0	Bipolar disorder	1 257	42.4	Obsessive-compulsive disorders	1 207	44.1
8	Obsessive-compulsive disorders	2 098	44.8	Dementia and other degenerative and hereditary CNS disorders	1 210	45.6	Diabetes mellitus	1 074	47.0
9	Road traffic accidents	2 015	47.5	Chronic obstructive pulmonary disease	1 150	48.6	Rheumatoid arthritis	1 053	49.8
10	Diabetes mellitus	1 946	50.1	Cerebrovascular disease	1 127	51.6	Alcohol use	882	52.2
Developing Regions									
	All Causes	397 347		All Causes	196 854		All Causes	200 493	
1	Unipolar major depression	41 031	10.3	Unipolar major depression	14 682	7.5	Unipolar major depression	26 348	13.1
2	Iron-deficiency anaemia	20 968	15.6	Falls	12 445	13.8	Iron-deficiency anaemia	11 541	18.9
3	Falls	20 274	20.7	Iron-deficiency anaemia	9 427	18.6	Falls	7 830	22.8
4	Chronic obstructive pulmonary disease	12 954	24.0	Alcohol use	8 704	23.0	Congenital anomalies	6 063	25.8
5	Congenital anomalies	12 071	27.0	Chronic obstructive pulmonary disease	7 207	26.7	Chronic obstructive pulmonary disease	5 747	28.7
6	Bipolar disorder	11 636	29.9	Congenital anomalies	6 009	29.7	Bipolar disorder	5 689	31.5
7	Protein-energy malnutrition	9 714	32.4	Bipolar disorder	5 947	32.7	Chlamydia	5 225	34.1
8	Alcohol use	9 658	34.8	Protein-energy malnutrition	4 923	35.2	Osteoarthritis	5 124	36.7
9	Conditions arising during the perinatal period	9 263	37.1	Schizophrenia	4 840	37.7	Obstructed labour	5 072	39.2
10	Schizophrenia	9 184	39.4	Conditions arising during the perinatal period	4 691	40.1	Protein-energy malnutrition	4 791	41.6

hampered by differences in methods and definitions (Romieu and Robine 1994). Available cross-sectional estimates of health expectancies have not been useful in evaluating the compression of morbidity or opposing hypotheses. A number of authors have examined trends in health expectancies for a specific country, thereby hoping to minimize methodological and definitional differences (Crimmins et al. 1989, Manton et al. 1993, Mathers 1994, Robine 1994, Roos et al. 1993, Wilkins et al. 1994). Recent evidence from France suggests that a compression of morbidity is occurring (Robine 1994) but similar studies in Australia (Mathers 1994) are more equivocal. Studies have suggested that the prevalence of disability in the United States is rising (Murray and Chen 1992). Interpretation of trends over time, particularly when measurements are based on self-reported disability, may be affected by changes in the perception of illness, the willingness to take on the sick role and the cost to the individual of missing work or school (Chirikos 1986, Johansson 1991, 1992, Mechanic 1986, Verbrugge 1984).

The Global Burden of Disease Study has provided an excellent opportunity to examine the cross-sectional relationship between life expectancy and the prevalence of various forms of disability. Despite the uncertainty associated with particular estimates, the GBD has produced a uniquely standardized database which can be used to explore the compression of morbidity hypothesis, as well as other opposing hypotheses. The results clearly demonstrate that populations with higher mortality have a higher prevalence of disability. The proportion of the expected lifespan lived with disability declines as life expectancy rises, from a high of nearly 15 per cent in SSA to around 8 per cent in EME. At age 60, evidence for compression is even more marked: in SSA males are expected to spend about 53 per cent of their remaining lifetime with a disability, a figure more than twice as high as in EME (22 per cent). In other words, if the cross-sectional regional patterns observed can be generalized to temporal trends, a one-year improvement in life expectancy would appear to be accompanied by slightly more than a one year improvement in Disability-Adjusted Life Expectancy (DALE). The regional patterns of DALE and life expectancy are consistent with the compression of morbidity hypothesis. However, more definitive evidence from time series data on DALE, based on observed measures of non-fatal health outcomes, is required before the compression hypothesis can be confirmed.

Information on the burden of non-fatal health outcomes has been presented in this study using a variety of indicators. As a summary measure of the burden of disability from all causes in a population, Disability-Adjusted Life Expectancy has a number of advantages. Chiefly, it is relatively easy to explain the concept of a lifespan without disability to a non-technical audience. The utility of such "transparency" in the health policy debate should not be underestimated. Second, DALE is easy to calculate using the Sullivan method which relies on prevalence data. An alternative would be the multi-state life table method of calculating DALE, which uses data on incidence and remission of disability to calculate a period health expectation (Crimmins et al. 1993). Since estimates of the incidence and duration of each disabling sequela have been developed as part of the GBD, it would be technically feasible to estimate DALE using the multi-state life table method. While it would be scientifically interesting to do so, it is unlikely that our estimates by region based on the Sullivan method would differ much from estimates based on the multi-state life table approach.

Estimating the expectation of life lived with different classes of disability is another useful method to summarize information on disability from all causes. These expectations can be used to calculate a variety of Disability-Free Life Expectancies (DFLE). Clearly, the threshold used to define the level of disability included in estimates of DFLE has a significant effect on the estimate. This methodological issue alone may explain the wide variation in cross-sectional results reported in national studies. Romieu and Robine (1994) provide an example of a difference in DFLE that largely reflects differences in definition; they report that DFLE at birth for males in the United States in 1985 was 51.9 yet for males in Switzerland in 1988–89 it was 67.1.

It is interesting to note that the value of DALE consistently falls between DFLE-IV and DFLE-V in all regions. While DALE and the expectation of life in different classes of disability are useful summary measures for a population, Years Lived with Disability (YLDs), Years of Life Lost (YLLs) and their sum, DALYs, are preferable when the burden of non-fatal health outcomes and premature mortality needs to be decomposed into the burden attributable to various diseases, injuries or exposures. This is analogous to the relative utility of life expectancy and cause-specific death rates as measures of mortality. Using a composite measure such as DALYs also facilitates direct comparisons between the measurement of the burden of disease and the cost-effectiveness analysis of different interventions.

Overall, the burden of disability is dominated by a relatively short list of causes. Collectively, neuro-psychiatric conditions are estimated to account for 28 per cent of all YLDs. Maternal conditions, sexually transmitted diseases and HIV, conditions largely related to sexual activity, explain 6–7 per cent of global YLDs, 2.5 per cent in developing countries and 7.3 per cent in developed regions. According to the estimates reported here, five other conditions account for a substantial amount of disability: anaemia, falls, road traffic accidents, COPD and osteoarthritis.

The necessity of analysing non-fatal health outcomes, in addition to mortality, is underscored by the very different ranking of diseases and injuries, depending on the nature of the health outcome. Of the ten leading causes of YLDs in the world, six of them (unipolar major depression, alcohol use, bipolar disorder, osteoarthritis, schizophrenia and obsessive-compulsive disorder) rank below 60th in a similar comparison of Years of Life Lost from premature mortality. Avoiding premature death, and obtaining the data required to develop policies and strategies to do so, is a priority for public health. So, too, is the avoidance of disability; better data on both are required.

Although life expectancy for females exceeds that for males in all regions, some studies have claimed that the prevalence of disability is higher among females than males (e.g. Rahman et al. 1994). In four regions, EME, FSE, LAC and SSA, males not only live shorter lives than females, on average, but they also spend a higher proportion of their life disabled. In four other regions, China, OAI, MEC and India, females live longer but spend a higher proportion of their life disabled than do males. However, the combined effect of life expectancy and the prevalence of severity-weighted disability is such that in *all* regions, Disability-Adjusted Life Expectancy is higher for females than for males.

Many of the estimates presented here have wide confidence intervals. Since we have integrated various estimation methods, and utilized several data sources to derive an internally consistent epidemiological profile, a statistical 95 per cent confidence interval cannot be defined. Nevertheless, the degree of uncertainty of the estimates varies from disease to disease, across age groups and between regions. How should the degree of uncertainty associated with an estimate alter the way in which decision-makers interpret these results? According to economic theory, when making decisions about programmes and policies today, decision-makers should treat certain estimates in a similar fashion.[6] Where there are wide confidence intervals, decision-makers may be willing to invest resources to acquire more information and narrow the uncertainty associated with an estimate. Priority conditions for acquiring further information should be those which are major public health concerns with a large degree of uncertainty associated with them (e.g. tobacco-related disease in developing countries).

The total volume of YLDs may be affected by two potential sources of bias. First, the approximation method used to estimate YLDs from residual diseases may be inaccurate. If the set of diseases and injuries that have been estimated are representative of the relationship between YLDs and YLLs for all conditions, then the estimates may not be biased. The set of conditions which have been evaluated may not be representative, however, since it does not include idiopathic disabilities, for which, by definition, there is no known cause. Take, for example, disability due to blindness. Disability from blindness is included in the estimated burden of disease via a series of blinding conditions including trachoma, onchocerciasis, glaucoma, cataract, congenital disorders, perinatal conditions, diabetes, and neurological damage from malaria, road traffic accidents and other trauma. Some idiopathic causes of blindness, such as macular degeneration, may not be included, but are fortunately not likely to be large. The approximation method may also capture some of the idiopathic forms of disability to the extent that some multi-causal or idiopathic deaths are included in the residual categories.

While the residual approximation method for YLDs could bias YLDs downwards, the problem of co-disability may bias the results upwards. The Global Burden of Disease Study estimates are built up from a disease perspective. Severity-weighted disability prevalence, DALE and YLDs are based on the total number of disabling sequelae for each class. By implication, we assume that the severity weight for a co-disability is simply the sum of the disability weights for the various disabling sequelae. Further research is required to better define the extent of dependent and independent co-disability in different populations. Disability weights for combinations of disabilities could also be developed by expanding the application of the methods discussed in Chapter 1 in this volume (Murray 1996).

The philisophy of the GBD represents an interesting mix of the ethos of applied demography and the focus of descriptive epidemiology. Reflecting their training, most epidemiologists are only willing to make statements about the descriptive epidemiology of a condition when these statements are strongly supported by empirical data. For example, many epidemiologists would undoubtedly prefer to leave blank the tables in this study which have been derived from weak data sources. Demographers, on the other hand, generally accept that, irrespective of the data that are available, it is important to try and estimate mortality, fertility or other population parameters, depending on the study. An estimate is nearly always generated; only the magnitude of the confidence interval is in question. For studies attempting to demonstrate causality, or for formal evaluations of the impact of a programme or an intervention, epidemiological rigour is both essential and laudable. However, for descriptive epidemiology where the objective is to assess the probable or even approximate magnitude of disease or injury so as to inform current policy debates and planning exercises, approximate estimates are better than no estimates. For example, if the estimate of annual lung cancer mortality in a population is somewhere between 100 000 and 300 000, the magnitude of this mortality is still sufficiently large to suggest that urgent public health measures are required to control the epidemic despite the fact that we cannot measure it more reliably. We conclude that there is a need for a greater infusion of demographic ethos into the epidemiological estimation process in order to better inform health policies and planning.

The quantification of non-fatal health outcomes and their contribution to the burden of disease and injury is, as this chapter has hopefully reinforced, still under development. To reduce the uncertainty of estimates and accelerate the effective incorporation of disability information into the public health planning process, the underlying database needs to be strengthened. We have reviewed and used a variety of data and information sources to estimate YLDs and related parameters, including health services data, disease and injury registries, community-based research and cross-sectional surveys. Given the conceptual basis for YLDs (see Murray 1996, Chapter 1 in this volume), with the emphasis on mapping the disabling sequelae of disease and injury, one of the more useful information bases for guiding prevention strategies to reduce non-fatal health outcomes may be prospective follow-up studies of incident cases. Reliable information is required about the incidence of disease and injury, about the likelihood of incurring sequelae, and about the severity and duration of these sequelae. Very few datasets of this type were available to inform estimates of YLDs for 1990 but such prospective data are urgently required if the measures used here are to be improved and be made more useful for promoting public health.

A registry to ensure the prospective follow-up of incident cases may not be feasible in many countries because of financial constraints. Valuable information of a dynamic nature on incident cases could also be obtained from a case-history taken at the time of admission to a hospital or another health facility. Retrospective cohorts of patients with injuries severe enough to be admitted to an emergency ward or hospital could be constructed for road traffic accidents, intentional violence and a number of other injuries in many settings. Much more information can be collected and analysed from settings where the coverage of hospitalization is complete and injuries are dual E- and N-coded. In addition, prospective studies of the short-term and long-term consequences of cohorts of individuals with different natures of injury may also need to be undertaken.

The probable magnitude of the burden of disease and injury which is *not* due to premature mortality, and the very substantial uncertainty about the size and disease/injury contributions to this pattern, require that research and database development be urgently undertaken to quantify non-fatal health outcomes more reliably. Research is required to improve the basic disease model used in this study; furthermore, extensive empirical work is necessary to create and field-test new instruments for collecting data and information on disability. In parallel, procedures for a more systematic identification, evaluation and use of existing data sources, studies and other information on disability should be actively promoted in order to make better use of what is already known.

NOTES

1   As discussed in Murray and Lopez (1996a), the only exception to this statement is adult mortality in SSA where the database is quite weak and as a result there is substantial disagreement about levels of adult mortality.

2   DISMOD, the computer programme that has been developed to test for internal consistency of epidemiological estimates, requires, as input, instantaneous incidence, remission and case-fatality rates. These are sometimes described in the epidemiological literature as "forces" or "densities" and should be distinguished from population incidence or remission rates.

3   One exception is the study of traumatic brain injury in Johannesburg (Brown and Nell 1991, 1992, Nell and Brown 1991). A more general study of non-fatal injuries has also been undertaken in South Africa (Butchart and Brown 1991, Butchart et al. 1991a, 1991b).

4   The E/N code matrix approach to the disabling sequealae of injuries was first developed and applied in the study of the National Burden of Disease of Mauritius (Gareeboo H et al. (1995).

5   YLDs[0,0] are YLDs that have been calculated using a discount rate of zero and uniform age-weights.

6   The following example may help explain this principle of decision-theory. Imagine that you are presented with two options. In option A you will receive $1000; option B is a gamble. In this gamble you have a 50 per cent chance of recieving $0 and a 50 per cent chance of receiving $2000. The expected value of the gamble is $1000 equal to the value of option A. Many individuals will prefer to take option A. These individuals can be described as *risk-averse*. One explanation of this behaviour is that the individual's utility level as a function of consumption dollars is concave. In other words, the utility of an extra $2000 is not twice as great as the utility of an extra $1000. Other individuals may be *risk-prone* and choose option B. This can also be explained by the shape of their utility function. These principles can also be applied to social decisions. However, as there is no strong argument for society to be risk- averse, a social decision-maker should be indifferent between A and B (Arrow and Lind 1970). While there are some difficulties in the application of these concepts to the health sector, in general, the idea that decision-makers should be risk neutral and treat a certain outcome as equally important to an uncertain outcome with the same expectation holds true. One obvious exception would be cases where the consequences of a problem are not a simple linear function of the magnitude of the problem. For example, if an infectious disease is more prevalent than expected, this may have implications for secondary transmission and the expected magnitude of the health problem in the future.

BIBLIOGRAPHY

Alter G, Riley JC (1989) Frailty, sickness and death: models of morbidity and mortality in historical populations. *Population Studies* 43:25–45.

Arrow KJ, Lind RC (1970) Uncertainty and the evaluation of public investment decisions. *American Economic Review* 60:364–78.

Barendregt JJ, Bonneux L, van der Maas PJ (1995) Health expectancy: from population health indicator to a tool for policy making. Paper presented at REVES 8, October 5–7 1995.

Brown DSO, Nell V (1991) The epidemiology of traumatic brain injury in Johannesburg. I. methodological issues in a developing country context. *Social Science and Medicine*, 33:283–287.

Brown DSO, Nell V (1992) Diffuse traumatic brain injury in Johannesburg: A concurrrent prospective study. *Archives of Physical Medicine and Rehabilitation*, 73:758–770.

Butchart A, Brown DSO (1991) Non-fatal injuries due to interpersonal violence in Johannesburg-Soweto: incidence, determinants and consequences. *Forensic Science International*, 52:35–51.

Butchart A et al. (1991a) The epidemiology of non-fatal trauma in Johannesburg-Soweto. I. methodology and materials. *South African Medical Journal*, 78:466–471.

Butchart A et al. (1991b) The epidemiology of non-fatal trauma in Johannesburg-Soweto. II. incidence and determinants. *South African Medical Journal*, 78:472–479.

Chirikos TN. (1986) Accounting for the historical rise in work-disability prevalence. *Milbank Memorial Fund Quarterly/Health and Society* 64:271–301.

Crimmins EM (1990) Are Americans healthier as well as longer-lived? *Journal of Internal Medicine*, 22:89–92.

Crimmins EM, Saito Y, Ingegneri D (1989) Changes in life expectancy and disability-free life expectancy in the United States. *Population and Development Review* 15:235–267.

Crimmins EM, Saito Y, Hayward MD (1993) Sullivan and multistate methods of estimating active life expectancy: two methods, two answers. In, Robine JM et al. (eds) Calculation of health expectancies: harmonization, concensus achieved and future perspectives. London: John Libbey Eurotext.

Feldman J (1983) Work ability of the aged under conditions of improving mortality. *Milbank Memorial Fund Quarterly/Health and Society* 61:430–444.

Fries JF (1980) Aging, natural death, and the compression of morbidity. *New England Journal of Medicine* 303(3):130–5.

Fries JF (1989) The compression of morbidity: near or far? *Milbank Quarterly* 67(2):208–32.

Fries JF, Green LW, Levine S (1989) Health promotion and the compression of morbidity. *Lancet* 1:481–483.

Gareeboo H et al. (1995) *The national burden of disease of Mauritius*. Report to the government of Mauritius.

Gruenberg EM (1977) The failure of success. *Milbank Quarterly/Health and Society* 55:3–24.

Halpert BP, Zimmerman MK (1986) The health status of the 'old-old': a reconsideration. *Social Science and Medicine* 22(9):893–9.

Johansson SR (1991) The health transition: the cultural inflation of morbidity during the decline of mortality. *Health Transition Review* 1:39–68.

Johansson SR (1992) Measuring the cultural inflation of morbidity during the decline of mortality. *Health Transition Review* 2:78–89.

Kramer M (1980) The rising pandemic of mental disorders and associated chronic diseases and disabilities. *Acta Pyschiatrica Scandinavica* 62(Supplement 285):282–297.

Leibson CL et al. (1992) The compression of morbidity hypothesis: promise and pitfalls of using record-linked data bases to assess secular trends in morbidity and mortality. *Millbank Quarterly* 70(1):127–54.

Leigh JP, Fries JF (1994) Education, geneder and the compression of morbidity. *International Journal of Aging and Human Development* 39(3):233–46.

Lozano R et al. (1996) Disability from injuries: new methods based on dual ICD-9 coding of injury, hospitalization and deaths. In: Murray CJL, Lopez AD, eds. *The global burden of injuries: mortality and disability from suicide, violence, war and unintentional injuries.* Cambridge, Harvard University Press.

Manton KG (1982) Changing concepts of morbidity and mortality in the elderly popluation, *Milbank Quarterly/Health and Society,* 60:183–244.

Manton KG, Corder LS, Stallard E (1993) Estimates of change in chronic disability and institutional incidence and prevalence rates in the US elderly population from the 1982, 1984 and 1989 National Long Term Care Survey. *Journal of Gerontology* 48(4):S153–S166.

Mathers C (1994) Health expectancies in Australia 1993: preliminary results. In, Mathers C, McCallum J, Robine JM (eds). *Advances in health expectancies.* Canberra: Australian Institute of Health and Welfare.

Mathers C, McCallum J, Robine JM, eds. (1994) *Advances in health expectancies.* Canberra: Australian Institute of Health and Welfare.

Mechanic D (1986) The concept of illness behaviour: culture, situation and personal predisposition. *Psychological Medicine* 16:1–7.

Murray CJL (1996) Rethinking DALYs. In: Murray CJL, Lopez AD, eds. *The global burden of disease: a comprehensive assessment of mortality and disability from diseases, injuries and risk factors in 1990 and projected to 2020.* Cambridge, Harvard University Press.

Murray CJL, Chen LC (1992) Understanding morbidity change. *Population and Development Review* 18(3):481–503.

Murray CJL, Lopez AD (1994) Global and regional cause-of-death patterns in 1990. *Bulletin of the World Health Organization,* 72:447–480.

Murray CJL, Lopez AD (1994) Quantifying disability: data, methods and results. *Bulletin of the World Health Organization,* 72:481–494

Murray CJL, Lopez AD, eds. (1994) *Global comparative assessments in the health sector.* World Health Organization, Geneva.

Murray CJL, Lopez AD (1996a) Estimating causes of death: methods and global and regional applications for 1990. In: Murray CJL, Lopez AD, eds. *The global burden of disease: a comprehensive assessment of mortality and disability from diseases, injuries and risk factors in 1990 and projected to 2020.* Cambridge, Harvard University Press.

Murray CJL, Lopez AD (1996b) *Global health statistics: a compendium of incidence, prevalence and mortality estimates for over 200 conditions.* Cambridge, Harvard University Press.

Murray CJL, Lopez AD, Jamison DT (1994) The global burden of disease in 1990: summary results, sensitivity analysis and future directions. *Bulletin of the World Health Organization,* 72:495–509

Nell V, Brown DSO (1991) The epidemiology of traumatic brain injury in Johannesburg. II. morbidity, mortality and etiology. *Social Sciences and Medicine,* 33:289–296.

Olshansky SJ et al. (1991) Trading off longer life for worsening health: the expansion of morbidity hypothesis. *Journal of Aging and Health* 3:194–216.

Rahman O et al. (1994) Gender differences in adult health: an international comparison, *Gerontologist*, 34(4):463–469.

Robine JM (1994) Disability-free life expectancy trends in France: 1981–1991, international comparison. In, Mathers C, McCallum J, Robine JM (eds). *Advances in health expectancies*. Canberra: Australian Institute of Health and Welfare.

Robine JM, Brouard N, Colvez A (1987) Les indicateurs d'esperance de vie sans incapacite (EVSI): des indicateurs globaux de l'etat de sante des populations. *Revue Epidemiologique de Sante Publique* 35:206–224.

Romieu I, Robine JM (1994) World atlas of health expectancy calculations. In, Mathers C, McCallum J, Robine JM (eds). *Advances in health expectancies*. Canberra: Australian Institute of Health and Welfare.

Roos NP, Havens B, Black C (1993) Living longer but doing worse: assessing health status in elderly persons at two points in time in Manitoba, Canada 1971 and 1983. *Social Science and Medicine* 36(3):273–82.

Shephard D, Zeckhauser R (1980) Long-term efforts of interventions to improve surivival of mixed populations. *Journal of Chronic Diseases* 33:413–433.

Schneider EL, Brody JA (1983) Aging, natural death, and the compression of morbidity: another view. *New England Journal of Medicine* 309(14):854–6.

Shibuya K, Murray CJL (1996) Poliomyelitis. In : Murray CJL, Lopez AD, eds. *The global epidemiology of infectious diseases*. Cambridge, Harvard University Press.

Sullivan DF (1971) A single index of mortality and morbidity. *HSMHA Health Reports* 86:347–354.

van Ginneken JK (1994) Potential of the Global Burden of Disease project for determining health expectancy. In, Mathers C, McCallum J, Robine JM (eds). *Advances in health expectancies*. Canberra: Australian Institute of Health and Welfare.

Verbrugge L (1984) Longer life but worsening health? Trends in health and mortality of middle-aged and older persons. *Milbank Memorial Fund Quarterly/Health and Society* 62:475–519.

Wilkins R, Chen J, Ng E (1994) Changes in health expectancy in Canada from 1986 to 1991. In, Mathers C, McCallum J, Robine JM (eds.) *Advances in health expectancies*. Canberra: Australian Institute of Health and Welfare.

World Bank (1993) *World Development Report 1993: investing in health*. New York, Oxford University Press for the World Bank.

Zwi A (1996) War. In: Murray CJL, Lopez AD, eds. *The global burden of injuries: mortality and disability from suicide, violence, war, and unintentional injuries*. Cambridge, Harvard University Press.

Chapter 5

THE GLOBAL BURDEN OF DISEASE IN 1990: FINAL RESULTS AND THEIR SENSITIVITY TO ALTERNATIVE EPIDEMIOLOGICAL PERSPECTIVES, DISCOUNT RATES, AGE-WEIGHTS AND DISABILITY WEIGHTS

CHRISTOPHER J. L. MURRAY
ALAN D. LOPEZ

In this chapter, we present the final results of the Global Burden of Disease Study (GBD) by age, sex, cause and region. The sensitivity of the main conclusions of the study to alternative assumptions for the discount rate, age-weights and disability weights, as well as to the choice of an incidence or a prevalence perspective, is also analysed. When considering the results of this study, it is important to keep in mind the three primary objectives of the exercise. First among these was our desire to infuse information about non-fatal health outcomes into debates on international health policy, which have been all too often focused on mortality (particularly in children). We also wished to decouple epidemiological assessment from advocacy, and, in so doing, to develop objective estimates of mortality and disability from each condition, solely on the basis of available evidence. This objective stems from our observation that evaluations of the burden of specific diseases or injuries, both at the national and at the international levels, are frequently produced by groups advocating particular policy changes, while what decision-makers require are independent, objective and competent evaluations. Finally, we sought to quantify the burden of disease using a measure that could also be used for cost-effectiveness analyses; for this the Disability-Adjusted Life Year (DALY) was developed, a composite measure of time lost due to premature mortality and time lived with disability. The advantages of using a common metric for burden assessment and economic appraisal of intervention options, in our opinion, far outweigh the analytical and conceptual complexity surrounding the derivation of DALYs.

Regardless of the metric preferred, the focus of attention in the public health debate should be the estimates which have been produced for the Global Burden of Disease Study. Whether one chooses to use as a metric deaths, Years of Life Lost (YLLs), health-adjusted expectancies, Years Lived with Disability (YLDs), DALYs or simply incidences and prevalences, the utility of the information summarized in these indices will be limited much more by the reliability of the underlying data sources, than by the choice of metric. As the twentieth century draws to a close, we still do not know reliably the levels of adult mortality in sub-Saharan Africa, or the main causes of death in much of the developing world, much less the descriptive epidemiology of the disabling sequelae of diseases and injuries.

Despite these massive lacunae in our basic epidemiological understanding, we have produced estimates for 483 sequelae of 107 diseases and injuries, for five age groups, eight regions and both sexes. We have done so (not always with great confidence) on the basis of our adherence to the "ethos of applied demography," namely the belief that making estimates on the basis of, at times, poor data is more useful than not making estimates at all. This is only true, however, if the estimates are plausible. Since we cannot know, on the basis of available data, whether our estimates are indeed accurate, it is critical that they at least be plausible and internally consistent. These principles have guided the estimation of demographic parameters for populations in the developing world for decades and have yielded much useful information for population planning and social development.

This chapter brings together the main results and conclusions of the Global Burden of Disease Study. We have had to be selective in choosing from among tens of thousands of individual results in order to present the findings in a manner which is useful for an overview of the state of the world's health. A wealth of detail that will be of interest to selected readers is provided in the Annex Tables of this volume.

METHODS

The focus of this section is on the methods used to estimate the total burden attributable to selected diseases that act as risk factors for other diseases, and the methods used to investigate the sensitivity of the GBD results to changes in critical social preferences incorporated into the indicators of burden. For the detailed methods used to estimate causes of death by age, sex and region, interested readers are referred to Chapter 3 in this volume (Murray and Lopez 1996c). For the detailed methods used to develop internally consistent estimates of the epidemiology of each condition, readers are referred to the disease specific chapters contained in Volumes III–VIII of the *Global Burden of Disease and Injury Series*, and, for an overview, to Chapter 4 in this volume (Murray and Lopez 1996d). The construction and justification of Years of Life Lost (YLLs), Years Lived with Disability (YLDs) and Disability-Adjusted Life Years (DALYs) are discussed in Chapter 1 in this volume (Murray 1996).

DISEASES AS RISK FACTORS FOR OTHER DISEASES

The true impact of a disease on mortality is sometimes poorly reflected in the tabulations of mortality by underlying cause of death, as estimated by Murray and Lopez (1996c) in Chapter 3 in this volume. One example is diabetes mellitus, which, in addition to its own direct sequelae, contributes to increased risks of death from ischaemic heart disease and cerebrovascular disease (McKeigue and King 1996). One can analyse these diseases in the same way as one analyses risk factors (e.g. tobacco use), by estimating the total reduction in burden that would occur if such causes were eliminated. "Attributable burden" for a disease estimated in this way would be greater than the burden assigned to it solely through the arbitrary ICD-9 conventions used in the primary GBD tabulations. We have estimated such total burdens for a short list of causes for which this attributable burden effect is important and well-studied. This list includes: tuberculosis, hepatitis B and hepatitis C, sexually transmitted diseases, Chagas disease, onchocerciasis, trachoma, diabetes mellitus, unipolar major depression, glaucoma and cataract. A brief review of the methods for calculating attributable burdens for diseases is given here; further details about these interactions are presented in the disease-specific chapters in Volumes III–VIII of the *Global Burden of Disease and Injury Series*.

Tuberculosis. The estimates of deaths and DALYs from tuberculosis included in the primary tabulations do not include the burden of tuberculosis among individuals that are HIV sero-positive. All deaths and opportunistic infections among HIV sero-positive individuals have been included in the estimates for HIV in the primary tabulations. Separate estimates of tuberculosis/HIV co-infection and the number of cases and deaths occurring in this population have been developed (Kumaresan et al. 1996). The distribution of tuberculosis cases among HIV sero-positives individuals, by age, sex and region, is provided in the tabulations for tuberculosis published in *Global Health Statistics* (Murray and Lopez 1996e).

Hepatitis B and hepatitis C. Chronic hepatitis B increases the risk of developing cirrhosis of the liver and liver cancer (Beasley et al. 1981). The primary GBD tabulations of the burden of hepatitis B and hepatitis C do not include the burdens of cirrhosis and liver cancer caused by previous hepatitis B infection; these are included in the estimates for cirrhosis and liver cancer, respectively. The fractions of cirrhosis and liver cancer deaths that can be attributed to hepatitis B have been estimated by Kane et al. (1996) on the basis of sero-prevalence data on hepatitis B, case-series of cirrhosis, and long-term risks of developing cirrhosis and liver cancer in chronic active hepatitis B individuals. Because of the limitations of the underlying community-based data, we have not estimated attributable fractions of cirrhosis for hepatitis C. Given that the distribution of hepatitis B and C often coincide, we suspect that the attributable fractions for liver cancer and cirrhosis due to hepatitis B may include a component due to hepatitis C. Estimates of the incidence, prevalence and death from cirrhosis and liver cancer due to hepatitis B are provided in detail in *Global Health Statistics* (Murray and Lopez 1996e).

Sexually transmitted diseases. In the GBD primary tabulations, some of the burden of sexually transmitted diseases (STDs) has been included in the estimates of burden from other causes, according to ICD-9 conventions. The contributions of chlamydia and gonorrhoea to the burden from ectopic pregnancy are included in maternal conditions; the contribution of chlamydia to the burden from neonatal pneumonia is included in lower respiratory infections; and the contributions of syphilis, chlamydia and gonorrhoea to the burden from low birth weight are included in the category of conditions arising during the perinatal period. Each of these outcomes has been evaluated by Berkley et al. (1996a). We have reaggregated all of these outcomes into composite estimates of the burden of each sexually transmitted disease. In addition, Berkley et al. (1996b) have estimated the total burden attributable to unsafe sex, which includes some of the burden of HIV, hepatitis B, maternal conditions and cervical cancer, in addition to the burden of sexually transmitted diseases—see Murray and Lopez 1996f, Chapter 6 in this volume.

Chagas disease. Individuals infected with Chagas disease who have developed cardiopathy have an increased risk of death, largely due to cardiovascular diseases (Mota et al. 1990). Mortality attributable to Chagas disease has been calculated using estimates of the relative risk of death among those infected with Chagas, derived from an ordinary differential equation model developed to quantify the impact of Chagas disease on disability and mortality (Moncayo and Myoshi 1996).

Blindness. A number of studies suggest that the risk of death for blind individuals is two to three times higher than the risk of death for non-blind individuals (Evans et al. 1996). Evans et al. (1996) have compiled an overview of the overall burden of disease attributable to all blinding conditions; this chapter is included in Volume IX of this series. In addition, we have also estimated, using the same approach, the burden attributable to four major blinding conditions: trachoma, onchocerciasis, glaucoma and cataract.

Diabetes mellitus. It has long been recognized that the burden of diabetes is poorly reflected in tabulations of underlying causes of death based on ICD coding rules (Bild and Stevenson 1992, Bisi et al. 1993, Fuller 1993, Jougla et al. 1992, Sasaki et al. 1994). We have therefore estimated the number of deaths and DALYs attributable to diabetes based on relative risks for cardiovascular causes of death, as reviewed by McKeigue and King (1996).

Unipolar major depression. Unipolar major depression is closely linked with suicide, as most individuals who commit suicide are also clinically depressed. To get a better indication of the true magnitude of the total burden attributable to unipolar major depression, we have combined DALYs from suicide with DALYs from unipolar major depression.

A number of other conditions also increase the risk of death from other diseases. For example, schistosomiasis may increase the risk of colon cancer and bladder cancer. Human papilloma virus is thought to cause a substantial share of cervical cancer. And diarrhoea increases the risk of death from lower respiratory infection in children. However, we have not included estimates of the burden attributable to these conditions in this chapter because we were unable to locate sufficient evidence on the relative risk of death from other causes due to these conditions to generate credible estimates.

Sensitivity Analysis Methods

Although the terms sensitivity analysis and uncertainty analysis are often used interchangeably, sensitivity analysis, as employed in this study, refers to the effect of changes in individual or social preferences which have been incorporated into the analysis of a study. Examples of preferences included in our sensitivity analysis are the discount rate, age-weights and health-state preferences. Uncertainty analysis, on the other hand, is the study of the effect of varying certain parameters included in the analysis. Examples of such parameters used in our study include incidence, prevalence, duration of disease and mortality. The uncertainty surrounding the precise values of these parameters can be reduced through further measurement. For uncertainty analysis, we may *ex ante* be able to define a probability distribution of different values for a parameter. This is in sharp contrast to sensitivity analysis, where it is not meaningful to speak of a probability distribution of a social preference, such as the discount rate. Clearly, the results of the GBD would be affected by changing the estimates of incidence, duration, or average age of onset of a condition. If the true prevalence of cataract is actually half of what we have estimated, then the burden is likely also to be half of what we have estimated. We will not pursue further the self-evident importance of the contribution of uncertainty in parameter estimates to uncertainty in the results. This has been emphasized in the introductory remarks to this chapter, and indeed throughout the study. Rather, the focus of this chapter is on measuring the effects of changes in epidemiological perspective, discount rate, age-weights and disability weights.

In the GBD, DALYs have been constructed using an incidence perspective (Murray 1996): the years of life lost due to mortality incident in a year are combined with the years of life expected to be lived with disability (due to diseases or injuries) incident in the same year. In the literature on Disability-Free Life Expectancy, this indicator has been calculated using either an incidence or prevalence-based perspective (Bebbington 1991, Crimmins et al. 1993, Robine and Ritchie 1991, Sullivan 1971). Using a similar framework, DALYs may be calculated using a prevalence-based perspective. While YLLs cannot, in practice, be measured in a prevalence framework—what is the notion of prevalence of dead individuals?—YLDs can.

We have calculated YLDs using the point prevalence of each condition and a duration of one year. For the disability severity weights, we have used the same set of age-specific disability weights as used for incidence-based DALYs. Incidence-based DALYs are calculated using the average age of onset, which is an output of the internal consistency analysis, derived using DISMOD (see Murray and Lopez 1996d, Chapter 4 in this volume for a more complete description). To calculate prevalence-based DALYs, we would need to estimate the average age of prevalent cases within each age group. The average age of prevalent cases for conditions with long average durations will be higher than the average age of onset. For example, a condition with a constant incidence rate of 1 per 1000 in the age group 15–44 in EME will have an *average age of onset* of 29.8, while the *average age of a prevalent case* will be closer to 36. DISMOD has not been designed to estimate the average age of prevalent cases within each age group, although this would not be technically difficult. We have, therefore, approximated prevalence-based DALYs by assuming that the average age of a prevalent case equals the average age of onset. When non-uniform age-weights are used as in the calculation of YLDs for this study, estimates of prevalence DALYs will be biased toward those conditions that have a long duration and an average age of onset that is not near the midpoint of the age-range. These prevalence-based YLDs are combined with YLLs to give prevalence-based DALYs. The prevalences by age, sex and region used for these computations are reported in detail in *Global Health Statistics,* the second volume in this series.

Murray (1996) in Chapter 1 in this volume provides generalized formulas for YLLs and YLDs so that the discount rate, r, and the age-weighting modulation factor, K, can be varied. When K is set equal to one, then the DALYs include age-weighting of the form:

$$Cxe^{-\beta x}$$

where C is a constant equal to 0.1658 and β is a parameter that controls the shape of the age-weighting function, such that the maximum value of the function is at $1/\beta$ (for the GBD, β has been set equal to 0.04). When K is set equal to zero, the age-weights are equivalent at all ages. To distinguish DALYs based on different parameter assumptions, a standard notation of the form "DALYs[r,K]", has been used where the first entry in brackets, r, is the discount rate and the second entry, K, is the age-weighting modulation factor. For the present sensitivity analysis, we have chosen the following five combinations of the discount rate and the age-weighting modulation factor: DALYs[0,0], DALYs[0,1], DALYs[0.03,0], DALYs[0.1,0] and DALYs[0.1,1]. Including the *standard* form of DALYs where r is 0.03 and K equals 1 (DALYs[0.03,1]), these six variants of DALYs define the boundaries of the plausible range of combinations of discounting and age-weighting. In testing the sensitivity of DALYs to age-weighting, we have altered K but have not varied β in the age-weighting function. Changes in β have virtually no effect on the results of the burden of disease and are not reported further here.

For each of the combinations of r and K, we have recalculated the results of the entire study. Each iteration of the study generates approximately 100 000 results. Simple aggregate measures of burden, such as the percentage distribution by age, sex, YLDs and YLLs, and cause Group, have been used to investigate the effects of changing r and K. In addition, we have examined changes in the total DALYs estimated for each disease and the rank order of each disease in terms of DALYs under these various assumptions. The relationship between various iterations of DALYs[r, K] and standard DALYs by condition have been measured using Pearson's correlation coefficients and Spearman's rank order correlation coefficients. These correlation coefficients have been estimated using the results for the 96 conditions listed in Table 5.2.[1] This list excludes summary categories such as all cardiovascular diseases, infectious and parasitic diseases and Group totals. Including these summary categories would tend to inflate the correlation coefficients; they have, therefore, been excluded.

For the development of severity weights for each disabling sequela, we have used the person-trade-off (PTO) method. In the limited number of applications of this approach thus far undertaken, the ordinal ranks of the 22 indicator conditions used to define the seven classes of disability severity are consistently preserved across cultures (Murray 1996). Other methods for health state preference measurement, such as the visual analogue method (also called rating scales), appear to generate much more severe disability weights for mild conditions than does the person-trade-off method (Eddy 1991, Nord 1991, 1993). Torrance (1986) has noted that visual analogue results are a power transformation of preference measurements derived from other methods, such as the standard gamble, time-trade-off and, we hypothesize, the person-trade-off method. We have explored the sensitivity of the results to changes in the scaling of the disability classes as if a visual analogue scale, such as the Quality of Well-Being scale, had been used (Kaplan and Anderson 1988, Richardson 1994). The median weight for each of the seven classes has been transformed using a function of the form:

$$DW_{i,VA} = DW_{i,PTO}^{\frac{1}{\beta}}$$

where $DW_{i,VA}$ is the visual analogue equivalent disability weight for class i and $DW_{i,PTO}$ is the standard disability weight based on the PTO for class i. Using a value of β equal to 1.225, the transformed disability severity weights for each class are close to, or in the range of the next highest class. Figure 5.1 illustrates that the relative increase in the disability weight caused by this power transformation is greatest for class I disability and declines thereafter. As the transformed disability weights are higher for every class, we can expect that this change will have a substantial effect on the volume of YLDs compared to YLLs. We have only tested this extreme transformation, in which the value of β was set to 1.225, and have not tested a series of intermediate transformations with values of β between

Figure 5.1   Effects of a power transformation of the disability weight for
each class to represent a visual analogue scale (where β
equals 1.225)

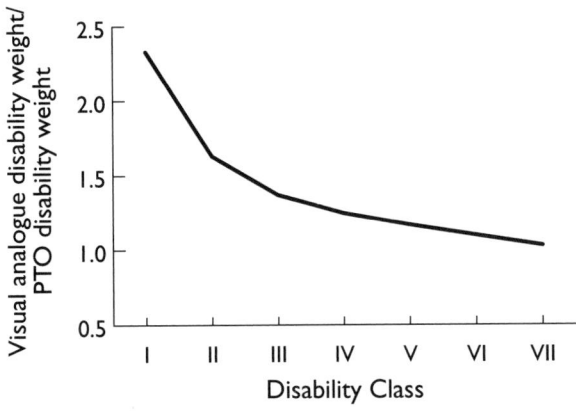

1 and 1.225. Summary measures and the rank orders of diseases have been
used to explore the overall effects of transforming the disability weights.

RESULTS

PATTERNS AND LEVELS OF DALYS

In terms of overall burden of disease, sub-Saharan Africa and India were
the two regions with the largest contributions, accounting for 21.4 per cent
and 20.9 per cent of the global total burden, respectively (see Figure 5.2).
The significant health gains achieved in China over the last few decades
are reflected by the fact that China accounts for only 15.1 per cent of the
global burden, while it has 21.5 per cent of the world's population. The
two developed regions, EME and FSE, in which Group I conditions (communicable, maternal, perinatal and nutritional) have, to a large extent,
been eliminated, together account for only 11.7 per cent of the global
burden of disease, while having about twice that share of the global population. Nearly, nine tenths of the global burden of disease occurs in developing regions where only one in ten health care dollars are spent
(Murray et al. 1994).

When population size is taken into account and crude YLL and YLD
rates are calculated (see Figure 5.3), the comparatively poor health profile of SSA becomes even more apparent. For every 1000 population living in the region, about 579 DALYs were incurred, compared with 124
DALYs per 1000 population in EME. Over three-quarters of the burden
of disease in SSA in 1990 was due to premature mortality (the remainder

Figure 5.2   Estimated distribution of DALYs by region, 1990

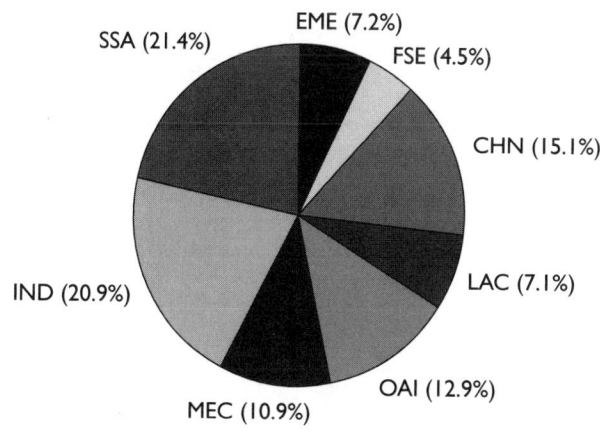

Figure 5.3   YLD and YLL rates by region, 1990

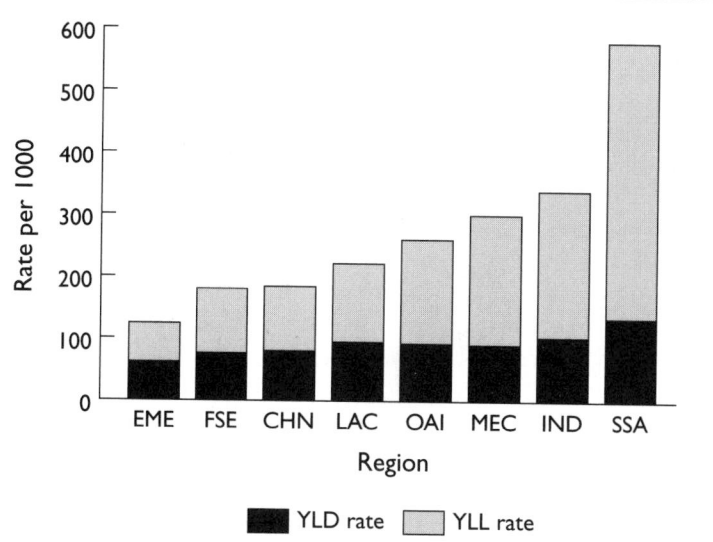

being attributable to disability); in India, MEC and OAI the proportion of burden due to premature mortality was only slightly lower (65–69 per cent). In FSE, China and LAC, 57–58 per cent of overall burden is due to YLLs, while in EME burden is roughly equally attributable to premature death and disability. The ratio of the highest YLL rate (observed in SSA) to the lowest YLL rate (in EME) is 7.1 to 1, whereas the same ratio for YLDs is 2.2 to 1. That is, there is much greater regional variation in the rate of premature mortality than in non-fatal health outcomes.

Figure 5.4   Percentage contribution of DALYs by age group to total DALYs, by region, 1990

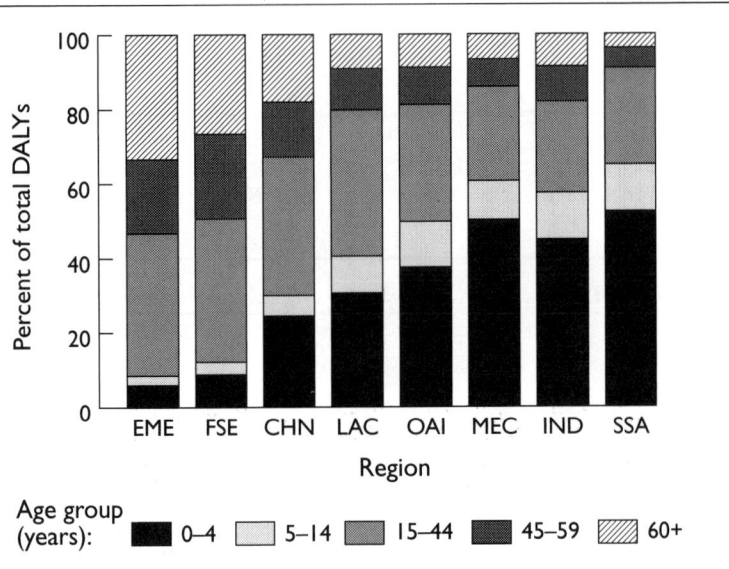

The age-distribution of DALYs differs dramatically across regions (Figure 5.4). In SSA, 52 per cent of burden is still due to mortality and disability originating in the age group 0–4 years. In contrast, in EME and FSE, only 6 and 9 per cent, respectively, of burden occurs in children aged 0–4 years. At the other end of the age spectrum, in EME one-third of burden occurs in the population over 60 years of age while in FSE just over one-quarter of total burden occurs in this age group. In China, 18 per cent of burden occurs in those aged over age 60; in all other regions less than 10 per cent of burden occurs in this age group. Forty-one per cent of global burden occurs in adults (aged 15–59), ranging from 31 per cent in SSA to 71 per cent in FSE. This large absolute and relative contribution to disease burden emphasizes the urgent need for global public health action to promote health and to prevent disease and injury among young adults.

The sex ratios (male/female) of crude YLL and YLD rates are shown in Figure 5.5. The rate of YLDs is similar for both sexes in all regions, with the male rates being 3–6 per cent higher in EME, FSE and LAC, and 2–5 per cent lower in OAI, MEC, India and SSA. In China, YLD rates are nearly equal for the two sexes. This relative uniformity in disability levels for the two sexes contrasts sharply with the marked variation across regions in mortality. In EME, and particularly, in FSE, rates of YLLs are 50–65 per cent higher for males than for females, while in LAC they are approximately 33 per cent higher for males. Much of the excess male mortality in LAC, as captured by the YLL rates, is due to

Figure 5.5   Male to female ratio of YLD and YLL rates, by region, 1990

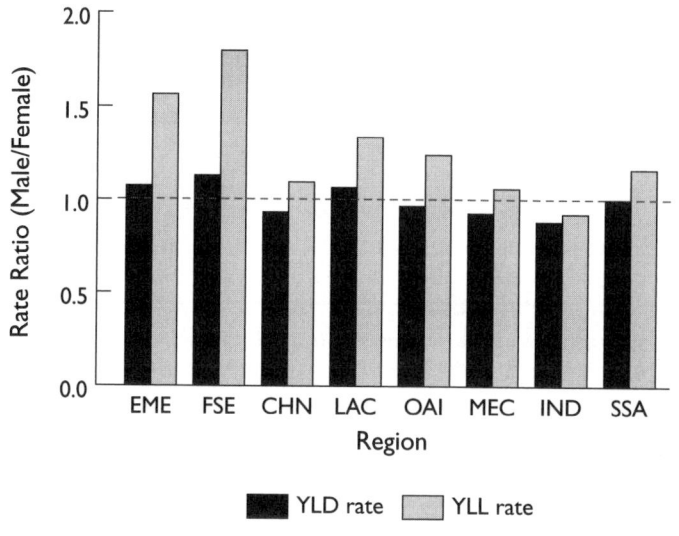

Figure 5.6   Groups I, II and III as a percentage of total DALYs, by region, 1990

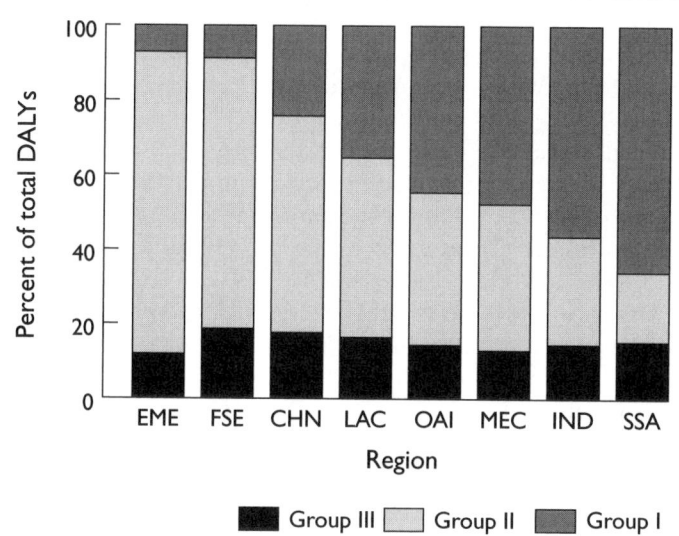

extremely high male death rates due to injuries. India is the only region for which the YLL rates are higher among females than among males.

The contribution of the three major Groups of causes to overall disease and injury burden differs dramatically across regions (see Figure 5.6).[2] As expected, Group I (communicable, maternal, perinatal and nutritional conditions) is the dominant cause of burden in SSA (66 per cent) but is of much less importance in EME (7 per cent). Even in China, where mortality rates are much closer to those of the developed regions, Group I conditions still account for one-quarter of burden. In LAC, OAI and MEC, burden from Group I ranges between 35 and 48 per cent of total burden. The pattern for Group II (noncommunicable diseases) is approximately the inverse of Group I. More than eight out of ten DALYs in EME are due to Group II causes, whereas just under one in five DALYs in SSA are due to Group II. Group III (injuries) remains an important source of burden in all regions, accounting for 12 to 19 per cent of total burden.

Figure 5.7 shows the relationship between the crude DALY rate and income per capita (measured in International dollars) by region and cause Group. This relationship appears to be reasonably strong and is largely driven by the strength of the association between Group I crude DALY rates and income per capita. Group II crude DALY rates are similar for most regions, except for India, where they are slightly lower, and FSE, where they are considerably higher. The crude Group II DALY rates are relatively constant because regions with younger age-structures have higher age-specific Group II DALY rates, while regions with older age-structures, such as EME, have lower age-specific Group II DALY rates. There is a slightly stronger relationship between Group III DALY rates and income per capita. China, OAI, MEC, LAC and FSE have similar Group III DALY rates, while the rate for India slightly exceeds this cluster. The outliers are SSA, where the rates are more than twice as high as in other regions, and EME, where the rates are about half the level observed in other regions.

Table 5.1 provides a regional breakdown of DALYs according to the second level of disaggregation within each Group. Globally, 23 per cent of DALYs are caused by infectious and parasitic diseases, but this proportion varies enormously from 2.7 per cent in FSE to 43 per cent in SSA. Respiratory infections contribute about 1.4 per cent of DALYs in EME, compared with 10.7 per cent in MEC, while DALYs from maternal conditions vary from 0.3 per cent in EME to 3.2 per cent in SSA. Among Group II causes, cancers, on average, account for approximately 5 per cent of global burden; however, this figure rises to 14 per cent in developed regions. Worldwide, neuro-psychiatric conditions account for 11 per cent of DALYs; their contribution is substantially higher in developed regions, where they comprise 22 per cent of total DALYs. Other major categories of burden include cardiovascular diseases, accounting for one in ten DALYs worldwide, and respiratory and digestive diseases, each accounting for over 3 per cent of global burden. In the developed regions, musculo-skeletal diseases are also major causes of burden, causing just under 5 per cent of DALYs. Unintentional injuries cause more than one in ten DALYs in every region except MEC, EME and SSA. Intentional injuries vary much

Figure 5.7   Relationships between DALY rates and income per capita, by broad cause Group, 1990

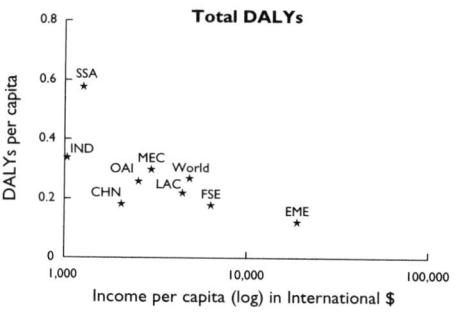

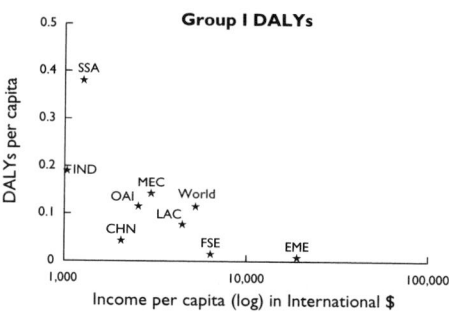

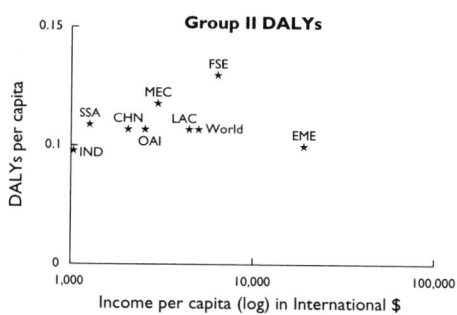

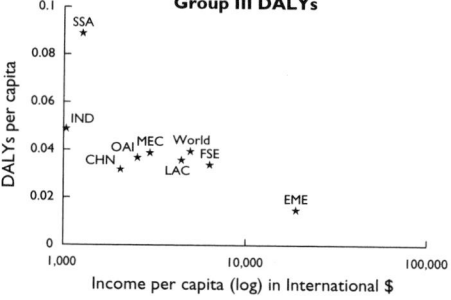

more, ranging from 1.5 per cent of DALYs in India to over 6 per cent in SSA and MEC.

The rank order of 96 conditions in terms of their contribution to DALYs for the world, developing and developed regions, for both sexes combined, is shown in Table 5.2. As may have been expected, the three leading causes of DALYs in 1990 were lower respiratory infections, diarrhoeal diseases and conditions arising during the perinatal period (low birth weight and birth asphyxia/birth trauma). Tuberculosis, measles and congenital anomalies are also among the ten leading causes of DALYs worldwide. Perhaps more surprisingly, unipolar major depression, ischaemic heart disease and cerebrovascular disease are ranked fourth, fifth, and sixth, respectively. Road traffic accidents are also among the leading causes of DALYs globally, accounting for 2.4 per cent of all DALYs. The ten leading causes of DALYs for males and females listed in Table 5.2 differ only slightly. Maternal causes of death are listed in this table by sub-cause, such as maternal haemorrhage or obstructed labour. If all maternal causes were to be combined, maternal conditions would occupy the fourth rank among causes of DALYs in females.

The rankings for developed regions (EME and FSE) are quite different from the global rankings: alcohol use, osteoarthritis, lung cancer, dementia, suicide and COPD are all among the leading causes of DALYs in EME and FSE, with the top three causes of burden being ischaemic heart disease, unipolar major depression and cerebrovascular diseases. The leading causes of DALYs in developing regions are similar to the global ranking, except that malaria enters the list as the seventh most important cause of burden.

A major advantage of the Global Burden of Disease Study is the availability of disaggregated estimates, which allows the assessment of major causes of death and DALYs within different periods of the life cycle. Table 5.3 lists the ten leading causes of DALYs from conditions which arise at ages 0–4 years. The composition of leading causes at the global level is very much what one would expect, with perinatal causes, acute respiratory infections, diarrhoeal diseases, measles, malaria and protein energy malnutrition contributing the most to disease burden at these ages. While this is hardly surprising, given what is known about the causes of disease in young children, the GBD methods permit a more objective, comparative assessment of the magnitude of major health problems at these (and other) ages. As disease levels and patterns at these ages are predominant in the developing world, the relative order of leading causes of DALYs is similar for developing regions and for the world. Moreover, there is little difference in the leading causes of DALYs between males and females at these ages, reflecting the nearly equivalent risks for infectious diseases incurred by both sexes. Interestingly, in developed regions, both road traffic accidents and war are among the leading causes of DALYs at these young ages.

Table 5.1 Percentage distribution of DALYs among specific causes (level two categories), 1990

Group/cause	Region										
	EME	FSE	IND	CHN	OAI	SSA	LAC	MEC	Developed	Developing	World
All Causes	100.0	100.0	100.0	100.0	100.0	100.0	100.0	100.0	100.0	100.0	100.0
I. Communicable, maternal, perinatal and nutritional conditions	7.1	8.8	56.4	24.2	44.7	65.9	35.3	47.7	7.8	48.7	43.9
A. Infectious and parasitic diseases	2.8	2.7	28.9	7.5	22.3	42.5	17.6	20.2	2.7	25.6	22.9
B. Respiratory infections	1.4	2.0	11.9	5.9	8.7	10.5	4.9	10.7	1.6	9.4	8.5
C. Maternal conditions	0.3	0.9	2.6	1.3	2.3	3.2	1.7	2.4	0.6	2.4	2.2
D. Conditions arising during the perinatal period	1.8	2.2	8.8	4.9	6.9	6.5	7.4	9.7	1.9	7.3	6.7
E. Nutritional deficiencies	0.9	1.0	4.2	4.6	4.5	3.2	3.7	4.7	0.9	4.1	3.7
II Noncommunicable diseases	81.0	72.6	29.0	58.2	40.9	18.8	48.2	39.3	77.7	36.1	40.9
A. Malignant neoplasms	15.0	11.7	2.5	8.7	5.1	2.1	4.5	2.4	13.7	4.0	5.1
B. Other neoplasms	0.9	0.6	0.1	0.4	0.3	0.2	0.5	0.2	0.8	0.2	0.3
C. Diabetes mellitus	2.4	1.1	0.8	0.5	0.7	0.2	1.5	1.0	1.9	0.7	0.8
E. Neuro-psychiatric conditions	25.1	17.2	7.0	14.2	10.8	4.0	15.9	8.7	22.0	9.0	10.5
F. Sense organ diseases	0.1	0.1	1.1	1.0	1.0	0.7	0.6	0.6	0.1	0.8	0.8
G. Cardiovascular diseases	18.6	23.2	8.2	11.0	10.1	3.9	8.0	11.1	20.4	8.3	9.7
H. Respiratory diseases	4.8	4.8	2.7	10.7	2.7	2.6	4.0	4.2	4.8	4.3	4.4
I. Digestive diseases	4.4	4.4	2.2	4.9	4.7	1.8	3.8	4.2	4.4	3.3	3.4
J. Genito-urinary diseases	1.1	1.6	0.7	1.2	1.1	0.9	1.2	2.0	1.3	1.1	1.1
L. Musculo-skeletal diseases	4.2	4.4	0.5	1.7	1.2	0.4	3.1	0.6	4.3	1.0	1.4
M. Congential anomalies	2.2	2.2	2.9	3.0	2.3	1.3	2.7	2.7	2.2	2.4	2.4
N. Oral conditions	0.9	0.8	0.4	0.5	0.7	0.1	1.0	0.9	0.8	0.5	0.5
III Injuries	11.9	18.7	14.6	17.6	14.4	15.4	16.4	13.0	14.5	15.2	15.1
A. Unintentional injuries	8.7	12.9	13.0	12.9	12.1	9.3	11.9	6.8	10.3	11.1	11.0
B. Intentional injuries	3.2	5.8	1.5	4.7	2.3	6.0	4.5	6.2	4.2	4.1	4.1

Table 5.2 Causes of DALYs (percentage of total) in descending order, 1990

	World			Developed Regions			Developing Regions		
Rank	Disease or Injury	DALYs (thousands)	% of Total	Disease or Injury	DALYs (thousands)	% of Total	Disease or Injury	DALYs (thousands)	% of Total
	All Causes	1 379 238		All Causes	160 994		All Causes	1 218 244	
1	Lower respiratory infections	112 898	8.2	Ischaemic heart disease	15 950	9.9	Lower respiratory infections	110 506	9.1
2	Diarrhoeal diseases	99 633	7.2	Unipolar major depression	9 780	6.1	Diarrhoeal diseases	99 168	8.1
3	Conditions arising during the perinatal period	92 313	6.7	Cerebrovascular disease	9 425	5.9	Conditions arising during the perinatal period	89 193	7.3
4	Unipolar major depression	50 810	3.7	Road traffic accidents	7 064	4.4	Unipolar major depression	41 031	3.4
5	Ischaemic heart disease	46 699	3.4	Alcohol use	6 446	4.0	Tuberculosis	37 930	3.1
6	Cerebrovascular disease	38 523	2.8	Osteoarthritis	4 681	2.9	Measles	36 498	3.0
7	Tuberculosis	38 426	2.8	Trachea, bronchus and lung cancers	4 587	2.9	Malaria	31 705	2.6
8	Measles	36 520	2.7	Dementia and other degenerative and hereditary CNS disorders	3 816	2.4	Ischaemic heart disease	30 749	2.5
9	Road traffic accidents	34 317	2.5	Self-inflicted injuries	3 768	2.3	Congenital anomalies	29 441	2.4
10	Congenital anomalies	32 921	2.4	Congenital anomalies	3 480	2.2	Cerebrovascular disease	29 099	2.4
11	Malaria	31 706	2.3	Chronic obstructive pulmonary disease	3 365	2.1	Road traffic accidents	27 253	2.2
12	Chronic obstructive pulmonary disease	29 136	2.1	Conditions arising during the perinatal period	3 120	1.9	Chronic obstructive pulmonary disease	25 771	2.1
13	Falls	26 680	1.9	Schizophrenia	3 106	1.9	Falls	24 232	2.0
14	Iron-deficiency anaemia	24 613	1.8	Diabetes mellitus	3 022	1.9	Iron-deficiency anaemia	23 465	1.9
15	Protein-energy malnutrition	20 957	1.5	Bipolar disorder	2 543	1.6	Protein-energy malnutrition	20 758	1.7
16	War	20 019	1.5	Falls	2 448	1.5	War	18 868	1.6
17	Self-inflicted injuries	18 967	1.4	Lower respiratory infections	2 392	1.5	Tetanus	17 513	1.4
18	Tetanus	17 517	1.3	Cirrhosis of the liver	2 345	1.5	Violence	15 632	1.3
19	Violence	17 472	1.3	Colon and rectum cancers	2 298	1.4	Self-inflicted injuries	15 199	1.3
20	Alcohol use	16 661	1.2	Obsessive-compulsive disorder	2 098	1.3	Drownings	14 819	1.2
21	Drownings	15 697	1.1	Stomach cancer	2 084	1.3	Pertussis	13 353	1.1
22	Bipolar disorder	14 257	1.0	Drug use	2 053	1.3	Bipolar disorder	11 714	1.0

Table 5.2 (continued)

		World		Developed Regions			Developing Regions		
Rank	Disease or Injury	DALYs (thousands)	% of Total	Disease or Injury	DALYs (thousands)	% of Total	Disease or Injury	DALYs (thousands)	% of Total
23	Pertussis	13 403	1.0	Breast cancer	1 930	1.2	Fires	11 424	0.9
24	Osteoarthritis	13 278	1.0	Violence	1 840	1.1	Cirrhosis of the liver	10 837	0.9
25	Cirrhosis of the liver	13 182	1.0	Asthma	1 734	1.1	Alcohol use	10 214	0.8
26	Schizophrenia	12 798	0.9	Rheumatoid arthritis	1 426	0.9	HIV	9 864	0.8
27	Fires	11 875	0.9	HIV	1 308	0.8	Schizophrenia	9 692	0.8
28	HIV	11 172	0.8	Poisonings	1 181	0.7	Inflammatory heart diseases	9 172	0.8
29	Diabetes mellitus	11 103	0.8	War	1 151	0.7	Asthma	9 042	0.7
30	Asthma	10 775	0.8	Inflammatory heart diseases	1 150	0.7	Osteoarthritis	8 597	0.7
31	Inflammatory heart diseases	10 322	0.8	Iron-deficiency anaemia	1 149	0.7	Obsessive-compulsive disorder	8 114	0.7
32	Obsessive-compulsive disorder	10 213	0.7	Panic disorder	996	0.6	Diabetes mellitus	8 080	0.7
33	Trachea bronchus and lung cancers	8 871	0.6	Lymphomas and multiple myeloma	949	0.6	Nephritis and nephrosis	7 886	0.7
34	Nephritis and nephrosis	8 607	0.6	Leukaemia	900	0.6	Cataracts	7 443	0.6
35	Dementia and other degenerative and hereditary CNS disorders	8 500	0.6	Epilepsy	884	0.6	Syphilis	6 586	0.5
36	Stomach cancer	7 694	0.6	Drownings	877	0.6	Chlamydia	6 524	0.5
37	Cataracts	7 510	0.5	Pancreas cancer	871	0.5	Obstructed labour	6 076	0.5
38	Chlamydia	7 169	0.5	Nephritis and nephrosis	721	0.5	Liver cancer	6 039	0.5
39	Syphilis	6 596	0.5	Prostate cancer	682	0.4	Bacterial meningitis and meningococcaemia	5 833	0.5
40	Liver cancer	6 550	0.5	Dental caries	647	0.4	Rheumatic heart disease	5 645	0.5
41	Obstructed labour	6 462	0.5	Chlamydia	645	0.4	Stomach cancer	5 610	0.5
42	Poisonings	6 455	0.5	Edentulism	644	0.4	Maternal sepsis	5 311	0.4
43	Bacterial meningitis and meningococcaemia	6 242	0.5	Mouth and oropharynx cancers	596	0.4	Poisonings	5 274	0.4
44	Rheumatic heart disease	6 191	0.5	Parkinson disease	574	0.4	Abortion	4 928	0.4
45	Drug use	5 675	0.4	Ovary cancer	565	0.4	Gonorrhoea	4 788	0.4
46	Maternal sepsis	5 452	0.4	Rheumatic heart disease	545	0.3	Dementia and other degenerative and hereditary CNS disorders	4 684	0.4

Table 5.2 (continued)

		World		Developed Regions			Developing Regions		
Rank	Disease or Injury	DALYs (thousands)	% of Total	Disease or Injury	DALYs (thousands)	% of Total	Disease or Injury	DALYs (thousands)	% of Total
47	Epilepsy	5 350	0.4	Bladder cancer	519	0.3	Epilepsy	4 466	0.4
48	Abortion	5 097	0.4	Liver cancer	510	0.3	Trachea bronchus and lung cancers	4 285	0.4
49	Gonorrhoea	4 909	0.4	Tuberculosis	496	0.3	Lymphatic filariasis	3 997	0.3
50	Panic disorder	4 766	0.4	Diarrhoeal diseases	465	0.3	Vitamin A deficiency	3 838	0.3
51	Colon and rectum cancers	4 617	0.3	Oesophagus cancer	461	0.3	Panic disorder	3 770	0.3
52	Leukaemia	4 567	0.3	Fires	452	0.3	Leukaemia	3 667	0.3
53	Dental caries	4 313	0.3	Peptic ulcer	442	0.3	Dental caries	3 665	0.3
54	Breast cancer	4 210	0.3	Bacterial meningitis and meningoccocaemia	409	0.3	Drug use	3 622	0.3
55	Lymphatic filariasis	3 997	0.3	Post-traumatic stress disorder	387	0.2	Maternal haemorrhage	3 531	0.3
56	Vitamin A deficiency	3 838	0.3	Obstructed labour	386	0.2	Poliomyelitis	3 368	0.3
57	Mouth and oropharynx cancers	3 743	0.3	Cervix uteri cancer	378	0.2	Mouth and oropharynx cancers	3 148	0.3
58	Oesophagus cancer	3 578	0.3	Multiple sclerosis	357	0.2	Oesophagus cancer	3 117	0.3
59	Maternal haemorrhage	3 564	0.3	Melanoma and other skin cancers	349	0.2	Glaucoma	2 478	0.2
60	Poliomyelitis	3 371	0.2	Corpus uteri cancer	318	0.2	Cervix uteri cancer	2 476	0.2
61	Rheumatoid arthritis	3 286	0.2	Benign prostatic hypertrophy	317	0.2	Peptic ulcer	2 323	0.2
62	Lymphomas and multiple myeloma	3 104	0.2	Protein-energy malnutrition	199	0.1	Colon and rectum cancers	2 319	0.2
63	Cervix uteri cancer	2 854	0.2	Abortion	170	0.1	Breast cancer	2 280	0.2
64	Edentulism	2 787	0.2	Maternal sepsis	141	0.1	Lymphomas and multiple myeloma	2 154	0.2
65	Peptic ulcer	2 766	0.2	Otitis media	132	0.1	Edentulism	2 143	0.2
66	Gonorrhoea	2 578	0.2	Gonorrhoea	121	0.1	Leishmaniasis	2 091	0.2
67	Glaucoma	2 163	0.2	Glaucoma	100	0.1	Hepatitis B and hepatitis C	2 045	0.2
68	Hepatitis B and hepatitis C	2 136	0.2	Hepatitis B and hepatitis C	91	0.1	Otitis media	2 031	0.2
69	Leishmaniasis	2 092	0.2	Upper respiratory infections	79	0.1	Rheumatoid arthritis	1 860	0.2
70	Post-traumatic stress disorder	1 945	0.1	Cataracts	67	0.0	Trichuriasis	1 788	0.2
71	Benign prostatic hypertrophy	1 818	0.1	Appendicitis	54	0.0	Ascariasis	1 750	0.1
72	Trichuriasis	1 788	0.1	Periodontal disease	52	0.0	Appendicitis	1 709	0.1

Table 5.2 (continued)

	World			Developed Regions			Developing Regions		
Rank	Disease or Injury	DALYs (thousands)	% of Total	Disease or Injury	DALYs (thousands)	% of Total	Disease or Injury	DALYs (thousands)	% of Total
73	Appendicitis	1 763	0.1	Pertussis	50	0.0	Hypertensive disorders of pregnancy	1 707	0.1
74	Ascariasis	1 750	0.1	Iodine deficiency	41	0.0	Post-traumatic stress disorder	1 558	0.1
75	Hypertensive disorders of pregnancy	1 731	0.1	Maternal haemorrhage	33	0.0	Iodine deficiency	1 520	0.1
76	Pancreas cancer	1 577	0.1	Hypertensive disorders of pregnancy	25	0.0	Schistosomiasis	1 519	0.1
77	Iodine deficiency	1 562	0.1	Measles	22	0.0	Benign prostatic hypertrophy	1 500	0.1
78	Schistosomiasis	1 519	0.1	Syphilis	10	0.0	Ancylostomiasis and necatoriasis	1 484	0.1
79	Ancylostomiasis and necatoriasis	1 484	0.1	Poliomyelitis	4	0.0	Trypanosomiasis	1 467	0.1
80	Trypanosomiasis	1 467	0.1	Tetanus	3	0.0	Upper respiratory infections	1 233	0.1
81	Multiple sclerosis	1 417	0.1	Malaria	2	0.0	Multiple sclerosis	1 061	0.1
82	Ovary cancer	1 403	0.1	Leprosy	1	0.0	Trachoma	1 024	0.1
83	Prostate cancer	1 345	0.1	Leishmaniasis	1	0.0	Onchocerciasis	884	0.1
84	Upper respiratory infections	1 311	0.1	Diphtheria	1	0.0	Ovary cancer	838	0.1
85	Bladder cancer	1 215	0.1	Japanese encephalitis	<1	0.0	Dengue	750	0.1
86	Parkinson disease	1 050	0.1	Schistosomiasis	<1	0.0	Japanese encephalitis	744	0.1
87	Trachoma	1 024	0.1	Trypanosomiasis	<1	0.0	Pancreas cancer	707	0.1
88	Onchocerciasis	884	0.1	Trachoma	<1	0.0	Bladder cancer	696	0.1
89	Dengue	750	0.1	Vitamin A deficiency	<1	0.0	Prostate cancer	663	0.1
90	Japanese encephalitis	744	0.1	Ancylostomiasis and necatoriasis	<1	0.0	Chagas disease	641	0.1
91	Corpus uteri cancer	644	0.1	Dengue	<1	0.0	Parkinson disease	476	0.0
92	Chagas disease	641	0.1	Trichuriasis	<1	0.0	Leprosy	382	0.0
93	Melanoma and other skin cancers	565	0.0	Ascariasis	<1	0.0	Diphtheria	360	0.0
94	Leprosy	384	0.0	Onchocerciasis	<1	0.0	Corpus uteri cancer	325	0.0
95	Diphtheria	361	0.0	Chagas disease	<1	0.0	Melanoma and other skin cancers	216	0.0
96	Periodontal disease	255	0.0	Lymphatic filariasis	<1	0.0	Periodontal disease	203	0.0

Table 5.3 Ten leading causes of DALYs at ages 0–4 years, 1990

Rank	Both Sexes — Disease or Injury	DALYs (thousands)	Cumulative %	Males — Disease or Injury	DALYs (thousands)	Cumulative %	Females — Disease or Injury	DALYs (thousands)	Cumulative %
	World								
	All Causes	518,790		All Causes	268,786		All Causes	250,003	
1	Conditions arising during the perinatal period	92,308	17.8	Conditions arising during the perinatal period	47,501	17.7	Conditions arising during the perinatal period	44,806	17.9
2	Lower respiratory infections	90,691	35.3	Lower respiratory infections	46,813	35.1	Lower respiratory infections	43,877	35.5
3	Diarrhoeal diseases	85,903	51.8	Diarrhoeal diseases	45,163	51.9	Diarrhoeal diseases	40,740	51.8
4	Measles	30,876	57.8	Measles	15,948	57.8	Measles	14,928	57.7
5	Congenital anomalies	29,580	63.5	Congenital anomalies	14,932	63.4	Congenital anomalies	14,648	63.6
6	Malaria	23,211	68.0	Malaria	12,661	68.1	Malaria	10,549	67.8
7	Protein-energy malnutrition	20,002	71.8	Protein-energy malnutrition	9,919	71.8	Protein-energy malnutrition	10,083	71.9
8	Tetanus	14,092	74.5	Tetanus	7,192	74.5	Tetanus	6,900	74.6
9	Pertussis	11,986	76.8	Pertussis	6,187	76.8	Pertussis	5,799	76.9
10	Falls	6,657	78.1	Falls	3,335	78.0	Falls	3,321	78.3
	Developed Regions								
	All Causes	11,349		All Causes	6,329		All Causes	5,020	
1	Congenital anomalies	3,146	27.7	Congenital anomalies	1,811	28.6	Congenital anomalies	1,469	29.3
2	Conditions arising during the perinatal period	3,117	55.2	Conditions arising during the perinatal period	1,677	55.1	Conditions arising during the perinatal period	1,306	55.3
3	Lower respiratory infections	696	61.3	Lower respiratory infections	395	61.4	Lower respiratory infections	301	61.3
4	Bacterial meningitis and meningococcaemia	261	63.6	Bacterial meningitis and meningococcaemia	144	63.6	Diarrhoeal diseases	121	63.7

Table 5.3 (continued)

	Both Sexes			Males			Females		
Rank	Disease or Injury	DALYs (thousands)	Cumulative %	Disease or Injury	DALYs (thousands)	Cumulative %	Disease or Injury	DALYs (thousands)	Cumulative %
Developed Regions (continued)									
5	Diarrhoeal diseases	257	65.9	Diarrhoeal diseases	136	65.8	Bacterial meningitis and meningococcaemia	117	66.0
6	War	225	67.9	Falls	118	67.6	War	113	68.3
7	Falls	197	69.6	War	113	69.4	Protein-energy malnutrition	81	69.9
8	Protein-energy malnutrition	166	71.1	Road traffic accidents	95	70.9	Falls	79	71.4
9	Road traffic accidents	160	72.5	Protein-energy malnutrition	85	72.3	Road traffic accidents	65	72.7
10	Dementia and other degenerative and hereditary CNS disorders	119	73.5	Drownings	72	73.4	Dementia and other degenerative and hereditary CNS disorders	58	73.9
Developing Regions									
	All Causes	507,440		All Causes	262,457		All Causes	244,983	
1	Lower respiratory infections	89,995	17.7	Lower respiratory infections	46,418	17.7	Lower respiratory infections	43,577	17.8
2	Conditions arising during the perinatal period	89,191	35.3	Conditions arising during the perinatal period	45,691	35.1	Conditions arising during the perinatal period	43,500	35.5
3	Diarrhoeal diseases	85,646	52.2	Diarrhoeal diseases	45,027	52.3	Diarrhoeal diseases	40,619	52.1
4	Measles	30,863	58.3	Measles	15,940	58.3	Measles	14,923	58.2
5	Congenital anomalies	26,434	63.5	Congenital anomalies	13,255	63.4	Congenital anomalies	13,179	63.6
6	Malaria	23,211	68.1	Malaria	12,661	68.2	Malaria	10,549	67.9
7	Protein-energy malnutrition	19,836	72.0	Protein-energy malnutrition	9,835	71.9	Protein-energy malnutrition	10,002	72.0
8	Tetanus	14,092	74.7	Tetanus	7,192	74.7	Tetanus	6,900	74.8
9	Pertussis	11,948	77.1	Pertussis	6,168	77.0	Pertussis	5,780	77.2
10	Falls	6,460	78.4	Falls	3,217	78.3	Falls	3,243	78.5

The similarity of the major causes of DALYs for males and females at the younger ages is in marked contrast to the very considerable sex differences at older ages (see Table 5.4). For example, among young adults aged 15–44 years, maternal conditions and anaemia (3rd rank) are major causes of DALYs for women, but not for men. Unipolar major depression is the leading cause of DALYs among women in both the developed and developing regions, with two other neuro-psychiatric conditions (bipolar disorder and schizophrenia) also among the top causes of DALYs at these ages. Suicide (4th rank) and war (10th rank) are major public health issues for young women as well, particularly in developing countries. For men aged 15–44, road traffic accidents are the major cause of DALYs in this age group, being the second leading cause in both developed and developing regions. This finding for developing regions is perhaps surprising and reinforces the need for dramatically increased efforts to improve traffic safety everywhere and particularly among young men. Alcohol use, which underlies a substantial proportion of traffic accidents in both developed and developing regions, is the leading cause of DALYs in men at these ages in developed countries, and a major cause (5th rank) in developing countries. The concentration of neuro-psychiatric causes, injuries and, in developing countries, tuberculosis, as major causes of DALYs among young adults is a public health priority which must be given much greater prominence in global health debates. DALYs at these young adult ages, similar to DALYs during childhood, represent a considerable drain on society.

Table 5.5 provides estimates of the total burden attributable to each of eight diseases, taking into account deaths and disability from these diseases which in the primary tabulations had been assigned to other categories. The largest difference between burden directly attributed to a disease, and total burden from a disease, occurs for hepatitis B and hepatitis C.[3] Globally, only 16 per cent of the burden associated with hepatitis B and hepatitis C is actually assigned to hepatitis B and hepatitis C in the primary tabulations. In these tabulations, hepatitis B and hepatitis C directly cause 2.1 million DALYs but, if the attributable fractions estimated for cirrhosis and liver cancer are taken into account, hepatitis B and hepatitis C are estimated to account for 13.3 million DALYs. In Table 5.2, hepatitis B and hepatitis C ranked 69th out of the 96 conditions listed; taking into account the attributable burden, hepatitis B rises to 25th place in the rank list of global causes of burden. In 1990 hepatitis B and hepatitis C are estimated to have caused 819 thousand deaths; most of these deaths occur in the population aged over 40.

After taking into consideration the higher risks of cardiovascular disease and death among diabetics, diabetes rises from the 29th most important cause of global burden to 14th. Diabetes accounts for 571 thousand deaths in the primary GBD tabulations of causes of death, whereas the total number of deaths attributed to diabetes in 1990 was closer to 1.3 million. The effect of incorporating attributable burden into our estimates of

DALYs is even more dramatic in developed regions, where diabetes rises from 14th to the second most significant cause of burden, after ischaemic heart disease. Only an estimated 42 per cent of the global burden of diabetes is captured in the primary tabulations of directly coded disease.

A similar fraction of the burden of Chagas disease is captured in the primary tabulations. In LAC, the only region with endemic Chagas, this disease rises from 92nd to 76th rank as a cause of burden. Most of this extra burden is due to the elevated risk of cardiovascular death in those infected with *T.cruzi,* the parasite that causes Chagas disease. For tuberculosis, the estimates of the total burden of disease in Table 5.5 include the contribution from HIV sero-positive individuals with tuberculosis. In 1990, tuberculosis in HIV sero-positive individuals is estimated to have contributed only four per cent of the total burden of tuberculosis; the only exception was observed in EME, where this fraction was estimated to be 23 per cent. Given the course of the HIV epidemic and its interaction with tuberculosis, the burden of tuberculosis in HIV sero-positive individuals is expected to grow dramatically between 1990 and 2005.

Somewhat tentatively, we have estimated the total burden of four important blinding conditions based on the assumption that blind individuals have a similar elevation in the relative risk of death across various causes of blindness and across regions. The results of these calculations suggest that a large number of deaths may be attributable to blinding conditions: 1.1 million due to cataract, 330 thousand from glaucoma, 103 thousand from trachoma and 19 thousand from onchocerciasis. If these crude estimates are approximately correct, cataract would rise from the 37th to the 18th most important cause of global DALYs.

Finally, we have combined the DALYs from unipolar major depression and the DALYs from suicide to estimate the total burden attributable to depression. These calculations are based on the assumption that everyone that commits suicide is clinically depressed, which may result in a slight overestimate of the impact of depression. The combined sum accounts for 5.1 per cent of total burden, making it the fourth most important cause of global burden.

Sensitivity Analysis Results

Changing from an incidence to a prevalence perspective for the calculation of YLDs and DALYs does not appear to significantly alter the results in terms of condition-specific burden, as illustrated in Figure 5.8. For this diagram, conditions have been ranked in ascending order, with the largest contributors to global burden in the top right-hand corner of the figure. There are three diseases for which YLDs and DALYs change notably depending on the perspective taken, namely poliomyelitis, congenital anomalies and schizophrenia. Poliomyelitis becomes more important as a cause of disease burden in terms of prevalence-based DALYs because of the recent decline in the incidence of poliomyelitis. Schizophrenia is more important in terms of prevalence-based DALYs because, in the approxi-

Table 5.4   Ten leading causes of DALYs at ages 15–44 years, 1990

	Both Sexes			Males			Females		
Rank	Disease or Injury	DALYs (thousands)	Cumula- tive %	Disease or Injury	DALYs (thousands)	Cumula- tive %	Disease or Injury	DALYs (thousands)	Cumula- tive%
World									
	All Causes	419,144		All Causes	217,153		All Causes	201,991	
1	Unipolar major depression	42,972	10.3	Road traffic accidents	15,554	7.2	Unipolar major depression	27,651	13.7
2	Tuberculosis	19,673	14.9	Unipolar major depression	15,321	14.2	Tuberculosis	8,736	18.0
3	Road traffic accidents	19,625	19.6	Alcohol use	13,096	20.2	Iron-deficiency anaemia	7,508	21.7
4	Alcohol use	14,848	23.2	Violence	11,040	25.3	Self-inflicted injuries	7,095	25.2
5	Self-inflicted injuries	14,645	26.7	Tuberculosis	10,937	30.4	Bipolar disorder	6,453	28.4
6	Bipolar disorder	13,189	29.8	War	7,899	34.0	Obstructed labour	6,419	31.6
7	War	13,134	32.9	Self-inflicted injuries	7,550	37.5	Chlamydia	5,964	34.6
8	Violence	12,955	36.0	Bipolar disorder	6,736	40.6	Schizophrenia	5,896	37.5
9	Schizophrenia	12,542	39.0	Schizophrenia	6,646	43.6	Maternal sepsis	5,367	40.1
10	Iron-deficiency anaemia	12,511	42.0	Falls	5,098	46.0	War	5,235	42.7
Developed Regions									
	All Causes	61,707		All Causes	36,943		All Causes	24,764	
1	Unipolar major depression	7,574	12.3	Alcohol use	4,677	12.7	Unipolar major depression	4,910	19.8
2	Alcohol use	5,477	21.2	Road traffic accidents	4,167	23.9	Schizophrenia	1,450	25.7
3	Road traffic accidents	5,304	29.7	Unipolar major depression	2,664	31.1	Road traffic accidents	1,137	30.3
4	Schizophrenia	3,028	34.7	Self-inflicted injuries	2,072	36.8	Bipolar disorder	1,106	34.7
5	Self-inflicted injuries	2,641	38.9	Schizophrenia	1,578	41.0	Obsessive-compulsive disorders	933	38.5

Table 5.4　(continued)

Rank	Both Sexes – Disease or Injury	DALYs (thousands)	Cumulative %	Males – Disease or Injury	DALYs (thousands)	Cumulative %	Females – Disease or Injury	DALYs (thousands)	Cumulative %
Developed Regions (continued)									
6	Bipolar disorder	2,241	42.6	Drug use	1,404	44.8	Alcohol use	801	41.7
7	Drug use	1,829	45.5	Violence	1,196	48.1	Osteoarthritis	783	44.9
8	Obsessive-compulsive disorders	1,652	48.2	Ischaemic heart disease	1,160	51.2	Chlamydia	599	47.3
9	Osteoarthritis	1,634	50.9	Bipolar disorder	1,135	54.3	Self-inflicted injuries	569	49.6
10	Violence	1,507	53.3	HIV	911	56.7	Rheumatoid arthritis	549	51.8
Developing Regions									
	All Causes	357,437		All Causes	180,211		All Causes	177,227	
1	Unipolar major depression	35,398	9.9	Unipolar major depression	12,658	7.0	Unipolar major depression	22,740	12.8
2	Tuberculosis	19,451	15.3	Road traffic accidents	11,387	13.3	Tuberculosis	8,703	17.7
3	Road traffic accidents	14,321	19.4	Tuberculosis	10,747	19.3	Iron-deficiency anaemia	7,135	21.8
4	War	12,382	22.8	Violence	9,844	24.8	Self-inflicted injuries	6,526	25.5
5	Iron-deficiency anaemia	12,033	26.2	Alcohol use	8,420	29.4	Obstructed labour	6,033	28.9
6	Self-inflicted injuries	12,004	29.5	War	7,448	33.6	Chlamydia	5,364	31.9
7	Violence	11,448	32.7	Bipolar disorder	5,601	36.7	Bipolar disorder	5,347	34.9
8	Bipolar disorder	10,948	35.8	Self-inflicted injuries	5,478	39.7	Maternal sepsis	5,226	37.8
9	Schizophrenia	9,514	38.5	Schizophrenia	5,068	42.5	War	4,934	40.6
10	Alcohol use	9,371	41.1	Iron-deficiency anaemia	4,898	45.3	Abortion	4,856	43.4

Table 5.5a   Total attributable burden for Chagas disease, 1990

	Deaths			
	Both sexes (thousands)	**Males** (thousands)	**Females** (thousands)	**Direct/** total
EME	0.0	0.0	0.0	
FSE	0.0	0.0	0.0	
IND	0.0	0.0	0.0	
CHN	0.0	0.0	0.0	
OAI	0.0	0.0	0.0	
SSA	0.0	0.0	0.0	
LAC	49.2	28.0	21.2	0.39
MEC	0.0	0.0	0.0	
World	49.2	28.0	21.2	0.39

	DALYs			
	Both sexes (millions)	**Males** (millions)	**Females** (millions)	**Direct/** total
EME	0.0	0.0	0.0	
FSE	0.0	0.0	0.0	
IND	0.0	0.0	0.0	
CHN	0.0	0.0	0.0	
OAI	0.0	0.0	0.0	
SSA	0.0	0.0	0.0	
LAC	1.6	0.9	0.7	0.40
MEC	0.0	0.0	0.0	
World	1.6	0.9	0.7	0.40

Table 5.5b   Total attributable burden for hepatitis B and hepatitis C, 1990

	Deaths			
	Both sexes (thousands)	**Males** (thousands)	**Females** (thousands)	**Direct/** total
EME	26.9	17.9	9.0	0.14
FSE	30.6	18.3	12.3	0.05
IND	97.3	66.5	30.7	0.18
CHN	379.5	264.0	115.5	0.09
OAI	157.4	111.6	45.8	0.12
SSA	69.4	47.2	22.2	0.22
LAC	17.9	11.4	6.5	0.25
MEC	39.7	22.7	17.1	0.32
World	818.7	559.6	259.1	0.13

	DALYs			
	Both sexes (millions)	**Males** (millions)	**Females** (millions)	**Direct/** total
EME	0.3	0.2	0.1	0.16
FSE	0.4	0.3	0.2	0.09
IND	1.8	1.2	0.6	0.19
CHN	5.7	4.1	1.6	0.11
OAI	2.6	1.9	0.7	0.15
SSA	1.2	0.8	0.4	0.25
LAC	0.4	0.2	0.1	0.33
MEC	0.7	0.4	0.3	0.35
World	13.3	9.2	4.1	0.16

Table 5.5c   Total attributable burden for tuberculosis, 1990

	Deaths			
	Both sexes (thousands)	Males (thousands)	Females (thousands)	Direct/ total
EME	14.6	10.0	4.6	1.00
FSE	23.0	19.1	3.9	1.00
IND	751.8	502.0	249.8	1.00
CHN	277.7	173.4	104.3	1.00
OAI	319.9	163.0	156.9	1.00
SSA	385.6	185.5	200.1	1.00
LAC	77.9	44.2	33.8	1.00
MEC	109.0	68.6	40.4	1.00
World	1959.6	1165.8	793.7	1.00
	DALYs			
	Both sexes (millions)	Males (millions)	Females (millions)	Direct/ total
EME	0.2	0.1	<0.1	0.77
FSE	0.4	0.3	0.1	1.00
IND	13.8	8.7	5.0	1.00
CHN	4.2	2.4	1.7	1.00
OAI	5.5	2.8	2.7	1.00
SSA	11.4	5.9	5.4	0.90
LAC	2.0	1.1	0.9	0.90
MEC	2.6	1.6	0.9	1.00
World	39.8	23.1	16.8	0.96

Table 5.5d   Total attributable burden for diabetes mellitus, 1990

	Deaths			
	Both sexes (thousands)	Males (thousands)	Females (thousands)	Direct/ total
EME	730.0	336.8	393.2	0.20
FSE	339.4	112.3	227.1	0.09
IND	473.7	239.9	233.8	0.22
CHN	212.6	107.3	105.3	0.28
OAI	332.8	158.2	174.6	0.18
SSA	98.3	42.1	56.1	0.24
LAC	263.7	131.4	132.3	0.34
MEC	308.6	151.4	157.1	0.20
World	2758.9	1279.4	1479.6	0.21
	DALYs			
	Both sexes (millions)	Males (millions)	Females (millions)	Direct/ total
EME	5.2	2.6	2.6	0.45
FSE	2.4	1.0	1.4	0.28
IND	5.3	2.7	2.6	0.43
CHN	2.2	1.1	1.1	0.50
OAI	3.6	1.7	1.9	0.37
SSA	1.1	0.5	0.6	0.46
LAC	2.9	1.4	1.4	0.50
MEC	3.6	1.8	1.8	0.40
World	26.3	12.9	13.4	0.42

Table 5.5e   Total attributable burden for cataracts, 1990

	Deaths			
	Both sexes (thousands)	**Males** (thousands)	**Females** (thousands)	**Direct/** total
EME	5.0	2.7	2.3	0.01
FSE	5.9	3.2	2.8	0.00
IND	341.1	166.6	174.5	0.00
CHN	154.6	76.1	78.5	0.04
OAI	166.2	83.1	83.1	0.00
SSA	238.6	116.0	122.6	0.00
LAC	75.9	38.1	37.8	0.00
MEC	117.1	58.2	58.9	0.00
World	1104.4	544.0	560.4	0.01

	DALYs			
	Both sexes (millions)	**Males** (millions)	**Females** (millions)	**Direct/** total
EME	<0.1	<0.1	<0.1	0.51
FSE	<0.1	<0.1	<0.1	0.44
IND	5.5	2.6	2.9	0.44
CHN	2.2	1.1	1.1	0.47
OAI	2.8	1.4	1.4	0.41
SSA	4.2	2.0	2.2	0.37
LAC	1.1	0.5	0.5	0.42
MEC	1.9	0.9	1.0	0.42
World	17.9	8.6	9.2	0.42

Table 5.5f   Total attributable burden for glaucoma, 1990

	Deaths			
	Both sexes (thousands)	**Males** (thousands)	**Females** (thousands)	**Direct/** total
EME	9.8	4.5	5.3	0.01
FSE	4.7	1.9	2.8	0.00
IND	69.7	39.6	30.1	0.00
CHN	85.3	30.7	54.6	0.07
OAI	58.8	21.3	37.5	0.00
SSA	76.9	32.6	44.3	0.00
LAC	11.6	4.9	6.7	0.00
MEC	13.7	5.9	7.8	0.00
World	330.5	141.4	189.1	0.02

	DALYs			
	Both sexes (millions)	**Males** (millions)	**Females** (millions)	**Direct/** total
EME	0.1	0.1	0.1	0.52
FSE	<0.1	<0.1	<0.1	0.46
IND	1.3	0.7	0.5	0.45
CHN	1.6	0.5	1.1	0.52
OAI	1.2	0.4	0.8	0.42
SSA	1.1	0.5	0.7	0.34
LAC	0.2	<0.1	0.1	0.45
MEC	0.2	<0.1	0.1	0.43
World	5.8	2.3	3.5	0.44

Table 5.5g   Total attributable burden for onchocerciasis, 1990

	Deaths			
	Both sexes (thousands)	**Males** (thousands)	**Females** (thousands)	**Direct/** total
EME	0.0	0.0	0.0	
FSE	0.0	0.0	0.0	
IND	0.0	0.0	0.0	
CHN	0.0	0.0	0.0	
OAI	0.0	0.0	0.0	
SSA	18.6	11.8	6.8	0.00
LAC	0.0	0.0	0.0	0.00
MEC	0.0	0.0	0.0	
World	18.6	11.8	6.8	0.00

	DALYs			
	Both sexes (millions)	**Males** (millions)	**Females** (millions)	**Direct/** total
EME	0.0	0.0	0.0	
FSE	0.0	0.0	0.0	
IND	0.0	0.0	0.0	
CHN	0.0	0.0	0.0	
OAI	0.0	0.0	0.0	
SSA	1.2	0.7	0.5	0.76
LAC	0.0	0.0	0.0	0.87
MEC	0.0	0.0	0.0	
World	1.2	0.7	0.5	0.76

Table 5.5h   Total attributable burden for trachoma, 1990

Deaths				
	Both sexes (thousands)	**Males** (thousands)	**Females** (thousands)	**Direct/** total
EME	0.0	0.0	0.0	
FSE	0.0	0.0	0.0	
IND	2.6	0.8	1.8	0.00
CHN	35.9	10.7	25.2	0.00
OAI	4.6	1.4	3.3	0.00
SSA	36.1	9.7	26.4	0.00
LAC	0.0	0.0	0.0	
MEC	24.0	7.0	17.0	0.00
World	103.1	29.4	73.7	0.00

	DALYs			
	Both sexes (millions)	**Males** (millions)	**Females** (millions)	**Direct/** total
EME	0.0	0.0	0.0	
FSE	0.0	0.0	0.0	
IND	<0.1	<0.1	<0.1	0.54
CHN	0.6	0.2	0.5	0.55
OAI	<0.1	<0.1	<0.1	0.51
SSA	0.8	0.2	0.6	0.47
LAC	0.0	0.0	0.0	
MEC	0.5	0.1	0.3	0.53
World	2.0	0.6	1.4	0.51

Table 5.5i   Total attributable burden for unipolar major depresssion, 1990

	Deaths			
	Both sexes (thousands)	**Males (thousands)**	**Females (thousands)**	**Direct/ total**
EME	112.1	80.7	31.3	0.00
FSE	80.5	61.9	18.7	0.00
IND	99.0	53.6	45.4	0.00
CHN	343.1	159.2	183.9	0.00
OAI	67.0	40.3	26.7	0.00
SSA	15.7	12.9	2.8	0.00
LAC	22.5	15.7	6.8	0.00
MEC	46.4	32.1	14.3	0.00
World	786.2	456.4	329.9	0.00

	DALYs			
	Both sexes (millions)	**Males (millions)**	**Females (millions)**	**Direct/ total**
EME	8.8	3.9	4.9	0.76
FSE	4.7	2.4	2.4	0.66
IND	10.9	4.4	6.5	0.74
CHN	21.1	8.0	13.1	0.62
OAI	8.6	3.4	5.2	0.78
SSA	5.0	1.9	3.1	0.91
LAC	4.8	1.8	2.9	0.88
MEC	5.9	2.5	3.3	0.77
World	69.8	28.3	41.5	0.73

Table 5.5j   Total attributable burden for sexually transmitted diseases, 1990

	Deaths			
	Both sexes (thousands)	**Males (thousands)**	**Females (thousands)**	**Direct/ total**
EME	1.4	0.5	0.8	0.52
FSE	2.5	1.2	1.3	0.14
IND	119.4	50.6	68.9	0.57
CHN	1.3	0.6	0.7	0.49
OAI	77.7	35.8	42.0	0.57
SSA	171.0	75.3	95.7	0.52
LAC	20.6	9.7	10.9	0.60
MEC	19.4	9.4	10.0	0.72
World	413.3	183.0	230.3	0.56

	DALYs			
	Both sexes (millions)	**Males (millions)**	**Females (millions)**	**Direct/ total**
EME	0.4	<0.1	0.4	0.94
FSE	0.5	<0.1	0.4	0.83
IND	7.4	2.7	4.8	0.75
CHN	0.1	<0.1	0.1	0.82
OAI	5.2	1.9	3.3	0.77
SSA	9.1	3.5	5.6	0.68
LAC	1.5	0.5	1.1	0.79
MEC	1.0	0.4	0.6	0.81
World	25.3	9.1	16.2	0.74

Note to Table 5.5: When no value appears in the "Direct/total" column, it indicates that there are no deaths or DALYs attributed to this condition or set of conditions in that region.

Figure 5.8   Relationship between the rank order of causes of global
DALYs calculated using an incidence or a prevalence
perspective, 1990 (highest rank is the largest cause)

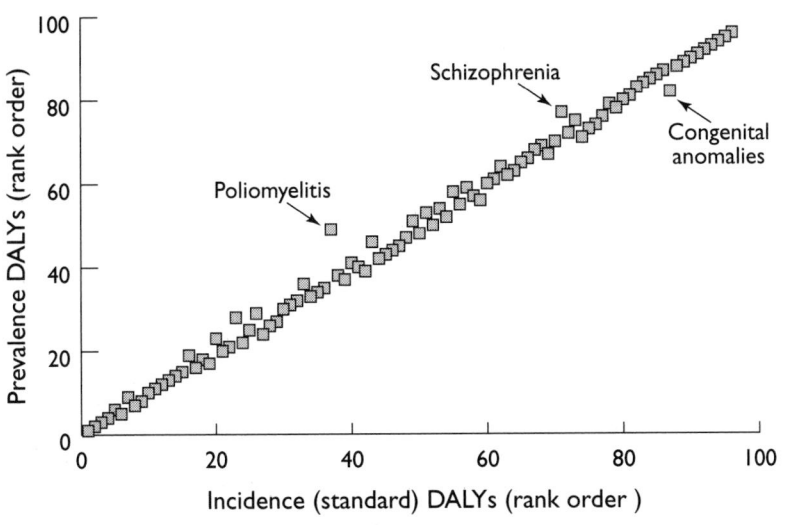

mation of prevalence DALYs, we have assumed that the average age of a
prevalent case equals the average age of onset. For schizophrenia, the
estimate of prevalence DALYs within the age group 15–44 years is strongly
affected by this limitation of the method, because the average age of onset in that age group is low (less than 22 years) and because the illness has
a long duration. Congenital anomalies are all incident at birth. An incidence perspective will yield a larger volume of YLDs, because the size of
the 1990 birth cohort is larger than the average birth cohort of the world
in the past, which was used to generate the prevalent cases of congenital
anomalies. Pearson's correlation coefficient between prevalence-based and
incidence-based DALYs by condition is 0.997, as is the Spearman's rank
order correlation coefficient, indicating the very close agreement of disease rankings derived from the two different perspectives.

   Table 5.6 indicates, nonetheless, that some subtle changes do arise by
shifting to a prevalence perspective. The share of YLDs in the global burden increases from 34.2 per cent for incidence-based DALYs to 34.9 per
cent for prevalence-based DALYs, and in developed regions, it increases
from 46.8 per cent to 50.2 per cent, respectively. Shifting to a prevalence
perspective changes the apparent age-distribution of burden. In incidence-
based YLDs, burden is ascribed to the age of onset whereas in prevalence-
based YLDs it is ascribed to the age at which the disability is lived. In both
forms, YLLs are assigned to the age at which death occurs. Changing perspective reduces the proportion of global DALYs assigned to the age group

Table 5.6   Comparison of the effects of changing the discount rate (r), the age-weighting modulation factor (K), the epidemiological perspective and the disability weights on the composition of DALYs (as percentages of total DALYs)

	Preva-lence DALYs	Visual analogue DALYs	DALYs[r,K]					
			$r=0$ $K=0$	$r=0$ $K=1$	$r=0.03$ $K=0$	$r=0.03$ $K=1$	$r=0.1$ $K=0$	$r=0.1$ $K=1$
			World					
By outcome								
Total YLD	34.9	39.2	22.1	24.4	30.3	34.2	41.7	47.3
Total YLL	65.1	60.8	77.9	75.6	69.7	65.8	58.3	52.7
By cause								
Group I	44.4	44.3	50.5	53.5	41.1	43.8	33.0	33.7
Group II	40.0	40.9	34.8	30.8	45.2	41.0	56.0	53.1
Group III	15.6	14.9	14.7	15.6	13.7	15.2	11.0	13.2
By sex								
All males	52.3	52.1	52.0	52.4	52.2	52.4	51.7	51.9
All females	47.7	47.9	48.0	47.6	47.8	47.6	48.3	48.1
By age group								
0–4	31.8	34.9	46.5	49.9	34.1	37.6	23.8	21.1
5–14	9.3	10.3	9.1	10.4	8.0	9.9	6.9	9.3
15–44	33.5	32.5	21.7	24.5	24.7	30.3	26.4	38.5
45–59	11.7	11.0	9.6	7.8	12.9	10.7	14.3	13.7
60+	13.7	11.3	13.0	7.4	20.4	11.5	28.6	17.3
			Developed Regions					
By outcome								
Total YLD	50.2	52.4	34.0	41.1	37.7	46.8	43.7	54.0
Total YLL	49.8	47.6	66.0	58.9	62.3	53.2	56.3	46.0
By cause								
Group I	8.1	8.1	8.7	10.1	6.9	7.7	6.1	6.3
Group II	76.6	78.2	76.1	72.1	81.2	77.8	85.5	83.0
Group III	15.2	13.7	15.2	17.9	11.9	14.5	8.4	10.7
By sex								
All males	55.5	55.5	54.9	57.2	53.7	56.2	52.0	54.7
All females	44.5	44.5	45.1	42.8	46.3	43.8	48.0	45.3
By age group								
0–4	4.6	5.7	8.5	10.7	4.9	7.1	3.1	2.8
5–14	2.7	3.2	2.4	3.4	1.9	2.9	1.8	2.7
15–44	36.5	40.3	28.6	39.4	25.3	38.3	22.9	38.7
45–59	21.1	21.2	21.0	20.3	20.9	21.0	18.3	20.1
60+	35.0	29.6	39.5	26.1	47.0	30.8	53.8	35.7

0–4 years from 37.6 per cent to 31.8 per cent, and increases the burden attributed to the age group over 60 years from 11.5 per cent to 13.7 per cent.

The effects of varying the discount rate, r, and the age-weighting modulation factor, K, on the overall pattern of burden are also summarized in Table 5.6. Changes in the discount rate and the age-weights appear to have little or no effect on the proportions of burden in males and females. For example, the proportion of all DALYs in males ranges from 51.7 per cent

Table 5.6   (continued)

	Prevalence DALYs	Visual analogue DALYs	DALYs[r,K]					
			r=0 K=0	r=0 K=1	r=0.03 K=0	r=0.03 K=1	r=0.1 K=0	r=0.1 K=1
				Developing Regions				
By outcome								
Total YLD	32.8	37.3	20.6	22.8	29.1	32.5	41.3	46.1
Total YLL	67.2	62.7	79.4	77.2	70.9	67.5	58.7	53.9
By cause								
Group I	49.5	49.2	55.5	57.8	46.8	48.6	38.8	38.7
Group II	34.9	35.8	29.8	26.8	39.2	36.1	49.6	47.7
Group III	15.7	15.0	14.7	15.4	14.1	15.2	11.5	13.6
By sex								
All males	51.8	51.6	51.7	52.0	51.9	51.9	51.7	51.4
All females	48.2	48.4	48.3	48.0	48.1	48.1	48.3	48.6
By age group								
0–4	35.6	38.9	51.1	53.7	39.0	41.7	28.3	24.5
5–14	10.3	11.3	9.9	11.1	9.0	10.8	8.1	10.6
15–44	33.0	31.4	20.9	23.1	24.6	29.3	27.1	38.4
45–59	10.4	9.6	8.3	6.6	11.5	9.3	13.4	12.6
60+	10.7	8.8	9.8	5.6	16.0	8.9	23.1	14.0

when r equals 10 per cent and K equals zero (DALYs[0.1,0]), to 52.4 per cent when r equals zero and K equals one (DALYs[0,1]), extremely different scenarios. Changes in the discount rate do have an important effect on the proportion of burden due to YLDs, on the age distribution of burden and on the distribution of burden by broad cause Group. When the discount rate is set to zero, YLDs account for less than one-quarter of burden. When the discount rate is set to 10 per cent, YLDs account for more than 40 per cent of burden. Likewise, a low discount rate enhances the importance of burden from disease or injury in children 0–4 years old, while a high discount rate augments the importance of burden in the age groups 45–59 years and over 60. Because of the differences in the Group structure of burden by age, these age effects also influence the overall distribution of DALYs by broad cause Group. When the discount rate is set equal to zero, Group I causes account for more than half of all burden, but when the discount rate is 10 per cent, Group I accounts for only one-third of burden. The proportion of DALYs due to Group III (injuries) is less affected by changes in the discount rate.

The effects of introducing non-uniform age-weights are much smaller in magnitude than the effects of changing the discount rate. Age-weighting in the standard formulation of DALYs enhances the importance of disability, because much disability occurs during adulthood, for which age-weights are greatest. Irrespective of the discount rate, the introduction of age-weights raises the proportion of burden due to YLDs: age-weights raise the proportion of YLDs by 2.3 percentage points from 22.1 to 24.4 per cent when the discount rate is set equal to zero, by 4.0 percentage points when r equals 3 per cent, and by 5.7 percentage points when *r* equals 10 per cent.

The effect of age-weighting on the age distribution of burden is the opposite of that of the discount rate (when the discount rate is less than ten per cent). Age-weighting at low to moderate discount rates increases the proportion of burden due to death or disability in children. This finding is in keeping with the observations of Barendregt et al. (1996) and Murray and Lopez (1996a) that age-weighting actually increases the importance of deaths in children and adolescents because of the effect of integrating under the age-weighting curve (including the adult years which are age-weighted more heavily by such functions) when calculating the number of DALYs due to childhood or adolescent deaths and long-term disabilities. When the discount rate is as high as ten per cent, age-weighting tends to increase the importance of burden arising at ages 15–44 years and decreases the importance of burden at ages 0–4, 45–59 and 60 years and over. The effects of age-weighting on the Group distribution of burden follows from these effects on the age distribution of burden. The importance of Group I is enhanced with age-weighting when the discount rate is less than 10 per cent, and the importance of Group II is decreased. The effects on Group III are relatively minor.

Given the interaction of the discount rate and the number of YLLs from deaths at each age, we might expect that the sex ratios of YLLs[0,0] rates might differ from the sex ratio of YLLs[0.03, 1] rates (see Table 5.7). The effect of removing age-weights and using a discount rate of zero is not uniform on the male-female ratio of YLD rates but uniformly decreases the male-female ratio of YLL rates. Nevertheless, YLL[0,0] rates are higher for women only in India, and are higher for males in all other regions.

There are two variants of DALYs which probably have the largest constituencies: the standard form, where the discount rate equals three per cent and age-weighting is used, and DALYs[0,0] where the discount rate is zero and uniform age-weights are used. Table 5.8 provides estimates of DALYs[0,0] according to the second level of cause disaggregation within a Group. Comparing these results with those in Table 5.1, it is apparent that the most important effect of using a zero discount rate and uniform age-weights is a substantial reduction in the proportion of global burden attributed to neuro-psychiatric conditions. Figure 5.9 shows the relationship of the rank orders for each disease or injury in terms of its contribution to global burden calculated using DALYs[0,0] and standard DALYs.

Table 5.7   Male to female YLD and YLL ratios

	EME	FSE	CHN	LAC	OAI	MEC	IND	SSA	World
YLD ratio	0.977	1.030	0.931	1.070	0.994	0.947	0.940	1.039	0.981
YLL ratio	1.409	1.599	1.023	1.273	1.200	1.016	0.902	1.133	1.093

Table 5.8 Percentage distribution of DALYs[0,0] according to specific causes (level two categories) with no discounting and uniform age-weights, 1990

Group/cause	Region										
	EME	FSE	IND	CHN	OAI	SSA	LAC	MEC	Developed	Developing	World
All Causes	100.0	100.0	100.0	100.0	100.0	100.0	100.0	100.0	100.0	100.0	100.0
I. Communicable, maternal, perinatal and nutritional conditions	7.9	9.8	62.7	28.0	50.8	72.0	42.9	55.3	8.7	55.5	50.5
A. Infectious and parasitic diseases	2.6	2.6	31.8	8.2	25.0	46.3	20.5	23.8	2.6	29.0	26.2
B. Respiratory infections	1.8	2.6	14.5	8.2	11.0	12.4	6.7	13.0	2.1	11.7	10.7
C. Maternal conditions	0.3	0.6	1.9	1.0	1.7	2.5	1.4	1.8	0.4	1.8	1.7
D. Conditions arising during the perinatal period	2.6	3.1	11.0	7.0	9.2	7.8	10.4	12.2	2.8	9.4	8.7
E. Nutritional deficiencies	0.7	0.8	3.6	3.7	3.9	3.0	3.9	4.5	0.7	3.6	3.3
II. Noncommunicable diseases	79.5	70.9	23.8	53.0	35.0	14.2	40.3	32.3	76.1	29.8	34.8
A. Malignant neoplasms	17.9	13.3	2.5	9.8	5.4	2.1	5.1	2.4	16.1	4.1	5.4
B. Other neoplasms	0.9	0.6	0.1	0.4	0.2	0.1	0.4	0.2	0.8	0.2	0.3
C. Diabetes mellitus	2.5	1.0	0.7	0.5	0.7	0.2	1.5	0.9	1.9	0.6	0.8
E. Neuro-psychiatric conditions	16.5	10.8	3.7	7.8	5.8	1.8	8.8	4.6	14.3	4.6	5.6
F. Sense organ diseases	0.1	0.1	0.7	0.8	0.7	0.4	0.5	0.4	0.1	0.6	0.6
G. Cardiovascular diseases	23.10	27.72	8.29	12.5	10.9	3.9	9.0	11.4	24.9	8.6	10.4
H. Respiratory diseases	4.7	4.5	2.1	10.4	2.3	1.9	3.5	3.5	4.6	3.7	3.8
I. Digestive diseases	4.6	4.3	1.9	4.8	4.3	1.5	3.6	3.6	4.5	2.9	3.1
J. Genito-urinary diseases	1.3	1.6	0.7	1.2	1.1	0.8	1.2	1.7	1.4	1.0	1.1
L. Musculo-skeletal diseases	4.2	4.0	0.4	1.6	1.0	0.3	2.7	0.5	4.1	0.8	1.2
M. Congenital anomalies	1.7	2.0	2.4	2.3	1.8	0.7	2.0	2.0	1.8	1.8	1.8
N. Oral conditions	0.73	0.6	0.2	0.5	0.5	0.1	0.6	0.7	0.7	0.4	0.4
III. Injuries	12.6	19.2	13.6	18.9	14.3	13.8	16.9	12.4	15.2	14.7	14.7
A. Unintentional injuries	9.1	13.0	12.1	13.9	12.0	8.3	12.2	6.4	10.7	10.7	10.7
B. Intentional injuries	3.5	6.2	1.5	5.0	2.3	5.5	4.7	6.0	4.5	4.0	4.1

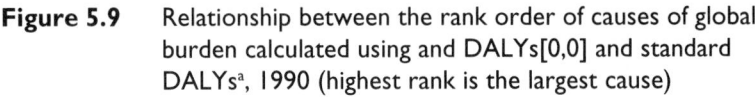

Figure 5.9   Relationship between the rank order of causes of global
burden calculated using and DALYs[0,0] and standard
DALYs[a], 1990 (highest rank is the largest cause)

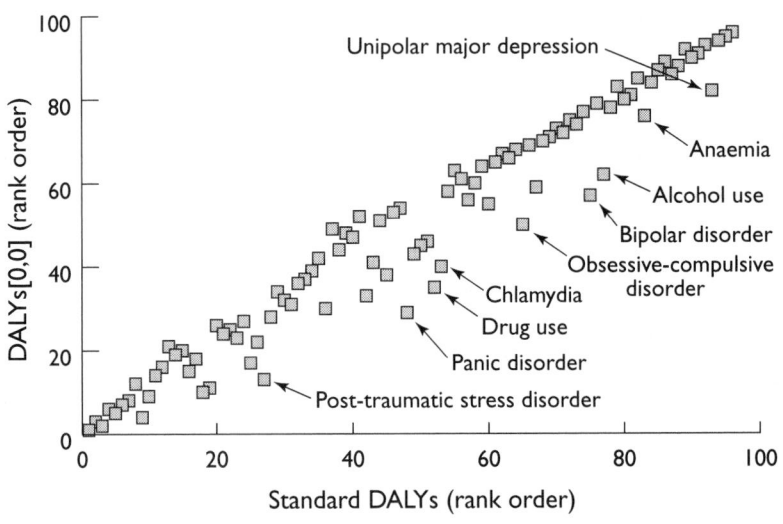

[a]   Standard DALYs are DALYs[0.03,1].

As in Figure 5.8, conditions have been ranked in ascending order, so that
the largest contributors to global burden are in the top right-hand corner
of the figure. The Pearson's correlation coefficient between DALYs[0,0]
and standard DALYs for these 96 conditions is 0.975, and the Spearman's
rank order correlation coefficient is practically indentical (0.974). The conditions for which ranks increase the most due to the introduction of discounting and age-weighting are labelled and, as already suggested by the
results in Table 5.8, include many of the neuro-psychiatric conditions,
which predominantly affect adults (i.e. unipolar major depression, post-
traumatic stress disorder, obsessive-compulsive disorders, drug use, alcohol use, bipolar disorder and panic disorder), as well as chlamydia which
largely affects adults as well.

For readers interested in more details, Annex Table 9 provides the
complete breakdowns for DALYs by age, sex, cause and region as used
in the GBD. In addition, we have presented the same level of detail for
DALYs[0,0] in Annex Table 10, for the convenience of those readers who
prefer measures of burden with a zero discount rate and uniform age-
weights.

The effects of changing disability weights are also summarized in Table 5.6. As expected, transforming the disability weights to a visual analogue scale raises the per cent of global DALYs due to YLDs from 30.3
per cent in standard DALYs to 39.2 per cent in the visual analogue DALYs.

Figure 5.10   Relationship between the rank order of causes of global
burden calculated using standard DALYs and visual analogue
DALYs[a], 1990 (highest rank is largest cause)

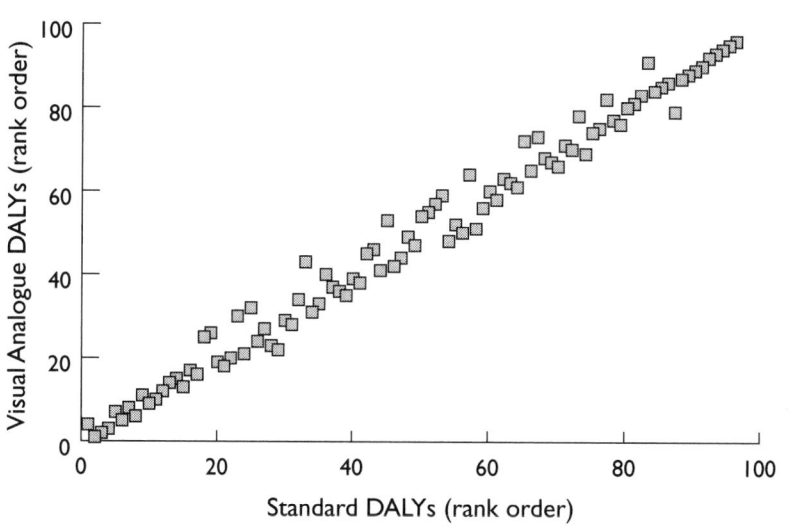

[a]   Standard DALYs are DALYs[0.03,1].

In developed regions, YLDs increase from 46.8 per cent to 52.4 per cent, and in developing regions from 32.5 per cent to 37.3 per cent. The transformation of disability weights has only minor effects on the distribution of global DALYs by age, sex and Group. The most significant of these minor changes is the slight enhancement of the importance of burden in the age group 15–44 years. The effect on the rank order of conditions, as shown in Figure 5.10, is also minor. Pearson's correlation coefficient by condition is 0.992, as is Spearman's rank order correlation coefficient.

DISCUSSION AND CONCLUSIONS

The approach taken in this study is based on the premise that an uncertain estimate of the burden of a disease or injury is preferable to no estimate. Frequently, the lack of an estimate is equated with zero burden, causing a potentially important health problem to disappear from the health policy dialogue. Given the differences in available epidemiological information between populations, the degree of uncertainty associated with each estimate varies by disease, region and even age and sex. For example, much more extensive community-based information is now available on neonatal tetanus than on adult tetanus. We have presented our best estimate for each condition without providing ranges or a quantitative assessment of the uncertainty associated with the estimate. We have done so for two reasons: first, in a study of this magnitude and complexity, providing a range of estimates for every figure would be extraordinarily difficult, particularly given the interlocked nature of cause-of-death estimates. Second, decision-makers, in the absence of better information, will generally choose to use the best estimate, giving little consideration to a range around the estimate.

If the best estimate of the burden of two conditions is 500 thousand DALYs, but one condition causes between 200 and 800 thousand DALYs and the other causes between 450 and 550 thousand DALYs, which condition should be considered more important? Some individuals might choose to attach greater importance to the condition with the wider uncertainty interval while others might be more concerned about the condition having less uncertainty. Economic theory suggests that social decision-makers should be equally concerned with both (Arrow and Lind 1970). Where there is substantial uncertainty, and narrowing the range of uncertainty would change our perception of priorities and ultimately affect policy choice, there is a significant value in collecting further information. Conditions that are estimated to have a surprisingly large or surprisingly small burden, and for which estimates are substantially uncertain, should be a priority for acquiring new epidemiological data.

This objective review of the contribution of different diseases and injuries to global health status has yielded a number of surprisingly large estimates for conditions or clusters of conditions, others that are surprisingly small, and many important modifications of past assessments of the magnitude of certain health problems. Perhaps the most surprising finding is the estimate that neuro-psychiatric conditions account for 10.5 per cent of the global burden of disease and injury and that unipolar major depression is the fourth most important cause of DALYs, after lower respiratory infections, diarrhoeal diseases and conditions arising during the perinatal period. Even in developing regions, neuro-psychiatric conditions account for 9.0 per cent of burden; in developed regions, the contribution is as high as 22.0 per cent. Another surprise is the uniformly large role played by injuries, which account for 14.5 per cent of burden in developed regions and slightly more (15.2 per cent) in developing regions. The pattern of injury burden by specific cause, however, varies dramatically across regions. Finally, the relatively poor health profile of FSE males in 1990 is worth noting. More alarmingly, recent trends and the projections presented in Chapter 7 in this volume (Murray and Lopez 1996b) suggest that this regional anomaly is unlikely to improve.

Without systematic comparative information, our perceptions of the magnitude of health problems may be heavily influenced by recent trends and popular portrayals. In 1990, HIV ranked 28th in terms of its contribution to the global burden of disease, but this contribution is expected to rise rapidly. Various projection scenarios (see Murray and Lopez 1996b, Chapter 7 in this volume) suggest that HIV will enter the ten leading causes of global burden early in the next century. The estimates of the magnitude of some major causes of burden have been substantially revised from those presented in previous analyses and preliminary versions of the GBD. Such revisions do not alter the fact that these conditions are major public health problems, although the 30–50 per cent reduction in the estimated magnitude of diseases such as malaria and tuberculosis is important for planning and evaluation purposes.

The importance of some diseases—such as hepatitis B, diabetes and many blinding conditions—increases dramatically when the full burden associated with these conditions is examined rather than just the burden listed in our primary tabulations. As is the case for various risk factors, interpretation of attributable burden estimates which include components of other diseases must take into account the fact that attributable burden estimates do not sum to one-hundred per cent. The same death from ischaemic heart disease may be "attributable" to diabetes, hypercholesterolemia, smoking and physical inactivity; i.e. the death would not have occurred if any one of these contributing factors were removed. As attributable estimates of burden are not bounded, and there is no "competition" between alternative causes for a fixed number of deaths or DALYs, there are fewer built-in checks on the validity of these claims.

The results of this study suggest that the epidemiological transition has progressed substantially in a number of developing regions. Despite the increased weight attached to deaths at younger ages in the computation of DALYs, Group II conditions—which occur primarily in older populations—already cause more disease burden than Group I conditions

Figure 5.11   Ratio of DALYs from Group II to Group I, by region, 1990

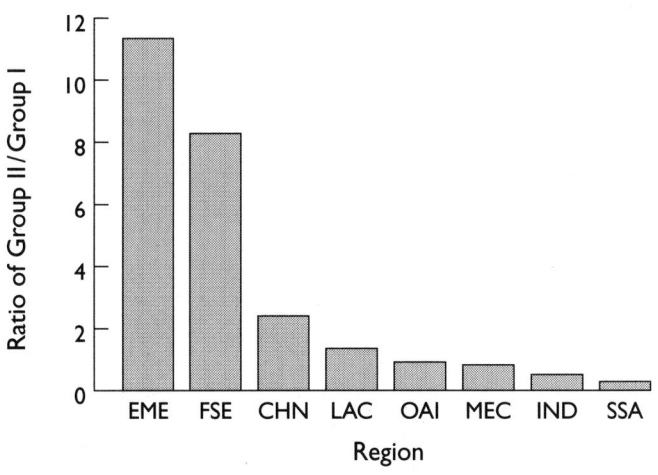

in China and LAC, while OAI and MEC are close to this transition point (see Figure 5.11). EME and FSE have essentially completed the epidemiological transition, whereas SSA remains in an early phase of this process. The ten leading causes of DALYs in all developing regions combined already include ischaemic heart disease and cerebrovascular disease. Clearly, research and debate about health policy in regions such as China, LAC and other parts of the developing world need to address the challenges posed by the epidemiological transition now, not several decades hence.

The array of health status indicators presented in the Global Burden of Disease Study points to a consistent pattern of differences in health status between males and females. The smallest male-female differences occur in India, where life expectancy for females is only slightly higher than for males (58.3 years compared with 57.3 years). Disability-Adjusted Life Expectancy in India is 50.9 for females and 50.3 for males. Females live slightly longer but live a greater proportion of their lifespan with disability (12.7 per cent compared with 11.8 per cent). Bearing in mind the longer standard life expectancy for females used in the calculation of DALYs, YLL rates are higher for females than for males.

In the low mortality regions, the comparative health situation for males is much worse than for females. The life expectancy of females at birth is substantially greater, Disability-Adjusted Life Expectancy at birth is greater for females than for males, and the percentage of the lifespan lived with disability is higher for men than women. YLL and YLD rates are higher for males than for females. These differences appear to be substantially greater than those expected purely on the basis of biological differences in maximum lifespan and health potential. Much of the difference can be explained by the combined effects of tobacco, alcohol and other addictions or exposures. Indeed, our projections suggest (see Murray and Lopez 1996b, Chapter 7 in this volume) that the male-female gap in health status is likely to widen in high income regions over the next few decades, contrary to what is commonly believed. Narrowing this gap will remain a major challenge for health policy into the twenty-first century.

Over the last two to three decades, international health policy has focused on lowering child mortality and improving the health conditions of children. This focus has been appropriate and highly successful in bringing about substantial reductions in child mortality. As a result, in regions such as China, LAC and OAI, the burden of disease incident in adults (aged 15–59) already exceeds the burden of disease incident in children. Health policies focusing on cost-effective reductions of the burden of disease in adults have been poorly researched and formulated. One of the first substantial reviews of adult health policy options in developing countries (Feachem et al. 1992) highlighted the need for further analysis of and attention to the rising burden of adult ill-health. The projections presented in Chapter 7 in this volume (Murray and Lopez 1996b) imply that by the year 2020, adult burden at ages 15–59 will exceed the burden of disease

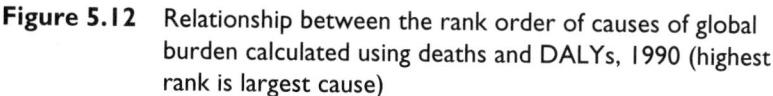

Figure 5.12   Relationship between the rank order of causes of global burden calculated using deaths and DALYs, 1990 (highest rank is largest cause)

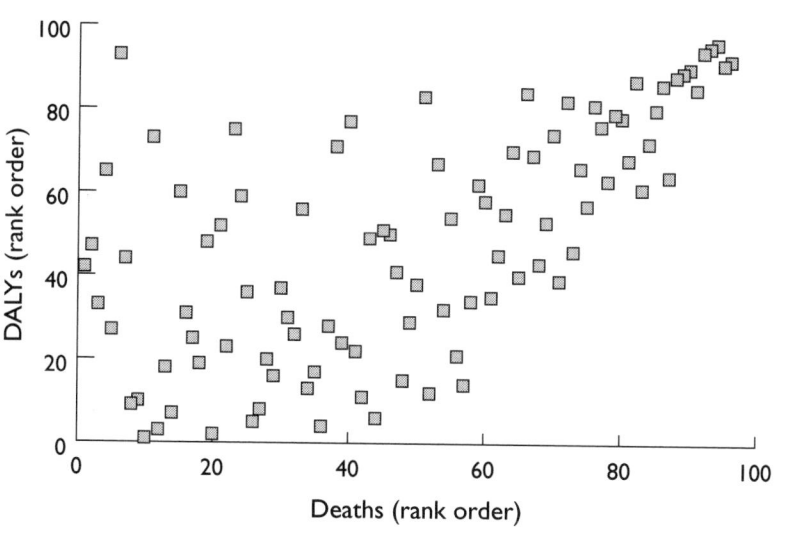

among young children (0–4 years) in all regions, reaffirming the growing need for more effective adult health policies.

Do these extensive efforts to quantify non-fatal health outcomes change our perception of the relative importance of different health problems? Would the priority attached to different health problems be the same if we examined only deaths, or only deaths in children by cause? Figure 5.12 shows a scatterplot of the rank order of all detailed conditions in the Global Burden of Disease Study in terms of deaths compared with the rank order in terms of DALYs. The Spearman's rank order correlation coefficient is only 0.63. More importantly, there are 14 conditions which are in the top half of the rank order list of causes of DALYs but are in the bottom half of the rank order list of causes of death. One of these conditions—unipolar major depression—is in the ten leading causes of burden but in the bottom ten causes of death. Not surprisingly, the relationship between the rank order of child deaths and the rank order of DALYs by cause is even weaker; the Spearman's rank order correlation coefficient is 0.45.

The overall rankings of various conditions in terms of their contribution to global burden are largely insensitive to alternative assumptions about the discount rate and age-weighting. The major effect of discounting and age-weighting is to enhance the importance of neuro-psychiatric conditions and sexually transmitted diseases. While disease ranks are largely unaffected, the share of burden due to disability, the age-distribution of burden and the distribution by broad cause Group are sensitive to the discount rate but largely unaffected by age-weighting. Although the results of specific cost-effectiveness studies may be sensitive to the social preferences incorporated in DALYs, we conclude that the uncertainty of underlying epidemiological assessments is vastly more important than these social preferences when interpreting the results of burden of disease analysis.

Disease and injury rankings are largely unaffected by transformations of the disability severity weights which inflate the weights of mild conditions, in the manner of visual analogue scales. These transformations, however, substantially increase the importance of YLDs relative to YLLs and substantially reduce Disability-Adjusted Life Expectancy (DALE). Clearly, for these composite measures of population health status and for cost-effectiveness analyses of interventions targeted at mild conditions, the method of preference measurement does matter. While the absolute values of DALE would change, however, it is doubtful that transforming the disability weights would alter the regional rankings of DALE. As with discounting and age-weighting, health state preferences will probably have a greater influence on the results of cost-effectiveness analysis than on the results of burden of disease analysis.

The similarity of disease rankings derived from prevalence-based and incidence-based DALYs raises several questions. The close relationship is perhaps not surprising given the extensive efforts in this study to develop internally consistent estimates of incidence and prevalence for each condition. The main differences arise for conditions where there is a recognized secular trend (for example, poliomyelitis), and this trend has been incorporated into the internal consistency analysis using DisMod. Given the close correspondence between the results of the two approaches, we might conclude that prevalence-based DALYs are preferable to incidence-based DALYs because they may be easier to calculate. Several considerations suggest that we should be cautious in coming to this conclusion. YLLs cannot meaningfully be calculated using a prevalence-based approach, so prevalence-based DALYs contain a fundamental inconsistency. Perhaps more importantly, using prevalence-based DALYs may lead some analysts to bypass the critical steps of developing internally consistent epidemiological estimates of incidence, duration, prevalence and mortality, except for those conditions where the available information is in terms of incidence, such as for most cancers. Finally, many convenient cross-sectional data sources on prevalence are based on self-reported health status. Our study has been constructed primarily from data based on observed rather than self-reported health status. There are many reasons to be concerned with self-reported information when making intercommunity or intertemporal comparisons for the same community—see Murray 1996, Chapter 1 in this volume for a more complete discussion of this point.

Future efforts at comprehensive assessment of the burden of disease could be improved through advances in several areas. First, the analytical tools that have been used to facilitate the internal consistency analysis could be improved. For example, DISMOD could be extended to include algorithms that would provide possible combinations of incidence, remission and case-fatality rates which are consistent with a particular set of prevalence, death and/or other information, such as the likely relationship between these rates and age. Second, the use of existing data sources could be improved. It is likely that there are many useful sources of information on the epidemiology of specific conditions that were not available to the authors of the disease and injury chapters and were not, therefore, incorporated in the final estimates shown here. Greater efforts at identifying and compiling such studies and other routinely collected information, and making them available to a broad audience, would be most valuable. Information which has been collected could be made more useful by encouraging the publication and dissemination of age and sex-specific results in all cases. Often potentially useful information could not be incorporated in this study when, for example, highly age-dependent phenomena had been reported using crude rates. Based on our experience in the GBD, we believe that the vital registration systems in many countries are an under-utilized source of information on the health status of the population that could be more constructively employed, albeit with care. In SSA, India, and OAI, as well as in certain communities of LAC and MEC, better information on the causes of death by age and sex is urgently needed. A sample registration scheme combined with a validated method for the attribution of causes of death to meaningful categories could be implemented in a number of populations. In areas such as in China, where most individuals have some contact with health services prior to death, the approach to cause-attribution is based on individual medical records and on reliable disease surveillance in well-defined populations. In many parts of SSA, verbal autopsy methods may be the only alternative; current efforts at validating adult verbal autopsy instruments may provide some reasonable approaches, at least for selected causes.

Progress in estimating the burden of non-fatal health outcomes could be made in at least four areas: improved methods for measuring deliberative preferences for health states, better and more widely-used instruments for measuring the incidence and/or prevalence of a number of important conditions, valid and reliable instruments for measuring disability at the individual level to be used in cross-sectional surveys in many different populations, and cohort studies on the medium and long-term disabling sequelae of specific injuries and diseases. Further details about these approaches are described in Chapter 4 in this volume (Murray and Lopez 1996d).

Looking back over this study, three observations seem particularly notable. If one term were to be used to describe this study, it might well be "meta-synthesis", in other words the construction of a comprehensive and comparable view of health problems using all available sources of information.[4] We believe that the estimates that emerge from a meta-synthesis approach to estimating death and disability from different conditions are superior to estimates that emerge from examination of specific health conditions in isolation. The GBD approach allows many more types of information to be incorporated into the analysis. It also avoids the tendency to assume that if there are no data, or if the data available are weak, then there is no problem. By considering an extensive range of diseases and injuries, there is more "competition" for deaths and disability and therefore less illness to ascribe to conditions with a vocal constituency.

The heavy emphasis on internal consistency in this study also provides a very clear idea of what aspects of the descriptive epidemiology of each condition are well understood and where. Many sources of information, for example routinely collected service data, may not be useful for estimating the burden of disease. Such insights can help prioritize efforts to gather more health information. In various national applications, these methods have helped identify gaps in the health information system and areas where currently collected information is not being used (see, for example, Lozano et al. 1995).

Social values play a prominent role in any dialogue about health problems and health priorities. Using DALYs, the social preferences incorporated into the analysis are made explicit. The effects of changing preferences are easily explored and understood, as illustrated in this chapter. Given the inevitable ethical dimension to any health policy dialogue, we believe that the information base for our understanding of the descriptive epidemiology of various health problems and the social values that influence our perception of these problems should be laid bare for the public to debate and deliberate. By making our assumptions and methods explicit, we hope that they will be topics for further debate, leading ultimately to their improvement. Future iterations of this study will no doubt be undertaken and such debates will make these estimates more reliable.

NOTES

1 The exact breakdown of conditions shown in Table 5.2 is somewhat arbitrary because we have not included the breakdown for conditions arising during the perinatal period into low birth weight and birth asphyxia/birth trauma, nor have we shown the breakdown of congenital anomalies into the ten detailed categories. The detailed categories within conditions arising during the perinatal period and congenital anomalies have not been projected and, to maintain consistency in the rank lists of conditions for 1990 and 2020, we have used the aggregate categories. For all other conditions, we have reported DALYs at the level of disaggregation that has been used for the epidemiological evaluations.

2 A complete description of the GBD cause classification system is provided in Chapter 3 in this volume and summarized in Table 3.1 (Murray and Lopez 1996c).

3 The estimates in the primary tabulations are actually for hepatitis B and hepatitis C combined. The vast majority of this burden, as estimated, is from

hepatitis B. The attributable burden for liver cancer and cirrhosis has been estimated for hepatitis B alone.

4   To our knowledge, the term meta-synthesis has been first used in the context of health status assessment by Michael Wolfson. We are grateful to him for pointing out the applicability of this term for the GBD.

BIBLIOGRAPHY

Arrow KJ, Lind RC (1970) Uncertainty and the evaluation of public investment decisions. *American Economic Review* 60:364–78.

Barendregt JJ, Bonneux L, Van der Maas PJ (1996) DALYs: the age-weights on balance. *Bulletin of the World Health Organization* 74(4):439-443.

Beasley RP et al. (1981) Hepatocellular carcinoma and hepatitis B virus. A prospective study of 22 707 men in Taiwan. *Lancet* 2(8526):1129–33.

Bebbington AC. (1991) The expectation of life without disability in England and Wales: 1976–88. *Population Trends* 66:26–29.

Berkley S et al. (1996a) Sexually transmitted diseases. In: Murray CJL, Lopez AD, eds. *Health dimensions of sex and reproduction: the global burden of sexually transmitted diseases, HIV, maternal conditions, perinatal disorders and congenital anomalies.* Cambridge, Harvard University Press.

Berkley S et al. (1996b) Unsafe sex. In: Murray CJL, Lopez AD, eds. *Quantifying global health risks: the burden of disease attributalbe to selected risk factors.* Cambridge, Harvard University Press.

Bild DE, Stevenson JM (1992) Frequency of recording of diabetes on US death certificates: analysis of the 1986 National Mortality Followback Survey. *Journal of Clinical Epidemiology* 45(3):275–81.

Bisi H et al. (1993) Study in necropsy material of "cause-specific mortality" in diabetics, in Sao Paulo-Brasil. *Revista Paulista de Medicine* 111(1):299–304.

Crimmins EM, Saito Y, Hayward MD (1993) Sullivan and multistate methods of estimating active life expectancy: two methods, two answers. In, Robine JM et al. (eds) *Calculation of health expectancies: harmonization, consensus achieved and future perspectives.* London: John Libbey Eurotext.

Eddy DM (1991) Oregon's methods: did cost-effectiveness analysis fail? *Journal of the American Medical Association* 266:2135–2141.

Evans TG, Thylerfors B, Ranson K (1996) Blindness. In: Murray CJL, Lopez AD, eds. *Quantifying global health risks: the burden of disease attributalbe to selected risk factors.* Cambridge, Harvard University Press.

Feachem RGA et al., eds. (1992) *The health of adults in the developing world.* New York, Oxford University Press for the World Bank.

Frenk J et al. (1989) Health transition in middle-income countries: new challenges for health care. *Health policy and planning,* 4(1):29–39.

Fuller JH (1993) Mortality trends and causes of death in diabetic patients. *Diabete et Metabolisme* 19:96–9.

Jougla E et al. (1992) Death certificate coding practices related to diabetes in European countries—the 'EURODIAB Subarea C' Study. *International Journal of Epidemiology* 21(2):343–51

Kane M, Schatz G, Halder S (1996) Hepatitis B In: Murray CJL, Lopez AD, eds. *The global epidemiology of infectious diseases* Cambridge, Harvard University Press.

Kaplan RM, Anderson JP (1988) A general health model: update and applications. *Health Services Research* 23:203–35.

Kumaresan J et al. (1996) Tuberculosis. In: Murray CJL, Lopez AD, eds. *The global epidemiology of infectious diseases* Cambridge, Harvard University Press.

Lozano R et al. (1995) Burden of disease assessment and health system. Reform results of a study in Mexico. *Journal of international development*, 7(3):555-563.

McKeigue P, King H (1996) Diabetes mellitus. In: Murray CJL, Lopez AD, eds. *Global perspectives on non-communicalbe diseases: the epidemiology of cancers, cardiovascular diseases, diabetes mellitus, respiratory disorders and other major conditions.* Cambridge, Harvard University Press.

Moncayo A, Myoshi C (1996) Chagas disease. In: Murray CJL, Lopez AD, eds. *The global epidemiology of infectious diseases* Cambridge, Harvard University Press.

Mota EA et al. (1990) A nine year prospective study of Chagas' disease in a defined rural population in Northest Brazil. *American Journal of Tropical Medicine and Hygiene* 42(5):429–440.

Murray CJL (1996) Rethinking DALYs. In: Murray CJL, Lopez AD (eds). *The global burden of disease: a comprehensive assessment of mortality and disability from diseases, injuries, and risk factors in 1990 and projected to 2020.* Cambridge, Harvard University Press.

Murray CJL, Govindaraj R, Musgrove P (1994) National health expenditures: a global analysis. *Bulletin of the World Health Organization* 72(4):623–627.

Murray CJL, Lopez AD (1996a) The incremental effect of age-weighting on YLLs, YLDs and DALYs: a response *Bulletin of the World Health Organization* 74(4):445-446.

Murray CJL, Lopez AD (1996b) Alternative visions of the future: projecting mortality and disability, 1990–2020. In: Murray CJL, Lopez AD (eds). *The global burden of disease: a comprehensive assessment of mortality and disability from diseases, injuries, and risk factors in 1990 and projected to 2020.* Cambridge, Harvard University Press.

Murray CJL, Lopez AD (1996c) Estimating causes of death: methods and global and regional applications for 1990. In: Murray CJL, Lopez AD (eds). *The global burden of disease: a comprehensive assessment of mortality and disability from diseases, injuries, and risk factors in 1990 and projected to 2020.* Cambridge, Harvard University Press.

Murray CJL, Lopez AD (1996d) Global and regional patterns of disability in 1990: incidence, prevalence, disability-free life expectancy, disability-adjusted life expectancy and Years Lived with Disability. In: Murray CJL, Lopez AD (eds).

The global burden of disease: a comprehensive assessment of mortality and disability from diseases, injuries, and risk factors in 1990 and projected to 2020. Cambridge, Harvard University Press.

Murray CJL, Lopez AD (1996e) *Global health statistics: a compendium of incidence, prevalence and mortality estimates for over 200 conditions.* Cambridge, Harvard University Press.

Murray CJL, Lopez AD (1996f) Quantifying the burden of disease and injury attributable to ten major risk factors. In: Murray CJL, Lopez AD, eds. *The global burden of disease: a comprehensive assessment of mortality and disability from diseases, injuries, and risk factors in 1990 and projected to 2020.* Cambridge, Harvard University Press.

Nord E (1991) The validity of a visual analogue scale in determining social utility weights for health states. *International Journal of Health Planning and Management* 6:234–242.

Nord E (1993) Unustified use of the Quality of Well-Being scale in priority setting in Oregon. *Health Policy* 24:45–53.

Richardson J (1994) Cost utility analysis: what should be measured. *Social Science and Medicine* 39(1):7–21.

Robine JM, Ritchie K (1991) Healthy life expectancy: evaluation of a new global indicator for change in population health. *British Medical Journal* 302:457–460.

Sasaki A, Kamado K, Uehara M (1994) Changes in causes of death in diabetic patients based on death certificates during a 30-year period in Osaka District, Japan, with special reference to cancer mortality. *Diabetes Research and Clinical Practice* 24(2):1033–12.

Sullivan DF(1971) A single index of mortality and morbidity. *HSMHA Health Reports* 86:347–354.

Torrance GW (1986) Measurement of health-state utilities for economic appraisal: a review. *Journal of health economics,* 5:1-30.

World Health Organization (1996) *World Health Report 1996:* World Health Organization, Geneva

Chapter 6

QUANTIFYING THE BURDEN OF DISEASE AND INJURY ATTRIBUTABLE TO TEN MAJOR RISK FACTORS

CHRISTOPHER J. L. MURRAY
ALAN D. LOPEZ

Reliable information about the descriptive epidemiology of diseases and injuries is an important element of any public health strategy aimed at reducing the burden of ill health. Over the past two centuries, medical statisticians have accumulated data on the incidence, prevalence and mortality of numerous diseases (and, to a lesser extent, injuries) in various parts of the world. The systems which have been established to generate data on the health status of populations globally have ranged from elaborate vital registration procedures now operational in all developed countries and in an increasing number of countries in the developing world to simple prevalence surveys of small population groups. As confidence in the reliability of these data on diseases and injuries has increased, so too has their usefulness for health policy formulation. Basic epidemiological statistics, and estimates for larger populations based on these statistics, have been widely used to justify public health action to combat causes of ill health, as diverse as malaria, tuberculosis, HIV infection, road traffic accidents and maternal conditions.

Many diseases or injuries are caused by infection with a single pathogen, or by an isolated violent event without any known precursor. Numerous cases of disease or injury do, however, arise from a prior or current exposure to a hazard of some sort. These cases of disease or injury would probably not have occurred in the absence of these exposures. It is important to identify and to quantify reliably such exposures in order to ensure that they receive the same consideration as diseases and injuries in health policy debates. For each disease or injury, a choice may need to be made between the prevention and treatment of the disease or injury itself, and the prevention or reduction of various exposures which may be the underlying causes of the disease or injury. Reliable estimates of the contribution of various exposures to the overall burden of disease and injury are thus required for a balanced and comprehensive assessment of the causes of ill health in populations.

For the Global Burden of Disease Study (GBD), assessments of the burden attributable to each of the following ten major risk factors have been undertaken by experts in each field: malnutrition, poor water supply, sanitation and personal and domestic hygiene practices, unsafe sex, tobacco, alocohol, occupation, hypertension, physical inactivity, illicit drugs and air pollution (Berkley et al. 1996, Donoghoe et al. 1996, Hong et al. 1996, Huttly 1996, Koplan and Pratt 1996, Leigh et al. 1996, Mason et al. 1996, Murray and Lopez 1996b, Murray and Lopez 1996d, Nichols and Elliott 1996). Volume IX of the *Global Burden of Disease and Injury Series*, entitled *Quantifying Global Health Risks: The Burden of Disease Attributable to Selected Risk Factors*, provides in more detail assessments of these risk factors in a series of chapters authored by these experts. The purpose of the present summary chapter is to provide a brief synopsis of this work, highlighting the results and their implications, rather than the methods. In this sense, this chapter does not represent our own original work on the burden attributable to various risk factors, but rather provides an interpretation of the results calculated by others, and our attempt to convert these results into estimates of attributable deaths and Disability-Adjusted Life Years (DALYs). This chapter begins with a discussion of some general issues in the definition of attributable burden, followed by a brief review of specific methodological limitations in the ten risk factor analyses and an overview of the main results and their implications.

DEFINING ATTRIBUTABLE BURDEN

Beaglehole et al. (1993) provide a definition of the traditional epidemiological concept of an *attributable fraction* as follows: "When an exposure is believed to be a cause of a given disease, the attributable fraction is the proportion of the disease in the specific population that would be eliminated in the absence of the exposure" (p. 29). The classical formula (Miettenen 1974) for computing the attributable fraction of a disease or injury due to an exposure is:

$$AF = \frac{P(RR-1)}{P(RR-1)+1}$$

where, for a given disease or injury, AF is the fraction of the burden that is attributable to a specific exposure, P is the proportion of the population exposed, and RR is the relative risk of death in the exposed population compared with an unexposed population. The simple concept of an attributable fraction requires elaboration and qualification, and the use of this familiar formula entails a number of assumptions. The application of the concept of attributable fraction and its formula is straightforward only when exposure is a simple dichotomous variable, with no allowance for variations in intensity, duration or the time lag of exposure. In reality, however, risk (as measured by RR) is dependent on dose, duration and other parameters which affect exposure both quantitatively and qualitatively.

The mechanisms through which risk factors affect health also vary greatly. Tobacco is a uniquely hazardous exposure, with virtually all of its public health impact reflected in the health consequences for the individual smoker. Alcohol is an example of a more complex exposure. To begin with, the effects are apparent both for the individual drinker and for social units (e.g. families, communities) or other groups (e.g. colleagues, road users). The hazard function for alcohol is also complex in that alcohol, in small quantities, appears to reduce the risk of death, but, at higher quantities, appears to increase the risk of death (for a recent review, see Anderson 1993, Poikolainen 1995). Abstainers from alcohol may be very different from drinkers with regard to a variety of personal and social characteristics related to health status, thereby confounding the comparisons between non-drinkers and drinkers. Thus, while lifelong non-smokers might be the appropriate comparison group for assessing the hazards associated with tobacco, lifelong abstainers from alcohol are not necessarily the appropriate comparison group for estimating the burden due to alcohol. An alternative comparison group might be drinkers with the lowest relative risk (up to one drink per day for women and one or two drinks per day for men) (English et al. 1995).

An important distinction needs to be made between the *current* burden of disease attributable to *past* exposure to a risk factor and the *future* burden that may arise from *current* exposure to that risk factor. Much of the literature on attributable risk, such as the estimates of smoking-attributable mortality by Peto et al. (1994), is based on estimating current burden attributable to past exposure. Calculating future burden due to current exposure is inherently more complicated, given secular trends in diseases, expected socio-economic changes and likely advances in technology. On the other hand, the future burden of disease and injury due to current exposure is more important for public health planning and prevention than the current burden due to past exposures, since the latter cannot be altered. For some risk factors, such as poor water supply, sanitation and hygiene, and alcohol use, the time lag between exposure and burden is likely to be very short. In these cases, the difference between current burden due to past exposure and future burden due to current exposure is likely to be less significant. For others, such as tobacco, hypertension and malnutrition, the time lags are longer. In this chapter, the focus is on estimating current burden due to past exposure, as this is likely to be more reliably estimated.

When analysing the burden attributable to a risk factor in a population, the notion of exposure needs to be qualified. Generally, population exposure to a risk factor is calculated by comparing current levels of exposure to some reference level. Four types of reference population distributions can be used:

1. *Zero exposure for the entire population.* This is the method used to estimate tobacco-attributable burden and fits closest to the textbook definition of an attributable fraction.

2. *A population distribution of exposure achieved in a real population.* The real population could be taken from an intervention trial or could be a population that has low levels of exposure to a particular risk factor. Using this type of reference, the calculation of attributable burden incorporates some notion of the technical feasibility of reducing exposure. Most of the estimates of attributable burden published in the *World Development Report 1993: Investing in Health* were based on using such a "feasible" reference population (World Bank 1993). "Feasibility" was not clearly defined, but appeared to imply an exposure level that could be achieved with existing technology and at reasonable cost. Such estimates of attributable burden are related to health-sector cost-effectiveness analyses in which a cluster of activities that are not currently being delivered are recommended because they are cost-effective. In sectoral cost-effectiveness exercises, only interventions that cost less than some threshold cost per unit health gain are recommended. "Feasible" attributable burden estimates differ in that an explicit cost-effectiveness threshold is not specified.

3. *An arbitrary reference distribution.* A good example of such an arbitrary reference distribution emerges from the research on alcohol-attributable burden. Low levels of alcohol intake lead to a decrease in mortality, while higher levels of consumption contribute to a rise in mortality for some causes. Rather than using a zero reference distribution, in which some of the harmful effects of alcohol will be offset by the benefits, some researchers have defined an arbitrary reference distribution where no one consumes *harmful* amounts of alcohol. All individuals that otherwise consume harmful levels are assumed to consume the amount of alcohol that minimizes mortality for some causes. The proportion of the population that abstains is assumed to be constant (English et al. 1995). Such a distribution is unlikely ever to be achieved in a real population, since instruments of public policy that discourage harmful use of alcohol are also likely to affect alcohol consumption among light drinkers (Holman and English 1996).

4. *An arbitrary reference point.* This concept is similar to an arbitrary reference distribution, the main difference being the underlying assumption that the entire population will have exactly the same level of exposure at some arbitrary point. The arbitrary reference point may be an official standard, such as for levels of pollution that are legally permitted, or may be chosen to minimize risk, such as a blood pressure cutoff point. Clearly, there is no population in which every individual will have exactly the same level of exposure; attributable burden based on such arbitrary reference points is, therefore, an abstract notion.

In order to provide an objective standard against which to evaluate the various approaches and estimates of the health effects of different exposures, we have chosen to define attributable burden (for a specific risk factor, population and time) as *the difference between currently observed burden and the burden that would be observed if past levels of exposure had been equal to a specified reference distribution of exposure.* It would be highly desirable, for the sake of comparability, to standardize the choice of a reference exposure distribution however, for this first effort at global assessment of the burden of disease and injury attributable to major risk factors, we have not been able to do so. In most cases, as noted below, we have used zero exposure as the reference, except for risk factors such as hypertension, for which such a concept is meaningless.

In this discussion of attributable burden, we have been using the terms "exposure" and "risk factor" interchangeably. In fact, one can distinguish at least three different types of risk factors for which "exposure" has different meanings. First, some risk factors are true exposures, such as tobacco, alcohol, physical inactivity, unsafe sex and air pollution. Other risk factors, such as blood pressure or nutritional status, are physiological states, not true exposures. Such risk factors are themselves complex functions of other true exposures. For example, an individual's blood pressure is likely to be a function of heredity, as well as salt intake, other dietary practices and other exposures. A low weight-for-height or a low height-for-age is a function of dietary intake, exposure to infectious diseases, possibly heredity, and other factors. Because the "exposure" is a physiological state which in turn is a complex function of other exposures, it is difficult to define a meaningful reference distribution. For example, while we can hypothesize about a population where no child is less than 2 standard deviations below the reference population mean weight-for-age, the nature of the exposures required to achieve this physiological state are uncertain. Attributable burden estimates for such risk factors are thus of a different nature than attributable burden estimates for a simple exposure where the reference distribution is fully specified. A third type of risk factor relates to social states, e.g. unemployment, poverty, or social inequality. Social states are similar to physiological states in that they are not simple exposures. The determinants of an individual's social state are complex; estimates of their attributable burden, therefore, would be interesting, but difficult to interpret. It is well known, for example, that individuals in lower social classes in the developed countries smoke more than the better educated, a fact which might account for a considerable proportion of the differential in disease between these groups (Marmot 1995, Pierce et al. 1989, Vagëro and Lundberg 1995) in this chapter we do not attempt to quantify the disease burden attributable to social states.

It is also critical to keep in mind that the sum of attributable burden is unbounded. Death and disability from many diseases and injuries can be caused by multiple factors acting simultaneously, and the same event can legitimately be attributed to many underlying causes. For example, imagine a model of disease causation that requires the coincidence of three factors such as hypertension, alcohol and smoking. If any one of the three is not present, a death will be averted. Using our formal definition of attributable burden, that death is fully attributable to all three risk factors. Because attributable burden is theoretically unbounded, the plausibility of an estimate is its only constraint.[1] The sum of attributable fractions can exceed one-hundred per cent for a given cause or for mortality from all causes. Because there are no bounds on the sum of attributable fractions, there is also no internal incentive on the part of advocates or analysts to limit their claims. For this reason, one must interpret the estimates of attributable burden with caution.

METHODS AND MATERIALS

Estimates of attributable burden can be divided into four categories, defined by the methods used: direct estimation, and three variants of the attributable fraction approach. An example of the direct estimation method is the assessment of burden attributable to occupational exposures and hazards. For the assessment of occupation-related injuries, Leigh et al. (1996) used a legally-mandated registration system to measure directly the number of injuries from occupational risks. The attributable fraction of all occupational injuries is calculated by comparing occupation-related injuries to all injuries for an age group. Similar registration systems employing medico-legal definitions are used to estimate the attributable fraction for occupation-related diseases, though there is likely to be more uncertainty associated with identification of an occupational disease than with an occupational injury.

The other nine studies summarized in this chapter used variants of the traditional attributable-fraction method. In theory, the attributable burden from a risk factor is defined by the following equation:

$$AB = \sum AF_j B_j \quad \text{where} \quad AF_j = \frac{P(RR_j - 1)}{P(RR_j - 1) + 1}$$

AB is the attributable burden for a given risk factor and population, AF_j is the fraction of the burden from cause j, B_j is the estimated population-level burden from cause j, P is the prevalence of the exposure, and RR_j is the relative risk of disease or injury for cause j in the exposed group compared to the unexposed group. To estimate attributable burden, it is necessary to know the relative risks for each cause of death and disability related to the exposure, the levels of exposure, and the burden of disease due to each cause of death and disability in a given population.

Relative risks of death or disability for individuals at different levels of exposure compared to some reference level of exposure are usually estimated from case-control or prospective studies. For example, Figure 6.1 shows the relative risk of death from all causes for males and females

Figure 6.1   Relationship of all-cause mortality to alcohol intake based
on pooled results of 16 cohort studies

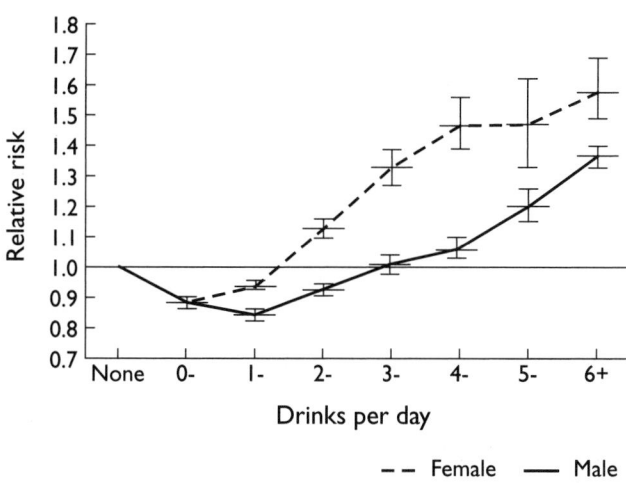

Source: English et al. (1995)

Note: Vertical bars reflect 95 per cent confidence intervals.

according to different levels of alcohol intake per day, based on the pooled results of 16 cohort studies (English et al. 1995). The relative risk of death from alcohol intake as shown in this figure is the ratio of the risk of death among individuals drinking a certain number of drinks per day compared to individuals who do not drink at all. The usual practice in the literature on attributable burden is to assume that relative risks are general i.e. those studied in one population can be applied to many other populations, albeit with caution. However, there is clear evidence from the two American Cancer Society Cancer Prevention Study prospective studies (CPS-I and CPS-II, respectively) on the risks of smoking in the United States that relative risks can change.[2] In fact, if the impact of an exposure on mortality risk is not simply multiplicative, then we would expect relative risks to change depending on other risk factors and on the levels of exposure.

Despite these concerns, the major determinant of variation (among different populations) in the attributable burdens due to a particular risk factor is not usually differences in relative risk, but rather differences in the population distribution of exposure levels. Once this population distribution is determined, the population-attributable burden is calculated by estimating what the level of mortality or disability would be if the distribution of the population by exposure level were shifted to the reference distribution. Estimating the population distribution of exposure for particular risk factors, therefore, is the major challenge in deriving attributable burden at least for those exposures for which the relative risk does not change dramatically over time.

Another important consideration in estimating attributable burden is the suitability of the available measures of exposure. For many exposures, such as cigarette smoking, relative risk is a function of the duration, intensity and type of exposure. Frequently, survey or consumption data are available only for current exposure status, such as the proportion of the population who are current smokers, the proportion who drank a certain number of drinks in the last two weeks, etc. Current exposure status measures are then used as proxies for cumulative past exposures. However, for most risk factors, current exposure, as summarized by a single index, is likely to be a very poor indicator of cumulative exposure over an individual's lifetime. Creative methods have been employed to overcome the difficulties of measuring past exposure. For example, Peto, Lopez and their colleagues estimate cumulative past exposure to smoking based on observed lung cancer rates, because in most countries lung cancer in excess of non-smoker lung cancer rates is due almost entirely to the cumulative effects of smoking (Peto et al. 1994). Unfortunately, for many of the risk factors discussed in this chapter, the measures of exposure are current-status measures and are often quite poor. For others, it is virtually impossible to measure the population distribution by exposure status at one moment in time or even over a period of time; an example of this problem is the measurement of blood alcohol levels used to estimate the impact of alcohol consumption on road traffic accidents. Individuals can move quite rapidly between exposure states (e.g. various phases of intoxication), creating enormous difficulties in estimating the average population distribution of exposure.

Where data on the population distribution of exposure are completely lacking, as is often the case, some have estimated the burden of a risk factor by taking the fraction of current burden attributable to a risk factor in one population and applying it to other populations. Implicitly, this practice is based on the assumption that both the relative risks and the population distributions of exposure are identical across the populations studied, which is unlikely to be the case. An example of this type of approach is the regional estimates of DALYs attributable to alcohol, published in the *World Development Report 1993* (World Bank 1993). This indiscriminate use of attributable fractions is difficult to justify, since it is highly *unlikely* that the population distributions of exposure for most risk factors are identical across all communities. Even cruder variants of this approach are used, not taking into consideration the structure of burden by cause, i.e. using estimates of the overall attributable fraction of burden from all causes calculated for one population and simply applying them to another.

The more plausible approach, involving measuring relative risks and population distribution of exposure, is certainly the preferred method for many risk factors. This framework assumes that the harm from exposure occurs only in the exposed i.e. the harm is internalized. However, for selected risk factors, such as alcohol and drug use, exposure may indirectly affect individuals who are not exposed. A road traffic accident caused by a drunk driver who collides with another person or vehicle is perhaps the most vivid example. An individual under the influence of drugs or alcohol may commit violent acts against other individuals. The resulting attributable burden will not be captured in the "relative risk and exposure" framework outlined earlier. When externalities such as these exist, the relative risk and exposure method needs to be extended. The estimates for alcohol and drugs included in this study do not take externalities into account explicitly, since we have no reliable way of knowing how common these are in different regions.

In evaluating claims on attributable burden for various risk factors, a critical question is whether a causal relationship has been established. Various criteria for demonstrating causality have been proposed, including strength of the association, consistency of effect, specificity, temporal relationship, biological gradient, biological plausibility, coherence of evidence, experimental evidence and reasoning by analogy (Hill 1965). For some risk factor-disease relationships, such as smoking and lung cancer, all of the relevant criteria for causality have been met. For other risk factors, such as air pollution, malnutrition and some occupational injuries, these strict causality criteria have not been fully met. Consequently, the degree of confidence in attributable burden estimates for different risk factors will vary, being greatest for those exposures for which causality has been reliably demonstrated, notably tobacco and alcohol. However, even when strict causality criteria have not been established, the weight of evidence regarding the impact of risk factors may still be substantial. In these cases, the estimates of attributable burden are at least interesting from a public health point of view, provided that they are not exaggerated.

BRIEF REVIEW OF METHODS USED FOR SPECIFIC RISK FACTORS

Table 6.1 provides a summary of various methodological aspects of the analyses of burden attributable to the ten major risk factors. This summary of methods and limitations is briefly discussed for each risk factor below.

MALNUTRITION

Mason et al. (1996) have developed estimates of the burden of disease attributable to the physiological state of undernutrition. Using data from 55 studies on the relative risk of mortality as a function of the standard deviation (SD) of nutritional status, they estimated the relative risk per SD for each region. The proportion of the population who were more than two SDs below the mean in a population distribution of weight-for-age

Table 6.1 Summary of methodological differences in the procedures used to estimate the attributable burden from ten major risk factors

Risk Factor	Type of Risk Factor		Relative Risk Controlled for Confounding	Measure of Exposure	Reference Distribution of Exposure	Time Lag from Exposure to Burden
	Exposure	Physiological State				
Malnutrition		■		Population less than 2 SDs weight-for-age based on extensive national surveys	Population weight-for-age higher than minus 2 SDs	Intermediate
Poor water, sanitation, and hygiene	■			Based on the theoretical fecal-oral route of transmission	Zero	Short
Unsafe Sex	■			Based on theoretical model of transmission of STDs and on contraceptive demand surveys for maternal conditions	Zero	Short to Long
Alcohol (disease)	■		■	Indexed on alcohol consumption, non-hepatitis B cirrhosis and alcohol dependence syndrome	Zero	Long
Alcohol (injury)	■			Indexed on estimate of consumption patterns based on small-scale studies	Zero	Short
Occupation (disease)	■			Registration data for EME, FSE and LAC and constant rates for all other regions	Zero	Long
Occupation (injury)	■			Registration data for EME and constant rates for all other regions	Zero	Short
Tobacco	■		■	Indexed on lung cancer	Zero	Long
Hypertension		■		Population surveys of blood pressure	Systolic blood pressure of 110mm Hg	Long
Physical inactivity	■		■	Population surveys of activity patterns	Regular physical activity	Long
Illicit drugs	■			Small-scale studies	Zero	Short to Intermediate
Air pollution	■			Monitoring systems in urban areas for most regions	WHO Guidelines	Short to Long

Note: For alcohol use and occupational exposures, different methods and characteristics apply depending on whether the burden arises from a disease or injury. These characteristics are, therefore, listed separately in the table.

was used to estimate the attributable fraction of child mortality in each region. Similar calculations were undertaken for morbidity, which clearly shows lower relative risks and attributable fractions. No attempt was made to calculate the burden attributable to mild undernutrition, i.e. the population between one and two SDs below the mean.

Mason et al. (1996) were unable to find studies on the relative risk of mortality from undernutrition for adults and thus calculated the burden of disease attributable to undernutrition for the population aged 5 44 years by assuming that the relative risks for children aged 0-4 years were applicable to this adolescent and adult population as well. Unfortunately, no convincing evidence has been collected to support this relationship; in fact recent studies suggest that significantly underweight adult women have lower mortality than heavier women (Manson et al. 1995). We have, therefore, only included the attributable burden estimated for children in the summary tables prepared for this chapter.

POOR WATER SUPPLY, SANITATION AND PERSONAL AND DOMESTIC HYGIENE PRACTICES

Huttly (1996) has reviewed the extensive literature on the role of poor water, sanitation and hygiene practices in causing diarrhoea, ascariasis, trichuriasis and dracunculiasis. Attributable fractions for each condition have been based largely on the theoretical effects of interrupting the faecal-oral route of transmission for diarrhoea and intestinal helminths. The estimates presented in this chapter are thus based on a reference distribution with zero exposure to poor water, sanitation or hygiene practices. Huttly has also estimated attributable fractions using a feasible reference distribution based on population intervention studies (Huttly 1996).

UNSAFE SEX

Berkley et al. (1996) have estimated the burden attributable to unsafe sex by using an attributable fraction approach for selected causes. One hundred per cent of the burden of sexually transmitted diseases, as reported in the GBD, has been assigned to this exposure, in addition to the burden of sexually transmitted diseases that appears under other categories in the primary GBD tabulations, such as ectopic pregnancy. The estimates also include fractions of HIV, hepatitis B and cervical cancer (caused by human papilloma virus) that can be attributed to sexual transmission.

Berkley et al. (1996) chose to estimate the burden of maternal conditions attributable to unsafe sex by first estimating the proportion of "unwanted births" based on the results of various contraceptive demand surveys. The maternal risks associated with unwanted fertility were then included in the estimates of attributable burden. (One-hundred per cent of abortions were included and the unwanted fertility method was used for other forms of maternal mortality and disability as well).

Tobacco

To estimate the burden attributed to tobacco, we have used a modification of the method first proposed by Peto and Lopez (Peto et al. 1994). Relative risks of death from lung cancer for smokers versus lifelong non-smokers, upper aero-digestive cancers, other cancers, chronic obstructive pulmonary disease (COPD), cardiovascular diseases, and other medical causes were taken from the second American Cancer Society Cancer Prevention Study (CPS-II), a prospective study with follow-up restricted to the years 1984-1988. In the case of tobacco use, self-reports are historically inaccurate. Moreover, current prevalence is not a good proxy for cumulative exposure, which largely determines relative risk for various diseases. Peto et al. (1994) recognized that, in developed countries at least, non-smoker lung cancer rates are low, stable and similar for men and women. Excess lung cancer incidence over and above this level is then an excellent biological assay of cumulative past exposure to the effects of tobacco. This excess lung cancer rate was then used as a guide to estimating what proportion of various other smoking-related diseases should be attributed to smoking. To do this, first a Smoking Impact Ratio (SIR) was calculated, defined as:

$$SIR = \frac{C_{LC} - N_{LC}}{S_{LC} - N_{LC}}$$

where C_{LC} is the observed lung cancer rate in a given age group in a population, N_{LC} is the non-smoker lung cancer rate observed in the CPS-II study population, and S_{LC} is the smoker lung cancer rate in CPS-II.

To correct for potential confounding of the estimated relative risks for smokers, the excess risk due to tobacco from all diseases other than lung cancer was halved so that:

$$RR^* = 1 + \frac{RR - 1}{2}$$

This modified relative risk and the SIR were then used in the classical attributable risk formula to estimate the attributable fraction for each age-sex group for all smoking-related cause. In causes other than lung cancer, the SIR is used in the attributable fraction formula as a surrogate for the prevalence of exposure.

This basic approach has been used to calculate tobacco-attributable mortality by region, using the cause-of-death results from the GBD. Because non-smoker lung cancer rates are higher in China and OAI than in the United States (Parkin et al. 1994), we have used an alternative method for these two regions. Preliminary results from a large case-control study in China were used to estimate the attributable fractions for China and OAI (R. Peto, personal communication, 1996). In addition, deaths from tobacco chewing among women in India were estimated using the attributable fractions reported by Notani et al. (1989). Further details on the application of these methods are provided in Murray and Lopez (1996d).

The attributable burden from tobacco has also been projected to the year 2020 using two methods. First, the projection model described in Chapter 7 in this volume (Murray and Lopez 1996b) includes a smoking impact variable defined as the lung-cancer rate minus the non-smoker lung cancer rate for each age group based on evidence from CPS-II and other studies. The impact of smoking can be estimated by setting the smoking intensity variable equal to zero for each time period and recalculating projected mortality and burden. In addition to this econometric approach to estimating the future burden of tobacco, the method described above was also applied to the projected mortality rates. Projected SIRs were calculated using the projected lung cancer rates from the GBD and the estimated attributable fractions applied to the projected death rates of each tobacco-related cause see Chapter 7 in this volume for a discussion of how lung cancer rates were projected on the basis of current levels of tobacco consumption (Murray and Lopez 1996b).

ALCOHOL

For the analysis of attributable burden due to alcohol, Murray and Lopez (1996a) have separated the health effects of alcohol into three components: the deleterious effect of alcohol on injuries, the deleterious effect of alcohol on disease, and the protective effect of alcohol on ischaemic heart disease. The reference distribution used for assessing the burden of alcohol from all three components was zero consumption.

The analysis of the fraction of injury mortality attributable to alcohol was based on the extensive review of published studies and clinical case series on the effects of alcohol on disease and injury, published by English et al. (1995). For EME, we have used the results of this meta-analysis to estimate the attributable fraction for each form of injury. For other regions, these attributable fractions were simply scaled to reflect different regional levels of consumption and estimated differences in drinking patterns, using similar principles to those suggested by Peto and Lopez for tobacco (Peto et al. 1994).

Deaths and disability from various diseases attributable to alcohol consumption have been estimated separately. For EME, the attributable fractions estimated in the meta-analysis by English et al. (1995) were used. For other regions, we have scaled these attributable fractions to reflect differences in alcohol consumption. Our estimates of alcohol consumption have been based on estimated per capita consumption by country, cirrhosis death rates (excluding cirrhosis deaths attributed to hepatitis B) and deaths coded to alcohol dependence. In all regions, we estimated what fraction of cirrhosis of the liver was attributable to hepatitis B, and then applied the scaled attributable fractions for alcohol to the non-hepatitis B cirrhosis rate.

There is consistent evidence from large-scale prospective studies, including the British Doctor's Study (Doll et al. 1994), CPS-I (Boffetta and Garfinkel 1990), CPS-II (Thun et al. 1995), and from case-control studies (e.g. Jackson et al. 1991), that after correcting for smoking, alcohol con-

Figure 6.2   Multivariate relative risks and 95 per cent confidence
                   intervals for coronary heart disease mortality according to
                   alcohol intake: preliminary results from CPS-II, United
                   States

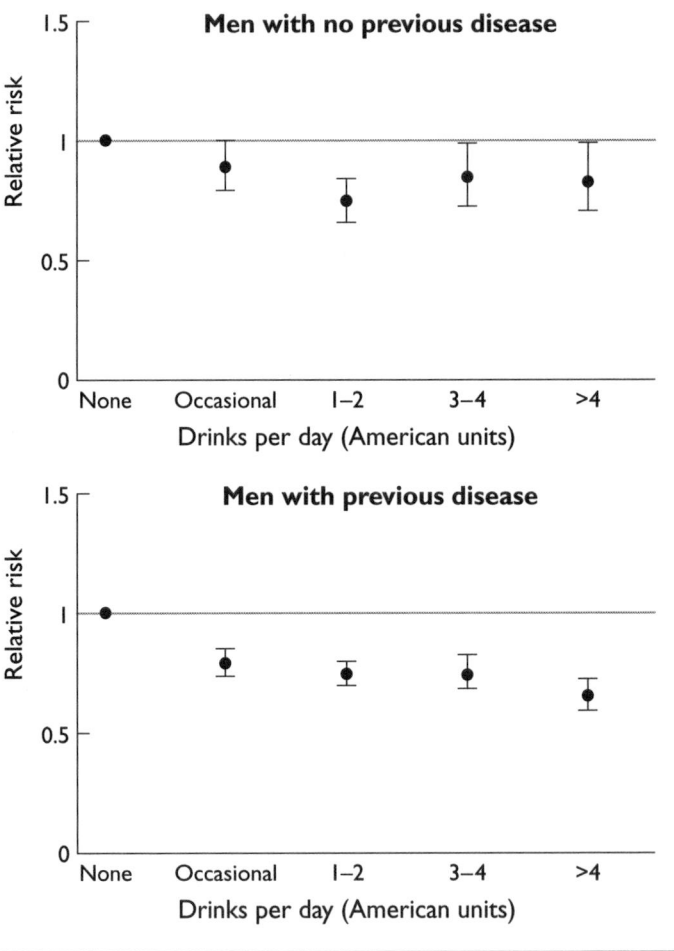

Source: Thun et al. (1995)

sumption exerts a protective effect on cardiovascular death at all levels of
consumption.[3] Figure 6.2 shows this relationship for males with and without previous disease based on data from CPS-II (see Thun et al. 1995). The
protective effect of alcohol was estimated for each region using the relative risk of death from ischaemic heart disease and scaled estimates of the
proportion of the population that abstains from drinking.

OCCUPATION

To estimate the injury burden attributable to occupational exposures, Leigh et al. (1996) used direct reports on occupation-related injuries in Scandinavia to arrive at minimum occupational injury rates for each region. The incidence rates were scaled based on small-scale published studies and other registration sources. For occupational diseases, data from reporting systems were available for the United States, Canada, Australia, Sweden, Denmark, the United Kingdom, Switzerland, Luxembourg, Hungary, Mexico and China (selected causes only). For most of the working population in countries without registration systems, the reported rates from Canada and Australia were used to estimate occupational disease death rates. By inference, the reference distribution of exposure is defined as a population without occupational injuries or diseases.

HYPERTENSION

Nichols and Elliott (1996) reviewed over 50 population-based studies (including a number of multi-centre studies) to estimate the distributions of systolic and diastolic blood pressure by region, age and sex. Relative risks of death for different levels of blood pressure were estimated using logistic regression analysis of data from 18 studies. The reference distribution used was a systolic blood pressure of 110mm Hg. Relative risks were estimated for ischaemic heart disease, cerebrovascular disease, cardiovascular disease (which includes ischaemic heart disease and cerebrovascular disease) and all-cause mortality. There are three ways we could estimate the burden attributable to hypertension based on their results: using the attributable fractions for all-cause mortality, using the attributable fractions for cardiovascular diseases (thus ignoring deaths from other causes attributable to hypertension), or using the attributable fractions for ischaemic heart disease and cerebrovascular disease to estimate the burden of each due to hypertension. Given the regional variation in cause-of-death structure, we have opted for the third method, so that our estimates of attributable burden due to hypertension are based on the attributable fractions for ischaemic heart disease and cerebrovascular disease, as estimated by Nichols and Elliott (1996).

PHYSICAL INACTIVITY

Pratt and Koplan (1996) have analysed the burden of disease attributable to physical inactivity, using a standard attributable risk approach. Age- and sex-specific relative risks for ischaemic heart disease, colon cancer and diabetes have been estimated based on a review of published studies. To control for confounding, the excess risk from inactivity has been halved in developing regions, a similar correction to that used for tobacco. The prevalence of inactivity has been estimated based on a review of population-based surveys of physical activity levels for each region. The reference distribution of exposure is a population where one hundred per cent of individuals are physically active on a regular basis. Because only three important causes related to inactivity have been evaluated, and because excess risk has been halved for developing countries, the estimates of burden attributable to inactivity are probably conservative.

ILLICIT DRUGS

The global burden of illicit drugs has been estimated by Donoghoe et al. (1996) based on estimated population-attributable fractions for HIV, hepatitis B, conditions arising during the perinatal period, protein-energy malnutrition, drug use, road traffic accidents, poisonings, self-inflicted injuries and violence. The attributable fractions for each region have been based on a review of the published literature about the health hazards of illicit drug use (see English et al. 1995) and, in the absence of local prevalence studies, on the estimated number of illicit drug users in each region. The reference distribution used was zero consumption of illicit drugs. Because of the great difficulties in reliably estimating prevalence of illicit drug use, and of reliably quantifying its health effects, the estimates for this risk factor may well be too low.

AIR POLLUTION

Hong et al. (1996) have analysed the burden attributable to air pollution by focusing on the contribution of total suspended particulates (TSP) and sulphur dioxide. For both of these air pollutants, there is an extensive literature on the relative risk of death from pneumonia, COPD, cardiovascular causes and all-cause mortality. Data are available on TSP and sulphur dioxide for urban areas in all regions except MEC and SSA. A traditional attributable fraction method was used to estimate the attributable fraction of deaths from pneumonia, COPD, cardiovascular diseases and all causes combined. The reference distribution used was the WHO Air Quality Guidelines for TSP and sulphur dioxide.

RESULTS

Estimates of attributable burden from various risk factors are bound to be very approximate due to the fact that a substantial amount of scientific research in different parts of the world is required before the impact of a particular risk factor can be reliably quantified. For some exposures, such as tobacco, this science is reasonably well advanced, whereas for others, knowledge of the health effects of exposures in different epidemiological environments is much less developed. Comparisons between the attributable burden from different risk factors are thus strongly affected by the extent of the underlying research, quite apart from basic data considerations which are required to assess the exposures of different populations to various hazards.

Table 6.2 provides an overview of the estimated contribution of the ten major risk factors to the global burden of disease in 1990. Malnutrition

Table 6.2 Global burden of disease and injury attributable to selected risk factors, 1990

Risk factor	Deaths (thousands)	As % of total deaths	YLLs (thousands)	As % of total YLLs	YLDs (thousands)	As % of total YLDs	DALYs (thousands)	As % of total DALYs
Malnutrition	5 881	11.7	199 486	22.0	20 089	4.2	219 575	15.9
Poor water supply sanitation and personal and domestic hygiene	2 668	5.3	85 520	9.4	7 872	1.7	93 392	6.8
Unsafe sex	1 095	2.2	27 602	3.0	21 100	4.5	48 702	3.5
Tobacco	3 038	6.0	26 217	2.9	9 965	2.1	36 182	2.6
Alcohol	774	1.5	19 287	2.1	28 400	6.0	47 687	3.5
Occupation	1 129	2.2	22 493	2.5	15 394	3.3	37 887	2.7
Hypertension	2 918	5.8	17 665	1.9	1 411	0.3	19 076	1.4
Physical inactivity	1 991	3.9	11 353	1.3	2 300	0.5	13 653	1.0
Illicit drugs	100	0.2	2 634	0.3	5 834	1.2	8 467	0.6
Air pollution	568	1.1	5 625	0.6	1 630	0.3	7 254	0.5

Source: Authors' estimates are based on data and information contained in individual chapters of Volume IX of the *Global Burden of Disease and Injury Series.*

is, not surprisingly, the risk factor responsible for the greatest loss of DALYs (about 16 per cent) globally, followed by the combination of poor water supply, poor sanitation and poor personal hygiene (collectively about 7 per cent). Unsafe sex and alcohol use each cause approximately 3.5 per cent of burden while occupational hazards and tobacco are each estimated to cause between 2.0 and 3.0 per cent of DALYs worldwide, roughly equivalent to the burden of measles or tuberculosis. Of the ten risk factors evaluated, air pollution and illicit drug use appear to be the least significant, each causing about 0.5 per cent of global DALYs. Nevertheless, these exposures are estimated to cause as much burden as stomach cancer, liver cancer or syphilis.

Notwithstanding the possibility that the sum of the attributable fractions for any disease or injury could exceed one hundred per cent, the combination of all ten risk factors included here accounts for approximately 40 per cent of deaths and DALYs worldwide in 1990. In the developed regions, the pattern of risk factors is substantially different from the global pattern. The leading risk factor in EME and FSE in 1990 was tobacco, accounting for 12 per cent of total burden in these regions, closely followed by alcohol, which accounts for an estimated 10 per cent. Three risk factors hypertension, occupation and physical inactivity each appear to explain 4 to 5 per cent of burden. The two leading risk factors in developing regions malnutrition and poor water, sanitation and hygiene are the least important in the developed regions.

Summary results from the application of the methods described in Table 6.1 are shown in Tables 6.3–6.12. A very brief overview of some of the major findings for each risk factor is given below.

Table 6.3   Burden of disease and injury attributable to malnutrition, 1990

Region	Deaths (thousands)	As % of total deaths	YLLs (thousands)	As % of total YLLs	YLDs (thousands)	As % of total YLDs	DALYs (thousands)	As % of total DALYs
EME	0.0	0.0	0	0.0	0	0.0	0	0.0
FSE	0.0	0.0	0	0.0	0	0.0	0	0.0
IND	1 722.0	18.4	58 086	29.0	6 450	7.4	64 536	22.4
CHN	278.0	3.1	9 366	7.9	1 781	2.0	11 147	5.3
OAI	679.0	12.3	23 037	20.1	2 721	4.3	25 758	14.5
SSA	2 619.0	31.9	89 305	39.4	7 129	10.4	96 434	32.7
LAC	135.0	4.5	4 540	8.1	520	1.2	5 059	5.1
MEC	447.0	9.8	15 152	14.4	1 489	3.3	16 641	11.0
World	**5 881.0**	**11.7**	**199 486**	**22.0**	**20 089**	**4.2**	**219 575**	**15.9**
Developed regions	*0.0*	*0.0*	*0*	*0.0*	*0*	*0.0*	*0*	*0.0*
Developing regions	*5 881.0*	*14.9*	*199 486*	*24.3*	*20 089*	*5.1*	*219 575*	*18.0*

Source: Authors' estimates are based on data and information given in Mason et al. (1996).

Table 6.4   Burden of disease and injury attributable to poor water supply, sanitation and personal and domestic hygiene, 1990

Region	Deaths (thousands)	As % of total deaths	YLLs (thousands)	As % of total YLLs	YLDs (thousands)	As % of total YLDs	DALYs (thousands)	As % of total DALYs
EME	1.1	0.0	8	0.0	92	0.2	101	0.1
FSE	2.4	0.1	75	0.2	53	0.2	128	0.2
IND	839.9	9.0	25 993	13.0	1 470	1.7	27 463	9.5
CHN	81.4	0.9	1 975	1.7	2 256	2.5	4 231	2.0
OAI	354.3	6.4	11 693	10.2	1 499	2.4	13 192	7.4
SSA	875.6	10.7	28 781	12.7	1 088	1.6	29 870	10.1
LAC	135.3	4.5	4 254	7.6	929	2.2	5 183	5.3
MEC	378.2	8.3	12 740	12.1	484	1.1	13 224	8.8
World	**2 668.2**	**5.3**	**85 520**	**9.4**	**7 872**	**1.7**	**93 392**	**6.8**
Developed regions	*3.5*	*0.0*	*83*	*0.1*	*146*	*0.2*	*229*	*0.1*
Developing regions	*2 664.7*	*6.7*	*85 436*	*10.4*	*7 726*	*1.9*	*93 163*	*7.6*

Source: Authors' estimates are based on data and information given in Huttly (1996).

Table 6.5   Burden of disease and injury attributable to unsafe sex, 1990

Region	Deaths (thousands)	As % of total deaths	YLLs (thousands)	As % of total YLLs	YLDs (thousands)	As % of total YLDs	DALYs (thousands)	As % of total DALYs
EME	53.6	0.8	1 271	2.6	687	1.4	1 957	2.0
FSE	33.1	0.9	756	2.1	613	2.3	1 369	2.2
IND	222.5	2.4	5 755	2.9	5 769	6.6	11 525	4.0
CHN	42.6	0.5	684	0.6	196	0.2	879	0.4
OAI	134.3	2.4	3 838	3.3	4 047	6.4	7 885	4.4
SSA	482.9	5.9	12 226	5.4	6 918	10.1	19 144	6.5
LAC	73.9	2.5	2 003	3.6	1 642	3.9	3 645	3.7
MEC	51.6	1.1	1 070	1.0	1 228	2.7	2 298	1.5
World	**1 094.5**	**2.2**	**27 602**	**3.0**	**21 100**	**4.5**	**48 702**	**3.5**
Developed regions	*86.8*	*0.8*	*2 026*	*2.4*	*1 300*	*1.7*	*3 326*	*2.1*
Developing regions	*1 007.7*	*2.5*	*25 576*	*3.1*	*19 800*	*5.0*	*45 376*	*3.7*

Source: Authors' estimates are based on data and information given in Berkley et al. (1996).

Table 6.6 Burden of disease and injury attributable to tobacco use, 1990

Region	Deaths (thousands)	As % of total deaths	YLLs (thousands)	As % of total YLLs	YLDs (thousands)	As % of total YLDs	DALYs (thousands)	As % of total DALYs
EME	1 062.6	14.9	7 967	16.0	3 640	7.4	11 607	11.7
FSE	514.7	13.6	5 869	16.3	1 934	7.4	7 803	12.5
IND	128.9	1.4	1 366	0.7	353	0.4	1 719	0.6
CHN	820.2	9.2	5 752	4.9	2 326	2.6	8 078	3.9
OAI	222.9	4.0	1 996	1.7	643	1.0	2 638	1.5
SSA	77.9	0.9	927	0.4	290	0.4	1 217	0.4
LAC	99.4	3.3	952	1.7	388	0.9	1 340	1.4
MEC	111.1	2.4	1 387	1.3	392	0.9	1 779	1.2
World	**3 037.6**	**6.0**	**26 217**	**2.9**	**9 965**	**2.1**	**36 182**	**2.6**
Developed regions	*1 577.3*	*14.5*	*13 836*	*16.2*	*5 574*	*7.4*	*19 410*	*12.1*
Developing regions	*1 460.4*	*3.7*	*12 381*	*1.5*	*4 391*	*1.1*	*16 772*	*1.4*

Source: Authors' estimates are based on data and information given in Murray and Lopez (1996d).

Table 6.7 Burden of disease and injury attributable to alcohol use, 1990

Region	Deaths (thousands)	As % of total deaths	YLLs (thousands)	As % of total YLLs	YLDs (thousands)	As % of total YLDs	DALYs (thousands)	As % of total DALYs
EME	83.8	1.2	2 537	5.1	7 667	15.6	10 204	10.3
FSE	53.0	1.4	2 063	5.7	3 130	11.9	5 193	8.3
IND	112.9	1.2	2 723	1.4	1 974	2.3	4 697	1.6
CHN	114.1	1.3	2 118	1.8	2 737	3.0	4 856	2.3
OAI	97.4	1.8	1 862	1.6	3 191	5.1	5 053	2.8
SSA	170.7	2.1	4 435	2.0	3 169	4.6	7 603	2.6
LAC	136.1	4.5	3 319	5.9	6 201	14.7	9 520	9.7
MEC	5.6	0.1	229	0.2	437	1.0	666	0.4
World	**773.6**	**1.5**	**19 287**	**2.1**	**28 400**	**6.0**	**47 687**	**3.5**
Developed regions	*136.8*	*1.3*	*4 601*	*5.4*	*10 797*	*14.3*	*15 398*	*9.6*
Developing regions	*636.8*	*1.6*	*14 686*	*1.8*	*17 603*	*4.4*	*32 289*	*2.7*

Source: Authors' estimates are based on data and information given in Murray and Lopez (1996a).

Table 6.8 Burden of disease and injury attributable to occupation, 1990

Region	Deaths (thousands)	As % of total deaths	YLLs (thousands)	As % of total YLLs	YLDs (thousands)	As % of total YLDs	DALYs (thousands)	As % of total DALYs
EME	154.0	2.2	2 826	5.7	2 144	4.4	4 971	5.0
FSE	76.2	2.0	1 409	3.9	951	3.6	2 359	3.8
IND	185.2	2.0	3 671	1.8	2 159	2.5	5 830	2.0
CHN	247.1	2.8	4 937	4.2	3 295	3.6	8 232	3.9
OAI	148.1	2.7	3 060	2.7	1 940	3.1	5 001	2.8
SSA	111.8	1.4	2 323	1.0	1 537	2.2	3 860	1.3
LAC	97.7	3.2	1 973	3.5	1 708	4.1	3 681	3.7
MEC	109.2	2.4	2 294	2.2	1 659	3.6	3 954	2.6
World	**1 129.3**	**2.2**	**22 493**	**2.5**	**15 394**	**3.3**	**37 887**	**2.7**
Developed regions	*230.1*	*2.1*	*4 235*	*4.9*	*3 095*	*4.1*	*7 330*	*4.6*
Developing regions	*899.1*	*2.3*	*18 258*	*2.2*	*12 299*	*3.1*	*30 557*	*2.5*

Source: Authors' estimates are based on data and information given in Leigh et al. (1996).

Table 6.9   Burden of disease and injury attributable to hypertension, 1990

Region	Deaths (thousands)	As % of total deaths	YLLs (thousands)	As % of total YLLs	YLDs (thousands)	As % of total YLDs	DALYs (thousands)	As % of total DALYs
EME	789.0	11.1	3 471	7.0	411	0.8	3 882	3.9
FSE	616.8	16.3	3 440	9.6	256	1.0	3 696	5.9
IND	369.1	3.9	2 568	1.3	130	0.1	2 697	0.9
CHN	288.4	3.2	1 934	1.6	144	0.2	2 077	1.0
OAI	57.8	1.0	440	0.4	40	0.1	480	0.3
SSA	203.1	2.5	1 789	0.8	128	0.2	1 917	0.6
LAC	242.5	8.1	1 674	3.0	134	0.3	1 808	1.8
MEC	351.3	7.7	2 351	2.2	169	0.4	2 520	1.7
World	**2 918.0**	**5.8**	**17 665**	**1.9**	**1 411**	**0.3**	**19 076**	**1.4**
Developed regions	*1 405.7*	*12.9*	*6 911*	*8.1*	*667*	*0.9*	*7 577*	*4.7*
Developing regions	*1 512.3*	*3.8*	*10 754*	*1.3*	*745*	*0.2*	*11 499*	*0.9*

Source: Authors' estimates are based on data and information given in Nichols and Elliott (1996).

Table 6.10   Burden of disease and injury attributable to physical inactivity, 1990

Region	Deaths (thousands)	As % of total deaths	YLLs (thousands)	As % of total YLLs	YLDs (thousands)	As % of total YLDs	DALYs (thousands)	As % of total DALYs
EME	833.1	11.7	3 860	7.8	862	1.8	4 722	4.8
FSE	266.2	7.0	1 482	4.1	249	0.9	1 731	2.8
IND	338.1	3.6	2 377	1.2	447	0.5	2 824	1.0
CHN	229.1	2.6	1 383	1.2	260	0.3	1 643	0.8
OAI	63.2	1.1	464	0.4	106	0.2	570	0.3
SSA	4.6	0.1	38	0.0	8	0.0	46	0.0
LAC	117.6	3.9	796	1.4	173	0.4	969	1.0
MEC	139.7	3.1	954	0.9	195	0.4	1 149	0.8
World	**1 991.5**	**3.9**	**11 353**	**1.3**	**2 300**	**0.5**	**13 653**	**1.0**
Developed regions	*1 099.2*	*10.1*	*5 343*	*6.2*	*1 110*	*1.5*	*6 453*	*4.0*
Developing regions	*892.2*	*2.3*	*6 011*	*0.7*	*1 190*	*0.3*	*7 200*	*0.6*

Source: Authors' estimates are based on data and information given in Pratt and Koplan (1996).

Table 6.11   Burden of disease and injury attributable to illicit drug use, 1990

Region	Deaths (thousands)	As % of total deaths	YLLs (thousands)	As % of total YLLs	YLDs (thousands)	As % of total YLDs	DALYs (thousands)	As % of total DALYs
EME	28.8	0.4	717	1.4	1 598	3.3	2 315	2.3
FSE	9.3	0.2	226	0.6	568	2.2	794	1.3
IND	7.4	0.1	192	0.1	112	0.1	305	0.1
CHN	16.8	0.2	443	0.4	209	0.2	652	0.3
OAI	9.2	0.2	250	0.2	927	1.5	1 177	0.7
SSA	7.8	0.1	223	0.1	382	0.6	605	0.2
LAC	16.0	0.5	449	0.8	1 140	2.7	1 589	1.6
MEC	4.9	0.1	134	0.1	898	2.0	1 031	0.7
World	**100.3**	**0.2**	**2 634**	**0.3**	**5 834**	**1.2**	**8 467**	**0.6**
Developed regions	*38.2*	*0.3*	*943*	*1.1*	*2 166*	*2.9*	*3 108*	*1.9*
Developing regions	*62.1*	*0.2*	*1 691*	*0.2*	*3 668*	*0.9*	*5 359*	*0.4*

Source: Authors' estimates are based on data and information given in Donoghoe et al. (1996).

Table 6.12 Burden of disease and injury attributable to air pollution, 1990

Region	Deaths (thousands)	As % of total deaths	YLLs (thousands)	As % of total YLLs	YLDs (thousands)	As % of total YLDs	DALYs (thousands)	As % of total DALYs
EME	65.1	0.9	310	0.6	169	0.3	478	0.5
FSE	209.9	5.5	1 320	3.7	627	2.4	1 948	3.1
IND	85.7	0.9	1 267	0.6	186	0.2	1 453	0.5
CHN	67.9	0.8	549	0.5	353	0.4	903	0.4
OAI	38.5	0.7	600	0.5	74	0.1	674	0.4
SSA	23.4	0.3	490	0.2	43	0.1	532	0.2
LAC	33.6	1.1	377	0.7	98	0.2	476	0.5
MEC	43.8	1.0	711	0.7	79	0.2	790	0.5
World	**567.9**	**1.1**	**5 625**	**0.6**	**1 630**	**0.3**	**7 254**	**0.5**
Developed regions	*275.0*	*2.5*	*1 630*	*1.9*	*796*	*1.1*	*2 426*	*1.5*
Developing regions	*292.9*	*0.7*	*3 995*	*0.5*	*833*	*0.2*	*4 828*	*0.4*

Source: Authors' estimates are based on data and information given in Hong et al. (1996).

MALNUTRITION

Even limiting the estimates of the burden of disease due to malnutrition to its effects in children, the attributable fraction is a staggering 33 per cent in SSA. In India, where rates of weight-for-height malnutrition are also high but the relative risk of death is lower than in SSA, nearly one-quarter of all disease and injury burden is attributed to malnutrition. In OAI and MEC, malnutrition is less important but still accounts for 10 per cent of DALYs, whereas in LAC and China the role of malnutrition in explaining the burden of disease is much smaller. These estimates are *not* attributable fractions for low caloric intake or low protein intake; nor are they the attributable fractions for infectious disease episodes that contribute to the physiological state of a low weight-for-age child. Rather, they indicate the magnitude of the health gains that might be achieved if, through some unspecified means, the nutritional status of children could be improved such that no child had a weight-for-age more than 2 SDs below the reference population mean. Taking into account the extent to which other socio-economic determinants of health status correlate with nutritional status (e.g. maternal education), these estimates may be biased upwards.

POOR WATER SUPPLY, SANITATION AND PERSONAL AND DOMESTIC HYGIENE

Exposure to poor water and poor sanitation greatly increases the risk of diarrhoeal diseases, and it is through this mechanism that most of the DALYs from this risk factor (which includes personal hygiene) arise. Apparently, and perhaps not surprisingly, the significance of this risk factor in different regions is very similar to that of malnutrition. Thus, the largest proportionate impact on DALYs is in SSA and India, where unsafe water, poor sanitation and personal hygiene are estimated to have caused about 10 per cent of DALYs in 1990. In other developing countries, the impact of this exposure is less important, especially in China (2 per cent of DALYs), and its impact is virtually negligible in EME and FSE.

UNSAFE SEX

In SSA, unsafe sex is estimated to account for over 6 per cent of total disease and injury burden in the region, and between 4 and 5 per cent of regional DALYs in India and OAI. Unlike poor water supply and poor sanitation, unsafe sex is an important risk factor in EME and FSE, accounting for two or more per cent of DALYs in each region. The low attributable fraction from unsafe sex in China may be a reasonable estimate for 1990, but recent trends in the prevalence of sexually transmitted diseases suggest that the burden may have increased since then. Given the strong age-dependence of sexual activity, the impact of this exposure is particularly evident among women of child-bearing age. Thus, in women aged 15-44 years, unsafe sex is estimated to account for 1 per cent of DALYs in China and ranging from 6 per cent in EME to over 30 per cent in SSA.

TOBACCO

Decades of research on the health effects of tobacco have demonstrated that tobacco is a uniquely hazardous product, causing over two dozen diseases, many of which are of major public health concern, including ischaemic heart disease, stroke, and lung cancer. This research has also demonstrated that there is a long delay (typically three to four decades) between the onset of persistent smoking and the development of its full health effects (Lopez et al. 1994). Hence tobacco-attributable DALYs in 1990 largely reflect the health consequences of smoking prior to 1990. The magnitude of the effect on mortality of the massive increase in cigarette consumption in developing countries, particularly during the 1970s and 1980s, will not be experienced for several decades, and will most likely be greatest in the 2020s or 2030s.

Nevertheless, tobacco was already a major cause of DALYs in 1990 in EME and FSE, where cigarette smoking has been widespread for many years. Tobacco is estimated to have caused about 1.8 million deaths in 1990 in these two regions combined.[4] This represents approximately 15 per cent of all deaths in EME and FSE, and about 12 per cent of DALYs, thus making tobacco the most important cause of DALYs in these two regions. Tobacco is not yet a major cause of DALYs in developing regions, simply because populations in these regions have not been smoking long enough to experience the full health effects. As 50 per cent of men in developing regions are currently smokers, and cigarette consumption is steadily rising in these countries (Collishaw and Lopez 1996), tobacco is predicted to be one of the major causes of deaths and DALYs early in the next century.

Because the epidemiology of smoking is well understood, knowledge about current levels of cigarette consumption provides a reasonable guide to the quantification of future health effects. Based on the methods of Peto and Lopez (Peto et al. 1994), future smoking-attributable mortality from

Figure 6.3   DALYs attributable to HIV, tobacco and diarrhoea, 1990 to 2020

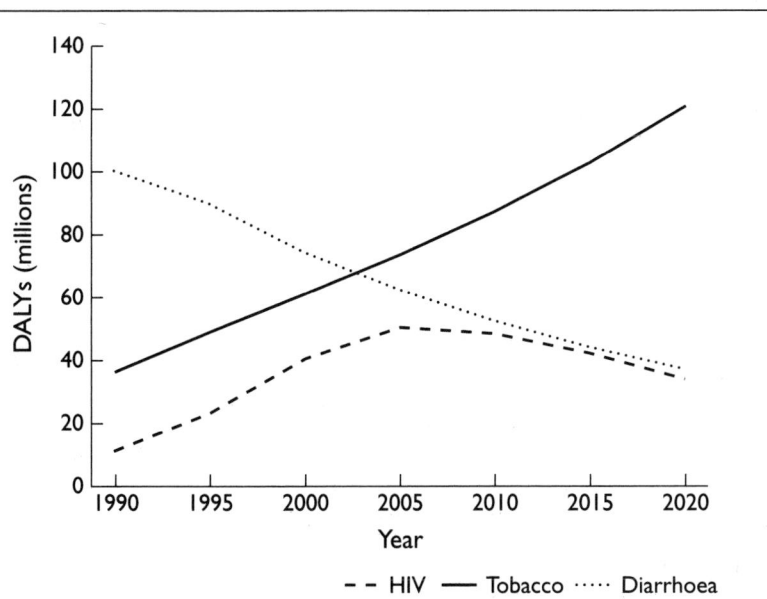

lung cancer and other diseases can be estimated. Figure 6.3 shows how tobacco-attributable deaths and DALYs are predicted to change between now and the year 2020. Annual tobacco-attributable mortality is expected to increase from three million deaths in 1990 to 8.4 million in 2020, with virtually all of this annual increase (4.7 million out of 5.4 million deaths) expected to occur in developing countries. Global DALYs attributed to tobacco are projected to rise from just under 40 million in 1990 (2.6 per cent of all DALYs) to 120 million in 2020 (just under 10 per cent of all DALYs). Indeed, as Figure 6.3 illustrates, by 2020, tobacco is projected to be an even greater cause of DALYs lost than HIV and is projected to exceed DALYs from diarrhoea within the next decade or so (see Murray and Lopez 1996b, Chapter 7 in this volume for more details on projection methods and assumptions). This is, however, just one scenario for HIV and the true impact of the disease may be much greater if assumptions about incidence used here prove to be too optimistic.

ALCOHOL

It is widely recognized that alcohol use can bring both benefits and harms to individuals and, through the externalities described earlier, to society as well. The evidence suggests that alcohol significantly reduces the risk of ischaemic heart disease (and ischaemic stroke) but increases risk for several other diseases (including upper aero-digestive cancers, cirrhosis of the liver, pancreatitis and alcoholic psychoses), and is a major cause of injuries, both intentional and unintentional (see, for example, Anderson et al. 1993). In societies where ischaemic heart disease is common, and injuries and violence are less common, alcohol may prevent about as many deaths as it causes. In populations where the converse is true, i.e. in much of the developing world, alcohol can be expected to have a net detrimental effect on mortality. The net impact of alcohol in terms of Years of Life Lost (YLLs) is more likely to be detrimental because its harmful and protective effects are typically experienced at very different ages (harm tends to be concentrated at younger adult ages and protective effects at older ages). In all regions, alcohol has a net detrimental effect in terms of Years Lived with Disability (YLDs). To illustrate the combined effect of alcohol in different societies, the estimated age-pattern of mortality caused by alcohol is shown in Figure 6.4 for males in EME and SSA, two regions with very different epidemiological profiles. The estimated numbers of deaths caused (and averted) by alcohol are shown for the three broad component causes described earlier in this chapter. In EME, alcohol probably averts almost as many deaths as it causes. However, most of these averted deaths would have occurred at older ages, since ischaemic heart disease is comparatively rare in those aged under 50. As a result, the number of DALYs averted is substantially smaller than the number of DALYs caused by alcohol, particularly from injuries at young adult ages. While the estimated proportion of deaths due to alcohol use is relatively small in EME (about 1 per cent), the contribution of alcohol to DALYs is large (10 per cent), due to the young ages of death and the large number of YLDs attributable to alcohol.

A very different pattern is evident in sub-Saharan Africa, where ischaemic heart disease is still relatively uncommon and hence the protective effect of alcohol is only of marginal public health significance. Conversely, alcohol is a major determinant of death and disability from injuries, quite apart from the social pathologies it causes, such as crime, domestic discord and unemployment, none of which are reflected in DALYs (Parry et al. 1996). As a result, proportionate mortality from alcohol is higher in SSA than in EME (2 versus 1 per cent). The impact of alcohol is even greater in LAC, where almost 5 per cent of deaths and 10 per cent of DALYs are estimated to be attributable to its use. Globally, alcohol is estimated to have caused about three-quarters of a million more deaths than it averted, with more than 80 per cent of this excess mortality occurring in developing countries.

OCCUPATION

Occupational hazards include exposures which lead to disease (e.g. asbestos-induced mesotheliomas) and injury (e.g. falls, drownings, industrial accidents). Over one million people (mostly males) are estimated to have died in 1990 from occupational exposures. The estimated contribution of occupational hazards to DALYs is relatively invariant across regions, being marginally greater in those with better developed health care systems (EME, FSE, China, LAC). However, since attributable burden for this exposure in developing regions is extrapolated from direct observation and monitoring of cases at the workplace in developed regions, it is quite probable that the true impact of occupation as a risk factor has been underestimated in most developing regions.

HYPERTENSION

High blood pressure has been identified as a major risk factor for major cardiovascular diseases, including ischaemic heart disease and stroke (Nichols and Elliott 1996). Although prevalence studies suggest that hy-

Figure 6.4 Deaths attributable to, and averted by, alcohol use, males, EME and SSA, 1990

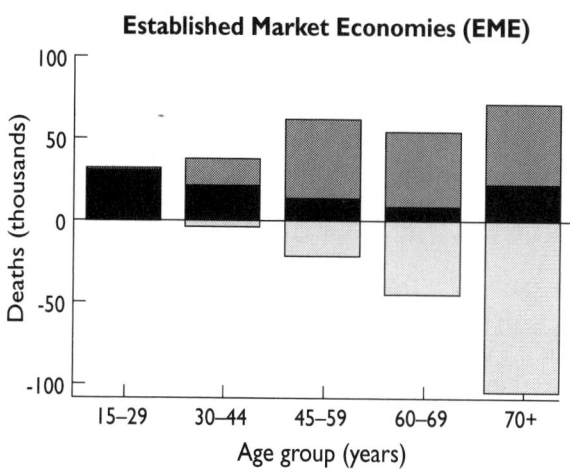

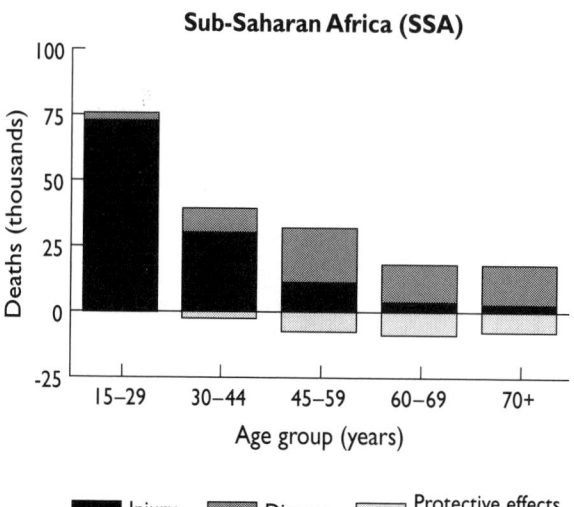

pertension is common among adults in all regions of the world, its public health consequences are greater in wealthier populations. Almost 13 per cent of deaths in EME and FSE are estimated to be due to hypertension. These are observed primarily at older ages, so that between 4 and 6 per cent of DALYs lost in EME and FSE, respectively, in 1990 were attributable to hypertension, substantially more than is estimated for the developing world. Of the developing regions, the largest proportion of DALYs attributable to hypertension in 1990 was 2 per cent (for LAC). The global estimate of 1.4 per cent of all DALYs is thus driven in large part by the comparatively high contributions of EME and FSE.

Physical Inactivity

Physical inactivity is a major cause of burden in the developed countries where the prevalence of a sedentary lifestyle or irregular activity levels is high. Indeed, in EME, physical inactivity is estimated to be a greater cause of burden than hypertension. In other regions, physical inactivity is much less important. The estimates for developing countries, however, are likely to be very conservative, since excess risks for inactivity have been halved, in order to avoid exaggeration of the attributable burden since relatively little is known about the effects of physical inactivity in these populations.

Illicit Drugs

This is one of the most difficult risk factors to quantify, simply because it is extremely difficult to conduct scientific research on an exposure which is illegal. Prospective studies of health hazards from drug use are hampered by the fact that drug users are notoriously difficult to follow up; hence, cohorts can quickly become effectively useless for mortality research. Respondents who use drugs may give evasive and incorrect answers to questionnaires and the population sampled may not be very representative of the general population.

As a result, the attributable burden estimates for illicit drug use are particularly problematic and must be interpreted with great caution. The available data on use and health effects suggest that about 100 000 people died from drug use in 1990, mostly young men. About 30 per cent of these deaths occurred in EME alone, where illicit drug use is estimated to be a significant cause of disease and injury burden (2.3 per cent of DALYs). Of the other regions, only in LAC (1.6 per cent) and FSE (1.2 per cent) do the estimated attributable fractions for drug use exceed 1 per cent of all DALYs. In all regions, more of the burden from drug use arises from YLDs than YLLs, reflecting the substantial social disability associated with drug use.

Air pollution

Exposure to particulates causes respiratory and cardiovascular diseases, resulting in about 500 000 deaths a year. Of these, 210 000 are estimated to occur in FSE, where air pollution accounts for about 3.1 per cent of all

DALYs. In all other regions, the contribution of air pollution to total DALYs is much lower, typically 0.5 per cent or less.

DISCUSSION

Estimating the burden of disease and injury attributable to various exposures or risk factors is intrinsically problematic. Much of the uncertainty is related to the conceptual difficulties in defining what exposures are avoidable. Some would argue that the theoretical contribution of exposure is what matters, irrespective of which might or might not be feasible to avoid. In the case of tobacco, any exposure is hazardous and hence the theoretically appropriate comparison is with a zero exposure population, although there are no known populations (with the exception of specific religious groups) where this has been, or is likely to be, achieved. Even where the conceptual framework for assessing attributable burden has been adequately defined, lack of data, particularly on hazards in developing countries, make quantification of attributable burden extremely difficult. In this case, it is very important to be conservative in estimating attributable fractions due to exposures or risk factors, particularly in view of the likelihood that exposure to different hazards may act synergistically to increase risk.

There are major obstacles to quantifying reliably the burden of ill-health due to risk factors. However, in order to ensure that these exposures are given the same consideration as disease and injury in the public health policy debate, it is essential that estimates of their current and future public health impact be made. In this chapter we have interpreted and summarized the first results of a comparative assessment of the impact of ten major health hazards in 1990. We have done so fully aware of the uncertainties around both the science and the information base required to estimate attributable burden. These results must be seen as approximate, but they are nonetheless provocative. What they suggest is that some exposures, particularly malnutrition, poor water and other hygiene-related factors, remain a major cause of disease burden, accounting for as much, if not more, of the global burden of disease as more widely-publicized health problems, such as malaria, measles, tuberculosis and maternal conditions. Other risk factors, particularly occupational exposures, alcohol, unsafe sex and tobacco, also accounted for a significant number of DALYs globally in 1990, and deserve a commensurate response from the global public-health community. In particular, DALYs attributable to tobacco are projected to triple between 1990 and 2020. The epidemic of tobacco-induced disease has become a global public health emergency, requiring concerted action at all levels of the health system.

Despite the very real and substantial methodological problems in calculating comparable and reliable estimates of burden attributable to various exposures, we remain convinced that such quantification must be attempted if epidemiology is to contribute effectively to the improvement of public health. Effective advocacy, health promotion and disease prevention require plausible information about the causes of disease and injury. Public health will be better served if we know not only that a particular exposure is hazardous, but also the comparative magnitude of that hazard compared with other health concerns. In this chapter, we have made a first attempt to estimate the probable magnitude of certain major health hazards in the early 1990s. This is a difficult undertaking, often going beyond the limits of what good data and science can irrefutably support. The estimates presented here are thus approximate, but have been presented nonetheless to stimulate urgently needed research about hazards of various exposures in various populations, and to focus debate about appropriate policy responses.

NOTES

1 Estimates of causes of death on the other hand, are constrained to sum to the total number of deaths estimated for a given population group.

2 For example, between CPS-I (1959 65) and CPS-II (1982 88), the relative risk of lung cancer for current smokers compared with lifelong non-smokers increased from 11.4 to 22.4 for males, and from 2.7 to 11.9 for females, reflecting rising hazards with longer exposure (in this case, duration of smoking) (U.S. Department of Health and Human Services 1989).

3 There is also evidence to suggest (see Doll et al. 1994) that alcohol is also protective for ischaemic stroke, but increases the risk of suffering a haemorrhagic stroke at higher intake levels. Since disaggregated estimates of stroke could not be made from the available data for all regions in the GBD, we have not been able to include the beneficial effects of alcohol on stroke in our estimates. The extent to which the opposing effects of alcohol on stroke counter-balance one another would obviously depend on consumption levels and patterns, and on the relative importance of ischaemic versus haemorrhagic stroke in different regions.

4 These estimates differ slightly from the regional totals estimated by Peto et al. (1994) for 1990 in view of differences in the country composition of regions and adjustments made in the GBD to cause-of-death data from countries (see Murray and Lopez 1996c, Chapter 3 in this volume).

BIBLIOGRAPHY

Anderson P et al. (1993) The risk of alcohol. *Addiction* 88:1493–1508.

Beaglehole R, Bonita R, Kjellstrom T (1993) *Basic epidemiology*. Geneva: World Health Organization.

Berkley S et al. (1996) Unsafe sex. In: Murray CJL, Lopez AD, eds. *Quantifying global health risks: the burden of disease attributable to selected risk factors*. Cambridge, Harvard University Press.

Boffetta P and Garfinkel L (1990) Alcohol drinking and mortality among men enrolled in an American Cancer Society Prospective Study. *Epidemiology,* 1:342–438.

Collishaw NE and Lopez AD (1996) The tobacco epidemic: a global public health emergency. *Tobacco Alert.* Geneva, World Health Organization.

Doll R et al. (1994) Mortality in relation to consumption of alcohol: 13 years' observations on male British doctors. *British Medical* Journal, 309:911–918.

Donoghoe M et al. (1996) Illicit drugs. In: Murray CJL, Lopez AD, eds. *Quantifying global health risks: the burden of disease attributable to selected risk factors.* Cambridge, Harvard University Press.

English DR et al. (1995) *The quantification of drug caused morbidity and mortality in Australia.* Commonwealth Department of Human Services and Health, Canberra, Australia.

Hill AB (1965) The environment and disease: association or causation. *Proceedings of the Royal Society of Medicine,* 58:295–300.

Holman CDJ and English DR (1996) Ought low alcohol intake be promoted for health reasons? *Journal of the Royal Society of Medicine,* 89:123–129.

Hong CJ et al. (1996) Air pollution. In: Murray CJL, Lopez AD, eds. *Quantifying global health risks: the burden of disease attributable to selected risk factors.* Cambridge, Harvard University Press.

Huttly S (1996) Water, sanitation and personal hygiene. In: Murray CJL, Lopez AD, eds. *Quantifying global health risks: the burden of disease attributable to selected risk factors.* Cambridge, Harvard University Press.

Jackson R, Saragg R and Beaglehole R (1991) Alcohol consumption and risk of coronary heart disease. *British Medical Journal,* 303:211–216.

Koplan JP and Pratt M (1996) Physical inactivity. In: Murray CJL, Lopez AD, eds. *Quantifying global health risks: the burden of disease attributable to selected risk factors.* Cambridge, Harvard University Press.

Leigh J et al. (1996) Occupational hazards. In: Murray CJL, Lopez AD, eds. *Quantifying global health risks: the burden of disease attributable to selected risk factors.* Cambridge, Harvard University Press.

Lopez AD, Collishaw NE and Piha T (1994) A descriptive model of the cigarette epidemic in developed countries. *Tobacco Control,* 3:242–247.

Manson JE et al. (1995) Body weight and mortality among women, *New England Journal of Medicine,* 333:677–685.

Marmot M (1995) Social differentials in mortality: the Whitehall Studies. pp. 143–260 in Lopez AD, Caselli G and Valkonen T, eds. *Adult Mortality in Developed Countries: from Description to Explanation.* Oxford: Clarendon Press.

Mason JB et al. (1996) Undernutrition. In: Murray CJL, Lopez AD, eds. *Malnutrition and the burden of disease: the global epidemiology of protein-energy malnutrition, anaemias and viatamin deficiencies.* Cambridge, Harvard University Press.

Miettenen OS (1974) Proportion of disease caused or prevented by a given exposure, trail or intervention. *American Journal of Epidemiology,* 99:325–332.

Murray CJL and Lopez AD (1996a) Alcohol. In: Murray CJL, Lopez AD, eds. *Quantifying global health risks: the burden of disease attributable to selected risk factors.* Cambridge, Harvard University Press.

Murray CJL and Lopez AD (1996b) Alternative visions of the future: projecting mortality and disability, 1990 2020. In: Murray CJL, Lopez AD, eds. *The global burden of disease: a comprehensive assessment of mortality and disability from diseases, injuries, and risk factors in 1990 and projected to 2020.* Cambridge, Harvard University Press.

Murray CJL and Lopez AD (1996c) Estimating causes of death: methods and global and regional applications for 1990. In: Murray CJL , Lopez AD, eds. *The global burden of disease: a comprehensive assesment of mortality and disability from diseases, injuries, and risk factors in 1990 and projected to 2020.* Cambridge, Harvard University Press.

Murray CJL and Lopez AD (1996d) Tobacco. In: Murray CJL, Lopez AD, eds. *Quantifying global health risks: the burden of disease attributable to selected risk factors.* Cambridge, Harvard University Press.

Nichols SR and Elliott P (1996) Hypertension. In: Murray CJL, Lopez AD, eds. *Quantifying global health risks: the burden of disease attributable to selected risk factors.* Cambridge, Harvard University Press.

Notani PN, Jayant K and Sanghvi LD (1989) Assessment of morbidity and mortality due to tobacco usage in India: pp. 63 78. In: Sanghvi LD and Notani PN, eds. *Tobacco and Health: the Indian Scene* Bombay, International Union Against Cancer (UICC).

Parkin DM et al. (1994) At least one in seven cases of cancer is caused by smoking: global estimates for 1985. *International Journal of Cancer,* 59:494–504.

Parry C et al. (1996) Alcohol attributable fractions for trauma in South Africa. *Curationis,* 19:1–5.

Peto R et al. (1994) *Mortality from smoking in developed countries 1950 2000.* Oxford: Oxford University Press.

Pierce JP et al. (1989) Trends in cigarette smoking in the United States: educational differences are increasing *Journal of the American Medical Association,* 261:56–60.

Poikolainen J (1995) Alcohol and mortality: a review. *Journal of Clinical Epidemiology,* 48(4):455–465.

Pratt M and Koplan J (1996) Physical inactivity. In: Murray CJL, Lopez AD, eds. *Quantifying global health risks: the burden of disease attributable to selected risk factors.* Cambridge, Harvard University Press.

Thun M et al. (1995) Alcohol and Mortality in the American Cancer Society Cancer Prevention Study-II (CPS-II). Paper presented at the WHO working group on Alcohol and Health: Implications for Public Health Policy, Oslo, 9-13 October 1995.

U.S. Department of Health and Human Services (1989) *Reducing the Health Consequences of Smoking: 25 Years of Progress. A Report of the Surgeon General U.S. Department of Health and Human Services, Public Health Service, Centers for Disease Control, Center for Chronic Disease Prevention and Health Promotion, Office on Smoking and Health.* DHHS Publication No. (CDC) 89 8411.

Chapter 7

ALTERNATIVE VISIONS OF THE FUTURE: PROJECTING MORTALITY AND DISABILITY, 1990–2020

CHRISTOPHER J. L. MURRAY
ALAN D. LOPEZ

Future health scenarios that are likely, probable or merely possible can play an important role in shaping public policy. The extensive literature on health projections (see, for example, Bezold 1994, Garrett 1993, Taket 1993) provides one indication of the strong interest on the part of the scientific and public health communities in defining and quantifying future health scenarios. As part of the Global Burden of Disease Study (GBD), a variety of alternative scenarios of future burden of disease and injury have been developed which may have important public policy implications.

In this chapter, we begin by briefly reviewing some of the prior efforts at projecting future health status, focusing on the strengths and weaknesses of the various approaches. Based on this review, we outline the approach we have taken to develop projections of mortality and disability over the period 1990–2020 by age, sex, region and cause. We have opted to use a set of simple models where age-, sex- and cause-specific mortality rates are a function of socio-economic variables. The parameter estimates for these models have been derived using a panel of empirical age-, sex- and cause-specific mortality rates covering the period 1950–1990 from countries with good vital registration systems. Crude assumptions about the relationship between incidence and duration of disability and mortality have been used to generate the various projections of time lived with disability based on the mortality projections.

APPROACHES TO HEALTH PROJECTIONS

There is an extensive literature on the projection or forecasting of all-cause mortality rates and cause-specific mortality rates for cancers, coronary heart disease, HIV, Down syndrome and many others conditions (see, for example, Anderson and May 1992, Aoki et al. 1987, Bulutao 1993, Capocaccia et al. 1995, Gautrin et al. 1990, Kessler et al. 1991, McNown and Rogers 1989, Nilsson et al. 1991, Olshansky 1987, Ruwaard et al.

1994, Shiraishi and Arimoto 1982, Steele and Stratford 1995, Weinstein 1987, World Health Organization 1986). These approaches can be distinguished by at least three important characteristics. Some researchers project only all-cause mortality, with or without subsequent disaggregation into component causes. Other authors have projected individual causes or clusters of causes, in theory obtaining all-cause mortality as the aggregate of the individual cause projections. Another critical distinction is between those methods based on the extrapolation of past trends and those based on relationships between mortality and a set of independent variables (and necessarily projections of these independent variables). Finally, some authors have developed methods for projecting mortality in all age groups simultaneously (e.g. logit models), while others have assumed that the relationships between mortality rates and the independent variables will vary by age and sex.

ALL-CAUSE MORTALITY PROJECTIONS

For many years, demographers at the United Nations Population Division, the World Bank, the Population Council and many national census bureaus or statistical offices have produced population projections (e.g. Bongaarts 1994, Bos et al. 1994, United Nations 1995). Such projections are an essential aid to national and international planning and development activities. Assumptions about future trends in fertility and mortality are, of course, required for these projections. Of the two, projections of fertility rates are a much more important determinant of future population size and age-distribution than are mortality projections. The United Nations and World Bank population projections are based on simple assumptions about the likely increase in life expectancy at birth during each five-year period.[1]

Except in unusual cases of war or disaster, increases in life expectancy are assumed to occur in all countries irrespective of the health and social development policies that a country pursues, and unrelated to the rate of economic growth. With the onset of the HIV epidemic, the UN and the World Bank have arbitrarily reduced the assumed growth rates in life expectancy for countries with high sero-prevalence of HIV. These simple, mechanistic projections of life expectancy can be used in conjunction with a model life table to produce projections of age-specific mortality rates; for example, the UN Population Division uses the UN model life tables (United Nations 1982), and the World Bank generally uses the Coale and Demeny model life tables (Coale et al. 1983, Coale and Guo 1989).

In his seminal analysis of mortality patterns, Preston (1976) developed a series of linear models relating cause-specific mortality to all-cause mortality. This was the first study to quantify the intuitive notion that the cause structure of mortality is closely related to the overall level of mortality. This study has influenced much of the subsequent demographic work on estimates and projections of causes of death, which has utilized more recent datasets to develop models relating cause-specific mortality to all-cause mortality for a given age-sex group (e.g. Lopez and Hull 1985, for child mortality). For example, Bulutao (1993) produced projections of mortality by cause by starting with World Bank projections of life expectancy, and using Coale and Demeny model life tables to generate projections of all-cause mortality for specific age groups. He then modified the regression equations derived by Hakulinen et al. (1986), using Preston's approach to predict mortality from seven major clusters of causes: infections, neoplasms, circulatory diseases, complications of pregnancy, perinatal conditions, injuries, and other and unknown causes. More detailed causes were also projected by developing regression equations, based on vital registration data from countries in the Established Market Economies (EME) and in Latin America and the Caribbean (LAC), describing detailed cause-specific mortality rates as a function of each of the nine major cause-clusters.[2]

The all-cause mortality projection approach, exemplified by Bulutao (1993), has a number of limitations. First, future trends in all-cause mortality are assumed to continue as in the past, while in reality, past trends undoubtedly reflect the combined consequences of differential cause-specific trends. As the composition of causes of death will change in the future, the trend in all-cause mortality is expected to change as well. Second, the age-pattern of mortality change in this type of approach is governed by the age-patterns of mortality in Europe from the end of the 19th century to the middle of the 20th century, as captured in the Coale and Demeny model life tables (Coale et al. 1983). Changes in mortality patterns due to such causes as road traffic accidents, tobacco, and the HIV epidemic are not adequately reflected in these models.[3] Third, regression models relating cause-of-death structure to the mortality level from all causes combined are often confounded by trends in the proportion of deaths coded to ill-defined categories. Typically, the category "Symptoms, signs and ill-defined conditions" declines in both absolute and relative terms with development and, consequently, with all-cause mortality. As a result, spurious trends emerge in other causes of death.[4] For example, Bulutao (1993) projects steady increases, even in developed countries, in death rates from cancers and circulatory conditions, despite overwhelming evidence that, over the past 50 years, age-specific mortality rates from cardiovascular diseases have been declining (admittedly with occasional increases, although not sufficient to offset the declining trend).

CAUSE-SPECIFIC PROJECTIONS

Many authors have projected the incidence or mortality from diseases or injuries based on the extrapolation of past trends. In some cases extrapolations have been based on more sophisticated curve-fitting procedures, such as gamma distributions for HIV incidence (Chin et al. 1992, Chin and Lwanga 1991). Age-period-cohort models, which are another approach to projecting past trends, have been popular with demographers for projecting incidence or mortality from a condition (e.g. Osmond and Barker 1991, Caselli 1996). Lopez and Hakama (1986) argue that age- and cause-specific projections are likely to be more plausible than all-cause mortality projections. Nevertheless, such projections are founded on two basic assumptions, namely that trends in the real determinants of health (such as the prevalence of smoking) will continue in the future, and that the relationships between these determinants and the incidence or mortality from specific diseases will be approximately the same in the future. Both of these assumptions may well turn out to be false, thereby invalidating such mechanistic approaches.

More complicated forecasts of the incidence or mortality from a condition or a cluster of conditions based on multivariate risk factor models have been developed (Anderson and May 1988, 1992, Dowd and Manton 1990, Gunning-Schepers 1989, Manton and Stallard 1988, Pekkanen et al. 1992, Weinstein 1987). For example, Trolley (World Bank 1994) has developed a model to forecast coronary heart disease, stroke, lung cancer, chronic respiratory diseases, cirrhosis, and traffic accidents for Chile. The key variables in the model include hypertension, cholesterol, smoking and alcohol. The projected effect of risk factor changes on disease (and injury) rates was based on epidemiological studies carried out in the United States (e.g. Multiple Risk Factor Intervention Trial Research Group 1982). The model predicted a doubling of coronary heart disease death rates between 1990 and 2030, based on projections of risk factor profiles. The strength of this type of approach lies in the careful attempts to incorporate current knowledge about the determinants of disease incidence and severity. Because of the wealth of prospective epidemiological studies on coronary heart disease, these projection methods are perhaps most elaborated for forecasting coronary heart disease. Through a direct modelling of the known proximate determinants of incidence and mortality, these types of models can also be used to evaluate the potential impact of different policy options, such as drug therapy for elevated cholesterol levels.

The richness of data on risk factors for coronary heart disease and cancers, however, also underlies a potential weakness of these forecasting models. Many of the classic risk factors for coronary heart disease and other noncommunicable diseases, such as hypertension, elevated cholesterol, smoking and sedentary lifestyle, are thought to be income-elastic — that is to say, their prevalence rises as income per capita rises. Not surprisingly, risk factor models for Chile (World Bank 1994) and China (World Bank 1990) suggest major increases in age-specific death rates from coronary heart disease and other noncommunicable diseases. Recent evidence, however, runs counter to this type of prediction. In many EME countries, coronary heart disease has declined since the early 1970s, and less than half of this decline appears to be explicable by changes in the classic risk factors (Goldman and Cook 1984). Even more puzzling, age-specific death rates from all noncommunicable causes have been declining in most countries where they have been reliably monitored for the last half century or more. Clearly, other important determinants of incidence and mortality for these conditions must be changing at a rate fast enough to substantially alter past trends and quite possibly alter future trends as well. To put the limitation of these models in another way, few of them have been validated by demonstrating their ability to predict past trends over two or three decades.

There is a simpler alternative to multivariate risk factor models using parameters derived from epidemiological studies. Multivariate models can be developed using parameter estimates based on the analysis of time-series or panel data of incidence and mortality rates. In this type of model, the direct causal chain from distal determinants, such as socio-economic status, through to proximate determinants of health outcomes, such as cholesterol levels, blood pressure, tobacco use, or access to appropriate medical therapy, is not specified. Rather, the relationships between distal determinants and health outcomes are quantified using past observations of mortality rates. Such models cannot be utilized to forecast the impact of specific health policies, such as those designed to lower cholesterol or raise levels of physical activity, because the causal chain linking these factors to health outcomes has not been specified. On the other hand, these models are reasonably satisfactory in predicting past trends for the countries included in the analysis.

For the Global Burden of Disease Study, we have opted to develop age-, sex- and cause-specific multivariate models based on an extremely limited set of distal socio-economic determinants of mortality, along with one extremely powerful risk factor, namely tobacco use. We considered that this approach was the most reasonable compromise between our desire to develop validated models for major causes of death, and the issue of excessive complexity, given our objective of projecting multiple causes for different age-sex groups in eight regions of the world.

METHODS

The projection method which we have used involves twelve separate analytical or computational steps. Below, a brief outline of the overall approach is presented. In subsequent sections, more complete detail is provided. The steps in the projection procedure were as follows:

1. Parsimonious regression equations for nine major cause-clusters, for 14 different age-sex groups, were estimated from a panel of vital registration data from 47 countries. The regression equations relate age-, sex- and cause-specific mortality rates to four distal determinants of mortality: income per capita, human capital, smoking intensity and time.

2. For each cause-cluster in each age-sex group, a choice was made between using the final parsimonious regression equation or an alternative assumption, such as stable (constant) rates.

3. Model predictions of age-, sex- and cause-specific mortality rates in 1990 for each of the nine clusters of causes were compared for each region with the results of the Global Burden of Disease Study for that year. A series of scalars were then derived so that projected values for 1990 were identical to the 1990 GBD results. We have crudely assumed that these scalars would remain constant over the period 1990–2020.

4. Baseline, pessimistic and optimistic projections of income per capita, human capital and smoking intensity were developed.

5. Regression equations were developed relating age- and sex-specific mortality rates from 98 detailed causes to the age- and sex-specific mortality rates from corresponding cause-clusters, based on vital registration data from 67 countries.

6. For each detailed cause in each age-sex group, a choice was made between using the regression equation or an alternative assumption, based on criteria of R^2 and significance of the x-coefficient.

7. Age-, sex- and cause-specific mortality rates were projected for 1995, 2000, 2005, 2010, 2015 and 2020 for eight regions.

8. Separate projections were elaborated for HIV.

9. Projected tuberculosis mortality rates were modified in India and SSA, due to the expected interaction of tuberculosis and HIV.

10. Projections of Years of Life lived with Disability (YLDs) were developed based on the ratio of YLDs to Years of Life Lost due to premature mortality (YLLs) in the GBD results for 1990. (Please refer to Murray 1996, Chapter 1 in this volume for an in-depth description of those measures.) For those conditions where there is little or no mortality, alternative assumptions were used.

11. Population projections for each region were developed based on World Bank projections of fertility and the results of our mortality projection model.

12. Baseline, optimistic and pessimistic projections of the numbers of deaths, YLLs, YLDs and DALYs for each condition were made using the projected rates and population projections.

PARSIMONIOUS EQUATIONS FOR NINE MAJOR CAUSE CLUSTERS

As with the cause-of-death analysis for 1990 (see Murray and Lopez 1996, Chapter 3 in this volume), we have developed separate projection models for males and females and for seven age groups: 0–4 years, 5–14, 15–29, 30–44, 45–59, 60–69, and 70 years and over. Causes of death have been divided into nine clusters of causes: Group I (communicable, maternal, perinatal and nutritional conditions) excluding HIV, malignant neoplasms, cardiovascular diseases, digestive diseases, chronic respiratory diseases, other Group II diseases (noncommunicable), road traffic accidents, other unintentional injuries, and intentional injuries.[5] Deaths from these nine cause groups sum to total mortality in each age-sex group. We have chosen these clusters of causes because mortality trends over the past 40 years in countries with good vital registration data suggest that the more specific causes within each cluster have followed a similar time-trend. There are some obvious exceptions to this, such as the rise of tuberculosis in EME over the last 5–10 years and the HIV epidemic, both of which are addressed in more detail below. Other clear exceptions include the change in the composition of cardiovascular disease deaths and cancer deaths with socio-economic development — an attempt is made to capture these effects through detailed cause regressions as described below. In general, however, an examination of vital registration data for the last four decades suggests that these nine clusters of causes appear to capture much of the dominant trends in cause-specific mortality rates.

A panel dataset based on vital registration data from 47 countries for the years 1950–1990 was used to develop the regression equations. For many countries, the data series was incomplete. In total, 1394 observation-years were available. The dataset includes most countries of Europe, North America, Australia, New Zealand and Japan, as well as a number of Latin American and Asian countries with good vital registration. We have included almost all data on causes of death that can be considered broadly reliable or comparable. By including time-series and cross-sectional data in a panel, the predictive models need to explain both cross-sectional variation and variation within a country over time. In order to estimate mortality from a cluster of causes over a long period of time, causes of death coded according to the 6th, 7th, 8th and 9th Revisions of the International Classification of Diseases (ICD) must be analysed and, hence, a mapping of the ICD codes for each of the nine cause-clusters across the four revisions of the ICD was developed.

Even though the dataset is extensive — even dropping observations based on only a very small number of deaths, the number of observations in nearly all age-sex-cause-clusters was generally in excess of 600 — it does not include many observations from populations with high rates of mortality. As such, the application of predictive equations based on this dataset to regions such as sub-Saharan Africa is obviously highly tentative, and the results must be interpreted with great caution.

We have assumed that there is a general relationship between mortality rates for the nine major cause-clusters and a limited set of socio-economic variables of the form:

$$M_{a,k,i} = f(HC, Y, SI, T) \qquad (1)$$

where $M_{a,k,i}$ is the mortality rate in age group a and sex k from cause i, HC is a variable measuring human capital, Y is income per capita, SI is smoking intensity, and T is time. This basic functional relationship implies an unspecified set of hypotheses about proximate determinants of mortality rates, and the relationship between these proximate determinants and the more distal socio-economic determinants reflected in the equation above. While all the pathways through which these socio-economic variables can influence mortality rates have not been described, the regression results presented below indicate that a considerable proportion of the variance in age-, sex- and cause-specific mortality rates can be explained by this limited set of distal determinants.

Income per capita, measured in International dollars, and adjusted for differences in purchasing power not captured in official exchange rates, is used as a general proxy for many aspects of development. Estimates of income per capita in international dollars have been prepared by Summers and Heston (1991).[6] Equally importantly, research has consistently shown that education is an important distal determinant of health status (Cleland and van Ginneken 1988, Caldwell 1979). We have chosen to reflect levels of education using the average number of years of schooling of the population above the age of 25. This variable has been labelled "human capital" and has been estimated for 98 countries since 1950 by Barro and Lee (1993).

One critical determinant of malignant neoplasms, cardiovascular diseases and chronic respiratory diseases in adults that is not well reflected by the income or education variables is cumulative exposure to smoking. Smoking prevalence rates from community surveys are notoriously poor measures of the overall health impact of smoking, since they do not reflect other important factors affecting exposure including duration, type, amount and mode of smoking. Following the approach of Peto et al. (1992), we have used observed lung cancer rates minus non-smoker lung cancer rates for each age and sex group to calculate a variable labelled as "smoking intensity."[7] As smoking is the primary determinant of population variation in lung cancer rates (except in China and OAI), estimated lung cancer rates minus non-smoker lung cancer rates may be a near perfect biological assay of the cumulative exposure to tobacco. This smoking intensity variable was used as one of the independent variables in the predictive equations for malignant neoplasms, cardiovascular diseases and chronic respiratory diseases for males and females aged 30 years and older.

The fourth independent variable used in the projections is time itself. Technology has profoundly changed in the health sector over the last 50 years and continues to change with substantial investments in research and development. Obtaining a measurement of technical change is not only difficult (such data are usually not available) but also controversial.

We have opted to use calendar year as a proxy measure of the impact of technological change on health status.

Log linear regression was used to test the validity of equation (1). The simplest form of equation (1), used for causes of death where smoking is not a major risk factor, is the following:

$$\ln M_{a,k,i} = C_{a,k,i} + \beta_1 \ln Y + \beta_2 \ln HC + \beta_3 T \qquad (2)$$

where $C_{a,k,i}$ is a constant term, $M_{a,k,i}$ is the mortality level for age group a, sex k, and cause i, and Y, HC and T denote GDP per capita, human capital and time, respectively. In this form, the elasticity of the mortality rate with respect to GDP per capita and human capital is constant, as is the rate of change of mortality. Hence, mortality is assumed to change at a constant rate over time with, for instance, a 1 per cent change in per-capita income leading to a β_1 per cent change in the mortality rate for the particular age-cause group. To introduce further non-linearity into the relationship between age-, sex- and cause-specific mortality and these independent variables, we included the squared term for the log of GDP per capita. For example, for road traffic accidents among males aged 30 to 44 years, we obtained the following relationship:

$$\ln M_{a,k,RTA} = -31.7 + 8.3 \ln Y + 0.122 \ln HC + 0.0059 T - 0.489 (\ln Y)^2$$

In this particular case, it requires only simple algebra to demonstrate that, all other things remaining constant, road traffic accident mortality for males ages 30 to 44 would tend to increase as income per capita rises to a level around $5200, but thereafter, would decline.

To estimate the equations of this form, we have used a variety of econometric approaches. The detailed econometric analysis underlying the results summarized here is reported elsewhere (Acharya and Murray 1996). In brief, the panel dataset used does not have an identical series of observation years for each country. Ordinary least squares (OLS) regression results from the pooled dataset could be biased because of auto-correlation and heteroscedasticity. While any given country's time series may suffer from auto-correlation, it is unlikely that the entire panel will be so affected. Acharya and Murray (1996) detected serialized correlation within a cross-sectional time series which produces heteroscedasticity since each error term would be correlated with a cross-sectional unit. The Parks method was used to correct the serialized correlation. The subset of the panel dataset on which the Parks method could be applied was much smaller than the entire dataset since the same set of observation-years is required for each country. OLS estimates for this subset yielded parameter estimates similar to the Parks method with no changes in the signs of the estimates. Because much information was lost on moderate to high mortality populations when the subset of data was used, we chose to use the OLS regression estimates based on the entire dataset for the final set of parameter estimates.

Parsimonious equations were developed based on two criteria. First, if the sign for a variable was consistent with our prior hypothesis, but the parameter estimate was not significant at the 1 per cent level, we opted to maintain this variable in the equation. If the sign of a parameter estimate was the opposite of our prior hypothesis, and the parameter estimate was not statistically significant at the 5 per cent level, we opted to exclude the variable. When more than one variable was to be excluded according to these criteria, both variables were dropped only if an F-test for the combination of variables was not significant. Table 7.1 summarizes the final parsimonious regression equations for each of the nine cause-clusters for the fourteen age-sex groups that were used to project death rates.

In general, these equations explain most of the variance in Group I mortality but explain rather little of the variance in intentional injuries (and road traffic accidents in children). It is also important to point out that, for males and females aged 70 and above, the R^2 for many cause-clusters was generally lower than for other age groups, probably reflecting poorer quality of coding of causes of death or the smaller range of variation in mortality rates between countries at these older ages. The R^2 for cardiovascular diseases among women ranged from 48 per cent to 69 per cent between the ages of 15 and 69, whereas for males in the same age groups, the R^2 values were lower, typically on the order of 12 to 63 per cent. Of the variance explained by the limited set of independent variables in the equations for cardiovascular diseases, the most important determinant was smoking intensity — if smoking intensity was to be excluded, the R^2 for age groups 30–44, 45–59 and 60 years and over would fall to 9.5 per cent, 3.5 per cent and 15.2 per cent, respectively. Given the size of the panel used to fit these equations, a surprising proportion of the variation for Group I and Group II causes across countries over four decades was explained with only four independent variables. The procedure appears to be less powerful for Group III causes, perhaps because there is much less temporal variation in these causes except for road traffic accidents.

SELECTION OF PREDICTIVE EQUATIONS OR ALTERNATIVE ASSUMPTIONS

Examination of Table 7.1 indicates that for some cause-clusters in some age-sex groups, the R^2 for the regression equation is low — for example, the R^2 for road traffic accidents among males aged 0–4 years was 0.03. Not surprisingly, projections of rates based on equations with poor predictive power could lead to counter-intuitive results — such as the projection of rapid rises in female intentional injury rates concurrent with declines in male rates. For causes where the R^2 was less than 10 per cent, we have chosen not to use the parsimonious regression equations. Rather, our projections are based on the simple assumption that the age-sex-specific mortality rate will stay constant for these causes.

Table 7.1 Parsimonious regression equations for nine cause-clusters based on a 47-country panel dataset, 1950–1990

Cause-cluster	Sex	Age group	Constant	lnHC	lnY	(lnY)²	Year	lnSI	R² (%)
Group I									
	M	0–4	13.47	-0.23	-0.44		-0.03		72
	M	5–14	11.30	-1.14	-0.64		-0.03		78
	M	15–29	12.58	-1.24	-0.67		-0.03		76
	M	30–44	13.51	-1.25	-0.67		-0.04		75
	M	45–59	13.03	-1.12	-0.56		-0.03		75
	M	60–69	11.77	-0.90	-0.39		-0.02		65
	M	70+	8.07	-0.46	0.00		-0.01		22
	F	0–4	13.67	-0.35	-0.46		-0.03		71
	F	5–14	11.17	-1.21	-0.60		-0.03		77
	F	15–29	14.24	-1.42	-0.73		-0.04		78
	F	30–44	14.90	-1.40	-0.72		-0.05		79
	F	45–59	12.01	-1.23	-0.51		-0.03		71
	F	60–69	11.26	-0.97	-0.40		-0.02		64
	F	70+	7.71	-0.42	0.02		-0.01		20
Malignant neoplasms									
	M	0–4	-13.41	0.42	3.83	-0.24	-0.01		17
	M	5–14	-4.28	-0.19	1.65	-0.10			16
	M	15–29	-1.07	0.08	0.94	-0.06	0.00		12
	M	30–44	-1.42		1.23	-0.08	0.00	0.05	36
	M	45–59	0.98	-0.06	1.02	-0.06		0.01	56
	M	60–69	1.39	0.05	1.15	-0.07		0.00	55
	M	70+	1.15	0.10	1.36	-0.08	0.00	0.00	55
	F	0–4	-16.55	0.35	4.44	-0.28			12
	F	5–14	-3.36	-0.16	1.41	-0.08	-0.01		37
	F	15–29	-1.25	-0.20	1.08	-0.07	0.00		37
	F	30–44	-2.12	-0.17	1.54	-0.09		0.04	18
	F	45–59	1.06		1.08	-0.06	-0.01	0.01	33
	F	60–69	1.39	0.04	1.17	-0.07	-0.01	0.00	30
	F	70+	0.17		1.59	-0.09	-0.01	0.00	26
Cardiovascular diseases									
	M	0–4	-13.81	-0.43	4.35	-0.28	0.01		13
	M	5–14	4.86	-1.31	0.16	-0.04			59
	M	15–29	6.00	-0.75	-0.07	-0.02	-0.01		62
	M	30–44	0.15		1.13	-0.07	-0.01	0.02	12
	M	45–59	1.20	-0.17	1.10	-0.06		0.00	13
	M	60–69	1.40	0.02	1.35	-0.08		0.00	27
	M	70+	4.04	0.28	1.10	-0.07	-0.01	0.00	23

Table 7.1   (continued)

Cause-cluster	Sex	Age group	Regression coefficients						R²(%)
			Constant	ln*HC*	ln*Y*	(ln*Y*)²	Year	ln*SI*	
Cardiovascular diseases (continued)									
	F	0–4	-5.21	-0.47	2.41	-0.16			11
	F	5–14	5.06	-1.24	0.26	-0.04	-0.01		59
	F	15–29	5.71	-1.04	0.26	-0.04	-0.01		69
	F	30–44	-1.55	-0.76	1.87	-0.13		0.11	53
	F	45–59	-4.41		2.87	-0.19	-0.02	0.02	49
	F	60–69	0.26	0.02	2.01	-0.13	-0.02	0.00	48
	F	70+	2.85	0.25	1.42	-0.09	-0.01		26
Digestive diseases									
	M	0–4	0.43	−0.22	1.93	−0.15	−0.03		45
	M	5–14	9.70	-1.31	-0.77	0.02	-0.02		54
	M	15–29	9.70	-1.14	-0.91	0.03	0.00		57
	M	30–44	5.69	-1.00	0.06	-0.02			29
	M	45–59	2.92	-0.82	0.74	-0.06	0.02		34
	M	60–69	0.97	-0.68	1.36	-0.10	0.01		35
	M	70+	1.95	-0.59	1.16	-0.08	0.01		34
	F	0–4	1.66	-0.27	1.52	-0.12	-0.03		41
	F	5–14	6.23	-1.22	-0.07	-0.02	-0.02		50
	F	15–29	8.02	-1.26	-0.62	0.02	-0.01		51
	F	30–44	9.95	-1.10	-1.13	0.05			33
	F	45–59	7.00	-0.79	-0.30	0.00	0.00		32
	F	60–69	1.33	-0.58	1.29	-0.09			41
	F	70+	1.20	-0.36	1.26	-0.08			16
Respiratory diseases									
	M	0–4	-15.97	-1.03	5.57	-0.36			28
	M	5–14	-0.21	-0.80	0.85	-0.07			32
	M	15–29	-0.80	-0.60	0.70	-0.05			24
	M	30–44	-8.21	-0.64	2.78	-0.18	0.01	0.03	34
	M	45–59	-6.36	-0.29	2.71	-0.18	0.00	0.01	26
	M	60–69	-0.36	-0.20	1.43	-0.10	0.01	0.00	28
	M	70+	2.23	-0.10	0.95	-0.08	0.02	0.00	32
	F	0–4	-12.98	-1.03	5.06	-0.33	-0.02		32
	F	5–14	12.13	-0.80	-2.07	0.10			35
	F	15–29	-4.22	-0.56	1.53	-0.10			21
	F	30–44	-6.53	-0.92	2.26	-0.15	0.01	0.19	33
	F	45–59	-7.47	-0.55	2.75	-0.19	0.02	0.04	46
	F	60–69	-1.82	-0.33	1.73	-0.14	0.02	0.01	46
	F	70+	-2.94		2.21	-0.17	0.02	0.00	34

Table 7.1   (continued)

Cause-cluster	Sex	Age group	Constant	lnHC	lnY	(lnY)²	Year	lnSI	R² (%)
Other Group II									
	M	0–4	-6.87	0.47	3.25	-0.20	-0.01		29
	M	5–14	5.29	-0.87	0.17	-0.03	-0.01		68
	M	15–29	8.71	-0.65	-0.84	0.04	-0.01		56
	M	30–44	1.91	-0.59	0.88	-0.06	-0.01		37
	M	45–59	2.37	-0.62	1.05	-0.07	-0.01		47
	M	60–69	2.14	-0.66	1.38	-0.09	-0.01		53
	M	70+	6.91	-0.53	0.36	-0.03	-0.01		35
	F	0–4	-7.24	0.54	3.26	-0.20	-0.01		30
	F	5–14	5.81	-0.97	0.04	-0.02	-0.01		66
	F	15–29	3.58	-0.89	0.63	-0.05	-0.02		65
	F	30–44	4.38	-0.75	0.60	-0.05	-0.02		62
	F	45–59	0.09	-0.59	1.66	-0.11	-0.01		55
	F	60–69	-2.93	-0.64	2.52	-0.16	-0.01		49
	F	70+	3.89	-0.73	0.83	-0.04			21
Road traffic accidents									
	M	0–4	**8.24**	**-0.11**	**-1.84**	**0.12**	**0.00**		3
	M	5–14	-17.66	0.09	4.53	-0.25	-0.01		17
	M	15–29	-9.47	0.15	2.64	-0.13	0.00		29
	M	30–44	-21.26	-0.21	5.82	-0.34	0.00		12
	M	45–59	-31.75	-0.12	8.32	-0.49	0.01		19
	M	60–69	-38.99	-0.08	10.01	-0.58	0.00		23
	M	70+	-38.78	0.03	9.82	-0.57	0.00		30
	F	0–4	**12.04**	**-0.06**	**-2.79**	**0.18**	**0.00**		5
	F	5–14	-13.26	0.12	3.21	-0.17	0.00		14
	F	15–29*	1.03	0.29	-0.57	0.07	0.01		52
	F	30–44	-5.19	0.02	1.23	-0.06	0.01		18
	F	45–59	-11.88	-0.01	2.98	-0.16	0.01		14
	F	60–69	-19.84	-0.12	4.99	-0.28	0.00		16
	F	70+	-26.16	0.23	6.52	-0.37	0.01		18
Other unintentional injuries									
	M	0–4	-5.23	0.70	2.45	-0.16	-0.02		15
	M	5–14	5.74	-0.25	-0.05	-0.02	-0.02		49
	M	15–29	3.56	-0.33	0.49	-0.05	0.00		32
	M	30–44	-1.49	-0.25	1.56	-0.11	0.00		22
	M	45–59	-0.18		1.22	-0.09	0.00		15
	M	60–69	-2.96		1.90	-0.13	0.00		20
	M	70+	-0.11	0.32	1.16	-0.07	0.00		13

Table 7.1   (continued)

Cause-cluster	Sex	Age group	Constant	lnHC	lnY	(lnY)²	Year	lnSI	R²(%)
Other unintentional injuries (continued)									
	F	0–4	-3.26	0.69	1.93	-0.13	-0.02		15
	F	5–14	11.16	-0.65	-1.48	0.07	-0.01		47
	F	15–29	7.77	-0.52	-0.94	0.03	0.01		32
	F	30–44	9.21	-0.28	-1.42	0.06	0.01		23
	F	45–59	*6.78*		*-0.90*	*0.04*	*0.00*		9
	F	60–69	*-3.44*	*0.28*	*1.69*	*-0.11*	*-0.01*		10
	F	70+	-9.85	0.62	3.28	-0.19	-0.01		39
Intentional injuries									
	M	0–4	*-5.17*	*0.67*	*1.52*	*-0.10*	*0.00*		8
	M	5–14	*-2.06*	*-0.10*	*0.72*	*-0.05*	*0.01*		16
	M	15–29	*24.82*	*-0.45*	*-5.21*	*0.30*	*0.02*		18
	M	30–44	*20.79*	*-0.23*	*-4.06*	*0.23*	*0.01*		13
	M	45–59	*7.23*	*0.07*	*-0.71*	*0.03*	*0.00*		5
	M	60–69	*-5.79*	*0.06*	*2.36*	*-0.15*			6
	M	70+	*-6.95*	*0.21*	*2.54*	*-0.15*			4
	F	0–4	*4.68*	*0.84*	*-0.70*	*0.02*	*-0.01*		13
	F	5–14	*-0.01*	*-0.10*	*0.09*	*-0.01*	*0.01*		8
	F	15–29	*23.99*	*-0.14*	*-5.28*	*0.31*	*0.01*		13
	F	30–44	*21.03*	*0.49*	*-4.76*	*0.29*	*0.00*		24
	F	45–59	*6.59*	*0.82*	*-1.39*	*0.08*			30
	F	60–69	*-2.98*	*0.85*	*0.96*	*-0.05*	*0.00*		26
	F	70+	*-13.65*	*0.86*	*3.47*	*-0.22*	*0.01*		18

Note: Bold italics indicate that constant rates were used in lieu of the regression equations to make projections.

* For EME and FSE, the regression coefficients used were -35.93, 0.19, 7.73, -0.39, and 0.00, respectively.

In addition, for all age-sex groups, we have chosen to use constant rates for intentional injuries despite R² values as high as 0.30 for females aged 45–59 years. Initial projections for those age groups with an R² greater than 0.10 generated implausibly rapid rises in the intentional injury rate — for some regions, a 300 per cent increase was predicted. Using the regression equations for some age groups and constant rates for others also generated implausible age-patterns of intentional injury deaths, and hence constant rates were used for all age-sex groups.

COMPARISON OF MODEL-BASED PROJECTIONS FOR 1990 WITH GBD 1990 ESTIMATES

These equations can be used to predict mortality rates by cause and age for each region using 1990 region-specific values for income per capita, human capital, smoking intensity and year. When this was done, the predictions did not agree exactly with the GBD estimates of mortality rates by cause in 1990, since very different approaches have been used. We have, therefore, estimated a series of age-, sex-, cause- and region-specific scalars such that:

$$M_{a,k,i,r} = \kappa_{a,k,i,r} \, M^*_{a,k,i,r} \qquad (4)$$

where $M_{a,k,i,r}$ is the age-, sex-, cause- and region-specific death rate in 1990, $M^*_{a,k,i,r}$ is the predicted death rate for cause i at age a and sex k in region r based on the regression equation in 1990, and $\kappa_{a,k,i,r}$ is the age-, sex-, cause- and region-specific scalar. For EME, which comprises the majority of the panel dataset, the scalars range from 0.2 for Group I at ages 0–4, to 2.1 for Group I at ages 30–44, with an average scalar of 0.99. Overall, as expected, the projection equations were least reliable for SSA, where scalars ranged from 0.19 for digestive diseases among males ages 0–4 years, to 15 for Group I causes among females aged 5–14 years. For SSA overall, the median scalar was 1.7. Typically, the scalars for Group I were substantially greater than one—in SSA, the average Group I scalar was 6.1. In other words, the regression equations are relatively poor predictors of Group I mortality in high mortality populations. This result is not surprising given the lack of data included in the panel dataset from high mortality populations.

To make projections, we have held the set of scalars $\kappa_{a,k,i,r}$ constant during the period of the projections. For example, if the death rate from cancers in India in 1990 for males aged 45–59 years was half that predicted by the regression equation, we have assumed that the death rate in the future will also be half that predicted by the equation based on changes in income, education and smoking. A consequence of the large scalars for Group I in regions such as SSA is that we may overestimate future Group I mortality in these regions. Alternative assumptions, such as forcing the scalars to converge towards 1 over time would yield substantially smaller projections of Group I mortality in 2020 than the constant scalar assumption used here. Since the results of the projection exercise (and epidemiological transition theory) suggest a steady shift towards Group II conditions over time, we have opted to preserve the rather conservative assumption that the regional scalars will remain constant. Readers should bear in mind that our projections of Group I mortality, especially for SSA and possibly India, may well be overly pessimistic.

PROJECTIONS OF GDP PER CAPITA, HUMAN CAPITAL AND SMOKING INTENSITY

For each independent variable, we have generated baseline, pessimistic and optimistic projections. Many more scenarios are clearly possible and each scenario will lead to a different set of projections of mortality by cause. The methods and assumptions which we have used to define these three scenarios are described below.

- *Income per capita*. In the baseline scenario, GDP per capita is projected to increase in each region according to the forecasts of the World Bank (1995) up to 2004. Income per capita in China is predicted to grow at 6.6 per cent per year, while in Latin America and the Caribbean (LAC), it is expected to grow at only 1.9 per cent per year. World Bank forecasts for SSA are even lower, with growth per year in income per capita expected to be only 0.9 per cent. Beyond the year 2004, we have assumed that growth rates will tend towards the mean rate observed in EME over the past 40 years. Figure 7.1 illustrates the baseline projections of income per capita by region. It is interesting to note that according to these assumptions, the gap in income per capita between developing regions and EME is expected to widen in both absolute and relative terms. Only for China is the relative gap in income per capita compared with EME expected to diminish substantially.

  For the optimistic scenario, the growth rate in income per capita was assumed to be approximately 40 per cent higher than the baseline projection, except for EME, where a growth rate of 3 per cent was assumed. In the pessimistic scenario, growth rates only slightly higher than the lowest trend in income per capita observed over the past 3 decades for a given region were assumed. For example, the growth rate

Figure 7.1   Baseline projections of GDP per capita by region, 1990–2020

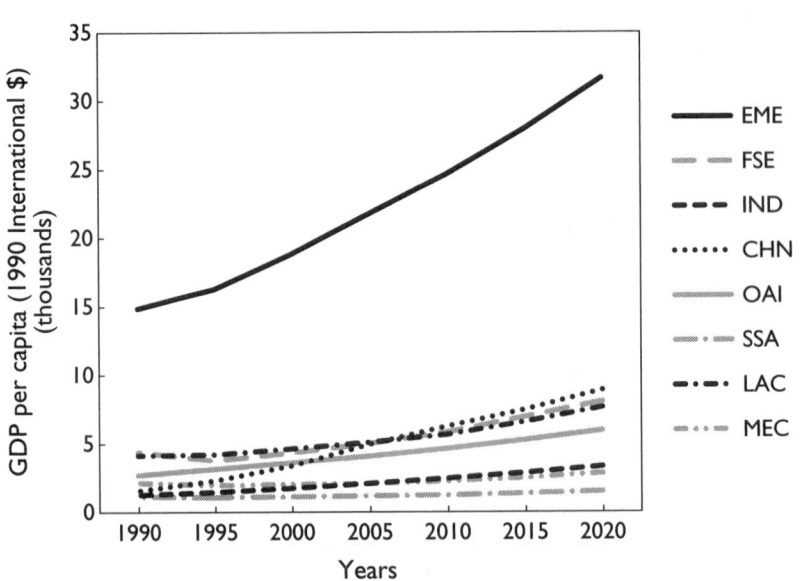

in LAC according to the pessimistic scenario was assumed to be slightly higher than that in the debt-ridden years, while for SSA the growth rate of the late 1980s-early 1990s was used to define the trend.

• *Human capital.* Barro and Lee (1993) estimated human capital for 98 countries for each five-year period from 1950 to 1990. Aggregating the available country-specific estimates for each region, we have estimated the growth rates of human capital between each five-year period from 1960 to 1990 for the eight regions. In this dataset, there is a clear relationship between the growth rate in human capital by region and the level of human capital already achieved. This relationship is described by an equation of the following form:

$$r = 0.043 - 0.004HC \qquad (5)$$

where r is the growth rate in human capital, and HC is the level of human capital. The R^2 for this relationship is 0.77. Baseline projections of human capital were then calculated using this equation for all regions. For the pessimistic projection, we arbitrarily modified the equation so that the coefficient for HC was 0.005 (i.e. a 25 per cent slower change for a given level of HC), and for the optimistic projection this coefficient was set equal to 0.003.

• *Smoking intensity.* To project smoking intensity to the year 2020, we have examined the relationship between the estimated number of cigarettes consumed per adult in the United Kingdom from 1900 to 1990 and the smoking intensity calculated for a more recent period. Figure 7.2 (for males aged 70 and over) illustrates that there is a predictable time lag between levels of cigarette consumption and the smoking impact variable. To project smoking intensity, we have assumed that the *time course* of the smoking epidemic observed in the United Kingdom will be repeated in each region. Estimates of per capita (adult) cigarette consumption in each country were used to obtain regional estimates in 1990.[8] These were further sub-divided into male and female cigarette consumption using sex-specific estimates of smoking prevalence and daily consumption per smoker. Based on these estimates, the timing of the cigarette epidemic in the United Kingdom was used to estimate the implied smoking intensity thirty years after a given level of cigarette consumption per capita had been reached. This figure was then used as the projected value of smoking intensity in 2020 for each region. For the intervening years, we have assumed that current smoking intensity will increase, or decrease, in a linear fashion towards the projected value in 2020.

As the future course of the smoking intensity variable is largely determined by current smoking patterns, we have not elaborated different optimistic and pessimistic scenarios. We do not want to suggest however, that reducing smoking prevalence or intensity of use would have no effect on smoking-attributable mortality over the next 30 years—the epidemiological evidence suggests that vascular disease risks decline substantially within 1–2 years after cessation (US Department of Health and Human Services 1989). Rather, the smoking intensity variable is entirely based on lung cancer risks which are much less responsive, over the short term, to changes in smoking levels. In particular, lung cancer levels in 2020 will be largely determined by current levels of cigarette consumption. One possibility to define optimistic and pessimistic scenarios would be to assume lower or higher proportionate mortality, respectively, for diseases other than lung cancer which are caused by smoking. However, we believe that the hazards of tobacco use in developing countries are not yet sufficiently well understood to construct meaningful scenarios about the proportionate mortality due to smoking from other causes associated with a given level of lung cancer.

REGRESSION EQUATIONS FOR DETAILED CAUSES

A time-series analysis of the socio-economic determinants of more specific causes of death is severely constrained by the difficulties of comparing cause-of-death data coded according to the different revisions of the International Classification of Diseases. We have, therefore, not attempted to model the relationship between GDP per capita, human capital, smoking

Figure 7.2   Trends for cigarette consumption and smoking intensity in the United Kingdom among males, aged 70 years and over, 1900–1990

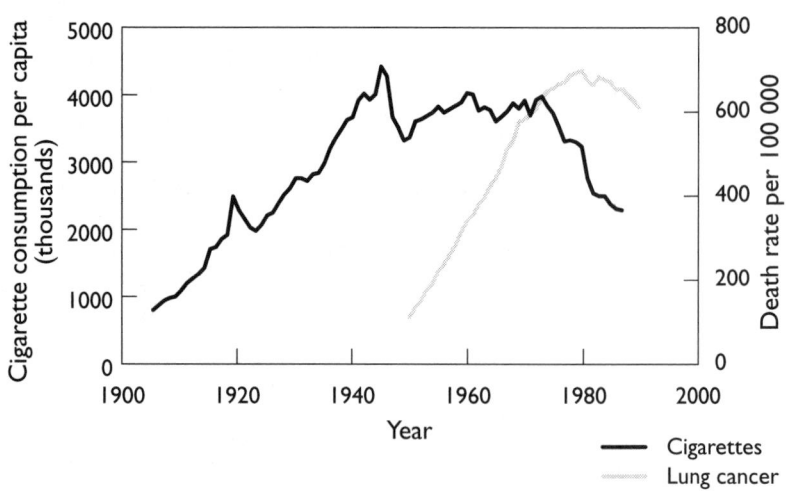

Note: Consumption is per adult (15 years and over). Death rates are age-standardized.

Source: Cigarette consumption estimates are from Wald and Nicolaides-Bowman (1991)

intensity and time, and more specific causes of death such as tuberculosis, liver cancer or peptic ulcer disease. To generate projections of these detailed causes, we have used a variant of the Preston cause-of-death model approach. More specifically, we have examined the relationship between the age-sex-specific mortality rate from a detailed cause and the age-sex-specific mortality rate from the cause-cluster to which the detailed cause belongs. The parameters defining these relationships have been estimated using a restricted dataset of ICD-9 data circa 1990 for 67 countries.

To avoid predicting negative mortality rates for detailed causes as cause-cluster mortality rates decline to low levels, the following log relationships were estimated:

$$\ln M_{a,k,i,d} = \beta_{a,k,i,d} \ln M_{a,k,i} + C_{a,k,i,d} \qquad (6)$$

where $M_{a,k,i,d}$ is the mortality rate from specific cause d within cause group i for age group a and sex k, $M_{a,k,i}$ is the mortality rate for cause group i within age group a and sex k, and $\beta_{a,k,i,d}$ is the coefficient from the OLS regression. These constant elasticity regressions provide estimates of the per centage change in death rates from a specific cause d for a given per centage change in the mortality rate for a broader cause-cluster i.

SELECTION OF PREDICTIVE EQUATIONS OR ALTERNATIVE ASSUMPTIONS FOR DETAILED CAUSES

As the dataset for evaluating the relationship between detailed causes and cause-cluster mortality rates is smaller and covers a much less extensive range of mortality rates, the disease and injury rates predicted by detailed cause regressions may well be unreliable at higher overall levels of mortality. We have, therefore, chosen to use the regression results only when the relationship was reasonably strong as measured by an R^2 greater than 0.25 and an x-coefficient with a p-value <0.001. Not many causes met these criteria, as Table 7.2 indicates.

To project mortality from all of the detailed causes, a two-step procedure was employed. First, for detailed causes with an equation in Table 7.2, scalars were estimated to adjust the predicted values for 1990 to match the GBD estimates for each detailed cause in 1990 by region. In this case, the scalar was simply the ratio of the GBD estimate for a detailed cause in a region to the predicted value for that detailed cause based on a robust equation. These region-specific scalars were used to predict the cause-specific mortality rate based on the projected mortality rate for the broader cause-cluster for each time period in the projection. For these causes, the projected mortality rate can be expressed as follows:

$$M_{a,k,i,d,r} = S_{a,k,i,r}\, e^{\,\beta_{a,k,i,d} M_{a,k,i,r} + C_{a,k,i,d}} \qquad (7)$$

where $M_{a,k,i,d,r}$ is the projected mortality rate for cause d in cause-cluster i for age a, sex k and in region r, $S_{a,k,i,d,r}$ is an age-, sex-, region- and cause-

Table 7.2 Results of regressions of age-sex-specific mortality from detailed causes on the respective cause-cluster. Results are shown only when the $R^2 \geq 0.25$ and the p-value for beta $\leq$ 0.001

Cause-cluster	Detailed cause	Sex	Age group	R^2	Inter-cept	Intercept p-value	Beta	Beta p-value
Group I								
	Respiratory infections	M	5–14	0.61	-1.55	0.0001	0.890	0.0001
	Respiratory infections	M	15–29	0.51	-1.38	0.0001	0.875	0.0001
	Respiratory infections	M	30–44	0.42	-1.33	0.0001	0.869	0.0001
	Respiratory infections	M	45–59	0.31	-0.83	0.0001	0.892	0.0001
	Respiratory infections	M	60–69	0.35	-0.42	0.0908	0.904	0.0001
	Respiratory infections	M	70+	0.99	-0.24	0.0001	0.983	0.0001
	Respiratory infections	F	5–14	0.58	-1.58	0.0001	0.874	0.0001
	Respiratory infections	F	15–29	0.38	-2.09	0.0001	0.795	0.0001
	Respiratory infections	F	30–44	0.43	-1.71	0.0001	0.832	0.0001
	Respiratory infections	F	45–59	0.43	-1.05	0.0001	0.893	0.0001
	Respiratory infections	F	60–69	0.55	-0.47	0.0017	0.924	0.0001
	Respiratory infections	F	70+	0.90	-0.23	0.0118	0.987	0.0001
	Maternal conditions	F	15–29	0.47	-2.00	0.0001	0.895	0.0001
	Maternal conditions	F	30–44	0.37	-2.38	0.0001	0.895	0.0001
Malignant neoplasms								
	Mouth and oropharynx cancer	M	70+	0.25	-3.55	0.0001	0.828	0.0001
	Oesophagus cancer	M	70+	0.28	-3.14	0.0001	0.832	0.0001
	Stomach cancer	M	60–69	0.29	-2.11	0.0001	0.940	0.0001
	Stomach cancer	M	70+	0.48	-1.75	0.0001	0.901	0.0001
	Stomach cancer	F	70+	0.38	-2.15	0.0001	0.915	0.0001
	Colon and rectum cancer	M	70+	0.33	-2.37	0.0001	0.903	0.0001
	Colon and rectum cancer	F	70+	0.38	-2.02	0.0001	0.916	0.0001
	Breast cancer	F	45–59	0.31	-1.66	0.0001	0.978	0.0001
	Breast cancer	F	70+	0.38	-2.27	0.0001	0.910	0.0001
	Prostate cancer	M	70+	0.65	-1.68	0.0001	0.929	0.0001
	Bladder cancer	M	70+	0.36	-2.85	0.0001	0.875	0.0001
	Lymphomas	M	0–4	0.57	-2.16	0.0001	0.840	0.0001
	Lymphomas	M	5–14	0.28	-3.91	0.0001	0.732	0.0001
	Lymphomas	M	15–29	0.26	-2.93	0.0001	0.833	0.0001
	Lymphomas	F	0–4	0.55	-2.51	0.0001	0.822	0.0001
	Leukaemia	M	0–4	0.69	-1.37	0.0001	0.897	0.0001
	Leukaemia	M	5–14	0.73	-1.11	0.0001	0.917	0.0001
	Leukaemia	M	15–29	0.32	-2.21	0.0001	0.870	0.0001
	Leukaemia	F	0–4	0.75	-1.25	0.0001	0.910	0.0001
	Leukaemia	F	5–14	0.55	-1.67	0.0001	0.878	0.0001
	Leukaemia	F	15–29	0.26	-2.54	0.0001	0.797	0.0001

Table 7.2   (continued)

Cause-cluster Detailed cause	Sex	Age group	R^2	Intercept	Intercept p-value	Beta	Beta p-value
Cardiovascular diseases							
Ischaemic heart disease	M	45–59	0.26	-1.14	0.0078	1.022	0.0001
Ischaemic heart disease	M	60–69	0.40	-0.79	0.0291	0.970	0.0001
Ischaemic heart disease	M	70+	0.70	-0.79	0.0004	0.941	0.0001
Ischaemic heart disease	F	60–69	0.36	-0.54	0.0985	0.890	0.0001
Ischaemic heart disease	F	70+	0.72	-0.91	0.0001	0.929	0.0001
Cerebrovascular disease	M	0–4	0.34	-3.45	0.0001	0.722	0.0001
Cerebrovascular disease	M	5–14	0.38	-3.17	0.0001	0.766	0.0001
Cerebrovascular disease	M	15–29	0.26	-2.20	0.0001	0.869	0.0001
Cerebrovascular disease	M	45–59	0.60	-1.16	0.0001	0.900	0.0001
Cerebrovascular disease	M	60–69	0.87	-1.04	0.0001	0.925	0.0001
Cerebrovascular disease	M	70+	0.87	-0.86	0.0001	0.933	0.0001
Cerebrovascular disease	F	0–4	0.31	-3.93	0.0001	0.716	0.0001
Cerebrovascular disease	F	5–14	0.37	-3.28	0.0001	0.758	0.0001
Cerebrovascular disease	F	30–44	0.31	-1.38	0.0001	0.875	0.0001
Cerebrovascular disease	F	45–59	0.49	-0.92	0.0001	0.919	0.0001
Cerebrovascular disease	F	60–69	0.91	-0.99	0.0001	0.951	0.0001
Cerebrovascular disease	F	70+	0.98	-0.77	0.0001	0.942	0.0001
Other Group II							
Diabetes mellitus	M	70+	0.60	-1.24	0.0001	0.925	0.0001
Diabetes mellitus	F	45–59	0.34	-1.96	0.0001	1.072	0.0001
Diabetes mellitus	F	60–69	0.42	-1.34	0.0001	1.037	0.0001
Diabetes mellitus	F	70+	0.82	-0.93	0.0001	0.941	0.0001
Neuro-psychiatric conditions	M	5–14	0.41	-1.73	0.0001	0.871	0.0001
Neuro-psychiatric conditions	M	15–29	0.29	-1.24	0.0001	0.970	0.0001
Neuro-psychiatric conditions	M	30–44	0.28	-1.29	0.0001	0.953	0.0001
Neuro-psychiatric conditions	M	70+	0.30	-1.61	0.0001	0.869	0.0001
Neuro-psychiatric conditions	F	5–14	0.46	-1.65	0.0001	0.875	0.0001
Neuro-psychiatric conditions	F	15–29	0.32	-1.38	0.0001	0.869	0.0001
Neuro-psychiatric conditions	F	30–44	0.32	-1.68	0.0001	0.862	0.0001
Neuro-psychiatric conditions	F	70+	0.30	-1.60	0.0001	0.852	0.0001
Intentional injuries							
Self-inflicted injuries	M	5–14	0.72	-1.75	0.0001	0.882	0.0001
Self-inflicted injuries	M	15–29	0.81	-0.68	0.0001	0.956	0.0001
Self-inflicted injuries	M	30–44	0.70	-0.93	0.0001	0.957	0.0001
Self-inflicted injuries	M	45–59	0.77	-0.77	0.0001	0.971	0.0001
Self-inflicted injuries	M	60–69	0.76	-0.83	0.0001	0.954	0.0001
Self-inflicted injuries	F	5–14	0.62	-2.77	0.0001	0.807	0.0001
Self-inflicted injuries	F	15–29	0.72	-0.95	0.0001	0.945	0.0001
Self-inflicted injuries	F	30–44	0.77	-0.81	0.0001	0.961	0.0001

Table 7.2　　(continued)

Cause-cluster	Detailed cause	Sex	Age group	R²	Inter-cept	Intercept p-value	Beta	Beta p-value
Intentional injuries (continued)								
	Self-inflicted injuries	F	45–59	0.76	-0.88	0.0001	0.953	0.0001
	Self-inflicted injuries	F	60–69	0.81	-0.86	0.0001	0.949	0.0001
	Self-inflicted injuries	F	70+	0.74	-1.25	0.0001	0.919	0.0001
	Violence	M	0–4	0.81	0.25	0.111	0.893	0.0001
	Violence	M	5–14	0.64	-2.43	0.0001	0.829	0.0001
	Violence	M	15–29	0.61	-1.95	0.0001	0.873	0.0001
	Violence	M	30–44	0.63	-1.85	0.0001	0.871	0.0001
	Violence	M	45–59	0.59	-2.28	0.0001	0.839	0.0001
	Violence	M	60–69	0.59	-2.73	0.0001	0.803	0.0001
	Violence	M	70+	0.57	-3.17	0.0001	0.769	0.0001
	Violence	F	0–4	0.81	0.21	0.1888	0.893	0.0001
	Violence	F	5–14	0.67	-2.17	0.0001	0.841	0.0001
	Violence	F	15–29	0.66	-2.00	0.0001	0.859	0.0001
	Violence	F	30–44	0.59	-2.34	0.0001	0.835	0.0001
	Violence	F	45–59	0.59	-2.89	0.0001	0.792	0.0001
	Violence	F	60–69	0.53	-3.71	0.0001	0.727	0.0001
	Violence	F	70+	0.58	-3.33	0.0001	0.756	0.0001

specific scalar, and the remaining variables are as defined in equation (6).

Second, the residual mortality rate for a cause-cluster remaining after subtracting the projected mortality for those detailed causes with a robust equation was distributed among the rest of the detailed causes in the cause-cluster. These deaths were distributed according to their relative proportionate distribution in the GBD estimates for 1990.

PROJECTING AGE-, SEX- AND CAUSE-SPECIFIC MORTALITY RATES, 1990–2020

Using the cause-cluster regression results and alternative assumptions for selected causes, the projections of the independent variables, and the equations for detailed causes, mortality rates for eight regions, 98 causes, and fourteen age-sex groups were projected from the base year 1990 to 1995, 2000, 2005, 2010, 2015 and 2020. To screen for data entry errors or mistakes in the computer code, we examined graphs of each of these age-specific rates over the period 1990–2020 (10 976 graphs in all). Computational errors revealed by this exercise were corrected. A final set of projected age-, sex-, cause- and region-specific rates were then generated. In a limited number of cases, implausible projections led to a re-examination of the panel dataset, resulting in the exclusion of some outliers and new parameter estimates for projection equations.[9]

PROJECTING HIV INCIDENCE AND MORTALITY

Given that mortality from HIV infection has only recently begun to dominate mortality patterns, and then only at some ages in some countries, the experience of countries with good vital registration data embodied in the predictive equations described above cannot adequately reflect the dynamics of the HIV epidemic. There is an extensive literature on alternative projections of incidence and mortality from the HIV epidemic (see, for example, Anderson 1993, Anderson et al. 1991, Anderson and May 1988, Brookmeyer and Damiano 1989, Chin et al. 1992, Chin and Lwanga 1991, Karon et al. 1988). For the purpose of the GBD, the projections prepared by the Global Programme on AIDS (GPA) of the World Health Organization were used, with some modifications.[10] Low-Beer et al. (1996) provide more detail on the development of the GPA projection model and the justification for the particular parameters used in their model. In brief, the GPA based their predictions on EPIMODEL, a software program developed by WHO, which fits a gamma distribution to reported AIDS cases and generates predictions of HIV incidence, cumulative incidence, AIDS incidence and mortality. The results of these projections by region and year were kindly made available by GPA/WHO for the GBD.

In the GPA projections, as a consequence of the gamma distribution used in EPIMODEL, HIV incidence in all regions is predicted to decline to zero soon after the peak in HIV incidence has been achieved. As a result, these predictions would suggest that in the year 2020 there would be essentially little or no HIV incidence anywhere. Based on the infectious disease modeling literature (e.g. Anderson and May 1992, Bailey 1957), we believe that this is too optimistic a scenario. We have, therefore, modified the GPA projections so that for our baseline scenario, the number of incident cases per year is assumed to stabilize once incidence has fallen to one-half of peak incidence—Figure 7.3 illustrates the baseline projections of incidence and mortality by region. As no region, except EME, is near the point where incidence is half of peak incidence, we do not know at what incidence level the HIV epidemic will actually stabilize in each region. Undoubtedly, the equilibrium incidence level will depend on a number of factors, including prevention policies, that will vary across regions. The choice of an equilibrium value for incidence that is 50 per cent of peak incidence is entirely arbitrary and does not take into account advances that may be achieved in behaviour modification or technological breakthroughs such as a vaccine or more effective chemotherapy. However, as it is not yet known what effect these developments may have, an arbitrary scalar has been applied to guess the future course of the epidemic. To estimate mortality from HIV, we have used the same assumptions as included in the GPA projection model regarding the time distribution for the progression from HIV to AIDS, and the distribution of deaths from AIDS over time.

Figure 7.3   Baseline projections of HIV incidence and mortality, by
region, 1990–2020

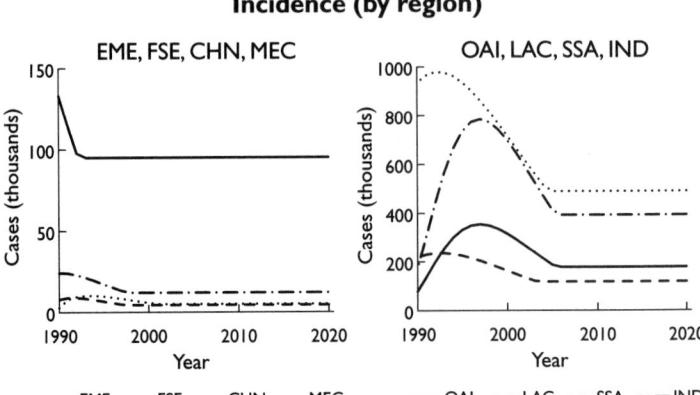

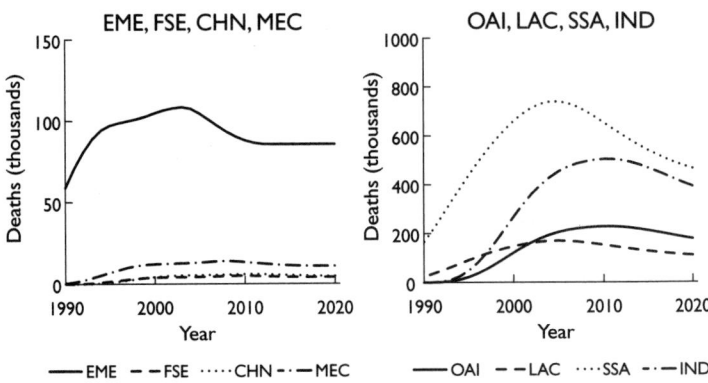

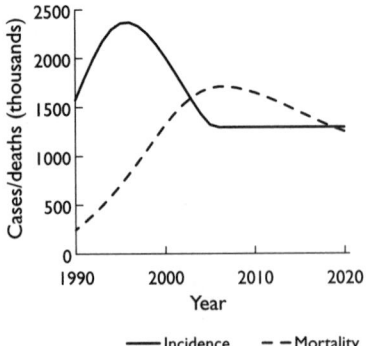

Note: Incidence and mortality for EME, FSE, CHN and MEC are shown on the left while OAI, LAC, SSA and
IND are shown on the right. They have been grouped this way to reflect differences in orders of
magnitude of incidence and mortality.

There is no objective basis on which to judge if the GPA estimates of the magnitude and timing of peak incidence are correct. Low-Beer et al. (1996) refer to evidence suggesting that HIV incidence has peaked in the United States, Uganda and Thailand, at least in selected groups that have been monitored closely. Furthermore, the projected peak incidences for most regions appear to be plausible. The pace and magnitude of the projected epidemic in India, OAI and China, which is often justified with reference to Thailand, may be overly pessimistic. For example, GPA has assumed that the time from first onset of the epidemic to peak incidence in India and OAI will be only 9 years whereas in SSA, the time from first onset to peak incidence was 13 years. Whether the more rapid unfolding of the epidemic in India and OAI as forecasted by GPA is reasonable, given the regional differences in the prevalence of other STDs remains uncertain.

For the pessimistic projections, we have assumed that equilibrium incidence will be attained at a level which is 75 per cent of peak incidence, and for the optimistic projections, we have assumed that incidence will fall to only 20 per cent of peak incidence before stabilizing. Clearly, given the uncertainty about many aspects of sexual behaviour in different regions and the relevant transmission parameters, the peak incidence forecasted by GPA may well be too high or too low. Consequently, considerable caution is required when interpreting these HIV projections, particularly for the years beyond 2005.

MODIFICATIONS OF TUBERCULOSIS PROJECTIONS

Because of the powerful interaction between tuberculosis and HIV infection in regions such as SSA, about one-third of HIV-positive individuals are expected to die from tuberculosis (Kumaresan et al. 1996). The increased case-load due to tuberculosis in HIV-positives is likely to influence the annual risk of infection of tuberculosis for HIV-negatives in the community. An elevated annual risk of infection will, over a period of years, lead to higher incidence and higher mortality from tuberculosis in HIV-negatives. Mathematical models of tuberculosis have been developed which have attempted to project the impact of HIV on tuberculosis (Bermejo et al. 1992, Schulzer et al. 1992). Some of these projections are frankly alarmist. For the purpose of the GBD, conservative assumptions were used to capture the likely impact of HIV on tuberculosis incidence and mortality in HIV-negatives. Thus, for the baseline projections, we assumed that the expected 2 per cent annual decline in mortality in SSA will be arrested, and that mortality will remain constant until 2010, and then begin to decline at a rate of 1 per cent per year. In India, it was assumed that mortality will remain constant until 2000, and then decline at 2 per cent per year. For the optimistic scenario, the trend in tuberculosis in India generated by the model was not modified, and in SSA, mortality was assumed to remain constant to 2000, and then to decline by 2 per cent a year. In the pessimistic scenario, the death rate in India is held constant while in SSA, mortality is assumed to increase by 1 per cent a year up to 2000, and then to remain constant.

PROJECTING YEARS LIVED WITH DISABILITY

From the projections of mortality by cause, it is a simple matter to calculate projected Years of Life Lost (YLLs). However, in order to project DALYs, it is also necessary to project Years Lived with Disability (YLDs). Ideally, projection models for each cause of disability should have been developed. However, given the paucity of information on disability trends, this would have been a major undertaking with very little confidence in the final results. Therefore, to project YLDs a much cruder approach was adopted. Firstly, causes of death and disability were divided into three distinct categories, and a different method to approximate YLDs was employed in each case, as outlined below.

- For those causes where the ratio of YLDs to YLLs was less than 10 in all regions, as estimated in the 1990 GBD results, YLDs were estimated by assuming that the age-, sex- and region-specific ratio of YLDs to YLLs as estimated for 1990 would hold constant in the future.

- For selected causes where there is considerable disability but little mortality—for example, sexually transmitted diseases—a decline in age-sex-specific rates has been predicted as income and education rise. We have assumed that the age-specific YLD rates for the component diseases of the tropical cluster of conditions and trachoma will decline at the same pace as Group I mortality, excluding HIV. For helminths, sexually transmitted diseases and anaemia, we have assumed that the pace of decline is slower than that for Group I as a whole.[11] Cataract is assumed to decline at the same rate as Group II mortality.

- The remaining causes include those largely disabling conditions for which there is no clear evidence of a temporal trend in age-sex-specific rates. Included in this set of conditions are bipolar disorder, unipolar major depression, drug dependence, schizophrenia, alcohol use, Alzheimer's and other dementias, Parkinson disease, multiple sclerosis, post-traumatic stress disorder, panic disorder, obsessive-compulsive disorder, rheumatoid arthritis, osteoarthritis, benign prostatic hypertrophy, dental caries, periodontal disease, edentulism and glaucoma. For these conditions, we have assumed that age-sex-specific YLD rates will remain constant over the period 1990–2020.

We recognize that the approach taken to projecting YLDs is extremely crude and hence the projections of DALYs are likely to be even more unreliable than projections of deaths. Much more research is required to generate robust and plausible methods to project YLDs from various conditions and to collect the requisite datasets to do so.

POPULATION PROJECTIONS

To maintain consistency with previous versions of the GBD already published, we have used World Bank estimates of 1990 population sizes and mortality rates by five-year age group in 1990 for each region. To elaborate projections of mortality and disability, population projections for each region for the baseline, optimistic and pessimistic projection scenarios were required. These were calculated as follows:

- Cause-specific mortality projections were first aggregated to obtain estimates of all-cause mortality in each of the seven age groups for each region.

- Mortality rates for these seven age groups were then used to estimate mortality rates for each five-year age group, using the ratio of the five-year age group mortality rate to the larger age band mortality rate, based on the World Bank estimates of mortality by region for 1990.

- World Bank projections of the crude birth rate for each region were used in the baseline, optimistic and pessimistic scenarios in order to project the size of the birth cohort for each year from 1990–2020.

- Population projections for each five-year age group were then obtained using the projected birth and death rates, and an assumption of no net migration between regions. While inter-regional migration is likely to occur, we have not developed separate projections of such population movements. As a result, our estimates are slightly lower for EME than the population projections for EME developed by the World Bank for the *World Development Report 1993*. Annex Table 11 provides details of our population projections for the baseline scenario, by region, for five-year age groups for the years 2000, 2010 and 2020.

FINAL PROJECTIONS

The projected rates of YLLs and YLDs, incorporating the projections of HIV and the modifications for tuberculosis, were applied to these projected populations to generate projected numbers of deaths, YLLs, YLDs, and DALYs for each of the three scenarios. Annex Tables 12–21 provide complete detail by age, sex, cause and region for deaths and DALYs for the baseline scenario for 2000, 2010 and 2020, and for the optimistic and pessimistic scenarios in 2020.

RESULTS

Before attempting to summarize the voluminous projections of disease and injury at different ages, in various regions, and for males and females separately, it is important first to reflect on what projections such as these actually represent. Baseline estimates of death, disability and DALYs in 1990 have been projected into the future based on an explicit set of assumptions and methods, which offer but one approach in a virtually infinite set of possible scenarios. The results of this exercise, however plausible they might appear and however correct (or incorrect) they might ultimately prove to be, are nothing more than the numerical consequences of the assumptions and methods employed. In the preceding sections of this chapter we have tried to be as transparent as possible about what assumptions have been made to define the three basic scenarios, and about what methods, or mix of methods, were used in different cases. The reader can judge how appropriate these methodological approaches might be and how they might be improved to produce more reliable projections. For the present, the methods and assumptions described here have resulted in a set of projections which must be taken as being merely indicative of probable future scenarios. We do not claim that these results are necessarily reliable predictions of the future. They do, however, represent the most comprehensive set of health status projections ever prepared, to our knowledge, and, in providing different visions of the future, may prove useful for guiding health policy choices designed to ensure that this future does, or does not occur as predicted.

All-Cause Mortality

The disease and injury patterns implied by these projections suggest many avenues for discussion. Perhaps the most meaningful starting point is an examination of how overall levels of mortality are projected to change. Figure 7.4 shows the number of deaths projected by age for the world in the three scenarios compared with the number of deaths by age in 1990. In all three scenarios, there is a dramatic shift in number of deaths from young ages to older ages. The difference between the absolute number of deaths in the optimistic and pessimistic scenarios appears to be less impressive than the difference in death rates in these scenarios because of the compensating effect of mortality rates on projected population numbers.

The projection methods generate mortality rates for seven age groups; for the population projections, we have estimated mortality rates for 5-year age groups using the simple approximation method described above. These mortality rates have been used to calculate life expectancy by region and sex in 2020 for the three scenarios (Figure 7.5). Figure 7.5 also shows for comparison estimates of life expectancy in 1990. In females, life expectancy at birth in all three scenarios is projected to increase in all regions, with the largest gains expected in SSA, India and OAI. Of note, life expectancy for EME females may nearly approach 90 years in the optimistic scenario—this projection appears all the more plausible considering that Asian women in the United States already have a life expectancy over 86 years. The smallest gain is projected for FSE. Comparison of female and male projected life expectancy highlights the much lower life expectancy of males in 1990 in all regions except India and the far smaller gains projected in all regions for males as compared with

Figure 7.4   Global number of deaths by age and sex: baseline, optimistic and pessimistic scenarios compared with 1990 estimates

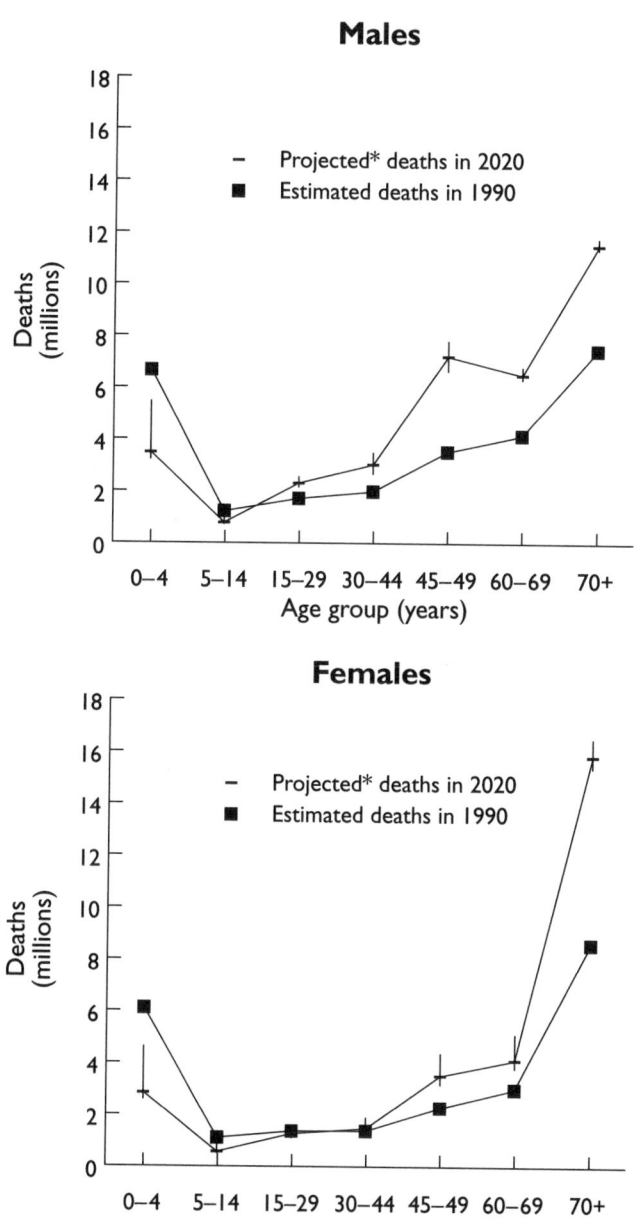

Males

Females

* Projected deaths are for the baseline scenario. The range of deaths suggested by the optimistic and pessimistic scenarios is reflected by the size of the vertical bars around each point.

Figure 7.5 Projected life expectancy at birth in 2020, by region: baseline, optimistic and pessimistic scenarios, compared with 1990 estimates

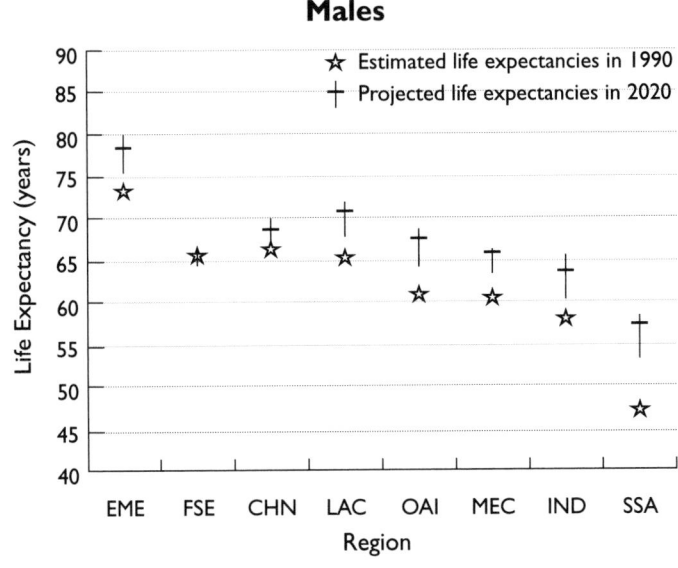

Males

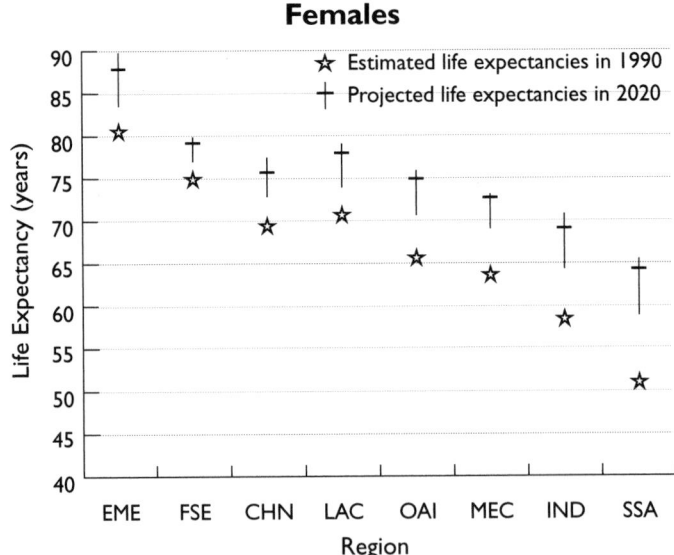

Females

Note: The stars in the figure denote life expectancies at birth in 1990. Baseline life expectancies projected for 2020 appear as a horizontal bar crossed by a vertical bar that gives upper and lower limits defined by the optimistic and pessimistic projection scenarios.

females (see Table 7.3) The much smaller improvements in male mortality are in large part due to the greater impact of the tobacco epidemic in males. Even in EME, where the sex differential in life expectancy at birth in 1990 was 7.1 years, the gap between males and females is projected to widen further. Males in FSE are the only group for which no improvement in life expectancy is projected between 1990 and 2020; however, as their life expectancy in 1995 has dropped as much as 5 years, some gain is forecasted between 1995 and 2020.

Table 7.3   Projected change in life expectancy at birth by sex and region, 1990–2020

Region	Increase (in years) in life expectancy at birth from 1990 to 2020		
	Male	Female	Female minus male gain
Baseline scenario			
EME	5.1	7.3	2.2
FSE	-0.1	4.1	4.2
CHN	2.3	6.3	4.0
LAC	5.5	7.2	1.7
OAI	6.6	9.2	2.6
MEC	5.3	8.9	3.6
IND	5.6	10.6	5.0
SSA	10.2	13.3	3.1
Optimistic scenario			
EME	6.7	9.1	2.5
FSE	0.7	4.8	4.2
CHN	3.6	8.1	4.5
LAC	6.7	8.3	1.6
OAI	7.7	10.2	2.5
MEC	5.7	9.4	3.7
IND	7.5	12.3	4.7
SSA	11.2	14.5	3.3
Pessimistic scenario			
EME	2.1	2.9	0.8
FSE	-1.2	2.0	3.2
CHN	0.3	3.3	3.0
LAC	2.4	3.1	0.8
OAI	3.2	4.9	1.7
MEC	2.8	5.3	2.5
IND	2.2	5.8	3.6
SSA	5.9	7.8	1.9

We have also compared our projections with the UN projections of life expectancy in 2020 for similar regions (United Nations 1995).[12] In general, the UN projections for females fall within the range of our projections of female life expectancy at birth. The notable exceptions are observe in EME and India. In EME, as noted above, we project substantial increases in life expectancy whereas the UN projections show only small gains. This difference is not surprising as the UN model assumes that life expectancy at birth increases by less than 0.1 years per calendar year after a life expectancy of 82.5 years for females has been reached. For males, however, there are marked differences in the all-cause mortality rates generated by our cause-specific approach and the demographic approach of the UN. In all regions except EME, our projections of male life expectancy are lower than those projected by the UN—in some regions such as India, FSE, and MEC, the difference in life expectancy at birth between our optimistic projection and the UN projections is greater than 3.5 years. Mechanistic projections of male life expectancy, such as those made by the UN, do not adequately reflect the impact of the epidemic of tobacco-related mortality, and the likely trends in cause-specific mortality including HIV.

Risks of death during three broad periods of the life cycle have been estimated for the three major groups of causes in 2020 for the baseline scenario, as illustrated in Figure 7.6. The top histogram shows the probability of death between birth and age 15, the middle histogram shows the probability of death between age 15 and age 60 and the bottom histogram shows the probability of death between ages 60 and 70.[13] In this scenario, risks of death in children and adolescents are expected to be dramatically lower by 2020 for both males and females as compared to 1990. Although the highest probabilities of death at these ages will still be in SSA, followed by India, mortality risks will have fallen by about two-thirds compared to 1990. Among adult women, the risk of death between ages 15 and 60 is projected to decline in all regions, with a major reduction of Group I mortality risk due largely to lower rates of maternal mortality and tuberculosis. The risk of death from Group II diseases as a whole is also projected to decline but not by as much as Group I. Group III mortality risks in the baseline scenario remain roughly constant through to 2020.

For males, the projected changes in the risk of death between ages 15 and 60 are more complex. Only modest reductions in the risk of death in this age group are projected for EME, LAC, OAI, MEC and India. All-cause mortality risks are actually projected to increase in FSE, China and India. The increase in FSE and China is entirely due to a projected rise in Group II, largely due to the impact of tobacco. Remarkably, FSE is projected to have the highest adult male risk of death, higher even than SSA in 2020. In India, Group II risk of death between ages 15 and 60 is projected to increase as well.

In terms of number of deaths by cause, the projections are more or less consistent with what might be expected on the basis of knowledge about the epidemiological transition. Thus, world-wide annual mortality from the general category of communicable, maternal, perinatal and nutritional conditions (Group I) is expected to decline from 17.2 million in 1990 to 10.3 million in 2020 (8.2 million in the optimistic and 16.9 million in the pessimistic scenarios). (Figures in parentheses in the following discussion

Figure 7.6   Regional probabilities of death, by age, sex and broad cause Group, 2020 (baseline scenario)

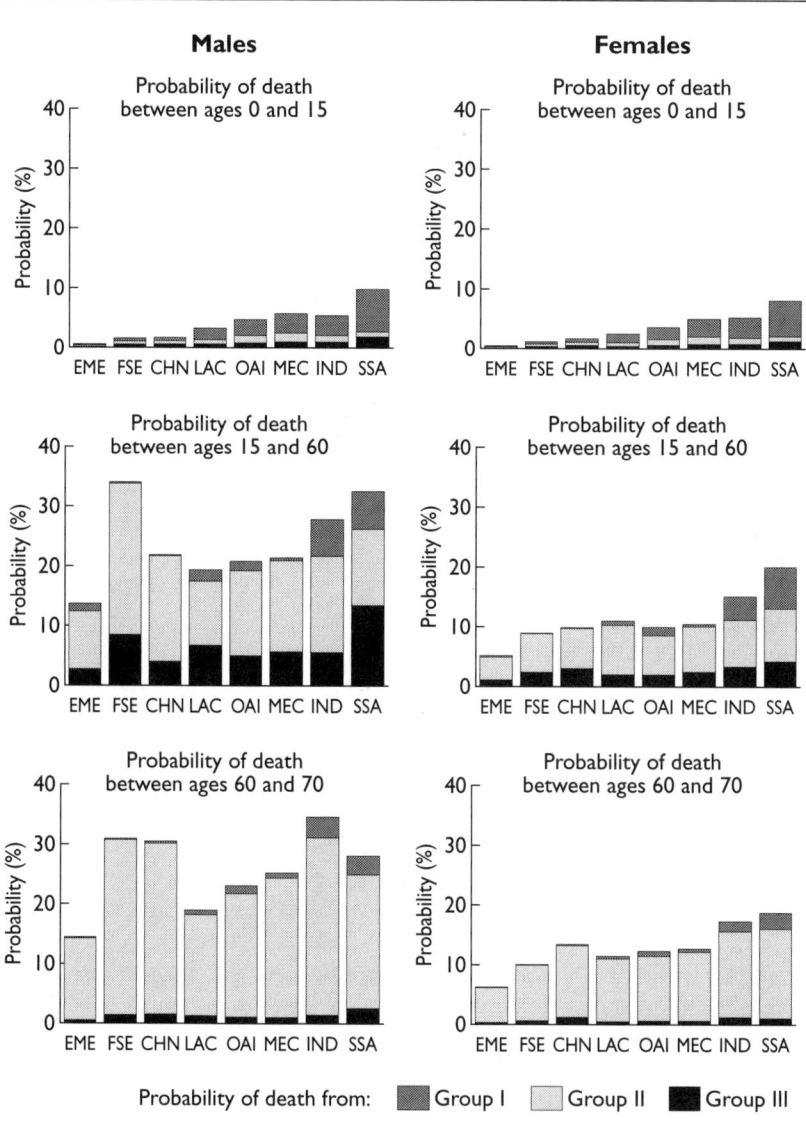

Probability of death from: ▨ Group I   ▧ Group II   ■ Group III

show the range bounded by the optimistic and pessimistic estimates.) Conversely, a very large *increase* in deaths from noncommunicable diseases (Group II) is expected, with annual mortality rising from an estimated 28.1 million deaths in 1990 to 49.7 (48.0–53.0) million in 2020, an increase of 77 per cent. The projected increase in Group II deaths is expected to be larger for males (91 per cent) than for females (61 per cent), consistent with what has been observed in industrialized countries during their mortality transition. Interestingly, deaths from injuries (Group III) are also projected to increase dramatically under the assumptions outlined earlier, rising from 5.1 million in 1990 to 8.4 (8.2–8.4) million in 2020. However, given the inherent difficulty in projecting deaths from injuries, these projections are even more uncertain than those for Groups I and II. Increases in the absolute number of deaths due to Group III are largely determined by the projected changes in population size and age structure, and, in particular, by an increase in the number of men at young adult ages, where the risk of injury death is highest.

In terms of proportionate mortality, Group II causes are projected to increase from 55 per cent of all deaths world-wide in 1990 to 73 (68–74) per cent in 2020. In other words, by 2020, three out of four deaths which occur each year will be due to non-communicable diseases, if these projections prove to be correct. Proportionate mortality from injuries is also expected to rise, albeit marginally, from 10 per cent in 1990 to 12 (11–13) per cent in 2020.

The contribution of major causes of death to these baseline projections of trends in mortality is shown in Figure 7.7. Large declines in mortality between 1990 and 2020 are expected for all of the principal Group I causes including infectious and parasitic diseases (9.3 to 6.5 million), respiratory infections (4.4 to 2.5 million), maternal causes (454 to 72 thousand), perinatal conditions (2.4 to 0.9 million) and nutritional disorders (0.6 to 0.3 million). Deaths from cancer, on the other hand, are projected to more than double between 1990 and 2020, rising to 12.3 million by 2020. Directly coded diabetes deaths are projected to rise by 32 per cent to about 753 thousand in 2020. In absolute terms, however, the largest projected increase in mortality is for cardiovascular diseases, which, under the baseline scenario, are expected to increase from 14 million deaths in 1990 to 23 million in 2020. At this level, cardiovascular diseases would account for more than one-third of all deaths world-wide. Deaths from chronic respiratory diseases are expected to double over the period, and by 2020 might well account for over 6 million deaths a year. The steady rise in injury deaths from nearly every cause of injury is the product of small projected changes in highest risks with rising population growth, particularly in those age groups at risk for injuries. Figure 7.8 also illustrates that, in the pessimistic scenario, there would be much less change in the absolute number of Group I deaths expected in the next 30 years. Relative changes in Group II and Group III are similar in all three scenarios.

Figure 7.7 Baseline projections of deaths from Group I, Group II and Group III causes, world, 1990–2020

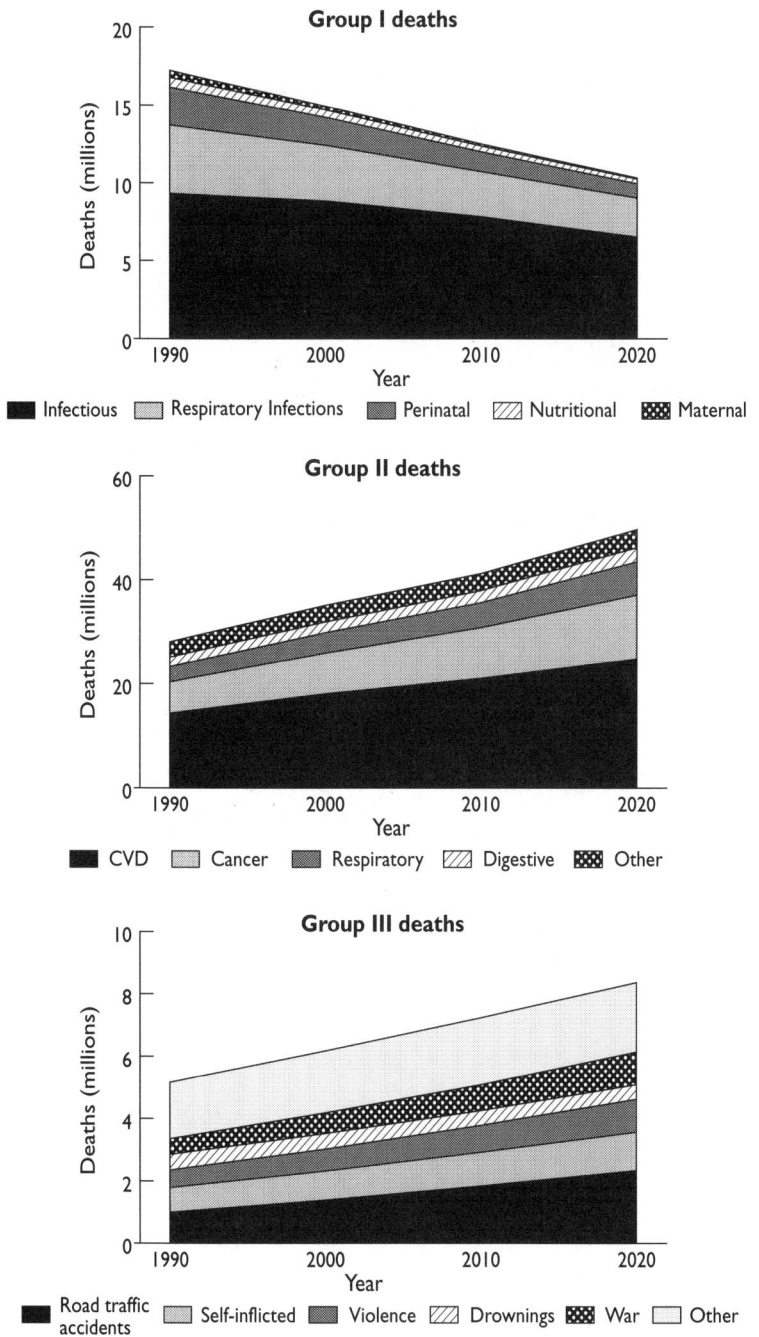

Figure 7.8 Pessimistic projections of deaths from Group I causes, world, 1990–2020

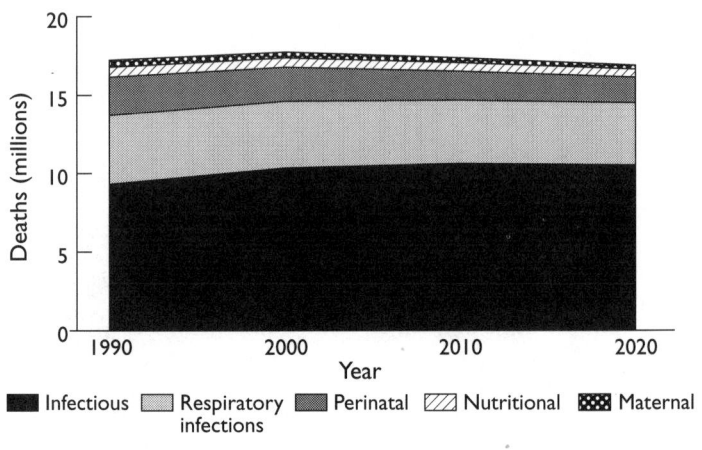

Another way to assess the projected changes in mortality is to examine the expected changes in the leading causes of death. Table 7.4 lists the ten leading causes of death according to the baseline scenario for males, females and both sexes combined as projected for 2020 for the world and for developing and developed regions. For comparison, Tables 7.5 and 7.6 show the ten leading causes of death for the optimistic and pessimistic scenarios, respectively. The three leading causes of death in all three scenarios are projected to be ischaemic heart disease, cerebrovascular disease and COPD, accounting collectively for one out of every three deaths. Lower respiratory infections remain a leading cause of death in all scenarios as do tuberculosis, road traffic accidents, lung cancer and stomach cancer. Figure 7.9 illustrates the change in the ranking of various causes of death between 1990 and 2020, according to the baseline projections. Diarrhoeal diseases, perinatal conditions, measles and malaria are all projected to substantially decline in importance. On the other hand, five causes of death among the fifteen highest in 2020 are projected to have moved up five or more places in the rankings, namely lung cancer, stomach cancer, war, liver cancer and HIV.

It is of some interest to examine how mortality from the various leading sites of cancer is expected to change over the next three decades, given the different etiology for different sites of the disease. Globally, lung cancer in 1990 is estimated to have been the cause of about 945 thousand deaths, 523 thousand of which occurred in EME and FSE. By 2020, the annual death toll from the disease world-wide is expected to more than double, rising to about 2.4 million deaths. Moreover, most (82 per cent) of this increase in lung cancer deaths is projected to occur in developing countries, and most of this among males who began smoking in large numbers

Figure 7.9   Change in rank order of deaths for the 15 leading causes,
world, 1990–2020

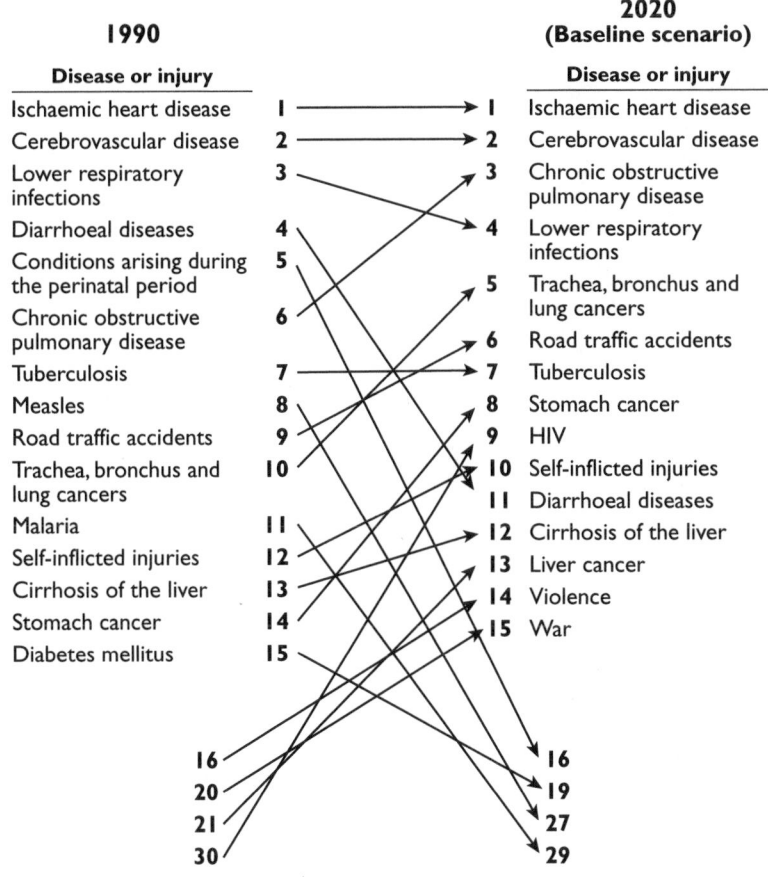

in recent decades. Stomach cancer is projected to be the second leading site of cancer mortality in 2020, causing about 1.6 million deaths world-wide, up from 750 thousand in 1990. Other leading sites of cancer in 2020 are projected to include the liver (1.2 million deaths), colon/rectum (832 thousand) and oesophagus (823 thousand). In developing countries, lung cancer is projected to be the leading cause of cancer deaths in 2020, causing 1.6 million deaths that year (up from 420 thousand in 1990), followed by stomach cancer (1.3 million), liver cancer (1.1 million), oesophageal cancer (753 thousand) and cancer of the mouth and oropharynx (566 thousand).

The pace of epidemiological transition is likely to be very different in different regions of the world. For example, in SSA, Group I causes accounted for an estimated 5.3 million deaths in 1990, or two-thirds of all

Table 7.4   Ten leading causes of death in 2020 (baseline scenario)

	Both Sexes			Males			Females		
Rank	Disease or injury	Deaths (thousands)	Cumulative %	Disease or injury	Deaths (thousands)	Cumulative %	Disease or injury	Deaths (thousands)	Cumulative %
World									
	All causes	68 337		All causes	38 788		All causes	29 549	
1	Ischaemic heart disease	11 107	16.3	Ischaemic heart disease	6 077	15.7	Ischaemic heart disease	5 030	17.0
2	Cerebrovascular disease	7 698	27.5	Cerebrovascular disease	3 977	25.9	Cerebrovascular disease	3 721	29.6
3	Chronic obstructive pulmonary disease	4 726	34.4	Chronic obstructive pulmonary disease	2 620	32.7	Chronic obstructive pulmonary disease	2 107	36.7
4	Lower respiratory infections	2 472	38.1	Lower respiratory infections	1 809	37.3	Lower respiratory infections	1 197	40.8
5	Trachea, bronchus and lung cancers	2 415	41.6	Trachea, bronchus and lung cancers	1 623	41.5	Tuberculosis	986	44.1
6	Road traffic accidents	2 338	45.0	Road traffic accidents	1 310	44.9	Road traffic accidents	715	46.5
7	Tuberculosis	2 296	48.4	Tuberculosis	1 275	48.2	Trachea, bronchus and lung cancers	606	48.6
8	Stomach cancer	1 588	50.7	Lower respiratory infections	1 069	50.9	Diarrhoeal diseases	550	50.5
9	HIV	1 250	52.5	Stomach cancer	885	53.2	HIV	522	52.2
10	Self-inflicted injuries	1 229	54.3	Liver cancer	841	55.4	Stomach cancer	519	54.0
				Violence					
Developed regions									
	All causes	13 505		All causes	7 345		All causes	6 160	
1	Ischaemic heart disease	3 259	24.1	Ischaemic heart disease	1 730	23.6	Ischaemic heart disease	1 529	24.8
2	Cerebrovascular disease	1 705	36.8	Cerebrovascular disease	760	33.9	Cerebrovascular disease	945	40.2
3	Trachea, bronchus and lung cancers	804	42.7	Trachea, bronchus and lung cancers	577	41.8	Trachea, bronchus and lung cancers	227	43.8
4	Chronic obstructive pulmonary disease	551	46.8	Chronic obstructive pulmonary disease	345	46.5	Lower respiratory infections	219	47.4
5	Lower respiratory infections	429	50.0	Stomach cancer	217	49.4	Chronic obstructive pulmonary disease	206	50.7

Table 7.4 (Continued)

	Both Sexes			Males			Females		
Rank	Disease or injury	Deaths (thousands)	Cumulative %	Disease or injury	Deaths (thousands)	Cumulative %	Disease or injury	Deaths (thousands)	Cumulative %
Developed Regions (continued)									
6	Colon and rectum cancers	364	52.7	Lower respiratory infections	210	52.3	Breast cancer	183	53.7
7	Stomach cancer	332	55.1	Colon and rectum cancers	198	55.0	Colon and rectum cancers	167	56.4
8	Self-inflicted injuries	234	56.9	Self-inflicted injuries	171	57.3	Diabetes mellitus	149	58.8
9	Diabetes mellitus	228	58.5	Prostate cancer	163	59.5	Stomach cancer	115	60.7
10	Road traffic accidents	221	60.2	Cirrhosis of the liver	155	61.6	Dementia and other degenerative and hereditary CNS disorders	109	62.5
Developing regions									
	All causes	54 832		All causes	31 443		All causes	23 390	
1	Ischaemic heart disease	7 848	14.3	Ischaemic heart disease	4 347	13.8	Ischaemic heart disease	3 501	15.0
2	Cerebrovascular disease	5 993	25.2	Cerebrovascular disease	3 217	24.1	Cerebrovascular disease	2 776	26.8
3	Chronic obstructive pulmonary disease	4 175	32.9	Chronic obstructive pulmonary disease	2 275	31.3	Chronic obstructive pulmonary disease	1 901	35.0
4	Tuberculosis	2 273	37.0	Road traffic accidents	1 475	36.0	Tuberculosis	979	39.1
5	Road traffic accidents	2 117	40.9	Tuberculosis	1 294	40.1	Lower respiratory infections	978	43.3
6	Lower respiratory infections	2 043	44.6	Lower respiratory infections	1 231	44.0	Road traffic accidents	642	46.1
7	Trachea, bronchus and lung cancers	1 611	47.5	Trachea, bronchus and lung cancers	1 065	47.4	Diarrhoeal diseases	548	48.4
8	Stomach cancer	1 256	49.8	Stomach cancer	853	50.1	HIV	509	50.6
9	Diarrhoeal diseases	1 208	52.0	Liver cancer	832	52.8	Self-inflicted injuries	454	52.5
10	HIV	1 160	54.1	Violence	795	55.3	War	426	54.4

Table 7.5   Ten leading causes of death in 2020 (optimistic scenario)

Rank	Both Sexes — Disease or injury	Deaths (thousands)	Cumulative %	Males — Disease or injury	Deaths (thousands)	Cumulative %	Females — Disease or injury	Deaths (thousands)	Cumulative %
World									
	All causes	64 635		All causes	36 867		All causes	27 768	
1	Ischaemic heart disease	11 208	17.3	Ischaemic heart disease	6 191	16.8	Ischaemic heart disease	5 017	18.1
2	Cerebrovascular disease	7 708	29.3	Cerebrovascular disease	4 024	27.7	Cerebrovascular disease	3 684	31.3
3	Chronic obstructive pulmonary disease	3 946	35.4	Chronic obstructive pulmonary disease	2 282	33.9	Chronic obstructive pulmonary disease	1 664	37.3
4	Trachea, bronchus and lung cancers	2 452	39.2	Trachea, bronchus and lung cancers	1 838	38.9	Lower respiratory infections	1 095	41.3
5	Road traffic accidents	2 421	42.9	Road traffic accidents	1 651	43.4	Road traffic accidents	770	44.0
6	Lower respiratory infections	2 261	46.4	Lower respiratory infections	1 166	46.5	Trachea, bronchus and lung cancers	614	46.3
7	Stomach cancer	1 570	48.8	Stomach cancer	1 053	49.4	Tuberculosis	601	48.4
8	Tuberculosis	1 317	50.9	Tuberculosis	861	51.7	Self-inflicted injuries	523	50.3
9	Self-inflicted injuries	1 242	52.8	Violence	846	54.0	Stomach cancer	517	52.2
10	Liver cancer	1 149	54.6	Self-inflicted injuries	719	56.0	Breast cancer	493	53.9
Developed regions									
	All causes	12 826		All causes	6 999		All causes	5 827	
1	Ischaemic heart disease	3 220	25.1	Ischaemic heart disease	1 722	24.6	Ischaemic heart disease	1 497	25.7
2	Cerebrovascular disease	1 688	38.3	Cerebrovascular disease	763	35.5	Cerebrovascular disease	925	41.6
3	Trachea, bronchus and lung cancers	814	44.6	Trachea, bronchus and lung cancers	585	43.9	Trachea, bronchus and lung cancers	229	45.5
4	Chronic obstructive pulmonary disease	461	48.2	Chronic obstructive pulmonary disease	299	48.1	Lower respiratory infections	203	49.0
5	Lower respiratory infections	395	51.3	Stomach cancer	210	51.1	Breast cancer	175	52.0

Table 7.5 (Continued)

	Both Sexes			Males			Females		
Rank	Disease or injury	Deaths (thousands)	Cumulative %	Disease or injury	Deaths (thousands)	Cumulative %	Disease or injury	Deaths (thousands)	Cumulative %
Developed Regions (continued)									
6	Colon and rectum cancers	352	54.0	Lower respiratory infections	192	53.9	Chronic obstructive pulmonary disease	162	54.8
7	Stomach cancer	322	56.5	Colon and rectum cancers	191	56.6	Colon and rectum cancers	160	57.5
8	Self-inflicted injuries	236	58.4	Self-inflicted injuries	172	59.1	Diabetes mellitus	126	59.7
9	Road traffic accidents	206	60.0	Prostate cancer	159	61.3	Stomach cancer	112	61.6
10	Diabetes mellitus	194	61.5	Road traffic accidents	135	63.3	Dementia and other degenerative and hereditary CNS disorders	95	63.2
Developing regions									
	All causes	51 809		All causes	29 868		All causes	21 941	
1	Ischaemic heart disease	7 988	15.4	Ischaemic heart disease	4 469	15.0	Ischaemic heart disease	3 519	16.0
2	Cerebrovascular disease	6 019	27.0	Cerebrovascular disease	3 261	25.9	Cerebrovascular disease	2 758	28.6
3	Chronic obstructive pulmonary disease	3 485	33.8	Chronic obstructive pulmonary disease	1 983	32.5	Chronic obstructive pulmonary disease	1 502	35.5
4	Road traffic accidents	2 215	38.0	Road traffic accidents	1 515	37.6	Lower respiratory infections	891	39.5
5	Lower respiratory infections	1 866	41.6	Trachea, bronchus and lung cancers	1 253	41.8	Road traffic accidents	699	42.7
6	Trachea, bronchus and lung cancers	1 638	44.8	Lower respiratory infections	974	45.1	Tuberculosis	596	45.4
7	Tuberculosis	1 298	47.3	Stomach cancer	843	47.9	Diarrhoeal diseases	490	47.7
8	Stomach cancer	1 248	49.7	Liver cancer	810	50.6	Self-inflicted injuries	459	49.7
9	Diarrhoeal diseases	1 089	51.8	Violence	800	53.3	War	428	51.7
10	Liver cancer	1 077	53.9	Tuberculosis	702	55.6	Stomach cancer	406	53.5

Table 7.6   Ten leading causes of death in 2020 (pessimistic scenario)

		Both Sexes			Males			Females	
Rank	Disease or injury	Deaths (thousands)	Cumula-tive %	Disease or injury	Deaths (thousands)	Cumula-tive %	Disease or injury	Deaths (thousands)	Cumula-tive %
World									
	All causes	78 144		All causes	43 254		All causes	34 890	
1	Ischaemic heart disease	11 891	15.2	Ischaemic heart disease	6 257	14.5	Ischaemic heart disease	5 633	16.1
2	Cerebrovascular disease	8 314	25.9	Cerebrovascular disease	4 100	23.9	Cerebrovascular disease	4 214	28.2
3	Chronic obstructive pulmonary disease	4 744	31.9	Chronic obstructive pulmonary disease	2 637	30.0	Chronic obstructive pulmonary disease	2 107	34.3
4	Lower respiratory infections	3 921	36.9	Lower respiratory infections	2 026	34.7	Lower respiratory infections	1 895	39.7
5	Tuberculosis	3 275	41.1	Tuberculosis	1 897	39.1	Tuberculosis	1 378	43.6
6	Trachea, bronchus and lung cancers	2 345	44.1	Trachea, bronchus and lung cancers	1 764	43.2	Diarrhoeal diseases	1 020	46.6
7	Diarrhoeal diseases	2 204	47.0	Road traffic accidents	1 387	46.4	Conditions arising during the perinatal period	759	48.7
8	Road traffic accidents	1 934	49.4	Diarrhoeal diseases	1 183	49.1	HIV	731	50.8
9	HIV	1 755	51.7	Stomach cancer	1 072	51.6	Trachea, bronchus and lung cancers	581	52.5
10	Stomach cancer	1 624	53.8	HIV	1 024	54.0	Diabetes mellitus	561	54.1
Developed regions									
	All causes	15 032		All causes	7 996		All causes	7 036	
1	Ischaemic heart disease	3 728	24.8	Ischaemic heart disease	1 920	24.0	Ischaemic heart disease	1 808	25.7
2	Cerebrovascular disease	1 954	37.8	Cerebrovascular disease	841	34.5	Cerebrovascular disease	1 113	41.5
3	Trachea, bronchus and lung cancers	778	43.0	Trachea, bronchus and lung cancers	561	41.5	Lower respiratory infections	261	45.2
4	Chronic obstructive pulmonary disease	536	46.5	Chronic obstructive pulmonary disease	328	45.6	Trachea, bronchus and lung cancers	217	48.3
5	Lower respiratory infections	512	50.0	Lower respiratory infections	251	48.8	Breast cancer	213	51.3

Table 7.6 (Continued)

		Both Sexes			Males			Females	
Rank	Disease or injury	Deaths (thousands)	Cumula-tive %	Disease or injury	Deaths (thousands)	Cumula-tive %	Disease or injury	Deaths (thousands)	Cumula-tive %

Developed Regions (continued)

Rank	Disease or injury (Both Sexes)	Deaths (thousands)	Cumula-tive %	Disease or injury (Males)	Deaths (thousands)	Cumula-tive %	Disease or injury (Females)	Deaths (thousands)	Cumula-tive %
6	Colon and rectum cancers	401	52.6	Stomach cancer	229	51.6	Chronic obstructive pulmonary disease	209	54.3
7	Stomach cancer	359	55.0	Colon and rectum cancers	211	54.3	Colon and rectum cancers	190	57.0
8	Diabetes mellitus	251	56.7	Prostate cancer	174	56.5	Diabetes mellitus	156	59.2
9	Road traffic accidents	239	58.3	Road traffic accidents	168	58.6	Stomach cancer	130	61.1
10	Cirrhosis of the liver	230	59.8	Self-inflicted injuries	168	60.7	Dementia and other degenerative and hereditary CNS disorders	111	62.6

Developing regions

Rank	Disease or injury (Both Sexes)	Deaths (thousands)	Cumula-tive %	Disease or injury (Males)	Deaths (thousands)	Cumula-tive %	Disease or injury (Females)	Deaths (thousands)	Cumula-tive %
	All causes	63 112		All causes	35 258		All causes	27 854	
1	Ischaemic heart disease	8 162	12.9	Ischaemic heart disease	4 337	12.3	Ischaemic heart disease	3 825	13.7
2	Cerebrovascular disease	6 360	23.0	Cerebrovascular disease	3 259	21.5	Cerebrovascular disease	3 101	24.9
3	Chronic obstructive pulmonary disease	4 208	29.7	Chronic obstructive pulmonary disease	2 309	28.1	Chronic obstructive pulmonary disease	1 899	31.7
4	Lower respiratory infections	3 409	35.1	Tuberculosis	1 873	33.4	Lower respiratory infections	1 633	37.5
5	Tuberculosis	3 242	40.2	Lower respiratory infections	1 776	38.4	Tuberculosis	1 369	42.5
6	Diarrhoeal diseases	2 198	43.7	Road traffic accidents	1 220	41.9	Diarrhoeal diseases	1 017	46.1
7	Road traffic accidents	1 695	46.4	Trachea, bronchus and lung cancers	1 203	45.3	Conditions arising during the perinatal period	740	48.8
8	HIV	1 621	49.0	Diarrhoeal diseases	1 181	48.7	HIV	711	51.3
9	Conditions arising during the perinatal period	1 575	51.4	HIV	910	51.2	Road traffic accidents	476	53.0
10	Trachea, bronchus and lung cancers	1 567	53.9	Stomach cancer	843	53.6	Self-inflicted injuries	442	54.6

deaths in the region. By 2020, Group I deaths are projected to have declined by about 25 per cent, but will still claim 4.0 (3.4–6.5) million lives a year, or 39 (35–51) per cent of all deaths in the region. In contrast, in India for example, where Group I diseases in 1990 caused half of all deaths (4.8 million), considerable progress is expected in reducing mortality from these diseases. By 2020, Group I deaths in India are expected to amount to approximately 2.5 (1.5–4.0) million, or 22 (14–31) per cent of all deaths. What these projections emphasize, therefore, is that despite progress towards lower overall levels of mortality, there will remain a large burden of premature death in some regions of the developing world from largely preventable causes (Group I). Effective strategies and policies to hasten the reduction of death rates from these diseases must remain a priority for global public health action.

In China and in LAC, however, the predominance of non-communicable diseases, already apparent in 1990, will become even more evident over the next few decades. Group II causes claimed about 6.5 million lives in China in 1990 (about 75 per cent of all deaths), and this is projected to rise to 11.9 (11.0–12.9) million by 2020 (85 per cent of deaths). Deaths from chronic diseases (Group II) are expected to double in LAC by 2020, by which time they might well account for about 3.6 (3.4–3.9) million deaths, or 76 per cent of all deaths in the region. Mortality from noncommunicable diseases in EME is expected to rise both for males (from 3.1 million deaths in 1990 to 4.0 million in 2020) and for females (from 3.1 to 3.6 million deaths), due, in part, to the continued rise in smoking-attributable deaths. Smoking is also likely to be a major factor underlying the 56 per cent projected increase in male deaths from chronic diseases in FSE between 1990 and 2020.

A convenient index proposed by Frenk et al. (1989) for summarizing the combined effect of the demographic and epidemiological transition is the ratio of mortality from Group II causes to that from Group I causes (the higher the ratio, the greater the predominance of noncommunicable diseases and the further along a region is in the demographic and epidemiological transitions). The projected trends for these ratios are illustrated in Figure 7.10 for the period 1990–2020, for the total population (males and females combined). These figures show the ratio of death *numbers,* which are a function of both the age-distribution of the population and the cause-specific death rates. The impact of these two components is analysed separately later in this chapter.

Even between the two developed regions, EME and FSE, the path of demographic and epidemiological transitions over the next few decades is likely to be very different. In EME, the ratio of Group II to Group I deaths is expected to remain relatively constant (rising from 13 to 14 between 1990 and 2020). In FSE, Group I mortality is expected to decline by 50 per cent over the projection period, while Group II deaths, and death rates, are projected to continue to rise. As a result, we are projecting a dramatic rise in the ratio of Group II to Group I deaths in FSE, as shown in Figure 7.10.

Figure 7.10   Ratio of Group II to Group I deaths, by region, both sexes combined, 1990–2020

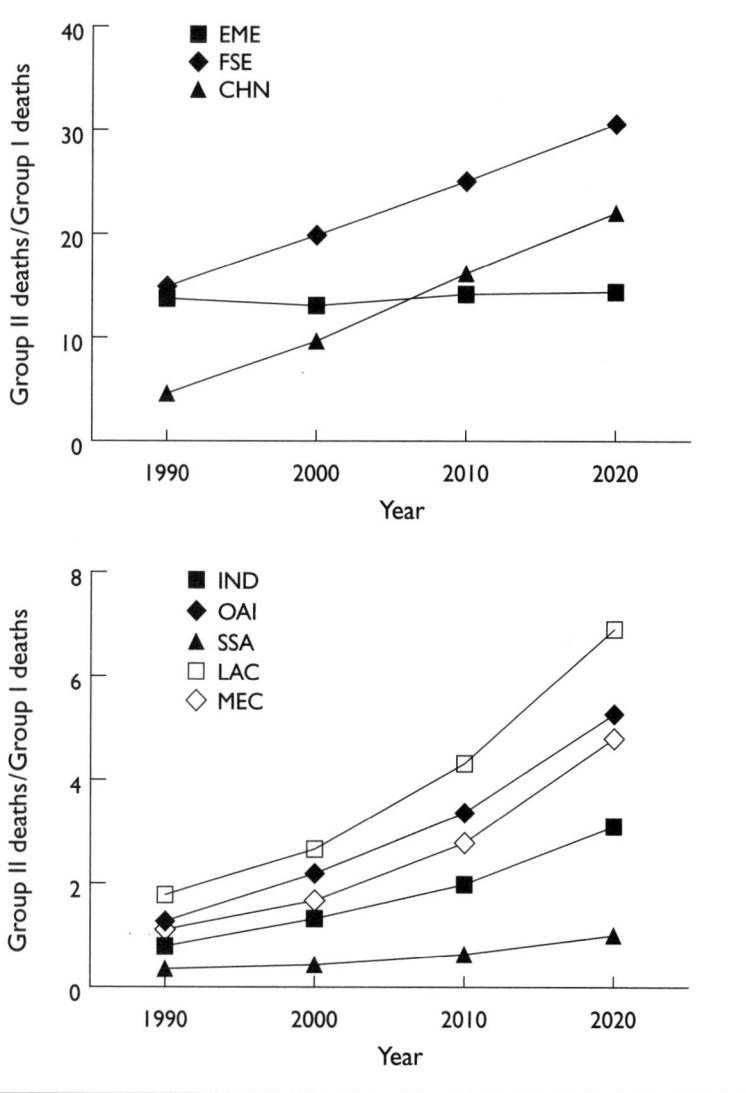

This epidemiological transition indicator is also expected to rise substantially in China, from 4.6 in 1990 to 22.0 in 2020. This marked increase in the ratio is due to three factors: very significant declines in projected Group I mortality both for males and females, stagnant Group II mortality rates for adult males, and an aging population.

The combined effects of the demographic and epidemiological transitions on the pattern of mortality for the other five regions are less extreme, as shown in Figure 7.10. In LAC, OAI and MEC, the ratio of Group II to

Group I deaths is projected to rise from under 2 to 6.9 in LAC, 5.3 in OAI and 4.8 in MEC. The two regions where the transition is expected to be much less rapid are India and SSA; in 2020 the ratio in India is expected to be around 3.1, while in SSA by 2020 Group II deaths are still not expected to exceed Group I deaths.

ADULT MORTALITY

In view of the increasing relative importance of deaths in middle age, it is of some interest to consider briefly how death rates from specific causes at ages 45–69 are expected to change. These projected trends are summarized below for each region. Much more detail is provided in Annex Tables 12–21.

EME. HIV mortality among males is projected to reach a peak level of about 27 per 100 000 at ages 45–59 around 1995, and thereafter to decline, but only slowly, to a level of about 20 per 100 000 in 2020. A similar pattern is expected for women, but at much reduced death rates compared to men. Ischaemic heart disease (IHD) mortality for men aged 60–69 years is projected to decline from around 520 per 100 000 to 400 per 100 000, and for women at these ages, from 210 per 100 000 to 85 per 100 000. Death rates from the disease among younger middle-aged women (45–59) are also projected to decline substantially, but not for men in this age group.

FSE. Death rates from HIV are projected to rise for both men and women, increasing by about four-fold between 1990 and 2020. However, the level of mortality from HIV is expected to remain comparatively low, with the highest maximum rates predicted for men aged 45–59 (0.4 per 100 000 in 2010). Cancer, ischaemic heart disease, stroke and chronic lung disease mortality rates are all projected to rise over the next few decades for men, but not for women (with the exception of COPD, for which a small absolute increase in death rates is projected under the baseline scenario).

India. Death rates from HIV are expected to rise dramatically. Among men, in both age groups 45–59 and 60–69, the death rate from the disease is expected to reach about 40–50 per 100 000 in 2010, declining to about 30–35 per 100 000 ten years later. This peak mortality level is substantially higher than for EME. HIV mortality among women is also expected to reach a peak in 2010–2015, but at a level about one-third that of men. Both cancer mortality and IHD death rates are projected to rise for men, but not for women. Death rates from injuries at these ages are expected to increase for both sexes.

China and OAI. Group I mortality is projected to decline sharply until about 2005 and to continue to decline at a slower pace thereafter. HIV deaths are assumed to follow a similar epidemic pattern to FSE. Total cancer mortality is projected to rise for men (substantially at ages 45–59), but to begin to decline after around 2000 for women. IHD and stroke death rates are projected to rise for men (particularly at ages 45–59), but to decline significantly for women. A slight increase in the already high death rates from COPD is expected for men, but not for women.

SSA. Group I mortality is projected to decline steadily, but at a slower rate than in other regions. HIV mortality is projected to increase for both sexes until about the year 2000, reaching levels of 70–85 per 100 000 for men and 35–55 per 100 000 for women. IHD and stroke are expected to decline for women, but not for men. Deaths from injuries, already about 4–5 times higher in SSA than EME, are not projected to decline before 2020.

LAC. Large declines are foreseen for Group I causes for both men and women. HIV mortality is expected to reach a maximum rate of around 40 per 100 000 in 2000 (5 per 100 000 for women), and to decline sharply thereafter. No significant changes are predicted in overall cancer mortality for either men or women. IHD and stroke rates are projected to remain constant for men, but to decline by 30–40 per cent for women.

MEC. HIV death rates are projected to remain low, and to reach a maximum of 2–6 per 100 000 for men in 2000–2005, before declining steadily until 2020 (and beyond). Cancer, IHD, stroke and COPD mortality are all expected to increase for men and to decrease for women, except for COPD among women (possibly for the same reasons as for LAC, but possibly reflecting other determinants of the disease as well).

YEARS OF LIFE LOST (YLLs)

These projections of mortality can also be viewed in terms of years of life lost (YLLs) due to premature death, giving greater weight to deaths at younger ages. A broad overview of projected trends in years of life lost is given in Table 7.7—see Murray and Lopez (1996), Chapter 3 in this volume for a comparison table for 1990. The projected pattern of change over the next few decades is very similar to what has been described for mortality. At the global level, YLLs from Group I diseases are expected to decline by 50 per cent, from 491 million years lost in 1990 to 241 million by 2020. Group II diseases are expected to cause many more YLLs in 2020 than in 1990, especially among men. Thus, YLLs for males from Group II causes are expected to rise by more than two thirds, from 153 million to 257 million. The rise in YLLs for females, however, is likely to be much more modest (130 million to 167 million). Similarly, injuries (Group III) are projected to cause 50 per cent more YLLs among males in 2020 than in 1990, and to rise from 45 million to 65 million among females. Overall, the number of years of life lost due to premature mortality is expected to decline from 907 million in 1990 to 859 million in 2020. Moreover, the relative share of different cause categories is likely to change substantially over the period, with the proportionate share of Group I diseases falling from 54 per cent to 28 per cent, while the share of Group II diseases might well rise from 30 per cent to almost 50 per cent. Perhaps most dramatically, YLLs from Group III are projected to increase from 15 per cent to 23 per cent in

2020. Figure 7.11 illustrates how the ten leading causes of YLLs for the world are expected to change between 1990 and 2020.

DISABILITY-ADJUSTED LIFE YEARS (DALYS)

Using the methods described earlier, it is also possible to project years lived with a disability (YLDs) and, therefore, the sum of YLLs and YLDs, namely Disability-Adjusted Life Years (DALYs). It should also be apparent from the description of methods that the projection of YLDs is likely to be even more unreliable than projections of mortality, since fixed-relational methods have largely been employed to estimate the amount of YLDs corresponding to a projected level of mortality. This added uncertainty must be kept in mind when interpreting the results for projected DALYs.

In 1990, an estimated 1.38 billion DALYs were lost due to disease and injury occurring in that year. The global total number of DALYs in 2020 is expected to remain relatively invariant, reaching 1.39 (1.30–1.69)

Table 7.7   Projected Years of Life Lost (YLLs) in 2020, by broad cause Group (baseline scenario)

	Group I	Group II	Group III	Total
YLLs (millions)				
EME	3.9	39.5	6.8	50.2
FSE	1.3	29.0	8.1	38.3
IND	49.7	72.6	29.1	151.3
CHI	6.4	97.5	26.0	129.9
OAI	21.9	55.5	19.3	96.7
SSA	117.6	49.0	67.2	233.8
LAC	11.0	30.4	14.4	55.9
MEC	28.7	50.4	24.3	103.5
World	240.5	423.8	195.2	859.5
Percentage of total				
EME	7.9	78.6	13.5	100.0
FSE	3.3	75.6	21.1	100.0
IND	32.8	48.0	19.2	100.0
CHI	4.9	75.1	20.0	100.0
OAI	22.7	57.4	19.9	100.0
SSA	50.3	21.0	28.7	100.0
LAC	19.7	54.5	25.8	100.0
MEC	27.8	48.7	23.5	100.0
World	28.0	49.3	22.7	100.0

Notes:

Group I: Communicable, maternal, perinatal and nutritional conditions
Group II: Noncommunicable diseases
Group III: Injuries

billion. (In the following discussion, the baseline value is given with the range bounded by the optimistic and pessimistic projections in parentheses.) The proportionate contribution from the three Groups, however, is expected to change significantly (see Table 7.8). Thus, in 2020, Group I causes are projected to account for 20.1 (17.2–29.4) per cent of global DALYs, less than half the percentage (43.9) in 1990. The contribution from Group II is projected to rise from 40.9 per cent to 59.7 (53.6–61.4) per cent. The relative contribution from injuries is also expected to rise from 15.1 per cent to 20.1 (17.0–21.4) per cent.

DALYs due to all of the major conditions included under Group I are expected to decline substantially over the next three decades. This includes the category of infectious and parasitic diseases (22.9 per cent of global DALYs in 1990, declining to 12.9 (10.4–18.0) per cent in 2020), mater-

Figure 7.11 Change in rank order of YLLs for the 15 leading causes, world, 1990–2020

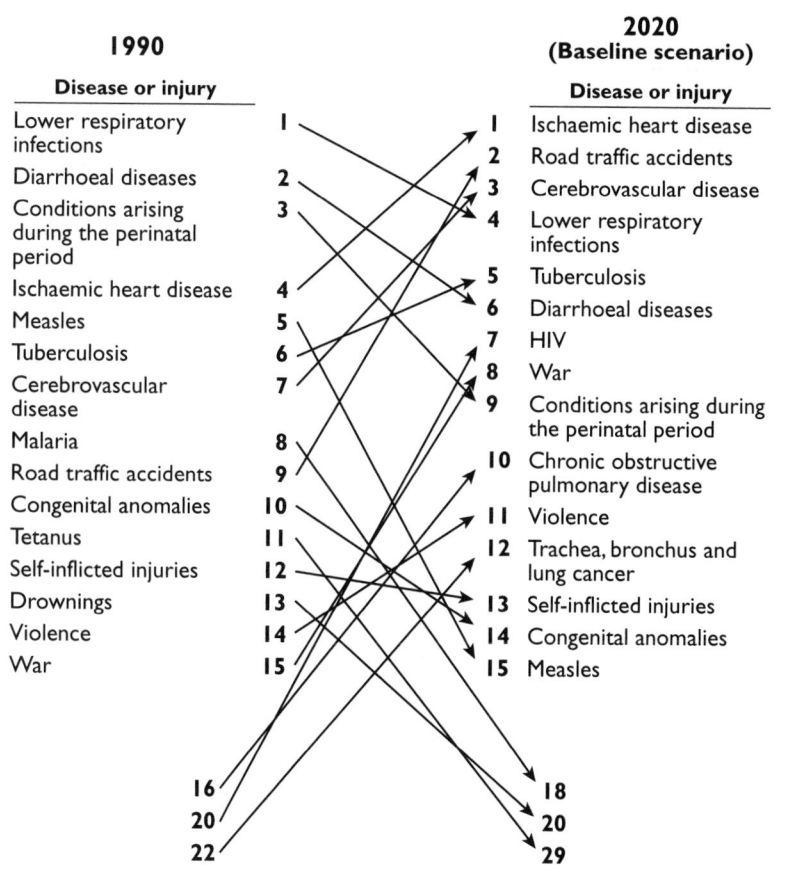

nal conditions (declining from 2.2 per cent down to 0.3 (0.3–0.9) per cent), and lower respiratory infections (falling from 8.5 per cent to 3.2 (3.0–4.8) per cent of global DALYs). Conversely, major increases in DALYs are expected from some of the leading noncommunicable diseases. Thus, DALYs from malignant neoplasms are expected to almost double as a share of global DALYs from 5.1 per cent to 9.9 (10.5–18.0) per cent in 2020. The proportionate share of the global burden of disease due to neuro-psychiatric conditions is projected to rise from 10.5 per cent in 1990 to 14.7 (12.2–15.7) per cent in 2020, slightly more than the increase predicted for cardiovascular diseases, (11.1 per cent to 14.7 (13.7–15.4) per cent). Chronic respiratory diseases are also likely to increase in relative importance as a cause of DALYs world-wide, rising from 4.4 per cent in 1990 to 7.3 (6.5–6.7) per cent in 2020. Both unintentional and intentional injuries are projected to increase as a share of global DALYs, rising from 11.1 per cent to 13.0 (11.3–13.8) per cent, and from 4.1 per cent to 7.1 (5.7–7.6) per cent, respectively.

Table 7.8　　Projected Disability-Adjusted Life Years (DALYs) in 2020, by broad cause Group (baseline scenario)

	Group I	Group II	Group III	Total
DALYs (millions)				
EME	5.0	82.1	9.8	97.0
FSE	1.9	50.6	11.0	63.5
IND	57.8	133.7	45.3	236.7
CHI	9.5	175.0	36.1	220.7
OAI	27.4	110.0	28.6	166.0
SSA	131.0	105.1	93.4	329.6
LAC	13.5	73.3	20.8	107.6
MEC	33.3	100.0	34.4	167.7
WORLD	279.5	829.8	279.6	1 388.8
Percentage of total				
EME	5.2	84.7	10.1	100.0
FSE	3.0	79.7	17.4	100.0
IND	24.4	56.5	19.1	100.0
CHI	4.3	79.3	16.4	100.0
OAI	16.5	66.3	17.2	100.0
SSA	39.8	31.9	28.3	100.0
LAC	12.6	68.1	19.3	100.0
MEC	19.9	59.6	20.5	100.0
WORLD	20.1	59.7	20.1	100.0

Notes:

Group I:　Communicable, maternal, perinatal and nutritional conditions
Group II:　Noncommunicable diseases
Group III:　Injuries

Figure 7.12 Change in rank order of DALYs for the 15 leading causes, world, 1990–2020

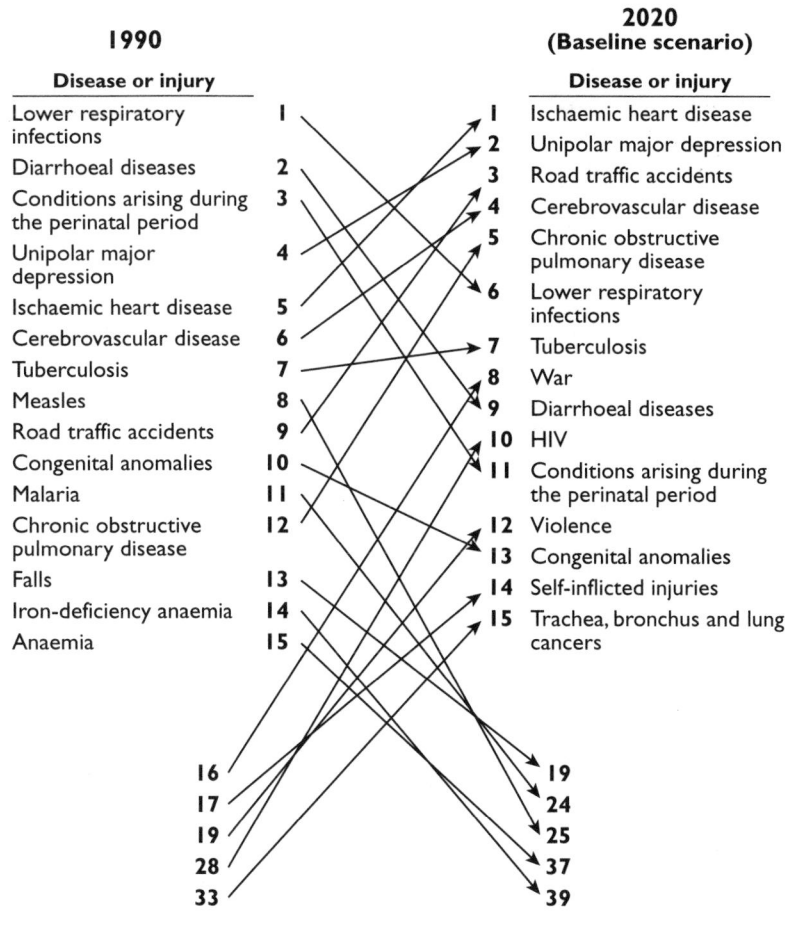

1990				2020 (Baseline scenario)
Disease or injury				Disease or injury
Lower respiratory infections	1		1	Ischaemic heart disease
			2	Unipolar major depression
Diarrhoeal diseases	2		3	Road traffic accidents
Conditions arising during the perinatal period	3		4	Cerebrovascular disease
			5	Chronic obstructive pulmonary disease
Unipolar major depression	4			
			6	Lower respiratory infections
Ischaemic heart disease	5			
Cerebrovascular disease	6		7	Tuberculosis
Tuberculosis	7		8	War
Measles	8		9	Diarrhoeal diseases
Road traffic accidents	9		10	HIV
Congenital anomalies	10		11	Conditions arising during the perinatal period
Malaria	11			
Chronic obstructive pulmonary disease	12		12	Violence
			13	Congenital anomalies
Falls	13		14	Self-inflicted injuries
Iron-deficiency anaemia	14		15	Trachea, bronchus and lung cancers
Anaemia	15			

16	19
17	24
19	25
28	37
33	39

Tables 7.9–7.11 show the ten leading causes of DALYs for males, females and for both sexes combined for the world and for developing and developed regions, according to the baseline, optimistic and pessimistic scenarios. Globally, the leading contributor to the burden of disease is ischaemic heart disease followed by unipolar major depression and road traffic accidents. Despite 30 years of decline projected for total Group I death and DALY rates, four Group I conditions are nonetheless expected to remain among the ten leading causes of DALYs in 2020: lower respiratory infections, tuberculosis, diarrhoeal diseases and HIV. In developing regions, these four causes are also the only Group I conditions expected to remain in the ten leading causes of DALYs. The principal differences between the optimistic and pessimistic scenarios is that suicide

Table 7.9 Ten leading causes of DALYs in 2020 (baseline scenario)

	Both Sexes			Males			Females		
Rank	Disease or injury	DALYs (thousands)	Cumulative %	Disease or injury	DALYs (thousands)	Cumulative %	Disease or injury	DALYs (thousands)	Cumulative %
World									
	All causes	1 388 836		All causes	796 144		All causes	592 692	
1	Ischaemic heart disease	82 325	5.9	Ischaemic heart disease	53 238	6.7	Unipolar major depression	51 075	8.6
2	Unipolar major depression	78 662	11.6	Road traffic accidents	49 719	12.9	Ischaemic heart disease	29 087	13.5
3	Road traffic accidents	71 240	16.7	Cerebrovascular disease	36 819	17.6	Cerebrovascular disease	24 573	17.7
4	Cerebrovascular disease	61 392	21.1	Chronic obstructive pulmonary disease	33 023	21.7	Chronic obstructive pulmonary disease	24 563	21.8
5	Chronic obstructive pulmonary disease	57 587	25.3	Unipolar major depression	27 587	25.2	Road traffic accidents	21 520	25.4
6	Lower respiratory infections	42 692	28.4	Violence	25 274	28.3	Lower respiratory infections	19 508	28.7
7	Tuberculosis	42 515	31.4	War	23 934	31.4	Tuberculosis	19 414	32.0
8	War	41 315	34.4	Lower respiratory infections	23 184	34.3	War	17 381	34.9
9	Diarrhoeal diseases	37 097	37.1	Tuberculosis	23 101	37.2	Diarrhoeal diseases	16 445	37.7
10	HIV	36 317	39.7	Diarrhoeal diseases	20 652	39.8	Conditions arising during the perinatal period	16 070	40.4
Developed regions									
	All causes	160 534		All causes	95 126		All causes	65 408	
1	Ischaemic heart disease	17 997	11.2	Ischaemic heart disease	12 316	12.9	Unipolar major depression	6 423	9.8
2	Cerebrovascular disease	9 875	17.4	Cerebrovascular disease	5 568	18.8	Ischaemic heart disease	5 681	18.5
3	Unipolar major depression	9 825	23.5	Trachea, bronchus and lung cancers	5 508	24.6	Cerebrovascular disease	4 307	25.1
4	Trachea, bronchus and lung cancers	7 253	28.0	Alcohol use	5 211	30.1	Osteoarthritis	3 416	30.3
5	Road traffic accidents	6 852	32.3	Road traffic accidents	4 812	35.1	Dementia and other degenerative and hereditary CNS disorders	3 414	35.5

Table 7.9 (Continued)

	Both Sexes			Males			Females		
Rank	Disease or injury	DALYs (thousands)	Cumulative %	Disease or injury	DALYs (thousands)	Cumulative %	Disease or injury	DALYs (thousands)	Cumulative %
Developed Regions (continued)									
6	Alcohol use	6 088	36.1	Unipolar major depression	3 401	38.7	Road traffic accidents	2 039	38.7
7	Osteoarthritis	5 580	39.5	Chronic obstructive pulmonary disease	3 164	42.0	Chronic obstructive pulmonary disease	1 746	41.3
8	Dementia and other degenerative and hereditary CNS disorders	5 506	43.0	Self-inflicted injuries	2 935	45.1	Trachea, bronchus and lung cancers	1 746	44.0
9	Chronic obstructive pulmonary disease	4 910	46.0	Osteoarthritis	2 164	47.4	Breast cancer	1 733	46.6
10	Self-inflicted injuries	3 879	48.4	Dementia and other degenerative and hereditary CNS disorders	2 092	49.6	Diabetes mellitus	1 360	48.7
Developing regions									
	All causes	1 228 302		All causes	701 018		All causes	527 284	
1	Unipolar major depression	68 837	5.6	Road traffic accidents	44 907	6.4	Unipolar major depression	44 652	8.5
2	Road traffic accidents	64 388	10.8	Ischaemic heart disease	40 922	12.2	Ischaemic heart disease	23 406	12.9
3	Ischaemic heart disease	64 328	16.1	Cerebrovascular disease	31 252	16.7	Chronic obstructive pulmonary disease	22 817	17.2
4	Chronic obstructive pulmonary disease	52 677	20.4	Chronic obstructive pulmonary disease	29 859	21.0	Cerebrovascular disease	20 266	21.1
5	Cerebrovascular disease	51 518	24.6	Unipolar major depression	24 185	24.4	Road traffic accidents	19 481	24.8
6	Violence	42 364	28.0	Tuberculosis	23 911	27.8	Tuberculosis	19 382	28.4
7	War	41 107	31.4	War	23 285	31.1	Lower respiratory infections	18 766	32.0
8	Tuberculosis	40 190	34.6	War	22 982	34.4	War	16 905	35.2
9	Lower respiratory infections	36 960	37.6	Lower respiratory infections	22 341	37.6	Diarrhoeal diseases	16 379	38.3
10	Diarrhoeal diseases	33 962	40.4	Diarrhoeal diseases	20 581	40.5	HIV	15 605	41.3

Table 7.10 Ten leading causes of DALYs in 2020 (optimistic scenario)

	Both Sexes			Males			Females		
Rank	Disease or injury	DALYs (thousands)	Cumulative %	Disease or injury	DALYs (thousands)	Cumulative %	Disease or injury	DALYs (thousands)	Cumulative %
World									
	All causes	1 295 628		All causes	745 946		All causes	549 682	
1	Ischaemic heart disease	81 574	6.3	Ischaemic heart disease	53 319	7.1	Unipolar major depression	51 296	9.3
2	Unipolar major depression	79 028	12.4	Road traffic accidents	51 950	14.1	Ischaemic heart disease	28 255	14.5
3	Road traffic accidents	75 592	18.2	Cerebrovascular disease	36 346	19.0	Road traffic accidents	23 642	18.8
4	Cerebrovascular disease	59 739	22.8	Chronic obstructive pulmonary disease	27 798	22.7	Cerebrovascular disease	23 393	23.0
5	Chronic obstructive pulmonary disease	46 924	26.5	Unipolar major depression	27 732	26.4	Chronic obstructive pulmonary disease	19 126	26.5
6	War	41 489	29.7	Violence	25 387	29.8	War	17 461	29.7
7	Lower respiratory infections	37 943	32.6	War	24 028	33.1	Lower respiratory infections	17 172	32.8
8	Diarrhoeal diseases	33 127	35.2	Lower respiratory infections	20 771	35.8	Congenital anomalies	16 222	35.8
9	Congenital anomalies	32 022	37.6	Alcohol use	20 269	38.6	Osteoarthritis	14 645	38.4
10	Violence	31 408	40.0	Trachea, bronchus and lung cancers	20 159	41.3	Diarrhoeal diseases	14 510	41.1
Developed regions									
	All causes	150 195		All causes	88 883		All causes	61 312	
1	Ischaemic heart disease	17 385	11.6	Ischaemic heart disease	11 965	13.5	Unipolar major depression	6 437	10.5
2	Unipolar major depression	9 853	18.1	Trachea, bronchus and lung cancers	5 566	19.7	Ischaemic heart disease	5 420	19.3
3	Cerebrovascular disease	9 510	24.5	Cerebrovascular disease	5 448	25.9	Cerebrovascular disease	4 063	26.0
4	Trachea, bronchus and lung cancers	7 322	29.3	Alcohol use	5 197	31.7	Osteoarthritis	3 432	31.6
5	Road traffic accidents	6 692	33.8	Road traffic accidents	4 640	36.9	Dementia and other degenerative and hereditary CNS disorders	3 393	37.1

Table 7.10 (Continued)

Rank	Both Sexes: Disease or injury	DALYs (thousands)	Cumulative %	Males: Disease or injury	DALYs (thousands)	Cumulative %	Females: Disease or injury	DALYs (thousands)	Cumulative %
Developed Regions (continued)									
6	Alcohol use	6 068	37.8	Unipolar major depression	3 416	40.8	Road traffic accidents	2 052	40.4
7	Osteoarthritis	5 610	41.6	Self-inflicted injuries	2 949	44.1	Trachea, bronchus and lung cancers	1 756	43.3
8	Dementia and other degenerative and hereditary CNS disorders	5 478	45.2	Chronic obstructive pulmonary disease	2 657	47.1	Breast cancer	1 643	46.0
9	Chronic obstructive pulmonary disease	3 991	47.9	Osteoarthritis	2 179	49.5	Schizophrenia	1 347	48.2
10	Self-inflicted injuries	3 896	50.5	Dementia and other degenerative and hereditary CNS disorders	2 085	51.9	Chronic obstructive pulmonary disease	1 334	50.4
Developing regions									
	All causes	1 145 433		All causes	657 063		All causes	488 370	
1	Unipolar major depression	69 175	6.0	Road traffic accidents	47 309	7.2	Unipolar major depression	44 859	9.2
2	Road traffic accidents	68 900	12.1	Ischaemic heart disease	41 354	13.5	Ischaemic heart disease	22 835	13.9
3	Ischaemic heart disease	64 189	17.7	Cerebrovascular disease	30 898	18.2	Road traffic accidents	21 591	18.3
4	Cerebrovascular disease	50 228	22.0	Chronic obstructive pulmonary disease	25 141	22.0	Cerebrovascular disease	19 330	22.2
5	Chronic obstructive pulmonary disease	42 933	25.8	Unipolar major depression	24 316	25.7	Chronic obstructive pulmonary disease	17 792	25.9
6	War	40 362	29.3	Violence	24 020	29.4	War	16 984	29.4
7	Lower respiratory infections	36 536	32.5	War	23 378	32.9	Lower respiratory infections	16 506	32.7
8	Diarrhoeal diseases	33 016	35.4	Lower respiratory infections	20 030	36.0	Congenital anomalies	15 501	35.9
9	Congenital anomalies	30 465	38.0	Diarrhoeal diseases	18 559	38.8	Diarrhoeal diseases	14 456	38.9
10	Conditions arising during the perinatal period	30 123	40.7	Conditions arising during the perinatal period	16 292	41.3	Conditions arising during the perinatal period	13 831	41.7

Table 7.11   Ten leading causes of DALYs in 2020 (pessimistic scenario)

Rank	Both Sexes — Disease or injury	DALYs (thousands)	Cumulative %	Males — Disease or injury	DALYs (thousands)	Cumulative %	Females — Disease or injury	DALYs (thousands)	Cumulative %
	World								
	All causes	1 687 661		All causes	940 102		All causes	747 559	
1	Ischaemic heart disease	89 958	5.3	Ischaemic heart disease	54 572	5.8	Unipolar major depression	50 240	6.7
2	Lower respiratory infections	79 010	10.0	Lower respiratory infections	42 081	10.3	Lower respiratory infections	36 929	11.7
3	Unipolar major depression	77 439	14.6	Road traffic accidents	42 029	14.8	Ischaemic heart disease	35 385	16.4
4	Diarrhoeal diseases	69 872	18.7	Cerebrovascular disease	38 458	18.8	Diarrhoeal diseases	31 978	20.7
5	Cerebrovascular disease	69 290	22.8	Diarrhoeal diseases	37 894	22.9	Cerebrovascular disease	30 831	24.8
6	Chronic obstructive pulmonary disease	64 638	26.7	Chronic obstructive pulmonary disease	37 783	26.9	Conditions arising during the perinatal period	29 391	28.7
7	Conditions arising during the perinatal period	62 208	30.4	Tuberculosis	33 255	30.4	Chronic obstructive pulmonary disease	26 855	32.3
8	Tuberculosis	60 032	33.9	Conditions arising during the perinatal period	32 817	33.9	Tuberculosis	26 777	35.9
9	Road traffic accidents	58 450	37.4	HIV	28 733	37.0	HIV	22 454	38.9
10	HIV	51 187	40.4	Unipolar major depression	27 200	39.9	War	16 815	41.2
	Developed regions								
	All causes	178 475		All causes	104 250		All causes	74 225	
1	Ischaemic heart disease	20 574	11.5	Ischaemic heart disease	13 401	12.9	Ischaemic heart disease	7 173	9.7
2	Cerebrovascular disease	11 549	18.0	Cerebrovascular disease	6 075	18.7	Unipolar major depression	6 376	18.3
3	Unipolar major depression	9 751	23.5	Trachea, bronchus and lung cancers	5 418	23.9	Cerebrovascular disease	5 474	25.6
4	Trachea, bronchus and lung cancers	7 125	27.5	Alcohol use	5 240	28.9	Osteoarthritis	3 358	30.2
5	Road traffic accidents	7 039	31.4	Road traffic accidents	5 132	33.8	Dementia and other degenerative and hereditary CNS disorders	3 322	34.6

Table 7.11 (Continued)

	Both Sexes			Males			Females		
Rank	Disease or injury	DALYs (thousands)	Cumula-tive %	Disease or injury	DALYs (thousands)	Cumula-tive %	Disease or injury	DALYs (thousands)	Cumula-tive %
Developed Regions (continued)									
6	Alcohol use	6 129	34.8	Chronic obstructive pulmonary disease	3 389	37.1	Breast cancer	2 069	37.4
7	Osteoarthritis	5 495	37.9	Unipolar major depression	3 375	40.3	Road traffic accidents	1 908	40.0
8	Dementia and other degenerative and hereditary CNS disorders	5 407	40.9	HIV	2 955	43.2	Chronic obstructive pulmonary disease	1 856	42.5
9	Chronic obstructive pulmonary disease	5 245	43.9	Self-inflicted injuries	2 912	45.9	Diabetes mellitus	1 709	44.8
10	Self-inflicted injuries	3 847	46.0	Osteoarthritis	2 137	48.0	Trachea, bronchus and lung cancers	1 707	47.1
Developing regions									
	All causes	1 509 186		All causes	835 852		All causes	673 334	
1	Lower respiratory infections	76 852	5.1	Ischaemic heart disease	41 171	4.9	Unipolar major depression	43 863	6.5
2	Diarrhoeal diseases	69 622	9.7	Lower respiratory infections	40 915	9.8	Lower respiratory infections	35 937	11.9
3	Ischaemic heart disease	69 383	14.3	Diarrhoeal diseases	37 764	14.3	Diarrhoeal diseases	31 858	16.6
4	Unipolar major depression	67 688	18.8	Road traffic accidents	36 898	18.8	Conditions arising during the perinatal period	28 547	20.8
5	Conditions arising during the perinatal period	60 223	22.8	Chronic obstructive pulmonary disease	34 395	22.9	Ischaemic heart disease	28 212	25.0
6	Tuberculosis	59 747	26.7	Tuberculosis	33 025	26.8	Tuberculosis	26 722	29.0
7	Chronic obstructive pulmonary disease	59 393	30.7	Cerebrovascular disease	32 383	30.7	Cerebrovascular disease	25 358	32.7
8	Cerebrovascular disease	57 741	34.5	Conditions arising during the perinatal period	31 677	34.5	Chronic obstructive pulmonary disease	24 999	36.5
9	Road traffic accidents	51 411	37.9	HIV	25 778	37.6	HIV	21 883	39.7
10	HIV	47 660	41.1	Unipolar major depression	23 825	40.4	War	16 341	42.1

and violence are expected to move into the ten leading causes of DALYs in the optimistic scenario, whereas conditions arising during the perinatal period remains in the pessimistic scenario. In developed regions, osteoarthritis, dementia and breast cancer are all expected to be leading causes of burden in 2020 for women. Figure 7.12 shows the change in DALY ranks from 1990–2020.

Some of the major changes expected in the relative contribution of various broad cause Groups to DALYs in each region are summarized below. Much more detail on projected DALYs, by age, sex and cause, is provided in Annex Tables 12–21.

EME. The total number of DALYs is expected to decrease slightly, from 98.8 million in 1990 to 97.0 million in 2020. By 2020, Group I diseases are expected to contribute only about 5.2 per cent of DALYs in this region, with HIV as the largest single Group I cause. Very little change in the percentage contribution of most major disease groups is expected, with neuro-psychiatric conditions (25.4 per cent), cardiovascular diseases (19.4 per cent), malignant neoplasms (17.3 per cent) and unintentional injuries (6.9 per cent) projected to be the largest causes of DALYs in 2020.

FSE. Total DALYs in this region are also projected to increase marginally from 62.2 million to 63.5 million in 2020. Group I diseases are expected to account for less than 3 per cent of DALYs in 2020. As for EME, no major changes are predicted in the principal causes of DALYs, with the exception of malignant neoplasms, which are projected to rise from 11.7 per cent to 16.1 per cent, and cardiovascular diseases, for which a modest rise (23.2 per cent to 26.1 per cent) is expected. Otherwise, the leading causes of DALYs are expected to be very similar to those for EME, with large contributions expected in 2020 from neuro-psychiatric disorders (16.4 per cent), unintentional injuries (11.6 per cent) and chronic respiratory diseases (8.1 per cent).

India. Due to the large expected declines in morbidity and mortality from Group I (communicable) diseases, the overall number of DALYs is expected to decline substantially, falling from 287.7 million in 1990 to 236.7 million in 2020. Large absolute and relative declines in DALYs are expected for all Group I conditions, most notably the broad category of infectious and parasitic diseases (28.9 per cent in 1990, compared to 17.3 per cent in 2020) and respiratory infections (11.9 per cent in 1990 and 3.2 per cent in 2020). Significant increases in DALYs are projected for all of the major noncommunicable diseases, especially for malignant neoplasms (2.5 per cent up to 7.1 per cent), neuro-psychiatric conditions (7.0 per cent up to 12.6 per cent), cardiovascular diseases (8.1 per cent up to 18.4 per cent) and chronic respiratory diseases (2.6 per cent up to 6.4 per cent). Unintentional injuries are also expected to rise as a proportion of DALYs (13.0 per cent up to 16.4 per cent), but not so much in absolute terms (37.5 million DALYs in 1990 rising to a projected 38.7 million in 2020).

China. Further rapid progress is expected in China towards the conquest of infectious diseases and other Group I conditions. For Group I as a whole, the proportionate contribution to total DALYs in China is expected to decline from 24.2 per cent in 1990 to less than 5 per cent in 2020. Conversely, major increases in DALYs (in both absolute and relative terms) are predicted for the major noncommunicable diseases including malignant neoplasms (up from 8.7 per cent of DALYs in 1990 to 18.7 per cent in 2020 and rising, in absolute terms, from 18.1 million DALYs in 1990 to 41.4 million in 2020), cardiovascular diseases (11.0 per cent and 22.9 million DALYs in 1990, up to 16.3 per cent and 36.0 million DALYs in 2020), and respiratory diseases (10.7 per cent and 22.3 million DALYs, rising to 16.3 per cent and 36.0 million DALYs). No major changes are projected in the number of DALYs from unintentional (slight decline) and intentional (slight increase) injuries, nor for the total number of DALYs (208.4 million in 1990, up to 220.7 million in 2020) due to these compensating trends for Group I and Group II diseases.

OAI. The projected trends for this region are very similar to those for China, although the reduction in Group I DALYs is expected to be less impressive (16.5 per cent of DALYs in 2020 are still expected to arise from Group I diseases). Neuro-psychiatric conditions are expected to increase from 10.8 per cent of DALYs in 1990 to 17.4 per cent in 2020, similar to what is expected for cardiovascular diseases. DALYs due to cancer are expected to double between 1990 and 2020 (from 9.0 million to 19.3 million or 11.6 per cent of projected DALYs in 2020). No major changes are expected in total DALYs for the region, declining marginally from 177.7 million to 166.0 million in 2020.

SSA. Total DALYs in the region are expected to rise from 295.3 million to 329.6 million. In absolute terms, DALYs from Group I conditions are expected to decline substantially, from 194.6 million in 1990 to 131.0 million in 2020. Nonetheless, the category of communicable, maternal, perinatal and nutritional conditions is still expected to account for about 42.5 per cent of DALYs in 2020. Large increases in DALYs due to injuries are foreseen, due primarily to demographic factors. Thus, DALYs from Group III are expected to more than double over the period, increasing from 45.3 million to 93.4 million, representing almost 28.3 per cent of all DALYs in 2020. This projected trend largely explains the overall increase in DALYs projected for the region.

LAC. A small increase in total DALYs, from 98.3 million to 108 million, is expected. As elsewhere in the developing world, Group I DALYs are projected to decline, decreasing from 35.3 per cent of all DALYs in 1990 to 12.6 per cent in 2020. DALYs from the major noncommunicable diseases are expected to increase, with the proportions roughly doubling for malignant neoplasms (from 4.5 per cent to 8.5 per cent) and increasing for cardiovascular diseases (7.9 per cent up to 13.2 per cent). DALYs from neuro-psychiatric conditions are also expected to increase (from 15.9 per cent in 1990 to 21.6 per cent in 2020). Injuries are projected to account for one-fifth of DALYs in 2020, up from 16.4 per cent in 1990.

MEC. Total DALYs are expected to increase by 11 per cent to 167.7 million in 2020. Group I DALYs are projected to decline from 48 per cent of all DALYs to 20 per cent by 2020. Neuro-psychiatric (14.9 per cent) and cardiovascular diseases (17.7 per cent) are the only two major categories among Group II conditions which are projected to account for more than 10 per cent of DALYs in 2020.

DEMOGRAPHIC VERSUS EPIDEMIOLOGICAL CHANGE

The results presented thus far have described projected changes in the absolute (and proportionate) amount of DALYs expected under the various scenarios. Such changes may arise, of course, due to real changes in disease and injury rates (i.e. in the risk of incurring disease or injury), due to demographic change which alters the age-distribution of the population, or due to a combination of both factors. In view of the strong age-dependence of risks for various conditions, substantial changes in projected age structure may have a very significant impact on the number of DALYs ascribed to a given disease or injury. Road traffic accidents are a good example of this. In populations where road traffic accident deaths are high, there is a concentration of mortality among young adult males (ages 15–29 years). If the population of young men increases dramatically, then the number of DALYs due to road traffic accidents will rise as well, even though there may be no projected increase in rates (or risk) of mortality.

Figure 7.13 illustrates the projected growth in the size of the population of each five-year age group from 1990 to 2020. The expected growth rate in the adult population is dramatic. Over the 30 year period, the male population of the world aged 45–59 is projected to increase by 102 per cent and females of the same age group by 108 per cent. Even if all age-specific death and DALY rates were to remain constant, the differential growth rate of different age groups would by itself lead to a major change in the composition of the burden of disease. To further analyse the relative impact of demographic and epidemiological change on the projected number of DALYs from Groups I, II and III for each region, we have calculated two hypothetical alternatives. First, we have calculated the expected number of DALYs in 2020, given 1990 age-specific DALY rates and the projected 2020 population, and, second, we have calculated the expected number of DALYs given 2020 projected age-specific rates and the 1990 population. The difference between the DALYs expected with 1990 rates and 2020 population compared to 1990 DALYs is a measure of the change in burden expected solely on the basis of population growth and distribution, labelled as *demographic* change in Figure 7.14. The difference between DALYs expected with 2020 rates applied to 1990 population compared with 1990 DALYs is a measure of the change in burden expected solely on the basis of changing age-specific DALY rates, labelled *epidemiological* change in Figure 7.14.

In almost all cases, demographic and epidemiological factors are operating in opposing directions in the determination of DALYs in 2020. Thus, in all regions, the risk of premature death or disability from an injury (Group III) is projected to decline, thereby reducing DALYs. Conversely, in every region, demographic change is expected to result in a shift of more and more people into the age groups at highest risk of injury, thereby increasing DALYs. Depending on the relative size of the two counteracting components, the net effect on projected DALYs from Group III is either to increase them (India, OAI, SSA, LAC and MEC) or to decrease them (EME, FSE and China).

For Group I diseases and conditions, for which substantial declines in risk are expected to lead to large declines in DALYs, the effect will be attenuated in all regions, except FSE, by demographic changes leading to an increase in population at the ages of highest risk for these diseases (primarily at ages 0–4 years). For Group II (noncommunicable diseases), demographic changes in all regions will tend to increase DALYs, while epidemiological changes will tend to reduce Group II DALYs, most significantly in EME.

DISCUSSION

The findings of this projection study raise many (perhaps unexpected) issues for health policy. It is worth briefly stepping back from the morass of detailed results to highlight several general findings which we believe have particular relevance for public health policy over the next three

Figure 7.13   Projected change in global population by age and sex, 1990–2020

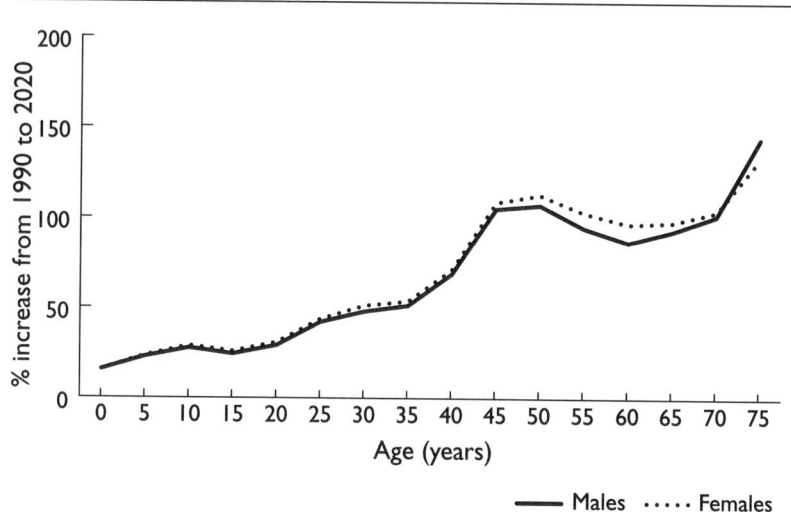

Figure 7.14   Decomposition of projected change in DALYs into
demographic and epidemiological components, 1990–2020

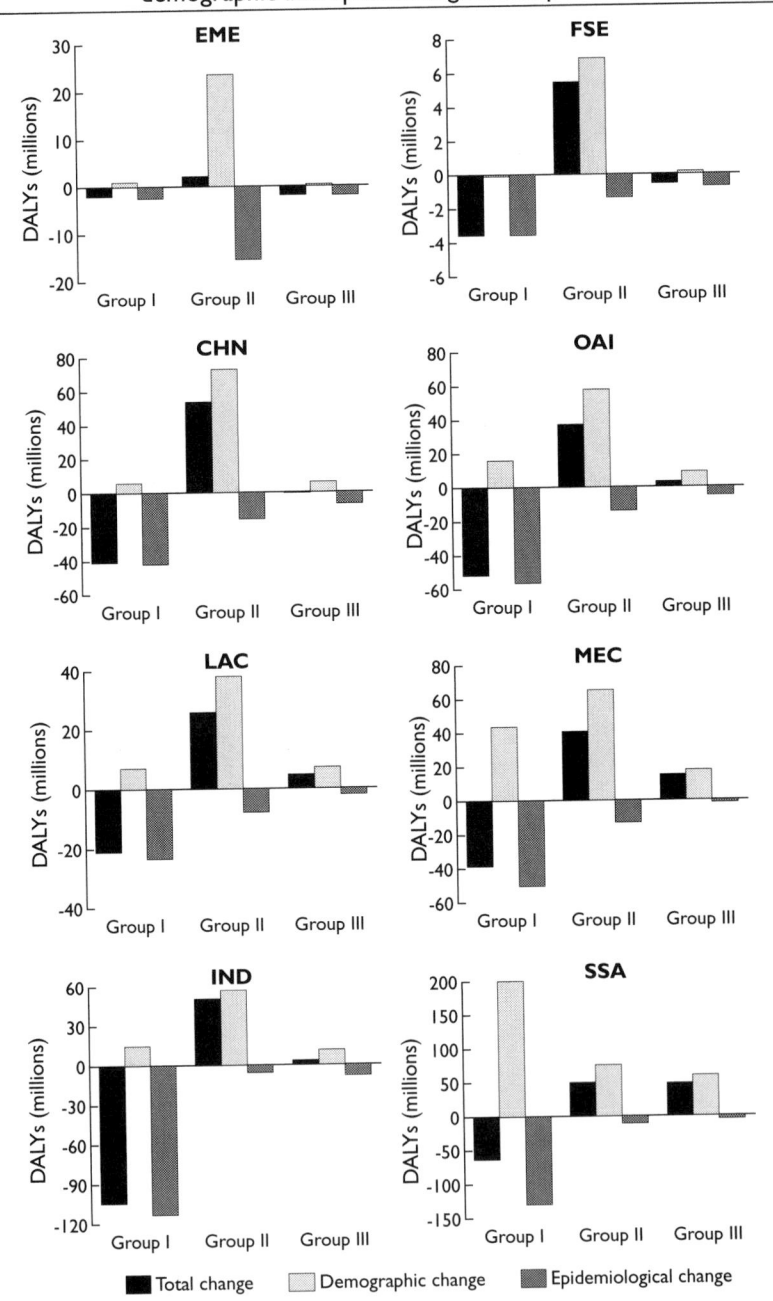

Note:

The difference between total change in DALYs for a Group from 1990 to 2020 and the sum of the demographic and epidemiological components, as calculated in this figure, is due to the interaction between demographic and epidemiological change.

decades. (Figures in parentheses in the following discussion give the range of results bounded by the pessimistic and the optimistic scenarios.)

1. In all three scenarios, there is a substantial shift in the expected age-pattern of mortality from younger to older ages. In 1990, 29.9 per cent of deaths occurred at ages under 15. This figure is expected to decline to only 11.1 (10.8–15.3) per cent in 2020.

2. Driving this shift in the age-pattern of death and DALYs is a major relative decline predicted in the burden of communicable, maternal, perinatal and nutritional conditions which is manifested in all three scenarios. Group I deaths are expected to fall from 34.2 per cent to 15.0 (12.7–21.6) per cent in 2020 and Group I DALYs from 43.9 per cent of all DALYs in 1990 to 20.1 (17.2–29.4) per cent in 2020.

3. Despite the overall decline in Group I, the HIV epidemic is projected to rise dramatically, causing some 1.7 million deaths in 2006 — in the optimistic scenario annual mortality peaks at 1.7 million deaths in 2006, and in the pessimistic scenario at 1.9 million deaths in 2012. Based on the assumptions presented in this chapter, HIV will still cause 1.2 (0.8–1.8) million deaths and 2.6 (1.8–3.0) per cent of all DALYs in 2020. Given that in 1980, the global burden due to HIV was very minor, the epidemic is an unprecedented reversal of human health progress. The HIV epidemic underscores the potential for other new diseases to emerge or known diseases to recrudesce and radically alter future health patterns. Nevertheless, despite the HIV epidemic, we foresee general progress over the next few decades in improving overall human health.

4. Due largely to the demographic transition brought about by declining fertility rates, the number of individuals aged 15–59 is likely to increase by 52 per cent from 3.1 billion in 1990 to 4.8 billion in 2020. As a consequence, the burden of selected neuro-psychiatric conditions is expected to rise from 10.5 per cent of DALYs in 1990 to 14.7 (12.2–15.7) per cent in 2020. The most dramatic relative increases are projected for OAI, MEC, SSA and India. A similar effect is seen for injuries which are expected to rise from 15.1 per cent of DALYs in 1990 to 20.1 (17.0–21.4) per cent in 2020. The largest increase in the relative share of DALYs due to injuries is expected to occur in SSA, from 15.4 per cent in 1990 to 28.3 (21.9–30.4) per cent in 2020.

5. The demographic and epidemiological transitions are expected to proceed rapidly in nearly all regions. The ratio of Group II to Group I DALYs globally is projected to increase from 0.93 in 1990 to 3.0 (1.8–3.6) in 2020. Only in SSA do we predict that the burden of Group I will not be less than that for Group II by 2020. It is worth noting that if the Barker hypothesis were correct, the likely growth in certain Group II conditions such as diabetes mellitus, hypertension,

COPD and associated cardiovascular diseases could be much greater than already projected (Barker and Martyn 1992, Barker et al. 1991).

6.   Despite the dramatic effects of the smoking epidemic, death and DALY rates from all Group II conditions combined are expected to decrease in many age groups and all regions. Notable exceptions are the substantial increases expected for FSE males, aged 45–69, and for Indian males in the same age group. In China, DALY rates from these diseases are expected to remain constant between 1990 and 2020. Overall trends in Group II death and DALY rates are determined by the counteracting effects of the secular decline in Group II rates and the increase brought about by the smoking epidemic.

7.   Life expectancy at birth for females is projected to increase in all regions, ranging from an additional 13.3 years in SSA to 4.1 years in FSE. Expected gains in male life expectancy, by contrast, are projected to be much smaller, ranging from 10.2 years in SSA to a small decline in male life expectancy of 0.1 years in FSE. The male-female gap in life expectancy is therefore projected to increase in all regions. In EME, female gains are projected to exceed male gains by 2.2 years; thus, even in this low mortality region, the male-female gap in life expectancy could well continue to widen, far beyond likely biological differences in potential life span.

The baseline, optimistic and pessimistic scenarios which we have presented here offer three possible visions of future mortality and disability. There are, however, many other possible, albeit less probable, scenarios that could be envisaged, particularly for Group I conditions. The decline of Group I which is predicted under all three scenarios is implicitly based on the presumption that socio-economic development will decrease disease incidence and severity, and/or that research and development will guarantee the availability of antibiotics effective against resistant strains of major pathogens. New antibiotics may not be discovered, and drug resistance may become so significant for tuberculosis, malaria, the pneumococcus or other pathogens that mortality rates could increase. Such a scenario is possible. But we believe it is not highly probable. In vitro drug resistance of certain bacteria—for example, methicillin-resistant *S. aureus*—has been detected for many years, but because of many factors, including differences between in vitro resistance and treatment failure and the continued development of novel antibiotics, there has not been a significant increase in mortality directly attributable to the development of drug resistance in any population with reliable data on mortality trends. Possible but improbable scenarios may still be important inputs to policy formulation. Society should be willing to reduce the risks or consequences of unlikely but potentially disastrous outcomes just as some individuals are willing to purchase fire extinguishers and smoke detectors for their homes because of a small, but real, risk of fire.

Any projection exercise is by its nature an exercise in conjecture with wide confidence intervals. Nevertheless, some aspects of our study entail more uncertainty than others. First, the timing and magnitude of the peak in HIV incidence was based on estimates developed by the former WHO Global Programme on AIDS. Alternative projections with higher or lower peak incidences occurring sooner or later are entirely credible. Second, death rates and YLD rates for intentional injuries are assumed to remain constant from 1990–2020 since we were unable to identify significant relationships between income, education and time with these injury death rates, based on the datasets available. The panel dataset, however, included some examples of countries such as Hungary where injury death rates have changed significantly over a short period of time. Injury death rates in a given region may well increase or decrease by 2020. For war in particular, the assumption of constant rates combined with substantial adult population growth yields projections that are highly speculative. Third, there are specific relationships between Group I conditions and Group II conditions—such as hepatitis B and liver cancer, and human papilloma virus and cervical cancer—that have not been modelled directly. We might expect that those Group II conditions that are partially related to Group I causes may decrease at a faster rate than other Group II conditions. As a result, our projections for such conditions may well be overestimated. Finally, the entire set of projections of YLDs is based on either fixed-relational models or arbitrary assumptions about rates of decline which are highly unsatisfactory for making projections.

There are several clear avenues that can be pursued to improve the reliability of the various projection scenarios. More detailed data on causes of death collected in countries or regions with good vital registration will improve the cause-of-death models. We have endeavoured to include all available and reliable cause-of-death data; time-series data on the Newly Independent States would be one very valuable addition to the panel dataset. An expanded set of independent variables might be explored in an attempt to identify more powerful predictors of mortality patterns across countries and over time, particularly for injuries. Perhaps, most importantly, there is a need to develop condition-specific projection models for years of life lived with a disability, at the very least for sexually transmitted diseases, neuro-psychiatric conditions, nutritional deficiencies and the intestinal helminths.

Despite the evident uncertainties, projections are useful, provided that they are transparent, and provided that they are interpreted with a degree of caution commensurate with their uncertainty. Health services planning, health promotion and disease prevention programmes all require some idea of the future burden of disease and injury in order to guide the health policy process. Decisions and choices need to be made today in order to cope with expected disease burden in the future. Projections provide the information support for these decisions and choices.

The results presented in this chapter provide a comprehensive view of the future. Death and disability from dozens of diseases and injuries have been projected for eight regions, for several age groups, and for each sex separately. As such, these projections may meet the needs of health planners in many different fields of public health. This being their strength, it is also their major disadvantage. Focused, detailed projections of a specific disease or injury in a given population may be more reliable than the more generic methods employed here, simply because more information about the disease or injury is usually available to guide projections.

We recognize these uncertainties in these projections and we urge those who use them to exercise great caution in their application. It is extremely important to keep in mind what the projections constitute, namely three visions of the future which are nothing more than the numerical consequences of the set of assumptions and methods used to generate these visions. Perhaps these methods and assumptions will ultimately prove to be reasonable, perhaps not. In making the results available to the public health community, we hope that the methods and assumptions will be challenged, re-thought and re-applied several times over to enhance their utility. There is a clear need for projections of this nature, and we are very much aware that the research reported here is, or should be seen as, the first step in a more continuous and exhaustive effort to preview the future. Subsequent research will, we hope, expand and improve on our efforts; nonetheless, the results presented here provide a starting point for a reasoned debate on health policies designed to anticipate possible future health scenarios.

NOTES

1 Based on an analysis of past global trends in life expectancy, the UN Population Division assumes for most countries that male life expectancy at birth will increase by 2.5 years during each five-year period until life expectancy at birth reaches 60 years, after which the quinquennial gain is assumed to decline reaching 0.4 years at a life expectancy of 77.5. Female life expectancy is assumed to increase by 2.5 years during each five calendar years until a life expectancy at birth of 65 years is attained, and then the rate of increase declines gradually to a gain of 0.4 years when a life expectancy of 82.5 years is attained (United Nations 1995). The World Bank has employed similar assumptions but distinguishes between countries with low and high levels of primary school enrolment (Bos et al. 1994).

2 Bulutao (1993) also reports estimates of mortality for selected causes in 1985 based exclusively on the regression models which he developed. This approach yielded global estimates of mortality from tuberculosis (844 thousand), malaria (146 thousand) and measles (421 thousand). These estimates are extraordinarily low and are not consistent with more exhaustive efforts at estimating cause of death structure. He also estimates 9 million deaths, or nearly 20 per cent of all global mortality, as being due to unspecified causes. This large ill-defined

category in his estimates is a simple consequence of the fact that no attempt was made to deal with deaths that are coded to Chapter XVI in ICD-9 (Symptoms, signs and ill-defined conditions). As this category is larger in developing countries, Bulutao's models predict a large share of mortality in developing countries due to the unspecified category. This study epitomizes the problems associated with the uncritical use of regression models based on vital registration data to estimate mortality by cause.

3   All-cause mortality projections have been developed for different age groups (e.g. McNown and Rogers 1989), but to date this type of all-cause mortality projection has not, to our knowledge, been used to project cause-specific mortality.

4   It is possible to try and correct for the trends in "Symptoms, signs and ill-defined conditions" when developing cause of death regression models — see Murray and Lopez 1996, Chapter 3 in this volume.

5   For a full description of the GBD classification system for diseases and injuries see Murray and Lopez 1996, Chapter 3 in this volume.

6   The most recent publication of their methods is Summers R, Heston A. The Penn World Tables Mark 5.0. An expanded set of international comparisons 1950–1988. *Quarterly Journal of Economics* May 1991. These estimates are periodically revised and released on diskette by Summers and Heston; for this analysis, we have used Penn World Tables Mark 5.5.

7   Non-smoker lung cancer rates for all regions, except China and OAI, have been assumed to equal the non-smoker lung cancer rates recorded in the CPS-II (1984–88) follow-up survey in the United States, as discussed in Parkin et al. 1994. For China, the age-specific non-smoker lung cancer rate in women was estimated on the basis of econometric analyses to equal 1.7 per 100 000 at ages 30–44, 22.0 at ages 45–59, 64.1 at ages 60–69 and 125.8 at ages 70 years and over. For OAI, we have estimated non-smoker lung cancer rates in women based on the assumption that there is currently little smoking-attributable mortality in women in the region — the estimated rates are 1.3 (30–44), 12.2 (45–59), 47.1 (60–69) and 89.9 (70 and over).

8   Collishaw NE, Lopez AD (1996) The tobacco epidemic: a global health emergency. *Tobacco Alert,* Geneva, World Health Organization.

9   For example, the equation for road traffic accidents in females aged 15–29 yielded a projected doubling of the death rate in EME and FSE which did not appear to be plausible or consistent with recent trends. Examination of a scatterplot of the female road traffic accident rates at these ages against income per capita suggested that the regression equation was not capturing a downturn in the death rate at the highest levels of income. For EME and FSE, we therefore re-estimated the equation for countries with higher levels of income per capita. This revised equation was used for projecting EME and FSE death rates from road traffic accidents.

10 As of 1 January 1996, the GPA has ceased to exist and has been replaced by UNAIDS. At the time of writing, revised projections from UNAIDS have not been released.

11 YLD rates for sexually transmitted diseases are assumed to decline at 50 per cent of the overall Group I (excluding HIV) YLD rate, whereas rates for helminths and anaemia are assumed to decline at 75 per cent of the Group I rate. Leprosy is assumed to decline at 5 per cent per year based on recent trends.

12 The UN Population Division publishes life expectancy estimates by country and for regional aggregates that are different from the regions used for this study. From this information we have attempted to reconstruct comparable regional estimates of life expectancy for our regions by weighting UN estimates of life expectancy by UN estimates of population for each country. The World Bank (1993) also published projections for the World Development Report 1993 regions used in this book for 2000 and 2030 but for both sexes combined.

13 In standard demographic notation, an age interval represented as 0–4 years includes everyone aged zero up to age 4.99. When representing a probability of death, the standard notation is $_xq_a$ where a is the beginning age of the interval and x is the length of the interval so that $_xq_a$ is the probability of death between age a and age $a+x$. In Figure 7.6, the top histogram shows $_{15}q_0$, the middle histogram $_{45}q_{15}$ and the bottom histogram $_{10}q_{60}$.

BIBLIOGRAPHY

Acharya A and Murray C (1996) An econometric model for forecasting age and cause-specific mortality rates. Harvard Center for Population and Development Studies Working Paper.

Anderson RM (1993) AIDS: trends, predictions, controversy. *Nature*, 363:393–394.

Anderson RM et al. (1991) The spread of HIV-1 in Africa: sexual contact patterns and the predicted demographic impact of AIDS. *Nature*, 352:581–587.

Anderson RM, May RM (1988) Epidemiological parameters of HIV transmission. *Nature*, 333(6173):514–519.

Anderson RM, May RM (1992) *Infectious diseases of humans. Dynamics and control*. Oxford, Oxford University Press.

Aoki N, Kasagi F, Horibe H (1987) Projection of mortality from cerebrovascular disease, 1985 through 2000 A.D., in Japan. *Japanese circulation journal*, 51:138–143.

Bailey C (1957) *The mathematical theory of epidemics*. London, Charles Griffin.

Barker DJP, Martyn CN (1992) The maternal and fetal origins of cardiovascular disease. *Journal of epidemiology and community health*, 46:8–11.

Barker DJP et al. (1991) Fetal and placental size and risk of hypertension in adult life. *British medical journal*, 301:259–262.

Barro RJ, Lee JW (1993) *Economic growth in a cross-section of countries. NBER Working Paper*. Cambridge, NBER.

Bermejo A et al. (1992) Tuberculosis incidence in developing countries with high prevalence of HIV infection. *AIDS*, 6:1203–1206.

Bezold C (1994) Health care: thinking ahead. *World health forum*, 15(2):189–192.

Bongaarts J (1994) Population policy options in the developing world. *Science*, 263(5148):771–776.

Bos E et al. (1994) *World population projections. Estimates and projections with related demographic statistics*. Baltimore, Johns Hopkins University Press.

Brookmeyer R, Damiano A (1989) Statistical methods for short-term projections of AIDS incidence. *Statistics in medicine*, 8:23–24.

Bulutao R (1993) Mortality by cause, 1970–2015. In: Gribble JN, Preston SH, eds. *The epidemiological transition. Policy and planning implications for developing countries. Workshop proceedings*. Washington DC, National Academy Press.

Bulutao R, Bos E (1989) *Projecting mortality for all countries. Policy, planning and research working papers*. Washington DC, World Bank.

Caldwell JC (1979) Education as a factor in mortality decline: an examination of Nigerian data. *Population studies*, 41:5–30.

Capocaccia R et al. (1995) Estimation and projections of stomach cancer trends in Italy. *Cancer causes and control*, 6: 339–346.

Caselli G (1996) Future longevity among the elderly. In: Caselli G, Lopez AD, eds. *Health and mortality among elderly populations*. Oxford, Clarendon Press.

Chin J et al. (1992) The global epidemiology of the HIV/AIDS pandemic and its projected demographic impact in Africa. *World health statistics quarterly*, 45(2-3):220–227.

Chin J, Lwanga S (1991) Estimation and projection of adult AIDS cases: a simple epidemiological model. *Bulletin of the World Health Organization*, 69:399–406.

Cleland JG, van Ginneken J (1988) Maternal education and child survival in developing countries. *Social science and medicine*, 27:1357–1368.

Coale A, Demeny P, Vaughn B (1983) *Regional model life tables and stable populations. Second edition*. New York, Academic Press.

Coale A, Guo G (1989) Revised regional model life tables at very low levels of mortality. *Population index*, 55(4):613–643.

Dowd JE, Manton KG (1990) Forecasting chronic disease risks in developing countries. *International journal of epidemiology*, 19(4):1019–1036.

Frenk J et al. (1989) Health transition in middle income countries: new challenges for health care. *Health policy and planning*, 4(1):29–39.

Garrett MJ (1993) A way through the maze: what futurists do and how they do it. *Futures*, April:254–274.

Gautrin D et al. (1990) Canadian projections of cases suffering from Alzheimer's disease and Senile Dementia of Alzheimer type over the period 1986–2031. *Canadian journal of psychiatry*, 35:162–165.

Gnanasekaran KS (1975)Mortality trends and projections for Canada and the provinces, 1950–1986. In: *Technical report on population projections for Canada and the provinces, 1972–2001*. Ottawa, Statistics Canada.

Goldman L, Cook EF (1984) The decline in ischaemic heart disease mortality rates: an analysis of the comparative effects of medical interventions and changes in lifestyle. *Annals of internal medicine*, 101:825–36.

Gunning-Schepers LJ (1989) The health benefits of prevention. A simulation approach. *Health Policy*, July 12(1-2):1–255.

Hakulinen T et al. (1986) Global and regional mortality patterns by cause of death in 1980. *International Journal of Epidemiology,* 15:226-233

Heligman L, Pollard JH (1980) The age pattern of mortality. *Journal of the institute of actuaries,* 107(1(434)):49–80.

Karon J, Dondero T, Curran J (1988) The projected incidence of AIDS and estimated prevalence of HIV infection in the United States. *AIDS,* 1:542–550.

Kessler LG et al. (1991) Projections of the breast cancer burden to U.S. women: 1990–2000. *Preventive medicine,* 20:170–182.

Kumaresan JA et al. (1996) Tuberculosis. In: Murray CJL, Lopez AD, eds. *The global epidemiology of infectious diseases.* Cambridge, Harvard Universtiy Press.

Lopez AD, Hakama M (1986) Approaches to the projection of health status. In: World Health Organization, *Health projections in Europe. Methods and applications.* Copenhagen, World Health Organization.

Lopez AD, Hull TH (1983) A note on estimating the cause-of-death structure in high mortality populations. *Population Bulletin of the United Nations,* 14:66–70

Low-Beer D et al. (1996) HIV. In: Murray CJL, Lopez AD, eds. *Health dimensions of sex and reproduction: the global burden of sexually transmitted diseases, HIV, maternal conditions, perinatal disorders, and congenital anomalies.* Cambridge, Harvard University.

Manton KG, Stallard E (1988) *Chronic disease modelling.* London, Griffin.

McNown R, Rogers A (1989) Forecasting mortality: a parameterized time series approach. *Demography,* 26(4):645–660.

Multiple risk factor intervention trial research group (1982) Multiple risk facter intervention trial. *Journal of the American Medical Association,* 248:1465–77.

Murray CJL (1996) Rethinking DALYs. In: Murray CJL, Lopez AD, eds. *The global burden of disease: a comprehensive assessment of mortality and disability from diseases, injuries and risk factors in 1990 and projected to 2020.* Cambridge, Harvard University Press.

Murray CJL, Lopez AD (1996) Estimating causes of death: methods and global and regional applications for 1990. In: Murray CJL, Lopez AD, eds. *The global burden of disease: a comprehensive assessment of mortality and disability from diseases, injuries and risk factors in 1990 and projected to 2020.* Cambridge, Harvard University Press.

Nilsson R et al. (1991) Increased hip-fracture incidence in the county of Ostergotland, Sweden, 1940–1986, with forecasts up to the year 2000: an epidemiological study. *International journal of epidemiology,* 20(4):1018–1024.

Olshansky SJ (1987) Simultaneous/multiple cause-delay (SIMCAD): an epidemiological approach to projecting mortality. *Journal of gerontology,* 42(4):358–365.

Osmond C (1985) Using age, period and cohort models to estimate future mortality rates. *International journal of epidemiology,* 14:124–129.

Osmond C, Barker DJP (1991) Ischaemic heart disease in England and Wales around the year 2000. *Journal of epidemiology and community health,* 45:71–72.

Patrick DL et al. (1994) Measuring preferences for health states worse than death. *Medical decision making,* 14(1):9-18

Pekkanen J et al. (1992) Risk factor dynamics, mortality and life expectancy differences between eastern and western Finland. *International journal of epidemiology,* 21(2):406–419.

Peto R et al. (1992) Mortality from tobacco in developed countries: indirect estimation from national vital statistics. *Lancet,* 339:1268–1278.

Ruwaard D et al. (1994) *Public health status and forecasts. The health status of the Dutch population over the period 1950–2010.* The Hague, Sdu Uitgeverij Plantijnstraat.

Schulzer M et al. (1992) An estimate of the future size of the tuberculosis problem in sub-Saharan Africa resulting from HIV infection. *Tubercle and lung disease,* 73:52–58.

Shiraishi M, Arimoto H (1982) Prediction of the future incidence of cancer in Japan. *Japanese journal of clinical oncology,* 12:65–72.

Steele J, Stratford B (1995) The United Kingdom population with Down Syndrome: present and future projections. *American journal on mental retardation,* 99(6):664–682.

Taket A (1993) *Health futures in support of health for all. Report of an international consultation convened by the World Health Organization Geneva, 19–23 July 1993.* Geneva, World Health Organization.

United Nations (1982) *United Nations model life tables for developing countries.* New York, United Nations.

United Nations (1995) *World population prospects. The 1994 revision.* New York, United Nations.

US Department of Health and Human Services (1989) Reducing the health consequences of smoking: 25 years of progress. A report of the Surgeon General. Washington, DC, Government Printing Office.

Wald N, Nicolaides-Bouman A (1991) *UK smoking statistics. Second Edition.* Oxford, Oxford University Press.

Weinstein MC (1987) Forecasting coronary heart disease incidence, mortality, and cost: the Coronary Heart Disease Policy Model. *American journal of public health,* 77(11):1417–1426.

World Bank (1990) *China. Long-term issues and options in the health transition.* Washington DC, World Bank.

World Bank (1994) *Chile. The adult health policy challenge.* Washington DC, World Bank.

World Bank (1995) *Global economic prospects and the developing countries.* Washington DC, World Bank.

World Health Organization (1986) *Health projections in Europe. Methods and applications.* Copenhagen, WHO.

Annex Tables

Annex Table 1. States or territories included in the Global Burden of Disease Study, by demographic region

Demographically developed regions		Demographically developing regions
Established market economies (EME)	Formerly socialist economies of Europe (FSE)	India (IND)
		China (CHN)
		Other Asia and islands (OAI)
Andorra	Albania	
Australia	Belarus	
Austria	Bosnia and Herzegovina	American Samoa
Belgium	Bulgaria	Bangladesh
Bermuda	Croatia	Bhutan
Canada	Czech Republic	Brunei Darussalam
Channel Islands	Estonia	Cambodia
Denmark	Hungary	Cook Islands
Faeroe Islands	Latvia	Federated States of Micronesia
Finland	Lithuania	Fiji
France	Macedonia,The Former Yugoslav	French Polynesia
Germany	Republic of	Guam
Gibraltar	Moldova	Hong Kong
Greece	Poland	Indonesia
Greenland	Romania	Johnston Island
Holy See	Russian Federation	Kiribati
Iceland	Slovakia	Korea, Democratic People's Republic of
Ireland	Slovenia	Korea, Republic of
Isle of Man	Ukraine	Lao People's Democratic Republic
Italy	Yugoslavia	Macao
Japan		Malaysia
Liechtenstein		Maldives
Luxembourg		Marshall Islands
Monaco		Mauritius
Netherlands		Midway Island
New Zealand		Mongolia
Norway		Myanmar
Portugal		Nauru
San Marino		Nepal
Spain		New Caledonia
St. Pierre and Miquelon		Niue
Sweden		Northern Mariana Islands
Switzerland		Palau
United Kingdom		Papua New Guinea
United States		Philippines
		Pitcairn Island
		Reunion
		Seychelles
		Singapore
		Solomon Islands
		Sri Lanka
		Taiwan
		Thailand
		Tokelau Island
		Tonga
		Tuvalu
		Vanuatu
		Viet Nam
		Wake Island
		Wallis and Futuna Islands
		Western Samoa

Annex Table 1, continued.

Sub-Saharan Africa (SSA)	Latin America and the Caribbean (LAC)	Middle Eastern crescent (MEC)
Angola	Anguilla	Afghanistan
Ascension	Antigua and Barbuda	Algeria
Benin	Argentina	Armenia
Botswana	Aruba	Azerbaijan
Burkina Faso	Bahamas	Bahrain
Burundi	Barbados	Cyprus
Cameroon	Belize	Egypt
Cape Verde	Bolivia	Former Spanish Sahara
Central African Republic	Brazil	Georgia
Chad	British Virgin Islands	Iran, Islamic Republic of
Comoros	Cayman Islands	Iraq
Congo	Chile	Israel
Côte d'Ivoire	Colombia	Jordan
Djibouti	Costa Rica	Kazakhstan
Equatorial Guinea	Cuba	Kuwait
Eritrea	Dominica	Kyrgyzstan
Ethiopia	Dominican Republic	Lebanon
Gabon	Ecuador	Libyan Arab Jamahiriya
Gambia	El Salvador	Malta
Ghana	French Guiana	Morocco
Guinea	Grenada	Oman
Guinea-Bissau	Guadeloupe	Pakistan
Kenya	Guatemala	Qatar
Lesotho	Guyana	Saudi Arabia
Liberia	Haiti	Syrian Arab Republic
Madagascar	Honduras	Tajikistan
Malawi	Jamaica	Tunisia
Mali	Martinique	Turkey
Mauritania	Mexico	Turkmenistan
Mayotte	Montserrat	United Arab Emirates
Mozambique	Netherlands Antilles	Uzbekistan
Namibia	Nicaragua	West Bank and Gaza Strip
Niger	Panama	Yemen
Nigeria	Paraguay	
Rwanda	Peru	
São Tomé and Principe	Puerto Rico	
Senegal	St. Kitts and Nevis	
Sierra Leone	St. Lucia	
Somalia	St. Vincent and the Grenadines	
South Africa	Suriname	
St. Helena	Trindad and Tobago	
Sudan	Turks and Caicos Islands	
Swaziland	Uruguay	
Tanzania	U.S. Virgin Islands	
Togo	Venezuela	
Tristan da Cunha		
Uganda		
Zaire		
Zambia		
Zimbabwe		

Annex Table 2. Cause groups, diseases and injuries, and sequelae included in the Global Burden of Disease Study and the set of sequelae for which data are presented in this volume

GBD Classification Code	Cause group, disease, injury, or sequela
I	Communicable, maternal, perinatal, and nutritional conditions
IA	Infectious and parasitic diseases
IA1	Tuberculosis
IA1-1	HIV sero-negative cases
IA1-2	HIV sero-positive cases
IA2	Sexually transmitted diseases excluding HIV
IA2a	Syphilis
IA2a-1	Congenital syphilis
IA2a-2	Low birth weight
IA2a-3	Primary
IA2a-4	Secondary
IA2a-5	Tertiary – cardiovascular
IA2a-6	Tertiary – gummas
IA2a-7	Tertiary – neurologic
IA2b	Chlamydia
IA2b-1	Ophthalmia neonatorum
IA2b-2	Low birth weight
IA2b-3	Corneal scar – blindness
IA2b-4	Corneal scar – low vision
IA2b-5	Cervicitis
IA2b-6	Neonatal pneumonia
IA2b-7	Pelvic inflammatory disease
IA2b-8	Ectopic pregnancy
IA2b-9	Tubo-ovarian abscess
IA2b-10	Chronic pelvic pain
IA2b-11	Infertility
IA2b-12	Symptomatic urethritis
IA2b-13	Epididymitis
IA2b-14	Stricture
IA2c	Gonorrhoea
IA2c-1	Ophthalmia neonatorum
IA2c-2	Low birth weight
IA2c-3	Corneal scar – blindness
IA2c-4	Corneal scar – low vision
IA2c-5	Cervicitis
IA2c-6	Pelvic inflammatory disease
IA2c-7	Ectopic pregnancy
IA2c-8	Tubo-ovarian abscess
IA2c-9	Chronic pelvic pain
IA2c-10	Infertility
IA2c-11	Symptomatic urethritis
IA2c-12	Epididymitis
IA2c-13	Stricture
IA3	HIV
IA3-1	Cases
IA3-2	AIDS
IA4	Diarrhoeal diseases
IA4-1	Episodes

Annex Table 2, continued.

GBD Classification Code	Cause group, disease, injury, or sequela
IA5	Childhood-cluster diseases
IA5a	Pertussis
IA5a-1	Episodes
IA5a-2	Mental retardation
IA5b	Poliomyelitis
IA5b-1	Lameness
IA5c	Diphtheria
IA5c-1	Episodes
IA5c-2	Neurological complications
IA5c-3	Myocarditis
IA5d	Measles
IA5d-1	Episodes
IA5e	Tetanus
IA5e-1	Episodes
IA6	Bacterial meningitis and meningococcaemia
IA6-1	All forms – episodes
IA6-2	Streptococcus pneumoniae – episodes
IA6-3	Haemophilus influenzae – episodes
IA6-4	Neisseria meningitidis – episodes
IA6-5	Meningococcaemia without meningitis – episodes
IA6-6	Deafness
IA6-7	Seizure disorder
IA6-8	Motor deficit
IA6-9	Mental retardation
IA7	Hepatitis B and hepatitis C
IA7-1	Episodes
IA7-2	Cirrhosis of the liver – symptomatic cases
IA7-3	Hepatoma
IA8	Malaria
IA8-1	Episodes
IA8-2	Anaemia
IA8-3	Neurological sequelae
IA9	Tropical-cluster diseases
IA9a	Trypanosomiasis
IA9a-1	Episodes
IA9b	Chagas disease
IA9b-1	Infection
IA9b-2	Cardiomyopathy without congestive heart failure
IA9b-3	Cardiomyopathy with congestive heart failure
IA9b-4	Megaviscera
IA9c	Schistosomiasis
IA9c-1	Infection
IA9d	Leishmaniasis
IA9d-1	Visceral
IA9d-2	Cutaneous
IA9e	Lymphatic filariasis
IA9e-1	Hydrocele > 15 cm0
IA9e-2	Bancroftian lymphoedema
IA9e-3	Brugian lymphoedema
IA9f	Onchocerciasis
IA9f-1	Blindness

Annex Table 2, continued.

GBD Classification Code	Cause group, disease, injury, or sequela
IA9f-2	Itching
IA9f-3	Low vision
IA10	Leprosy
IA10-1	Cases
IA10-2	Disabling leprosy
IA11	Dengue
IA11-1	Dengue haemorrhagic fever
IA12	Japanese encephalitis
IA12-1	Episodes
IA12-2	Cognitive impairment
IA12-3	Neurological sequelae
IA13	Trachoma
IA13-1	Blindness
IA13-2	Low vision
IA14	Intestinal nematode infections
IA14a	Ascariasis
IA14a-1	High intensity infection
IA14a-2	Cotemporaneous cognitive deficit
IA14a-3	Cognitive impairment
IA14a-4	Intestinal obstruction
IA14b	Trichuriasis
IA14b-1	High intensity infection
IA14b-2	Cotemporaneous cognitive deficit
IA14b-3	Massive dysentery syndrome
IA14b-4	Cognitive impairment
IA14c	Ancylostomiasis and necatoriasis
IA14c-1	High intensity infection
IA14c-2	Anaemia
IA14c-3	Cognitive impairment
IB	Respiratory infections
IB1	Lower respiratory infections
IB1-1	Episodes
IB1-2	Chronic sequelae
IB2	Upper respiratory infections
IB2-1	Episodes
IB2-2	Pharyngitis
IB3	Otitis media
IB3-1	Episodes
IB3-2	Deafness
IC	Maternal conditions
IC1	Maternal haemorrhage
IC1-1	Episodes
IC1-2	Sheehan syndrome
IC1-3	Severe anaemia
IC2	Maternal sepsis
IC2-1	Episodes
IC2-2	Infertility
IC3	Hypertensive disorders of pregnancy
IC3-1	Episodes
IC3-2	Neurological sequelae
IC4	Obstructed labour
IC4-1	Episodes

Annex Table 2, continued.

GBD Classification Code	Cause group, disease, injury, or sequela
IC4-2	Stress incontinence
IC4-3	Rectovaginal fistula
IC5	Abortion
IC5-1	Episodes
IC5-2	Infertility
ID	Conditions arising during the perinatal period
ID1	Low birth weight
ID1-1	All sequelae
ID2	Birth asphyxia and birth trauma
ID2-1	All sequelae
IE	Nutritional deficiencies
IE1	Protein-energy malnutrition
IE1-1	Wasting
IE1-2	Stunting
IE1-3	Developmental disability
IE2	Iodine deficiency
IE2-1	Goitre – grade 0
IE2-2	Goitre – grade 1
IE2-3	Goitre – grade 2
IE2-4	Mild developmental disability
IE2-5	Cretinoidism
IE2-6	Cretinism
IE3	Vitamin A deficiency
IE3-1	Xerophthalmia
IE3-2	Corneal scar
IE4	Iron-deficiency anaemia
IE4-1	All forms
IE4-2	Mild
IE4-3	Moderate
IE4-4	Severe
IE4-5	Very severe
IE4-6	Cognitive impairment
II	Noncommunicable diseases
IIA	Malignant neoplasms
IIA1	Mouth and oropharynx cancers
IIA1-1	Cases
IIA2	Oesophagus cancer
IIA2-1	Cases
IIA3	Stomach cancer
IIA3-1	Cases
IIA4	Colon and rectum cancers
IIA4-1	Cases
IIA5	Liver cancer
IIA5-1	Cases
IIA6	Pancreas cancer
IIA6-1	Cases
IIA7	Trachea, bronchus and lung cancers
IIA7-1	Cases
IIA8	Melanoma and other skin cancers
IIA8-1	Cases
IIA9	Breast cancer
IIA9-1	Cases

Annex Table 2, continued.

GBD Classification Code	Cause group, disease, injury, or sequela
IIA10	Cervix uteri cancer
IIA10-1	Cases
IIA11	Corpus uteri cancer
IIA11-1	Cases
IIA12	Ovary cancer
IIA12-1	Cases
IIA13	Prostate cancer
IIA13-1	Cases
IIA14	Bladder cancer
IIA14-1	Cases
IIA15	Lymphomas and multiple myeloma
IIA15-1	Cases
IIA16	Leukaemia
IIA16-1	Cases
IIB	Other neoplasms
IIC	Diabetes mellitus
IIC-1	Cases
IIC-2	Diabetic foot
IIC-3	Neuropathy
IIC-4	Retinopathy – blindness
IIC-5	Amputation
IID	Endocrine disorders
IIE	Neuro-psychiatric conditions
IIE1	Unipolar major depression
IIE1-1	Depressive episodes
IIE2	Bipolar disorder
IIE2-1	Cases
IIE3	Schizophrenia
IIE3-1	Cases
IIE4	Epilepsy
IIE4-1	Cases
IIE5	Alcohol use
IIE5-1	Alcohol dependence syndrome
IIE6	Dementia and other degenerative and hereditary CNS disorders
IIE6-1	Cases
IIE7	Parkinson disease
IIE7-1	Cases
IIE8	Multiple sclerosis
IIE8-1	Cases
IIE9	Drug use
IIE9-1	Dysfunctional and harmful drug use
IIE10	Post-traumatic stress disorder
IIE10-1	Cases
IIE11	Obsessive-compulsive disorders
IIE11-1	Cases
IIE12	Panic disorder
IIE12-1	Cases
IIF	Sense organ diseases
IIF1	Glaucoma
IIF1-1	Blindness
IIF2	Cataracts
IIF2-1	Blindness

Annex Table 2, continued.

GBD Classification Code	Cause group, disease, injury, or sequela
IIG	Cardiovascular diseases
IIG1	Rheumatic heart disease
IIG1-1	Congestive heart failure
IIG2	Ischaemic heart disease
IIG2-1	Acute myocardial infarction
IIG2-2	Angina pectoris
IIG2-3	Congestive heart failure
IIG3	Cerebrovascular disease
IIG3-1	First-ever stroke
IIG4	Inflammatory heart diseases
IIG4-1	Myocarditis
IIG4-2	Pericarditis
IIG4-3	Endocarditis
IIG4-4	Cardiomyopathy
IIH	Respiratory diseases
IIH1	Chronic obstructive pulmonary disease
IIH1-1	Symptomatic cases
IIH2	Asthma
IIH2-1	Cases
III	Digestive diseases
III1	Peptic ulcer
III1-1	Cases
III2	Cirrhosis of the liver
III2-1	Symptomatic Cases
III3	Appendicitis
III3-1	Episodes
IIJ	Genito-urinary diseases
IIJ1	Nephritis and nephrosis
IIJ1-1	Acute glomerulonephritis
IIJ1-2	End-stage renal disease
IIJ2	Benign prostatic hypertrophy
IIJ2-1	Symptomatic cases
IIK	Skin diseases
IIL	Musculo-skeletal diseases
IIL1	Rheumatoid arthritis
IIL1-1	Cases
IIL2	Osteoarthritis
IIL2-1	Hip
IIL2-2	Knee
IIM	Congenital anomalies
IIM1	Abdominal wall defect
IIM1-1	Cases
IIM2	Anencephaly
IIM2-1	Cases
IIM3	Anorectal atresia
IIM3-1	Cases
IIM4	Cleft lip
IIM4-1	Cases
IIM5	Cleft palate
IIM5-1	Cases
IIM6	Oesophageal atresia
IIM6-1	Cases

Annex Table 2, continued.

GBD Classification Code	Cause group, disease, injury, or sequela
IIM7	Renal agenesis
IIM7-1	Cases
IIM8	Down syndrome
IIM8-1	Cases
IIM9	Congenital heart anomalies
IIM9-1	Cases
IIM10	Spina bifida
IIM10-1	Cases
IIN	Oral conditions
IIN1	Dental caries
IIN1-1	Episodes
IIN2	Periodontal disease
IIN2-1	Episodes
IIN3	Edentulism
IIN3-1	Cases
III	Injuries
IIIA	Unintentional injuries
IIIA1	Road traffic accidents
IIIA1-1	Episodes
IIIA1-2	Fractured skull – short term
IIIA1-3	Fractured skull – long term
IIIA1-4	Fractured face bones
IIIA1-5	Fractured vertebral column
IIIA1-6	Injured spinal cord
IIIA1-7	Fractured rib or sternum
IIIA1-8	Fractured pelvis
IIIA1-9	Fractured clavicle, scapula, or humerus
IIIA1-10	Fractured radius or ulna
IIIA1-11	Fractured hand bones
IIIA1-12	Fractured femur – short term
IIIA1-13	Fractured femur – long term
IIIA1-14	Fractured patella, tibia, or fibula
IIIA1-15	Fractured ankle
IIIA1-16	Fractured foot bones
IIIA1-17	Other dislocation
IIIA1-18	Dislocated shoulder, elbow, or hip
IIIA1-19	Sprains
IIIA1-20	Intracranial injury – short term
IIIA1-21	Intracranial injury – long term
IIIA1-22	Internal injuries
IIIA1-23	Open wound
IIIA1-24	Injury to eyes
IIIA1-25	Amputated thumb
IIIA1-26	Amputated finger
IIIA1-27	Amputated arm
IIIA1-28	Amputated toe
IIIA1-29	Amputated foot
IIIA1-30	Amputated leg
IIIA1-31	Crushing
IIIA1-32	Burns < 20% – short term
IIIA1-33	Burns < 20% – long term
IIIA1-34	Burns > 20% and < 60% – short term

Annex Table 2, continued.

GBD Classification Code	Cause group, disease, injury, or sequela	
IIIA1-35		Burns > 20% and < 60% – long term
IIIA1-36		Burns > 60% – short term
IIIA1-37		Burns > 60% – long term
IIIA1-38		Injured nerves
IIIA1-39		Poisoning
IIIA1-40		Residual
IIIA2	Poisonings	
IIIA2-1		Episodes
IIIA3	Falls	
IIIA3-1		Episodes
IIIA3-2		Fractured skull – short term
IIIA3-3		Fractured skull – long term
IIIA3-4		Fractured face bones
IIIA3-5		Fractured vertebral column
IIIA3-6		Injured spinal cord
IIIA3-7		Fractured rib or sternum
IIIA3-8		Fractured pelvis
IIIA3-9		Fractured clavicle, scapula, or humerus
IIIA3-10		Fractured radius or ulna
IIIA3-11		Fractured hand bones
IIIA3-12		Fractured femur – short term
IIIA3-13		Fractured femur – long term
IIIA3-14		Fractured patella, tibia, or fibula
IIIA3-15		Fractured ankle
IIIA3-16		Fractured foot bones
IIIA3-17		Other dislocation
IIIA3-18		Dislocated shoulder, elbow, or hip
IIIA3-19		Sprains
IIIA3-20		Intracranial injury – short term
IIIA3-21		Intracranial injury – long term
IIIA3-22		Internal injuries
IIIA3-23		Open wound
IIIA3-24		Injury to eyes
IIIA3-25		Amputated thumb
IIIA3-26		Amputated finger
IIIA3-27		Amputated arm
IIIA3-28		Amputated toe
IIIA3-29		Amputated foot
IIIA3-30		Amputated leg
IIIA3-31		Crushing
IIIA3-32		Burns < 20% – short term
IIIA3-33		Burns < 20% – long term
IIIA3-34		Burns > 20% and < 60% – short term
IIIA3-35		Burns > 20% and < 60% – long term
IIIA3-36		Burns > 60% – short term
IIIA3-37		Burns > 60% – long term
IIIA3-38		Injured nerves
IIIA3-39		Poisoning
IIIA4-40		Residual
IIIA4	Fires	
IIIA4-1		Episodes
IIIA4-2		Fractured skull – short term

Annex Table 2, continued.

GBD Classification Code	Cause group, disease, injury, or sequela
IIIA4-3	Fractured skull – long term
IIIA4-4	Fractured face bones
IIIA4-5	Fractured vertebral column
IIIA4-6	Injured spinal cord
IIIA4-7	Fractured rib or sternum
IIIA4-8	Fractured pelvis
IIIA4-9	Fractured clavicle, scapula, or humerus
IIIA4-10	Fractured radius or ulna
IIIA4-11	Fractured hand bones
IIIA4-12	Fractured femur – short term
IIIA4-13	Fractured femur – long term
IIIA4-14	Fractured patella, tibia, or fibula
IIIA4-15	Fractured ankle
IIIA4-16	Fractured foot bones
IIIA4-17	Other dislocation
IIIA4-18	Dislocated shoulder, elbow, or hip
IIIA4-19	Sprains
IIIA4-20	Intracranial injury – short term
IIIA4-21	Intracranial injury – long term
IIIA4-22	Internal injuries
IIIA4-23	Open wound
IIIA4-24	Injury to eyes
IIIA4-25	Amputated thumb
IIIA4-26	Amputated finger
IIIA4-27	Amputated arm
IIIA4-28	Amputated toe
IIIA4-29	Amputated foot
IIIA4-30	Amputated leg
IIIA4-31	Crushing
IIIA4-32	Burns < 20% – short term
IIIA4-33	Burns < 20% – long term
IIIA4-34	Burns > 20% and < 60% – short term
IIIA4-35	Burns > 20% and < 60% – long term
IIIA4-36	Burns > 60% – short term
IIIA4-37	Burns > 60% – long term
IIIA4-38	Injured nerves
IIIA4-39	Poisoning
IIIA4-40	Residual
IIIA5	Drownings
IIIA5-1	Episodes
IIIA5-2	Quadriplegia
IIIA6	Other unintentional injuries
IIIA6-1	Episodes
IIIA6-2	Fractured skull – short term
IIIA6-3	Fractured skull – long term
IIIA6-4	Fractured face bones
IIIA6-5	Fractured vertebral column
IIIA6-6	Injured spinal cord
IIIA6-7	Fractured rib or sternum
IIIA6-8	Fractured pelvis
IIIA6-9	Fractured clavicle, scapula, or humerus
IIIA6-10	Fractured radius or ulna

Annex Table 2, continued.

GBD Classification Code	Cause group, disease, injury, or sequela
IIIA6-11	Fractured hand bones
IIIA6-12	Fractured femur – short term
IIIA6-13	Fractured femur – long term
IIIA6-14	Fractured patella, tibia, or fibula
IIIA6-15	Fractured ankle
IIIA6-16	Fractured foot bones
IIIA6-17	Other dislocation
IIIA6-18	Dislocated shoulder, elbow, or hip
IIIA6-19	Sprains
IIIA6-20	Intracranial injury – short term
IIIA6-21	Intracranial injury – long term
IIIA6-22	Internal injuries
IIIA6-23	Open wound
IIIA6-24	Injury to eyes
IIIA6-25	Amputated thumb
IIIA6-26	Amputated finger
IIIA6-27	Amputated arm
IIIA6-28	Amputated toe
IIIA6-29	Amputated foot
IIIA6-30	Amputated leg
IIIA6-31	Crushing
IIIA6-32	Burns < 20% – short term
IIIA6-33	Burns < 20% – long term
IIIA6-34	Burns > 20% and < 60% – short term
IIIA6-35	Burns > 20% and < 60% – long term
IIIA6-36	Burns > 60% – short term
IIIA6-37	Burns > 60% – long term
IIIA6-38	Injured nerves
IIIA6-39	Poisoning
IIIA6-40	Residual
IIIB	Intentional injuries
IIIB1	Self-inflicted injuries
IIIB1-1	Episodes
IIIB1-2	Fractured skull – short term
IIIB1-3	Fractured skull – long term
IIIB1-4	Fractured face bones
IIIB1-5	Fractured vertebral column
IIIB1-6	Injured spinal cord
IIIB1-7	Fractured rib or sternum
IIIB1-8	Fractured pelvis
IIIB1-9	Fractured clavicle, scapula, or humerus
IIIB1-10	Fractured radius or ulna
IIIB1-11	Fractured hand bones
IIIB1-12	Fractured femur – short term
IIIB1-13	Fractured femur – long term
IIIB1-14	Fractured patella, tibia, or fibula
IIIB1-15	Fractured ankle
IIIB1-16	Fractured foot bones
IIIB1-17	Other dislocation
IIIB1-18	Dislocated shoulder, elbow, or hip
IIIB1-19	Sprains
IIIB1-20	Intracranial injury – short term

Annex Table 2, continued.

GBD Classification Code	Cause group, disease, injury, or sequela
IIIB1-21	Intracranial injury – long term
IIIB1-22	Internal injuries
IIIB1-23	Open wound
IIIB1-24	Injury to eyes
IIIB1-25	Amputated thumb
IIIB1-26	Amputated finger
IIIB1-27	Amputated arm
IIIB1-28	Amputated toe
IIIB1-29	Amputated foot
IIIB1-30	Amputated leg
IIIB1-31	Crushing
IIIB1-32	Burns < 20% – short term
IIIB1-33	Burns < 20% – long term
IIIB1-34	Burns > 20% and < 60% – short term
IIIB1-35	Burns > 20% and < 60% – long term
IIIB1-36	Burns > 60% – short term
IIIB1-37	Burns > 60% – long term
IIIB1-38	Injured nerves
IIIB1-39	Poisoning
IIIB1-40	Residual
IIIB2	Violence
IIIB2-1	Episodes
IIIB2-2	Fractured skull – short term
IIIB2-3	Fractured skull – long term
IIIB2-4	Fractured face bones
IIIB2-5	Fractured vertebral column
IIIB2-6	Injured spinal cord
IIIB2-7	Fractured rib or sternum
IIIB2-8	Fractured pelvis
IIIB2-9	Fractured clavicle, scapula, or humerus
IIIB2-10	Fractured radius or ulna
IIIB2-11	Fractured hand bones
IIIB2-12	Fractured femur – short term
IIIB2-13	Fractured femur – long term
IIIB2-14	Fractured patella, tibia, or fibula
IIIB2-15	Fractured ankle
IIIB2-16	Fractured foot bones
IIIB2-17	Other dislocation
IIIB2-18	Dislocated shoulder, elbow, or hip
IIIB2-19	Sprains
IIIB2-20	Intracranial injury – short term
IIIB2-21	Intracranial injury – long term
IIIB2-22	Internal injuries
IIIB2-23	Open wound
IIIB2-24	Injury to eyes
IIIB2-25	Amputated thumb
IIIB2-26	Amputated finger
IIIB2-27	Amputated arm
IIIB2-28	Amputated toe
IIIB2-29	Amputated foot
IIIB2-30	Amputated leg
IIIB2-31	Crushing

Annex Table 2, continued.

GBD Classification Code	Cause group, disease, injury, or sequela	
IIIB2-32		Burns < 20% – short term
IIIB2-33		Burns < 20% – long term
IIIB2-34		Burns > 20% and < 60% – short term
IIIB2-35		Burns > 20% and < 60% – long term
IIIB2-36		Burns > 60% – short term
IIIB2-37		Burns > 60% – long term
IIIB2-38		Injured nerves
IIIB2-39		Poisoning
IIIB2-40		Residual
IIIB3	War	
IIIB3-1		Episodes
IIIB3-2		Fractured skull – short term
IIIB3-3		Fractured skull – long term
IIIB3-4		Fractured face bones
IIIB3-5		Fractured vertebral column
IIIB3-6		Injured spinal cord
IIIB3-7		Fractured rib or sternum
IIIB3-8		Fractured pelvis
IIIB3-9		Fractured clavicle, scapula, or humerus
IIIB3-10		Fractured radius or ulna
IIIB3-11		Fractured hand bones
IIIB3-12		Fractured femur – short term
IIIB3-13		Fractured femur – long term
IIIB3-14		Fractured patella, tibia, or fibula
IIIB3-15		Fractured ankle
IIIB3-16		Fractured foot bones
IIIB3-17		Other dislocation
IIIB3-18		Dislocated shoulder, elbow, or hip
IIIB3-19		Sprains
IIIB3-20		Intracranial injury – short term
IIIB3-21		Intracranial injury – long term
IIIB3-22		Internal injuries
IIIB3-23		Open wound
IIIB3-24		Injury to eyes
IIIB3-25		Amputated thumb
IIIB3-26		Amputated finger
IIIB3-27		Amputated arm
IIIB3-28		Amputated toe
IIIB3-29		Amputated foot
IIIB3-30		Amputated leg
IIIB3-31		Crushing
IIIB3-32		Burns < 20% – short term
IIIB3-33		Burns < 20% – long term
IIIB3-34		Burns > 20% and < 60% – short term
IIIB3-35		Burns > 20% and < 60% – long term
IIIB3-36		Burns > 60% – short term
IIIB3-37		Burns > 60% – long term
IIIB3-38		Injured nerves
IIIB3-39		Poisoning
IIIB3-40		Residual

Annex Table 3.

Age-specific disability weights for untreated and treated forms of sequelae included in the Global Burden of Disease Study

	Untreated form					Treated form				
	Age group (years)					Age group (years)				
Sequela	0-4	5-14	15-44	45-59	60+	0-4	5-14	15-44	45-59	60+
Tuberculosis										
HIV sero-negative cases	0.294	0.294	0.264	0.274	0.274	0.294	0.294	0.264	0.274	0.274
HIV sero-positive cases	0.294	0.294	0.264	0.274	0.274	0.294	0.294	0.264	0.274	0.274
Syphilis										
Congenital syphilis	0.315	0.315	0.315	0.315	0.315	0.315	0.315	0.315	0.315	0.315
Low birth weight	0.000	0.000	0.000	0.000	0.000	0.000	0.000	0.000	0.000	0.000
Primary	0.015	0.015	0.015	0.014	0.014	0.015	0.015	0.015	0.014	0.014
Secondary	0.048	0.048	0.048	0.048	0.044	0.048	0.048	0.048	0.048	0.044
Tertiary -- Cardiovascular	0.196	0.196	0.196	0.196	0.196	0.196	0.196	0.196	0.196	0.196
Tertiary -- Gummas	0.102	0.102	0.102	0.102	0.094	0.102	0.102	0.102	0.102	0.094
Tertiary -- Neurologic	0.283	0.283	0.283	0.283	0.283	0.283	0.283	0.283	0.283	0.283
Chlamydia										
Ophthalmia neonatorum	0.180	0.000	0.000	0.000	0.000	0.180	0.000	0.000	0.000	0.000
Low birth weight	0.000	0.000	0.000	0.000	0.000	0.000	0.000	0.000	0.000	0.000
Corneal scar -- Blindness	0.600	0.600	0.600	0.600	0.600	0.493	0.491	0.488	0.488	0.488
Corneal scar -- Low vision	0.223	0.245	0.245	0.245	0.245	0.223	0.245	0.245	0.245	0.245
Cervicitis	0.049	0.049	0.049	0.049	0.049	0.049	0.049	0.049	0.049	0.049
Neonatal pneumonia	0.280	0.280	0.276	0.276	0.280	0.280	0.280	0.276	0.276	0.280
Pelvic inflammatory disease	0.420	0.420	0.420	0.420	0.420	0.169	0.169	0.169	0.169	0.169
Ectopic pregnancy	0.000	0.549	0.549	0.549	0.000	0.000	0.549	0.549	0.549	0.000
Tubo-ovarian abscess	0.000	0.549	0.549	0.549	0.000	0.000	0.549	0.549	0.549	0.000
Chronic pelvic pain	0.122	0.122	0.122	0.122	0.122	0.122	0.122	0.122	0.122	0.122
Infertility	0.180	0.180	0.180	0.180	0.180	0.180	0.180	0.180	0.180	0.180
Symptomatic urethritis	0.067	0.067	0.067	0.067	0.067	0.067	0.067	0.067	0.067	0.067
Epididymitis	0.167	0.167	0.167	0.167	0.167	0.167	0.167	0.167	0.167	0.167
Stricture	0.151	0.151	0.151	0.151	0.151	0.151	0.151	0.151	0.151	0.151
Gonorrhoea										
Ophthalmia neonatorum	0.180	0.000	0.000	0.000	0.000	0.180	0.000	0.000	0.000	0.000
Low birth weight	0.000	0.000	0.000	0.000	0.000	0.000	0.000	0.000	0.000	0.000
Corneal scar -- Blindness	0.600	0.000	0.000	0.000	0.000	0.600	0.000	0.000	0.000	0.000
Corneal scar -- Low vision	0.223	0.245	0.245	0.245	0.245	0.223	0.245	0.245	0.245	0.245
Cervicitis	0.049	0.049	0.049	0.049	0.049	0.049	0.049	0.049	0.049	0.049
Pelvic inflammatory disease	0.169	0.169	0.169	0.169	0.169	0.169	0.169	0.169	0.169	0.169
Ectopic pregnancy	0.000	0.549	0.549	0.549	0.000	0.000	0.549	0.549	0.549	0.000
Tubo-ovarian abscess	0.000	0.549	0.549	0.549	0.000	0.000	0.549	0.549	0.549	0.000
Chronic pelvic pain	0.122	0.122	0.122	0.122	0.122	0.122	0.122	0.122	0.122	0.122
Infertility	0.180	0.180	0.180	0.180	0.180	0.180	0.180	0.180	0.180	0.180
Symptomatic urethritis	0.067	0.067	0.067	0.067	0.067	0.067	0.067	0.067	0.067	0.067
Epididymitis	0.167	0.167	0.167	0.167	0.167	0.167	0.167	0.167	0.167	0.167
Stricture	0.151	0.151	0.151	0.151	0.151	0.151	0.151	0.151	0.151	0.151
HIV										
Cases	0.123	0.123	0.136	0.136	0.136	0.123	0.123	0.136	0.136	0.136
AIDS	0.505	0.505	0.505	0.505	0.505	0.505	0.505	0.505	0.505	0.505
Diarrhoeal diseases -- Episodes	0.119	0.094	0.086	0.086	0.088	0.119	0.094	0.086	0.086	0.088
Pertussis										
Episodes	0.178	0.166	0.156	0.156	0.156	0.000	0.000	0.000	0.000	0.000
Mental retardation	0.469	0.483	0.483	0.486	0.485	0.394	0.420	0.451	0.466	0.468
Poliomyelitis -- Lameness	0.369	0.369	0.369	0.369	0.369	0.369	0.369	0.369	0.369	0.369
Diphtheria										
Episodes	0.231	0.230	0.230	0.230	0.230	0.231	0.230	0.230	0.230	0.230
Neurological complications	0.078	0.078	0.078	0.078	0.078	0.078	0.078	0.078	0.078	0.078
Myocarditis	0.323	0.323	0.323	0.323	0.323	0.323	0.323	0.323	0.323	0.323
Measles -- Episodes	0.152	0.152	0.152	0.152	0.152	0.152	0.152	0.152	0.152	0.152
Tetanus -- Episodes	0.640	0.640	0.610	0.604	0.612	0.640	0.640	0.610	0.604	0.612
Bacterial meningitis, meningococcaemia										
Episodes	0.616	0.616	0.613	0.613	0.613	0.616	0.616	0.613	0.613	0.613
Haemophilus influenzae -- Episodes	0.616	0.616	0.613	0.613	0.613	0.616	0.616	0.613	0.613	0.613
Neisseria meningitidis -- Episodes	0.616	0.616	0.613	0.613	0.613	0.616	0.616	0.613	0.613	0.613

Annex Table 3, continued.   **Age-specific disability weights for untreated and treated forms of sequelae included in the Global Burden of Disease Study**

Sequela	Untreated form Age group (years)					Treated form Age group (years)				
	0-4	5-14	15-44	45-59	60+	0-4	5-14	15-44	45-59	60+
Meningococcaemia without meningitis --										
Episodes	0.152	0.152	0.152	0.152	0.152	0.152	0.152	0.152	0.152	0.152
Deafness	0.233	0.227	0.216	0.215	0.213	0.175	0.169	0.168	0.168	0.168
Seizure disorder	0.099	0.150	0.150	0.150	0.150	0.041	0.065	0.065	0.065	0.065
Motor deficit	0.388	0.388	0.388	0.397	0.468	0.334	0.334	0.334	0.337	0.390
Mental retardation	0.469	0.483	0.483	0.486	0.485	0.394	0.420	0.451	0.466	0.468
Hepatitis B and hepatitis C -- Episodes	0.170	0.181	0.209	0.212	0.212	0.170	0.181	0.209	0.212	0.212
Malaria										
Episodes	0.211	0.195	0.172	0.172	0.172	0.211	0.195	0.172	0.172	0.172
Anaemia	0.012	0.012	0.012	0.013	0.012	0.012	0.012	0.012	0.013	0.012
Neurological sequelae	0.473	0.473	0.473	0.473	0.473	0.436	0.435	0.435	0.435	0.435
Trypanosomiasis -- Episodes	0.350	0.350	0.350	0.350	0.350	0.350	0.350	0.350	0.350	0.350
Chagas disease										
Infection	0.000	0.000	0.000	0.000	0.000	0.000	0.000	0.000	0.000	0.000
Cardiomyopathy without congestive heart failure	0.062	0.062	0.062	0.062	0.062	0.062	0.062	0.062	0.062	0.062
Cardiomyopathy with congestive heart failure	0.323	0.323	0.323	0.323	0.323	0.171	0.171	0.171	0.171	0.171
Megaviscera	0.240	0.240	0.240	0.240	0.240	0.240	0.240	0.240	0.240	0.240
Schistosomiasis -- Infection	0.005	0.005	0.006	0.006	0.006	0.005	0.005	0.006	0.006	0.006
Leishmaniasis										
Visceral	0.243	0.243	0.243	0.243	0.243	0.243	0.243	0.243	0.243	0.243
Cutaneous	0.023	0.023	0.023	0.023	0.023	0.023	0.023	0.023	0.023	0.023
Lymphatic filariasis										
Hydrocele >15 cm	0.066	0.070	0.075	0.075	0.075	0.066	0.070	0.075	0.075	0.075
Bancroftian lymphoedema	0.067	0.080	0.113	0.128	0.119	0.067	0.080	0.113	0.128	0.119
Brugian lymphoedema	0.064	0.080	0.113	0.128	0.119	0.064	0.080	0.113	0.128	0.119
Onchocerciasis										
Blindness	0.600	0.600	0.600	0.600	0.600	0.493	0.491	0.488	0.488	0.488
Itching	0.068	0.068	0.068	0.068	0.068	0.068	0.068	0.068	0.068	0.068
Low vision	0.223	0.245	0.245	0.245	0.245	0.223	0.245	0.245	0.245	0.245
Leprosy										
Cases	0.000	0.000	0.000	0.000	0.000	0.000	0.000	0.000	0.000	0.000
Disabling leprosy	0.153	0.153	0.153	0.153	0.153	0.153	0.153	0.153	0.153	0.153
Dengue										
Dengue haemorrhagic fever	0.211	0.195	0.172	0.172	0.172	0.211	0.195	0.172	0.172	0.172
Japanese encephalitis										
Episodes	0.616	0.616	0.613	0.613	0.613	0.616	0.616	0.613	0.613	0.613
Cognitive impairment	0.469	0.483	0.483	0.486	0.485	0.394	0.420	0.451	0.466	0.468
Neurological sequelae	0.388	0.388	0.388	0.397	0.468	0.334	0.334	0.334	0.337	0.390
Trachoma										
Blindness	0.600	0.600	0.600	0.600	0.600	0.493	0.491	0.488	0.488	0.488
Low Vision	0.223	0.245	0.245	0.245	0.245	0.223	0.245	0.245	0.245	0.245
Ascariasis										
High intensity infection	0.000	0.000	0.000	0.000	0.000	0.000	0.000	0.000	0.000	0.000
Cotemporaneous cognitive deficit	0.006	0.006	0.006	0.006	0.006	0.006	0.006	0.006	0.006	0.006
Cognitive impairment	0.463	0.463	0.463	0.463	0.463	0.463	0.463	0.463	0.463	0.463
Intestinal obstruction	0.024	0.024	0.024	0.024	0.024	0.024	0.024	0.024	0.024	0.024
Trichuriasis										
High intensity infection	0.000	0.000	0.000	0.000	0.000	0.000	0.000	0.000	0.000	0.000
Cotemporaneous cognitive deficit	0.006	0.006	0.006	0.006	0.006	0.006	0.006	0.006	0.006	0.006
Massive dysentery syndrome	0.138	0.116	0.114	0.114	0.129	0.138	0.116	0.114	0.114	0.129
Cognitive impairment	0.024	0.024	0.024	0.024	0.024	0.024	0.024	0.024	0.024	0.024
Ancylostomiasis and necatoriasis										
High intensity infection	0.000	0.000	0.000	0.000	0.000	0.000	0.000	0.000	0.000	0.000
Anaemia	0.024	0.024	0.024	0.024	0.024	0.024	0.024	0.024	0.024	0.024
Cognitive impairment	0.024	0.024	0.024	0.024	0.024	0.024	0.024	0.024	0.024	0.024
Lower respiratory infections										
Episodes	0.280	0.280	0.276	0.276	0.280	0.280	0.280	0.276	0.276	0.280
Chronic sequelae	0.099	0.099	0.099	0.099	0.099	0.099	0.099	0.099	0.099	0.099

Annex Table 3, continued.	**Age-specific disability weights for untreated and treated forms of sequelae included in the Global Burden of Disease Study**

	Untreated form					Treated form				
	Age group (years)					Age group (years)				
Sequela	0-4	5-14	15-44	45-59	60+	0-4	5-14	15-44	45-59	60+
Upper respiratory infections										
Episodes	0.000	0.000	0.000	0.000	0.000	0.000	0.000	0.000	0.000	0.000
Pharyngitis	0.070	0.070	0.070	0.070	0.070	0.070	0.070	0.070	0.070	0.070
Otitis media										
Episodes	0.023	0.023	0.023	0.023	0.023	0.023	0.023	0.023	0.023	0.023
Deafness	0.233	0.227	0.216	0.215	0.213	0.175	0.169	0.168	0.168	0.168
Maternal haemorrhage										
Episodes	0.000	0.000	0.000	0.000	0.000	0.000	0.000	0.000	0.000	0.000
Sheehan syndrome	0.065	0.065	0.065	0.065	0.065	0.065	0.065	0.065	0.065	0.065
Severe anaemia	0.087	0.087	0.093	0.090	0.087	0.087	0.087	0.093	0.090	0.087
Maternal sepsis										
Episodes	0.000	0.000	0.000	0.000	0.000	0.000	0.000	0.000	0.000	0.000
Infertility	0.000	0.000	0.180	0.000	0.000	0.000	0.000	0.180	0.000	0.000
Hypertensive disorders of pregnancy										
Episodes	0.000	0.000	0.000	0.000	0.000	0.000	0.000	0.000	0.000	0.000
Neurological sequelae	0.388	0.388	0.388	0.397	0.468	0.388	0.388	0.388	0.397	0.468
Obstructed labour										
Episodes	0.000	0.000	0.000	0.000	0.000	0.000	0.000	0.000	0.000	0.000
Stress incontinence	0.025	0.025	0.025	0.025	0.033	0.025	0.025	0.025	0.025	0.033
Rectovaginal fistula	0.000	0.000	0.430	0.000	0.000	0.000	0.000	0.430	0.000	0.000
Abortion										
Episodes	0.000	0.000	0.000	0.000	0.000	0.000	0.000	0.000	0.000	0.000
Infertility	0.000	0.000	0.180	0.000	0.000	0.000	0.000	0.180	0.000	0.000
Low birth weight -- All sequelae	0.291	0.291	0.291	0.291	0.291	0.256	0.256	0.256	0.256	0.256
Birth asphyxia and birth trauma -- All sequelae	0.381	0.381	0.381	0.381	0.381	0.334	0.334	0.334	0.334	0.334
Protein-energy malnutrition										
Wasting	0.053	0.000	0.000	0.000	0.000	0.053	0.000	0.000	0.000	0.000
Stunting	0.002	0.000	0.000	0.000	0.000	0.002	0.000	0.000	0.000	0.000
Developmental disability	0.024	0.024	0.024	0.024	0.024	0.024	0.024	0.024	0.024	0.024
Iodine deficiency										
Goitre -- grade 0	0.000	0.000	0.000	0.000	0.000	0.000	0.000	0.000	0.000	0.000
Goitre -- grade 1	0.001	0.001	0.001	0.001	0.001	0.001	0.001	0.001	0.001	0.001
Goitre -- grade 2	0.025	0.025	0.025	0.025	0.025	0.025	0.025	0.025	0.025	0.025
Mild developmental disability	0.006	0.006	0.006	0.006	0.006	0.006	0.006	0.006	0.006	0.006
Cretinoidism	0.255	0.255	0.255	0.255	0.255	0.255	0.255	0.255	0.255	0.255
Cretinism	0.804	0.804	0.804	0.804	0.804	0.804	0.804	0.804	0.804	0.804
Vitamin A deficiency										
Xerophthalmia	0.000	0.000	0.000	0.000	0.000	0.000	0.000	0.000	0.000	0.000
Corneal scar	0.274	0.282	0.282	0.282	0.282	0.274	0.282	0.282	0.282	0.282
Iron-deficiency anaemia										
Mild	0.000	0.000	0.000	0.000	0.000	0.000	0.000	0.000	0.000	0.000
Moderate	0.011	0.011	0.011	0.012	0.012	0.011	0.011	0.011	0.012	0.012
Severe	0.087	0.087	0.093	0.090	0.087	0.087	0.087	0.093	0.090	0.087
Very severe	0.241	0.244	0.255	0.252	0.252	0.241	0.244	0.255	0.252	0.252
Cognitive impairment	0.024	0.024	0.024	0.024	0.024	0.024	0.024	0.024	0.024	0.024
Cancers -- Preterminal										
Mouth and oropharynx	0.145	0.145	0.145	0.145	0.145	0.090	0.090	0.090	0.090	0.090
Oesophagus	0.217	0.217	0.217	0.217	0.217	0.217	0.217	0.217	0.217	0.217
Stomach	0.217	0.217	0.217	0.217	0.217	0.217	0.217	0.217	0.217	0.217
Colon and rectum	0.217	0.217	0.217	0.217	0.217	0.217	0.217	0.217	0.217	0.217
Liver	0.239	0.239	0.239	0.239	0.239	0.239	0.239	0.239	0.239	0.239
Pancreas	0.301	0.301	0.301	0.301	0.301	0.237	0.237	0.237	0.237	0.237
Trachea, bronchus and lung	0.146	0.146	0.146	0.146	0.146	0.146	0.146	0.146	0.146	0.146
Melanoma and other skin	0.045	0.045	0.045	0.045	0.045	0.045	0.045	0.045	0.045	0.045
Breast	0.069	0.069	0.069	0.069	0.069	0.086	0.086	0.086	0.086	0.086
Cervix uteri	0.066	0.066	0.066	0.066	0.066	0.075	0.075	0.075	0.075	0.075
Corpus uteri	0.066	0.066	0.066	0.066	0.066	0.099	0.104	0.104	0.096	0.079
Ovary	0.081	0.081	0.081	0.081	0.081	0.097	0.097	0.097	0.084	0.059
Prostate	0.113	0.113	0.113	0.113	0.113	0.134	0.134	0.134	0.134	0.134

Annex Table 3, continued. **Age-specific disability weights for untreated and treated forms of sequelae included in the Global Burden of Disease Study**

Sequela	Untreated form Age group (years)					Treated form Age group (years)				
	0-4	5-14	15-44	45-59	60+	0-4	5-14	15-44	45-59	60+
Bladder	0.085	0.085	0.085	0.085	0.085	0.087	0.087	0.087	0.087	0.085
Lymphomas and multiple myeloma	0.089	0.089	0.089	0.089	0.089	0.057	0.057	0.057	0.057	0.057
Leukaemia	0.098	0.098	0.108	0.112	0.112	0.083	0.083	0.093	0.097	0.097
Cancers -- Terminal	0.809	0.809	0.809	0.809	0.809	0.809	0.809	0.809	0.809	0.809
Diabetes mellitus										
Cases	0.012	0.012	0.012	0.012	0.012	0.033	0.033	0.033	0.033	0.033
Diabetic foot	0.137	0.137	0.137	0.137	0.137	0.129	0.129	0.129	0.129	0.129
Neuropathy	0.078	0.078	0.078	0.078	0.078	0.064	0.064	0.064	0.064	0.064
Retinopathy -- Blindness	0.600	0.600	0.600	0.600	0.600	0.493	0.491	0.488	0.488	0.488
Amputation	0.155	0.155	0.155	0.155	0.155	0.068	0.068	0.068	0.068	0.068
Unipolar major depression -- episodes	0.600	0.600	0.600	0.600	0.600	0.302	0.302	0.302	0.302	0.302
Bipolar disorder -- Cases	0.583	0.583	0.583	0.583	0.583	0.383	0.383	0.383	0.383	0.383
Schizophrenia -- Cases	0.627	0.627	0.627	0.645	0.667	0.351	0.351	0.351	0.351	0.351
Epilepsy -- Cases	0.099	0.150	0.150	0.150	0.150	0.041	0.065	0.065	0.065	0.065
Alcohol --	0.180	0.180	0.180	0.180	0.180	0.180	0.180	0.180	0.180	0.180
Alcohol dependence syndrome	0.180	0.180	0.180	0.180	0.180	0.180	0.180	0.180	0.180	0.180
Dementia -- Cases	0.627	0.627	0.627	0.645	0.667	0.627	0.627	0.627	0.645	0.667
Parkinson disease -- Cases	0.392	0.392	0.392	0.392	0.406	0.316	0.316	0.316	0.316	0.332
Multiple sclerosis -- Cases	0.410	0.410	0.410	0.420	0.437	0.410	0.410	0.410	0.420	0.437
Drug use --										
Dysfunctional and harmful drug use	0.252	0.252	0.250	0.250	0.250	0.252	0.252	0.250	0.250	0.250
Post-traumatic stress disorder -- Cases	0.105	0.105	0.108	0.108	0.108	0.105	0.105	0.108	0.108	0.108
Obsessive-compulsive disorders --										
Cases	0.129	0.129	0.129	0.129	0.129	0.080	0.080	0.080	0.080	0.080
Panic disorder -- Cases	0.173	0.173	0.173	0.173	0.173	0.091	0.091	0.091	0.091	0.091
Glaucoma -- Blindness	0.600	0.600	0.600	0.600	0.600	0.600	0.600	0.600	0.600	0.600
Cataracts -- Blindness	0.600	0.600	0.600	0.600	0.600	0.493	0.491	0.488	0.488	0.488
Rheumatic heart disease --										
Congestive heart failure	0.323	0.323	0.323	0.323	0.323	0.171	0.171	0.171	0.171	0.171
Ischaemic heart disease										
Acute myocardial infarction	0.491	0.491	0.491	0.491	0.491	0.395	0.395	0.395	0.395	0.395
Angina pectoris	0.227	0.227	0.227	0.227	0.227	0.095	0.095	0.095	0.095	0.095
Congestive heart failure	0.323	0.323	0.323	0.323	0.323	0.171	0.171	0.171	0.171	0.171
Cerebrovascular disease --										
First-ever stroke	0.262	0.262	0.262	0.268	0.301	0.224	0.224	0.224	0.224	0.258
Inflammatory heart diseases										
Myocarditis	0.323	0.323	0.323	0.323	0.323	0.171	0.171	0.171	0.171	0.171
Pericarditis	0.323	0.323	0.323	0.323	0.323	0.171	0.171	0.171	0.171	0.171
Endocarditis	0.323	0.323	0.323	0.323	0.323	0.171	0.171	0.171	0.171	0.171
Cardiomyopathy	0.323	0.323	0.323	0.323	0.323	0.171	0.171	0.171	0.171	0.171
COPD -- Symptomatic cases	0.428	0.428	0.428	0.428	0.428	0.388	0.388	0.388	0.388	0.388
Asthma -- Cases	0.099	0.099	0.099	0.099	0.099	0.059	0.059	0.059	0.059	0.059
Peptic ulcer -- Cases	0.115	0.115	0.115	0.115	0.115	0.003	0.003	0.003	0.003	0.003
Cirrhosis of the liver --										
Symptomatic cases	0.330	0.330	0.330	0.330	0.330	0.330	0.330	0.330	0.330	0.330
Appendicitis -- Episodes	0.463	0.463	0.463	0.463	0.463	0.463	0.463	0.463	0.463	0.463
Nephritis and nephrosis										
Acute glomerulonephritis	0.082	0.082	0.104	0.104	0.104	0.107	0.107	0.107	0.096	0.096
End-stage renal disease	0.082	0.082	0.104	0.104	0.104	0.107	0.107	0.107	0.096	0.096
Benign prostatic hypertrophy --										
Symptomatic cases	0.038	0.038	0.038	0.038	0.038	0.038	0.038	0.038	0.038	0.038
Rheumatoid arthritis -- Cases	0.233	0.233	0.233	0.233	0.233	0.174	0.174	0.174	0.174	0.174
Osteoarthritis										
Hip	0.156	0.156	0.156	0.156	0.156	0.108	0.108	0.108	0.108	0.108
Knee	0.156	0.156	0.156	0.156	0.156	0.108	0.108	0.108	0.108	0.108

Annex Table 3, continued. **Age-specific disability weights for untreated and treated forms of sequelae included in the Global Burden of Disease Study**

Sequela	Untreated form Age group (years)					Treated form Age group (years)				
	0-4	5-14	15-44	45-59	60+	0-4	5-14	15-44	45-59	60+
Congenital anomalies										
Abdominal wall defect -- Cases	0.850	0.000	0.000	0.000	0.000	0.850	0.000	0.000	0.000	0.000
Anencephaly -- Cases	0.850	0.000	0.000	0.000	0.000	0.850	0.000	0.000	0.000	0.000
Anorectal atresia -- Cases	0.850	0.000	0.000	0.000	0.000	0.850	0.000	0.000	0.000	0.000
Cleft lip -- Cases	0.098	0.000	0.000	0.000	0.000	0.016	0.000	0.000	0.000	0.000
Cleft palate -- Cases	0.231	0.000	0.000	0.000	0.000	0.015	0.000	0.000	0.000	0.000
Oesophageal atresia -- Cases	0.850	0.000	0.000	0.000	0.000	0.850	0.000	0.000	0.000	0.000
Renal agenesis -- Cases	0.850	0.000	0.000	0.000	0.000	0.850	0.000	0.000	0.000	0.000
Down syndrome -- Cases	0.593	0.593	0.593	0.593	0.593	0.593	0.593	0.593	0.593	0.593
Congenital heart anomalies -- Cases	0.323	0.323	0.323	0.323	0.323	0.323	0.323	0.323	0.323	0.323
Spina bifida -- Cases	0.593	0.593	0.593	0.593	0.593	0.593	0.593	0.593	0.593	0.593
Dental caries -- Episodes	0.081	0.081	0.081	0.081	0.081	0.081	0.081	0.081	0.081	0.081
Periodontal disease -- Episodes	0.001	0.001	0.001	0.001	0.001	0.001	0.001	0.001	0.001	0.001
Edentulism -- Cases	0.061	0.061	0.061	0.061	0.061	0.001	0.001	0.001	0.001	0.001
Drownings										
Episodes	0.000	0.000	0.000	0.000	0.000	0.000	0.000	0.000	0.000	0.000
Quadriplegia	0.005	0.005	0.005	0.005	0.005	0.005	0.005	0.005	0.005	0.005
Poisoning -- Episodes	0.611	0.611	0.607	0.607	0.607	0.611	0.611	0.607	0.607	0.607
Fractures										
Skull -- Short term	0.431	0.431	0.431	0.431	0.431	0.431	0.431	0.431	0.431	0.431
Skull -- Long term	0.411	0.411	0.411	0.410	0.395	0.350	0.350	0.350	0.350	0.404
Face bones	0.223	0.223	0.223	0.223	0.223	0.223	0.223	0.223	0.223	0.223
Vertebral column	0.266	0.266	0.266	0.266	0.266	0.266	0.266	0.266	0.266	0.266
Injured spinal cord	0.725	0.725	0.725	0.725	0.725	0.725	0.725	0.725	0.725	0.725
Fractures										
Rib or sternum	0.199	0.199	0.199	0.199	0.199	0.199	0.199	0.199	0.199	0.199
Pelvis	0.247	0.247	0.247	0.247	0.247	0.247	0.247	0.247	0.247	0.247
Clavicle, scapula, or humerus	0.153	0.153	0.137	0.137	0.137	0.153	0.153	0.137	0.137	0.137
Radius or ulna	0.180	0.180	0.180	0.180	0.180	0.180	0.180	0.180	0.180	0.180
Hand bones	0.100	0.100	0.100	0.100	0.100	0.100	0.100	0.100	0.100	0.100
Femur -- Short term	0.372	0.372	0.372	0.372	0.372	0.372	0.372	0.372	0.372	0.372
Femur -- Long term	0.272	0.272	0.272	0.272	0.272	0.272	0.272	0.272	0.272	0.272
Patella, tibia, or fibula	0.271	0.271	0.271	0.271	0.271	0.271	0.271	0.271	0.271	0.271
Ankle	0.196	0.196	0.196	0.196	0.196	0.196	0.196	0.196	0.196	0.196
Foot bones	0.077	0.077	0.077	0.077	0.077	0.077	0.077	0.077	0.077	0.077
Dislocated shoulder, elbow, or hip	0.074	0.074	0.074	0.074	0.074	0.074	0.074	0.074	0.074	0.074
Sprains	0.064	0.064	0.064	0.064	0.064	0.064	0.064	0.064	0.064	0.064
Intracranial injury										
Short term	0.359	0.359	0.359	0.359	0.359	0.359	0.359	0.359	0.359	0.359
Long term	0.359	0.359	0.359	0.359	0.359	0.359	0.359	0.359	0.359	0.359
Internal injuries	0.000	0.000	0.000	0.000	0.000	0.208	0.208	0.208	0.208	0.208
Open wound	0.108	0.108	0.108	0.108	0.108	0.108	0.108	0.108	0.108	0.108
Injury to eyes	0.354	0.354	0.354	0.354	0.354	0.301	0.300	0.299	0.299	0.299
Amputations										
Thumb	0.165	0.165	0.165	0.165	0.165	0.165	0.165	0.165	0.165	0.165
Finger	0.102	0.102	0.102	0.102	0.102	0.102	0.102	0.102	0.102	0.102
Arm	0.102	0.102	0.102	0.102	0.102	0.102	0.102	0.102	0.102	0.102
Toe	0.078	0.078	0.078	0.078	0.078	0.064	0.064	0.064	0.064	0.064
Foot	0.300	0.300	0.300	0.300	0.300	0.300	0.300	0.300	0.300	0.300
Leg	0.300	0.300	0.300	0.300	0.300	0.300	0.300	0.300	0.300	0.300
Crushing	0.218	0.218	0.218	0.218	0.218	0.218	0.218	0.218	0.218	0.218
Burns										
<20% -- Short term	0.186	0.186	0.186	0.186	0.186	0.158	0.158	0.158	0.158	0.158
<20% -- Long term	0.041	0.041	0.041	0.041	0.041	0.011	0.011	0.011	0.011	0.011
>20% and <60% -- Short term	0.469	0.469	0.469	0.469	0.469	0.441	0.441	0.441	0.441	0.441
>20% and <60% -- Long term	0.255	0.255	0.255	0.255	0.255	0.255	0.255	0.255	0.255	0.255
>60% -- Short term	0.469	0.469	0.469	0.469	0.469	0.441	0.441	0.441	0.441	0.441
>60% -- Long term	0.255	0.255	0.255	0.255	0.255	0.255	0.255	0.255	0.255	0.255
Injured nerves	0.078	0.078	0.078	0.078	0.078	0.064	0.064	0.064	0.064	0.064

Annex Table 4. **Estimated proportions of cases receiving treatment for each sequela, by region, 1990**

Sequela	Region							
	EME	FSE	IND	CHN	OAI	SSA	LAC	MEC
Chlamydia								
Corneal scar -- Blindness	0.80	0.65	0.30	0.30	0.30	0.05	0.50	0.40
Pelvic inflammatory disease	0.74	0.49	0.25	0.49	0.25	0.25	0.49	0.49
Gonorrhoea								
Corneal scar -- Blindness	0.80	0.65	0.30	0.30	0.30	0.05	0.50	0.40
Pelvic inflammatory disease	0.74	0.49	0.25	0.49	0.25	0.25	0.49	0.49
Pertussis								
Episodes	0.90	0.70	0.20	0.20	0.20	0.10	0.50	0.40
Mental retardation	0.90	0.70	0.20	0.20	0.20	0.10	0.50	0.40
Bacterial meningitis, meningococcaemia								
Seizure disorder	0.90	0.70	0.20	0.20	0.20	0.10	0.50	0.40
Motor deficit	0.90	0.70	0.20	0.20	0.20	0.10	0.50	0.40
Mental retardation	0.90	0.70	0.20	0.20	0.20	0.10	0.50	0.40
Malaria -- Neurological sequelae	0.80	0.65	0.30	0.30	0.30	0.05	0.50	0.40
Chagas disease -- Cardiomyopathy								
with congestive heart failure	0.90	0.80	0.20	0.50	0.25	0.10	0.35	0.35
Onchocerciasis -- Blindness	0.80	0.65	0.30	0.30	0.30	0.05	0.50	0.40
Japanese encephalitis								
Cognitive impairment	0.90	0.70	0.20	0.20	0.20	0.10	0.50	0.40
Neurological sequelae	0.90	0.70	0.20	0.20	0.20	0.10	0.50	0.40
Trachoma -- Blindness	0.80	0.65	0.30	0.30	0.30	0.05	0.50	0.40
Low birth weight -- All sequelae	0.80	0.60	0.15	0.20	0.15	0.05	0.35	0.30
Birth asphyxia and birth trauma --								
All sequelae	0.80	0.60	0.15	0.20	0.15	0.05	0.35	0.30
Cancers -- Preterminal	0.90	0.80	0.20	0.30	0.25	0.10	0.45	0.40
Diabetes mellitus								
Cases	0.30	0.20	0.05	0.10	0.08	0.03	0.15	0.13
Diabetic foot	0.80	0.70	0.20	0.30	0.25	0.15	0.40	0.35
Neuropathy	0.80	0.70	0.20	0.30	0.25	0.15	0.40	0.35
Retinopathy -- Blindness	0.80	0.65	0.30	0.30	0.30	0.05	0.50	0.40
Amputation	0.80	0.65	0.30	0.30	0.30	0.05	0.50	0.40
Unipolar major depression -- Episodes	0.35	0.25	0.10	0.05	0.10	0.05	0.15	0.10
Bipolar disorder -- Cases	0.35	0.25	0.10	0.05	0.10	0.05	0.15	0.10
Schizophrenia -- Cases	0.80	0.70	0.20	0.30	0.25	0.20	0.55	0.45
Epilepsy -- Cases	0.80	0.70	0.20	0.50	0.25	0.10	0.40	0.35
Parkinson disease -- Cases	0.80	0.70	0.20	0.30	0.25	0.20	0.55	0.45
Obsessive-compulsive disorders -- Cases	0.15	0.05	0.00	0.00	0.00	0.00	0.10	0.03
Panic disorder -- Cases	0.25	0.15	0.05	0.05	0.05	0.03	0.20	0.15
Cataracts -- Blindness	0.80	0.65	0.30	0.30	0.30	0.05	0.50	0.40
Rheumatic heart disease --								
Congestive heart failure	0.90	0.80	0.20	0.50	0.35	0.15	0.60	0.50
Ischaemic heart disease								
Acute myocardial infarction	0.90	0.80	0.20	0.50	0.35	0.15	0.60	0.50
Angina pectoris	0.90	0.80	0.20	0.50	0.35	0.15	0.60	0.50
Congestive heart failure	0.90	0.80	0.20	0.50	0.35	0.15	0.60	0.50
Cerebrovascular disease								
First-ever stroke	0.90	0.80	0.20	0.50	0.35	0.15	0.60	0.50

Annex Table 4, continued. **Estimated proportions of cases receiving treatment for each sequela, by region, 1990**

Sequela	Region							
	EME	FSE	IND	CHN	OAI	SSA	LAC	MEC
Inflammatory heart diseases								
Myocarditis	0.90	0.80	0.20	0.50	0.35	0.15	0.60	0.50
Pericarditis	0.90	0.80	0.20	0.50	0.35	0.15	0.60	0.50
Endocarditis	0.90	0.80	0.20	0.50	0.35	0.15	0.60	0.50
Cardiomyopathy	0.90	0.80	0.20	0.50	0.35	0.15	0.60	0.50
COPD -- Symptomatic cases	0.90	0.80	0.20	0.50	0.40	0.10	0.50	0.45
Asthma -- Cases	0.95	0.90	0.45	0.65	0.55	0.20	0.65	0.55
Peptic ulcer -- Cases	0.90	0.80	0.65	0.70	0.65	0.20	0.75	0.70
Nephritis and nephrosis --								
End-stage renal disease	0.80	0.60	0.30	0.40	0.35	0.20	0.65	0.50
Rheumatoid arthritis -- Cases	0.80	0.70	0.40	0.50	0.45	0.20	0.65	0.55
Osteoarthritis								
Hip	0.80	0.70	0.40	0.50	0.45	0.20	0.65	0.55
Knee	0.80	0.70	0.40	0.50	0.45	0.20	0.65	0.55
Cleft lip -- Cases	0.90	0.85	0.50	0.70	0.40	0.20	0.70	0.60
Cleft palate -- Cases	0.90	0.85	0.50	0.70	0.40	0.20	0.70	0.60
Edentulism -- Cases	0.90	0.90	0.20	0.40	0.30	0.15	0.50	0.40
Fractures								
Skull -- Long term	0.90	0.80	0.20	0.50	0.35	0.15	0.60	0.50
Femur -- Short term	0.95	0.95	0.70	0.90	0.85	0.60	0.80	0.80
Femur -- Long term	0.95	0.95	0.70	0.90	0.85	0.60	0.80	0.80
Internal injuries	0.90	0.80	0.40	0.70	0.75	0.35	0.75	0.65
Open wound	0.95	0.90	0.60	0.80	0.75	0.35	0.80	0.75
Injury to eyes	0.80	0.65	0.30	0.30	0.30	0.05	0.50	0.40
Burns								
<20% -- Short term	0.80	0.70	0.15	0.40	0.25	0.05	0.45	0.35
<20% -- Long term	0.80	0.70	0.15	0.40	0.25	0.05	0.45	0.35
>20% and <60% -- Short term	0.80	0.70	0.15	0.40	0.25	0.05	0.45	0.35
>20% and <60% -- Long term	0.80	0.70	0.15	0.40	0.25	0.05	0.45	0.35
>60% -- Short term	0.80	0.70	0.15	0.40	0.25	0.05	0.45	0.35
>60% -- Long term	0.80	0.70	0.15	0.40	0.25	0.05	0.45	0.35
Injured nerves	0.80	0.70	0.20	0.30	0.25	0.15	0.40	0.35

Annex Table 5a. Percentage of deaths in each broad cause Group at varying levels of mortality; based on simulations and the regression results from 67 countries, males, aged 0-4 years

Standard deviations from expectation	All-cause mortality rate for males, aged 0-4 years (deaths per 100 000)																			
	200	300	400	500	750	1000	1250	1500	1750	2000	2250	2500	2750	3000	3500	4000	4500	5000	5500	6000
Group I: Communicable, maternal, perinatal and nutritional conditions																				
+4	63.81	72.40	77.85	81.60	87.30	90.47	92.49	93.88	94.87	95.61	96.22	96.69	97.07	97.39	97.88	98.24	98.53	98.74	98.92	99.02
+3	59.67	68.16	73.67	77.54	83.57	87.05	89.33	90.94	92.13	93.04	93.78	94.37	94.86	95.28	95.94	96.44	96.85	97.16	97.43	97.62
+2	55.53	63.93	69.49	73.47	79.83	83.63	86.17	88.00	89.38	90.46	91.34	92.06	92.66	93.18	94.01	94.65	95.17	95.58	95.93	96.21
+1	51.39	59.69	65.31	69.40	76.10	80.20	83.01	85.06	86.63	87.88	88.90	89.74	90.46	91.07	92.07	92.85	93.48	94.00	94.44	94.80
Expectation	**47.26**	**55.46**	**61.13**	**65.33**	**72.36**	**76.78**	**79.85**	**82.13**	**83.89**	**85.30**	**86.46**	**87.43**	**88.25**	**88.96**	**90.13**	**91.06**	**91.80**	**92.42**	**92.95**	**93.40**
-1	43.12	51.22	56.95	61.26	68.63	73.36	76.69	79.19	81.14	82.72	84.02	85.11	86.05	86.86	88.20	89.26	90.12	90.84	91.45	91.99
-2	38.98	46.99	52.77	57.20	64.90	69.94	73.53	76.25	78.40	80.14	81.57	82.80	83.84	84.75	86.26	87.46	88.44	89.26	89.96	90.58
-3	34.84	42.75	48.59	53.13	61.16	66.51	70.37	73.31	75.65	77.56	79.13	80.48	81.64	82.65	84.32	85.67	86.76	87.69	88.47	89.18
-4	30.70	38.51	44.41	49.06	57.43	63.09	67.21	70.38	72.90	74.98	76.69	78.17	79.44	80.54	82.39	83.87	85.08	86.11	86.97	87.77
Group II: Noncommunicable diseases																				
+4	61.55	54.05	48.55	44.26	36.71	31.66	28.03	25.25	23.04	21.23	19.75	18.47	17.38	16.43	14.84	13.56	12.53	11.65	10.91	10.23
+3	57.11	49.76	44.44	40.35	33.22	28.51	25.15	22.60	20.58	18.93	17.58	16.42	15.43	14.57	13.13	11.99	11.06	10.28	9.61	9.01
+2	52.68	45.47	40.34	36.44	29.73	25.36	22.28	19.94	18.11	16.62	15.40	14.37	13.48	12.71	11.43	10.42	9.60	8.90	8.32	7.79
+1	48.24	41.19	36.24	32.53	26.24	22.22	19.40	17.29	15.65	14.32	13.23	12.31	11.53	10.85	9.73	8.85	8.13	7.53	7.02	6.57
Expectation	**43.81**	**36.90**	**32.14**	**28.62**	**22.75**	**19.07**	**16.52**	**14.64**	**13.18**	**12.02**	**11.06**	**10.26**	**9.58**	**8.99**	**8.03**	**7.27**	**6.66**	**6.15**	**5.72**	**5.35**
-1	39.38	32.61	28.04	24.70	19.26	15.93	13.65	11.99	10.72	9.71	8.89	8.21	7.63	7.13	6.33	5.70	5.19	4.77	4.42	4.13
-2	34.94	28.32	23.93	20.79	15.77	12.78	10.77	9.33	8.25	7.41	6.71	6.15	5.68	5.28	4.63	4.13	3.72	3.40	3.13	2.91
-3	30.51	24.03	19.83	16.88	12.28	9.63	7.90	6.68	5.79	5.10	4.54	4.10	3.73	3.42	2.93	2.56	2.25	2.02	1.83	1.69
-4	26.08	19.74	15.73	12.97	8.79	6.49	5.02	4.03	3.32	2.80	2.37	2.04	1.78	1.56	1.23	0.99	0.79	0.65	0.53	0.47
Group III: Injuries																				
+4	19.33	17.03	15.34	14.02	11.71	10.16	9.06	8.20	7.53	6.97	6.51	6.12	5.78	5.48	4.98	4.58	4.26	3.98	3.75	3.53
+3	16.73	14.69	13.19	12.03	10.00	8.66	7.70	6.96	6.38	5.90	5.51	5.17	4.88	4.62	4.20	3.86	3.58	3.34	3.14	2.96
+2	14.13	12.34	11.04	10.03	8.30	7.15	6.34	5.72	5.23	4.83	4.50	4.22	3.97	3.76	3.41	3.13	2.90	2.70	2.54	2.39
+1	11.53	9.99	8.89	8.04	6.59	5.65	4.98	4.48	4.08	3.76	3.49	3.26	3.07	2.90	2.62	2.40	2.22	2.07	1.94	1.82
Expectation	**8.93**	**7.65**	**6.74**	**6.05**	**4.89**	**4.15**	**3.63**	**3.24**	**2.93**	**2.69**	**2.48**	**2.31**	**2.17**	**2.04**	**1.84**	**1.67**	**1.54**	**1.43**	**1.33**	**1.25**
-1	6.33	5.30	4.59	4.06	3.18	2.64	2.27	1.99	1.78	1.62	1.48	1.36	1.27	1.18	1.05	0.94	0.86	0.79	0.73	0.68
-2	3.73	2.95	2.44	2.07	1.48	1.14	0.91	0.75	0.63	0.55	0.47	0.41	0.36	0.32	0.26	0.22	0.18	0.15	0.12	0.11
-3	1.13	0.61	0.29	0.08	–	–	–	–	–	–	–	–	–	–	–	–	–	–	–	–
-4	–	–	–	–	–	–	–	–	–	–	–	–	–	–	–	–	–	–	–	–

Note: A dash (–) is used when the value at a given number of standard deviations below the expectation would be negative.

Annex Table 5b. Percentage of deaths in each broad cause Group at varying levels of mortality; based on simulations and the regression results from 67 countries, males, aged 5-14 years

Standard deviations from expectation	All-cause mortality rate for males, aged 5-14 years (deaths per 100 000)																			
	25	30	40	50	75	100	125	150	175	200	250	300	350	400	450	500	550	600	650	700
Group I: Communicable, maternal, perinatal and nutritional conditions																				
+4	13.49	16.38	22.01	27.34	39.33	49.48	57.96	65.14	71.22	76.45	84.62	90.78	95.49	99.16	101.93	104.18	105.96	107.38	108.53	109.48
+3	11.62	14.10	18.95	23.55	33.96	42.85	50.37	56.79	62.29	67.06	74.67	80.53	85.10	88.75	91.59	93.95	95.87	97.46	98.79	99.91
+2	9.76	11.83	15.89	19.76	28.59	36.22	42.77	48.44	53.36	57.68	64.72	70.27	74.71	78.33	81.25	83.72	85.79	87.54	89.04	90.35
+1	7.89	9.56	12.83	15.97	23.21	29.59	35.18	40.10	44.44	48.30	54.77	60.01	64.32	67.91	70.92	73.49	75.70	77.62	79.30	80.78
Expectation	**6.02**	**7.28**	**9.77**	**12.18**	**17.84**	**22.97**	**27.59**	**31.75**	**35.51**	**38.91**	**44.82**	**49.76**	**53.93**	**57.50**	**60.58**	**63.26**	**65.62**	**67.70**	**69.56**	**71.22**
-1	4.16	5.01	6.71	8.39	12.47	16.34	19.99	23.40	26.58	29.53	34.87	39.50	43.54	47.08	50.24	53.03	55.53	57.78	59.81	61.65
-2	2.29	2.74	3.64	4.60	7.10	9.71	12.40	15.06	17.65	20.15	24.92	29.25	33.15	36.67	39.90	42.80	45.45	47.86	50.07	52.09
-3	0.42	0.46	0.58	0.81	1.72	3.08	4.80	6.71	8.73	10.76	14.97	18.99	22.76	26.25	29.57	32.57	35.36	37.94	40.33	42.52
-4	–	–	–	–	–	–	–	–	–	1.38	5.02	8.74	12.37	15.83	19.23	22.35	25.28	28.02	30.59	32.96
Group II: Noncommunicable diseases																				
+4	61.88	62.55	63.37	63.80	64.21	64.20	63.94	63.49	62.90	62.21	60.54	58.73	56.87	55.05	53.21	51.49	49.84	48.28	46.79	45.41
+3	57.66	58.26	58.94	59.24	59.29	58.90	58.28	57.53	56.68	55.77	53.81	51.82	49.88	48.03	46.23	44.56	42.98	41.50	40.12	38.83
+2	53.44	53.96	54.50	54.68	54.36	53.60	52.63	51.57	50.46	49.34	47.08	44.92	42.89	41.01	39.24	37.62	36.12	34.73	33.44	32.26
+1	49.22	49.66	50.07	50.11	49.44	48.30	46.98	45.61	44.24	42.90	40.35	38.01	35.90	33.99	32.25	30.68	29.26	27.96	26.77	25.68
Expectation	**45.00**	**45.37**	**45.64**	**45.55**	**44.51**	**43.00**	**41.33**	**39.65**	**38.02**	**36.47**	**33.61**	**31.11**	**28.90**	**26.97**	**25.26**	**23.75**	**22.40**	**21.18**	**20.09**	**19.11**
-1	40.78	41.07	41.21	40.98	39.59	37.70	35.68	33.69	31.80	30.03	26.88	24.20	21.91	19.95	18.27	16.81	15.53	14.41	13.42	12.53
-2	36.56	36.77	36.78	36.42	34.66	32.40	30.03	27.73	25.58	23.59	20.15	17.29	14.92	12.93	11.29	9.87	8.67	7.64	6.74	5.95
-3	32.34	32.48	32.35	31.85	29.74	27.10	24.38	21.77	19.36	17.16	13.42	10.39	7.93	5.91	4.30	2.94	1.81	0.86	0.07	–
-4	28.12	28.18	27.92	27.29	24.81	21.80	18.72	15.81	13.15	10.72	6.69	3.48	0.93	–	–	–	–	–	–	–
Group III: Injuries																				
+4	66.82	65.67	63.69	61.98	58.45	55.55	53.01	50.74	48.66	46.77	43.34	40.36	37.75	35.44	33.38	31.54	29.88	28.39	27.03	25.76
+3	62.36	61.09	58.92	57.05	53.25	50.17	47.53	45.20	43.12	41.23	37.89	35.06	32.61	30.46	28.58	26.91	25.41	24.07	22.86	21.74
+2	57.90	56.51	54.14	52.13	48.05	44.79	42.05	39.67	37.57	35.69	32.45	29.75	27.46	25.49	23.77	22.27	20.94	19.75	18.69	17.72
+1	53.44	51.93	49.37	47.20	42.85	39.42	36.37	34.13	32.02	30.16	27.01	24.44	22.31	20.51	18.97	17.63	16.46	15.43	14.52	13.70
Expectation	**48.98**	**47.35**	**44.59**	**42.28**	**37.65**	**34.04**	**31.09**	**28.60**	**26.47**	**24.62**	**21.56**	**19.14**	**17.16**	**15.53**	**14.16**	**12.99**	**11.99**	**11.11**	**10.35**	**9.68**
-1	44.51	42.77	39.82	37.35	32.45	28.66	25.60	23.07	20.92	19.09	16.12	13.83	12.02	10.55	9.35	8.35	7.51	6.80	6.18	5.65
-2	40.05	38.19	35.04	32.43	27.25	23.28	20.12	17.53	15.37	13.55	10.68	8.52	6.87	5.58	4.55	3.72	3.04	2.48	2.01	1.63
-3	35.59	33.61	30.27	27.50	22.05	17.91	14.64	12.00	9.83	8.01	5.23	3.22	1.72	0.60	–	–	–	–	–	–
-4	31.13	29.03	25.49	22.58	16.85	12.53	9.16	6.46	4.28	2.48	–	–	–	–	–	–	–	–	–	–

Note: A dash (-) is used when the value at a given number of standard deviations below the expectation would be negative.

Annex Table 5c. Percentage of deaths in each broad cause Group at varying levels of mortality; based on simulations and the regression results from 67 countries, males, aged 15-29 years

Standard deviations from expectation	All-cause mortality rate for males, aged 15-29 years (deaths per 100 000)																			
	100	125	150	175	200	225	250	275	300	325	350	375	400	450	500	550	600	650	700	750
Group I: Communicable, maternal, perinatal and nutritional conditions																				
+4	16.03	18.05	19.90	21.58	23.13	24.56	25.91	27.17	28.37	29.50	30.57	31.60	32.59	34.44	36.15	37.75	39.25	40.65	41.97	43.26
+3	12.95	14.56	16.04	17.38	18.62	19.76	20.84	21.85	22.80	23.70	24.56	25.39	26.18	27.66	29.02	30.30	31.50	32.62	33.69	34.71
+2	9.86	11.07	12.18	13.18	14.11	14.96	15.76	16.52	17.24	17.91	18.55	19.17	19.76	20.87	21.90	22.86	23.75	24.60	25.40	26.17
+1	6.77	7.58	8.31	8.98	9.59	10.16	10.69	11.19	11.67	12.12	12.54	12.95	13.34	14.08	14.77	15.41	16.01	16.58	17.11	17.63
Expectation	**3.69**	**4.09**	**4.45**	**4.78**	**5.08**	**5.36**	**5.62**	**5.87**	**6.10**	**6.32**	**6.53**	**6.74**	**6.93**	**7.30**	**7.64**	**7.96**	**8.26**	**8.55**	**8.83**	**9.09**
-1	0.60	0.60	0.59	0.58	0.57	0.56	0.55	0.54	0.53	0.53	0.52	0.52	0.51	0.51	0.51	0.51	0.52	0.53	0.54	0.55
-2	-	-	-	-	-	-	-	-	-	-	-	-	-	-	-	-	-	-	-	-
-3	-	-	-	-	-	-	-	-	-	-	-	-	-	-	-	-	-	-	-	-
-4	-	-	-	-	-	-	-	-	-	-	-	-	-	-	-	-	-	-	-	-
Group II: Noncommunicable diseases																				
+4	60.94	59.72	58.71	57.85	57.10	56.43	55.82	55.27	54.77	54.31	53.87	53.47	53.09	52.40	51.77	51.21	50.69	50.21	49.76	49.35
+3	53.75	52.52	51.51	50.65	49.91	49.25	48.65	48.11	47.62	47.17	46.75	46.35	45.99	45.32	44.71	44.17	43.67	43.21	42.79	42.39
+2	46.57	45.33	44.32	43.46	42.72	42.06	41.48	40.95	40.47	40.03	39.62	39.24	38.88	38.23	37.66	37.13	36.66	36.22	35.82	35.44
+1	39.39	38.14	37.12	36.27	35.53	34.88	34.31	33.79	33.32	32.89	32.49	32.12	31.78	31.15	30.60	30.10	29.64	29.23	28.84	28.49
Expectation	**32.21**	**30.94**	**29.92**	**29.07**	**28.34**	**27.70**	**27.14**	**26.63**	**26.17**	**25.75**	**25.36**	**25.01**	**24.67**	**24.07**	**23.54**	**23.06**	**22.63**	**22.23**	**21.87**	**21.54**
-1	25.02	23.75	22.73	21.88	21.15	20.52	19.97	19.47	19.02	18.61	18.24	17.89	17.57	16.99	16.48	16.02	15.61	15.24	14.90	14.58
-2	17.84	16.56	15.53	14.68	13.96	13.34	12.80	12.31	11.87	11.47	11.11	10.77	10.46	9.91	9.42	8.99	8.60	8.25	7.92	7.63
-3	10.66	9.36	8.33	7.49	6.78	6.16	5.62	5.15	4.72	4.33	3.98	3.66	3.36	2.83	2.36	1.95	1.58	1.25	0.95	0.68
-4	3.47	2.17	1.14	0.30	-	-	-	-	-	-	-	-	-	-	-	-	-	-	-	-
Group III: Injuries																				
+4	92.91	94.22	95.32	96.26	97.11	97.87	98.57	99.23	99.84	100.41	100.95	101.47	101.97	102.90	103.76	104.57	105.33	106.04	106.71	107.36
+3	85.71	86.91	87.89	88.74	89.48	90.14	90.74	91.29	91.81	92.29	92.74	93.17	93.58	94.33	95.03	95.67	96.27	96.83	97.36	97.87
+2	78.51	79.59	80.47	81.21	81.84	82.40	82.91	83.36	83.78	84.17	84.53	84.87	85.18	85.77	86.29	86.78	87.22	87.63	88.01	88.37
+1	71.31	72.28	73.05	73.68	74.21	74.67	75.07	75.43	75.76	76.05	76.32	76.56	76.79	77.20	77.56	77.88	78.16	78.42	78.66	78.87
Expectation	**64.11**	**64.97**	**65.62**	**66.15**	**66.58**	**66.94**	**67.24**	**67.50**	**67.73**	**67.93**	**68.10**	**68.26**	**68.40**	**68.63**	**68.82**	**68.98**	**69.11**	**69.22**	**69.30**	**69.38**
-1	56.91	57.65	58.20	58.62	58.94	59.20	59.41	59.57	59.70	59.81	59.89	59.96	60.00	60.07	60.09	60.08	60.05	60.01	59.95	59.88
-2	49.71	50.34	50.78	51.09	51.31	51.47	51.57	51.64	51.68	51.69	51.68	51.65	51.61	51.50	51.35	51.19	51.00	50.80	50.60	50.38
-3	42.51	43.03	43.36	43.56	43.68	43.73	43.74	43.71	43.65	43.57	43.47	43.35	43.22	42.93	42.62	42.29	41.95	41.60	41.25	40.89
-4	35.31	35.71	35.93	36.03	36.05	36.00	35.91	35.78	35.62	35.45	35.25	35.04	34.83	34.37	33.88	33.39	32.89	32.39	31.89	31.39

Note: A dash (-) is used when the value at a given number of standard deviations below the expectation would be negative.

Annex Table 5d. Percentage of deaths in each broad cause Group at varying levels of mortality; based on simulations and the regression results from 67 countries, males, aged 30-44 years

Standard deviations from expectation	All-cause mortality rate for males, aged 30-44 years (deaths per 100 000)																			
	200	225	250	300	350	400	450	500	550	600	650	700	750	800	850	900	950	1000	1050	1100
Group I: Communicable, maternal, perinatal and nutritional conditions																				
+4	13.72	14.94	16.12	18.34	20.42	22.37	24.22	25.97	27.63	29.23	30.75	32.21	33.62	34.96	36.26	37.53	38.74	39.92	41.05	42.18
+3	11.29	12.29	13.26	15.08	16.78	18.39	19.90	21.34	22.71	24.03	25.28	26.49	27.65	28.76	29.84	30.89	31.89	32.87	33.81	34.75
+2	8.86	9.64	10.39	11.82	13.15	14.40	15.59	16.72	17.79	18.83	19.81	20.76	21.68	22.56	23.42	24.25	25.04	25.82	26.57	27.31
+1	6.43	6.99	7.53	8.55	9.51	10.42	11.27	12.09	12.87	13.63	14.35	15.04	15.72	16.36	16.99	17.60	18.19	18.77	19.33	19.88
Expectation	**4.00**	**4.34**	**4.67**	**5.29**	**5.87**	**6.43**	**6.96**	**7.47**	**7.96**	**8.43**	**8.88**	**9.32**	**9.75**	**10.16**	**10.57**	**10.96**	**11.35**	**11.72**	**12.09**	**12.45**
-1	1.57	1.69	1.80	2.03	2.24	2.44	2.65	2.84	3.04	3.23	3.41	3.60	3.78	3.96	4.14	4.32	4.50	4.67	4.85	5.01
-2	-	-	-	-	-	-	-	-	-	-	-	-	-	-	-	-	-	-	-	-
-3	-	-	-	-	-	-	-	-	-	-	-	-	-	-	-	-	-	-	-	-
-4	-	-	-	-	-	-	-	-	-	-	-	-	-	-	-	-	-	-	-	-
Group II: Noncommunicable diseases																				
+4	84.52	84.28	84.06	83.67	83.31	82.99	82.70	82.43	82.18	81.95	81.73	81.52	81.33	81.15	80.97	80.81	80.64	80.49	80.34	80.20
+3	78.61	78.30	78.01	77.49	77.03	76.61	76.23	75.87	75.55	75.24	74.96	74.69	74.43	74.19	73.96	73.74	73.52	73.32	73.12	72.94
+2	72.71	72.32	71.96	71.31	70.74	70.23	69.76	69.32	68.92	68.54	68.19	67.85	67.54	67.23	66.95	66.67	66.40	66.15	65.90	65.67
+1	66.80	66.34	65.91	65.14	64.46	63.85	63.29	62.77	62.29	61.84	61.42	61.02	60.64	60.28	59.93	59.60	59.28	58.98	58.68	58.40
Expectation	**60.89**	**60.35**	**59.86**	**58.96**	**58.17**	**57.46**	**56.82**	**56.22**	**55.66**	**55.14**	**54.65**	**54.18**	**53.74**	**53.32**	**52.92**	**52.53**	**52.16**	**51.81**	**51.46**	**51.13**
-1	54.99	54.37	53.80	52.79	51.89	51.08	50.35	49.67	49.03	48.44	47.88	47.35	46.85	46.37	45.91	45.47	45.04	44.63	44.24	43.86
-2	49.08	48.39	47.75	46.61	45.61	44.70	43.88	43.11	42.40	41.74	41.11	40.52	39.95	39.41	38.89	38.40	37.92	37.46	37.02	36.59
-3	43.18	42.41	41.70	40.44	39.32	38.32	37.41	36.56	35.77	35.04	34.34	33.68	33.05	32.45	31.88	31.33	30.80	30.29	29.80	29.32
-4	37.27	36.42	35.65	34.26	33.04	31.94	30.94	30.01	29.15	28.34	27.57	26.85	26.16	25.50	24.87	24.26	23.68	23.12	22.58	22.05
Group III: Injuries																				
+4	59.31	59.82	60.27	61.03	61.65	62.18	62.64	63.05	63.41	63.73	64.02	64.29	64.54	64.77	64.98	65.18	65.37	65.55	65.71	65.87
+3	53.26	53.69	54.07	54.71	55.23	55.66	56.04	56.36	56.65	56.91	57.13	57.34	57.53	57.71	57.86	58.01	58.15	58.28	58.40	58.51
+2	47.21	47.56	47.87	48.39	48.80	49.14	49.43	49.68	49.89	50.08	50.25	50.39	50.53	50.64	50.75	50.84	50.93	51.01	51.08	51.15
+1	41.16	41.43	41.67	42.07	42.38	42.63	42.83	43.00	43.14	43.26	43.36	43.44	43.52	43.58	43.63	43.67	43.71	43.74	43.77	43.79
Expectation	**35.11**	**35.31**	**35.48**	**35.75**	**35.95**	**36.11**	**36.22**	**36.31**	**36.38**	**36.43**	**36.47**	**36.49**	**36.51**	**36.51**	**36.51**	**36.50**	**36.49**	**36.47**	**36.45**	**36.42**
-1	29.05	29.18	29.28	29.43	29.53	29.59	29.62	29.63	29.62	29.61	29.58	29.55	29.50	29.45	29.40	29.33	29.27	29.20	29.14	29.06
-2	23.00	23.05	23.08	23.11	23.10	23.07	23.02	22.95	22.87	22.79	22.69	22.60	22.49	22.39	22.28	22.16	22.05	21.94	21.82	21.70
-3	16.95	16.92	16.88	16.79	16.67	16.55	16.41	16.27	16.12	15.96	15.81	15.65	15.48	15.32	15.16	15.00	14.83	14.67	14.50	14.34
-4	10.90	10.79	10.69	10.47	10.25	10.03	9.81	9.58	9.36	9.14	8.92	8.70	8.48	8.26	8.04	7.83	7.61	7.40	7.19	6.98

Note: A dash (-) is used when the value at a given number of standard deviations below the expectation would be negative.

Annex Table 5e. Percentage of deaths in each broad cause Group at varying levels of mortality; based on simulations and the regression results from 67 countries, males, aged 45-59 years

Standard deviations from expectation	All-cause mortality rate for males, aged 45-59 years (deaths per 100 000)																			
	600	675	750	825	900	975	1050	1125	1200	1275	1350	1425	1500	1575	1650	1725	1800	1875	1950	2100
Group I: Communicable, maternal, perinatal and nutritional conditions																				
+4	21.52	23.19	24.79	26.32	27.77	29.15	30.48	31.76	32.98	34.17	35.31	36.41	37.47	38.50	39.51	40.49	41.43	42.35	43.25	44.98
+3	16.87	18.18	19.44	20.63	21.77	22.86	23.91	24.91	25.87	26.81	27.71	28.57	29.41	30.23	31.02	31.79	32.54	33.27	33.98	35.35
+2	12.22	13.17	14.08	14.95	15.78	16.57	17.33	18.06	18.77	19.45	20.10	20.74	21.35	21.95	22.53	23.10	23.65	24.19	24.71	25.72
+1	7.57	8.16	8.73	9.27	9.78	10.28	10.76	11.21	11.66	12.09	12.50	12.91	13.30	13.68	14.05	14.41	14.76	15.10	15.44	16.09
Expectation	**2.92**	**3.15**	**3.37**	**3.58**	**3.79**	**3.99**	**4.18**	**4.37**	**4.55**	**4.73**	**4.90**	**5.07**	**5.24**	**5.40**	**5.56**	**5.72**	**5.87**	**6.02**	**6.17**	**6.46**
-1	-	-	-	-	-	-	-	-	-	-	-	-	-	-	-	-	-	-	-	-
-2	-	-	-	-	-	-	-	-	-	-	-	-	-	-	-	-	-	-	-	-
-3	-	-	-	-	-	-	-	-	-	-	-	-	-	-	-	-	-	-	-	-
-4	-	-	-	-	-	-	-	-	-	-	-	-	-	-	-	-	-	-	-	-
Group II: Noncommunicable diseases																				
+4	115.89	116.45	117.01	117.55	118.08	118.60	119.10	119.59	120.06	120.53	120.98	121.42	121.85	122.27	122.68	123.08	123.46	123.84	124.21	124.93
+3	108.35	108.74	109.12	109.49	109.85	110.20	110.55	110.88	111.20	111.52	111.83	112.13	112.42	112.70	112.98	113.25	113.51	113.76	114.01	114.49
+2	100.81	101.02	101.23	101.43	101.62	101.81	101.99	102.17	102.34	102.51	102.67	102.83	102.98	103.13	103.28	103.42	103.55	103.68	103.81	104.06
+1	93.27	93.30	93.33	93.36	93.39	93.42	93.44	93.46	93.48	93.50	93.52	93.54	93.55	93.56	93.58	93.59	93.60	93.60	93.61	93.62
Expectation	**85.73**	**85.59**	**85.44**	**85.30**	**85.16**	**85.03**	**84.89**	**84.76**	**84.63**	**84.50**	**84.37**	**84.24**	**84.12**	**84.00**	**83.88**	**83.76**	**83.64**	**83.52**	**83.41**	**83.18**
-1	78.19	77.87	77.55	77.24	76.93	76.63	76.34	76.05	75.77	75.49	75.22	74.95	74.69	74.43	74.18	73.93	73.68	73.44	73.21	72.75
-2	70.66	70.15	69.66	69.18	68.70	68.24	67.79	67.34	66.91	66.48	66.06	65.65	65.25	64.86	64.48	64.10	63.73	63.36	63.01	62.31
-3	63.12	62.44	61.77	61.11	60.47	59.85	59.23	58.63	58.05	57.47	56.91	56.36	55.82	55.29	54.78	54.27	53.77	53.28	52.81	51.87
-4	55.58	54.72	53.88	53.05	52.25	51.45	50.68	49.93	49.19	48.46	47.76	47.06	46.39	45.73	45.08	44.44	43.82	43.20	42.60	41.44
Group III: Injuries																				
+4	37.02	37.03	37.03	37.03	37.03	37.02	37.02	37.01	37.00	36.99	36.98	36.97	36.96	36.95	36.94	36.92	36.91	36.90	36.88	36.86
+3	30.60	30.59	30.57	30.55	30.53	30.51	30.49	30.48	30.46	30.44	30.42	30.40	30.38	30.36	30.34	30.32	30.30	30.29	30.27	30.23
+2	24.19	24.15	24.11	24.07	24.04	24.01	23.97	23.94	23.91	23.88	23.86	23.83	23.80	23.78	23.75	23.72	23.70	23.67	23.65	23.60
+1	17.77	17.70	17.65	17.59	17.54	17.50	17.45	17.41	17.37	17.33	17.29	17.26	17.22	17.19	17.16	17.12	17.09	17.06	17.03	16.98
Expectation	**11.35**	**11.26**	**11.19**	**11.12**	**11.05**	**10.99**	**10.93**	**10.88**	**10.83**	**10.78**	**10.73**	**10.69**	**10.64**	**10.60**	**10.56**	**10.53**	**10.49**	**10.45**	**10.42**	**10.35**
-1	4.93	4.82	4.73	4.64	4.56	4.48	4.41	4.34	4.28	4.22	4.17	4.12	4.06	4.02	3.97	3.93	3.88	3.84	3.80	3.73
-2	-	-	-	-	-	-	-	-	-	-	-	-	-	-	-	-	-	-	-	-
-3	-	-	-	-	-	-	-	-	-	-	-	-	-	-	-	-	-	-	-	-
-4	-	-	-	-	-	-	-	-	-	-	-	-	-	-	-	-	-	-	-	-

Note: A dash (-) is used when the value at a given number of standard deviations below the expectation would be negative.

Annex Table 5f. Percentage of deaths in each broad cause Group at varying levels of mortality; based on simulations and the regression results from 67 countries, males, aged 60-69 years

Standard deviations from expectation	All-cause mortality rate for males, aged 60-69 years (deaths per 100 000)																			
	2000	2100	2200	2300	2400	2600	2800	3000	3200	3400	3600	3800	4000	4200	4400	4600	4800	5000	5300	5600
Group I: Communicable, maternal, perinatal and nutritional conditions																				
+4	28.59	28.96	29.31	29.64	29.96	30.57	31.14	31.68	32.19	32.67	33.12	33.56	33.98	34.37	34.75	35.12	35.47	35.81	36.30	36.76
+3	22.32	22.60	22.87	23.13	23.38	23.85	24.29	24.71	25.10	25.47	25.83	26.16	26.48	26.79	27.08	27.37	27.64	27.91	28.28	28.64
+2	16.04	16.24	16.43	16.61	16.79	17.12	17.44	17.73	18.01	18.28	18.53	18.76	18.99	19.21	19.42	19.62	19.81	20.00	20.27	20.52
+1	9.76	9.88	9.99	10.10	10.20	10.40	10.59	10.76	10.92	11.08	11.23	11.37	11.50	11.63	11.75	11.87	11.98	12.09	12.25	12.40
Expectation	**3.48**	**3.52**	**3.55**	**3.59**	**3.62**	**3.68**	**3.73**	**3.79**	**3.83**	**3.88**	**3.93**	**3.97**	**4.01**	**4.05**	**4.08**	**4.12**	**4.16**	**4.19**	**4.24**	**4.28**
-1	-	-	-	-	-	-	-	-	-	-	-	-	-	-	-	-	-	-	-	-
-2	-	-	-	-	-	-	-	-	-	-	-	-	-	-	-	-	-	-	-	-
-3	-	-	-	-	-	-	-	-	-	-	-	-	-	-	-	-	-	-	-	-
-4	-	-	-	-	-	-	-	-	-	-	-	-	-	-	-	-	-	-	-	-
Group II: Noncommunicable diseases																				
+4	122.37	122.55	122.74	122.91	123.09	123.44	123.78	124.10	124.42	124.73	125.02	125.31	125.59	125.86	126.13	126.38	126.63	126.87	127.23	127.56
+3	114.64	114.80	114.95	115.11	115.26	115.55	115.83	116.10	116.35	116.60	116.84	117.08	117.30	117.52	117.72	117.93	118.12	118.31	118.59	118.85
+2	106.90	107.04	107.17	107.30	107.42	107.66	107.88	108.09	108.29	108.48	108.67	108.84	109.01	109.17	109.32	109.47	109.61	109.75	109.95	110.14
+1	99.17	99.28	99.39	99.49	99.58	99.77	99.93	100.09	100.23	100.36	100.49	100.60	100.71	100.82	100.92	101.01	101.11	101.19	101.31	101.43
Expectation	**91.43**	**91.52**	**91.60**	**91.68**	**91.75**	**91.87**	**91.98**	**92.08**	**92.16**	**92.24**	**92.31**	**92.37**	**92.42**	**92.47**	**92.52**	**92.56**	**92.60**	**92.63**	**92.68**	**92.72**
-1	83.70	83.76	83.82	83.87	83.91	83.98	84.04	84.07	84.10	84.12	84.13	84.13	84.13	84.12	84.12	84.10	84.09	84.07	84.04	84.01
-2	75.97	76.01	76.04	76.06	76.08	76.09	76.09	76.07	76.04	76.00	75.95	75.90	75.84	75.78	75.71	75.65	75.58	75.51	75.40	75.30
-3	68.23	68.25	68.25	68.25	68.24	68.20	68.14	68.06	67.97	67.88	67.77	67.66	67.55	67.43	67.31	67.19	67.07	66.95	66.77	66.58
-4	60.50	60.49	60.47	60.44	60.41	60.31	60.19	60.06	59.91	59.75	59.59	59.42	59.25	59.08	58.91	58.74	58.56	58.39	58.13	57.87
Group III: Injuries																				
+4	24.35	23.92	23.52	23.15	22.79	22.14	21.54	21.00	20.51	20.05	19.63	19.24	18.87	18.53	18.22	17.91	17.63	17.36	16.98	16.63
+3	19.53	19.18	18.85	18.54	18.25	17.71	17.23	16.79	16.38	16.01	15.67	15.35	15.05	14.77	14.51	14.27	14.03	13.81	13.51	13.22
+2	14.72	14.44	14.18	13.94	13.71	13.29	12.91	12.57	12.25	11.97	11.70	11.45	11.22	11.01	10.81	10.62	10.44	10.27	10.03	9.81
+1	9.90	9.70	9.51	9.34	9.17	8.87	8.60	8.35	8.13	7.92	7.73	7.56	7.40	7.24	7.10	6.97	6.84	6.73	6.56	6.41
Expectation	**5.08**	**4.96**	**4.84**	**4.73**	**4.63**	**4.45**	**4.28**	**4.14**	**4.00**	**3.88**	**3.77**	**3.66**	**3.57**	**3.48**	**3.40**	**3.32**	**3.25**	**3.18**	**3.09**	**3.00**
-1	0.26	0.22	0.17	0.13	0.09	0.03	-	-	-	-	-	-	-	-	-	-	-	-	-	-
-2	-	-	-	-	-	-	-	-	-	-	-	-	-	-	-	-	-	-	-	-
-3	-	-	-	-	-	-	-	-	-	-	-	-	-	-	-	-	-	-	-	-
-4	-	-	-	-	-	-	-	-	-	-	-	-	-	-	-	-	-	-	-	-

Note: A dash (-) is used when the value at a given number of standard deviations below the expectation would be negative.

Annex Table 5g. Percentage of deaths in each broad cause Group at varying levels of mortality; based on simulations and the regression results from 67 countries, males, aged 70 years and over

Standard deviations from expectation	All-cause mortality rate for males, aged 70 years and over (deaths per 100 000)																			
	7000	7300	7600	7900	8200	8500	8800	9100	9400	9700	10000	10300	10600	10900	11200	11500	11800	12100	12400	12700
Group I: Communicable, maternal, perinatal and nutritional conditions																				
+4	54.52	54.03	53.57	53.12	52.70	52.29	51.90	51.52	51.16	50.81	50.48	50.16	49.85	49.55	49.26	48.98	48.70	48.44	48.18	47.93
+3	41.80	41.41	41.04	40.69	40.35	40.03	39.72	39.42	39.14	38.87	38.60	38.35	38.10	37.87	37.64	37.42	37.20	37.00	36.79	36.60
+2	29.08	28.79	28.52	28.26	28.01	27.77	27.54	27.33	27.12	26.92	26.73	26.54	26.36	26.19	26.02	25.86	25.70	25.55	25.41	25.26
+1	16.35	16.17	15.99	15.82	15.67	15.51	15.37	15.23	15.10	14.97	14.85	14.73	14.62	14.51	14.40	14.30	14.20	14.11	14.02	13.93
Expectation	**3.63**	**3.55**	**3.47**	**3.39**	**3.32**	**3.26**	**3.19**	**3.13**	**3.08**	**3.02**	**2.97**	**2.92**	**2.87**	**2.83**	**2.79**	**2.74**	**2.70**	**2.67**	**2.63**	**2.59**
-1	-	-	-	-	-	-	-	-	-	-	-	-	-	-	-	-	-	-	-	-
-2	-	-	-	-	-	-	-	-	-	-	-	-	-	-	-	-	-	-	-	-
-3	-	-	-	-	-	-	-	-	-	-	-	-	-	-	-	-	-	-	-	-
-4	-	-	-	-	-	-	-	-	-	-	-	-	-	-	-	-	-	-	-	-
Group II: Noncommunicable diseases																				
+4	148.27	148.03	147.79	147.55	147.33	147.11	146.90	146.69	146.49	146.30	146.11	145.92	145.75	145.57	145.40	145.24	145.08	144.92	144.77	144.62
+3	134.63	134.48	134.33	134.18	134.04	133.90	133.76	133.63	133.50	133.38	133.26	133.14	133.02	132.91	132.80	132.69	132.58	132.48	132.38	132.28
+2	120.99	120.93	120.87	120.81	120.75	120.69	120.63	120.57	120.52	120.46	120.40	120.35	120.30	120.24	120.19	120.14	120.09	120.04	119.99	119.95
+1	107.35	107.39	107.41	107.44	107.46	107.48	107.50	107.51	107.53	107.54	107.55	107.56	107.57	107.58	107.59	107.59	107.60	107.60	107.61	107.61
Expectation	**93.71**	**93.84**	**93.96**	**94.07**	**94.17**	**94.27**	**94.37**	**94.45**	**94.54**	**94.62**	**94.70**	**94.77**	**94.85**	**94.91**	**94.98**	**95.04**	**95.10**	**95.16**	**95.22**	**95.27**
-1	80.07	80.29	80.50	80.70	80.88	81.06	81.23	81.40	81.55	81.70	81.85	81.99	82.12	82.25	82.37	82.49	82.61	82.72	82.83	82.94
-2	66.43	66.75	67.04	67.32	67.59	67.85	68.10	68.34	68.57	68.78	69.00	69.20	69.39	69.58	69.77	69.95	70.12	70.28	70.44	70.60
-3	52.79	53.20	53.58	53.95	54.31	54.64	54.97	55.28	55.58	55.87	56.14	56.41	56.67	56.92	57.16	57.40	57.62	57.84	58.06	58.27
-4	39.15	39.65	40.13	40.58	41.02	41.43	41.84	42.22	42.59	42.95	43.29	43.62	43.94	44.25	44.56	44.85	45.13	45.40	45.67	45.93
Group III: Injuries																				
+4	25.03	24.85	24.67	24.50	24.33	24.18	24.03	23.88	23.75	23.61	23.48	23.36	23.24	23.12	23.01	22.90	22.80	22.70	22.60	22.50
+3	19.44	19.29	19.15	19.01	18.88	18.75	18.63	18.52	18.41	18.30	18.20	18.10	18.00	17.91	17.82	17.73	17.65	17.57	17.49	17.41
+2	13.84	13.73	13.62	13.52	13.42	13.33	13.24	13.15	13.07	12.98	12.91	12.83	12.76	12.69	12.62	12.56	12.50	12.43	12.37	12.32
+1	8.25	8.17	8.10	8.03	7.96	7.90	7.84	7.78	7.72	7.67	7.62	7.57	7.52	7.47	7.43	7.39	7.34	7.30	7.26	7.23
Expectation	**2.66**	**2.61**	**2.58**	**2.54**	**2.51**	**2.47**	**2.44**	**2.41**	**2.38**	**2.36**	**2.33**	**2.31**	**2.28**	**2.26**	**2.23**	**2.21**	**2.19**	**2.17**	**2.15**	**2.13**
-1	-	-	-	-	-	-	-	-	-	-	-	-	-	-	-	-	-	-	-	-
-2	-	-	-	-	-	-	-	-	-	-	-	-	-	-	-	-	-	-	-	-
-3	-	-	-	-	-	-	-	-	-	-	-	-	-	-	-	-	-	-	-	-
-4	-	-	-	-	-	-	-	-	-	-	-	-	-	-	-	-	-	-	-	-

Note: A dash (-) is used when the value at a given number of standard deviations below the expectation would be negative.

Annex Table 5h. Percentage of deaths in each broad cause Group at varying levels of mortality; based on simulations and the regression results from 67 countries, females, aged 0-4 years

Standard deviations from expectation	All-cause mortality rate for females, aged 0-4 years (deaths per 100 000)																			
	150	250	500	750	1000	1250	1500	1750	2000	2250	2500	2750	3000	3250	3500	3750	4000	4250	4500	4750
Group I: Communicable, maternal, perinatal and nutritional conditions																				
+4	57.85	69.47	82.45	87.98	91.00	92.90	94.19	95.11	95.78	96.35	96.77	97.13	97.41	97.66	97.85	98.05	98.20	98.32	98.46	98.56
+3	54.09	65.51	78.74	84.66	88.01	90.18	91.69	92.80	93.64	94.33	94.87	95.33	95.71	96.04	96.30	96.56	96.77	96.95	97.13	97.28
+2	50.32	61.55	75.04	81.34	85.03	87.47	89.20	90.50	91.50	92.32	92.98	93.54	94.01	94.41	94.76	95.07	95.34	95.58	95.81	96.00
+1	46.56	57.59	71.34	78.03	82.04	84.75	86.71	88.19	89.35	90.31	91.08	91.74	92.30	92.79	93.21	93.59	93.92	94.21	94.48	94.73
Expectation	**42.80**	**53.63**	**67.64**	**74.71**	**79.06**	**82.04**	**84.22**	**85.89**	**87.21**	**88.29**	**89.19**	**89.95**	**90.60**	**91.17**	**91.66**	**92.10**	**92.49**	**92.84**	**93.16**	**93.45**
-1	39.03	49.68	63.93	71.39	76.07	79.32	81.72	83.58	85.07	86.28	87.29	88.15	88.90	89.54	90.12	90.62	91.07	91.47	91.84	92.17
-2	35.27	45.72	60.23	68.07	73.09	76.61	79.23	81.28	82.93	84.26	85.40	86.36	87.20	87.92	88.57	89.13	89.64	90.10	90.51	90.90
-3	31.50	41.76	56.53	64.75	70.10	73.89	76.74	78.97	80.79	82.25	83.50	84.57	85.49	86.30	87.02	87.64	88.22	88.73	89.19	89.62
-4	27.74	37.80	52.82	61.43	67.12	71.17	74.25	76.67	78.65	80.24	81.61	82.77	83.79	84.67	85.47	86.16	86.79	87.36	87.87	88.34
Group II: Noncommunicable diseases																				
+4	65.05	55.53	41.77	34.04	28.97	25.37	22.65	20.51	18.77	17.37	16.16	15.13	14.23	13.46	12.75	12.16	11.60	11.09	10.65	10.23
+3	60.92	51.47	38.17	30.88	26.15	22.82	20.32	18.36	16.77	15.50	14.40	13.47	12.66	11.96	11.32	10.78	10.28	9.83	9.43	9.05
+2	56.78	47.41	34.58	27.71	23.33	20.27	17.99	16.21	14.78	13.62	12.64	11.80	11.08	10.45	9.89	9.41	8.96	8.56	8.21	7.88
+1	52.65	43.35	30.98	24.55	20.51	17.72	15.66	14.06	12.79	11.75	10.88	10.14	9.50	8.95	8.46	8.03	7.64	7.30	6.98	6.70
Expectation	**48.52**	**39.28**	**27.39**	**21.39**	**17.70**	**15.17**	**13.33**	**11.91**	**10.79**	**9.88**	**9.12**	**8.48**	**7.93**	**7.45**	**7.03**	**6.66**	**6.33**	**6.03**	**5.76**	**5.52**
-1	44.38	35.22	23.79	18.22	14.88	12.62	10.99	9.76	8.80	8.01	7.36	6.81	6.35	5.94	5.60	5.28	5.01	4.76	4.54	4.34
-2	40.25	31.16	20.20	15.06	12.06	10.07	8.66	7.61	6.80	6.13	5.60	5.15	4.77	4.44	4.17	3.91	3.69	3.50	3.32	3.16
-3	36.12	27.10	16.60	11.90	9.24	7.52	6.33	5.46	4.81	4.26	3.84	3.48	3.19	2.94	2.73	2.53	2.37	2.23	2.09	1.98
-4	31.98	23.04	13.01	8.73	6.42	4.97	4.00	3.31	2.81	2.39	2.08	1.82	1.62	1.43	1.30	1.16	1.06	0.97	0.87	0.80
Group III: Injuries																				
+4	18.57	15.63	11.52	9.31	7.89	6.91	6.16	5.58	5.10	4.73	4.40	4.13	3.88	3.68	3.49	3.33	3.18	3.04	2.92	2.81
+3	16.10	13.49	9.88	7.96	6.73	5.88	5.24	4.73	4.33	4.00	3.72	3.49	3.28	3.11	2.94	2.81	2.68	2.56	2.46	2.37
+2	13.63	11.35	8.25	6.61	5.57	4.85	4.31	3.89	3.55	3.28	3.05	2.85	2.68	2.53	2.40	2.28	2.18	2.08	2.00	1.92
+1	11.16	9.22	6.61	5.26	4.41	3.82	3.38	3.04	2.77	2.56	2.37	2.21	2.08	1.96	1.85	1.76	1.68	1.60	1.54	1.48
Expectation	**8.69**	**7.08**	**4.98**	**3.91**	**3.25**	**2.79**	**2.46**	**2.20**	**2.00**	**1.83**	**1.69**	**1.57**	**1.47**	**1.39**	**1.31**	**1.24**	**1.18**	**1.13**	**1.08**	**1.03**
-1	6.22	4.94	3.34	2.56	2.08	1.76	1.53	1.36	1.22	1.11	1.01	0.94	0.87	0.81	0.77	0.72	0.68	0.65	0.62	0.59
-2	3.75	2.81	1.71	1.20	0.92	0.73	0.60	0.51	0.44	0.38	0.34	0.30	0.27	0.24	0.22	0.20	0.18	0.17	0.15	0.14
-3	1.28	0.67	0.07	-	-	-	-	-	-	-	-	-	-	-	-	-	-	-	-	-
-4	-	-	-	-	-	-	-	-	-	-	-	-	-	-	-	-	-	-	-	-

Note: A dash (-) is used when the value at a given number of standard deviations below the expectation would be negative.

Annex Table 5i. Percentage of deaths in each broad cause Group at varying levels of mortality; based on simulations and the regression results from 67 countries, females, aged 5-14 years

Standard deviations from expectation	All-cause mortality rate for females, aged 5-14 years (deaths per 100 000)																			
	15	20	30	40	50	75	100	125	150	175	200	250	300	350	400	450	500	550	600	650
Group I: Communicable, maternal, perinatal and nutritional conditions																				
+4	12.55	16.77	24.67	31.79	38.17	51.26	61.12	68.82	74.88	79.75	83.77	89.66	93.82	96.82	99.03	100.73	102.02	103.02	103.81	104.41
+3	11.11	14.83	21.80	28.11	33.79	45.55	54.54	61.66	67.35	71.98	75.84	81.66	85.90	89.04	91.44	93.34	94.83	96.04	97.03	97.83
+2	9.66	12.89	18.94	24.43	29.40	39.83	47.97	54.50	59.82	64.21	67.92	73.67	77.97	81.26	83.85	85.94	87.65	89.06	90.25	91.25
+1	8.22	10.94	16.07	20.75	25.02	34.12	41.39	47.35	52.28	56.44	59.99	65.67	70.04	73.48	76.26	78.55	80.46	82.08	83.48	84.67
Expectation	**6.78**	**9.00**	**13.20**	**17.08**	**20.64**	**28.40**	**34.82**	**40.19**	**44.75**	**48.67**	**52.07**	**57.68**	**62.11**	**65.70**	**68.66**	**71.15**	**73.27**	**75.10**	**76.70**	**78.10**
-1	5.34	7.06	10.34	13.40	16.26	22.69	28.24	33.03	37.22	40.90	44.15	49.68	54.18	57.92	61.07	63.76	66.09	68.12	69.92	71.52
-2	3.90	5.12	7.47	9.72	11.88	16.97	21.66	25.87	29.68	33.13	36.22	41.69	46.25	50.14	53.48	56.36	58.90	61.14	63.14	64.94
-3	2.46	3.18	4.60	6.04	7.50	11.26	15.09	18.71	22.15	25.36	28.30	33.69	38.32	42.36	45.88	48.97	51.72	54.16	56.36	58.36
-4	1.02	1.24	1.74	2.36	3.12	5.55	8.51	11.56	14.62	17.58	20.37	25.70	30.39	34.58	38.29	41.58	44.53	47.18	49.58	51.78
Group II: Noncommunicable diseases																				
+4	67.96	68.96	69.81	70.07	70.07	69.48	68.29	66.81	65.15	63.43	61.74	58.34	55.20	52.30	49.68	47.31	45.15	43.19	41.39	39.74
+3	64.69	65.59	66.24	66.23	65.95	64.68	62.96	61.09	59.16	57.25	55.44	51.95	48.83	46.02	43.52	41.29	39.27	37.46	35.81	34.31
+2	61.41	62.23	62.66	62.40	61.83	59.88	57.64	55.37	53.17	51.08	49.13	45.56	42.45	39.74	37.36	35.26	33.40	31.73	30.23	28.87
+1	58.14	58.87	59.09	58.56	57.71	55.09	52.31	49.65	47.18	44.90	42.83	39.16	36.08	33.46	31.20	29.24	27.52	26.00	24.65	23.44
Expectation	**54.86**	**55.51**	**55.51**	**54.73**	**53.59**	**50.29**	**46.98**	**43.93**	**41.18**	**38.73**	**36.52**	**32.77**	**29.71**	**27.17**	**25.04**	**23.21**	**21.64**	**20.27**	**19.07**	**18.01**
-1	51.59	52.15	51.94	50.89	49.48	45.49	41.66	38.21	35.19	32.55	30.22	26.38	23.34	20.89	18.88	17.19	15.77	14.55	13.49	12.57
-2	48.31	48.79	48.37	47.06	45.36	40.69	36.33	32.49	29.20	26.37	23.92	19.99	16.97	14.61	12.72	11.16	9.89	8.82	7.91	7.14
-3	45.04	45.43	44.79	43.22	41.24	35.90	31.00	26.78	23.21	20.20	17.61	13.60	10.60	8.32	6.56	5.14	4.01	3.09	2.33	1.71
-4	41.76	42.06	42.06	39.39	37.12	31.10	25.67	21.06	17.22	14.02	11.31	7.21	4.23	2.04	0.40	–	–	–	–	–
Group III: Injuries																				
+4	52.32	49.60	45.48	42.34	39.79	34.90	31.28	28.41	26.06	24.08	22.38	19.62	17.46	15.72	14.30	13.08	12.07	11.18	10.43	9.73
+3	48.83	46.07	41.93	38.81	36.28	31.50	28.01	25.28	23.06	21.21	19.64	17.11	15.14	13.57	12.30	11.22	10.32	9.54	8.88	8.27
+2	45.34	42.54	38.38	35.27	32.78	28.10	24.74	22.15	20.06	18.34	16.89	14.59	12.82	11.42	10.30	9.36	8.58	7.90	7.33	6.81
+1	41.85	39.01	34.83	31.73	29.27	24.71	21.47	19.01	17.06	15.48	14.15	12.07	10.50	9.28	8.30	7.50	6.83	6.26	5.78	5.35
Expectation	**38.36**	**35.49**	**31.28**	**28.20**	**25.76**	**21.31**	**18.20**	**15.88**	**14.07**	**12.61**	**11.41**	**9.55**	**8.18**	**7.13**	**6.30**	**5.63**	**5.08**	**4.62**	**4.23**	**3.90**
-1	34.87	31.96	27.73	24.66	22.26	17.91	14.93	12.75	11.07	9.74	8.66	7.03	5.86	4.98	4.30	3.77	3.34	2.98	2.68	2.44
-2	31.37	28.43	24.18	21.12	18.75	14.51	11.67	9.61	8.07	6.87	5.92	4.51	3.54	2.83	2.30	1.91	1.59	1.34	1.13	0.98
-3	27.88	24.90	20.63	17.59	15.24	11.11	8.40	6.48	5.07	4.00	3.17	1.99	1.22	0.69	0.31	0.04	–	–	–	–
-4	24.39	21.37	17.08	14.05	11.73	7.71	5.13	3.35	2.07	1.13	0.43	–	–	–	–	–	–	–	–	–

Note: A dash (-) is used when the value at a given number of standard deviations below the expectation would be negative.

Annex Table 5j. Percentage of deaths in each broad cause Group at varying levels of mortality; based on simulations and the regression results from 67 countries, females, aged 15-29 years

Standard deviations from expectation	All-cause mortality rate for females, aged 15-29 years (deaths per 100 000)																			
	50	75	100	125	150	175	200	225	250	275	300	325	350	375	400	450	500	550	600	650
Group I: Communicable, maternal, perinatal and nutritional conditions																				
+4	20.60	31.51	41.30	49.97	57.43	63.94	69.61	74.57	78.80	82.53	85.88	88.68	91.27	93.46	95.51	98.80	101.42	103.55	105.24	106.68
+3	17.71	27.13	35.66	43.27	49.89	55.71	60.83	65.36	69.27	72.75	75.89	78.58	81.06	83.20	85.21	88.51	91.22	93.46	95.31	96.90
+2	14.82	22.75	30.02	36.56	42.34	47.49	52.06	56.15	59.74	62.97	65.90	68.47	70.85	72.95	74.91	78.23	81.02	83.38	85.38	87.12
+1	11.93	18.38	24.38	29.86	34.80	39.26	43.29	46.93	50.21	53.18	55.91	58.36	60.63	62.69	64.60	67.95	70.82	73.30	75.45	77.34
Expectation	**9.03**	**14.00**	**18.73**	**23.16**	**27.25**	**31.03**	**34.51**	**37.72**	**40.68**	**43.40**	**45.92**	**48.26**	**50.42**	**52.43**	**54.30**	**57.67**	**60.62**	**63.21**	**65.51**	**67.57**
-1	6.14	9.63	13.09	16.45	19.71	22.81	25.74	28.51	31.15	33.62	35.94	38.15	40.21	42.17	43.99	47.38	50.41	53.13	55.58	57.79
-2	3.25	5.25	7.45	9.75	12.16	14.58	16.97	19.30	21.62	23.84	25.95	28.04	29.99	31.91	33.69	37.10	40.21	43.05	45.65	48.01
-3	0.35	0.88	1.81	3.04	4.62	6.35	8.20	10.09	12.08	14.06	15.96	17.94	19.78	21.65	23.38	26.82	30.01	32.96	35.72	38.23
-4	-	-	-	-	-	-	-	0.88	2.55	4.28	5.97	7.83	9.56	11.39	13.08	16.54	19.81	22.88	25.79	28.46
Group II: Noncommunicable diseases																				
+4	75.09	75.71	75.58	75.19	74.66	74.01	73.26	72.43	71.50	70.51	69.53	68.44	67.40	66.30	65.26	63.11	61.02	59.03	57.11	55.33
+3	69.25	69.80	69.49	68.87	68.08	67.19	66.21	65.18	64.09	62.97	61.87	60.71	59.61	58.48	57.41	55.25	53.21	51.28	49.45	47.77
+2	63.41	63.88	63.40	62.55	61.51	60.36	59.16	57.93	56.68	55.43	54.21	52.99	51.82	50.65	49.55	47.40	45.40	43.54	41.80	40.21
+1	57.58	57.96	57.32	56.23	54.93	53.54	52.11	50.68	49.26	47.88	46.56	45.26	44.02	42.83	41.69	39.55	37.59	35.79	34.15	32.65
Expectation	**51.74**	**52.05**	**51.23**	**49.91**	**48.35**	**46.71**	**45.06**	**43.43**	**41.85**	**40.34**	**38.90**	**37.53**	**36.23**	**35.00**	**33.84**	**31.69**	**29.77**	**28.05**	**26.49**	**25.09**
-1	45.90	46.13	45.14	43.59	41.78	39.89	38.00	36.18	34.44	32.80	31.24	29.80	28.44	27.18	25.98	23.84	21.96	20.30	18.84	17.52
-2	40.07	40.21	39.05	37.27	35.20	33.06	30.95	28.93	27.03	25.26	23.59	22.07	20.64	19.35	18.12	15.99	14.15	12.56	11.19	9.96
-3	34.23	34.30	32.97	30.95	28.62	26.24	23.90	21.68	19.62	17.71	15.93	14.35	12.85	11.53	10.27	8.13	6.34	4.81	3.53	2.40
-4	28.39	28.38	26.88	24.63	22.05	19.41	16.85	14.42	12.21	10.17	8.27	6.62	5.06	3.70	2.41	0.28	-	-	-	-
Group III: Injuries																				
+4	63.31	57.93	53.60	49.97	46.82	44.06	41.60	39.40	37.40	35.59	33.93	32.41	31.00	29.71	28.50	26.35	24.47	22.81	21.35	19.99
+3	57.29	51.93	47.71	44.21	41.21	38.61	36.31	34.26	32.42	30.76	29.24	27.86	26.59	25.43	24.34	22.42	20.76	19.29	18.01	16.83
+2	51.27	45.94	41.82	38.45	35.61	33.16	31.02	29.12	27.44	25.92	24.55	23.31	22.17	21.14	20.18	18.49	17.04	15.78	14.67	13.67
+1	45.25	39.95	35.93	32.69	30.00	27.71	25.72	23.99	22.45	21.09	19.86	18.76	17.76	16.86	16.02	14.57	13.33	12.26	11.33	10.51
Expectation	**39.23**	**33.95**	**30.04**	**26.94**	**24.39**	**22.26**	**20.43**	**18.85**	**17.47**	**16.25**	**15.18**	**14.21**	**13.35**	**12.57**	**11.87**	**10.64**	**9.61**	**8.74**	**7.99**	**7.35**
-1	33.21	27.96	24.15	21.18	18.79	16.80	15.14	13.71	12.49	11.42	10.49	9.66	8.94	8.29	7.71	6.71	5.90	5.22	4.65	4.19
-2	27.19	21.96	18.25	15.42	13.18	11.35	9.84	8.58	7.50	6.59	5.80	5.11	4.52	4.00	3.55	2.78	2.18	1.70	1.31	1.03
-3	21.16	15.97	12.36	9.67	7.57	5.90	4.55	3.44	2.52	1.75	1.11	0.57	0.11	-	-	-	-	-	-	-
-4	15.14	9.97	6.47	3.91	1.97	0.45	-	-	-	-	-	-	-	-	-	-	-	-	-	-

Note: A dash (-) is used when the value at a given number of standard deviations below the expectation would be negative.

Annex Table 5k. Percentage of deaths in each broad cause Group at varying levels of mortality; based on simulations and the regression results from 67 countries, females, aged 30-44 years

Standard deviations from expectation	All-cause mortality rate for females, aged 30-44 years (deaths per 100 000)																			
	75	100	125	150	200	250	300	350	400	450	500	550	600	650	700	750	800	850	900	950
Group I: Communicable, maternal, perinatal and nutritional conditions																				
+4	8.27	13.15	18.41	23.94	35.22	46.17	56.33	65.58	73.80	81.00	87.25	92.70	97.50	101.56	105.04	108.13	110.63	112.94	114.70	116.30
+3	6.88	10.92	15.30	19.91	29.38	38.66	47.37	55.38	62.59	68.98	74.62	79.60	84.04	87.87	91.22	94.21	96.72	99.05	100.91	102.62
+2	5.49	8.69	12.18	15.88	23.54	31.15	38.40	45.17	51.37	56.97	61.99	66.50	70.58	74.19	77.39	80.30	82.81	85.15	87.13	88.95
+1	4.09	6.46	9.07	11.85	17.71	23.65	29.44	34.97	40.15	44.95	49.36	53.41	57.12	60.50	63.56	66.38	68.91	71.26	73.34	75.27
Expectation	**2.70**	**4.23**	**5.96**	**7.83**	**11.87**	**16.14**	**20.48**	**24.77**	**28.93**	**32.93**	**36.73**	**40.31**	**43.67**	**46.81**	**49.74**	**52.47**	**55.00**	**57.36**	**59.56**	**61.60**
-1	1.31	2.01	2.84	3.80	6.04	8.64	11.51	14.56	17.72	20.91	24.09	27.21	30.21	33.12	35.91	38.55	41.10	43.47	45.77	47.92
-2	–	–	–	–	0.20	1.13	2.55	4.36	6.50	8.90	11.46	14.11	16.75	19.43	22.08	24.63	27.19	29.57	31.99	34.25
-3	–	–	–	–	–	–	–	–	–	–	1.01	3.29	5.74	8.26	10.72	13.29	15.68	18.20	20.57	
-4	–	–	–	–	–	–	–	–	–	–	–	–	–	–	–	–	–	1.78	4.41	6.89
Group II: Noncommunicable diseases																				
+4	98.93	99.04	99.06	99.28	100.37	101.71	102.79	103.37	103.39	102.86	101.86	100.52	98.97	97.16	95.18	93.19	91.00	88.96	86.70	84.56
+3	93.63	93.80	93.74	93.73	94.01	94.32	94.35	93.97	93.17	91.96	90.44	88.69	86.82	84.80	82.68	80.60	78.42	76.37	74.20	72.15
+2	88.33	88.56	88.42	88.18	87.64	86.92	85.90	84.57	82.95	81.07	79.02	76.86	74.67	72.43	70.19	68.02	65.83	63.79	61.70	59.73
+1	83.03	83.31	83.10	82.64	81.28	79.53	77.46	75.17	72.72	70.18	67.59	65.03	62.52	60.07	57.70	55.44	53.25	51.20	49.20	47.32
Expectation	**77.74**	**78.07**	**77.78**	**77.09**	**74.92**	**72.13**	**69.02**	**65.77**	**62.50**	**59.28**	**56.17**	**53.20**	**50.37**	**47.71**	**45.20**	**42.86**	**40.66**	**38.61**	**36.70**	**34.91**
-1	72.44	72.82	72.46	71.54	68.56	64.74	60.58	56.37	52.27	48.39	44.75	41.37	38.22	35.35	32.71	30.28	28.08	26.02	24.19	22.49
-2	67.14	67.58	67.14	65.99	62.20	57.34	52.14	46.97	42.05	37.49	33.33	29.54	26.07	22.99	20.22	17.69	15.49	13.44	11.69	10.08
-3	61.84	62.34	61.82	60.44	55.83	49.95	43.69	37.57	31.83	26.60	21.91	17.70	13.92	10.62	7.73	5.11	2.91	0.85	–	–
-4	56.54	57.09	56.51	54.90	49.47	42.55	35.25	28.16	21.60	15.71	10.48	5.87	1.77	–	–	–	–	–	–	–
Group III: Injuries																				
+4	40.60	37.91	35.73	33.88	30.84	28.36	26.26	24.43	22.82	21.37	20.07	18.90	17.81	16.83	15.93	15.09	14.33	13.60	12.96	12.34
+3	35.34	32.86	30.86	29.18	26.43	24.20	22.32	20.69	19.25	17.98	16.83	15.80	14.85	13.99	13.21	12.48	11.83	11.21	10.66	10.13
+2	30.08	27.81	26.00	24.48	22.02	20.04	18.38	16.95	15.69	14.58	13.59	12.70	11.89	11.16	10.49	9.88	9.33	8.81	8.35	7.92
+1	24.82	22.75	21.13	19.78	17.62	15.89	14.44	13.21	12.13	11.18	10.34	9.60	8.92	8.32	7.78	7.28	6.83	6.42	6.05	5.71
Expectation	**19.56**	**17.70**	**16.26**	**15.08**	**13.21**	**11.73**	**10.50**	**9.46**	**8.57**	**7.79**	**7.10**	**6.50**	**5.96**	**5.48**	**5.06**	**4.68**	**4.33**	**4.03**	**3.75**	**3.50**
-1	14.30	12.64	11.40	10.39	8.80	7.57	6.56	5.72	5.01	4.39	3.86	3.40	3.00	2.65	2.34	2.07	1.84	1.63	1.45	1.28
-2	9.04	7.59	6.53	5.69	4.39	3.41	2.62	1.98	1.44	0.99	0.62	0.30	0.03	–	–	–	–	–	–	–
-3	3.78	2.54	1.66	0.99	–	–	–	–	–	–	–	–	–	–	–	–	–	–	–	–
-4	–	–	–	–	–	–	–	–	–	–	–	–	–	–	–	–	–	–	–	–

Note: A dash (-) is used when the value at a given number of standard deviations below the expectation would be negative.

Annex Table 5I. Percentage of deaths in each broad cause Group at varying levels of mortality; based on simulations and the regression results from 67 countries, females, aged 45-59 years

Standard deviations from expectation	All-cause mortality rate for females, aged 45-59 years (deaths per 100 000)																			
	325	350	400	450	500	550	600	650	700	750	800	850	900	1000	1100	1200	1300	1400	1500	1600
Group I: Communicable, maternal, perinatal and nutritional conditions																				
+4	12.97	14.11	16.37	18.63	20.86	23.06	25.23	27.36	29.46	31.52	33.53	35.50	37.44	41.18	44.77	48.21	51.50	54.65	57.68	60.56
+3	10.31	11.21	13.02	14.81	16.59	18.35	20.08	21.78	23.46	25.11	26.72	28.31	29.87	32.89	35.79	38.57	41.25	43.82	46.29	48.66
+2	7.65	8.32	9.66	11.00	12.32	13.63	14.93	16.20	17.46	18.70	19.92	21.12	22.30	24.59	26.80	28.94	31.00	32.98	34.91	36.75
+1	4.99	5.43	6.31	7.18	8.05	8.92	9.77	10.62	11.47	12.30	13.12	13.93	14.73	16.30	17.82	19.31	20.75	22.15	23.52	24.84
Expectation	**2.33**	**2.54**	**2.95**	**3.36**	**3.78**	**4.20**	**4.62**	**5.04**	**5.47**	**5.89**	**6.31**	**6.74**	**7.16**	**8.00**	**8.84**	**9.67**	**10.50**	**11.32**	**12.13**	**12.93**
-1	-	-	-	-	-	-	-	-	-	-	-	-	-	-	-	0.04	0.25	0.49	0.74	1.03
-2	-	-	-	-	-	-	-	-	-	-	-	-	-	-	-	-	-	-	-	-
-3	-	-	-	-	-	-	-	-	-	-	-	-	-	-	-	-	-	-	-	-
-4	-	-	-	-	-	-	-	-	-	-	-	-	-	-	-	-	-	-	-	-
Group II: Noncommunicable diseases																				
+4	110.83	110.93	111.29	111.82	112.49	113.27	114.12	115.02	115.94	116.88	117.82	118.76	119.68	121.47	123.16	124.76	126.26	127.65	128.95	130.14
+3	105.71	105.81	106.10	106.49	106.98	107.53	108.13	108.75	109.39	110.04	110.68	111.31	111.94	113.13	114.25	115.29	116.24	117.12	117.93	118.65
+2	100.60	100.69	100.90	101.16	101.49	101.79	102.14	102.49	102.84	103.19	103.54	103.87	104.19	104.79	105.33	105.81	106.23	106.60	106.91	107.16
+1	95.48	95.57	95.71	95.83	95.95	96.05	96.14	96.22	96.29	96.35	96.40	96.43	96.45	96.46	96.42	96.34	96.22	96.07	95.89	95.68
Expectation	**90.37**	**90.45**	**90.52**	**90.51**	**90.43**	**90.31**	**90.15**	**89.96**	**89.74**	**89.51**	**89.25**	**88.99**	**88.71**	**88.12**	**87.50**	**86.86**	**86.21**	**85.54**	**84.87**	**84.19**
-1	85.25	85.32	85.32	85.18	84.92	84.57	84.16	83.69	83.19	82.66	82.11	81.54	80.96	79.78	78.59	77.39	76.20	75.02	73.85	72.70
-2	80.14	80.20	80.13	79.85	79.40	78.83	78.16	77.43	76.65	75.82	74.97	74.10	73.22	71.45	69.67	67.91	66.18	64.49	62.83	61.22
-3	75.02	75.08	74.94	74.52	73.89	73.09	72.17	71.17	70.10	68.98	67.83	66.66	65.48	63.11	60.76	58.44	56.17	53.96	51.81	49.73
-4	69.91	69.96	69.74	69.19	68.37	67.35	66.18	64.90	63.55	62.13	60.69	59.22	57.74	54.77	51.84	48.96	46.16	43.44	40.79	38.24
Group III: Injuries																				
+4	25.82	25.07	23.76	22.64	21.67	20.81	20.05	19.37	18.75	18.18	17.67	17.19	16.74	15.95	15.25	14.62	14.06	13.56	13.09	12.67
+3	21.19	20.56	19.46	18.51	17.70	16.98	16.35	15.78	15.26	14.79	14.36	13.96	13.59	12.93	12.35	11.83	11.37	10.95	10.57	10.22
+2	16.56	16.04	15.15	14.38	13.73	13.15	12.64	12.18	11.77	11.39	11.05	10.73	10.44	9.91	9.45	9.04	8.68	8.35	8.05	7.77
+1	11.93	11.53	10.84	10.26	9.76	9.32	8.93	8.59	8.28	8.00	7.74	7.50	7.28	6.90	6.55	6.25	5.99	5.74	5.52	5.32
Expectation	**7.30**	**7.02**	**6.53**	**6.13**	**5.79**	**5.49**	**5.23**	**5.00**	**4.79**	**4.60**	**4.43**	**4.28**	**4.13**	**3.88**	**3.66**	**3.46**	**3.29**	**3.14**	**3.00**	**2.87**
-1	2.67	2.50	2.23	2.00	1.82	1.66	1.52	1.40	1.30	1.21	1.12	1.05	0.98	0.86	0.76	0.67	0.60	0.53	0.48	0.43
-2	-	-	-	-	-	-	-	-	-	-	-	-	-	-	-	-	-	-	-	-
-3	-	-	-	-	-	-	-	-	-	-	-	-	-	-	-	-	-	-	-	-
-4	-	-	-	-	-	-	-	-	-	-	-	-	-	-	-	-	-	-	-	-

Note: A dash (-) is used when the value at a given number of standard deviations below the expectation would be negative.

Annex Table 5m. Percentage of deaths in each broad cause Group at varying levels of mortality; based on simulations and the regression results from 67 countries; females, aged 60-69 years

Standard deviations from expectation	All-cause mortality rate for females, aged 60-69 years (deaths per 100 000)																			
	1000	1100	1200	1300	1400	1500	1600	1700	1800	2000	2200	2400	2600	2800	3000	3200	3400	3600	3800	4000
Group I: Communicable, maternal, perinatal and nutritional conditions																				
+4	15.64	16.52	17.36	18.16	18.93	19.67	20.38	21.07	21.73	23.00	24.19	25.31	26.38	27.40	28.37	29.30	30.20	31.06	31.89	32.71
+3	12.43	13.13	13.80	14.43	15.04	15.63	16.19	16.74	17.26	18.27	19.21	20.11	20.96	21.77	22.54	23.28	23.99	24.68	25.34	25.99
+2	9.23	9.74	10.23	10.70	11.15	11.59	12.00	12.40	12.79	13.54	14.24	14.90	15.53	16.13	16.71	17.26	17.79	18.30	18.79	19.28
+1	6.02	6.35	6.67	6.97	7.26	7.54	7.81	8.07	8.33	8.81	9.26	9.69	10.10	10.50	10.87	11.24	11.58	11.92	12.24	12.56
Expectation	**2.81**	**2.96**	**3.11**	**3.24**	**3.37**	**3.50**	**3.62**	**3.74**	**3.86**	**4.08**	**4.29**	**4.49**	**4.68**	**4.86**	**5.04**	**5.21**	**5.38**	**5.54**	**5.69**	**5.85**
-1	-	-	-	-	-	-	-	-	-	-	-	-	-	-	-	-	-	-	-	-
-2	-	-	-	-	-	-	-	-	-	-	-	-	-	-	-	-	-	-	-	-
-3	-	-	-	-	-	-	-	-	-	-	-	-	-	-	-	-	-	-	-	-
-4	-	-	-	-	-	-	-	-	-	-	-	-	-	-	-	-	-	-	-	-
Group II: Noncommunicable diseases																				
+4	109.67	109.77	109.92	110.10	110.30	110.53	110.78	111.03	111.29	111.83	112.38	112.92	113.47	114.00	114.52	115.02	115.52	116.00	116.47	116.93
+3	105.62	105.72	105.84	105.98	106.14	106.31	106.49	106.68	106.87	107.26	107.65	108.04	108.43	108.81	109.17	109.53	109.88	110.21	110.54	110.86
+2	101.57	101.66	101.75	101.86	101.97	102.09	102.20	102.32	102.45	102.69	102.93	103.16	103.39	103.61	103.83	104.03	104.23	104.42	104.61	104.79
+1	97.52	97.60	97.67	97.74	97.80	97.86	97.92	97.97	98.02	98.12	98.21	98.28	98.36	98.42	98.48	98.54	98.59	98.64	98.68	98.72
Expectation	**93.47**	**93.54**	**93.59**	**93.62**	**93.63**	**93.64**	**93.63**	**93.62**	**93.60**	**93.55**	**93.48**	**93.40**	**93.32**	**93.23**	**93.14**	**93.04**	**92.95**	**92.85**	**92.75**	**92.65**
-1	89.42	89.49	89.51	89.50	89.47	89.41	89.35	89.27	89.18	88.98	88.76	88.52	88.28	88.04	87.80	87.55	87.30	87.06	86.82	86.58
-2	85.38	85.43	85.43	85.38	85.30	85.19	85.06	84.91	84.75	84.41	84.03	83.64	83.25	82.85	82.45	82.05	81.66	81.27	80.89	80.51
-3	81.33	81.37	81.34	81.26	81.13	80.97	80.77	80.56	80.33	79.84	79.31	78.76	78.21	77.66	77.11	76.56	76.02	75.49	74.96	74.44
-4	77.28	77.31	77.26	77.14	76.96	76.74	76.49	76.21	75.91	75.27	74.59	73.89	73.18	72.47	71.76	71.06	70.38	69.70	69.03	68.37
Group III: Injuries																				
+4	16.29	15.51	14.84	14.23	13.69	13.21	12.77	12.37	12.00	11.35	10.78	10.30	9.86	9.47	9.13	8.81	8.52	8.26	8.02	7.79
+3	13.14	12.51	11.95	11.46	11.02	10.62	10.26	9.94	9.64	9.11	8.65	8.25	7.90	7.58	7.30	7.04	6.81	6.60	6.40	6.22
+2	10.00	9.50	9.07	8.69	8.34	8.04	7.76	7.50	7.27	6.86	6.51	6.20	5.93	5.69	5.47	5.28	5.10	4.94	4.79	4.64
+1	6.85	6.50	6.19	5.91	5.67	5.45	5.25	5.07	4.91	4.62	4.37	4.15	3.97	3.80	3.65	3.51	3.39	3.27	3.17	3.07
Expectation	**3.71**	**3.49**	**3.30**	**3.14**	**2.99**	**2.86**	**2.74**	**2.64**	**2.54**	**2.37**	**2.23**	**2.11**	**2.00**	**1.90**	**1.82**	**1.74**	**1.68**	**1.61**	**1.56**	**1.50**
-1	0.57	0.49	0.42	0.36	0.32	0.27	0.24	0.21	0.18	0.13	0.09	0.06	0.03	0.01	-	-	-	-	-	-
-2	-	-	-	-	-	-	-	-	-	-	-	-	-	-	-	-	-	-	-	-
-3	-	-	-	-	-	-	-	-	-	-	-	-	-	-	-	-	-	-	-	-
-4	-	-	-	-	-	-	-	-	-	-	-	-	-	-	-	-	-	-	-	-

Note: A dash (-) is used when the value at a given number of standard deviations below the expectation would be negative.

Annex Table 5n. Percentage of deaths in each broad cause Group at varying levels of mortality; based on simulations and the regression results from 67 countries, females, aged 70 years and over

Standard deviations from expectation	5250	5500	5750	6000	6250	6500	6750	7000	7250	7500	7750	8000	8250	8500	9000	9500	10000	10500	11000	11500
										All-cause mortality rate for females, aged 70 years and over (deaths per 100 000)										
Group I: Communicable, maternal, perinatal and nutritional conditions																				
+4	43.97	44.16	44.34	44.51	44.67	44.83	44.99	45.13	45.28	45.41	45.55	45.68	45.81	45.93	46.16	46.39	46.60	46.80	46.99	47.18
+3	33.96	34.10	34.24	34.37	34.49	34.61	34.72	34.83	34.94	35.04	35.15	35.24	35.34	35.43	35.61	35.77	35.93	36.09	36.23	36.37
+2	23.95	24.05	24.14	24.22	24.30	24.38	24.46	24.53	24.61	24.68	24.74	24.81	24.87	24.93	25.05	25.16	25.27	25.37	25.47	25.56
+1	13.94	13.99	14.03	14.08	14.12	14.16	14.20	14.24	14.27	14.31	14.34	14.37	14.40	14.44	14.49	14.55	14.60	14.65	14.70	14.75
Expectation	**3.93**	**3.93**	**3.93**	**3.93**	**3.93**	**3.93**	**3.94**	**3.94**	**3.94**	**3.94**	**3.94**	**3.94**	**3.94**	**3.94**	**3.94**	**3.94**	**3.94**	**3.94**	**3.94**	**3.94**
-1	-	-	-	-	-	-	-	-	-	-	-	-	-	-	-	-	-	-	-	-
-2	-	-	-	-	-	-	-	-	-	-	-	-	-	-	-	-	-	-	-	-
-3	-	-	-	-	-	-	-	-	-	-	-	-	-	-	-	-	-	-	-	-
-4	-	-	-	-	-	-	-	-	-	-	-	-	-	-	-	-	-	-	-	-
Group II: Noncommunicable diseases																				
+4	134.01	134.21	134.40	134.58	134.75	134.92	135.08	135.24	135.39	135.54	135.68	135.82	135.95	136.08	136.33	136.57	136.80	137.01	137.22	137.42
+3	124.05	124.21	124.36	124.50	124.64	124.77	124.90	125.02	125.14	125.25	125.37	125.47	125.58	125.68	125.88	126.06	126.24	126.41	126.57	126.72
+2	114.09	114.21	114.31	114.42	114.52	114.62	114.71	114.80	114.89	114.97	115.05	115.13	115.21	115.28	115.42	115.56	115.68	115.81	115.92	116.03
+1	104.13	104.20	104.27	104.34	104.40	104.47	104.52	104.58	104.63	104.69	104.74	104.79	104.83	104.88	104.97	105.05	105.13	105.20	105.27	105.34
Expectation	**94.17**	**94.20**	**94.23**	**94.26**	**94.29**	**94.31**	**94.34**	**94.36**	**94.38**	**94.40**	**94.42**	**94.44**	**94.46**	**94.48**	**94.51**	**94.54**	**94.57**	**94.60**	**94.62**	**94.65**
-1	84.21	84.20	84.19	84.18	84.17	84.16	84.15	84.14	84.13	84.12	84.11	84.10	84.09	84.08	84.06	84.04	84.01	83.99	83.97	83.95
-2	74.25	74.20	74.15	74.10	74.06	74.01	73.97	73.92	73.88	73.84	73.80	73.75	73.71	73.68	73.60	73.53	73.46	73.39	73.32	73.26
-3	64.29	64.20	64.11	64.02	63.94	63.86	63.78	63.70	63.63	63.55	63.48	63.41	63.34	63.28	63.15	63.02	62.90	62.79	62.68	62.57
-4	54.33	54.20	54.07	53.94	53.82	53.71	53.59	53.48	53.37	53.27	53.17	53.07	52.97	52.87	52.69	52.51	52.34	52.18	52.03	51.87
Group III: Injuries																				
+4	14.70	14.55	14.41	14.28	14.15	14.03	13.91	13.80	13.70	13.60	13.50	13.41	13.32	13.24	13.07	12.92	12.78	12.65	12.52	12.40
+3	11.50	11.38	11.27	11.16	11.06	10.96	10.87	10.78	10.70	10.61	10.54	10.46	10.39	10.32	10.19	10.07	9.96	9.85	9.75	9.65
+2	8.30	8.21	8.12	8.04	7.96	7.89	7.82	7.75	7.69	7.63	7.57	7.52	7.46	7.41	7.31	7.22	7.13	7.05	6.98	6.91
+1	5.10	5.04	4.98	4.92	4.87	4.82	4.77	4.73	4.69	4.65	4.61	4.57	4.53	4.50	4.43	4.37	4.31	4.26	4.21	4.16
Expectation	**1.90**	**1.87**	**1.83**	**1.81**	**1.78**	**1.75**	**1.73**	**1.70**	**1.68**	**1.66**	**1.64**	**1.62**	**1.60**	**1.58**	**1.55**	**1.52**	**1.49**	**1.46**	**1.44**	**1.41**
-1	-	-	-	-	-	-	-	-	-	-	-	-	-	-	-	-	-	-	-	-
-2	-	-	-	-	-	-	-	-	-	-	-	-	-	-	-	-	-	-	-	-
-3	-	-	-	-	-	-	-	-	-	-	-	-	-	-	-	-	-	-	-	-
-4	-	-	-	-	-	-	-	-	-	-	-	-	-	-	-	-	-	-	-	-

Note: A dash (-) is used when the value at a given number of standard deviations below the expectation would be negative.

Annex Table 6a. Deaths by age, sex and cause (thousands): Established Market Economies, 1990

Cause	Total	Male	Female	Males							Females						
				0-4	5-14	15-29	30-44	45-59	60-69	70+	0-4	5-14	15-29	30-44	45-59	60-69	70+
Population (millions)	798	390	407	26	53	94	90	66	34	26	25	51	90	89	68	41	44
All causes	7 121	3 659	3 462	60	14	114	187	468	742	2 075	45	9	39	87	244	448	2 590
I. Communicable, maternal, perinatal and nutritional conditions	453	237	216	31	1	8	24	19	22	133	22	1	3	6	6	13	166
A. Infectious and parasitic diseases	111	71	40	2	-	6	22	13	7	20	2	-	2	4	3	5	25
1. Tuberculosis	15	10	5	-	-	-	1	2	2	5	-	-	-	-	-	1	3
2. STDs excluding HIV	1	-	-	-	-	-	-	-	-	-	-	-	-	-	-	-	-
a. Syphilis	-	-	-	-	-	-	-	-	-	-	-	-	-	-	-	-	-
b. Chlamydia	-	-	-	-	-	-	-	-	-	-	-	-	-	-	-	-	-
c. Gonorrhoea	-	-	-	-	-	-	-	-	-	-	-	-	-	-	-	-	-
3. HIV	41	36	6	-	-	6	19	9	1	-	-	-	1	3	1	-	-
4. Diarrhoeal diseases	3	1	2	-	-	-	-	-	-	1	-	-	-	-	-	-	1
5. Childhood-cluster diseases	1	-	-	-	-	-	-	-	-	-	-	-	-	-	-	-	-
a. Pertussis	-	-	-	-	-	-	-	-	-	-	-	-	-	-	-	-	-
b. Poliomyelitis	-	-	-	-	-	-	-	-	-	-	-	-	-	-	-	-	-
c. Diphtheria	-	-	-	-	-	-	-	-	-	-	-	-	-	-	-	-	-
d. Measles	-	-	-	-	-	-	-	-	-	-	-	-	-	-	-	-	-
e. Tetanus	-	-	-	-	-	-	-	-	-	-	-	-	-	-	-	-	-
6. Bacterial meningitis*	5	2	2	1	-	-	-	-	-	-	1	-	-	-	-	-	-
7. Hepatitis B and hepatitis C	4	2	2	-	-	-	-	1	1	1	-	-	-	-	-	-	1
8. Malaria	-	-	-	-	-	-	-	-	-	-	-	-	-	-	-	-	-
9. Tropical-cluster diseases	-	-	-	-	-	-	-	-	-	-	-	-	-	-	-	-	-
a. Trypanosomiasis	-	-	-	-	-	-	-	-	-	-	-	-	-	-	-	-	-
b. Chagas disease	-	-	-	-	-	-	-	-	-	-	-	-	-	-	-	-	-
c. Schistosomiasis	-	-	-	-	-	-	-	-	-	-	-	-	-	-	-	-	-
d. Leishmaniasis	-	-	-	-	-	-	-	-	-	-	-	-	-	-	-	-	-
10. Leprosy	-	-	-	-	-	-	-	-	-	-	-	-	-	-	-	-	-
11. Dengue	-	-	-	-	-	-	-	-	-	-	-	-	-	-	-	-	-
12. Japanese encephalitis	-	-	-	-	-	-	-	-	-	-	-	-	-	-	-	-	-
13. Trachoma	-	-	-	-	-	-	-	-	-	-	-	-	-	-	-	-	-
14. Intestinal nematode infections	-	-	-	-	-	-	-	-	-	-	-	-	-	-	-	-	-
a. Ascariasis	-	-	-	-	-	-	-	-	-	-	-	-	-	-	-	-	-
b. Trichuriasis	-	-	-	-	-	-	-	-	-	-	-	-	-	-	-	-	-
c. Ancylostomiasis, necatoriasis	-	-	-	-	-	-	-	-	-	-	-	-	-	-	-	-	-
15. Other infectious and parasitic	42	19	24	1	-	-	1	1	3	12	-	-	1	1	1	3	19

Annex Table 6a, continued. Deaths by age, sex and cause (thousands): Established Market Economies, 1990

Cause	Total	Male	Female	Males							Females						
				0-4	5-14	15-29	30-44	45-59	60-69	70+	0-4	5-14	15-29	30-44	45-59	60-69	70+
B. Respiratory infections	**275**	**131**	**144**	2	-	1	2	6	13	107	1	-	1	1	3	7	131
1. Lower respiratory infections	272	129	142	2	-	1	2	5	13	106	1	-	1	1	3	7	129
2. Upper respiratory infections	3	1	2							1							1
3. Otitis media																	
C. Maternal conditions	**1**		**1**										1				
1. Maternal haemorrhage																	
2. Maternal sepsis																	
3. Hypertensive disorders*																	
4. Obstructed labour																	
5. Abortion																	
6. Other maternal																	
D. Perinatal conditions*	**46**	**27**	**19**	26							19						
1. Low birth weight	10	6	5	6							5						
2. Birth asphyxia and birth trauma	20	12	8	12							8						
3. Other perinatal	15	9	7	9							7						
E. Nutritional deficiencies	**21**	**8**	**12**						1	6						1	10
1. Protein-energy malnutrition	6	2	4						1	2						1	3
2. Iodine deficiency																	
3. Vitamin A deficiency																	
4. Iron-deficiency anaemia	14	6	8							4							6
II. Noncommunicable diseases	**6 223**	**3 125**	**3 099**	24	6	26	97	397	689	1 886	19	5	16	63	219	419	2 358
A. Malignant neoplasms	**1 762**	**977**	**785**	1	2	8	30	163	275	498	1	2	6	34	119	180	444
1. Mouth and oropharynx cancers	33	25	8				2	8	8	7				1	1	2	4
2. Oesophagus cancer	42	32	10				1	8	11	12					1	2	7
3. Stomach cancer	140	83	57				2	14	22	45			1	2	6	10	38
4. Colon and rectum cancers	208	103	105				3	15	27	58				2	11	21	71
5. Liver cancer	37	27	10				1	7	10	9					1	3	6
6. Pancreas cancer	85	43	42				1	8	13	22				1	4	9	28
7. Trachea, bronchus, lung cancers	379	279	100				6	50	93	130				3	17	31	50
8. Melanoma and other skin cancers	22	13	10				2	3	3	5				1	2	2	5
9. Breast cancer	134	-	134										1	11	32	32	58
10. Cervix uteri cancer	16	-	16											3	3	4	6
11. Corpus uteri cancer	24	-	24											1	3	6	14
12. Ovary cancer	41	-	41											2	9	12	19
13. Prostate cancer	92	92	-					3	16	74							
14. Bladder cancer	47	33	13					2	8	23					1	2	10
15. Lymphomas, multiple myeloma	79	42	38			1	3	7	10	19			1	2	4	8	23
16. Leukaemia	57	31	26	1	2	1	1	4	7	15	1	1	1	2	3	5	14
17. Other cancers	323	173	150	1	1	3	8	33	48	79	1	1	2	5	18	32	92

Annex Table 6a, continued. Deaths by age, sex and cause (thousands): Established Market Economies, 1990

Cause	Total	Male	Female	Males							Females						
				0-4	5-14	15-29	30-44	45-59	60-69	70+	0-4	5-14	15-29	30-44	45-59	60-69	70+
B. Other neoplasms	**36**	**18**	**18**	–	–	–	1	3	4	10	–	–	–	1	2	3	12
C. Diabetes mellitus	**145**	**57**	**88**	–	–	–	2	7	13	34	–	–	–	1	5	14	67
D. Endocrine disorders	**46**	**21**	**26**	1	–	1	1	2	4	11	1	–	1	1	2	3	17
E. Neuro-psychiatric conditions	**205**	**97**	**108**	1	1	6	9	12	14	54	1	1	2	3	6	10	84
2. Bipolar disorder	1	–	–	–	–	–	–	–	–	–	–	–	–	–	–	–	–
3. Schizophrenia	13	5	7	–	–	–	–	–	1	4	–	–	–	–	–	–	7
4. Epilepsy	7	4	3	–	–	1	–	1	1	1	–	–	–	–	–	1	1
5. Alcohol use	16	12	3	–	–	–	3	5	3	2	–	–	–	1	1	–	1
6. Dementia*	94	35	58	–	–	–	1	2	5	26	–	–	–	–	2	5	51
7. Parkinson disease	29	15	14	–	–	–	–	1	1	13	–	–	–	–	–	1	13
8. Multiple sclerosis	6	2	3	–	–	–	–	1	1	–	–	–	–	–	1	1	1
9. Drug use	4	3	1	–	–	2	1	–	–	–	–	–	1	–	–	–	–
13. Other neuro-psychiatric	36	18	17	1	1	2	2	2	3	7	1	1	1	1	–	2	11
F. Sense organ diseases	–	–	–	–	–	–	–	–	–	–	–	–	–	–	–	–	–
1. Glaucoma	–	–	–	–	–	–	–	–	–	–	–	–	–	–	–	–	–
2. Cataracts	–	–	–	–	–	–	–	–	–	–	–	–	–	–	–	–	–
G. Cardiovascular diseases	**3 175**	**1 491**	**1 684**	1	1	6	35	156	292	1 000	1	1	3	13	58	156	1 451
1. Rheumatic heart disease	20	6	14	–	–	–	–	1	2	3	–	–	–	–	2	3	9
2. Ischaemic heart disease	1 668	829	838	–	–	1	18	98	178	536	–	–	1	5	29	86	719
3. Cerebrovascular disease	788	322	467	–	–	1	6	24	47	242	–	1	1	4	15	36	410
4. Inflammatory heart diseases	65	33	32	–	–	1	3	6	5	17	–	–	–	1	3	3	25
5. Other cardiovascular	633	301	332	1	–	3	8	26	60	203	1	–	3	3	9	29	288
H. Respiratory diseases	**343**	**209**	**134**	1	–	1	3	13	39	152	1	–	1	2	8	20	102
1. COPD*	245	157	88	–	–	–	1	8	30	118	–	–	–	–	5	15	68
2. Asthma	22	10	12	–	–	1	1	1	2	5	–	–	1	1	1	2	7
3. Other respiratory	76	42	34	1	1	1	1	3	7	28	1	1	–	–	2	3	27
I. Digestive diseases	**305**	**163**	**142**	1	–	1	13	36	38	73	1	–	1	5	14	21	100
1. Peptic ulcer	31	16	15	–	–	–	–	2	3	11	–	–	–	–	1	1	13
2. Cirrhosis of the liver	117	77	39	–	–	1	9	26	22	19	–	–	–	3	9	11	16
3. Appendicitis	1	1	–	1	–	–	–	–	–	–	–	–	–	–	–	–	–
4. Other digestive	156	69	87	1	–	1	3	8	12	43	1	–	1	2	4	9	71
J. Genito-urinary diseases	**123**	**58**	**64**	–	–	–	1	4	8	44	–	–	–	1	3	7	54
1. Nephritis and nephrosis	80	39	41	–	–	–	1	3	6	28	–	–	–	1	2	5	34
2. Benign prostatic hypertrophy	4	4	–	–	–	–	–	–	–	3	–	–	–	–	–	–	–
3. Other genito-urinary	39	16	23	–	–	–	–	1	2	12	–	–	–	–	1	2	20
K. Skin diseases	**12**	**4**	**8**	–	–	–	–	–	–	3	–	–	–	–	–	–	7

Annex Table 6a, continued. Deaths by age, sex and cause (thousands): Established Market Economies, 1990

Cause	Total	Male	Female	Males							Females						
				0-4	5-14	15-29	30-44	45-59	60-69	70+	0-4	5-14	15-29	30-44	45-59	60-69	70+
L. Musculo-skeletal diseases	32	9	23	–	–	–	–	1	2	6	–	–	–	1	2	3	17
1. Rheumatoid arthritis	9	2	7	–	–	–	–	–	1	1	–	–	–	–	1	1	5
3. Other musculo-skeletal	23	7	16	–	–	–	–	1	1	4	–	–	–	1	1	2	12
M. Congenital anomalies	39	21	18	16	1	1	1	1	1	–	13	1	1	1	1	–	1
1. Abdominal wall defect	3	1	2	1	–	–	–	–	–	–	2	–	–	–	–	–	–
2. Anencephaly	–	–	–	–	–	–	–	–	–	–	–	–	–	–	–	–	–
3. Anorectal atresia	–	–	–	–	–	–	–	–	–	–	–	–	–	–	–	–	–
4. Cleft lip	–	–	–	–	–	–	–	–	–	–	–	–	–	–	–	–	–
5. Cleft palate	–	–	–	–	–	–	–	–	–	–	–	–	–	–	–	–	–
6. Oesophageal atresia	2	1	1	1	–	–	–	–	–	–	1	–	–	–	–	–	–
7. Renal agenesis	3	2	1	1	–	–	–	–	–	–	1	–	–	–	–	–	–
8. Down syndrome	16	9	7	6	1	1	1	1	1	–	4	1	1	1	1	–	–
9. Congenital heart anomalies	2	1	1	1	–	–	–	–	–	–	1	–	–	–	–	–	1
10. Spina bifida	–	1	–	1	–	–	–	–	–	–	–	–	–	–	–	–	–
11. Other congenital	13	7	5	6	–	–	–	–	–	–	4	–	–	–	–	–	–
N. Oral conditions	–	–	–	–	–	–	–	–	–	–	–	–	–	–	–	–	–
III. Injuries	*445*	*298*	*147*	*6*	*7*	*80*	*66*	*51*	*31*	*57*	*4*	*3*	*20*	*19*	*18*	*15*	*66*
A. Unintentional injuries	303	195	108	5	6	53	37	30	20	43	4	3	14	10	10	10	58
1. Road traffic accidents	131	94	37	1	3	38	19	13	8	11	1	2	11	6	5	4	8
2. Poisonings	13	9	4	–	–	2	4	1	1	1	–	–	–	1	1	1	1
3. Falls	70	30	39	–	–	2	3	4	4	18	–	–	–	1	1	2	35
4. Fires	11	6	4	1	–	1	1	1	1	1	1	–	–	1	–	–	2
5. Drownings	13	10	3	1	2	2	2	1	1	1	1	–	–	–	–	–	2
6. Other unintentional	65	45	20	2	1	8	9	9	6	11	1	–	1	2	2	2	11
B. Intentional injuries	143	104	39	1	1	27	29	21	11	14	1	–	7	9	8	5	8
1. Self-inflicted injuries	112	81	31	–	–	17	21	18	10	14	–	–	4	7	8	5	8
2. Violence	30	23	8	1	1	10	7	3	1	1	1	–	2	2	1	–	1
3. War	–	–	–	–	–	–	–	–	–	–	–	–	–	–	–	–	–

Notes:
Causes responsible for no deaths have been omitted from this table.
A dash (–) symbol indicates fewer than 500 deaths.
*IA6 is Bacterial meningitis and meningococcaemia; IC3 is Hypertensive disorders of pregnancy; ID is Conditions arising during the perinatal period; IIE6 is Dementia and other degenerative and hereditary CNS disorders; IIH1 is Chronic obstructive pulmonary disease.

Annex Table 6b. Deaths by age, sex and cause (thousands): Formerly Socialist Economies of Europe, 1990

Cause	Total	Male	Female	Males							Females						
				0-4	5-14	15-29	30-44	45-59	60-69	70+	0-4	5-14	15-29	30-44	45-59	60-69	70+
Population (millions)	*346*	*165*	*181*	*14*	*27*	*36*	*40*	*27*	*14*	*7*	*13*	*26*	*35*	*40*	*30*	*20*	*16*
All causes	*3 791*	*1 908*	*1 883*	*66*	*17*	*84*	*174*	*420*	*440*	*707*	*48*	*9*	*27*	*58*	*180*	*320*	*1 241*
I. Communicable, maternal, perinatal and nutritional conditions																	
A. Infectious and parasitic diseases	214	109	105	38	1	2	8	14	11	34	27	1	2	3	3	7	62
1. Tuberculosis	52	33	19	6	–	1	6	9	5	5	4	–	1	1	2	3	9
2. STDs excluding HIV	23	19	4	–	–	1	5	7	4	2	–	–	–	1	1	1	1
a. Syphilis	–	–	–	–	–	–	–	–	–	–	–	–	–	–	–	–	–
b. Chlamydia	–	–	–	–	–	–	–	–	–	–	–	–	–	–	–	–	–
c. Gonorrhoea	–	–	–	–	–	–	–	–	–	–	–	–	–	–	–	–	–
3. HIV	1	1	–	–	–	–	1	–	–	–	–	–	–	–	–	–	–
4. Diarrhoeal diseases	4	2	2	2	–	–	–	–	–	–	2	–	–	–	–	–	–
5. Childhood-cluster diseases	1	–	–	–	–	–	–	–	–	–	–	–	–	–	–	–	–
a. Pertussis	–	–	–	–	–	–	–	–	–	–	–	–	–	–	–	–	–
b. Poliomyelitis	–	–	–	–	–	–	–	–	–	–	–	–	–	–	–	–	–
c. Diphtheria	–	–	–	–	–	–	–	–	–	–	–	–	–	–	–	–	–
d. Measles	–	–	–	–	–	–	–	–	–	–	–	–	–	–	–	–	–
e. Tetanus	–	–	–	–	–	–	–	–	–	–	–	–	–	–	–	–	–
6. Bacterial meningitis*	6	4	3	2	–	–	–	1	1	–	1	–	–	–	1	–	1
7. Hepatitis B and hepatitis C	2	1	1	1	–	–	–	–	–	–	–	–	–	–	–	–	1
8. Malaria	–	–	–	–	–	–	–	–	–	–	–	–	–	–	–	–	–
9. Tropical-cluster diseases	–	–	–	–	–	–	–	–	–	–	–	–	–	–	–	–	–
a. Trypanosomiasis	–	–	–	–	–	–	–	–	–	–	–	–	–	–	–	–	–
b. Chagas disease	–	–	–	–	–	–	–	–	–	–	–	–	–	–	–	–	–
c. Schistosomiasis	–	–	–	–	–	–	–	–	–	–	–	–	–	–	–	–	–
d. Leishmaniasis	–	–	–	–	–	–	–	–	–	–	–	–	–	–	–	–	–
10. Leprosy	–	–	–	–	–	–	–	–	–	–	–	–	–	–	–	–	–
11. Dengue	–	–	–	–	–	–	–	–	–	–	–	–	–	–	–	–	–
12. Japanese encephalitis	–	–	–	–	–	–	–	–	–	–	–	–	–	–	–	–	–
13. Trachoma	–	–	–	–	–	–	–	–	–	–	–	–	–	–	–	–	–
14. Intestinal nematode infections	–	–	–	–	–	–	–	–	–	–	–	–	–	–	–	–	–
a. Ascariasis	–	–	–	–	–	–	–	–	–	–	–	–	–	–	–	–	–
b. Trichuriasis	–	–	–	–	–	–	–	–	–	–	–	–	–	–	–	–	–
c. Ancylostomiasis, necatoriasis	–	–	–	–	–	–	–	–	–	–	–	–	–	–	–	–	–
15. Other infectious and parasitic	15	6	9	2	–	–	1	1	–	2	1	–	–	–	1	1	6

Annex Table 6b, continued. Deaths by age, sex and cause (thousands): Formerly Socialist Economies of Europe, 1990

Cause	Total	Male	Female	Males							Females						
				0-4	5-14	15-29	30-44	45-59	60-69	70+	0-4	5-14	15-29	30-44	45-59	60-69	70+
B. Respiratory infections	114	51	63	10	1	1	2	5	5	27	8	-	1	1	1	4	48
1. Lower respiratory infections	113	51	62	10	1	1	2	5	5	27	7	1	1	1	1	4	48
2. Upper respiratory infections	1	-	-	-	-	-	-	-	-	-	-	-	-	-	-	-	-
3. Otitis media	-	-	-	-	-	-	-	-	-	-	-	-	-	-	-	-	-
C. Maternal conditions	2	-	2	-	-	-	-	-	-	-	-	-	1	1	-	-	-
1. Maternal haemorrhage	-	-	-	-	-	-	-	-	-	-	-	-	-	-	-	-	-
2. Maternal sepsis	-	-	-	-	-	-	-	-	-	-	-	-	-	-	-	-	-
3. Hypertensive disorders*	-	-	-	-	-	-	-	-	-	-	-	-	-	-	-	-	-
4. Obstructed labour	-	-	-	-	-	-	-	-	-	-	-	-	-	-	-	-	-
5. Abortion	1	-	1	-	-	-	-	-	-	-	-	-	1	-	-	-	-
6. Other maternal	1	-	1	-	-	-	-	-	-	-	-	-	-	1	-	-	-
D. Perinatal conditions*	36	22	14	22	-	-	-	-	-	-	14	-	-	-	-	-	-
1. Low birth weight	5	3	2	3	-	-	-	-	-	-	2	-	-	-	-	-	-
2. Birth asphyxia and birth trauma	9	5	3	5	-	-	-	-	-	-	3	-	-	-	-	-	-
3. Other perinatal	22	14	9	14	-	-	-	-	-	-	9	-	-	-	-	-	-
E. Nutritional deficiencies	9	3	6	-	-	-	-	-	-	2	-	-	-	-	-	-	2
1. Protein-energy malnutrition	2	1	1	-	-	-	-	-	-	-	-	-	-	-	-	-	-
2. Iodine deficiency	-	-	-	-	-	-	-	-	-	-	-	-	-	-	-	-	-
3. Vitamin A deficiency	-	-	-	-	-	-	-	-	-	-	-	-	-	-	-	-	-
4. Iron-deficiency anaemia	5	2	3	-	-	-	-	-	-	1	-	-	-	-	-	-	2
II. Noncommunicable diseases	3 188	1 511	1 677	18	5	16	79	335	404	653	14	4	10	38	158	300	1 153
A. Malignant neoplasms	650	370	280	1	2	5	20	117	126	100	1	1	4	18	63	82	111
1. Mouth and oropharynx cancers	17	14	3	-	-	-	1	7	4	2	-	-	-	-	1	1	1
2. Oesophagus cancer	10	8	2	-	-	-	-	4	3	2	-	-	-	-	-	-	2
3. Stomach cancer	101	59	42	-	-	1	3	18	20	17	-	-	-	2	8	12	20
4. Colon and rectum cancers	69	32	37	-	-	-	-	7	11	12	-	-	1	1	6	11	18
5. Liver cancer	21	11	10	-	-	-	1	3	4	3	-	-	-	1	3	3	5
6. Pancreas cancer	29	16	13	-	-	-	1	5	6	4	-	-	-	2	4	4	2
7. Trachea, bronchus, lung cancers	144	120	24	-	-	-	5	46	46	24	-	-	-	1	6	8	9
8. Melanoma and other skin cancers	8	4	5	-	-	1	1	1	1	1	-	-	-	1	1	1	2
9. Breast cancer	40	-	40	-	-	-	-	-	-	-	-	-	-	4	13	11	11
10. Cervix uteri cancer	15	-	15	-	-	-	-	-	-	-	-	-	-	2	4	4	5
11. Corpus uteri cancer	13	-	13	-	-	-	-	-	-	-	-	-	-	1	3	4	5
12. Ovary cancer	16	-	16	-	-	-	-	-	-	-	-	-	1	1	5	5	4
13. Prostate cancer	15	15	-	-	-	-	1	1	4	9	-	-	-	-	-	-	-
14. Bladder cancer	16	12	4	-	-	-	-	2	4	5	-	-	-	1	-	1	2
15. Lymphomas, multiple myeloma	16	9	7	-	-	1	1	3	2	2	-	-	1	1	1	2	2
16. Leukaemia	19	10	9	1	1	1	1	2	3	2	1	1	1	1	2	2	2
17. Other cancers	101	60	42	1	1	2	5	18	19	15	1	1	1	2	8	12	18

Annex Table 6b, continued. Deaths by age, sex and cause (thousands): Formerly Socialist Economies of Europe, 1990

Cause	Total	Male	Female	Males							Females						
				0-4	5-14	15-29	30-44	45-59	60-69	70+	0-4	5-14	15-29	30-44	45-59	60-69	70+
B. Other neoplasms	8	4	4	-	-	-	-	1	1	1	-	-	-	-	1	1	1
C. Diabetes mellitus	30	11	19	-	-	-	1	2	4	4	-	-	-	1	3	6	9
D. Endocrine disorders	4	2	2	-	-	-	1	-	-	-	-	-	-	1	-	-	-
E. Neuro-psychiatric conditions	70	32	37	2	1	2	4	6	6	10	1	1	1	2	3	5	23
2. Bipolar disorder	6	1	5	-	-	-	-	-	-	1	-	-	1	1	-	1	1
3. Schizophrenia	4	2	2	-	-	1	-	1	-	1	-	-	1	-	-	-	1
4. Epilepsy	6	4	3	-	-	1	1	1	-	-	-	-	1	1	1	-	-
5. Alcohol use	8	7	2	-	-	-	1	2	2	1	-	-	-	-	1	2	3
6. Dementia*	17	5	12	-	-	-	-	-	1	3	-	-	-	-	-	1	10
7. Parkinson disease	7	3	4	-	-	-	-	-	1	2	-	-	-	-	-	1	4
8. Multiple sclerosis	4	2	3	-	-	-	1	1	-	-	-	-	-	1	1	1	1
9. Drug use	-	-	-	-	-	-	-	-	-	-	-	-	-	-	-	-	-
13. Other neuro-psychiatric	16	9	8	1	1	1	1	1	1	2	1	1	1	1	1	1	3
F. Sense organ diseases	-	-	-	-	-	-	-	-	-	-	-	-	-	-	-	-	-
1. Glaucoma	-	-	-	-	-	-	-	-	-	-	-	-	-	-	-	-	-
2. Cataracts	-	-	-	-	-	-	-	-	-	-	-	-	-	-	-	-	-
G. Cardiovascular diseases	2 071	885	1 186	1	-	5	39	162	215	462	1	-	2	11	68	174	931
1. Rheumatic heart disease	25	10	15	-	-	1	2	5	2	1	-	-	-	1	6	5	2
2. Ischaemic heart disease	1 027	468	559	-	-	2	22	99	113	233	-	-	-	4	30	80	445
3. Cerebrovascular disease	639	239	400	-	-	1	6	37	61	133	-	-	-	3	25	64	307
4. Inflammatory heart diseases	39	19	20	-	-	1	3	5	3	7	-	-	1	1	2	2	14
5. Other cardiovascular	341	148	193	1	-	1	6	18	35	88	-	-	1	1	5	23	163
H. Respiratory diseases	158	96	62	-	-	1	2	18	27	48	-	-	-	1	5	11	44
1. COPD*	80	49	31	-	-	-	-	8	14	25	-	-	-	-	2	5	24
2. Asthma	8	3	4	-	-	-	1	1	1	1	-	-	-	-	1	1	2
3. Other respiratory	70	44	26	-	-	1	1	9	12	21	-	-	-	1	2	5	18
I. Digestive diseases	120	69	51	1	-	1	8	22	19	17	1	-	1	3	9	13	24
1. Peptic ulcer	14	10	5	-	-	-	1	3	3	3	-	-	-	-	1	1	3
2. Cirrhosis of the liver	52	33	19	-	-	-	4	12	10	6	-	-	-	1	5	6	6
3. Appendicitis	1	-	-	-	-	-	-	-	-	-	-	-	-	-	-	-	-
4. Other digestive	54	26	27	1	-	1	3	7	6	8	1	-	1	3	4	6	15
J. Genito-urinary diseases	45	25	19	-	-	1	2	5	6	11	-	-	1	2	4	5	7
1. Nephritis and nephrosis	20	11	9	-	-	1	2	3	2	3	-	-	1	1	2	2	3
2. Benign prostatic hypertrophy	6	6	-	-	-	-	-	-	1	5	-	-	-	-	-	-	-
3. Other genito-urinary	19	8	10	-	-	-	1	2	2	4	-	-	-	1	2	3	4
K. Skin diseases	2	1	1	-	-	-	-	-	-	-	-	-	-	-	-	-	-

Annex Table 6b, continued. Deaths by age, sex and cause (thousands): Formerly Socialist Economies of Europe, 1990

Cause	Total	Male	Female	Males 0-4	5-14	15-29	30-44	45-59	60-69	70+	Females 0-4	5-14	15-29	30-44	45-59	60-69	70+
L. Musculo-skeletal diseases	5	2	3	-	-	-	-	-	-	1	-	-	-	-	-	1	1
1. Rheumatoid arthritis	1	1	1	-	-	-	-	-	-	-	-	-	-	-	-	1	-
3. Other musculo-skeletal	4	1	3	-	-	-	-	-	-	1	-	-	-	-	1	-	1
M. Congenital anomalies	27	15	12	13	1	1	-	-	-	-	10	1	-	-	-	-	-
1. Abdominal wall defect	1	-	-	1	-	-	-	-	-	-	-	-	-	-	-	-	-
2. Anencephaly	-	-	-	-	-	-	-	-	-	-	-	-	-	-	-	-	-
3. Anorectal atresia	-	-	-	-	-	-	-	-	-	-	-	-	-	-	-	-	-
4. Cleft lip	-	-	-	-	-	-	-	-	-	-	-	-	-	-	-	-	-
5. Cleft palate	-	-	-	-	-	-	-	-	-	-	-	-	-	-	-	-	-
6. Oesophageal atresia	-	-	-	-	-	-	-	-	-	-	-	-	-	-	-	-	-
7. Renal agenesis	1	-	1	-	-	-	-	-	-	-	-	-	-	-	-	-	-
8. Down syndrome	-	1	-	-	-	-	-	-	-	-	-	-	-	-	-	-	-
9. Congenital heart anomalies	11	6	5	5	-	-	-	-	-	-	4	-	-	-	-	-	-
10. Spina bifida	2	1	1	1	-	-	-	-	-	-	1	-	-	-	-	-	-
11. Other congenital	10	6	4	5	-	-	-	-	-	-	4	-	-	-	-	-	-
N. Oral conditions	-	-	-	-	-	-	-	-	-	-	-	-	-	-	-	-	-
III. Injuries	389	288	101	9	11	65	87	71	25	19	7	5	15	17	18	13	26
A. Unintentional injuries	249	187	62	6	8	41	55	47	17	13	4	3	7	8	11	8	20
1. Road traffic accidents	91	71	20	1	3	22	21	14	5	4	1	1	4	3	4	3	4
2. Poisonings	45	34	11	1	-	3	12	13	4	1	1	-	1	2	3	2	2
3. Falls	29	16	13	-	-	2	3	4	2	4	-	-	1	-	1	1	10
4. Fires	8	5	3	-	-	1	3	1	1	1	-	1	1	-	-	-	1
5. Drownings	24	20	4	1	2	5	6	4	1	1	-	1	1	1	1	-	1
6. Other unintentional	54	42	12	3	2	8	12	11	4	2	2	1	1	2	2	2	3
B. Intentional injuries	140	101	39	3	2	24	32	24	9	6	3	1	8	8	7	5	6
1. Self-inflicted injuries	81	62	19	-	-	11	20	18	7	6	-	-	2	3	5	4	5
2. Violence	30	22	8	-	-	6	9	4	1	1	-	1	1	3	2	1	1
3. War	29	17	12	3	2	7	4	1	-	-	3	1	5	2	1	-	-

Notes:
Causes responsible for no deaths have been omitted from this table.
A dash (-) symbol indicates fewer than 500 deaths.
*IA6 is Bacterial meningitis and meningococcaemia; IC3 is Hypertensive disorders of pregnancy; ID is Conditions arising during the perinatal period; IIE6 is Dementia and other degenerative and hereditary CNS disorders; IIH1 is Chronic obstructive pulmonary disease.

Annex Table 6c. Deaths by age, sex and cause (thousands): India, 1990

Cause	Total	Male	Female	Males 0-4	5-14	15-29	30-44	45-59	60-69	70+	Females 0-4	5-14	15-29	30-44	45-59	60-69	70+
Population (millions)	*850*	*439*	*410*	*60*	*102*	*121*	*79*	*48*	*19*	*11*	*57*	*95*	*111*	*72*	*46*	*19*	*10*
All causes	*9 371*	*4 875*	*4 496*	*1 600*	*256*	*251*	*343*	*665*	*738*	*1 022*	*1 650*	*294*	*306*	*261*	*479*	*569*	*937*
I. Communicable, maternal, perinatal and nutritional conditions	*4 775*	*2 418*	*2 356*	*1 411*	*129*	*96*	*147*	*202*	*183*	*252*	*1 479*	*171*	*141*	*135*	*135*	*109*	*186*
A. Infectious and parasitic diseases	2 647	1 436	1 210	679	89	83	129	182	118	156	698	105	70	68	110	62	98
1. Tuberculosis	752	502	250	15	9	52	86	152	82	106	11	7	37	36	84	30	45
2. STDs excluding HIV	68	29	40	22	-	-	-	1	1	4	23	-	5	5	1	1	4
a. Syphilis	60	29	31	22	-	-	-	1	1	4	23	-	3	3	1	1	4
b. Chlamydia	6	-	6	-	-	-	-	-	-	-	-	-	3	3	-	-	-
c. Gonorrhoea	3	-	3	-	-	-	-	-	-	-	-	-	1	1	-	-	-
3. HIV	1																
4. Diarrhoeal diseases	922	446	476	355	23	7	11	10	17	24	378	32	9	9	9	14	25
5. Childhood-cluster diseases	513	257	256	211	25	5	8	4	2	2	207	29	7	6	4	1	2
a. Pertussis	80	40	39	37	3	-	-	-	-	-	36	3	-	-	-	-	-
b. Poliomyelitis	11	6	5	6	-	-	-	-	-	-	5	-	-	-	-	-	-
c. Diphtheria	4	2	2	2	-	-	-	-	-	-	2	-	-	-	-	-	-
d. Measles	206	103	103	89	14	-	-	-	-	-	88	14	-	-	-	-	-
e. Tetanus	212	105	107	77	8	5	8	3	2	2	76	11	6	6	4	1	2
6. Bacterial meningitis*	44	23	21	12	-	1	4	2	2	1	12	-	1	3	2	2	1
7. Hepatitis B and hepatitis C	17	10	8	1	1	1	1	2	1	2	1	1	1	1	1	1	2
8. Malaria	26	14	12	3	3	2	3	1	-	1	3	4	2	2	1	-	-
9. Tropical-cluster diseases	35	21	14	1	8	7	4	1	-	-	1	6	4	2	1	-	-
a. Trypanosomiasis																	
b. Chagas disease																	
c. Schistosomiasis																	
d. Leishmaniasis	35	21	14	1	8	7	4	1	-	-	1	6	4	2	1	-	-
10. Leprosy	1	1	-	-	-	-	-	-	-	-	-	-	-	-	-	-	-
11. Dengue	12	6	7	1	4	-	-	-	-	-	1	5	-	-	-	-	-
12. Japanese encephalitis	1	-	1	-	-	-	-	-	-	-	-	-	-	-	-	-	-
13. Trachoma	-	-	-														
14. Intestinal nematode infections	3	2	2	-	1	-	-	-	-	-	-	1	-	-	-	-	-
a. Ascariasis	1	1	1	-	1	-	-	-	-	-	-	1	-	-	-	-	-
b. Trichuriasis	1	-	1	-	-	-	-	-	-	-	-	-	-	-	-	-	-
c. Ancylostomiasis, necatoriasis	1	1	1	-	1	-	-	-	-	-	-	1	-	-	-	-	-
15. Other infectious and parasitic	251	127	124	57	15	7	10	9	13	17	61	19	4	4	7	11	18

Annex Table 6c, continued. Deaths by age, sex and cause (thousands): India, 1990

Cause	Total	Male	Female	Males							Females						
				0-4	5-14	15-29	30-44	45-59	60-69	70+	0-4	5-14	15-29	30-44	45-59	60-69	70+
B. Respiratory infections	1 229	599	629	372	33	10	15	18	61	90	405	58	11	10	18	44	83
1. Lower respiratory infections	1 195	588	607	363	32	10	15	18	61	89	386	57	10	10	18	44	82
2. Upper respiratory infections	12	6	6	4	–	–	–	–	–	1	4	–	–	–	–	–	1
3. Otitis media	12	5	6	5	–	–	–	–	–	–	6	1	–	–	–	–	–
C. Maternal conditions	115		115										57	54	4		
1. Maternal haemorrhage	28		28										14	13	1		
2. Maternal sepsis	18		18										9	9			
3. Hypertensive disorders*	14		14										7	6	1		
4. Obstructed labour	9		9										5	4			
5. Abortion	17		17										8	8	1		
6. Other maternal	29		29										14	14	1		
D. Perinatal conditions*	660	326	334	326							334						
1. Low birth weight	333	164	169	164							169						
2. Birth asphyxia and birth trauma	169	87	82	87							82						
3. Other perinatal	159	75	83	75							83						
E. Nutritional deficiencies	124	57	68	34	7	3	2	2	3	6	41	8	4	3	3	3	6
1. Protein-energy malnutrition	69	30	39	23	1	1	1	1	1	2	30	3	2	1	1	1	1
2. Iodine deficiency	6	3	3	2	1	–	–	–	–	–	2	1	–	–	–	–	–
3. Vitamin A deficiency	21	10	10	7	1	1	1	–	–	–	6	4	–	–	–	–	–
4. Iron-deficiency anaemia	29	13	16	2	4	1	–	1	2	3	3	3	2	2	2	2	2
II. Noncommunicable diseases	3 788	2 001	1 788	116	48	56	108	394	533	744	117	54	71	76	302	439	730
A. Malignant neoplasms	505	253	252	4	6	11	19	77	58	78	2	3	19	22	94	56	58
1. Mouth and oropharynx cancers	80	48	32	–	–	2	3	16	13	14	–	–	2	2	13	8	7
2. Oesophagus cancer	51	26	25	–	–	1	3	9	7	6	–	–	1	1	9	7	7
3. Stomach cancer	44	28	16	–	–	1	2	10	7	8	–	–	1	1	5	4	5
4. Colon and rectum cancers	21	11	10	–	–	1	1	3	3	3	–	–	1	1	3	3	2
5. Liver cancer	13	9	4	–	–	1	1	3	2	2	–	–	–	1	1	1	1
6. Pancreas cancer	8	4	3	–	–	–	–	2	1	1	–	–	–	–	1	1	1
7. Trachea, bronchus, lung cancers	35	29	6	–	–	1	1	10	8	9	–	–	–	1	2	1	2
8. Melanoma and other skin cancers	1	–	1								–	–	–	–	–	1	–
9. Breast cancer	35	–	35								–	–	3	4	14	7	7
10. Cervix uteri cancer	49	–	49								–	–	3	4	25	9	8
11. Corpus uteri cancer	3	–	3								–	–	–	1	1	1	–
12. Ovary cancer	12	–	12								–	–	1	2	4	3	2
13. Prostate cancer	12	12	–	–	–	–	–	1	5	6							
14. Bladder cancer	7	5	2	–	–	–	–	1	2	2	–	–	–	–	1	–	1
15. Lymphomas, multiple myeloma	18	11	7	–	1	1	2	3	2	2	–	1	1	1	2	1	1
16. Leukaemia	16	9	7	–	2	1	1	2	1	2	1	1	1	1	1	1	1
17. Other cancers	103	60	43	4	3	2	5	17	7	22	1	1	5	2	12	9	13

Annex Table 6c, continued. Deaths by age, sex and cause (thousands): India, 1990

Cause	Total	Male	Female	Males							Females						
				0-4	5-14	15-29	30-44	45-59	60-69	70+	0-4	5-14	15-29	30-44	45-59	60-69	70+
B. Other neoplasms	**5**	**3**	**2**	–	–	1	1	–	–	–	–	–	–	–	–	–	–
C. Diabetes mellitus	**104**	**49**	**55**	2	4	1	3	10	12	16	2	4	2	2	11	16	18
D. Endocrine disorders	**2**	**1**	**1**	–	–	–	–	–	–	–	–	–	–	–	–	–	–
E. Neuro-psychiatric conditions	**106**	**60**	**45**	6	5	4	8	9	12	16	7	4	5	3	3	8	15
2. Bipolar disorder	2	1	1	–	–	–	–	1	–	–	–	–	–	–	–	–	1
3. Schizophrenia	5	2	2	–	–	1	–	–	1	–	–	–	–	–	–	1	1
4. Epilepsy	13	8	5	1	1	1	2	1	1	1	1	1	2	1	–	1	1
5. Alcohol use	5	5	–	–	–	–	2	2	1	–	–	–	–	–	–	–	–
6. Dementia*	22	11	11	–	–	–	–	–	3	6	1	–	–	–	–	2	7
7. Parkinson disease	6	4	2	–	–	–	–	–	1	3	–	–	–	–	–	1	1
8. Multiple sclerosis	3	1	2	–	–	–	–	1	–	–	–	–	–	–	1	1	–
9. Drug use	–	–	–	–	–	–	–	–	–	–	–	–	–	–	–	–	–
13. Other neuro-psychiatric	49	28	21	5	4	2	3	3	6	5	6	3	3	1	1	4	4
F. Sense organ diseases	**–**	**–**	**–**	–	–	–	–	–	–	–	–	–	–	–	–	–	–
1. Glaucoma	–	–	–	–	–	–	–	–	–	–	–	–	–	–	–	–	–
2. Cataracts	–	–	–	–	–	–	–	–	–	–	–	–	–	–	–	–	–
G. Cardiovascular diseases	**2 266**	**1 165**	**1 100**	16	10	16	40	206	365	513	18	15	22	27	140	314	564
1. Rheumatic heart disease	70	29	41	–	1	5	6	10	5	2	–	2	7	8	15	7	3
2. Ischaemic heart disease	1 175	619	556	–	–	1	12	111	209	286	–	–	–	8	67	169	310
3. Cerebrovascular disease	448	227	220	3	2	1	4	32	73	112	3	2	3	3	20	68	121
4. Inflammatory heart diseases	83	41	42	3	2	4	4	11	7	10	3	4	4	3	9	7	12
5. Other cardiovascular	490	249	241	10	5	6	13	42	71	102	12	8	7	4	30	63	119
H. Respiratory diseases	**267**	**150**	**117**	8	7	2	5	22	42	64	10	7	4	4	19	24	47
1. COPD*	140	84	57	2	1	–	1	11	26	42	2	1	1	1	9	14	28
2. Asthma	20	11	9	–	1	–	1	2	2	4	–	1	–	1	2	2	3
3. Other respiratory	106	56	51	6	5	1	3	9	14	18	7	5	3	3	8	8	16
I. Digestive diseases	**255**	**171**	**84**	5	4	14	27	59	27	34	5	4	11	11	24	12	16
1. Peptic ulcer	42	27	15	–	–	2	3	8	6	8	–	–	2	2	4	3	4
2. Cirrhosis of the liver	151	108	44	1	1	8	16	41	18	23	2	2	5	5	15	6	9
3. Appendicitis	12	7	5	–	2	3	2	1	–	–	–	1	2	1	–	–	–
4. Other digestive	49	29	20	4	1	2	6	9	4	4	3	–	3	3	5	3	3
J. Genito-urinary diseases	**104**	**60**	**44**	2	6	2	3	10	15	21	1	10	3	3	7	8	11
1. Nephritis and nephrosis	91	48	43	2	6	2	3	9	10	14	1	10	3	3	7	7	11
2. Benign prostatic hypertrophy	11	11	–	–	–	–	–	–	4	6	–	–	–	–	–	–	–
3. Other genito-urinary	2	1	1	–	–	–	–	–	–	–	–	–	–	–	–	–	–
K. Skin diseases	**2**	**2**	**1**	–	–	–	–	–	–	–	–	–	–	–	–	–	–

Annex Table 6c, continued. Deaths by age, sex and cause (thousands): India, 1990

Cause	Total	Male	Female	Males							Females						
				0-4	5-14	15-29	30-44	45-59	60-69	70+	0-4	5-14	15-29	30-44	45-59	60-69	70+
L. Musculo-skeletal diseases	3																
1. Rheumatoid arthritis	2	1	1	–	–	–	–	1	–	–	–	–	–	–	1	1	–
3. Other musculo-skeletal	1	1		–	–	–	–	–	–	–	–	–	–	–	–	–	–
M. Congenital anomalies	170	85	85	72	5	3	2	1	1	1	70	6	3	2	2	1	1
1. Abdominal wall defect	1	1	–	1	–	–	–	–	–	–	1	–	–	–	–	–	–
2. Anencephaly	46	18	28	18	–	–	–	–	–	–	28	–	–	–	–	–	–
3. Anorectal atresia	1	1	–	1	–	–	–	–	–	–	–	–	–	–	–	–	–
4. Cleft lip	1	1	–	1	–	–	–	–	–	–	–	–	–	–	–	–	–
5. Cleft palate	1	1	–	–	–	–	–	–	–	–	–	–	–	–	–	–	–
6. Oesophageal atresia	1	1	–	1	–	–	–	–	–	–	–	–	–	–	–	–	–
7. Renal agenesis	2	1	1	1	–	–	–	–	–	–	1	1	1	–	–	–	–
8. Down syndrome	16	9	7	5	2	2	1	–	–	–	3	3	1	–	–	–	–
9. Congenital heart anomalies	57	30	27	24	3	1	1	1	1	–	19	1	1	1	–	1	–
10. Spina bifida	21	11	10	11	1	–	–	–	–	–	9	1	–	–	–	–	–
11. Other congenital	22	12	11	10	1	1	–	–	–	–	8	1	1	–	–	–	–
N. Oral conditions	–																
III. Injuries	808	456	352	73	79	99	88	69	22	26	55	69	94	50	43	21	20
A. Unintentional injuries	650	366	284	67	75	70	66	49	18	21	47	65	66	38	32	18	18
1. Road traffic accidents	174	124	50	17	19	33	26	17	5	7	5	14	7	6	10	4	4
2. Poisonings	30	16	14	5	3	3	3	2	1	–	3	2	4	3	2	–	–
3. Falls	46	30	16	4	8	3	4	5	3	4	4	4	1	1	2	2	3
4. Fires	124	37	87	9	4	8	8	6	1	2	8	12	36	17	6	4	4
5. Drownings	89	48	41	11	16	8	6	3	1	2	9	16	6	3	3	1	2
6. Other unintentional	187	112	75	22	25	16	19	17	7	7	19	17	11	7	8	6	6
B. Intentional injuries	158	90	68	6	4	29	22	19	4	5	7	4	28	12	11	3	2
1. Self-inflicted injuries	99	54	45	–	3	20	14	12	2	3	–	3	25	11	5	1	1
2. Violence	56	33	23	6	2	6	8	7	2	2	7	1	3	1	6	3	1
3. War	3	3	–	–	–	2	1	–	–	–	–	–	–	–	–	–	–

Notes:
Causes responsible for no deaths have been omitted from this table.
A dash (-) symbol indicates fewer than 500 deaths.
*IA6 is Bacterial meningitis and meningococcaemia; IC3 is Hypertensive disorders of pregnancy; ID is Conditions arising during the perinatal period;
IIE6 is Dementia and other degenerative and hereditary CNS disorders; IIH1 is Chronic obstructive pulmonary disease.

Annex Table 6d. Deaths by age, sex and cause (thousands): China, 1990

Cause	Total	Male	Female	Males 0-4	5-14	15-29	30-44	45-59	60-69	70+	Females 0-4	5-14	15-29	30-44	45-59	60-69	70+
Population (millions)	1 134	585	548	60	97	184	122	73	31	18	58	90	172	113	64	30	22
All causes	8 885	4 829	4 056	505	86	279	347	746	1 061	1 805	565	63	231	233	462	695	1 807
I. Communicable, maternal, perinatal and nutritional conditions	1 405	708	697	342	16	19	35	71	74	151	399	17	37	36	37	47	124
A. Infectious and parasitic diseases	544	315	229	61	9	14	33	65	60	75	66	9	11	23	31	35	54
1. Tuberculosis	278	173	104	3	1	7	18	47	46	53	3	2	7	15	24	24	30
2. STDs excluding HIV	1	-	-	-	-	-	-	-	-	-	-	-	-	-	-	-	-
a. Syphilis	1	-	-	-	-	-	-	-	-	-	-	-	-	-	-	-	-
b. Chlamydia	-	-	-	-	-	-	-	-	-	-	-	-	-	-	-	-	-
c. Gonorrhoea	-	-	-	-	-	-	-	-	-	-	-	-	-	-	-	-	-
3. HIV	-	-	-	-	-	-	-	-	-	-	-	-	-	-	-	-	-
4. Diarrhoeal diseases	93	44	48	22	1	2	1	2	5	11	28	1	1	1	1	2	14
5. Childhood-cluster diseases	53	28	25	24	2	1	1	-	-	-	22	2	1	-	-	-	-
a. Pertussis	17	9	8	8	1	-	-	-	-	-	8	1	-	-	-	-	-
b. Poliomyelitis	3	1	1	1	1	-	-	-	-	-	1	1	-	-	-	-	-
c. Diphtheria	-	-	-	1	-	-	-	-	-	-	1	-	-	-	-	-	-
d. Measles	15	8	7	6	1	1	-	-	-	-	6	1	-	-	-	-	-
e. Tetanus	18	10	8	8	1	1	-	-	-	-	7	-	-	-	-	-	-
6. Bacterial meningitis*	41	21	20	7	-	1	5	3	3	2	7	-	1	5	3	3	2
7. Hepatitis B and hepatitis C	34	23	12	2	-	3	5	7	2	4	2	-	1	1	1	3	3
8. Malaria	1	1	-	-	-	-	-	-	-	-	-	-	-	-	-	-	-
9. Tropical-cluster diseases	1	1	1	-	-	-	-	-	-	-	-	-	-	-	-	-	-
a. Trypanosomiasis	-	-	-	-	-	-	-	-	-	-	-	-	-	-	-	-	-
b. Chagas disease	-	-	-	-	-	-	-	-	-	-	-	-	-	-	-	-	-
c. Schistosomiasis	1	1	-	-	-	-	-	-	-	-	-	-	-	-	-	-	-
d. Leishmaniasis	-	-	-	-	-	-	-	-	-	-	-	-	-	-	-	-	-
10. Leprosy	-	-	-	-	-	-	-	-	-	-	-	-	-	-	-	-	-
11. Dengue	1	-	1	-	-	-	-	-	-	-	-	-	-	-	-	-	-
12. Japanese encephalitis	3	1	1	1	-	-	-	-	-	-	1	-	-	-	-	-	-
13. Trachoma	-	-	-	-	-	-	-	-	-	-	-	-	-	-	-	-	-
14. Intestinal nematode infections	7	4	3	-	-	-	-	-	-	-	-	-	-	-	-	-	-
a. Ascariasis	4	2	3	-	3	-	-	-	-	-	-	3	-	-	-	-	-
b. Trichuriasis	2	1	2	-	2	-	-	-	-	-	-	2	-	-	-	-	-
c. Ancylostomiasis, necatoriasis	-	-	1	-	1	-	-	-	-	-	-	1	-	-	-	-	-
15. Other infectious and parasitic	33	19	14	3	-	1	2	5	3	5	3	-	1	1	2	2	6

Annex Table 6d, continued. Deaths by age, sex and cause (thousands): China, 1990

Cause	Total	Male	Female	Males 0-4	5-14	15-29	30-44	45-59	60-69	70+	Females 0-4	5-14	15-29	30-44	45-59	60-69	70+
B. Respiratory infections	**474**	**229**	**245**	**132**	**4**	**3**	**2**	**5**	**12**	**71**	**159**	**4**	**3**	**2**	**3**	**9**	**64**
1. Lower respiratory infections	467	226	241	129	4	3	2	5	12	70	156	4	3	2	3	9	63
2. Upper respiratory infections	5	2	2	1	–	–	–	–	–	1	2	–	–	–	–	–	1
3. Otitis media	2	1	1	1	–	–	–	–	–	–	1	–	–	–	–	–	–
C. Maternal conditions	**30**		**30**										**20**	**8**	**2**		
1. Maternal haemorrhage	12		12										8	3	1		
2. Maternal sepsis	1		1										1				
3. Hypertensive disorders*	2		2										2	1			
4. Obstructed labour	–		–														
5. Abortion	3		3										2	1			
6. Other maternal	12		12										8	3	1		
D. Perinatal conditions*	**276**	**133**	**144**	**133**							**144**						
1. Low birth weight	46	24	22	24							22						
2. Birth asphyxia and birth trauma	147	67	80	67							80						
3. Other perinatal	83	41	42	41							42						
E. Nutritional deficiencies	**80**	**31**	**49**	**17**	**3**	**2**	**1**	**1**	**2**	**5**	**31**	**4**	**2**	**3**	**1**	**3**	**6**
1. Protein-energy malnutrition	38	14	24	8				1	1	4	19				1	1	3
2. Iodine deficiency	8	4	4	3	1						3	1					
3. Vitamin A deficiency	9	5	5	3	1	1					3	1	1				
4. Iron-deficiency anaemia	25	8	17	2	2	1		1	1	2	5	2	1	3	1	2	3
II. Noncommunicable diseases	**6 460**	**3 531**	**2 929**	**88**	**29**	**106**	**199**	**594**	**933**	**1 583**	**95**	**19**	**80**	**139**	**376**	**612**	**1 608**
A. Malignant neoplasms	**1 464**	**924**	**540**	**5**	**10**	**30**	**86**	**248**	**295**	**250**	**7**	**5**	**20**	**53**	**129**	**151**	**174**
1. Mouth and oropharynx cancers	36	25	11			1	5	7	7	5			1	2	3	3	2
2. Oesophagus cancer	189	129	60			1	6	31	47	44				1	12	25	23
3. Stomach cancer	319	209	110			1	9	55	78	66			2	9	22	34	43
4. Colon and rectum cancers	83	46	37			2	4	11	14	15			1	3	9	11	13
5. Liver cancer	293	213	80			6	41	77	56	34	1	1	2	10	23	22	24
6. Pancreas cancer	32	20	13			1	1	4	7	7					2	5	6
7. Trachea, bronchus, lung cancers	218	152	66			2	3	35	60	51			1	2	15	20	28
8. Melanoma and other skin cancers	1	1	–														
9. Breast cancer	26	–	26											6	8	5	6
10. Cervix uteri cancer	21	–	21											3	7	6	5
11. Corpus uteri cancer	6	–	6												3	1	1
12. Ovary cancer	10	–	10											2	3	2	2
13. Prostate cancer	5	5	–						2	3							
14. Bladder cancer	19	15	4				2	2	5	6						2	2
15. Lymphomas, multiple myeloma	23	15	8			3	2	3	4	3			1	1	3	2	1
16. Leukaemia	66	34	32	3	5	8	6	6	3	3	3	3	7	6	5	3	4
17. Other cancers	115	61	55	2	2	6	9	17	12	13	3	1	3	7	14	12	14

Annex Table 6d, continued. Deaths by age, sex and cause (thousands): China, 1990

Cause	Total	Male	Female	Males 0-4	5-14	15-29	30-44	45-59	60-69	70+	Females 0-4	5-14	15-29	30-44	45-59	60-69	70+
B. Other neoplasms	21	11	10	1	-	2	1	2	3	2	1	1	1	1	2	3	2
C. Diabetes mellitus	60	27	33	-	-	1	3	6	8	9	-	-	1	2	6	11	12
D. Endocrine disorders	14	5	9	2	-	-	1	1	1	2	2	-	1	1	1	1	3
E. Neuro-psychiatric conditions	98	53	46	2	2	14	10	5	5	14	2	1	7	7	5	6	18
2. Bipolar disorder	3	1	2	-	-	1	-	-	-	-	-	-	1	1	-	-	-
3. Schizophrenia	15	10	5	-	-	3	4	1	1	1	-	-	1	1	1	1	1
4. Epilepsy	12	7	5	-	-	3	1	1	1	1	-	-	2	1	1	-	1
5. Alcohol use	5	4	-	-	-	-	2	1	1	-	-	-	-	-	-	-	-
6. Dementia*	27	11	16	-	-	-	-	1	3	6	-	-	-	-	1	3	10
7. Parkinson disease	5	3	2	-	-	-	-	-	1	2	-	-	-	-	-	1	1
8. Multiple sclerosis	5	2	3	-	-	-	-	1	1	-	-	-	-	1	1	1	-
9. Drug use	-	-	-	-	-	-	-	-	-	-	-	-	-	-	-	-	-
13. Other neuro-psychiatric	26	14	12	1	1	6	2	1	1	2	1	1	3	3	1	1	2
F. Sense organ diseases	18	10	8	1	-	-	-	2	3	2	1	-	-	-	2	3	2
1. Glaucoma	6	4	3	-	-	-	-	2	1	1	-	-	-	-	1	1	1
2. Cataracts	6	3	2	-	-	-	-	-	1	1	-	-	-	-	-	1	1
G. Cardiovascular diseases	2 568	1 322	1 246	10	4	28	47	192	337	704	7	2	25	42	143	254	772
1. Rheumatic heart disease	163	69	94	-	1	10	7	13	12	26	1	1	9	11	19	17	37
2. Ischaemic heart disease	762	386	377	-	-	5	15	53	96	217	-	-	3	12	37	74	251
3. Cerebrovascular disease	1 272	672	601	2	2	7	18	98	186	359	2	1	5	13	71	137	372
4. Inflammatory heart diseases	66	33	33	2	1	4	3	7	5	11	1	1	4	4	6	4	13
5. Other cardiovascular	305	163	142	6	1	2	3	22	38	91	3	-	5	2	10	22	100
H. Respiratory diseases	1 530	789	741	10	1	5	10	67	204	491	14	1	2	10	47	138	530
1. COPD*	1 432	737	695	4	-	3	7	62	195	465	10	-	-	8	44	131	502
2. Asthma	35	19	16	-	1	1	2	3	4	8	-	-	1	1	3	3	8
3. Other respiratory	63	33	30	5	-	2	1	2	5	18	4	-	1	1	2	3	20
I. Digestive diseases	411	241	170	17	3	10	32	57	57	65	19	3	8	12	30	32	66
1. Peptic ulcer	33	19	14	-	-	1	2	3	4	9	-	-	-	-	2	3	9
2. Cirrhosis of the liver	187	123	64	-	1	4	24	37	34	23	1	1	2	6	17	18	19
3. Appendicitis	12	7	5	2	1	1	1	1	1	-	1	1	2	1	-	-	-
4. Other digestive	179	92	87	15	1	3	5	16	18	33	18	1	4	5	11	12	37
J. Genito-urinary diseases	124	73	50	2	1	5	9	8	14	28	2	1	5	8	8	11	16
1. Nephritis and nephrosis	99	57	42	2	1	5	9	7	11	17	2	1	5	7	7	8	12
2. Benign prostatic hypertrophy	7	7	-	-	-	-	-	1	2	6	-	-	-	-	-	-	-
3. Other genito-urinary	18	10	9	-	-	-	1	1	2	5	-	-	-	1	2	3	4
K. Skin diseases	12	7	5	-	1	1	-	1	1	2	-	1	1	-	-	1	2

Annex Table 6d, continued. Deaths by age, sex and cause (thousands): China, 1990

Cause	Total	Male	Female	Males 0-4	Males 5-14	Males 15-29	Males 30-44	Males 45-59	Males 60-69	Males 70+	Females 0-4	Females 5-14	Females 15-29	Females 30-44	Females 45-59	Females 60-69	Females 70+
L. Musculo-skeletal diseases	**36**	**17**	**19**	-	-	1	1	1	5	11	-	-	1	2	2	2	11
1. Rheumatoid arthritis	2	1	1	-	-	-	-	-	-	1	-	-	-	-	-	-	1
3. Other musculo-skeletal	34	16	18	-	-	1	1	1	4	10	-	-	1	2	2	2	11
M. Congenital anomalies	**105**	**51**	**54**	40	5	5	1	-	-	-	41	5	7	1	-	-	-
1. Abdominal wall defect	1	1	-	1	-	-	-	-	-	-	-	-	-	-	-	-	-
2. Anencephaly	39	15	24	15	-	-	-	-	-	-	24	-	-	-	-	-	-
3. Anorectal atresia	1	1	-	1	-	-	-	-	-	-	-	-	-	-	-	-	-
4. Cleft lip	1	-	1	-	-	-	-	-	-	-	1	-	-	-	-	-	-
5. Cleft palate	1	1	-	-	-	-	-	-	-	-	-	-	-	-	-	-	-
6. Oesophageal atresia	-	-	-	-	-	-	-	-	-	-	-	-	-	-	-	-	-
7. Renal agenesis	-	-	-	-	-	-	-	-	-	-	-	-	-	-	-	-	-
8. Down syndrome	12	6	7	3	-	-	-	-	-	-	3	1	-	-	-	-	-
9. Congenital heart anomalies	29	16	13	11	1	2	-	-	-	-	7	2	-	-	-	-	-
10. Spina bifida	12	7	5	6	1	-	-	-	-	-	4	1	-	-	-	-	-
11. Other congenital	9	5	4	3	1	1	-	-	-	-	2	1	1	-	-	-	-
N. Oral conditions	-	-	-	-	-	-	-	-	-	-	-	-	-	-	-	-	-
III. Injuries	**1 020**	**590**	**430**	75	42	154	113	81	54	71	71	27	114	58	50	36	75
A. Unintentional injuries	**626**	**400**	**226**	71	38	99	69	51	30	42	62	24	36	21	22	17	43
1. Road traffic accidents	135	97	38	4	6	27	28	17	9	7	3	5	9	6	8	3	4
2. Poisonings	65	38	27	5	2	7	7	9	3	6	2	2	9	5	2	3	4
3. Falls	65	32	33	2	2	6	4	4	5	10	4	1	1	1	3	5	18
4. Fires	24	14	10	3	1	2	2	1	-	5	2	1	1	1	1	1	4
5. Drownings	147	91	56	30	22	20	6	4	3	5	26	11	7	3	2	2	5
6. Other unintentional	190	128	62	26	7	37	23	16	9	10	27	4	8	6	6	3	9
B. Intentional injuries	**394**	**190**	**204**	9	3	55	44	30	24	29	9	3	78	36	28	19	32
1. Self-inflicted injuries	343	159	184	-	2	42	37	27	23	28	-	2	76	33	26	18	30
2. Violence	51	30	20	5	1	13	7	3	2	-	9	1	2	4	2	1	1
3. War	1	1	-	-	-	-	-	-	-	-	-	-	-	-	-	-	-

Notes:

Causes responsible for no deaths have been omitted from this table.

A dash (-) symbol indicates fewer than 500 deaths.

"IA6 is Bacterial meningitis and meningococcaemia; IC3 is Hypertensive disorders of pregnancy; ID is Conditions arising during the perinatal period; IIE6 is Dementia and other degenerative and hereditary CNS disorders; IIH1 is Chronic obstructive pulmonary disease.

Annex Table 6e. Deaths by age, sex and cause (thousands): Other Asia and Islands, 1990

Cause	Total	Male	Female	Males							Females						
				0-4	5-14	15-29	30-44	45-59	60-69	70+	0-4	5-14	15-29	30-44	45-59	60-69	70+
Population (millions)	*683*	*343*	*340*	*44*	*84*	*99*	*62*	*34*	*13*	*7*	*42*	*80*	*98*	*62*	*35*	*14*	*9*
All causes	5 534	3 044	2 490	901	230	209	248	398	421	637	716	172	158	184	278	314	668
I. Communicable, maternal, perinatal and nutritional conditions	2 190	1 161	1 029	747	82	38	42	70	78	104	586	72	61	74	70	54	112
A. Infectious and parasitic diseases	1 176	630	546	346	50	31	37	62	48	56	274	44	30	42	59	39	58
1. Tuberculosis	320	163	157	1	2	14	20	46	37	42	–	2	13	21	45	33	43
2. STDs excluding HIV	45	21	23	17	–	–	–	1	1	2	12	–	3	4	1	1	3
a. Syphilis	39	21	17	17	–	–	–	1	1	2	12	–	–	2	1	1	1
b. Chlamydia	4	–	4	–	–	–	–	–	–	–	–	–	2	2	–	–	–
c. Gonorrhoea	2	–	2	–	–	–	–	–	–	–	–	–	1	1	–	–	–
3. HIV	–	–	–	–	–	–	–	–	–	–	–	–	–	–	–	–	–
4. Diarrhoeal diseases	397	226	171	202	13	1	1	2	3	3	150	9	1	2	3	2	4
5. Childhood-cluster diseases	227	119	109	97	13	2	3	2	1	1	87	13	3	3	2	1	1
a. Pertussis	33	18	16	16	1	–	–	–	–	–	15	1	–	–	–	–	–
b. Poliomyelitis	3	2	1	2	–	–	–	–	–	–	1	–	–	–	–	–	–
c. Diphtheria	2	1	1	1	–	–	–	–	–	–	1	–	–	–	–	–	–
d. Measles	113	60	54	52	8	–	–	–	–	–	47	7	–	–	–	–	–
e. Tetanus	75	38	37	26	4	2	3	2	1	1	23	5	3	3	2	1	1
6. Bacterial meningitis*	24	13	12	6	–	–	3	2	1	1	5	–	–	3	2	1	1
7. Hepatitis B and hepatitis C	19	11	8	2	1	1	2	2	2	1	1	1	1	1	1	1	2
8. Malaria	77	41	37	5	12	10	7	4	2	1	5	10	8	7	4	1	1
9. Tropical-cluster diseases	3	2	1	–	–	–	–	–	–	–	–	–	–	–	–	–	–
a. Trypanosomiasis	–	–	–	–	–	–	–	–	–	–	–	–	–	–	–	–	–
b. Chagas disease	–	–	–	–	–	–	–	–	–	–	–	–	–	–	–	–	–
c. Schistosomiasis	1	1	–	–	–	–	–	–	–	–	–	–	–	–	–	–	–
d. Leishmaniasis	2	1	1	–	–	–	–	–	–	–	–	–	–	–	–	–	–
10. Leprosy	1	–	–	–	–	–	–	–	–	–	–	–	–	–	–	–	–
11. Dengue	7	3	4	1	2	–	–	–	–	–	1	3	–	–	–	–	–
12. Japanese encephalitis	1	1	1	–	–	–	–	–	–	–	–	–	–	–	–	–	–
13. Trachoma	–	–	–	–	–	–	–	–	–	–	–	–	–	–	–	–	–
14. Intestinal nematode infections	7	4	3	–	3	–	–	–	–	–	–	3	–	–	–	–	–
a. Ascariasis	3	2	1	–	2	–	–	–	–	–	–	1	–	–	–	–	–
b. Trichuriasis	3	1	1	–	1	–	–	–	–	–	–	1	–	–	–	–	–
c. Ancylostomiasis, necatoriasis	1	1	1	–	–	–	–	–	–	–	–	–	–	–	–	–	–
15. Other infectious and parasitic	48	26	22	15	3	1	1	2	1	3	11	3	1	1	1	1	3

Annex Table 6e, continued. Deaths by age, sex and cause (thousands): Other Asia and Islands, 1990

Cause	Total	Male	Female	Males							Females						
				0-4	5-14	15-29	30-44	45-59	60-69	70+	0-4	5-14	15-29	30-44	45-59	60-69	70+
B. Respiratory infections	552	307	245	189	28	6	4	6	28	46	140	24	5	4	6	13	51
1. Lower respiratory infections	543	302	241	185	27	6	4	6	28	46	138	24	5	4	6	13	51
2. Upper respiratory infections	6	3	3	2	1	–	–	–	–	–	1	–	–	–	–	–	–
3. Otitis media	3	2	1	2	–	–	–	–	–	–	1	–	–	–	–	–	–
C. Maternal conditions	52	–	52	–	–	–	–	–	–	–	–	–	24	26	2	–	–
1. Maternal haemorrhage	13	–	13	–	–	–	–	–	–	–	–	–	6	6	1	–	–
2. Maternal sepsis	8	–	8	–	–	–	–	–	–	–	–	–	4	4	–	–	–
3. Hypertensive disorders*	6	–	6	–	–	–	–	–	–	–	–	–	3	3	–	–	–
4. Obstructed labour	4	–	4	–	–	–	–	–	–	–	–	–	2	2	–	–	–
5. Abortion	7	–	7	–	–	–	–	–	–	–	–	–	3	4	–	–	–
6. Other maternal	14	–	14	–	–	–	–	–	–	–	–	–	6	7	1	–	–
D. Perinatal conditions*	331	184	147	184	–	–	–	–	–	–	147	–	–	–	–	–	–
1. Low birth weight	164	91	73	91	–	–	–	–	–	–	73	–	–	–	–	–	–
2. Birth asphyxia and birth trauma	77	43	34	43	–	–	–	–	–	–	34	–	–	–	–	–	–
3. Other perinatal	90	51	39	51	–	–	–	–	–	–	39	–	–	–	–	–	–
E. Nutritional deficiencies	79	40	39	28	5	2	1	1	1	2	25	4	2	2	2	1	3
1. Protein–energy malnutrition	41	21	19	19	–	–	–	–	–	2	17	–	–	–	–	–	2
2. Iodine deficiency	3	1	1	1	–	–	–	–	–	–	1	–	–	–	–	–	–
3. Vitamin A deficiency	18	9	8	6	3	–	–	–	–	–	5	3	–	–	–	–	–
4. Iron-deficiency anaemia	18	8	10	2	2	2	1	1	–	–	2	1	2	2	2	1	–
II. Noncommunicable diseases	2 785	1 499	1 286	99	90	53	125	285	327	520	85	71	52	84	194	252	548
A. Malignant neoplasms	640	361	280	7	18	8	30	90	103	105	7	12	12	30	69	71	79
1. Mouth and oropharynx cancers	68	42	26	–	–	1	3	6	15	17	–	–	1	2	3	9	11
2. Oesophagus cancer	22	15	7	–	–	–	1	4	5	5	–	–	–	–	1	2	4
3. Stomach cancer	57	37	20	–	–	1	2	12	11	11	–	–	1	2	5	6	6
4. Colon and rectum cancers	40	21	19	–	–	–	2	3	8	8	–	–	1	1	5	5	7
5. Liver cancer	67	49	18	1	1	1	5	19	11	11	1	–	–	2	4	5	6
6. Pancreas cancer	10	6	4	–	–	–	–	2	2	2	–	–	–	–	1	2	1
7. Trachea, bronchus, lung cancers	85	64	21	–	–	1	2	19	21	21	–	–	–	2	5	6	8
8. Melanoma and other skin cancers	2	1	1	–	–	–	–	–	–	1	–	–	–	–	–	–	1
9. Breast cancer	28	–	28	–	–	–	–	–	–	–	–	–	2	4	11	5	6
10. Cervix uteri cancer	33	–	33	–	–	–	–	–	–	–	–	–	2	4	14	6	7
11. Corpus uteri cancer	4	–	4	–	–	–	–	–	–	–	–	–	–	1	1	1	1
12. Ovary cancer	11	–	11	–	–	–	–	–	–	–	–	–	2	2	3	2	2
13. Prostate cancer	13	13	–	–	–	–	–	1	6	6	–	–	–	–	–	–	–
14. Bladder cancer	11	8	3	–	–	–	–	2	3	3	–	–	–	–	–	2	1
15. Lymphomas, multiple myeloma	25	15	10	–	1	1	2	3	4	4	–	–	1	1	2	3	3
16. Leukaemia	31	17	14	3	6	1	3	–	2	2	3	4	1	2	1	2	1
17. Other cancers	133	75	59	3	8	2	8	17	19	18	3	5	3	8	13	13	14

Annex Table 6e, continued. Deaths by age, sex and cause (thousands): Other Asia and Islands, 1990

Cause	Total	Male	Female	Males							Females						
				0-4	5-14	15-29	30-44	45-59	60-69	70+	0-4	5-14	15-29	30-44	45-59	60-69	70+
B. Other neoplasms	10	5	5	1	1	-	1	1	1	1	1	1	1	1	1	1	1
C. Diabetes mellitus	59	26	33	-	1	1	2	6	7	8	-	1	1	2	7	10	12
D. Endocrine disorders	9	4	5	1	1	-	-	-	-	1	1	1	-	-	1	1	1
E. Neuro-psychiatric conditions	69	40	30	2	3	5	7	7	5	10	2	3	3	2	4	5	11
2. Bipolar disorder	2	1	1	-	-	-	1	-	1	1	-	-	1	1	1	1	1
3. Schizophrenia	5	3	3	-	-	1	1	1	-	-	-	-	1	1	1	1	1
4. Epilepsy	9	5	3	1	1	1	1	1	-	1	-	1	1	1	-	-	-
5. Alcohol use	9	5	3	-	-	1	2	2	1	1	-	-	1	1	2	1	1
6. Dementia*	18	8	10	-	-	-	-	1	2	5	-	-	-	1	1	2	6
7. Parkinson disease	4	3	1	-	-	-	-	-	1	2	-	-	-	-	-	-	1
8. Multiple sclerosis	2	1	1	-	-	-	1	-	-	-	-	-	-	1	-	-	-
9. Drug use	2	2	-	-	-	1	1	-	-	-	-	-	-	-	-	-	-
13. Other neuro-psychiatric	23	13	10	2	3	2	2	2	1	2	2	2	1	1	1	1	2
F. Sense organ diseases	-	-	-	-	-	-	-	-	-	-	-	-	-	-	-	-	-
1. Glaucoma	-	-	-	-	-	-	-	-	-	-	-	-	-	-	-	-	-
2. Cataracts	-	-	-	-	-	-	-	-	-	-	-	-	-	-	-	-	-
G. Cardiovascular diseases	1 349	681	667	31	43	27	49	102	138	291	28	37	24	32	75	119	353
1. Rheumatic heart disease	10	5	6	-	-	1	-	1	1	2	-	-	-	1	1	1	3
2. Ischaemic heart disease	461	233	227	-	-	1	15	36	57	125	-	-	1	10	24	47	146
3. Cerebrovascular disease	390	190	200	4	8	6	11	29	46	87	4	6	4	7	24	42	114
4. Inflammatory heart diseases	82	43	39	6	10	5	6	6	3	7	6	9	4	4	5	3	8
5. Other cardiovascular	406	210	196	21	25	15	17	30	31	70	18	22	15	11	22	26	83
H. Respiratory diseases	148	87	61	10	4	2	3	9	17	41	8	3	2	2	5	10	31
1. COPD*	77	47	30	2	1	1	1	5	11	27	1	1	1	1	3	5	18
2. Asthma	18	10	8	2	1	1	1	2	1	2	2	1	1	-	-	1	3
3. Other respiratory	54	31	23	8	2	1	1	3	5	11	5	1	-	1	2	4	10
I. Digestive diseases	315	200	115	11	10	5	27	59	44	44	8	7	4	10	24	24	37
1. Peptic ulcer	24	14	9	-	1	-	-	3	4	6	-	-	-	1	1	2	5
2. Cirrhosis of the liver	131	95	36	1	1	2	17	37	22	15	1	1	1	4	11	9	9
3. Appendicitis	10	6	4	1	2	2	1	-	-	-	-	2	1	-	1	-	-
4. Other digestive	150	85	65	9	6	1	8	19	18	23	7	4	2	5	11	13	23
J. Genito-urinary diseases	98	48	50	8	3	2	4	8	9	14	1	3	3	4	9	11	19
1. Nephritis and nephrosis	85	41	44	8	3	2	4	7	8	9	1	3	3	4	8	9	17
2. Benign prostatic hypertrophy	1	1	-	-	-	-	-	-	-	1	-	-	-	-	-	-	-
3. Other genito-urinary	13	6	6	-	-	-	-	1	1	3	-	-	-	-	1	2	3
K. Skin diseases	2	1	1	-	-	-	-	-	-	-	-	-	-	-	-	-	-

Annex Table 6e, continued. Deaths by age, sex and cause (thousands): Other Asia and Islands, 1990

Cause	Total	Male	Female	Males							Females						
				0-4	5-14	15-29	30-44	45-59	60-69	70+	0-4	5-14	15-29	30-44	45-59	60-69	70+
L. Musculo-skeletal diseases	9	4	5	-	-	-	-	1	1	1	-	1	-	1	1	1	2
1. Rheumatoid arthritis	1	-	-	-	-	-	-	1	-	-	-	-	-	1	1	-	-
3. Other musculo-skeletal	8	3	5	-	-	-	-	1	1	1	-	1	-	-	1	1	2
M. Congenital anomalies	75	40	34	34	3	2	1	1	-	-	28	3	1	1	1	-	-
1. Abdominal wall defect	1	-	-	-	-	-	-	-	-	-	-	-	-	-	-	-	-
2. Anencephaly	19	8	12	8	-	-	-	-	-	-	12	-	-	-	-	-	-
3. Anorectal atresia	-	-	-	-	-	-	-	-	-	-	-	-	-	-	-	-	-
4. Cleft lip	1	1	-	1	-	-	-	-	-	-	-	-	-	-	-	-	-
5. Cleft palate	1	-	-	-	-	-	-	-	-	-	-	-	-	-	-	-	-
6. Oesophageal atresia	-	-	-	-	-	-	-	-	-	-	-	-	-	-	-	-	-
7. Renal agenesis	2	1	1	1	-	-	-	-	-	-	1	-	-	-	-	-	-
8. Down syndrome	6	4	2	3	-	-	-	-	-	-	2	-	-	-	-	-	-
9. Congenital heart anomalies	29	17	12	14	1	1	-	1	-	-	8	1	1	-	1	-	-
10. Spina bifida	6	3	3	3	1	-	-	-	-	-	1	1	-	-	-	-	-
11. Other congenital	10	6	4	5	1	-	-	-	-	-	3	1	-	-	-	-	-
N. Oral conditions	-	-	-	-	-	-	-	-	-	-	-	-	-	-	-	-	-
III. Injuries	559	384	175	54	58	117	81	44	16	13	45	28	46	25	14	9	8
A. Unintentional injuries	426	294	132	52	53	82	56	31	12	9	42	25	26	15	11	7	6
1. Road traffic accidents	133	94	39	13	14	29	21	11	4	3	12	7	7	5	4	3	2
2. Poisonings	36	19	16	2	3	6	4	3	1	1	2	3	6	3	1	1	1
3. Falls	34	25	9	4	2	6	6	4	2	1	3	1	1	1	1	1	1
4. Fires	10	6	4	2	1	1	1	-	-	-	2	1	1	-	-	-	-
5. Drownings	85	59	26	19	21	10	4	2	1	1	12	8	3	1	1	1	1
6. Other unintentional	128	91	37	12	13	30	20	11	4	2	12	6	7	5	3	2	2
B. Intentional injuries	133	90	43	3	5	35	25	13	4	4	3	3	20	10	4	2	2
1. Self-inflicted injuries	67	40	27	-	2	16	10	6	3	3	-	1	14	6	2	1	1
2. Violence	51	41	10	1	2	15	13	6	1	1	1	1	3	3	2	1	-
3. War	15	9	6	2	1	4	2	-	-	-	2	1	2	1	-	-	-

Notes:
Causes responsible for no deaths have been omitted from this table.
A dash (-) symbol indicates fewer than 500 deaths.
"IA6 is Bacterial meningitis and meningococcaemia; IC3 is Hypertensive disorders of pregnancy; ID is Conditions arising during the perinatal period; IIE6 is Dementia and other degenerative and hereditary CNS disorders; IIH1 is Chronic obstructive pulmonary disease.

Annex Table 6f. Deaths by age, sex and cause (thousands): Sub-Saharan Africa, 1990

Cause	Total	Male	Female	Males 0-4	5-14	15-29	30-44	45-59	60-69	70+	Females 0-4	5-14	15-29	30-44	45-59	60-69	70+
Population (millions)	*510*	*252*	*258*	*47*	*70*	*67*	*37*	*20*	*7*	*3*	*47*	*70*	*67*	*39*	*22*	*8*	*5*
All causes	*8 202*	*4 324*	*3 878*	*2 169*	*385*	*454*	*353*	*340*	*262*	*360*	*1 861*	*355*	*367*	*315*	*288*	*255*	*437*
I. Communicable, maternal, perinatal and nutritional conditions	*5 316*	*2 671*	*2 645*	*2 008*	*203*	*121*	*107*	*85*	*57*	*92*	*1 720*	*213*	*247*	*224*	*79*	*58*	*103*
A. Infectious and parasitic diseases	3 456	1 793	1 663	1 283	151	112	101	78	36	33	1 090	158	152	123	71	34	34
1. Tuberculosis	386	186	200	18	11	49	35	44	19	10	20	16	57	40	40	17	10
2. STDs excluding HIV	89	40	49	33				1	1	4	31		5	4	2	2	5
a. Syphilis	80	40	40	33				1	1	4	31			1	2	2	5
b. Chlamydia	5		5										3	2			
c. Gonorrhoea	4		4										2	1			
3. HIV	239	112	126	32	4	29	36	8	2	1	30	4	44	40	6	1	1
4. Diarrhoeal diseases	950	510	440	447	34	4	5	4	5	10	362	37	9	10	5	5	12
5. Childhood-cluster diseases	863	450	413	386	54	2	4	2	1	1	349	54	3	3	2	1	1
a. Pertussis	148	78	70	71	7						64	6					
b. Poliomyelitis	5	3	2	3							2						
c. Diphtheria	2	1	1	1							1						
d. Measles	576	300	276	257	43						233	43					
e. Tetanus	133	68	64	55	4	2	3	2	1	1	50	5	3	3	2	1	1
6. Bacterial meningitis*	26	13	13	9			2	1	1		8			2	1	1	1
7. Hepatitis B and hepatitis C	15	8	7	1	1	1	1	2	1	1	1	1	1	1	1	1	1
8. Malaria	732	392	340	325	29	16	11	7	3	1	263	29	21	14	8	3	2
9. Tropical-cluster diseases	62	33	29	1	10	8	6	6	1	1	1	9	8	5	4	1	1
a. Trypanosomiasis	47	24	24		6	6	4	5	1	1	1	7	7	5	4	1	1
b. Chagas disease																	
c. Schistosomiasis	4	2	1				1	1						1			
d. Leishmaniasis	11	7	4		3	2	1	1				2	1	1			
10. Leprosy																	
11. Dengue	1																
12. Japanese encephalitis																	
13. Trachoma																	
14. Intestinal nematode infections	2	1	1		1							1					
a. Ascariasis	1		1									1					
b. Trichuriasis																	
c. Ancylostomiasis, necatoriasis	1				1												
15. Other infectious and parasitic	92	48	43	30	7	2	3	2	1	2	25	7	3	3	2	1	2

Annex Table 6f, continued. Deaths by age, sex and cause (thousands): Sub-Saharan Africa, 1990

Cause	Total	Male	Female	Males 0-4	5-14	15-29	30-44	45-59	60-69	70+	Females 0-4	5-14	15-29	30-44	45-59	60-69	70+
B. Respiratory infections	1 023	545	478	407	45	7	5	6	20	56	329	38	10	6	6	23	66
1. Lower respiratory infections	1 006	536	470	399	44	7	5	6	20	56	323	37	9	6	6	23	65
2. Upper respiratory infections	10	5	5	4						1	3		1				1
3. Otitis media	7	4	3	3							3						
C. Maternal conditions	186		186									10	83	93			
1. Maternal haemorrhage	45		45									2	20	22			
2. Maternal sepsis	30		30									2	13	15			
3. Hypertensive disorders*	22		22									1	10	11			
4. Obstructed labour	15		15									1	7	7			
5. Abortion	25		25										11	13			
6. Other maternal	49		49									3	22	25			
D. Perinatal conditions*	503	258	245	258							245						
1. Low birth weight	249	127	122	127							122						
2. Birth asphyxia and birth trauma	164	82	82	82							82						
3. Other perinatal	90	49	41	49							41						
E. Nutritional deficiencies	148	74	74	60	8	1	1	1	1	3	56	8	3	2	1	1	3
1. Protein-energy malnutrition	102	52	50	47	1	1	1	1	1	2	44	1		1	1	1	2
2. Iodine deficiency	2	1	1	1							1						
3. Vitamin A deficiency	33	17	16	11	6						10	6					
4. Iron-deficiency anaemia	12	5	7	2						1	2		1	1			1
II. Noncommunicable diseases	1 864	934	930	63	64	47	112	204	186	258	65	75	36	49	192	187	325
A. Malignant neoplasms	429	239	190	4	11	8	26	66	59	66	4	11	6	14	57	45	53
1. Mouth and oropharynx cancers	23	14	9				1	2	5	6				1	1	3	4
2. Oesophagus cancer	23	17	6				1	7	4	5					2	2	2
3. Stomach cancer	32	19	13				1	7	5	6				1	5	3	4
4. Colon and rectum cancers	15	8	7					1	2	5					1	3	3
5. Liver cancer	56	41	15	1	4	3	9	16	6	2	1	3	1	1	5	2	2
6. Pancreas cancer	7	4	3					2	1	1					2		1
7. Trachea, bronchus, lung cancers	20	15	5				1	6	4	4				1		2	2
8. Melanoma and other skin cancers	8	3	5				1	1	1	1				1	1	1	2
9. Breast cancer	17		17											1	7	4	5
10. Cervix uteri cancer	33		33										1	2	13	8	9
11. Corpus uteri cancer	4		4												1	1	2
12. Ovary cancer	8		8											1	3	2	2
13. Prostate cancer	32	32						4	13	15							
14. Bladder cancer	14	9	5				1	2	3	3				1	1	1	2
15. Lymphomas, multiple myeloma	26	16	10		1	2	2	3	3	5	1	1	1	2	1	2	2
16. Leukaemia	9	4	5	1	1	2						2	1			1	1
17. Other cancers	102	56	46	2	5	1	8	15	12	13	2	5	2	2	13	9	10

Annex Table 6f, continued. Deaths by age, sex and cause (thousands): Sub-Saharan Africa, 1990

Cause	Total	Male	Female	Males 0-4	5-14	15-29	30-44	45-59	60-69	70+	Females 0-4	5-14	15-29	30-44	45-59	60-69	70+
B. Other neoplasms	10	5	5	–	2	–	1	1	1	1	–	2	1	–	1	1	1
C. Diabetes mellitus	23	10	13	–	1	–	1	2	2	3	–	1	–	–	3	4	4
D. Endocrine disorders	23	10	13	2	1	1	2	2	1	2	1	2	1	1	2	2	5
E. Neuro-psychiatric conditions	41	24	17	2	3	3	5	4	3	5	2	3	1	1	3	3	5
2. Bipolar disorder	1	1	1	–	–	–	–	–	–	–	–	–	–	–	–	–	–
3. Schizophrenia	1	–	1	–	–	–	1	1	–	–	–	–	1	1	1	–	–
4. Epilepsy	6	4	2	–	1	1	1	1	1	–	–	–	1	1	1	1	–
5. Alcohol use	5	3	1	–	–	1	1	1	1	–	–	–	–	1	1	1	–
6. Dementia*	8	4	4	–	–	–	–	–	1	2	–	–	–	–	–	1	2
7. Parkinson disease	2	1	1	–	–	–	–	–	–	1	–	–	–	–	–	–	1
8. Multiple sclerosis	1	1	1	–	–	–	–	–	–	–	–	–	1	–	–	–	–
9. Drug use	1	1	–	–	–	–	–	–	–	–	–	–	–	–	–	–	–
13. Other neuro-psychiatric	16	10	6	1	2	2	2	1	1	1	1	2	1	2	1	–	1
F. Sense organ diseases	–	–	–	–	–	–	–	–	–	–	–	–	–	–	–	–	–
1. Glaucoma	–	–	–	–	–	–	–	–	–	–	–	–	–	–	–	–	–
2. Cataracts	–	–	–	–	–	–	–	–	–	–	–	–	–	–	–	–	–
G. Cardiovascular diseases	815	344	471	11	19	17	39	74	70	114	13	27	15	21	89	101	203
1. Rheumatic heart disease	20	9	11	–	3	3	2	1	–	–	–	5	3	1	1	–	1
2. Ischaemic heart disease	209	92	117	–	–	1	10	22	23	36	–	–	1	5	23	30	55
3. Cerebrovascular disease	383	152	231	2	6	7	16	32	33	56	2	6	3	9	44	53	113
4. Inflammatory heart diseases	63	28	35	4	3	1	4	6	4	6	5	6	3	1	5	7	9
5. Other cardiovascular	140	63	77	5	7	5	7	14	9	16	2	11	5	4	17	12	25
H. Respiratory diseases	210	126	85	10	6	4	13	24	26	41	10	6	3	4	16	13	32
1. COPD*	102	63	39	2	1	1	3	13	16	27	3	1	–	1	8	8	19
2. Asthma	13	8	6	–	1	1	1	2	1	2	–	1	–	1	1	1	2
3. Other respiratory	95	55	40	8	4	3	9	11	9	12	8	4	2	2	8	5	11
I. Digestive diseases	153	92	60	4	9	8	18	22	15	15	4	12	5	5	11	11	13
1. Peptic ulcer	13	8	5	–	–	1	2	2	1	2	–	–	1	1	1	1	2
2. Cirrhosis of the liver	34	24	10	–	–	1	5	8	5	4	–	–	1	1	3	3	2
3. Appendicitis	14	8	5	–	4	2	5	8	–	–	–	3	1	1	3	–	2
4. Other digestive	92	53	40	4	5	3	10	12	9	10	4	8	3	3	6	7	8
J. Genito-urinary diseases	96	52	44	6	9	4	7	8	8	11	5	7	3	3	9	7	9
1. Nephritis and nephrosis	83	45	38	5	8	3	5	7	7	10	5	7	2	3	8	6	8
2. Benign prostatic hypertrophy	–	7	–	–	–	–	–	1	1	1	–	–	–	–	–	–	–
3. Other genito-urinary	12	7	6	1	1	1	1	1	1	1	1	1	1	1	2	1	1
K. Skin diseases	7	4	3	3	–	–	–	–	–	–	2	–	–	–	–	–	–

Annex Table 6f, continued. Deaths by age, sex and cause (thousands): Sub-Saharan Africa, 1990

Cause	Total	Male	Female	Males							Females						
				0-4	5-14	15-29	30-44	45-59	60-69	70+	0-4	5-14	15-29	30-44	45-59	60-69	70+
L. Musculo-skeletal diseases																	
1. Rheumatoid arthritis	1	-	-	-	-	-	-	-	-	-	-	-	-	-	-	-	-
3. Other musculo-skeletal	1	-	-	-	-	-	-	-	-	-	-	-	-	-	-	-	-
M. Congenital anomalies	**55**	**26**	**28**	20	3	1	1	1	-	-	22	3	1	-	1	-	-
1. Abdominal wall defect	12	5	7	5	-	-	-	-	-	-	7	-	-	-	-	-	-
2. Anencephaly	-	-	-	-	-	-	-	-	-	-	-	-	-	-	-	-	-
3. Anorectal atresia	-	-	-	-	-	-	-	-	-	-	-	-	-	-	-	-	-
4. Cleft lip	-	-	-	-	-	-	-	-	-	-	-	-	-	-	-	-	-
5. Cleft palate	-	-	-	-	-	-	-	-	-	-	-	-	-	-	-	-	-
6. Oesophageal atresia	-	-	-	-	-	-	-	-	-	-	-	-	-	-	-	-	-
7. Renal agenesis	2	1	1	1	-	-	-	-	-	-	1	-	-	-	-	-	-
8. Down syndrome	6	3	3	1	-	1	1	-	-	-	1	-	1	-	-	-	-
9. Congenital heart anomalies	21	10	10	7	1	-	-	1	-	-	7	1	-	-	1	-	-
10. Spina bifida	5	2	2	2	-	-	-	-	-	-	2	-	-	-	-	-	-
11. Other congenital	7	4	3	3	1	-	-	-	-	-	3	1	-	-	-	-	-
N. Oral conditions	-	-	-	-	-	-	-	-	-	-	-	-	-	-	-	-	-
III. Injuries	**1 022**	**718**	**303**	**98**	**118**	**286**	**134**	**51**	**19**	**11**	**76**	**67**	**84**	**41**	**17**	**9**	**8**
A. Unintentional injuries	534	375	158	67	93	110	59	27	11	8	47	53	27	13	8	4	6
1. Road traffic accidents	155	114	41	10	30	35	22	11	4	2	7	14	10	5	3	1	1
2. Poisonings	37	22	15	14	4	1	2	1	1	-	10	2	2	1	1	1	-
3. Falls	18	11	6	1	2	4	2	1	1	1	1	1	-	1	1	1	2
4. Fires	67	35	32	13	6	7	3	2	1	1	11	8	6	3	1	1	2
5. Drownings	91	66	25	16	33	10	4	2	1	1	8	13	2	1	-	-	-
6. Other unintentional	166	126	40	14	18	52	27	10	3	2	10	14	7	4	2	1	1
B. Intentional injuries	488	343	145	31	25	176	75	23	8	3	29	14	58	28	9	5	2
1. Self-inflicted injuries	16	13	3	-	1	6	3	1	1	-	-	-	2	1	-	-	-
2. Violence	205	176	29	4	8	105	39	14	4	2	2	3	13	6	3	1	1
3. War	268	154	114	27	16	65	32	8	4	1	27	11	43	22	5	4	1

Notes:
Causes responsible for no deaths have been omitted from this table.
A dash (-) symbol indicates fewer than 500 deaths.
*IA6 is Bacterial meningitis and meningococcaemia; IC3 is Hypertensive disorders of pregnancy; ID is Conditions arising during the perinatal period; IIE6 is Dementia and other degenerative and hereditary CNS disorders; IIH1 is Chronic obstructive pulmonary disease.

Annex Table 6g. Deaths by age, sex and cause (thousands): Latin America and the Caribbean, 1990

Cause	Total	Male	Female	Males 0-4	5-14	15-29	30-44	45-59	60-69	70+	Females 0-4	5-14	15-29	30-44	45-59	60-69	70+
Population (millions)	*444*	*222*	*223*	*29*	*52*	*64*	*40*	*22*	*9*	*5*	*28*	*51*	*63*	*41*	*23*	*10*	*7*
All causes	*3 009*	*1 654*	*1 355*	*403*	*73*	*154*	*167*	*228*	*218*	*411*	*306*	*55*	*99*	*112*	*170*	*176*	*437*
I. Communicable, maternal, perinatal and nutritional conditions	*943*	*511*	*432*	*340*	*19*	*30*	*27*	*29*	*24*	*42*	*251*	*22*	*40*	*33*	*22*	*18*	*45*
A. Infectious and parasitic diseases	473	262	211	144	12	26	23	22	17	16	112	14	21	20	16	12	16
1. Tuberculosis	78	44	34	1	1	11	6	10	9	6	1	2	9	6	6	5	4
2. STDs excluding HIV	12	6	6	5	-	-	-	-	-	-	4	-	1	1	-	-	1
a. Syphilis	11	6	5	5	-	-	-	-	-	-	4	-	1	1	-	-	1
b. Chlamydia	1	-	1	-	-	-	-	-	-	-	-	-	-	-	-	-	-
c. Gonorrhoea	-	-	-	-	-	-	-	-	-	-	-	-	-	-	-	-	-
3. HIV	29	23	6	1	-	10	9	3	1	-	1	-	2	2	1	1	-
4. Diarrhoeal diseases	153	86	67	76	2	1	1	1	1	4	54	3	2	1	2	1	4
5. Childhood-cluster diseases	91	48	43	44	3	-	-	-	-	-	39	3	2	-	-	-	-
a. Pertussis	17	9	8	9	-	-	-	-	-	-	8	1	-	-	-	-	-
b. Poliomyelitis	2	1	1	1	-	-	-	-	-	-	1	-	-	-	-	-	-
c. Diphtheria	-	-	-	-	-	-	-	-	-	-	-	-	-	-	-	-	-
d. Measles	52	27	25	24	2	-	-	-	-	-	22	3	-	-	-	-	-
e. Tetanus	20	11	10	10	-	-	-	-	-	-	9	-	-	-	-	-	-
6. Bacterial meningitis*	14	7	7	3	-	-	1	1	1	1	3	-	-	2	1	1	1
7. Hepatitis B and hepatitis C	4	2	2	1	-	-	-	-	-	-	1	-	1	-	-	-	-
8. Malaria	14	7	7	1	1	2	1	1	-	-	1	1	2	1	1	-	-
9. Tropical-cluster diseases	20	9	11	-	-	1	2	3	2	1	-	-	1	3	3	2	1
a. Trypanosomiasis	19	9	10	-	-	1	2	3	2	1	-	-	1	3	3	2	1
b. Chagas disease	-	-	-	-	-	-	-	-	-	-	-	-	-	-	-	-	-
c. Schistosomiasis	1	-	-	-	-	-	-	-	-	-	-	-	-	-	-	-	-
d. Leishmaniasis	1	-	-	-	-	-	-	-	-	-	-	-	-	-	-	-	-
10. Leprosy	1	-	-	-	-	-	-	-	-	-	-	-	-	-	-	-	-
11. Dengue	-	-	-	-	-	-	-	-	-	-	-	-	-	-	-	-	-
12. Japanese encephalitis	-	-	-	-	-	-	-	-	-	-	-	-	-	-	-	-	-
13. Trachoma	-	-	-	-	-	-	-	-	-	-	-	-	-	-	-	-	-
14. Intestinal nematode infections	2	1	1	-	1	-	-	-	-	-	-	1	-	-	-	-	-
a. Ascariasis	1	1	1	-	1	-	-	-	-	-	-	1	-	-	-	-	-
b. Trichuriasis	1	1	-	-	1	-	-	-	-	-	-	-	-	-	-	-	-
c. Ancylostomiasis, necatoriasis	-	-	-	-	-	-	-	-	-	-	-	-	-	-	-	-	-
15. Other infectious and parasitic	53	27	26	12	2	2	3	3	2	4	9	2	3	3	3	2	4

Annex Table 6g, continued. Deaths by age, sex and cause (thousands): Latin America and the Caribbean, 1990

Cause	Total	Male	Female	Males							Females						
				0-4	5-14	15-29	30-44	45-59	60-69	70+	0-4	5-14	15-29	30-44	45-59	60-69	70+
B. Respiratory infections	**180**	**97**	**83**	**58**	**4**	**2**	**3**	**5**	**5**	**19**	**41**	**5**	**4**	**4**	**4**	**4**	**21**
1. Lower respiratory infections	178	96	82	58	4	2	3	5	5	19	41	4	4	4	4	4	21
2. Upper respiratory infections	2	1	1	1	-	-	-	-	-	-	1	-	-	-	-	-	-
3. Otitis media	-	-	-	-	-	-	-	-	-	-	-	-	-	-	-	-	-
C. Maternal conditions	**19**		**19**	-	-	-	-	-	-	-	-	-	12	7	-	-	-
1. Maternal haemorrhage	5		5										3	2			
2. Maternal sepsis	2		2										1	1			
3. Hypertensive disorders*	3		3										2	1			
4. Obstructed labour	2		2										2	1			
5. Abortion	4		4										3	2			
6. Other maternal	4		4										2	1			
D. Perinatal conditions*	**196**	**115**	**81**	**115**	-	-	-	-	-	-	**81**	-	-	-	-	-	-
1. Low birth weight	29	16	12	16							12						
2. Birth asphyxia and birth trauma	91	54	37	54							37						
3. Other perinatal	76	44	31	44							31						
E. Nutritional deficiencies	**76**	**38**	**38**	**22**	**3**	**1**	**1**	**2**	**2**	**7**	**17**	**3**	**2**	**2**	**2**	**2**	**9**
1. Protein-energy malnutrition	52	27	25	18	1	-	1	1	1	5	13	1	1	1	1	1	6
2. Iodine deficiency	1	-	1	-							1						
3. Vitamin A deficiency	5	3	3	2	1						2	1					
4. Iron-deficiency anaemia	17	7	10	2	1					2	2	1	1	1	1	1	3
II. Noncommunicable diseases	**1 676**	**850**	**826**	**44**	**22**	**18**	**68**	**163**	**180**	**355**	**40**	**18**	**30**	**64**	**139**	**153**	**382**
A. Malignant neoplasms	**345**	**168**	**176**	**2**	**7**	**4**	**10**	**36**	**43**	**66**	**2**	**5**	**6**	**21**	**45**	**41**	**56**
1. Mouth and oropharynx cancers	12	9	4				1	3	2	3					1	1	1
2. Oesophagus cancer	10	7	3					2	2	3					1	1	2
3. Stomach cancer	38	22	15				1	5	7	9				1	3	4	7
4. Colon and rectum cancers	23	10	13				1	2	3	4				1	2	4	6
5. Liver cancer	6	3	3					1	1	1				1	1	1	1
6. Pancreas cancer	8	4	4					1	1	1					1	1	2
7. Trachea, bronchus, lung cancers	34	25	9				1	7	7	10				1	2	3	4
8. Melanoma and other skin cancers	3	1	2							1				1		1	1
9. Breast cancer	30	-	30											4	10	7	8
10. Cervix uteri cancer	25	-	25										1	4	9	5	6
11. Corpus uteri cancer	7	-	7												2	2	2
12. Ovary cancer	6	-	6											1	2	1	1
13. Prostate cancer	20	20	-					1	7	12							
14. Bladder cancer	8	6	2						2	3					1	1	2
15. Lymphomas, multiple myeloma	16	9	7			1	2	2	2	2				1	1	2	2
16. Leukaemia	13	7	6		2		1	1	1	1	1	2			1	1	1
17. Other cancers	86	45	41	1	3	1	3	9	9	18	1	2	2	6	10	8	10

Annex Table 6g, continued. Deaths by age, sex and cause (thousands): Latin America and the Caribbean, 1990

Cause	Total	Male	Female	Males 0-4	5-14	15-29	30-44	45-59	60-69	70+	Females 0-4	5-14	15-29	30-44	45-59	60-69	70+
B. Other neoplasms	9	4	5	-	1	1	-	1	1	1	-	1	-	1	1	1	1
C. Diabetes mellitus	89	35	53	-	1	1	3	8	10	14	-	1	1	2	11	15	23
D. Endocrine disorders	27	13	14	4	1	1	1	1	1	4	3	1	1	1	2	1	5
E. Neuro-psychiatric conditions	50	30	20	3	4	3	6	6	3	5	3	3	3	3	2	2	5
2. Bipolar disorder	1	1	-	-	-	-	1	-	-	-	-	-	-	-	-	-	-
3. Schizophrenia	4	2	2	-	-	-	1	1	-	-	-	-	-	-	1	-	1
4. Epilepsy	6	3	3	-	1	1	1	-	-	-	-	1	1	1	-	-	-
5. Alcohol use	11	10	1	-	-	1	3	4	1	1	-	-	-	-	1	-	-
6. Dementia*	8	4	4	-	-	-	-	-	1	2	-	-	-	-	-	1	2
7. Parkinson disease	2	1	1	-	-	-	-	-	1	1	-	-	-	-	-	1	1
8. Multiple sclerosis	2	1	1	-	-	-	1	-	-	-	-	-	-	-	-	-	-
9. Drug use	2	1	1	-	-	1	-	1	-	-	-	-	1	1	1	-	-
13. Other neuro-psychiatric	15	8	7	2	-	-	-	-	-	1	-	2	-	-	-	-	1
F. Sense organ diseases	1	-	-	-	-	-	-	-	-	-	-	-	-	-	-	-	-
1. Glaucoma	-	-	-	-	-	-	-	-	-	-	-	-	-	-	-	-	-
2. Cataracts	-	-	-	-	-	-	-	-	-	-	-	-	-	-	-	-	-
G. Cardiovascular diseases	789	395	394	4	3	5	25	73	88	196	3	3	9	23	55	69	232
1. Rheumatic heart disease	8	3	6	-	-	-	1	1	-	-	-	1	1	-	1	1	1
2. Ischaemic heart disease	348	179	169	-	-	1	10	34	42	92	-	-	1	7	22	31	107
3. Cerebrovascular disease	249	121	127	1	1	1	8	23	27	61	1	1	2	8	20	23	73
4. Inflammatory heart diseases	25	12	12	3	1	1	2	3	2	4	-	1	1	2	2	1	5
5. Other cardiovascular	160	80	80	3	2	2	5	13	17	40	2	1	3	4	10	13	47
H. Respiratory diseases	116	65	51	8	1	1	3	8	12	32	7	1	2	3	6	8	25
1. COPD*	61	36	25	2	-	-	1	4	8	21	2	-	-	1	3	5	15
2. Asthma	12	6	6	-	-	-	1	1	1	2	-	-	-	1	1	1	3
3. Other respiratory	44	24	20	6	1	1	1	3	4	9	5	1	1	2	2	2	7
I. Digestive diseases	140	85	55	3	2	2	15	25	16	21	2	1	3	6	11	10	21
1. Peptic ulcer	11	7	5	-	-	-	1	1	1	3	-	-	-	-	1	1	3
2. Cirrhosis of the liver	62	45	17	-	-	1	11	17	9	7	-	-	2	3	5	4	4
3. Appendicitis	2	1	1	-	-	1	-	-	-	-	-	-	-	-	-	-	-
4. Other digestive	65	33	32	3	1	1	4	7	6	11	2	1	2	3	5	6	14
J. Genito-urinary diseases	53	27	26	1	1	1	2	4	5	13	1	1	2	3	4	4	10
1. Nephritis and nephrosis	39	19	20	1	1	1	2	3	4	8	1	1	2	2	3	3	7
2. Benign prostatic hypertrophy	2	2	-	-	-	-	-	-	-	2	-	-	-	-	-	-	-
3. Other genito-urinary	12	6	7	-	-	-	1	1	1	3	-	-	1	1	1	1	3
K. Skin diseases	3	1	2	-	-	-	-	-	-	-	-	-	-	-	-	-	1

Annex Table 6q, continued. Deaths by age, sex and cause (thousands): Latin America and the Caribbean, 1990

Cause	Total	Male	Female	Males							Females						
				0-4	5-14	15-29	30-44	45-59	60-69	70+	0-4	5-14	15-29	30-44	45-59	60-69	70+
L. Musculo-skeletal diseases	9	3	6	-	-	-	-	-	-	1	-	-	1	1	1	1	2
1. Rheumatoid arthritis	1	-	1	-	-	-	-	-	-	-	-	-	-	-	1	1	1
3. Other musculo-skeletal	8	2	5	-	-	-	-	-	-	1	-	-	1	1	1	1	2
M. Congenital anomalies	43	21	22	18	2	1	-	-	-	-	18	2	1	-	-	-	-
1. Abdominal wall defect	1	-	-	-	-	-	-	-	-	-	-	-	-	-	-	-	-
2. Anencephaly	9	3	5	3	-	-	-	-	-	-	5	-	-	-	-	-	-
3. Anorectal atresia	-	-	-	-	-	-	-	-	-	-	-	-	-	-	-	-	-
4. Cleft lip	1	1	-	-	-	-	-	-	-	-	-	-	-	-	-	-	-
5. Cleft palate	1	-	-	-	-	-	-	-	-	-	-	-	-	-	-	-	-
6. Oesophageal atresia	-	-	-	-	-	-	-	-	-	-	-	-	-	-	-	-	-
7. Renal agenesis	1	-	-	1	-	-	-	-	-	-	1	-	-	-	-	-	-
8. Down syndrome	4	2	2	-	1	-	-	-	-	-	-	1	-	-	-	-	-
9. Congenital heart anomalies	15	8	7	6	-	-	-	-	-	-	5	1	-	-	-	-	-
10. Spina bifida	6	3	3	3	-	-	-	-	-	-	3	-	-	-	-	-	-
11. Other congenital	6	3	3	3	-	-	-	-	-	-	2	-	-	-	-	-	-
N. Oral conditions	-	-	-	-	-	-	-	-	-	-	-	-	-	-	-	-	-
III. Injuries	389	293	97	19	32	106	72	36	14	15	14	15	29	15	9	5	10
A. Unintentional injuries	248	178	70	16	27	52	39	23	10	12	12	13	17	9	6	4	9
1. Road traffic accidents	109	80	29	3	12	26	20	11	4	4	2	6	9	5	3	2	2
2. Poisonings	5	3	2	1	-	1	2	2	1	-	-	-	1	2	-	1	-
3. Falls	18	12	7	1	1	2	2	2	1	3	1	1	-	-	1	1	1
4. Fires	7	4	3	1	1	1	1	-	-	-	1	1	1	-	-	-	-
5. Drownings	28	22	6	3	6	8	4	2	-	-	2	2	1	1	-	-	-
6. Other unintentional	80	57	23	7	7	15	12	8	3	4	6	3	5	3	1	2	3
B. Intentional injuries	141	114	27	3	4	54	33	13	4	3	3	2	12	6	2	1	1
1. Self-inflicted injuries	22	16	7	-	-	6	4	3	1	1	-	-	3	2	1	1	-
2. Violence	102	89	13	1	3	44	27	10	2	1	1	1	6	3	1	-	1
3. War	17	10	7	2	1	4	2	1	-	-	2	1	3	1	-	-	-

Notes:
Causes responsible for no deaths have been omitted from this table.
A dash (-) symbol indicates fewer than 500 deaths.
*IA6 is Bacterial meningitis and meningococcaemia; IC3 is Hypertensive disorders of pregnancy; ID is Conditions arising during the perinatal period; IIE6 is Dementia and other degenerative and hereditary CNS disorders; IIH1 is Chronic obstructive pulmonary disease.

Annex Table 6h. Deaths by age, sex and cause (thousands): Middle Eastern Crescent, 1990

Cause	Total	Male	Female	Males 0-4	5-14	15-29	30-44	45-59	60-69	70+	Females 0-4	5-14	15-29	30-44	45-59	60-69	70+
Population (millions)	*503*	*256*	*247*	*41*	*65*	*70*	*44*	*22*	*9*	*5*	*40*	*62*	*66*	*41*	*22*	*10*	*6*
All causes	**4 553**	**2 399**	**2 154**	**955**	**158**	**165**	**163**	**252**	**270**	**437**	**908**	**141**	**135**	**121**	**172**	**209**	**468**
I. Communicable, maternal, perinatal and nutritional conditions	***1 945***	***980***	***964***	***789***	***46***	***21***	***20***	***26***	***37***	***40***	***752***	***46***	***40***	***39***	***21***	***25***	***40***
A. Infectious and parasitic diseases	**871**	**459**	**411**	**351**	**24**	**19**	**18**	**23**	**15**	**10**	**332**	**22**	**14**	**12**	**14**	**9**	**9**
1. Tuberculosis	109	69	40	5	3	15	13	17	11	6	3	2	9	6	9	6	5
2. STDs excluding HIV	14	7	7	6	-	-	-	-	-	-	6	-	-	-	-	-	-
a. Syphilis	14	7	7	6	-	-	-	-	-	-	6	-	-	-	-	-	-
b. Chlamydia	-	-	-	-	-	-	-	-	-	-	-	-	-	-	-	-	-
c. Gonorrhoea	-	-	-	-	-	-	-	-	-	-	-	-	-	-	-	-	-
3. HIV	1	1	-	-	-	-	-	-	-	-	-	-	-	-	-	-	-
4. Diarrhoeal diseases	424	217	208	206	7	-	1	1	1	1	196	8	1	-	1	1	1
5. Childhood-cluster diseases	236	120	116	109	10	-	-	-	-	-	104	9	1	-	-	-	-
a. Pertussis	52	27	26	25	2	-	-	-	-	-	24	2	-	-	-	-	-
b. Poliomyelitis	4	2	2	2	-	-	-	-	-	-	2	-	-	-	-	-	-
c. Diphtheria	1	1	1	1	-	-	-	-	-	-	1	-	-	-	-	-	-
d. Measles	96	49	47	43	6	-	-	-	-	-	41	6	-	-	-	-	-
e. Tetanus	83	42	41	39	2	-	-	-	-	-	37	1	-	-	-	-	-
6. Bacterial meningitis*	18	9	9	5	1	-	2	1	1	-	5	1	1	1	1	1	1
7. Hepatitis B and hepatitis C	13	7	6	1	1	-	1	2	1	1	1	1	1	-	-	1	1
8. Malaria	7	3	3	1	1	1	1	-	-	-	1	1	1	-	-	-	-
9. Tropical-cluster diseases	4	3	1	-	1	-	-	-	-	-	-	-	-	-	-	-	-
a. Trypanosomiasis	-	-	-	-	-	-	-	-	-	-	-	-	-	-	-	-	-
b. Chagas disease	-	-	-	-	-	-	-	-	-	-	-	-	-	-	-	-	-
c. Schistosomiasis	2	1	1	-	-	-	-	-	-	-	-	-	-	-	-	-	-
d. Leishmaniasis	2	1	1	1	1	-	1	-	-	-	-	-	-	-	-	-	-
10. Leprosy	-	-	-	-	-	-	-	-	-	-	-	-	-	-	-	-	-
11. Dengue	-	-	-	-	-	-	-	-	-	-	-	-	-	-	-	-	-
12. Japanese encephalitis	-	-	-	-	-	-	-	-	-	-	-	-	-	-	-	-	-
13. Trachoma	-	-	-	-	-	-	-	-	-	-	-	-	-	-	-	-	-
14. Intestinal nematode infections	1	1	-	-	-	-	-	-	-	-	-	-	-	-	-	-	-
a. Ascariasis	1	1	-	-	-	-	-	-	-	-	-	-	-	-	-	-	-
b. Trichuriasis	-	-	-	-	-	-	-	-	-	-	-	-	-	-	-	-	-
c. Ancylostomiasis, necatoriasis	-	-	-	-	-	-	-	-	-	-	-	-	-	-	-	-	-
15. Other infectious and parasitic	44	23	21	17	1	1	1	1	1	1	16	1	1	1	1	-	1

Annex Table 6h, continued. Deaths by age, sex and cause (thousands): Middle Eastern Crescent, 1990

Cause	Total	Male	Female	Males 0-4	Males 5-14	Males 15-29	Males 30-44	Males 45-59	Males 60-69	Males 70+	Females 0-4	Females 5-14	Females 15-29	Females 30-44	Females 45-59	Females 60-69	Females 70+
B. Respiratory infections	534	272	262	197	18	2	2	3	22	29	187	20	4	2	4	15	30
1. Lower respiratory infections	525	268	258	193	18	2	2	3	22	29	184	20	4	2	4	15	30
2. Upper respiratory infections	5	3	2	2							2						
3. Otitis media	3	2	2	2							1						
C. Maternal conditions	48		48										21	24	3		
1. Maternal haemorrhage	12		12										5	6	1		
2. Maternal sepsis	8		8										3	4			
3. Hypertensive disorders*	8		8										3	4			
4. Obstructed labour	4		4										2	2			
5. Abortion	4		4										2	2			
6. Other maternal	13		13										5	6	1		
D. Perinatal conditions*	395	201	194	201							194						
1. Low birth weight	199	101	98	101							98						
2. Birth asphyxia and birth trauma	94	48	46	48							46						
3. Other perinatal	102	52	50	52							50						
E. Nutritional deficiencies	96	48	49	40	4	1			1	1	39	4	2	1	1	1	1
1. Protein-energy malnutrition	63	32	31	30						1	29						1
2. Iodine deficiency	4	2	2	1													
3. Vitamin A deficiency	20	10	10	7	3						7	3					
4. Iron-deficiency anaemia	9	4	6	2							2		1	1	1		
II. Noncommunicable diseases	2 156	1 123	1 033	119	68	46	77	201	222	390	112	72	51	58	141	177	422
A. Malignant neoplasms	228	126	102	3	8	6	11	36	33	30	2	7	6	12	26	24	24
1. Mouth and oropharynx cancers	16	10	6			1	1	2	3	3					1	1	2
2. Oesophagus cancer	10	6	4					2	2	1					1	1	1
3. Stomach cancer	21	12	9			1	1	5	3	3				1	2	3	3
4. Colon and rectum cancers	13	6	7				1	1	2	2				1	1	2	2
5. Liver cancer	9	5	3			1	1	2	1	1					1	1	1
6. Pancreas cancer	5	3	2						1	1						1	2
7. Trachea, bronchus, lung cancers	30	24	6					10	6	6						2	2
8. Melanoma and other skin cancers	1	1						1									
9. Breast cancer	13		13										1	2	5	2	2
10. Cervix uteri cancer	8		8										1	1	3	2	2
11. Corpus uteri cancer	2		2												1	1	1
12. Ovary cancer	4		4											1	1	1	1
13. Prostate cancer	5	5						1	2	2							
14. Bladder cancer	10	8	2					2	2	2					1	2	2
15. Lymphomas, multiple myeloma	10	6	3	1	1	1	1	1		1	1	1	1		1	1	1
16. Leukaemia	14	7	7	1	2	1		1	1	1	1	2	1		1	1	1
17. Other cancers	59	33	26	2	4	2	3	8	8	7	2	4	2	4	6	5	4

Annex Table 6h, continued. Deaths by age, sex and cause (thousands): Middle Eastern Crescent, 1990

Cause	Total	Male	Female	Males							Females						
				0-4	5-14	15-29	30-44	45-59	60-69	70+	0-4	5-14	15-29	30-44	45-59	60-69	70+
B. Other neoplasms	6	3	3	-	1	1	-	1	-	-	-	1	-	-	1	-	-
C. Diabetes mellitus	61	28	33	1	2	1	3	7	7	8	1	2	1	2	7	10	11
D. Endocrine disorders	17	8	9	3	1	1	1	1	1	1	3	3	1	-	1	1	1
E. Neuro-psychiatric conditions	61	33	29	7	7	4	3	3	3	6	5	7	4	2	2	2	6
2. Bipolar disorder	1	-	1	-	-	-	-	-	-	-	-	-	-	-	1	-	-
3. Schizophrenia	4	2	2	-	-	-	-	1	-	1	-	-	-	-	1	1	-
4. Epilepsy	9	5	4	1	1	1	1	1	-	-	-	1	1	1	1	-	-
5. Alcohol use	1	1	-	-	-	1	-	-	-	-	-	-	-	-	-	-	-
6. Dementia*	10	4	5	-	-	-	-	-	1	3	-	-	-	-	1	1	3
7. Parkinson disease	3	2	1	-	-	-	-	-	1	1	-	-	-	-	-	-	1
8. Multiple sclerosis	1	1	1	-	-	-	-	-	-	-	-	-	-	-	-	-	-
9. Drug use	2	2	-	-	-	1	1	-	-	-	-	-	-	-	-	-	-
13. Other neuro-psychiatric	31	17	15	6	5	2	1	1	1	1	4	5	2	1	1	1	1
F. Sense organ diseases	-	-	-	-	-	-	-	-	-	-	-	-	-	-	-	-	-
1. Glaucoma	-	-	-	-	-	-	-	-	-	-	-	-	-	-	-	-	-
2. Cataracts	-	-	-	-	-	-	-	-	-	-	-	-	-	-	-	-	-
G. Cardiovascular diseases	1 295	658	637	34	33	22	39	109	137	285	29	34	26	27	75	113	332
1. Rheumatic heart disease	24	10	14	-	3	4	2	1	-	1	-	4	5	3	1	-	1
2. Ischaemic heart disease	610	319	291	-	-	3	18	59	77	161	-	-	2	11	34	60	182
3. Cerebrovascular disease	212	99	113	2	5	3	5	16	22	46	1	5	4	3	15	22	65
4. Inflammatory heart diseases	72	37	35	6	6	4	4	6	3	7	7	6	4	3	4	3	8
5. Other cardiovascular	377	194	184	26	19	8	9	27	35	71	21	19	11	7	21	28	78
H. Respiratory diseases	163	87	76	19	4	2	4	12	16	30	20	7	3	3	8	10	25
1. COPD*	74	42	32	4	1	-	1	6	10	20	5	1	-	1	4	6	15
2. Asthma	9	5	4	-	-	-	1	1	1	2	-	-	1	1	1	1	2
3. Other respiratory	79	40	40	14	3	1	2	5	5	8	15	5	2	2	3	3	8
I. Digestive diseases	152	85	67	18	6	4	10	20	14	13	20	5	4	5	12	10	12
1. Peptic ulcer	6	4	2	-	-	-	1	1	1	1	-	-	-	-	1	-	1
2. Cirrhosis of the liver	45	26	20	-	1	1	3	8	6	5	-	2	1	2	5	4	5
3. Appendicitis	5	3	2	-	1	1	1	-	-	-	-	1	1	-	-	-	-
4. Other digestive	97	53	44	17	4	2	5	10	7	7	20	2	2	3	6	5	6
J. Genito-urinary diseases	92	53	39	2	4	4	6	11	10	16	2	4	5	5	8	6	9
1. Nephritis and nephrosis	39	21	18	1	2	2	2	4	3	7	1	3	3	2	3	3	4
2. Benign prostatic hypertrophy	2	2	-	-	-	-	-	-	1	1	-	-	-	-	-	-	-
3. Other genito-urinary	51	30	21	1	1	2	4	8	6	8	1	1	2	3	5	4	5
K. Skin diseases	2	1	1	-	-	-	-	-	-	-	-	-	-	-	-	-	-

Annex Table 6h, continued. Deaths by age, sex and cause (thousands): Middle Eastern Crescent, 1990

Cause	Total	Male	Female	Males							Females						
				0-4	5-14	15-29	30-44	45-59	60-69	70+	0-4	5-14	15-29	30-44	45-59	60-69	70+
L. Musculo-skeletal diseases	2	1	1	-	-	-	-	-	-	-	-	-	-	-	-	-	-
1. Rheumatoid arthritis	-	-	1	-	-	-	-	-	-	-	-	-	-	-	-	-	-
3. Other musculo-skeletal	2	1	1	-	-	-	-	-	-	-	-	-	-	-	-	-	-
M. Congenital anomalies	76	39	37	33	3	2	1	1	-	-	30	3	1	1	1	-	-
1. Abdominal wall defect	1	1	-	1	-	-	-	-	-	-	-	-	-	-	-	-	-
2. Anencephaly	20	8	12	8	-	-	-	-	-	-	12	-	-	-	-	-	-
3. Anorectal atresia	-	-	-	-	-	-	-	-	-	-	-	-	-	-	-	-	-
4. Cleft lip	1	-	-	-	-	-	-	-	-	-	-	-	-	-	-	-	-
5. Cleft palate	1	-	-	-	-	-	-	-	-	-	-	-	-	-	-	-	-
6. Oesophageal atresia	1	1	1	1	-	-	-	-	-	-	-	-	-	-	-	-	-
7. Renal agenesis	2	1	1	1	-	-	-	-	-	-	1	-	-	-	-	-	-
8. Down syndrome	8	4	4	3	1	1	-	-	-	-	2	1	1	-	-	-	-
9. Congenital heart anomalies	29	16	13	13	1	1	-	1	-	-	9	1	1	1	1	-	-
10. Spina bifida	5	3	2	2	1	-	-	-	-	-	2	1	-	-	-	-	-
11. Other congenital	10	5	4	4	-	-	-	-	-	-	3	-	-	-	-	-	-
N. Oral conditions	-	-	-	-	-	-	-	-	-	-	-	-	-	-	-	-	-
III. Injuries	*452*	*296*	*156*	*46*	*44*	*98*	*65*	*26*	*10*	*7*	*44*	*23*	*44*	*24*	*10*	*6*	*6*
A. Unintentional injuries	198	142	57	23	23	39	33	14	5	4	20	10	10	6	4	2	3
1. Road traffic accidents	70	55	15	3	8	19	16	6	2	1	2	4	3	2	2	1	1
2. Poisonings	12	8	4	1	1	2	2	1	-	-	1	1	1	1	1	-	1
3. Falls	11	8	3	1	1	2	2	1	-	1	1	-	-	1	1	-	-
4. Fires	15	7	8	2	1	1	1	1	-	-	2	1	3	1	-	1	1
5. Drownings	28	20	8	6	6	5	2	1	-	-	5	2	1	-	-	-	-
6. Other unintentional	62	44	18	10	7	11	9	4	2	1	8	3	2	2	1	1	1
B. Intentional injuries	254	154	100	23	21	59	33	12	5	3	23	13	34	17	6	4	3
1. Self-inflicted injuries	46	32	14	-	8	10	7	4	2	2	-	4	4	2	2	1	1
2. Violence	39	25	14	6	2	8	6	2	1	1	6	2	3	2	1	-	-
3. War	169	97	72	17	10	41	21	5	3	1	17	7	27	14	3	3	1

Notes:

Causes responsible for no deaths have been omitted from this table.

A dash (-) symbol indicates fewer than 500 deaths.

*IA6 is Bacterial meningitis and meningococcaemia; IC3 is Hypertensive disorders of pregnancy; ID is Conditions arising during the perinatal period; IIE6 is Dementia and other degenerative and hereditary CNS disorders; IIH1 is Chronic obstructive pulmonary disease.

Annex Table 6i. Deaths by age, sex and cause (thousands): World, 1990

Cause	Total	Male	Female	Males							Females						
				0-4	5-14	15-29	30-44	45-59	60-69	70+	0-4	5-14	15-29	30-44	45-59	60-69	70+
Population (millions)	5 267	2 654	2 614	321	551	736	514	312	137	82	309	526	703	496	311	151	118
All causes	50 467	26 692	23 775	6 658	1 219	1 709	1 981	3 517	4 152	7 455	6 099	1 097	1 363	1 371	2 274	2 986	8 585
I. Communicable, maternal, perinatal and nutritional conditions	17 241	8 796	8 445	5 705	496	335	411	516	485	848	5 236	543	572	550	373	331	839
A. Infectious and parasitic diseases	9 329	4 999	4 331	2 872	336	292	369	453	306	371	2 578	352	301	293	306	199	302
1. Tuberculosis	1 960	1 166	794	43	26	149	184	325	209	230	39	31	133	125	209	117	140
2. STDs excluding HIV	230	104	126	84	–	1	1	3	4	11	77	1	13	13	4	5	13
a. Syphilis	204	104	101	84	–	1	1	3	4	11	77	–	1	2	4	4	13
b. Chlamydia	16	–	16	–	–	–	–	–	–	–	–	–	7	8	–	–	1
c. Gonorrhoea	9	–	9	–	–	–	–	–	–	–	–	–	5	3	–	1	–
3. HIV	312	173	138	34	5	44	64	20	4	2	32	5	47	45	7	2	1
4. Diarrhoeal diseases	2 946	1 533	1 414	1 311	81	16	20	20	32	53	1 169	90	24	24	20	25	61
5. Childhood-cluster diseases	1 985	1 022	963	870	108	11	16	8	4	4	808	111	14	15	8	3	4
a. Pertussis	347	180	167	166	14	–	–	–	–	–	153	14	–	–	–	–	–
b. Poliomyelitis	27	16	12	15	1	–	–	–	–	–	11	1	–	–	–	–	–
c. Diphtheria	11	5	5	5	–	–	–	–	–	–	4	1	–	–	–	–	–
d. Measles	1 058	547	512	471	74	1	1	–	–	–	437	73	1	1	–	–	–
e. Tetanus	542	274	267	214	19	10	16	8	3	4	202	23	13	14	8	3	4
6. Bacterial meningitis*	180	92	88	44	1	3	17	11	10	6	41	3	3	16	11	9	6
7. Hepatitis B and hepatitis C	108	64	44	8	4	6	11	17	8	11	6	3	6	5	6	8	10
8. Malaria	856	457	400	335	46	31	22	14	5	3	272	46	34	24	15	5	4
9. Tropical-cluster diseases	125	68	56	3	19	16	12	11	4	3	2	15	13	12	8	3	2
a. Trypanosomiasis	47	24	24	–	6	6	4	5	1	1	1	7	7	5	4	1	–
b. Chagas disease	19	9	10	–	–	–	2	5	1	1	–	–	1	3	3	2	1
c. Schistosomiasis	8	5	3	–	1	–	2	3	2	–	–	1	1	1	1	–	–
d. Leishmaniasis	50	31	20	2	12	9	5	1	–	1	2	8	6	3	1	–	1
10. Leprosy	3	2	1	–	–	–	–	–	–	–	–	–	–	–	–	–	–
11. Dengue	21	9	11	2	7	–	–	–	–	–	2	8	–	–	–	–	–
12. Japanese encephalitis	5	3	2	1	1	–	–	–	–	–	1	1	–	–	–	–	–
13. Trachoma	–	–	–	–	–	–	–	–	–	–	–	–	–	–	–	–	–
14. Intestinal nematode infections	22	11	11	–	9	1	–	–	–	1	–	9	1	–	–	–	1
a. Ascariasis	11	6	5	–	5	1	–	–	–	–	–	5	1	–	–	–	–
b. Trichuriasis	7	4	3	–	4	–	–	–	–	–	–	3	–	–	–	–	–
c. Ancylostomiasis, necatoriasis	4	2	2	–	–	–	–	–	–	1	–	–	–	–	–	–	1
15. Other infectious and parasitic	577	295	282	136	29	14	20	24	25	47	126	33	13	13	16	22	59

Annex Table 6i, continued. Deaths by age, sex and cause (thousands): World, 1990

Cause	Total	Male	Female	Males							Females						
				0-4	5-14	15-29	30-44	45-59	60-69	70+	0-4	5-14	15-29	30-44	45-59	60-69	70+
B. Respiratory infections	**4 380**	**2 232**	**2 148**	**1 366**	**132**	**33**	**35**	**53**	**168**	**445**	**1 271**	**149**	**37**	**30**	**46**	**121**	**494**
1. Lower respiratory infections	4 299	2 196	2 103	1 340	130	32	35	53	166	441	1 237	147	36	30	45	119	489
2. Upper respiratory infections	43	22	21	14	1	–	–	1	2	4	13	2	–	–	1	1	5
3. Otitis media	28	14	14	12	1	–	–	–	–	–	13	–	–	–	–	–	–
C. Maternal conditions	**454**	**–**	**454**								**–**	**10**	**219**	**214**	**11**	**–**	**–**
1. Maternal haemorrhage	114		114									2	56	53	3		
2. Maternal sepsis	68		68									2	32	33	2		
3. Hypertensive disorders*	57		57									1	27	27	1		
4. Obstructed labour	34		34									1	16	17	1		
5. Abortion	61		61									1	30	29	1		
6. Other maternal	121		121									3	59	56	3		
D. Perinatal conditions*	**2 443**	**1 266**	**1 177**	**1 266**							**1 177**						
1. Low birth weight	1 036	533	503	533							503						
2. Birth asphyxia and birth trauma	770	397	373	397							373						
3. Other perinatal	637	336	302	336							301						
E. Nutritional deficiencies	**634**	**299**	**335**	**201**	**28**	**10**	**7**	**9**	**12**	**32**	**210**	**32**	**15**	**13**	**11**	**11**	**43**
1. Protein-energy malnutrition	372	179	192	146	4	2	2	4	6	17	153	6	3	2	3	5	20
2. Iodine deficiency	23	12	11	9	2	1	–	–	–	–	9	2	1	–	–	–	–
3. Vitamin A deficiency	106	54	52	35	18	1	–	–	–	–	33	17	1	–	–	–	–
4. Iron-deficiency anaemia	129	52	76	12	5	6	4	5	6	15	14	7	10	10	8	7	21
II. Noncommunicable diseases	***28 141***	***14 573***	***13 569***	***572***	***332***	***368***	***864***	***2 573***	***3 475***	***6 388***	***547***	***317***	***345***	***572***	***1 721***	***2 540***	***7 526***
A. Malignant neoplasms	**6 024**	**3 418**	**2 605**	**28**	**62**	**79**	**232**	**833**	**992**	**1 192**	**27**	**46**	**79**	**202**	**601**	**651**	**999**
1. Mouth and oropharynx cancers	286	187	99	1	1	5	17	52	56	55	–	1	4	8	24	29	32
2. Oesophagus cancer	358	240	118	–	–	2	11	68	79	80	–	–	2	3	27	40	46
3. Stomach cancer	752	469	282	–	–	5	22	125	151	165	–	–	5	18	56	76	126
4. Colon and rectum cancers	472	237	235	1	2	3	13	44	69	106	1	1	3	10	37	60	124
5. Liver cancer	501	357	143	1	–	11	57	128	90	69	1	1	3	13	38	39	48
6. Pancreas cancer	183	100	84	–	–	1	4	23	31	40	–	–	1	2	12	23	46
7. Trachea, bronchus, lung cancers	945	708	237	–	–	5	20	182	245	255	–	–	2	8	50	74	104
8. Melanoma and other skin cancers	48	24	24	–	–	1	3	7	6	8	–	–	1	2	5	5	10
9. Breast cancer	322	–	322								–	–	9	38	101	73	101
10. Cervix uteri cancer	200	–	200								–	–	9	23	78	44	46
11. Corpus uteri cancer	64		64								–	–	1	3	15	17	27
12. Ovary cancer	107		107								–	1	5	11	29	27	33
13. Prostate cancer	193	193	–	–	–	–	–	13	51	127							
14. Bladder cancer	131	96	34	–	–	1	2	16	29	48	–	–	1	1	4	9	20
15. Lymphomas, multiple myeloma	214	123	90	4	11	8	13	23	28	36	2	6	4	7	14	20	37
16. Leukaemia	226	120	105	9	19	14	17	17	18	26	9	14	12	14	15	15	27
17. Other cancers	1 023	563	460	13	27	22	50	135	139	178	13	21	19	41	94	100	171

Annex Table 6i, continued. Deaths by age, sex and cause (thousands): World, 1990

Cause	Total	Male	Female	Males							Females						
				0-4	5-14	15-29	30-44	45-59	60-69	70+	0-4	5-14	15-29	30-44	45-59	60-69	70+
B. Other neoplasms	**106**	**54**	**51**	**3**	**6**	**4**	**5**	**10**	**10**	**16**	**3**	**5**	**4**	**5**	**8**	**9**	**18**
C. Diabetes mellitus	**571**	**244**	**328**	**4**	**10**	**5**	**18**	**48**	**63**	**96**	**4**	**9**	**7**	**12**	**51**	**86**	**158**
D. Endocrine disorders	**143**	**65**	**78**	**12**	**5**	**4**	**6**	**8**	**9**	**20**	**11**	**6**	**5**	**5**	**9**	**9**	**33**
E. Neuro-psychiatric conditions	**700**	**369**	**331**	**25**	**26**	**40**	**51**	**54**	**51**	**121**	**24**	**21**	**26**	**24**	**28**	**41**	**167**
2. Bipolar disorder	15	5	10	-	-	-	1	1	1	2	-	-	-	1	1	1	8
3. Schizophrenia	51	28	24	-	-	3	6	5	4	10	-	-	2	5	3	4	10
4. Epilepsy	68	40	28	2	5	9	10	7	4	4	3	3	8	5	3	2	4
5. Alcohol use	56	47	9	-	-	2	14	18	8	5	-	-	2	2	2	2	1
6. Dementia*	203	83	121	3	1	2	2	7	14	53	4	1	2	2	6	15	91
7. Parkinson disease	58	31	27	-	-	-	-	1	5	26	-	-	-	-	1	3	23
8. Multiple sclerosis	25	10	15	-	-	5	2	4	2	2	-	-	1	3	5	3	3
9. Drug use	11	9	2	-	-	5	3	-	-	-	-	-	1	1	-	-	-
13. Other neuro-psychiatric	212	116	96	20	20	19	13	12	13	20	18	17	13	8	6	10	25
F. Sense organ diseases	**20**	**11**	**9**	**1**	**-**	**1**	**-**	**2**	**3**	**3**	**1**	**-**	**-**	**1**	**2**	**3**	**2**
1. Glaucoma	6	4	3	-	-	-	-	-	1	1	-	-	-	-	1	1	1
2. Cataracts	6	4	2	-	-	-	-	-	1	1	-	-	-	-	1	1	1
G. Cardiovascular diseases	**14 327**	**6 942**	**7 385**	**108**	**114**	**127**	**313**	**1 073**	**1 642**	**3 565**	**100**	**119**	**126**	**197**	**704**	**1 300**	**4 839**
1. Rheumatic heart disease	340	141	199	-	8	23	20	31	23	35	1	12	25	27	46	34	55
2. Ischaemic heart disease	6 260	3 126	3 134	-	-	14	122	511	794	1 685	4	-	10	62	266	576	2 214
3. Cerebrovascular disease	4 381	2 022	2 359	14	24	27	75	291	496	1 095	13	21	22	52	233	444	1 574
4. Inflammatory heart diseases	495	247	249	21	23	22	29	49	33	70	25	25	21	20	36	29	93
5. Other cardiovascular	2 852	1 407	1 444	73	58	40	67	191	297	681	58	61	49	36	122	216	902
H. Respiratory diseases	**2 935**	**1 610**	**1 325**	**66**	**25**	**19**	**43**	**173**	**386**	**899**	**69**	**25**	**17**	**29**	**114**	**234**	**836**
1. COPD*	2 211	1 214	997	17	4	5	16	117	310	746	23	5	3	12	76	189	690
2. Asthma	137	71	66	1	4	4	8	12	15	28	1	2	3	6	11	13	29
3. Other respiratory	587	324	263	48	17	10	19	44	61	126	45	18	12	12	27	32	117
I. Digestive diseases	**1 851**	**1 107**	**744**	**60**	**34**	**47**	**152**	**300**	**231**	**284**	**60**	**32**	**37**	**56**	**136**	**134**	**289**
1. Peptic ulcer	175	105	71	-	1	4	11	24	23	42	1	1	3	4	11	12	40
2. Cirrhosis of the liver	779	529	250	5	5	19	89	186	126	101	3	6	11	25	71	62	71
3. Appendicitis	56	33	23	1	10	10	7	2	1	1	1	8	6	4	2	1	1
4. Other digestive	841	440	401	54	18	14	45	88	81	140	55	17	16	23	53	59	178
J. Genito-urinary diseases	**735**	**397**	**338**	**15**	**26**	**24**	**35**	**61**	**74**	**162**	**12**	**27**	**22**	**29**	**53**	**59**	**136**
1. Nephritis and nephrosis	536	281	255	13	23	20	27	46	51	101	11	24	18	23	40	44	96
2. Benign prostatic hypertrophy	32	32	-	3	-	-	-	1	7	24	-	-	-	-	-	-	-
3. Other genito-urinary	167	83	83	3	3	3	7	15	16	36	1	2	5	6	13	15	41
K. Skin diseases	**43**	**21**	**22**	**5**	**1**	**1**	**1**	**2**	**2**	**9**	**4**	**-**	**2**	**1**	**2**	**2**	**11**

Annex Table 6i, continued. Deaths by age, sex and cause (thousands): World, 1990

Cause	Total	Male	Female	Males 0-4	5-14	15-29	30-44	45-59	60-69	70+	Females 0-4	5-14	15-29	30-44	45-59	60-69	70+
L. Musculo-skeletal diseases	**97**	**37**	**60**	**1**	**2**	**2**	**2**	**4**	**8**	**19**	**1**	**1**	**4**	**5**	**7**	**9**	**34**
1. Rheumatoid arthritis	16	5	11	-	-	-	-	1	1	3	-	-	-	-	2	2	7
2. Other musculo-skeletal	81	32	49	1	2	1	1	3	7	16	1	1	4	4	6	6	27
M. Congenital anomalies	**589**	**299**	**290**	**244**	**22**	**16**	**7**	**5**	**2**	**3**	**232**	**23**	**16**	**6**	**6**	**3**	**3**
1. Abdominal wall defect	5	3	2	3							2						
2. Anencephaly	148	58	90	58							90						
3. Anorectal atresia	2	1	1	1							1						
4. Cleft lip	5	3	2	3							2						
5. Cleft palate	4	2	2	2							2						
6. Oesophageal atresia	3	2	1	2							1						
7. Renal agenesis	12	6	6	6							6						
8. Down syndrome	57	31	26	17	5	5	2	1			12	5	5	2	1	2	
9. Congenital heart anomalies	207	113	94	85	10	7	3	4	2	2	64	10	8	3	4	2	2
10. Spina bifida	59	31	28	28	3						23	3	1				
11. Other congenital	87	49	38	39	4	3	1	1			29	5	2	1			1
N. Oral conditions	**2**	**1**	**1**				1						1				
III. Injuries	**5 084**	**3 323**	**1 761**	**381**	**390**	**1 006**	**706**	**429**	**192**	**219**	**315**	**237**	**446**	**250**	**179**	**115**	**220**
A. Unintentional injuries	**3 233**	**2 137**	**1 096**	**307**	**324**	**546**	**413**	**274**	**121**	**151**	**238**	**196**	**202**	**122**	**104**	**70**	**164**
1. Road traffic accidents	999	730	269	51	95	230	173	100	42	39	32	53	61	39	38	21	24
2. Poisonings	242	148	94	29	12	24	33	31	11	9	19	10	24	15	10	6	8
3. Falls	292	165	127	13	16	26	25	26	18	41	13	8	5	6	13	12	74
4. Fires	265	113	152	31	14	22	18	13	5	11	27	25	47	23	11	7	13
5. Drownings	504	335	168	87	107	69	34	19	9	11	62	52	21	10	8	5	10
6. Other unintentional	932	645	286	96	80	176	130	86	38	41	84	48	44	30	28	19	35
B. Intentional injuries	**1 851**	**1 186**	**665**	**74**	**66**	**460**	**293**	**155**	**70**	**68**	**77**	**41**	**244**	**128**	**75**	**44**	**55**
1. Self-inflicted injuries	786	456	330	-	18	128	115	91	48	56	-	10	131	64	49	30	47
2. Violence	563	439	124	23	18	208	117	49	14	9	27	11	33	23	16	7	6
3. War	502	291	211	50	30	123	62	15	8	3	50	20	81	40	10	8	3

Notes:
Causes responsible for no deaths have been omitted from this table.
A dash (-) symbol indicates fewer than 500 deaths.
*IA6 is Bacterial meningitis and meningococcaemia; IC3 is Hypertensive disorders of pregnancy; ID is Conditions arising during the perinatal period; IIE6 is Dementia and other degenerative and hereditary CNS disorders; IIH1 is Chronic obstructive pulmonary disease.

Annex Table 7a. YLLs by age, sex and cause (thousands): Established Market Economies, 1990

Cause	Total	Male	Female	Males							Females						
				0-4	5-14	15-29	30-44	45-59	60-69	70+	0-4	5-14	15-29	30-44	45-59	60-69	70+
Population (millions)	798	390	407	26	53	94	90	66	34	26	25	51	90	89	68	41	44
All causes	49 674	29 804	19 871	2 010	516	3 807	4 480	6 820	6 397	5 773	1 515	332	1 313	2 120	3 729	4 144	6 717
I. Communicable, maternal, perinatal and nutritional conditions	4 367	2 718	1 650	1 026	24	255	583	273	186	370	744	24	100	134	95	122	430
A. Infectious and parasitic diseases	1 495	1 126	369	72	11	217	523	183	64	56	53	11	60	91	44	46	64
1. Tuberculosis	107	77	30	-	-	4	14	23	20	15	-	-	2	4	7	8	8
2. STDs excluding HIV	7	3	4	1	-	-	-	1	-	-	-	-	-	1	1	1	1
a. Syphilis	4	3	1	1	-	-	-	1	-	-	-	-	-	-	1	1	1
b. Chlamydia	1	-	1	1	-	-	-	-	-	-	-	-	-	1	-	-	-
c. Gonorrhoea	1	-	-	-	-	-	-	-	-	-	-	-	-	-	-	-	-
3. HIV	950	812	138	17	3	189	467	124	10	1	12	3	42	66	14	3	3
4. Diarrhoeal diseases	23	13	10	7	1	1	1	1	1	2	5	-	-	-	1	1	2
5. Childhood-cluster diseases	10	5	5	2	1	1	1	1	1	-	5	-	-	-	-	-	-
a. Pertussis	2	1	1	1	1	-	-	-	-	-	1	-	-	-	-	-	-
b. Poliomyelitis	3	2	1	-	1	1	1	1	1	-	1	1	-	-	-	-	-
c. Diphtheria	-	-	-	-	-	-	-	-	-	-	-	-	-	-	-	-	-
d. Measles	4	2	2	1	1	-	-	-	1	-	1	1	-	-	-	-	-
e. Tetanus	1	1	1	-	-	-	-	-	-	-	-	-	-	-	-	-	-
6. Bacterial meningitis*	90	51	39	27	3	6	6	5	3	1	20	4	4	3	3	2	2
7. Hepatitis B and hepatitis C	48	30	18	1	1	5	9	8	4	2	1	-	4	4	4	3	2
8. Malaria	2	1	1	-	-	-	-	-	-	-	-	-	-	-	-	-	-
9. Tropical-cluster diseases	1	1	-	-	-	-	1	-	-	-	-	-	-	-	-	-	-
a. Trypanosomiasis	-	-	-	-	-	-	-	-	-	-	-	-	-	-	-	-	-
b. Chagas disease	-	-	-	-	-	-	-	-	-	-	-	-	-	-	-	-	-
c. Schistosomiasis	-	-	-	-	-	-	-	-	-	-	-	-	-	-	-	-	-
d. Leishmaniasis	-	-	-	-	-	-	-	-	-	-	-	-	-	-	-	-	-
10. Leprosy	-	-	-	-	-	-	-	-	-	-	-	-	-	-	-	-	-
11. Dengue	-	-	-	-	-	-	-	-	-	-	-	-	-	-	-	-	-
12. Japanese encephalitis	-	-	-	-	-	-	-	-	-	-	-	-	-	-	-	-	-
13. Trachoma	-	-	-	-	-	-	-	-	-	-	-	-	-	-	-	-	-
14. Intestinal nematode infections	-	-	-	-	-	-	-	-	-	-	-	-	-	-	-	-	-
a. Ascariasis	-	-	-	-	-	-	-	-	-	-	-	-	-	-	-	-	-
b. Trichuriasis	-	-	-	-	-	-	-	-	-	-	-	-	-	-	-	-	-
c. Ancylostomiasis, necatoriasis	-	-	-	-	-	-	-	-	-	-	-	-	-	-	-	-	-
15. Other infectious and parasitic	257	133	124	17	3	11	24	20	24	35	12	3	7	12	14	27	49

Annex Table 7a, continued. YLLs by age, sex and cause (thousands): Established Market Economies, 1990

Cause	Total	Male	Female	Males 0-4	5-14	15-29	30-44	45-59	60-69	70+	Females 0-4	5-14	15-29	30-44	45-59	60-69	70+
B. Respiratory infections	**1 193**	**644**	**549**	**64**	**10**	**27**	**51**	**81**	**113**	**297**	**44**	**9**	**20**	**27**	**44**	**67**	**339**
1. Lower respiratory infections	1 162	626	536	55	9	26	50	80	112	295	38	8	19	26	43	67	335
2. Upper respiratory infections	26	15	11	8	1	1	1	1	1	2	4	1	1	-	1	1	3
3. Otitis media	5	3	2	2	-	-	-	-	-	-	1	-	-	-	-	-	-
C. Maternal conditions	**23**		**23**										**14**	**9**			
1. Maternal haemorrhage	3		3										2	2			
2. Maternal sepsis	2		2										1	1			
3. Hypertensive disorders*	11		11										6	5			
4. Obstructed labour	-		-														
5. Abortion	3		3										2	1			
6. Other maternal	3		3										3	1			
D. Perinatal conditions*	**1 533**	**887**	**646**	**885**	**1**	**1**					**644**	**1**					
1. Low birth weight	349	197	152	197							152						
2. Birth asphyxia and birth trauma	666	396	270	396	1						269	1					
3. Other perinatal	518	294	224	293		1					223						
E. Nutritional deficiencies	**124**	**61**	**63**	**4**	**3**	**10**	**9**	**9**	**9**	**16**	**4**	**3**	**7**	**7**	**7**	**9**	**27**
1. Protein-energy malnutrition	24	11	14	1	-	-	1	2	2	5	1	-	-	1	1	2	9
2. Iodine deficiency	-	-	-														
3. Vitamin A deficiency	-	-	-														
4. Iron-deficiency anaemia	94	47	47	4	3	10	7	6	6	11	3	3	6	6	5	7	17
II. Noncommunicable diseases	**37 403**	**21 187**	**16 216**	**786**	**225**	**871**	**2 319**	**5 796**	**5 945**	**5 244**	**635**	**177**	**528**	**1 524**	**3 356**	**3 881**	**6 115**
A. Malignant neoplasms	**12 985**	**7 246**	**5 739**	**39**	**83**	**261**	**727**	**2 379**	**2 372**	**1 384**	**32**	**62**	**186**	**821**	**1 819**	**1 668**	**1 151**
1. Mouth and oropharynx cancers	312	249	63			4	36	122	66	20			2	9	23	18	11
2. Oesophagus cancer	323	262	61			1	21	115	91	35				4	18	21	18
3. Stomach cancer	932	581	351			7	21	198	191	125			7	55	96	94	99
4. Colon and rectum cancers	1 296	688	608			7	60	221	234	161			6	55	173	190	184
5. Liver cancer	306	236	70	1	1	9	19	101	85	26	1	1	2	5	19	27	15
6. Pancreas cancer	553	311	242			2	28	111	110	60			1	15	66	87	72
7. Trachea, bronchus, lung cancers	2 771	2 037	734			6	134	729	804	362			4	61	254	286	130
8. Melanoma and other skin cancers	217	130	87	1		10	38	42	26	14			8	24	26	16	15
9. Breast cancer	1 228	-	1 228										14	268	497	300	149
10. Cervix uteri cancer	175	-	175										10	62	57	32	14
11. Corpus uteri cancer	162	-	162										2	17	50	57	37
12. Ovary cancer	346	-	346										9	45	136	107	48
13. Prostate cancer	386	386	-					43	134	205							
14. Bladder cancer	235	176	59			1	2	41	66	63				3	10	19	27
15. Lymphomas, multiple myeloma	643	375	268	2	9	45	70	105	90	54		3	23	37	67	77	59
16. Leukaemia	570	327	243	12	34	66	54	63	57	41	11	23	39	41	49	42	37
17. Other cancers	2 530	1 488	1 042	22	38	107	198	488	416	219	18	33	60	120	279	294	238
B. Other neoplasms	**286**	**154**	**132**	**7**	**9**	**16**	**23**	**39**	**33**	**27**	**6**	**7**	**11**	**19**	**30**	**28**	**31**

Annex Table 7a, continued. YLLs by age, sex and cause (thousands): Established Market Economies, 1990

Cause	Total	Male	Female	Males 0-4	5-14	15-29	30-44	45-59	60-69	70+	Females 0-4	5-14	15-29	30-44	45-59	60-69	70+
C. Diabetes mellitus	810	382	428	1	1	15	52	106	111	96	1	2	11	31	78	133	174
D. Endocrine disorders	401	201	200	37	17	28	27	23	38	31	32	13	22	21	36	31	45
E. Neuro-psychiatric conditions	1 564	933	631	54	37	186	209	179	119	149	42	28	71	85	95	92	219
2. Bipolar disorder	3	1	2	–	–	1	–	–	–	–	–	–	1	1	–	–	–
3. Schizophrenia	63	36	27	–	–	8	9	14	5	2	–	3	16	7	1	–	–
4. Epilepsy	131	84	47	3	5	27	28	10	7	4	3	4	3	17	9	4	7
5. Alcohol use	223	176	47	–	8	10	65	74	24	10	–	–	5	13	13	9	7
6. Dementia*	437	200	237	19	–	–	14	32	43	74	18	–	–	7	30	42	132
7. Parkinson disease	99	53	46	–	–	–	–	2	13	37	–	–	–	2	4	9	34
8. Multiple sclerosis	70	28	42	–	–	2	9	11	5	1	–	1	2	7	17	9	2
9. Drug use	108	89	19	–	–	58	29	1	–	1	–	–	12	6	–	–	–
13. Other neuro-psychiatric	430	266	164	32	24	78	55	35	22	20	21	19	31	26	21	17	29
F. Sense organ diseases	2	1	1	–	–	–	–	–	–	–	–	–	–	–	–	–	–
1. Glaucoma	–	–	–	–	–	–	–	–	–	–	–	–	–	–	–	–	–
2. Cataracts	–	–	–	–	–	–	–	–	–	–	–	–	–	–	–	–	–
G. Cardiovascular diseases	15 288	8 695	6 593	59	24	205	839	2 270	2 516	2 782	48	20	110	324	880	1 446	3 764
1. Rheumatic heart disease	141	51	91	–	–	3	9	15	14	8	–	–	4	10	25	29	23
2. Ischaemic heart disease	8 113	4 897	3 216	–	–	30	421	1 425	1 531	1 490	–	–	9	113	436	792	1 866
3. Cerebrovascular disease	3 424	1 645	1 779	9	6	42	150	356	409	672	7	5	31	107	236	330	1 063
4. Inflammatory heart diseases	504	314	190	11	5	44	71	91	44	48	13	4	17	27	39	25	64
5. Other cardiovascular	3 105	1 788	1 318	38	13	85	188	383	518	564	27	10	50	67	145	270	748
H. Respiratory diseases	1 768	1 096	671	28	13	46	62	186	338	423	19	8	32	42	116	189	266
1. COPD*	1 122	725	398	5	2	4	14	116	256	329	3	1	3	7	70	138	176
2. Asthma	191	97	95	2	7	18	16	20	18	15	1	4	14	17	21	19	18
3. Other respiratory	454	275	179	21	5	25	32	50	64	79	15	3	15	18	26	32	71
I. Digestive diseases	2 292	1 450	842	25	6	49	313	527	326	204	16	5	28	121	216	195	260
1. Peptic ulcer	159	96	62	1	–	3	12	26	25	29	1	–	–	4	9	14	33
2. Cirrhosis of the liver	1 238	867	371	1	1	20	220	380	192	53	1	1	10	79	141	99	41
3. Appendicitis	14	8	5	–	1	1	1	1	3	1	–	–	1	–	1	2	1
4. Other digestive	882	478	404	23	4	25	80	119	105	121	15	4	17	38	65	80	185
J. Genito-urinary diseases	592	308	284	8	2	12	33	57	69	122	8	2	9	21	43	62	139
1. Nephritis and nephrosis	408	219	188	7	1	9	25	44	51	78	7	1	6	13	30	43	87
2. Benign prostatic hypertrophy	12	12	–	–	–	–	–	–	2	10	–	–	–	–	–	–	–
3. Other genito-urinary	172	76	96	1	–	3	8	13	16	34	1	1	4	7	13	18	51
K. Skin diseases	50	20	30	1	–	1	3	3	4	8	–	–	1	2	3	4	19
L. Musculo-skeletal diseases	193	58	135	1	1	5	8	13	14	16	1	2	15	19	26	29	44
1. Rheumatoid arthritis	48	12	36	–	–	–	–	3	5	4	–	–	–	2	7	13	13
3. Other musculo-skeletal	145	46	99	1	1	5	7	10	9	12	1	2	14	18	19	16	31

Annex Table 7a, continued. YLLs by age, sex and cause (thousands): Established Market Economies, 1990

Cause	Total	Male	Female	Males 0-4	5-14	15-29	30-44	45-59	60-69	70+	Females 0-4	5-14	15-29	30-44	45-59	60-69	70+
M. Congenital anomalies	**1 171**	**643**	**528**	**522**	**31**	**46**	**22**	**12**	**6**	**3**	**430**	**28**	**31**	**17**	**12**	**6**	**3**
1. Abdominal wall defect	15	5	10	5	-	-	-	-	-	-	10	-	-	-	-	-	-
2. Anencephaly	87	35	52	35	-	-	-	-	-	-	52	-	-	-	-	-	-
3. Anorectal atresia	3	1	2	1	-	-	-	-	-	-	2	-	-	-	-	-	-
4. Cleft lip	17	8	9	8	-	-	-	-	-	-	9	-	-	-	-	-	-
5. Cleft palate	14	5	9	5	-	-	-	-	-	-	9	-	-	-	-	-	-
6. Oesophageal atresia	8	3	4	3	-	-	-	-	-	-	4	-	-	-	-	-	-
7. Renal agenesis	62	32	30	32	-	-	-	-	-	-	30	-	-	-	-	-	-
8. Down syndrome	70	39	31	26	-	2	1	5	2	1	20	2	1	1	5	1	1
9. Congenital heart anomalies	451	252	199	188	15	25	14	6	3	-	150	13	15	10	6	3	2
10. Spina bifida	60	28	32	21	3	3	1	-	-	-	26	2	2	-	-	-	-
11. Other congenital	385	233	152	197	10	18	7	1	1	1	120	10	13	5	-	2	1
N. Oral conditions	**2**	**1**	**1**	-	-	-	-	-	-	-	-	-	-	-	-	-	-
III. Injuries	***7 904***	***5 899***	***2 005***	***199***	***266***	***2 681***	***1 577***	***751***	***267***	***158***	***135***	***131***	***685***	***462***	***278***	***141***	***172***
A. Unintentional injuries	**5 134**	**3 813**	**1 321**	**180**	**236**	**1 777**	**888**	**440**	**173**	**118**	**117**	**115**	**456**	**243**	**149**	**91**	**151**
1. Road traffic accidents	2 961	2 201	760	46	125	1 282	458	192	67	30	34	73	366	149	78	39	21
2. Poisonings	266	199	67	3	3	74	90	21	5	2	2	3	22	25	10	4	3
3. Falls	435	279	156	7	7	54	66	63	33	49	4	3	8	13	16	19	92
4. Fires	183	116	67	22	14	27	27	15	7	4	17	12	12	11	7	4	5
5. Drownings	276	222	54	36	35	77	42	20	8	4	18	8	9	8	5	3	3
6. Other unintentional	1 014	796	218	66	52	262	205	129	52	30	42	17	39	38	32	22	28
B. Intentional injuries	**2 769**	**2 086**	**683**	**19**	**30**	**904**	**689**	**311**	**93**	**40**	**18**	**16**	**229**	**219**	**130**	**51**	**21**
1. Self-inflicted injuries	1 989	1 492	497	-	13	579	510	268	85	38	-	4	146	166	115	46	20
2. Violence	778	593	186	19	16	325	179	43	8	2	18	12	82	52	15	4	2
3. War	1	1	-	-	-	-	-	-	-	-	-	-	-	-	-	-	-

Notes:
Causes responsible for no deaths have been omitted from this table.
A dash (-) symbol indicates fewer than 500 YLLs.
*IA6 is Bacterial meningitis and meningococcaemia; IC3 is Conditions arising during the perinatal period; ID is Hypertensive disorders of pregnancy; ID is Conditions arising during the perinatal period;
IIE6 is Dementia and other degenerative and hereditary CNS disorders; IIH1 is Chronic obstructive pulmonary disease.

Annex Table 7b. YLLs by age, sex and cause (thousands): Formerly Socialist Economies of Europe, 1990

Cause	Total	Male	Female	Males							Females						
				0-4	5-14	15-29	30-44	45-59	60-69	70+	0-4	5-14	15-29	30-44	45-59	60-69	70+
Population (millions)	346	165	181	14	27	36	40	27	14	7	13	26	35	40	30	20	16
All causes	35 930	22 333	13 597	2 216	624	2 804	4 471	6 203	3 819	2 195	1 616	356	911	1 418	2 764	2 979	3 553
I. Communicable, maternal, perinatal and nutritional conditions	3 390	2 019	1 372	1 281	36	82	206	209	98	107	894	30	77	76	53	65	176
A. Infectious and parasitic diseases	878	596	281	193	13	48	148	131	47	17	146	11	22	27	26	26	25
1. Tuberculosis	352	305	47	2	–	30	124	109	32	7	1	1	7	13	13	8	4
2. STDs excluding HIV	6	4	2	–	–	–	2	1	–	–	–	–	–	2	–	–	–
a. Syphilis	1	1	1	–	–	–	–	–	–	–	–	–	–	–	–	–	–
b. Chlamydia	1	1	1	–	–	–	–	–	–	–	–	–	–	–	–	–	–
c. Gonorrhoea	–	–	–	–	–	–	–	–	–	–	–	–	–	–	–	–	–
3. HIV	31	17	14	10	2	2	3	1	–	–	10	–	1	1	1	–	–
4. Diarrhoeal diseases	129	70	59	66	1	1	1	1	–	–	56	1	1	1	–	–	–
5. Childhood-cluster diseases	13	7	6	3	1	1	1	1	–	–	3	1	1	1	–	–	–
a. Pertussis	1	1	–	–	–	–	–	–	–	–	–	–	–	–	–	–	–
b. Poliomyelitis	1	–	1	–	–	–	–	–	–	–	–	–	–	–	–	–	–
c. Diphtheria	1	1	–	–	–	–	–	–	–	–	–	–	–	–	–	–	–
d. Measles	9	5	4	–	–	–	1	1	–	–	1	1	–	–	–	–	–
e. Tetanus	2	1	1	–	–	–	–	–	–	–	2	–	–	–	–	–	–
6. Bacterial meningitis*	141	86	54	53	3	6	9	8	5	2	36	3	3	4	4	3	2
7. Hepatitis B and hepatitis C	35	19	16	7	2	3	2	2	1	–	5	1	4	3	1	1	–
8. Malaria	–	–	–	–	–	–	–	–	–	–	–	–	–	–	–	–	–
9. Tropical-cluster diseases	–	–	–	–	–	–	–	–	–	–	–	–	–	–	–	–	–
a. Trypanosomiasis	–	–	–	–	–	–	–	–	–	–	–	–	–	–	–	–	–
b. Chagas disease	–	–	–	–	–	–	–	–	–	–	–	–	–	–	–	–	–
c. Schistosomiasis	–	–	–	–	–	–	–	–	–	–	–	–	–	–	–	–	–
d. Leishmaniasis	–	–	–	–	–	–	–	–	–	–	–	–	–	–	–	–	–
10. Leprosy	–	–	–	–	–	–	–	–	–	–	–	–	–	–	–	–	–
11. Dengue	–	–	–	–	–	–	–	–	–	–	–	–	–	–	–	–	–
12. Japanese encephalitis	–	–	–	–	–	–	–	–	–	–	–	–	–	–	–	–	–
13. Trachoma	–	–	–	–	–	–	–	–	–	–	–	–	–	–	–	–	–
14. Intestinal nematode infections	1	–	–	–	–	–	–	–	–	–	–	–	–	–	–	–	–
a. Ascariasis	1	–	–	–	–	–	–	–	–	–	–	–	–	–	–	–	–
b. Trichuriasis	–	–	–	–	–	–	–	–	–	–	–	–	–	–	–	–	–
c. Ancylostomiasis, necatoriasis	–	–	–	–	–	–	–	–	–	–	–	–	–	–	–	–	–
15. Other infectious and parasitic	171	89	83	51	4	6	5	8	7	7	33	3	5	5	6	12	18

Annex Table 7b, continued. YLLs by age, sex and cause (thousands): Formerly Socialist Economies of Europe, 1990

Cause	Total	Male	Female	Males 0-4	Males 5-14	Males 15-29	Males 30-44	Males 45-59	Males 60-69	Males 70+	Females 0-4	Females 5-14	Females 15-29	Females 30-44	Females 45-59	Females 60-69	Females 70+
B. Respiratory infections	**1 146**	**644**	**503**	**337**	**19**	**29**	**54**	**72**	**47**	**85**	**258**	**17**	**17**	**17**	**22**	**34**	**138**
1. Lower respiratory infections	1 128	633	495	329	19	29	53	72	47	85	252	17	17	17	21	34	138
2. Upper respiratory infections	11	6	5	5	–	–	–	–	–	–	4	–	–	–	–	–	–
3. Otitis media	7	4	3	4	–	–	–	–	–	–	3	–	–	–	–	–	–
C. Maternal conditions	**63**		**63**								–	–	**35**	**28**	–	–	–
1. Maternal haemorrhage	6		6								–	–	3	3	–	–	–
2. Maternal sepsis	4		4								–	–	3	1	–	–	–
3. Hypertensive disorders*	9		9								–	–	5	4	–	–	–
4. Obstructed labour	1		1								–	–	–	–	–	–	–
5. Abortion	29		29								–	–	15	14	–	–	–
6. Other maternal	15		15								–	–	9	6	–	–	–
D. Perinatal conditions*	**1 218**	**738**	**480**	**738**							**480**						
1. Low birth weight	181	103	77	103							77						
2. Birth asphyxia and birth trauma	291	176	115	176							115						
3. Other perinatal	746	459	288	459							288						
E. Nutritional deficiencies	**85**	**41**	**44**	**13**	**3**	**4**	**5**	**6**	**4**	**5**	**10**	**3**	**3**	**4**	**6**	**6**	**13**
1. Protein-energy malnutrition	11	5	6	1	–	–	1	1	1	1	1	–	–	–	–	1	4
2. Iodine deficiency	–																
3. Vitamin A deficiency	–																
4. Iron-deficiency anaemia	36	16	20	2	2	3	2	3	2	3	2	2	2	2	3	3	6
II. Noncommunicable diseases	***24 271***	***13 849***	***10 422***	***617***	***192***	***538***	***2 025***	***4 947***	***3 502***	***2 029***	***479***	***146***	***338***	***935***	***2 426***	***2 795***	***3 303***
A. Malignant neoplasms	**6 601**	**3 910**	**2 691**	**43**	**76**	**154**	**512**	**1 727**	**1 089**	**309**	**32**	**50**	**118**	**441**	**962**	**768**	**319**
1. Mouth and oropharynx cancers	203	176	27	–	1	1	32	98	36	7	–	–	1	5	9	7	7
2. Oesophagus cancer	108	93	15	–	–	–	12	52	24	5	–	–	–	2	5	5	3
3. Stomach cancer	925	583	342	–	–	9	79	270	171	54	–	–	8	47	116	113	58
4. Colon and rectum cancers	570	282	288	–	–	8	36	108	92	39	–	–	5	32	98	100	53
5. Liver cancer	182	107	75	1	1	2	13	44	37	10	1	1	–	7	24	29	13
6. Pancreas cancer	259	159	101	–	–	–	22	73	49	14	–	–	–	9	33	40	18
7. Trachea, bronchus, lung cancers	1 498	1 274	224	–	–	7	124	672	396	73	–	–	5	28	89	77	24
8. Melanoma and other skin cancers	90	46	43	1	–	3	15	16	8	4	–	–	4	13	12	8	6
9. Breast cancer	456	–	456								–	–	–	109	206	104	30
10. Cervix uteri cancer	172	–	172								–	–	1	49	61	41	14
11. Corpus uteri cancer	119	–	119								–	–	–	15	46	41	14
12. Ovary cancer	176	–	176								–	–	–	31	79	47	11
13. Prostate cancer	85	85	–	–	–	–	–	19	34	29							
14. Bladder cancer	121	95	26	–	–	–	2	35	38	16	–	–	–	2	7	10	6
15. Lymphomas, multiple myeloma	234	143	91	5	14	26	32	39	21	5	3	5	17	17	23	19	6
16. Leukaemia	286	163	123	14	29	31	26	33	23	7	10	19	19	20	26	20	7
17. Other cancers	1 118	703	415	20	28	63	116	268	161	47	17	22	32	57	127	109	51
B. Other neoplasms	**109**	**55**	**54**	**5**	**5**	**7**	**12**	**17**	**7**	**2**	**4**	**4**	**6**	**12**	**17**	**9**	**3**

Annex Table 7b, continued. YLLs by age, sex and cause (thousands): Formerly Socialist Economies of Europe, 1990

Cause	Total	Male	Female	Males 0-4	5-14	15-29	30-44	45-59	60-69	70+	Females 0-4	5-14	15-29	30-44	45-59	60-69	70+
C. Diabetes mellitus	267	115	152	-	1	8	26	36	32	12	1	1	12	13	39	60	26
D. Endocrine disorders	71	35	36	10	3	6	7	5	3	1	9	3	5	5	7	5	1
E. Neuro-psychiatric conditions	817	475	342	57	51	77	115	94	49	33	43	37	48	54	47	45	67
2. Bipolar disorder	34	13	21	-	-	2	4	3	2	2	-	-	1	2	3	3	11
3. Schizophrenia	43	27	16	-	-	2	10	9	4	2	-	-	2	3	4	4	1
4. Epilepsy	130	81	49	4	9	23	27	12	4	1	4	6	17	12	6	4	4
5. Alcohol use	111	93	18	-	-	3	36	37	14	3	-	-	4	6	6	-	2
6. Dementia*	115	50	65	10	6	5	4	6	8	10	8	4	4	4	5	11	28
7. Parkinson disease	30	12	17	-	-	-	-	1	4	7	-	-	-	-	1	5	10
8. Multiple sclerosis	54	22	31	-	-	2	9	6	3	1	-	-	2	12	9	5	3
9. Drug use	1	1	-	-	-	1	-	-	-	-	-	-	-	-	-	-	-
13. Other neuro-psychiatric	300	176	124	43	35	39	25	19	10	6	32	27	21	15	11	10	8
F. Sense organ diseases	-	-	-	-	-	-	-	-	-	-	-	-	-	-	-	-	-
1. Glaucoma	-	-	-	-	-	-	-	-	-	-	-	-	-	-	-	-	-
2. Cataracts	-	-	-	-	-	-	-	-	-	-	-	-	-	-	-	-	-
G. Cardiovascular diseases	12 588	6 903	5 685	24	13	165	1 005	2 396	1 867	1 434	22	10	65	260	1 044	1 618	2 666
1. Rheumatic heart disease	345	159	185	-	2	17	50	67	20	3	-	2	9	34	90	44	7
2. Ischaemic heart disease	6 365	3 778	2 587	-	-	50	570	1 456	979	722	-	-	9	100	462	741	1 275
3. Cerebrovascular disease	3 657	1 696	1 961	4	3	36	167	540	533	414	3	3	19	78	383	596	879
4. Inflammatory heart diseases	366	229	137	5	3	26	71	75	27	23	6	2	9	21	37	22	39
5. Other cardiovascular	1 856	1 041	815	15	5	36	147	259	307	273	13	4	20	26	72	215	466
H. Respiratory diseases	1 092	738	354	10	4	19	60	259	236	148	7	3	14	26	77	101	126
1. COPD*	505	348	157	-	1	4	19	123	122	78	1	-	3	7	31	48	68
2. Asthma	75	37	39	1	3	5	7	7	7	4	1	2	4	7	9	9	7
3. Other respiratory	512	354	158	9	1	10	34	128	107	66	6	1	7	12	37	44	52
I. Digestive diseases	1 302	844	458	37	6	43	216	327	164	52	23	5	22	68	146	125	68
1. Peptic ulcer	143	111	33	-	-	6	27	45	24	8	1	-	1	4	9	11	7
2. Cirrhosis of the liver	604	405	199	2	1	12	103	182	87	18	1	2	7	34	80	57	18
3. Appendicitis	8	5	4	-	-	1	1	1	1	-	1	2	1	1	-	-	-
4. Other digestive	554	329	226	35	5	25	86	100	52	26	22	4	13	30	56	57	43
J. Genito-urinary diseases	451	248	203	4	5	29	54	71	49	36	3	4	22	37	65	51	21
1. Nephritis and nephrosis	248	141	107	2	4	23	40	43	20	9	2	3	15	24	32	22	9
2. Benign prostatic hypertrophy	28	28	-	-	-	-	-	1	10	16	-	-	-	-	-	-	-
3. Other genito-urinary	176	80	96	2	1	7	14	25	19	11	1	1	7	14	33	29	12
K. Skin diseases	29	14	14	2	-	3	3	4	2	1	2	-	3	3	3	3	1
L. Musculo-skeletal diseases	71	24	46	1	2	5	6	6	3	1	1	2	8	9	15	9	2
1. Rheumatoid arthritis	6	2	4	-	-	-	-	1	1	-	-	-	-	1	2	-	1
3. Other musculo-skeletal	65	23	42	1	2	5	6	6	3	1	1	2	8	8	13	8	2

Annex Table 7b, continued. YLLs by age, sex and cause (thousands): Formerly Socialist Economies of Europe, 1990

Cause	Total	Male	Female	Males							Females						
				0-4	5-14	15-29	30-44	45-59	60-69	70+	0-4	5-14	15-29	30-44	45-59	60-69	70+
M. Congenital anomalies	873	487	386	424	26	22	10	4	1	-	334	25	15	7	4	1	-
1. Abdominal wall defect	9	3	6	3	-	-	-	-	-	-	6	-	-	-	-	-	-
2. Anencephaly	26	10	16	10	-	-	-	-	-	-	16	-	-	-	-	-	-
3. Anorectal atresia	11	7	4	7	-	-	-	-	-	-	4	-	-	-	-	-	-
4. Cleft lip	11	7	4	7	-	-	-	-	-	-	4	-	-	-	-	-	-
5. Cleft palate	9	5	4	5	-	-	-	-	-	-	4	-	-	-	-	-	-
6. Oesophageal atresia	4	2	2	2	-	-	-	-	-	-	2	-	-	-	-	-	-
7. Renal agenesis	15	7	7	7	-	-	-	-	-	-	7	-	-	-	-	-	-
8. Down syndrome	33	19	14	12	3	1	1	2	-	-	9	1	6	5	3	-	-
9. Congenital heart anomalies	348	195	153	161	10	16	6	2	1	-	131	9	1	1	-	-	-
10. Spina bifida	76	37	40	32	3	1	1	-	-	-	35	3	-	-	-	-	-
11. Other congenital	340	201	140	184	9	4	3	-	-	-	118	13	8	1	-	-	-
N. Oral conditions	-	-	-	-	-	-	-	-	-	-	-	-	-	-	-	-	-
III. Injuries	8 269	6 466	1 804	318	397	2 185	2 240	1 047	219	60	243	180	496	407	284	119	74
A. Unintentional injuries	5 184	4 189	996	212	304	1 374	1 416	700	143	40	138	124	220	208	174	74	57
1. Road traffic accidents	2 089	1 706	383	34	109	751	542	211	48	12	20	55	128	84	58	25	12
2. Poisonings	864	680	184	32	14	109	297	194	31	4	23	10	28	49	53	16	5
3. Falls	339	256	83	10	14	58	87	55	19	13	7	5	9	12	12	11	28
4. Fires	144	103	42	16	7	21	33	19	5	3	13	5	5	7	6	4	3
5. Drownings	601	511	90	36	94	166	150	54	10	2	16	31	17	13	8	3	2
6. Other unintentional	1 147	934	214	85	66	269	308	166	32	7	59	18	33	43	37	15	8
B. Intentional injuries	3 085	2 277	808	105	93	811	824	347	76	20	105	55	276	200	111	45	17
1. Self-inflicted injuries	1 506	1 230	276	-	19	359	504	269	61	18	-	4	72	80	74	33	14
2. Violence	698	538	160	7	8	216	230	65	11	2	7	7	46	62	28	8	3
3. War	880	509	372	99	66	236	90	13	4	-	99	44	158	57	9	4	-

Notes:

Causes responsible for no deaths have been omitted from this table.

A dash (-) symbol indicates fewer than 500 YLLs.

*IA6 is Bacterial meningitis and meningococcaemia; IC3 is Hypertensive disorders of pregnancy; ID is Conditions arising during the perinatal period; IIE6 is Dementia and other degenerative and hereditary CNS disorders; IIH1 is Chronic obstructive pulmonary disease.

Annex Table 7c. YLLs by age, sex and cause (thousands): India, 1990

Cause	Total	Male	Female	Males							Females						
				0-4	5-14	15-29	30-44	45-59	60-69	70+	0-4	5-14	15-29	30-44	45-59	60-69	70+
Population (millions)	*850*	*439*	*410*	*60*	*102*	*121*	*79*	*48*	*19*	*11*	*57*	*95*	*111*	*72*	*46*	*19*	*10*
All causes	*200 059*	*99 566*	*100 493*	*53 378*	*9 591*	*8 405*	*8 362*	*9 923*	*6 432*	*3 475*	*56 219*	*11 056*	*10 322*	*6 519*	*7 478*	*5 375*	*3 524*
I. Communicable, maternal, perinatal and nutritional conditions	*132 921*	*64 129*	*68 791*	*47 067*	*4 817*	*3 203*	*3 579*	*3 016*	*1 591*	*856*	*50 392*	*6 436*	*4 763*	*3 367*	*2 101*	*1 032*	*701*
A. Infectious and parasitic diseases	*70 644*	*36 193*	*34 452*	*22 648*	*3 346*	*2 777*	*3 146*	*2 715*	*1 031*	*530*	*23 790*	*3 936*	*2 353*	*1 702*	*1 717*	*587*	*367*
1. Tuberculosis	12 564	8 022	4 542	488	346	1 741	2 108	2 267	711	361	377	269	1 241	897	1 305	281	171
2. STDs excluding HIV	1 919	791	1 128	729	–	12	12	15	11	12	795	8	155	118	22	14	15
a. Syphilis	1 659	791	868	729	–	12	12	15	11	12	795	–	13	12	18	14	15
b. Chlamydia	174	–	174								–	5	95	71	2	–	–
c. Gonorrhoea	86	–	86								–	3	47	35	1	–	–
3. HIV	17	11	6	5	1	2	3	–	–	–	5	1	–	–	–	–	–
4. Diarrhoeal diseases	28 557	13 584	14 973	11 850	845	250	271	143	145	80	12 863	1 210	311	218	145	134	93
5. Childhood-cluster diseases	17 056	8 436	8 619	7 029	952	183	198	53	13	7	7 052	1 107	222	162	56	14	7
a. Pertussis	2 706	1 350	1 356	1 230	120	–	1	–	–	–	1 234	123	–	–	–	–	–
b. Poliomyelitis	371	210	161	208	1	1	–	–	–	–	160	1	–	–	–	–	–
c. Diphtheria	150	75	75	65	8	4	2	–	–	–	66	9	3	2	–	–	–
d. Measles	7 056	3 501	3 555	2 969	525	–	–	–	–	–	3 005	544	–	–	–	–	–
e. Tetanus	6 772	3 300	3 472	2 557	298	178	195	52	13	7	2 588	432	217	160	55	13	7
6. Bacterial meningitis*	1 181	600	581	412	6	35	93	35	17	4	411	6	30	77	35	17	4
7. Hepatitis B and hepatitis C	346	190	156	44	28	32	36	33	12	6	37	28	35	23	16	11	6
8. Malaria	769	394	375	103	117	70	78	20	4	2	91	140	71	52	17	3	2
9. Tropical-cluster diseases	1 124	675	449	47	293	223	97	12	3	1	33	210	136	58	8	2	1
a. Trypanosomiasis																	
b. Chagas disease																	
c. Schistosomiasis																	
d. Leishmaniasis	1 124	675	449	47	293	223	97	12	3	1	33	210	136	58	8	2	1
10. Leprosy	13	6	6	–	–	1	1	2	2	–	–	1	1	1	1	2	–
11. Dengue	440	198	242	39	153	2	2	1	–	–	47	189	3	1	1	–	–
12. Japanese encephalitis	34	16	18	9	6	1	1	–	–	–	9	7	1	–	–	–	–
13. Trachoma	–	–	–														
14. Intestinal nematode infections	100	51	50	–	37	7	4	2	1	1	–	37	6	3	2	1	1
a. Ascariasis	52	26	26	–	26						–	26					
b. Trichuriasis	22	11	11	–	11						–	11					
c. Ancylostomiasis, necatoriasis	26	14	12	–		7	4	2	1	1	–		5	3	2	1	1
15. Other infectious and parasitic	6 524	3 218	3 306	1 893	564	218	242	132	112	57	2 069	722	140	90	109	108	68

478

Annex Table 7c, continued. YLLs by age, sex and cause (thousands): India, 1990

Cause	Total	Male	Female	Males							Females						
				0-4	5-14	15-29	30-44	45-59	60-69	70+	0-4	5-14	15-29	30-44	45-59	60-69	70+
B. Respiratory infections	**33 052**	**15 442**	**17 610**	12 405	1 223	329	374	269	535	307	13 810	2 181	357	252	279	419	312
1. Lower respiratory infections	32 011	15 114	16 897	12 120	1 200	323	370	267	530	304	13 156	2 141	350	250	276	415	309
2. Upper respiratory infections	321	152	170	121	12	3	4	3	5	3	132	22	4	3	3	4	3
3. Otitis media	395	176	219	164	10	3	-	-	-	-	199	17	-	-	-	-	-
C. Maternal conditions	**3 329**		**3 329**										1 926	1 346	57	-	-
1. Maternal haemorrhage	799		799										462	323	14		
2. Maternal sepsis	532		532										308	215	9		
3. Hypertensive disorders*	400		400										231	162	7		
4. Obstructed labour	267		267										155	108	5		
5. Abortion	495		495										286	200	8		
6. Other maternal	836		836										484	338	14		
D. Perinatal conditions*	**22 261**	**10 874**	**11 387**	10 874							11 387						
1. Low birth weight	11 225	5 475	5 750	5 475							5 750						
2. Birth asphyxia and birth trauma	5 690	2 889	2 801	2 889							2 801						
3. Other perinatal	5 346	2 510	2 836	2 510							2 836						
E. Nutritional deficiencies	**3 635**	**1 621**	**2 014**	1 140	248	97	60	32	25	19	1 405	319	127	67	49	25	22
1. Protein-energy malnutrition	2 071	876	1 194	760	38	20	25	11	14	8	1 027	108	16	12	9	13	10
2. Iodine deficiency	203	103	101	75	20	7	1				74	20	6	1			
3. Vitamin A deficiency	725	363	362	219	133	11					218	135	9				
4. Iron-deficiency anaemia	636	279	357	86	56	59	34	21	12	11	86	57	96	55	40	12	12
II. Noncommunicable diseases	**45 157**	**23 274**	**21 883**	**3 881**	**1 816**	**1 878**	**2 640**	**5 884**	**4 646**	**2 529**	**3 970**	**2 028**	**2 391**	**1 894**	**4 708**	**4 146**	**2 747**
A. Malignant neoplasms	**6 633**	**3 085**	**3 548**	131	206	373	453	1 148	508	266	63	108	631	538	1 461	529	217
1. Mouth and oropharynx cancers	955	533	423	2	4	54	66	246	113	48	2	4	61	52	133	75	27
2. Oesophagus cancer	554	271	283			22	27	130	61	30			33	28	86	60	28
3. Stomach cancer	514	312	202		1	34	41	148	59	29			33	28	47	38	16
4. Colon and rectum cancers	240	126	114		2	21	26	42	23	12			16	14	19	25	12
5. Liver cancer	145	98	46	1		11	14	44	16	10	1		7	6		8	6
6. Pancreas cancer	83	48	35			5	6	23	10	5			5	5	14	7	5
7. Trachea, bronchus, lung cancers	369	303	65		1	25	30	150	67	31			8	7	27	14	8
8. Melanoma and other skin cancers	15	7	8			1	1	3	1				1	1	3		1
9. Breast cancer	524		524										115	98	223	64	23
10. Cervix uteri cancer	715		715										115	98	386	89	27
11. Corpus uteri cancer	35		35										3	2	17	9	5
12. Ovary cancer	173		173										44	37	52	28	10
13. Prostate cancer	66	66						15	22	27					-		
14. Bladder cancer	60	46	14					18	12	9			1	1	5	3	3
15. Lymphomas, multiple myeloma	300	206	94	22	37	37	45	44	15	8	4	8	18	16	25	14	8
16. Leukaemia	369	215	154	40	67	34	41	23	7	4	20	39	34	29	22	7	3
17. Other cancers	1 516	853	663	64	94	125	151	261	102	55	35	52	137	117	199	86	37
B. Other neoplasms	**117**	**73**	**44**	9	14	19	21	6	3	1	5	3	16	12	5	2	1

Annex Table 7c, continued. YLLs by age, sex and cause (thousands): India, 1990

Cause	Total	Male	Female	Males							Females						
				0-4	5-14	15-29	30-44	45-59	60-69	70+	0-4	5-14	15-29	30-44	45-59	60-69	70+
C. Diabetes mellitus	1 391	663	728	70	162	37	84	148	109	53	70	158	54	62	168	149	67
D. Endocrine disorders	49	28	21	11	5	5	2	3	1	-	8	2	4	2	3	2	-
E. Neuro-psychiatric conditions	1 828	1 006	822	189	183	142	196	139	101	56	244	143	172	80	49	78	56
2. Bipolar disorder	20	10	10	-	-	1	3	2	2	2	-	-	1	4	1	2	4
3. Schizophrenia	50	30	20	-	-	5	8	10	4	3	-	-	3	4	4	5	4
4. Epilepsy	307	169	138	17	33	40	47	21	8	2	20	23	59	22	7	6	1
5. Alcohol use	90	85	6	-	-	4	44	29	7	1	-	-	1	1	1	1	-
6. Dementia*	199	91	108	11	5	10	10	16	19	22	23	7	10	10	14	20	25
7. Parkinson disease	33	22	12	-	-	-	-	2	9	10	-	-	-	-	2	5	5
8. Multiple sclerosis	50	22	28	-	-	3	8	8	3	1	-	-	2	11	10	4	1
9. Drug use	7	6	1	-	-	4	2	-	-	-	-	-	1	-	-	-	-
13. Other neuro-psychiatric	1 071	572	499	162	145	75	75	52	48	15	201	113	95	32	9	34	16
F. Sense organ diseases	1	1	-	1	-	-	-	-	-	-	1	-	-	-	-	-	-
1. Glaucoma	-	-	-														
2. Cataracts	-	-	-														
G. Cardiovascular diseases	20 302	10 416	9 886	534	374	547	973	3 068	3 177	1 743	606	578	745	683	2 191	2 963	2 121
1. Rheumatic heart disease	1 352	550	801	1	42	164	145	150	41	7	2	63	229	204	227	64	12
2. Ischaemic heart disease	8 850	4 783	4 068	-	-	34	301	1 655	1 819	973	-	-	45	212	1 047	1 600	1 164
3. Cerebrovascular disease	3 584	1 802	1 783	109	63	31	106	478	633	382	116	76	97	87	312	641	455
4. Inflammatory heart diseases	1 400	666	734	94	87	127	103	157	64	34	132	144	130	82	140	64	44
5. Other cardiovascular	5 116	2 615	2 500	330	182	190	318	628	620	347	357	295	245	98	465	595	446
H. Respiratory diseases	3 207	1 637	1 570	279	251	79	116	326	369	217	331	269	149	112	300	231	177
1. COPD*	1 237	683	554	64	40	13	29	166	229	143	84	48	20	23	140	133	106
2. Asthma	257	137	119	8	28	17	22	29	20	14	5	20	13	21	29	19	12
3. Other respiratory	1 713	816	897	207	183	50	65	131	120	60	242	201	116	68	131	79	58
I. Digestive diseases	4 233	2 704	1 529	170	156	483	662	877	239	117	187	143	377	270	378	111	62
1. Peptic ulcer	587	354	234	3	4	68	79	124	49	26	7	13	59	47	67	25	16
2. Cirrhosis of the liver	2 316	1 576	740	42	37	272	382	609	157	77	56	73	163	127	227	59	35
3. Appendicitis	371	213	158	8	63	89	43	8	2	-	8	53	60	29	6	2	-
4. Other digestive	958	561	397	117	52	54	158	137	31	13	117	5	95	67	78	26	10
J. Genito-urinary diseases	1 662	819	842	76	243	71	83	146	129	72	39	373	117	85	116	71	42
1. Nephritis and nephrosis	1 553	728	825	67	236	67	79	141	89	49	37	371	112	83	112	69	42
2. Benign prostatic hypertrophy	62	62	-	-	-	-	-	1	39	22	-	-	-	-	-	-	-
3. Other genito-urinary	46	29	17	10	7	3	4	3	1	1	2	2	5	2	4	3	1
K. Skin diseases	61	37	24	14	10	4	3	3	2	1	15	3	2	2	1	1	-
L. Musculo-skeletal diseases	41	21	21	2	7	3	2	2	3	2	1	4	3	2	9	2	1
1. Rheumatoid arthritis	23	9	13	1	1	1	1	2	2	1	1	-	2	2	8	1	1
3. Other musculo-skeletal	19	11	7	1	6	2	1	1	1	-	-	4	1	-	1	1	-

Annex Table 7c, continued. YLLs by age, sex and cause (thousands): India, 1990

Cause	Total	Male	Female	Males 0-4	5-14	15-29	30-44	45-59	60-69	70+	Females 0-4	5-14	15-29	30-44	45-59	60-69	70+
M. Congenital anomalies	**5 621**	**2 782**	**2 839**	**2 394**	**203**	**114**	**44**	**19**	**5**	**2**	**2 399**	**243**	**114**	**46**	**27**	**7**	**2**
1. Abdominal wall defect	43	23	19	23	-	-	-	-	-	-	19	-	-	-	-	-	-
2. Anencephaly	1 552	612	940	612	-	-	-	-	-	-	940	-	-	-	-	-	-
3. Anorectal atresia	22	12	10	12	-	-	-	-	-	-	10	-	-	-	-	-	-
4. Cleft lip	38	23	15	23	-	-	-	-	-	-	15	-	-	-	-	-	-
5. Cleft palate	30	15	15	15	-	-	-	-	-	-	15	-	-	-	-	-	-
6. Oesophageal atresia	29	16	13	16	-	-	-	-	-	-	13	-	-	-	-	-	-
7. Renal agenesis	82	41	40	41	-	-	-	-	-	-	40	-	-	-	-	-	-
8. Down syndrome	528	299	228	166	57	55	21	-	-	-	110	55	45	18	-	-	-
9. Congenital heart anomalies	1 840	970	870	793	97	41	16	17	5	2	664	116	42	17	22	6	2
10. Spina bifida	712	380	333	360	18	1	-	-	-	-	294	23	10	4	2	1	-
11. Other congenital	747	391	356	333	32	17	7	2	-	-	280	49	17	7	3	-	-
N. Oral conditions	**13**	**3**	**10**	**1**	**1**	**1**	**-**	**-**	**-**	**-**	**-**	**3**	**6**	**-**	**-**	**-**	**-**
III. Injuries	***21 981***	***12 162***	***9 819***	***2 430***	***2 958***	***3 323***	***2 142***	***1 023***	***195***	***89***	***1 857***	***2 592***	***3 168***	***1 258***	***669***	***198***	***77***
A. Unintentional injuries	**17 921**	**9 958**	**7 963**	**2 238**	**2 792**	**2 359**	**1 603**	**738**	**156**	**72**	**1 614**	**2 435**	**2 230**	**957**	**492**	**167**	**68**
1. Road traffic accidents	4 617	3 334	1 283	555	707	1 108	634	259	47	24	163	511	242	159	150	42	15
2. Poisonings	880	450	431	157	101	86	76	24	5	1	111	76	148	67	28	2	-
3. Falls	1 136	739	397	117	304	109	99	74	23	12	127	132	47	34	31	16	10
4. Fires	3 532	1 003	2 529	302	148	263	187	85	12	5	266	468	1 215	435	100	33	13
5. Drownings	2 711	1 457	1 254	359	613	273	146	49	11	6	301	591	201	86	53	14	8
6. Other unintentional	5 044	2 975	2 069	748	919	519	460	248	58	24	645	656	379	176	131	61	22
B. Intentional injuries	**4 060**	**2 204**	**1 856**	**192**	**167**	**964**	**540**	**285**	**39**	**17**	**243**	**157**	**938**	**301**	**177**	**31**	**8**
1. Self-inflicted injuries	2 637	1 324	1 313	-	106	677	330	183	38	9	-	105	851	266	83	5	3
2. Violence	1 328	784	544	192	61	215	186	101	21	8	243	53	87	35	95	26	5
3. War	95	95	-	-	-	72	23	-	-	-	-	-	-	-	-	-	-

Notes:
Causes responsible for no deaths have been omitted from this table.
A dash (-) symbol indicates fewer than 500 YLLs.
*IA6 is Bacterial meningitis and meningococcaemia; IC3 is Hypertensive disorders of pregnancy; ID is Conditions arising during the perinatal period;
IIE6 is Dementia and other degenerative and hereditary CNS disorders; IIH1 is Chronic obstructive pulmonary disease.

Annex Table 7d. YLLs by age, sex and cause (thousands): China, 1990

Cause	Total	Male	Female	Males							Females						
				0-4	5-14	15-29	30-44	45-59	60-69	70+	0-4	5-14	15-29	30-44	45-59	60-69	70+
Population (millions)	*1 134*	*585*	*548*	*60*	*97*	*184*	*122*	*73*	*31*	*18*	*58*	*90*	*172*	*113*	*64*	*30*	*22*
All causes	*117 882*	*63 494*	*54 388*	*16 952*	*3 222*	*9 335*	*8 379*	*10 977*	*9 187*	*5 442*	*19 072*	*2 370*	*7 758*	*5 743*	*7 143*	*6 508*	*5 795*
I. Communicable, maternal, perinatal and nutritional conditions	*33 328*	*15 691*	*17 637*	*11 469*	*584*	*650*	*848*	*1 043*	*640*	*456*	*13 461*	*641*	*1 243*	*887*	*565*	*442*	*399*
A. Infectious and parasitic diseases	9 795	5 309	4 486	2 039	326	468	785	951	515	226	2 212	339	380	576	480	326	174
1. Tuberculosis	3 482	2 023	1 459	91	20	232	437	687	396	159	99	69	244	359	365	228	96
2. STDs excluding HIV	9	4	5	1	-	1	1	1	-	-	1	-	2	2	-	-	-
a. Syphilis	6	4	2	1	-	1	1	1	-	-	1	-	1	-	-	-	-
b. Chlamydia	2	-	2	-	-	-	-	-	-	-	-	-	1	1	-	-	-
c. Gonorrhoea	1	-	1	-	-	-	-	-	-	-	-	-	-	1	-	-	-
3. HIV	-	-	-	-	-	-	-	-	-	-	-	-	-	-	-	-	-
4. Diarrhoeal diseases	2 113	978	1 135	736	53	54	31	26	44	34	953	45	23	29	19	22	43
5. Childhood-cluster diseases	1 764	922	842	800	74	21	18	5	1	1	757	61	12	8	3	1	-
a. Pertussis	572	294	278	272	22	-	-	-	-	-	257	21	-	-	-	-	-
b. Poliomyelitis	85	49	36	47	-	1	-	-	1	-	35	-	-	-	-	1	-
c. Diphtheria	7	4	3	3	-	-	-	-	-	-	3	-	-	-	-	-	-
d. Measles	509	260	250	217	32	6	3	1	-	-	209	31	6	3	1	-	-
e. Tetanus	590	315	275	261	19	14	15	4	1	-	253	9	6	5	1	-	-
6. Bacterial meningitis*	928	476	453	230	4	32	130	47	28	5	223	3	28	119	44	29	6
7. Hepatitis B and hepatitis C	607	415	192	62	12	86	120	107	18	11	51	11	42	29	22	28	9
8. Malaria	8	4	4	-	1	2	1	-	-	-	-	1	1	1	1	-	-
9. Tropical-cluster diseases	17	12	6	-	-	1	3	4	2	-	-	-	1	1	2	1	-
a. Trypanosomiasis	-	-	-	-	-	-	-	-	-	-	-	-	-	-	-	-	-
b. Chagas disease	-	-	-	-	-	-	-	-	-	-	-	-	-	-	-	-	-
c. Schistosomiasis	16	11	5	-	-	1	3	4	2	-	-	-	1	1	2	1	-
d. Leishmaniasis	1	1	-	-	-	-	-	-	-	-	-	-	-	1	-	-	-
10. Leprosy	1	-	-	-	-	-	-	-	-	-	-	-	-	-	-	-	-
11. Dengue	29	14	15	3	10	-	-	-	-	-	3	11	2	-	-	-	-
12. Japanese encephalitis	84	44	41	22	16	3	2	1	-	-	25	11	2	1	-	-	-
13. Trachoma	-	-	-	-	-	-	-	-	-	-	-	-	-	-	-	-	-
14. Intestinal nematode infections	245	128	118	-	121	3	2	1	-	-	-	112	3	2	1	-	-
a. Ascariasis	148	77	71	-	74	2	1	1	-	-	-	68	3	1	-	-	-
b. Trichuriasis	91	47	44	-	47	2	1	-	-	-	-	44	1	1	-	-	-
c. Ancylostomiasis, necatoriasis	6	3	3	-	-	2	-	-	-	-	-	-	1	1	-	-	-
15. Other infectious and parasitic	508	290	217	92	14	32	39	72	25	16	99	14	22	25	23	16	18

Annex Table 7d, continued. YLLs by age, sex and cause (thousands): China, 1990

Cause	Total	Male	Female	Males							Females						
				0-4	5-14	15-29	30-44	45-59	60-69	70+	0-4	5-14	15-29	30-44	45-59	60-69	70+
B. Respiratory infections	**11 153**	**5 129**	**6 024**	**4 421**	**160**	**106**	**44**	**80**	**104**	**214**	**5 371**	**163**	**110**	**43**	**44**	**88**	**205**
1. Lower respiratory infections	10 959	5 040	5 919	4 341	157	104	43	79	103	212	5 274	160	108	43	43	87	203
2. Upper respiratory infections	112	51	60	44	2	1	-	1	1	2	54	2	1	-	-	1	2
3. Otitis media	83	37	45	35	1	1	-	-	-	-	43	1	1	-	-	-	-
C. Maternal conditions	**913**		**913**										**686**	**199**	**28**		
1. Maternal haemorrhage	357		357										268	78	11		
2. Maternal sepsis	43		43										33	9	2		
3. Hypertensive disorders*	74		74										56	16	2		
4. Obstructed labour	13		13										10	3	-		
5. Abortion	76		76										57	17	2		
6. Other maternal	349		349										262	76	11		
D. Perinatal conditions*	**9 302**	**4 455**	**4 847**	**4 455**							**4 847**						
1. Low birth weight	1 556	818	738	818							738						
2. Birth asphyxia and birth trauma	4 946	2 245	2 701	2 245							2 701						
3. Other perinatal	2 800	1 393	1 408	1 393							1 408						
E. Nutritional deficiencies	**2 165**	**798**	**1 367**	**555**	**98**	**76**	**19**	**13**	**21**	**16**	**1 031**	**139**	**67**	**69**	**14**	**28**	**20**
1. Protein-energy malnutrition	1 012	324	688	285	3	8	3	5	9	11	654	3	10	1	3	6	10
2. Iodine deficiency	273	141	132	105	22	13	1	-	-	-	100	20	11	-	-	-	-
3. Vitamin A deficiency	329	169	160	109	52	8	-	-	-	-	105	48	7	-	-	-	-
4. Iron-deficiency anaemia	551	164	387	56	22	47	15	8	12	5	172	69	39	65	11	22	10
II. Noncommunicable diseases	**60 710**	**33 958**	**26 752**	**2 953**	**1 080**	**3 530**	**4 805**	**8 737**	**8 078**	**4 773**	**3 223**	**720**	**2 681**	**3 436**	**5 807**	**5 731**	**5 155**
A. Malignant neoplasms	**16 949**	**10 578**	**6 372**	**175**	**375**	**998**	**2 072**	**3 647**	**2 557**	**754**	**227**	**188**	**684**	**1 302**	**1 996**	**1 417**	**559**
1. Mouth and oropharynx cancers	509	347	162	7	8	39	124	98	57	15			28	46	52	29	7
2. Oesophagus cancer	1 694	1 170	524			19	156	460	403	132			20	21	180	230	73
3. Stomach cancer	3 051	1 950	1 101		8	38	223	810	672	199		8	76	225	340	316	136
4. Colon and rectum cancers	911	510	401		8	77	107	156	117	46		9	29	85	137	101	41
5. Liver cancer	3 852	2 904	949	7	24	186	979	1 126	481	101	7	22	52	237	352	202	76
6. Pancreas cancer	284	182	102			19	22	60	59	22			4	7	28	44	18
7. Trachea, bronchus, lung cancers	1 945	1 356	589	7	15	67	77	515	522	154			23	49	239	189	88
8. Melanoma and other skin cancers	13	8	5			1	2	2	2	1			1		2	1	1
9. Breast cancer	358		358										9	154	128	48	20
10. Cervix uteri cancer	253		253										15	62	102	57	17
11. Corpus uteri cancer	81		81										8	12	46	11	5
12. Ovary cancer	164		164										31	49	48	18	7
13. Prostate cancer	32	32						4	18	7							
14. Bladder cancer	148	117	31			8	9	29	51	19			1	2	7	15	6
15. Lymphomas, multiple myeloma	334	233	101		31	86	14	51	42	9			22	15	43	14	6
16. Leukaemia	1 566	828	738	98	188	271	144	89	27	9	105	97	251	160	82	30	12
17. Other cancers	1 753	939	814	56	93	185	213	247	106	39	109	44	115	178	212	111	45
B. Other neoplasms	**355**	**191**	**164**	**35**	**16**	**50**	**25**	**35**	**24**	**6**	**34**	**22**	**27**	**27**	**24**	**25**	**6**

Annex Table 7d, continued. YLLs by age, sex and cause (thousands): China, 1990

Cause	Total	Male	Female	Males							Females						
				0-4	5-14	15-29	30-44	45-59	60-69	70+	0-4	5-14	15-29	30-44	45-59	60-69	70+
C. Diabetes mellitus	634	295	339	8	14	28	63	85	69	28	8	13	36	42	97	103	40
D. Endocrine disorders	228	68	160	7	8	13	13	13	8	6	53	17	35	30	9	7	10
E. Neuro-psychiatric conditions	1 691	1 009	683	77	70	452	242	79	44	43	61	34	229	166	76	59	58
2. Bipolar disorder	19	8	12	-	-	3	2	1	1	1	-	-	2	2	2	2	4
3. Schizophrenia	297	198	99	-	-	87	86	11	6	7	-	-	38	35	15	7	3
4. Epilepsy	302	173	128	7	13	104	34	11	3	7	5	5	67	36	10	4	3
5. Alcohol use	96	88	8	-	-	14	55	16	3	2	-	-	2	3	2	1	2
6. Dementia*	228	107	121	15	9	20	8	18	17	19	14	4	14	11	19	26	33
7. Parkinson disease	23	12	11	-	-	-	-	1	4	7	-	-	-	-	2	3	6
8. Multiple sclerosis	77	34	43	-	-	4	12	12	5	1	-	-	4	16	16	6	1
9. Drug use	12	11	1	-	-	7	3	-	-	1	-	-	1	-	-	-	-
13. Other neuro-psychiatric	638	378	260	55	49	213	42	9	5	6	42	25	103	62	10	10	8
F. Sense organ diseases	230	117	113	28	-	13	4	36	28	7	18	9	10	14	29	26	6
1. Glaucoma	75	46	29	7	-	13	-	11	11	3	9	-	-	-	9	9	3
2. Cataracts	69	44	25	14	-	13	-	16	11	2	-	-	-	5	12	7	2
G. Cardiovascular diseases	19 698	10 416	9 282	326	148	951	1 127	2 818	2 922	2 123	241	82	854	1 041	2 212	2 375	2 477
1. Rheumatic heart disease	2 074	891	1 183	-	24	325	169	187	107	78	26	25	287	268	300	157	118
2. Ischaemic heart disease	5 265	2 806	2 459	-	-	181	367	775	830	653	-	-	97	295	571	691	805
3. Cerebrovascular disease	9 105	4 942	4 163	78	62	234	438	1 436	1 611	1 082	60	24	172	333	1 100	1 282	1 192
4. Inflammatory heart diseases	941	481	460	55	24	141	82	102	42	34	49	17	125	100	91	35	42
5. Other cardiovascular	2 314	1 297	1 017	193	38	70	70	317	332	276	106	16	172	45	150	209	319
H. Respiratory diseases	9 555	5 040	4 515	330	49	176	248	986	1 770	1 482	470	28	63	237	730	1 288	1 698
1. COPD*	8 469	4 424	4 045	141	7	90	179	912	1 691	1 403	325	5	10	189	676	1 229	1 611
2. Asthma	382	213	169	9	26	30	39	49	37	23	6	9	21	34	43	32	23
3. Other respiratory	704	403	301	180	16	56	31	25	41	54	139	14	32	14	11	26	64
I. Digestive diseases	5 610	3 324	2 286	558	126	334	778	840	492	196	630	102	278	300	465	300	210
1. Peptic ulcer	287	170	117	10	4	17	31	43	39	27	11	3	14	12	24	24	29
2. Cirrhosis of the liver	2 455	1 694	762	56	23	131	576	548	291	68	18	24	82	146	264	165	63
3. Appendicitis	344	203	140	5	54	91	43	8	3	-	5	41	58	28	5	2	-
4. Other digestive	2 523	1 256	1 267	487	44	96	129	240	160	101	597	34	123	114	172	109	118
J. Genito-urinary diseases	1 735	994	741	56	63	300	208	166	118	83	61	42	163	195	127	103	50
1. Nephritis and nephrosis	1 532	877	655	42	63	294	191	141	94	51	61	42	152	182	102	78	38
2. Benign prostatic hypertrophy	38	38	-	7	-	-	8	3	3	17	-	-	-	-	-	-	-
3. Other genito-urinary	165	79	86	7	-	6	9	22	21	15	-	-	11	13	26	24	12
K. Skin diseases	151	79	72	14	23	6	5	11	8	13	17	-	33	4	6	7	6
L. Musculo-skeletal diseases	320	132	188	-	16	24	5	16	40	31	9	9	39	47	29	21	35
1. Rheumatoid arthritis	16	7	9	-	1	1	1	1	1	2	-	-	2	2	1	1	2
3. Other musculo-skeletal	304	125	179	-	15	23	4	15	39	29	8	8	37	44	27	20	34

Annex Table 7d, continued. YLLs by age, sex and cause (thousands): China, 1990

Cause	Total	Male	Female	Males 0-4	5-14	15-29	30-44	45-59	60-69	70+	Females 0-4	5-14	15-29	30-44	45-59	60-69	70+
M. Congenital anomalies	**3 536**	**1 712**	**1 824**	**1 337**	**172**	**183**	**15**	**5**	**-**	**-**	**1 393**	**173**	**221**	**32**	**6**	**-**	**-**
1. Abdominal wall defect	23	13	10	13							10						
2. Anencephaly	1 314	506	808	506							808						
3. Anorectal atresia	5	3	2	3							2						
4. Cleft lip	24	15	9	15							9						
5. Cleft palate	19	10	9	10							9						
6. Oesophageal atresia	4	2	2	2							2						
7. Renal agenesis	18	9	9	9							9						
8. Down syndrome	413	189	223	92	36	54	4	2			93	43	74	11	3		
9. Congenital heart anomalies	989	552	437	376	76	91	7	2			230	64	123	18	2		
10. Spina bifida	419	233	186	197	34	2					144	39	2				
11. Other congenital	309	180	128	114	26	37	3	1			77	26	22	3			
N. Oral conditions	**16**	**4**	**12**	**1**	**1**	**2**					**-**	**2**	**9**				
III. Injuries	**23 845**	**13 846**	**9 999**	**2 530**	**1 559**	**5 155**	**2 726**	**1 196**	**468**	**213**	**2 389**	**1 009**	**3 834**	**1 420**	**771**	**335**	**241**
A. Unintentional injuries	**15 282**	**9 915**	**5 366**	**2 370**	**1 433**	**3 308**	**1 668**	**755**	**256**	**127**	**2 092**	**894**	**1 212**	**523**	**345**	**160**	**139**
1. Road traffic accidents	3 194	2 265	929	131	219	903	673	243	76	21	96	207	318	148	117	32	11
2. Poisonings	1 436	789	647	167	58	218	167	132	30	17	52	82	310	130	35	24	13
3. Falls	907	544	363	80	34	201	90	66	44	29	122	29	33	25	51	46	58
4. Fires	446	265	181	87	24	78	41	16	4	14	61	35	31	15	16	10	13
5. Drownings	4 424	2 771	1 653	1 018	819	681	149	66	23	15	864	402	250	68	33	20	16
6. Other unintentional	4 874	3 281	1 594	886	279	1 227	548	232	79	30	898	139	270	138	93	28	28
B. Intentional injuries	**8 563**	**3 930**	**4 633**	**160**	**126**	**1 847**	**1 058**	**441**	**212**	**86**	**296**	**114**	**2 622**	**897**	**426**	**175**	**101**
1. Self-inflicted injuries	7 140	3 063	4 078	-	89	1 407	882	402	198	85	-	65	2 545	806	401	165	97
2. Violence	1 404	849	555	160	37	426	172	39	14	1	296	50	78	92	25	10	4
3. War	19	19	-			14	4										

Notes:
Causes responsible for no deaths have been omitted from this table.
A dash (-) symbol indicates fewer than 500 YLLs.
*IA6 is Bacterial meningitis and meningococcaemia; IC3 is Hypertensive disorders of pregnancy; ID is Conditions arising during the perinatal period;
IIE6 is Dementia and other degenerative and hereditary CNS disorders; IIH1 is Chronic obstructive pulmonary disease.

Annex Table 7e. YLLs by age, sex and cause (thousands): Other Asia and Islands, 1990

Cause	Total	Male	Female	Males 0-4	5-14	15-29	30-44	45-59	60-69	70+	Females 0-4	5-14	15-29	30-44	45-59	60-69	70+
Population (millions)	683	343	340	44	84	99	62	34	13	7	42	80	98	62	35	14	9
All causes	114 592	63 732	50 860	30 406	8 614	6 984	6 026	5 926	3 666	2 109	24 443	6 445	5 351	4 620	4 359	2 979	2 662
I. Communicable, maternal, perinatal and nutritional conditions	61 364	32 667	28 697	25 220	3 079	1 284	1 028	1 034	677	345	20 024	2 697	2 065	1 867	1 090	508	447
A. Infectious and parasitic diseases	31 612	17 006	14 606	11 688	1 862	1 023	906	922	420	184	9 357	1 636	1 022	1 057	930	374	231
1. Tuberculosis	4 461	2 219	2 242	38	72	475	481	689	324	140	13	77	439	529	705	309	171
2. STDs excluding HIV	1 244	616	628	578	-	6	7	10	7	8	411	5	90	89	15	7	12
a. Syphilis	1 073	616	457	578	-	6	7	10	7	8	411	-	7	8	13	7	12
b. Chlamydia	113	-	113	-	-	-	-	-	-	-	-	3	55	53	2	-	-
c. Gonorrhoea	59	-	59	-	-	-	-	-	-	-	-	2	29	28	1	-	-
3. HIV	9	5	4	3	-	1	1	-	-	-	3	-	-	-	-	-	-
4. Diarrhoeal diseases	13 098	7 435	5 662	6 820	473	38	33	33	28	11	5 140	350	47	55	40	15	15
5. Childhood-cluster diseases	7 602	3 951	3 652	3 271	488	78	82	23	6	3	2 966	481	89	82	26	4	4
a. Pertussis	1 138	599	539	548	50	-	-	-	-	-	495	44	-	-	-	-	-
b. Poliomyelitis	111	65	46	61	1	2	1	-	-	-	43	4	1	1	-	-	-
c. Diphtheria	81	42	38	37	5	-	-	-	-	-	34	4	-	-	-	-	-
d. Measles	3 898	2 043	1 855	1 746	292	3	1	1	-	-	1 594	257	2	1	1	-	-
e. Tetanus	2 375	1 201	1 174	877	140	73	79	23	6	3	801	176	85	79	25	4	4
6. Bacterial meningitis*	606	311	294	197	5	4	65	26	12	2	180	4	3	67	28	10	3
7. Hepatitis B and hepatitis C	368	210	158	52	31	31	37	38	15	7	39	27	30	26	19	9	7
8. Malaria	2 277	1 203	1 074	183	432	344	162	65	15	3	167	377	279	166	70	12	5
9. Tropical-cluster diseases	65	41	25	1	11	15	9	3	1	-	1	7	8	6	2	1	1
a. Trypanosomiasis	-	-	-	-	-	-	-	-	-	-	-	-	-	-	-	-	-
b. Chagas disease	-	-	-	-	-	-	-	-	-	-	-	-	-	-	-	-	-
c. Schistosomiasis	7	4	3	-	-	-	1	2	1	-	-	-	-	-	1	1	1
d. Leishmaniasis	59	37	22	1	11	15	8	1	-	-	1	7	8	5	1	-	-
10. Leprosy	17	8	9	-	2	-	1	3	1	-	6	-	1	1	1	1	-
11. Dengue	252	119	133	25	91	1	1	1	-	-	29	101	2	1	-	-	-
12. Japanese encephalitis	45	26	19	14	9	1	1	-	-	-	11	6	1	1	-	-	-
13. Trachoma	-	-	-	-	-	-	-	-	-	-	-	-	-	-	-	-	-
14. Intestinal nematode infections	239	127	112	-	117	5	3	2	-	-	-	102	4	3	2	-	-
a. Ascariasis	117	62	54	-	61	1	-	-	-	-	-	53	-	-	2	-	-
b. Trichuriasis	104	55	48	-	55	-	-	-	-	-	-	48	-	-	-	-	-
c. Ancylostomiasis, necatoriasis	18	9	9	-	-	4	2	2	-	-	-	-	4	3	2	-	-
15. Other infectious and parasitic	1 329	735	594	507	131	24	25	28	10	10	393	99	30	33	22	6	13

Annex Table 7e, continued. YLLs by age, sex and cause (thousands): Other Asia and Islands, 1990

Cause	Total	Male	Female	Males 0-4	5-14	15-29	30-44	45-59	60-69	70+	Females 0-4	5-14	15-29	30-44	45-59	60-69	70+
B. Respiratory infections	**14 605**	**8 201**	**6 404**	**6 365**	**1 043**	**205**	**96**	**92**	**247**	**152**	**4 797**	**911**	**166**	**99**	**99**	**127**	**205**
1. Lower respiratory infections	14 351	8 058	6 293	6 251	1 024	201	95	91	244	151	4 711	894	163	98	98	126	203
2. Upper respiratory infections	146	82	64	64	10	2	1	1	2	2	48	9	2	1	1	1	2
3. Otitis media	108	61	47	51	8	2					38	7					
C. Maternal conditions	**1 497**		**1 497**										**801**	**664**	**33**		
1. Maternal haemorrhage	359		359										192	159	8		
2. Maternal sepsis	239		239										128	106	5		
3. Hypertensive disorders*	179		179										96	80	4		
4. Obstructed labour	120		120										64	53	3		
5. Abortion	199		199										107	88	4		
6. Other maternal	401		401										214	178	9		
D. Perinatal conditions*	**11 232**	**6 223**	**5 009**	**6 223**							**5 009**						
1. Low birth weight	5 562	3 067	2 494	3 067							2 494						
2. Birth asphyxia and birth trauma	2 620	1 445	1 176	1 445							1 176						
3. Other perinatal	3 050	1 711	1 339	1 711							1 339						
E. Nutritional deficiencies	**2 417**	**1 237**	**1 180**	**943**	**174**	**56**	**26**	**20**	**10**	**8**	**861**	**150**	**75**	**47**	**28**	**7**	**11**
1. Protein-energy malnutrition	1 312	687	625	656	14	4	2	5	4	2	597	11	5	4	4	2	3
2. Iodine deficiency	93	48	45	35	10	3					33	9	2				
3. Vitamin A deficiency	618	326	291	193	124	9					176	108	7				
4. Iron-deficiency anaemia	395	176	219	60	25	41	23	15	6	6	54	22	61	44	24	5	8
II. Noncommunicable diseases	***37 372***	***20 331***	***17 041***	***3 356***	***3 362***	***1 774***	***3 035***	***4 237***	***2 847***	***1 721***	***2 889***	***2 681***	***1 741***	***2 115***	***3 042***	***2 389***	***2 184***
A. Malignant neoplasms	**8 386**	**4 489**	**3 897**	**244**	**659**	**276**	**722**	**1 341**	**900**	**346**	**248**	**441**	**398**	**745**	**1 074**	**674**	**316**
1. Mouth and oropharynx cancers	694	413	282	7	18	31	82	94	131	51	8	15	29	53	48	87	41
2. Oesophagus cancer	221	149	72			5	14	71	42	16			4	8	29	21	10
3. Stomach cancer	615	391	223	1	2	23	60	178	92	36		1	19	36	82	58	28
4. Colon and rectum cancers	405	205	200	2	6	17	44	45	65	25	3	5	18	34	44	65	31
5. Liver cancer	842	631	211	9	24	48	125	297	92	36	7	12	16	30	74	48	23
6. Pancreas cancer	98	60	38			4	10	24	16	6	1	1	1	3	14	12	6
7. Trachea, bronchus, lung cancers	842	626	216	3	8	23	60	284	178	70	3	5	11	21	78	67	32
8. Melanoma and other skin cancers	28	12	15		1	1	3	4	2	1			2	3	4	4	2
9. Breast cancer	411		411								2	3	58	108	168	49	23
10. Cervix uteri cancer	471		471								2	1	55	104	225	58	28
11. Corpus uteri cancer	46		46											5	19	11	5
12. Ovary cancer	188		188									2	3	60	45	17	8
13. Prostate cancer	91	91				1	2	18	48	19							
14. Bladder cancer	95	67	27			2	6	24	25	10			1	2	6	11	5
15. Lymphomas, multiple myeloma	400	256	144	31	82	20	52	30	29	11	16	27	15	27	18	28	13
16. Leukaemia	804	443	361	85	224	26	69	16	16	6	90	156	26	48	16	17	8
17. Other cancers	2 135	1 144	992	105	292	75	196	254	163	58	106	196	108	203	204	122	53
B. Other neoplasms	**225**	**119**	**106**	**28**	**42**	**10**	**14**	**16**	**7**	**2**	**19**	**41**	**14**	**13**	**10**	**5**	**4**

Annex Table 7e, continued. YLLs by age, sex and cause (thousands): Other Asia and Islands, 1990

Cause	Total	Male	Female	Males 0-4	5-14	15-29	30-44	45-59	60-69	70+	Females 0-4	5-14	15-29	30-44	45-59	60-69	70+
C. Diabetes mellitus	664	302	362	10	28	23	58	94	62	28	10	27	34	39	106	97	48
D. Endocrine disorders	204	109	96	48	32	10	6	7	4	2	36	18	13	9	9	6	6
E. Neuro-psychiatric conditions	1 203	718	484	82	129	158	163	106	47	33	79	111	91	61	55	43	44
2. Bipolar disorder	13	7	7			1	2	2	1				1	1	1	1	3
3. Schizophrenia	60	37	24			6	10	12	5	3			3	4	6	7	5
4. Epilepsy	210	125	85	9	25	32	37	16	4	1	9	19	32	15	6	3	
5. Alcohol use	91	83	8			6	37	32	7	1			1	2	2	2	1
6. Dementia*	159	69	90	8	5	8	7	13	14	15	17	7	8	6	13	17	24
7. Parkinson disease	22	13	9					1	6	6					1	4	4
8. Multiple sclerosis	34	15	19			2	6	5	2				2	7	8	2	
9. Drug use	47	43	4		1	26	15	1					3	1			
13. Other neuro-psychiatric	567	328	239	65	99	77	49	24	9	6	54	85	42	25	17	8	7
F. Sense organ diseases	11	7	4	2		1					3						
1. Glaucoma																	
2. Cataracts	2		2	2							2						
G. Cardiovascular diseases	16 100	8 447	7 653	1 041	1 628	910	1 191	1 515	1 200	963	943	1 381	812	811	1 173	1 126	1 407
1. Rheumatic heart disease	126	53	73		8	11	10	9	7	7		12	15	13	13	9	10
2. Ischaemic heart disease	3 496	1 830	1 666			18	374	530	495	413			12	248	379	445	582
3. Cerebrovascular disease	3 895	2 018	1 877	135	312	196	255	435	397	288	123	237	130	167	370	398	453
4. Inflammatory heart diseases	1 943	1 027	916	197	361	183	144	92	27	23	218	323	144	102	71	25	33
5. Other cardiovascular	6 641	3 519	3 122	708	947	502	408	448	274	232	602	809	511	282	340	249	329
H. Respiratory diseases	1 870	1 064	806	341	168	59	73	134	151	137	271	124	58	61	78	90	125
1. COPD*	659	385	274	79	27	9	18	69	94	90	69	22	8	13	36	52	75
2. Asthma	259	142	117	4	26	27	34	25	16	10	3	17	20	26	24	16	11
3. Other respiratory	952	536	415	258	115	23	21	41	41	37	200	85	30	22	18	22	38
I. Digestive diseases	4 663	2 970	1 693	356	357	178	667	881	386	146	269	275	152	239	378	232	146
1. Peptic ulcer	237	148	88	6	11	9	26	45	30	20	5	8	8	9	20	18	20
2. Cirrhosis of the liver	1 846	1 346	501	34	46	64	414	545	194	49	23	42	33	98	176	94	34
3. Appendicitis	305	176	129	4	81	55	29	5	1		4	65	37	18	4	1	
4. Other digestive	2 275	1 300	974	311	220	50	198	285	160	77	237	160	73	114	180	119	92
J. Genito-urinary diseases	1 370	682	688	50	177	90	108	122	78	58	37	126	107	104	134	102	77
1. Nephritis and nephrosis	1 212	602	609	41	158	83	98	107	69	47	37	112	92	94	119	89	66
2. Benign prostatic hypertrophy	2	2								2							
3. Other genito-urinary	156	78	78	8	19	7	10	16	9	9		13	15	10	16	13	11
K. Skin diseases	49	25	24	9	7	2	2	3	1	1	7	7	3	2	2	1	1
L. Musculo-skeletal diseases	141	57	84	8	17	6	7	9	7	3	7	20	16	13	11	9	8
1. Rheumatoid arthritis	9	3	6					1	1	1			2	1	2	2	1
3. Other musculo-skeletal	132	53	78	8	17	6	6	7	6	3	7	20	14	12	9	7	8

Annex Table 7e, continued. YLLs by age, sex and cause (thousands): Other Asia and Islands, 1990

Cause	Total	Male	Female	Males							Females						
				0-4	5-14	15-29	30-44	45-59	60-69	70+	0-4	5-14	15-29	30-44	45-59	60-69	70+
M. Congenital anomalies	2 478	1 339	1 139	1 136	114	52	23	10	3	1	958	108	41	17	12	3	1
1. Abdominal wall defect	24	14	9	14							9						
2. Anencephaly	658	257	401	257							401						
3. Anorectal atresia	8	5	3	5							3						
4. Cleft lip	25	17	8	17							8						
5. Cleft palate	20	11	8	11							8						
6. Oesophageal atresia	16	10	6	10							6						
7. Renal agenesis	58	30	29	30							29						
8. Down syndrome	209	133	77	86	21	18	8				45	16	11	4			
9. Congenital heart anomalies	937	563	374	459	54	26	12	9	2		284	48	20	8	10	3	
10. Spina bifida	199	106	92	90	16					1	64	22	3		1		
11. Other congenital	324	193	130	158	23	8	3	1			98	22	6	2			
N. Oral conditions	8	2	6		1	1						2	4				
III. Injuries	15 856	10 734	5 122	1 831	2 173	3 926	1 963	655	143	43	1 530	1 068	1 545	639	227	82	32
A. Unintentional injuries	12 323	8 423	3 900	1 741	1 990	2 740	1 356	463	104	29	1 433	955	872	385	167	64	24
1. Road traffic accidents	3 741	2 623	1 118	429	510	977	503	156	37	10	394	256	247	127	63	24	7
2. Poisonings	983	511	472	67	95	199	93	44	11	3	61	99	214	64	23	9	3
3. Falls	879	638	241	134	93	192	141	60	13	4	103	41	46	25	16	6	4
4. Fires	306	168	138	67	28	40	24	7	2	1	70	30	24	9	3	2	1
5. Drownings	2 774	1 915	859	647	769	343	108	35	9	3	406	300	98	36	12	5	2
6. Other unintentional	3 639	2 568	1 071	398	494	989	486	162	32	8	400	229	244	124	49	18	7
B. Intentional injuries	3 533	2 311	1 222	90	183	1 186	608	192	39	14	97	113	673	254	60	18	7
1. Self-inflicted injuries	1 726	993	733	-	71	552	244	91	26	9	-	43	477	155	39	13	6
2. Violence	1 356	1 059	296	39	78	513	319	94	11	5	45	47	114	69	17	3	1
3. War	452	259	193	51	34	121	44	7	2	-	51	23	81	30	5	2	-

Notes:
Causes responsible for no deaths have been omitted from this table.
A dash (-) symbol indicates fewer than 500 YLLs.
*IA6 is Bacterial meningitis and meningococcaemia; IC3 is Hypertensive disorders of pregnancy; ID is Conditions arising during the perinatal period; IIE6 is Dementia and other degenerative and hereditary CNS disorders; IIH1 is Chronic obstructive pulmonary disease.

Annex Table 7f. YLLs by age, sex and cause (thousands): Sub-Saharan Africa, 1990

Cause	Total	Male	Female	Males 0-4	5-14	15-29	30-44	45-59	60-69	70+	Females 0-4	5-14	15-29	30-44	45-59	60-69	70+
Population (millions)	510	252	258	47	70	67	37	20	7	3	47	70	67	39	22	8	5
All causes	226 890	120 733	106 157	73 707	14 428	15 207	8 657	5 122	2 295	1 318	63 685	13 341	12 417	7 918	4 531	2 426	1 838
I. Communicable, maternal, perinatal and nutritional conditions	167 695	84 591	83 104	68 226	7 592	4 042	2 619	1 280	497	335	58 852	8 021	8 363	5 636	1 244	554	435
A. Infectious and parasitic diseases	110 145	57 079	53 066	43 594	5 640	3 752	2 482	1 180	312	119	37 310	5 941	5 138	3 090	1 120	322	145
1. Tuberculosis	9 434	4 385	5 049	618	398	1 650	858	660	165	36	677	587	1 938	1 009	633	166	40
2. STDs excluding HIV	2 595	1 183	1 413	1 122	-	9	10	16	12	14	1 069	8	164	107	26	17	21
a. Syphilis	2 343	1 183	1 160	1 122	-	9	10	16	12	14	1 069	-	14	16	22	17	21
b. Chlamydia	148		148								-	5	87	53	3	-	-
c. Gonorrhoea	105		105								-	3	62	38	2	-	-
3. HIV	7 020	3 230	3 791	1 085	163	957	873	127	20	4	1 032	169	1 477	1 002	95	13	3
4. Diarrhoeal diseases	31 393	16 895	14 498	15 199	1 290	147	117	61	42	38	12 379	1 374	317	245	81	49	52
5. Childhood-cluster diseases	29 560	15 341	14 219	13 121	2 023	69	87	29	7	4	11 955	2 040	102	85	27	7	4
a. Pertussis	5 093	2 667	2 427	2 421	246	1	1	-	-	-	2 186	241	-	1	-	-	-
b. Poliomyelitis	161	93	68	90	4	1	-	-	-	-	65	4	1	-	-	-	-
c. Diphtheria	63	33	30	29	4	-	-	-	-	-	26	4	-	-	-	-	-
d. Measles	19 923	10 339	9 584	8 724	1 613	2	1	-	-	-	7 979	1 601	2	1	-	-	-
e. Tetanus	4 319	2 209	2 110	1 857	160	66	86	28	7	4	1 699	193	98	84	26	7	4
6. Bacterial meningitis*	756	376	380	297	4	12	39	17	6	1	280	4	16	51	19	8	2
7. Hepatitis B and hepatitis C	301	160	142	39	26	20	27	30	11	6	29	25	31	24	15	11	6
8. Malaria	24 385	13 064	11 321	11 054	1 075	539	259	110	22	5	9 003	1 103	710	342	127	29	7
9. Tropical-cluster diseases	1 781	917	865	26	382	263	141	91	13	2	36	331	275	151	62	9	2
a. Trypanosomiasis	1 346	644	702	16	243	195	102	78	9	2	31	256	230	121	56	7	1
b. Chagas disease																	
c. Schistosomiasis	80	47	33	1	12	8	14	8	3	-	-	8	5	14	4	1	-
d. Leishmaniasis	356	226	129	9	128	60	24	4	-	-	4	66	40	16	3	-	-
10. Leprosy	7	4	3	-	1	1	1	-	-	-	-	-	1	1	-	-	-
11. Dengue	21	9	12	2	7	-	-	-	-	-	2	9	-	-	-	-	-
12. Japanese encephalitis	-	-	-	-	-	-	-	-	-	-	-	-	-	-	-	-	-
13. Trachoma	-	-	-	-	-	-	-	-	-	-	-	-	-	-	-	-	-
14. Intestinal nematode infections	58	28	30	-	21	3	2	1	-	-	-	21	4	2	1	-	-
a. Ascariasis	25	12	13	-	12	-	-	-	-	-	-	12	-	-	-	-	-
b. Trichuriasis	17	8	9	-	8	-	-	-	-	-	-	9	-	-	-	-	-
c. Ancylostomiasis, necatoriasis	16	7	9	-	-	3	2	1	-	-	-	-	4	2	1	-	-
15. Other infectious and parasitic	2 832	1 489	1 344	1 033	249	81	67	38	13	8	848	269	103	70	33	12	8

Annex Table 7f, continued. YLLs by age, sex and cause (thousands): Sub-Saharan Africa, 1990

Cause	Total	Male	Female	Males							Females						
				0-4	5-14	15-29	30-44	45-59	60-69	70+	0-4	5-14	15-29	30-44	45-59	60-69	70+
B. Respiratory infections	30 063	16 318	13 745	13 817	1 668	248	119	84	176	205	11 254	1 414	327	157	96	221	277
1. Lower respiratory infections	29 533	16 029	13 504	13 569	1 638	244	118	83	174	203	11 051	1 388	321	156	95	219	274
2. Upper respiratory infections	301	163	137	138	17	2	1		2	2	113	14	3	2	1	2	3
3. Otitis media	230	126	104	111	13	2					90	11	3				
C. Maternal conditions	5 530		5 530										2 803	2 346			
1. Maternal haemorrhage	1 327		1 327										673	563			
2. Maternal sepsis	883		883										448	375			
3. Hypertensive disorders*	665		665										337	282			
4. Obstructed labour	444		444										225	188			
5. Abortion	747		747										379	317			
6. Other maternal	1 464		1 464										742	621			
D. Perinatal conditions*	17 150	8 780	8 370	8 780							8 370						
1. Low birth weight	8 495	4 327	4 168	4 327							4 168						
2. Birth asphyxia and birth trauma	5 586	2 782	2 804	2 782							2 804						
3. Other perinatal	3 069	1 671	1 399	1 671							1 399						
E. Nutritional deficiencies	4 807	2 414	2 393	2 035	283	42	18	16	9	11	1 918	292	95	42	22	10	13
1. Protein-energy malnutrition	3 285	1 671	1 613	1 587	38	14	8	9	6	8	1 495	42	37	16	9	6	9
2. Iodine deficiency	57	28	29	21	6	1					21	6	2				
3. Vitamin A deficiency	1 160	587	572	369	209	9					347	213	12				
4. Iron-deficiency anaemia	306	127	178	58	30	17	10	7	3	3	55	31	45	26	14	4	4
II. Noncommunicable diseases	28 165	14 512	13 653	2 146	2 399	1 573	2 743	3 076	1 633	942	2 227	2 812	1 202	1 238	3 023	1 783	1 368
A. Malignant neoplasms	5 866	3 179	2 688	127	394	274	632	997	516	240	153	432	218	343	894	427	221
1. Mouth and oropharynx cancers	242	139	103	1	3	12	28	34	41	20	5	16	8	12	18	29	15
2. Oesophagus cancer	267	201	66			13	30	108	34	16			4	6	28	18	9
3. Stomach cancer	363	211	152		1	14	32	102	41	20		1	10	16	79	31	16
4. Colon and rectum cancers	152	82	69		1	8	19	21	22	10		2	6	9	17	24	13
5. Liver cancer	841	640	201	3	10	93	214	241	54	26	4	11	23	36	76	34	18
6. Pancreas cancer	82	47	35			4	8	23	8	4			3	4	18	7	4
7. Trachea, bronchus, lung cancers	216	164	53			9	21	84	34	16			3	5	27	12	6
8. Melanoma and other skin cancers	88	38	51			2	5	19	7	3			2	3	21	15	8
9. Breast cancer	219		219								1		23	36	103	36	19
10. Cervix uteri cancer	404		404										35	55	199	74	39
11. Corpus uteri cancer	37		37										2	3	16	10	6
12. Ovary cancer	110		110									13	11	18	42	15	8
13. Prostate cancer	239	239				2	5	67	113	54							
14. Bladder cancer	142	90	51			5	4	37	24	11			4	7	21	13	7
15. Lymphomas, multiple myeloma	580	342	238	44	159	21	49	34	23	11	39	125	12	19	20	15	8
16. Leukaemia	191	80	111	8	29	8	17	7	8	4	17	55	6	10	12	7	4
17. Other cancers	1 694	906	788	69	189	84	193	220	107	44	84	207	66	105	197	89	41
B. Other neoplasms	252	128	124	8	75	11	15	13	4	3	16	62	17	9	9	7	3

Annex Table 7f, continued. YLLs by age, sex and cause (thousands): Sub-Saharan Africa, 1990

Cause	Total	Male	Female	Males 0-4	5-14	15-29	30-44	45-59	60-69	70+	Females 0-4	5-14	15-29	30-44	45-59	60-69	70+
C. Diabetes mellitus	333	154	179	13	52	7	19	32	21	10	16	54	7	7	41	37	19
D. Endocrine disorders	439	218	221	67	31	33	38	34	10	6	41	62	27	20	36	17	20
E. Neuro-psychiatric conditions	810	494	316	59	112	109	110	59	25	18	64	103	39	24	40	25	21
2. Bipolar disorder	8	4	4	-	-	1	-	1	1	1	-	-	1	-	1	2	-
3. Schizophrenia	18	12	6	-	-	3	4	3	1	1	-	-	1	1	2	1	1
4. Epilepsy	142	92	50	7	22	22	29	10	2	1	7	18	14	5	3	1	1
5. Alcohol use	71	52	19	-	-	4	21	19	5	2	-	-	-	4	5	5	2
6. Dementia*	86	38	48	4	3	4	4	7	7	8	11	5	3	2	10	7	10
7. Parkinson disease	12	7	5	-	-	-	-	1	3	3	-	-	-	-	1	2	2
8. Multiple sclerosis	21	10	11	-	-	1	4	3	1	-	-	-	1	3	6	1	-
9. Drug use	20	19	1	-	-	11	7	-	-	-	-	-	1	-	-	-	-
13. Other neuro-psychiatric	432	260	172	48	86	63	39	15	5	3	45	80	19	9	11	4	4
F. Sense organ diseases	3	2	1	-	-	2	-	-	-	-	-	-	-	1	-	-	-
1. Glaucoma	-	-	-	-	-	-	-	-	-	-	-	-	-	-	-	-	-
2. Cataracts	-	-	-	-	-	-	-	-	-	-	-	-	-	-	-	-	-
G. Cardiovascular diseases	10 527	4 774	5 754	389	717	573	957	1 107	614	417	456	1 034	515	526	1 405	965	853
1. Rheumatic heart disease	607	279	328	1	118	102	45	10	2	-	2	181	92	31	17	4	1
2. Ischaemic heart disease	2 095	949	1 146	-	-	34	255	327	200	132	74	-	10	188	361	282	231
3. Cerebrovascular disease	4 244	1 900	2 344	65	232	233	394	480	293	203	140	232	141	167	687	502	475
4. Inflammatory heart diseases	1 190	512	678	101	116	48	100	86	39	22	165	209	86	36	79	63	40
5. Other cardiovascular	2 392	1 134	1 258	222	251	155	163	204	80	58	76	411	186	104	261	114	106
H. Respiratory diseases	3 084	1 798	1 287	355	225	141	327	369	231	149	352	216	100	101	256	128	134
1. COPD*	1 086	651	435	82	36	22	81	188	143	98	89	39	13	21	119	74	81
2. Asthma	219	133	85	10	27	26	32	20	11	7	5	15	13	17	17	10	8
3. Other respiratory	1 779	1 013	766	263	163	93	213	161	77	44	258	163	73	63	119	45	46
I. Digestive diseases	2 928	1 731	1 197	148	354	254	453	332	133	56	144	447	153	120	173	105	55
1. Peptic ulcer	189	131	57	-	-	26	55	34	10	6	-	-	6	11	22	9	10
2. Cirrhosis of the liver	520	369	151	-	30	49	120	114	43	14	-	15	23	29	49	25	10
3. Appendicitis	441	265	176	6	137	73	41	6	1	-	7	116	32	14	5	1	-
4. Other digestive	1 779	966	813	142	188	105	238	178	79	35	137	316	92	66	97	70	35
J. Genito-urinary diseases	1 898	1 040	858	195	330	119	161	118	74	41	157	278	94	75	148	67	40
1. Nephritis and nephrosis	1 669	913	756	181	286	115	135	99	61	36	155	247	73	68	123	56	34
2. Benign prostatic hypertrophy	2	2	-	-	-	-	-	-	-	2	-	-	-	-	-	-	-
3. Other genito-urinary	227	125	102	14	44	4	27	19	13	4	2	31	21	7	24	11	6
K. Skin diseases	205	122	82	113	-	2	4	3	-	-	73	-	2	1	4	1	1
L. Musculo-skeletal diseases	12	6	6	-	-	-	2	2	2	-	-	-	2	1	4	1	1
1. Rheumatoid arthritis	3	2	2	-	-	-	-	1	1	1	-	-	2	1	2	1	1
3. Other musculo-skeletal	8	4	4	-	-	-	2	1	1	-	-	-	2	1	1	1	-

Annex Table 7f, continued. YLLs by age, sex and cause (thousands): Sub-Saharan Africa, 1990

Cause	Total	Male	Female	Males 0-4	5-14	15-29	30-44	45-59	60-69	70+	Females 0-4	5-14	15-29	30-44	45-59	60-69	70+
M. Congenital anomalies	**1 799**	**865**	**933**	**673**	**107**	**47**	**25**	**10**	**3**	**1**	**753**	**122**	**27**	**11**	**15**	**4**	**1**
1. Abdominal wall defect	14	7	7	7	-	-	-	-	-	-	7	-	-	-	-	-	-
2. Anencephaly	410	154	255	154	-	-	-	-	-	-	255	-	-	-	-	-	-
3. Anorectal atresia	7	4	4	4	-	-	-	-	-	-	4	-	-	-	-	-	-
4. Cleft lip	12	7	5	7	-	-	-	-	-	-	5	-	-	-	-	-	-
5. Cleft palate	10	5	5	5	-	-	-	-	-	-	5	-	-	-	-	-	-
6. Oesophageal atresia	10	5	5	5	-	-	-	-	-	-	5	-	-	-	-	-	-
7. Renal agenesis	70	35	35	35	-	-	-	-	-	-	35	-	-	-	-	-	-
8. Down syndrome	205	115	91	50	29	23	12	-	-	-	41	29	11	9	-	-	-
9. Congenital heart anomalies	660	329	331	242	49	17	9	8	2	1	237	60	10	8	12	2	1
10. Spina bifida	162	79	83	72	6	-	-	-	-	-	71	8	-	1	-	-	-
11. Other congenital	239	126	113	92	21	7	4	2	-	-	89	24	4	-	1	-	-
N. Oral conditions	**9**	**2**	**6**	-	-	-	-	-	-	-	-	**4**	**2**	-	-	-	-
III. Injuries	***31 031***	***21 631***	***9 400***	***3 334***	***4 437***	***9 592***	***3 295***	***766***	***165***	***41***	***2 607***	***2 507***	***2 853***	***1 044***	***263***	***90***	***36***
A. Unintentional injuries	**16 459**	**11 438**	**5 021**	**2 277**	**3 489**	**3 685**	**1 453**	**412**	**93**	**29**	**1 612**	**1 981**	**903**	**332**	**126**	**40**	**27**
1. Road traffic accidents	4 668	3 387	1 281	326	1 128	1 172	551	164	37	8	227	524	347	120	50	10	3
2. Poisonings	1 206	711	496	471	149	46	26	14	4	1	349	75	53	13	4	1	1
3. Falls	416	292	124	30	66	123	38	22	9	4	33	39	15	16	6	1	10
4. Fires	2 060	1 059	1 001	455	236	243	82	31	8	5	392	319	187	64	23	10	7
5. Drownings	3 124	2 262	862	534	1 249	350	93	27	6	2	274	501	57	20	7	2	1
6. Other unintentional	4 985	3 728	1 257	461	661	1 752	663	154	29	9	337	523	244	100	37	11	5
B. Intentional injuries	**14 572**	**10 193**	**4 379**	**1 057**	**949**	**5 907**	**1 842**	**354**	**72**	**12**	**995**	**526**	**1 950**	**712**	**137**	**50**	**9**
1. Self-inflicted injuries	439	361	78	-	52	204	79	21	5	1	-	-	56	15	7	1	-
2. Violence	6 008	5 174	834	139	289	3 529	967	211	32	6	70	120	431	153	46	10	3
3. War	8 125	4 658	3 467	918	607	2 174	795	122	36	5	925	407	1 462	544	85	39	6

Notes:
Causes responsible for no deaths have been omitted from this table.
A dash (-) symbol indicates fewer than 500 YLLs.
ᵃIA6 is Bacterial meningitis and meningococcaemia; IC3 is Hypertensive disorders of pregnancy; ID is Conditions arising during the perinatal period; IIE6 is Dementia and other degenerative and hereditary CNS disorders; IIH1 is Chronic obstructive pulmonary disease.

Annex Table 7g. YLLs by age, sex and cause (thousands): Latin America and the Caribbean, 1990

Cause	Total	Male	Female	Males							Females						
				0-4	5-14	15-29	30-44	45-59	60-69	70+	0-4	5-14	15-29	30-44	45-59	60-69	70+
Population (millions)	*444*	*222*	*223*	*29*	*52*	*64*	*40*	*22*	*9*	*7*	*28*	*51*	*63*	*41*	*23*	*10*	*7*
All causes	**56 240**	**32 085**	**24 155**	**13 570**	**2 737**	**5 161**	**4 053**	**3 371**	**1 896**	**1 298**	**10 323**	**2 058**	**3 319**	**2 771**	**2 635**	**1 651**	**1 399**
I. Communicable, maternal, perinatal and nutritional conditions	**26 726**	**14 596**	**12 130**	**11 444**	**716**	**998**	**666**	**432**	**207**	**133**	**8 479**	**835**	**1 338**	**814**	**347**	**173**	**145**
A. Infectious and parasitic diseases	**13 224**	**7 304**	**5 920**	**4 867**	**466**	**885**	**564**	**326**	**144**	**52**	**3 768**	**530**	**716**	**492**	**249**	**114**	**50**
1. Tuberculosis	**1 599**	**855**	**745**	50	55	361	149	146	76	18	40	84	313	157	93	47	12
2. STDs excluding HIV	**364**	**181**	**182**	174		1	1	2	1	1	145	1	17	14	3	2	2
a. Syphilis	336	181	154	174		1	1	2	1	1	145		2	2	2	2	2
b. Chlamydia	19		19										10	8			
c. Gonorrhoea	9		9										5	4			
3. HIV	**790**	**623**	**167**	36	3	320	217	38	7	1	33	4	77	46	5	1	
4. Diarrhoeal diseases	**4 804**	**2 742**	**2 062**	2 567	88	24	20	20	11	11	1 808	106	61	36	24	13	14
5. Childhood-cluster diseases	**3 076**	**1 614**	**1 462**	1 475	126	6	3	3	1		1 311	132	11	4	3	1	
a. Pertussis	579	304	275	287	18						255	20					
b. Poliomyelitis	51	30	21	30							20						
c. Diphtheria	16	8	8	5	3						4	4					
d. Measles	1 758	916	842	822	92	2					734	102	1				
e. Tetanus	672	356	316	333	14	3	2	2	1		297	6	6	4	3	1	
6. Bacterial meningitis*	**344**	**170**	**173**	104	2	10	32	14	8	2	93	2	10	42	15	9	2
7. Hepatitis B and hepatitis C	**118**	**50**	**68**	19	15	7	4	3	1	1	14	16	20	11	5	1	
8. Malaria	**392**	**188**	**204**	33	49	67	26	11	3	1	29	55	70	34	12	3	1
9. Tropical-cluster diseases	**332**	**148**	**184**	7	9	18	45	48	17	5	5	6	28	73	52	17	4
a. Trypanosomiasis																	
b. Chagas disease	300	129	171	1	3	15	43	46	16	5	1	1	26	71	51	17	4
c. Schistosomiasis	10	5	5			1	2	1				1	1	2	1		
d. Leishmaniasis	23	14	9	6	6	1			1		3	4	1	1			
10. Leprosy	**7**	**4**	**3**			1	1	1	1				1	1	1	1	
11. Dengue	**1**		**1**														
12. Japanese encephalitis																	
13. Trachoma																	
14. Intestinal nematode infections	**84**	**40**	**45**		36	2	1	1				40	2	1	1		
a. Ascariasis	42	20	22		19							22	2				
b. Trichuriasis	35	16	19		16	2	1	1				19		1	1		
c. Ancylostomiasis, necatoriasis	7	3	4									4					
15. Other infectious and parasitic	**1 313**	**689**	**624**	402	84	70	66	39	18	12	291	85	107	73	36	17	14

Annex Table 7g, continued. YLLs by age, sex and cause (thousands): Latin America and the Caribbean, 1990

Cause	Total	Male	Female	Males							Females						
				0-4	5-14	15-29	30-44	45-59	60-69	70+	0-4	5-14	15-29	30-44	45-59	60-69	70+
B. Respiratory infections	**4 423**	**2 446**	**1 978**	**1 965**	**145**	**77**	**75**	**78**	**47**	**59**	**1 399**	**170**	**138**	**99**	**64**	**41**	**66**
1. Lower respiratory infections	4 371	2 419	1 953	1 944	143	75	74	77	46	59	1 383	167	135	97	63	40	66
2. Upper respiratory infections	44	24	20	20	1	1	1	1	–	–	14	2	1	1	1	1	1
3. Otitis media	8	2	5	1	1	–	–	–	–	–	2	1	1	1	–	–	–
C. Maternal conditions	**580**		**580**										5	404	169	2		
1. Maternal haemorrhage	141		141											98	41			
2. Maternal sepsis	48		48											33	14			
3. Hypertensive disorders*	93		93											65	27			
4. Obstructed labour	48		48											33	14			
5. Abortion	132		132											92	38			
6. Other maternal	120		120											83	35			
D. Perinatal conditions*	**6 593**	**3 860**	**2 733**	**3 859**	1						**2 732**	1					
1. Low birth weight	971	550	421	550							421						
2. Birth asphyxia and birth trauma	3 068	1 817	1 251	1 817							1 251						
3. Other perinatal	2 554	1 494	1 060	1 493	1						1 060						
E. Nutritional deficiencies	**1 905**	**987**	**919**	**754**	**104**	**36**	**27**	**28**	**16**	**21**	**579**	**128**	**80**	**54**	**31**	**18**	**21**
1. Protein-energy malnutrition	1 310	715	595	606	39	12	16	17	10	15	450	52	25	22	15	10	15
2. Iodine deficiency	47	24	23	19	3						18	4					
3. Vitamin A deficiency	178	90	87	62	25	3					56	28	3				
4. Iron-deficiency anaemia	357	151	205	63	37	18	10	11	6	6	49	44	50	30	16	8	6
II. Noncommunicable diseases	***19 098***	***9 673***	***9 425***	***1 493***	***830***	***613***	***1 641***	***2 409***	***1 567***	***1 120***	***1 356***	***661***	***1 016***	***1 583***	***2 156***	***1 430***	***1 223***
A. Malignant neoplasms	**4 062**	**1 824**	**2 237**	**75**	**247**	**130**	**255**	**534**	**375**	**209**	**69**	**181**	**217**	**508**	**703**	**379**	**180**
1. Mouth and oropharynx cancers	136	100	36	1	2	8	17	47	18	8	1	1	2	5	12	9	5
2. Oesophagus cancer	92	67	25			3	5	33	18	7				2	9	8	6
3. Stomach cancer	337	204	133			13	26	79	58	28			8	19	43	39	24
4. Colon and rectum cancers	209	97	111	1	2	9	17	34	23	14			7	15	36	35	18
5. Liver cancer	54	28	26		2	2	5	10	6	3			1	3	8	8	4
6. Pancreas cancer	70	36	33				4	15	11	5			1	3	11	11	7
7. Trachea, bronchus, lung cancers	314	230	85			12	24	100	63	30			5	11	31	25	12
8. Melanoma and other skin cancers	40	19	21		1	3	6	6	2	1			3	6	7	3	2
9. Breast cancer	390		390										43	99	162	62	25
10. Cervix uteri cancer	350		350										46	107	136	43	18
11. Corpus uteri cancer	70		70										4	10	32	17	7
12. Ovary cancer	84		84										11	25	24	13	5
13. Prostate cancer	119	119	–				2	19	60	37							
14. Bladder cancer	66	49	17		1	2	4	17	16	9			1	2	5	6	4
15. Lymphomas, multiple myeloma	267	158	109	14	42	19	38	27	12	6	9	26	10	22	20	15	8
16. Leukaemia	302	169	133	24	74	17	33	12	6	3	19	58	10	24	12	7	4
17. Other cancers	1 161	548	612	36	124	38	75	136	82	57	37	87	66	155	155	79	33
B. Other neoplasms	**170**	**81**	**89**	**13**	**25**	**10**	**12**	**12**	**7**	**3**	**12**	**18**	**15**	**16**	**16**	**8**	**4**

Annex Table 7g, continued. YLLs by age, sex and cause (thousands): Latin America and the Caribbean, 1990

Cause	Total	Male	Female	Males							Females						
				0-4	5-14	15-29	30-44	45-59	60-69	70+	0-4	5-14	15-29	30-44	45-59	60-69	70+
C. Diabetes mellitus	**872**	**361**	**511**	12	28	18	61	115	83	44	11	23	38	60	164	141	74
D. Endocrine disorders	**511**	**263**	**248**	131	33	20	36	20	11	12	103	25	33	30	27	14	16
E. Neuro-psychiatric conditions	**1 039**	**610**	**429**	102	134	89	148	92	29	16	89	103	107	65	36	16	15
2. Bipolar disorder	7	3	4	-	-	1	1	1	-	-	-	-	1	1	1	-	1
3. Schizophrenia	39	25	14	-	-	3	7	9	4	2	-	-	3	3	4	3	1
4. Epilepsy	162	82	80	9	24	20	20	7	1	1	7	16	36	12	5	1	3
5. Alcohol use	196	173	23	-	-	19	84	55	12	3	-	-	4	11	6	2	-
6. Dementia*	121	61	60	20	16	4	5	7	4	5	21	11	7	4	5	5	7
7. Parkinson disease	8	4	4	-	-	-	-	-	1	3	-	-	-	-	1	1	2
8. Multiple sclerosis	24	10	14	-	-	1	5	3	1	-	-	-	1	5	5	2	1
9. Drug use	55	35	20	-	-	20	13	1	1	-	-	-	12	7	1	-	-
13. Other neuro-psychiatric	428	217	211	73	94	21	14	9	4	2	60	76	45	18	8	3	1
F. Sense organ diseases	**21**	**12**	**9**	8	2	1	1	-	-	-	5	2	1	1	-	-	-
1. Glaucoma	-	-	-														
2. Cataracts	-	-	-														
G. Cardiovascular diseases	**6 819**	**3 502**	**3 317**	130	117	167	617	1 085	766	620	113	104	291	566	852	648	743
1. Rheumatic heart disease	163	52	111	1	13	11	13	9	3	1	1	19	27	32	22	7	2
2. Ischaemic heart disease	2 635	1 434	1 201	-	-	29	243	506	365	291	-	-	37	185	345	293	341
3. Cerebrovascular disease	2 112	1 044	1 067	11	22	43	194	343	238	191	9	20	81	204	303	217	233
4. Inflammatory heart diseases	377	185	191	24	24	25	46	40	14	12	25	22	37	45	34	12	15
5. Other cardiovascular	1 532	786	746	94	57	59	120	187	144	125	77	43	108	100	148	118	151
H. Respiratory diseases	**1 386**	**737**	**648**	253	53	38	72	114	106	101	222	41	64	71	94	76	79
1. COPD*	504	282	222	58	8	6	18	58	66	67	56	7	9	15	44	44	47
2. Asthma	149	76	73	3	13	8	22	13	9	7	3	9	9	15	17	11	9
3. Other respiratory	733	380	353	191	31	23	32	42	31	28	164	25	47	41	33	21	23
I. Digestive diseases	**1 918**	**1 206**	**712**	109	64	82	374	367	142	68	81	45	94	153	174	96	67
1. Peptic ulcer	107	66	41	1	2	6	15	20	12	10	1	1	4	7	10	8	9
2. Cirrhosis of the liver	904	660	245	9	10	36	260	247	76	22	7	9	25	70	84	37	13
3. Appendicitis	49	29	21	1	12	8	5	1	1	-	1	8	7	4	1	-	-
4. Other digestive	857	451	405	98	40	32	94	99	54	36	72	27	59	72	78	52	45
J. Genito-urinary diseases	**675**	**308**	**367**	47	39	32	50	58	41	41	37	40	77	73	67	40	33
1. Nephritis and nephrosis	520	244	276	34	34	28	43	48	32	25	27	33	56	53	52	31	24
2. Benign prostatic hypertrophy	8	8	-	-	-	-	-	1	1	5	-	-	-	-	-	-	-
3. Other genito-urinary	147	57	91	13	5	4	7	9	7	10	10	7	22	20	14	9	9
K. Skin diseases	**50**	**20**	**31**	6	4	2	2	3	2	2	6	3	8	5	3	2	3
L. Musculo-skeletal diseases	**141**	**38**	**102**	3	11	6	5	6	4	4	2	12	35	23	16	8	7
1. Rheumatoid arthritis	12	3	8	-	-	-	-	1	1	1	-	-	1	2	2	2	2
2. Other musculo-skeletal	127	34	93	3	10	5	4	5	3	3	2	11	34	21	13	6	5

Annex Table 7q, continued. YLLs by age, sex and cause (thousands): Latin America and the Caribbean, 1990

Cause	Total	Male	Female	Males 0-4	5-14	15-29	30-44	45-59	60-69	70+	Females 0-4	5-14	15-29	30-44	45-59	60-69	70+
M. Congenital anomalies	**1 432**	**710**	**722**	**603**	**73**	**20**	**9**	**3**	**1**	**1**	**606**	**63**	**34**	**12**	**5**	**1**	**1**
1. Abdominal wall defect	17	8	8	8	–	–	–	–	–	–	8	–	–	–	–	–	–
2. Anencephaly	288	113	175	113	–	–	–	–	–	–	175	–	–	–	–	–	–
3. Anorectal atresia	5	3	3	3	–	–	–	–	–	–	3	–	–	–	–	–	–
4. Cleft lip	21	12	9	12	–	–	–	–	–	–	9	–	–	–	–	–	–
5. Cleft palate	17	8	9	8	–	–	–	–	–	–	9	–	–	–	–	–	–
6. Oesophageal atresia	11	6	6	6	–	–	–	–	–	–	6	–	–	–	–	–	–
7. Renal agenesis	31	16	15	16	–	–	–	–	–	–	15	–	–	–	–	–	–
8. Down syndrome	134	71	63	48	14	5	2	2	–	–	39	12	7	2	3	–	–
9. Congenital heart anomalies	490	260	229	211	33	10	4	1	1	1	174	26	19	6	2	1	1
10. Spina bifida	213	105	108	91	12	2					91	12	3	1			
11. Other congenital	205	107	97	88	15	3	1				77	12	5	2	1		
N. Oral conditions	**3**	**1**	**2**									1					
III. Injuries	**10 416**	**7 816**	**2 601**	**632**	**1 191**	**3 550**	**1 746**	**530**	**121**	**46**	**488**	**562**	**965**	**374**	**132**	**48**	**31**
A. Unintentional injuries	**6 529**	**4 698**	**1 831**	**536**	**1 025**	**1 740**	**935**	**338**	**86**	**37**	**402**	**478**	**565**	**224**	**96**	**38**	**29**
1. Road traffic accidents	2 930	2 127	803	113	459	868	474	164	39	12	84	231	293	122	50	17	5
2. Poisonings	133	77	55	21	15	22	12	5	1	1	15	13	18	6	2	1	–
3. Falls	312	233	79	22	40	74	52	26	9	9	14	20	13	8	6	5	13
4. Fires	189	106	83	35	22	23	17	6	2	1	32	22	16	7	3	1	1
5. Drownings	883	683	200	99	216	252	86	24	4	9	63	76	45	11	4	1	–
6. Other unintentional	2 082	1 471	611	246	272	501	295	114	30	13	193	116	179	70	31	13	9
B. Intentional injuries	**3 887**	**3 118**	**770**	**96**	**166**	**1 810**	**810**	**192**	**35**	**8**	**86**	**84**	**400**	**150**	**36**	**10**	**2**
1. Self-inflicted injuries	540	363	177		17	188	100	41	12	4		13	104	40	14	4	1
2. Violence	2 825	2 454	371	37	110	1 481	659	142	21	4	27	45	202	76	17	4	1
3. War	522	300	222	59	39	141	51	8	2	–	59	26	94	35	5	2	–

Notes:
Causes responsible for no deaths have been omitted from this table.
A dash (-) symbol indicates fewer than 500 YLLs.
*IA6 is Bacterial meningitis and meningococcaemia; IC3 is Hypertensive disorders of pregnancy; ID is Conditions arising during the perinatal period; IIE6 is Dementia and other degenerative and hereditary CNS disorders; IIH1 is Chronic obstructive pulmonary disease.

Annex Table 7h. YLLs by age, sex and cause (thousands): Middle Eastern Crescent, 1990

Cause	Total	Male	Female	Males 0-4	5-14	15-29	30-44	45-59	60-69	70+	Females 0-4	5-14	15-29	30-44	45-59	60-69	70+
Population (millions)	*503*	*256*	*247*	*41*	*65*	*70*	*44*	*22*	*9*	*5*	*40*	*62*	*66*	*41*	*22*	*10*	*6*
All causes	**105 234**	**55 190**	**50 044**	**32 286**	**5 929**	**5 526**	**3 959**	**3 758**	**2 349**	**1 383**	**30 847**	**5 298**	**4 559**	**3 001**	**2 684**	**1 965**	**1 690**
I. Communicable, maternal, perinatal and nutritional conditions	**60 797**	**30 465**	**30 332**	**26 686**	**1 734**	**716**	**490**	**387**	**326**	**126**	**25 551**	**1 737**	**1 357**	**975**	**333**	**233**	**145**
A. Infectious and parasitic diseases	**27 542**	**14 340**	**13 202**	**11 864**	**910**	**624**	**441**	**342**	**129**	**30**	**11 282**	**827**	**469**	**289**	**217**	**88**	**31**
1. Tuberculosis	2 306	1 448	858	172	101	505	307	254	92	17	107	64	315	151	146	59	16
2. STDs excluding HIV	439	219	220	214	–	1	1	2	1	1	205	–	6	4	2	1	2
a. Syphilis	431	219	212	214	–	1	1	2	1	1	205	–	1	1	2	1	2
b. Chlamydia	6	–	6	–	–	–	–	–	–	–	–	–	3	2	–	–	–
c. Gonorrhoea	2	–	2	–	–	–	–	–	–	–	–	–	1	1	–	–	–
3. HIV	16	12	3	2	–	5	4	1	–	–	2	–	1	1	–	–	–
4. Diarrhoeal diseases	14 318	7 299	7 019	6 976	276	17	14	9	6	2	6 659	282	34	26	11	4	3
5. Childhood-cluster diseases	8 024	4 084	3 940	3 678	380	11	7	6	2	2	3 530	347	28	22	11	2	–
a. Pertussis	1 786	912	874	839	73	–	–	–	–	–	803	71	–	–	–	–	–
b. Poliomyelitis	127	73	54	72	–	–	–	–	–	–	54	–	–	–	–	–	–
c. Diphtheria	41	21	20	19	2	1	–	–	–	–	18	2	–	–	–	–	–
d. Measles	3 293	1 670	1 622	1 442	227	1	–	–	–	–	1 393	225	2	1	–	–	–
e. Tetanus	2 776	1 408	1 369	1 307	77	9	6	6	2	–	1 263	48	25	21	10	2	–
6. Bacterial meningitis*	486	247	239	170	3	8	41	16	8	1	165	3	9	36	17	8	2
7. Hepatitis B and hepatitis C	248	136	112	36	20	16	23	26	10	4	29	20	23	15	13	8	4
8. Malaria	204	102	102	21	39	23	13	5	1	–	21	38	25	11	5	1	–
9. Tropical-cluster diseases	109	70	40	15	30	7	10	6	2	–	10	15	5	7	2	1	–
a. Trypanosomiasis	–	–	–	–	–	–	–	–	–	–	–	–	–	–	–	–	–
b. Chagas disease	–	–	–	–	–	–	–	–	–	–	–	–	–	–	–	–	–
c. Schistosomiasis	43	30	13	–	7	5	10	6	2	–	–	–	3	7	2	1	–
d. Leishmaniasis	66	39	27	14	22	2	–	–	–	–	10	15	2	–	–	–	–
10. Leprosy	2	1	1	1	–	–	–	–	–	–	–	–	–	–	–	–	–
11. Dengue	–	–	–	–	–	–	–	–	–	–	–	–	–	–	–	–	–
12. Japanese encephalitis	–	–	–	–	–	–	–	–	–	–	–	–	–	–	–	–	–
13. Trachoma	–	–	–	–	–	–	–	–	–	–	–	–	–	–	–	–	–
14. Intestinal nematode infections	26	13	13	–	11	1	1	–	–	–	–	10	1	1	–	–	–
a. Ascariasis	21	11	11	–	11	–	–	–	–	–	–	10	1	–	–	–	–
b. Trichuriasis	–	–	–	–	–	–	–	–	–	–	–	–	–	–	–	–	–
c. Ancylostomiasis, necatoriasis	4	2	2	–	–	1	1	–	–	–	–	–	–	1	–	–	–
15. Other infectious and parasitic	1 365	708	657	580	50	31	21	17	6	3	555	47	23	14	11	4	3

Annex Table 7h, continued. YLLs by age, sex and cause (thousands): Middle Eastern Crescent, 1990

Cause	Total	Male	Female	Males 0-4	5-14	15-29	30-44	45-59	60-69	70+	Females 0-4	5-14	15-29	30-44	45-59	60-69	70+
B. Respiratory infections	15 355	7 765	7 591	6 659	674	71	40	38	191	91	6 356	749	120	55	61	141	109
1. Lower respiratory infections	15 085	7 628	7 457	6 539	662	70	40	38	189	90	6 242	736	118	54	60	139	108
2. Upper respiratory infections	154	78	76	67	7	1	-	-	2	1	64	7	1	1	1	-	1
3. Otitis media	117	59	58	53	5	1	-	-	-	-	51	6	1	-	-	-	-
C. Maternal conditions	1 364	-	1 364								-	2	711	605	45		
1. Maternal haemorrhage	336	-	336									1	175	149	11		
2. Maternal sepsis	225	-	225										117	100	7		
3. Hypertensive disorders*	225	-	225										117	100	7		
4. Obstructed labour	113	-	113										59	50	4		
5. Abortion	113	-	113										59	50	4		
6. Other maternal	352	-	352									1	184	156	12		
D. Perinatal conditions*	13 392	6 809	6 583	6 809							6 583						
1. Low birth weight	6 752	3 428	3 324	3 428							3 324						
2. Birth asphyxia and birth trauma	3 182	1 615	1 567	1 615							1 567						
3. Other perinatal	3 458	1 766	1 692	1 766							1 692						
E. Nutritional deficiencies	3 144	1 552	1 592	1 354	150	22	9	7	6	4	1 330	159	57	26	9	5	4
1. Protein-energy malnutrition	2 055	1 040	1 015	1 017	7	4	2	3	4	3	987	7	8	4	2	3	3
2. Iodine deficiency	122	61	61	48	11	2					47	11	2				
3. Vitamin A deficiency	714	347	367	228	113	6					237	123	7				
4. Iron-deficiency anaemia	253	103	149	61	19	10	6	4	2	-	59	18	39	22	7	2	2
II. Noncommunicable diseases	31 219	16 153	15 067	4 037	2 548	1 532	1 876	2 989	1 936	1 235	3 818	2 696	1 729	1 434	2 195	1 671	1 524
A. Malignant neoplasms	3 355	1 773	1 582	93	300	194	274	533	285	95	80	277	204	298	407	229	87
1. Mouth and oropharynx cancers	196	123	73	1	5	20	28	31	29	10	-	5	11	15	16	18	7
2. Oesophagus cancer	116	67	48	-	1	6	9	33	13	4	-	2	5	7	20	11	4
3. Stomach cancer	248	150	98	1	1	17	24	68	29	9	1	1	11	16	35	26	10
4. Colon and rectum cancers	144	73	71	-	2	12	17	18	18	6	1	3	9	13	14	23	9
5. Liver cancer	109	67	42	1	4	7	10	29	12	4	1	4	4	6	15	9	4
6. Pancreas cancer	55	34	21				6	16	6	2			2	2	9	6	2
7. Trachea, bronchus, lung cancers	348	278	70		5	22	32	143	56	19		5	1	9	26	17	7
8. Melanoma and other skin cancers	18	11	7			2	2	5	1				2	2	1	1	
9. Breast cancer	199	-	199										36	53	76	22	9
10. Cervix uteri cancer	121	-	121								1	2	19	27	53	15	6
11. Corpus uteri cancer	25	-	25								1	-	-	3	10	6	2
12. Ovary cancer	67	-	67								-	6	13	19	19	6	2
13. Prostate cancer	36	36	-			1	1	10	17	6							
14. Bladder cancer	110	86	23			1	13	35	21	7		1	2	3	9	6	3
15. Lymphomas, multiple myeloma	196	128	68	11	43	20	28	14	9	3	7	27	8	12	6	6	3
16. Leukaemia	334	169	164	20	79	21	29	10	8	3	22	88	14	20	8	9	3
17. Other cancers	1 034	551	483	57	157	52	74	122	66	22	44	133	62	91	90	47	16
B. Other neoplasms	136	66	70	8	25	11	8	8	3	2	6	25	16	9	9	3	1

Annex Table 7h, continued. YLLs by age, sex and cause (thousands): Middle Eastern Crescent, 1990

Cause	Total	Male	Female	Males 0-4	5-14	15-29	30-44	45-59	60-69	70+	Females 0-4	5-14	15-29	30-44	45-59	60-69	70+
C. Diabetes mellitus	798	379	420	31	72	28	64	97	61	25	29	71	39	42	108	91	41
D. Endocrine disorders	460	208	252	100	50	19	15	15	6	3	94	101	27	11	10	5	3
E. Neuro-psychiatric conditions	1 472	783	689	227	249	143	71	48	27	18	178	249	125	54	39	23	21
2. Bipolar disorder	10	4	6			1	1	1	1	1			1	1	1	1	1
3. Schizophrenia	45	21	24			3	5	7	3	1			3	6	9	3	1
4. Epilepsy	258	138	120	20	44	42	20	8	2	2	15	39	43	15	6	2	2
5. Alcohol use	12	11	1			1	5	4	1	1					1		
6. Dementia*	91	40	51	6	3	5	4	7	8	8	12	4	4	3	7	9	11
7. Parkinson disease	15	9	6					1	4	4				1	1	2	2
8. Multiple sclerosis	23	10	13			1	3	3	3				3	5	3	2	
9. Drug use	49	45	5		1	28	15	1					3	1	1		
13. Other neuro-psychiatric	969	505	464	200	201	62	16	16	7	3	151	205	69	23	9	4	4
F. Sense organ diseases	4	2	2			1							1				
1. Glaucoma																	
2. Cataracts																	
G. Cardiovascular diseases	15 002	7 768	7 234	1 146	1 234	724	940	1 626	1 196	902	991	1 264	861	675	1 174	1 068	1 201
1. Rheumatic heart disease	720	312	409	1	105	131	58	14	3		1	143	166	71	22	5	1
2. Ischaemic heart disease	4 776	2 617	2 158			103	450	884	670	511			125	274	536	566	657
3. Cerebrovascular disease	2 094	1 052	1 042	64	199	94	117	244	191	144	50	177	67	78	227	208	235
4. Inflammatory heart diseases	1 627	821	806	216	236	138	95	84	30	22	232	226	144	83	69	26	27
5. Other cardiovascular	5 785	2 967	2 818	866	694	257	220	401	304	225	708	717	359	169	320	263	281
H. Respiratory diseases	2 793	1 378	1 415	629	168	73	87	184	143	94	676	262	95	75	121	96	91
1. COPD*	861	449	412	145	26	12	22	94	89	62	171	47	13	16	56	55	54
2. Asthma	132	75	57		16	12	17	13	8	5	2	10	8	10	12	9	6
3. Other respiratory	1 800	854	945	481	126	49	48	77	46	27	503	205	74	49	52	32	30
I. Digestive diseases	3 105	1 662	1 443	605	218	145	232	293	126	42	679	188	137	123	182	91	43
1. Peptic ulcer	80	58	23		4	8	15	19	9	3	1	1	3	4	7	4	2
2. Cirrhosis of the liver	666	366	300	10	36	42	82	124	53	16	8	67	39	44	83	41	18
3. Appendicitis	144	84	60	3	38	27	13	2	1		3	31	17	8	2	2	
4. Other digestive	2 215	1 155	1 060	591	139	69	122	148	63	23	668	89	77	67	91	46	22
J. Genito-urinary diseases	1 493	797	697	80	120	134	158	170	84	50	64	135	159	119	126	60	34
1. Nephritis and nephrosis	697	337	359	45	67	60	58	57	30	21	37	99	87	49	49	24	14
2. Benign prostatic hypertrophy	9	9							3	4							
3. Other genito-urinary	787	450	337	35	52	74	100	113	50	26	27	37	72	70	77	36	20
K. Skin diseases	39	18	22	7	3	3	1	2	1	1	6	1	8	2	2	1	1
L. Musculo-skeletal diseases	52	25	28	6	7	4	4	2	1		4	5	8	5	3	1	1
1. Rheumatoid arthritis	1	1															
3. Other musculo-skeletal	51	24	27	5	7	4	3	2	1		4	5	8	5	3	1	1

Annex Table 7h, continued. YLLs by age, sex and cause (thousands): Middle Eastern Crescent, 1990

Cause	Total	Male	Female	Males							Females						
				0-4	5-14	15-29	30-44	45-59	60-69	70+	0-4	5-14	15-29	30-44	45-59	60-69	70+
M. Congenital anomalies	2 504	1 294	1 210	1 103	102	53	22	10	2	1	1 008	116	49	19	13	3	1
1. Abdominal wall defect	30	19	10	19	-	-	-	-	-	-	10	-	-	-	-	-	-
2. Anencephaly	659	258	401	258	-	-	-	-	-	-	401	-	-	-	-	-	-
3. Anorectal atresia	10	6	3	6	-	-	-	-	-	-	3	-	-	-	-	-	-
4. Cleft lip	22	13	9	13	-	-	-	-	-	-	9	-	-	-	-	-	-
5. Cleft palate	18	9	9	9	-	-	-	-	-	-	9	-	-	-	-	-	-
6. Oesophageal atresia	20	13	7	13	-	-	-	-	-	-	7	-	-	-	-	-	-
7. Renal agenesis	59	30	29	30	-	-	9	-	-	-	29	-	-	-	-	-	-
8. Down syndrome	263	144	119	87	25	22	9	-	-	-	61	31	19	8	11	-	-
9. Congenital heart anomalies	940	534	406	440	51	23	-	8	2	1	309	55	19	8	1	3	1
10. Spina bifida	154	86	68	79	6	-	-	1	-	-	56	7	3	1	1	-	-
11. Other congenital	330	182	148	148	20	8	3	-	-	-	113	23	7	3	-	-	-
N. Oral conditions	6	2	5	-	1	1	-	-	-	-	-	2	3	-	-	-	-
III. Injuries	13 218	8 572	4 646	1 563	1 647	3 278	1 593	382	86	22	1 478	864	1 473	593	156	61	21
A. Unintentional injuries	5 704	4 040	1 664	789	879	1 312	795	210	43	12	682	387	335	159	65	23	12
1. Road traffic accidents	1 963	1 542	421	92	308	636	395	90	17	4	80	144	101	60	25	8	3
2. Poisonings	321	203	118	50	21	51	55	22	4	1	46	17	29	15	8	3	1
3. Falls	306	217	90	50	55	54	38	14	3	2	43	23	10	7	3	2	2
4. Fires	436	196	240	75	40	46	26	8	2	1	76	42	89	23	6	2	1
5. Drownings	898	636	262	191	210	160	60	12	2	1	164	58	27	9	3	1	-
6. Other unintentional	1 780	1 247	533	331	245	365	221	65	15	5	273	103	80	46	20	8	4
B. Intentional injuries	7 514	4 532	2 982	774	768	1 966	798	172	43	10	796	476	1 138	434	91	38	9
1. Self-inflicted injuries	1 253	872	382	-	307	319	161	65	15	5	-	139	149	54	25	11	5
2. Violence	1 142	722	420	196	77	273	137	31	6	2	215	80	68	39	13	3	1
3. War	5 119	2 938	2 180	578	384	1 374	500	76	22	3	581	257	921	340	53	24	3

Notes:
Causes responsible for no deaths have been omitted from this table.
A dash (-) symbol indicates fewer than 500 YLLs.
*IA6 is Bacterial meningitis and meningococcaemia; IC3 is Hypertensive disorders of pregnancy; ID is Conditions arising during the perinatal period; IIE6 is Dementia and other degenerative and hereditary CNS disorders; IIH1 is Chronic obstructive pulmonary disease.

Annex Table 7i. YLLs by age, sex and cause (thousands): World, 1990

Cause	Total	Male	Female	Males							Females						
				0-4	5-14	15-29	30-44	45-59	60-69	70+	0-4	5-14	15-29	30-44	45-59	60-69	70+
Population (millions)	*5 267*	*2 654*	*2 614*	*321*	*551*	*736*	*514*	*312*	*137*	*82*	*309*	*526*	*703*	*496*	*311*	*151*	*118*
All causes	**906 501**	**486 937**	**419 565**	**224 525**	**45 661**	**57 230**	**48 387**	**52 101**	**36 041**	**22 992**	**207 721**	**41 256**	**45 949**	**34 110**	**35 323**	**28 028**	**27 178**
I. Communicable, maternal, perinatal and nutritional conditions	**490 588**	**246 875**	**243 713**	**192 420**	**18 581**	**11 230**	**10 020**	**7 674**	**4 223**	**2 726**	**178 397**	**20 422**	**19 305**	**13 756**	**5 829**	**3 127**	**2 877**
A. Infectious and parasitic diseases	**265 334**	**138 952**	**126 382**	**96 965**	**12 574**	**9 794**	**8 995**	**6 749**	**2 661**	**1 214**	**87 917**	**13 231**	**10 160**	**7 324**	**4 783**	**1 881**	**1 086**
1. Tuberculosis	**34 304**	**19 334**	**14 971**	**1 459**	**992**	**4 998**	**4 479**	**4 835**	**1 816**	**753**	**1 314**	**1 151**	**4 498**	**3 119**	**3 265**	**1 107**	**517**
2. STDs excluding HIV	**6 584**	**3 001**	**3 583**	**2 818**	-	**31**	**33**	**47**	**34**	**37**	**2 626**	**22**	**434**	**335**	**70**	**43**	**52**
a. Syphilis	5 852	2 998	2 854	2 818	-	30	32	46	34	37	2 626	-	37	40	58	42	52
b. Chlamydia	463	-	463								-	14	253	189	7	-	-
c. Gonorrhoea	263	-	263								-	8	145	106	4	-	-
3. HIV	**8 832**	**4 709**	**4 123**	**1 156**	**172**	**1 475**	**1 568**	**292**	**38**	**7**	**1 097**	**178**	**1 598**	**1 117**	**114**	**17**	**3**
4. Diarrhoeal diseases	**94 434**	**49 016**	**45 418**	**44 220**	**3 027**	**531**	**488**	**294**	**278**	**178**	**39 863**	**3 369**	**794**	**610**	**320**	**239**	**224**
5. Childhood-cluster diseases	**67 104**	**34 359**	**32 746**	**29 381**	**4 044**	**369**	**397**	**120**	**32**	**15**	**27 576**	**4 170**	**464**	**364**	**126**	**29**	**17**
a. Pertussis	11 878	6 127	5 750	5 598	529	-	-	-	-	-	5 231	520	-	-	-	-	-
b. Poliomyelitis	909	521	388	508	3	5	4	1	-	-	378	2	4	2	2	-	-
c. Diphtheria	360	184	177	159	22	2	1	-	-	-	150	23	4	-	-	-	-
d. Measles	36 450	18 737	17 713	15 923	2 783	18	8	3	2	-	14 918	2 761	22	8	3	1	-
e. Tetanus	17 508	8 790	8 718	7 192	708	345	384	116	30	15	6 900	864	436	352	121	28	16
6. Bacterial meningitis*	**4 532**	**2 318**	**2 214**	**1 490**	**30**	**113**	**414**	**168**	**85**	**18**	**1 407**	**30**	**105**	**399**	**165**	**86**	**22**
7. Hepatitis B and hepatitis C	**2 072**	**1 211**	**861**	**260**	**134**	**201**	**259**	**248**	**73**	**36**	**206**	**128**	**188**	**136**	**95**	**73**	**35**
8. Malaria	**28 038**	**14 957**	**13 081**	**11 394**	**1 712**	**1 045**	**539**	**212**	**45**	**11**	**9 311**	**1 714**	**1 156**	**606**	**231**	**48**	**15**
9. Tropical-cluster diseases	**3 430**	**1 861**	**1 568**	**96**	**725**	**528**	**304**	**162**	**38**	**8**	**85**	**570**	**453**	**295**	**129**	**31**	**7**
a. Trypanosomiasis	1 346	644	702	16	243	195	102	78	9	2	31	256	230	121	56	7	1
b. Chagas disease	300	129	171	1	3	15	43	46	16	5	1	1	26	71	51	17	1
c. Schistosomiasis	156	97	58	1	19	16	30	21	9	1	1	9	9	24	11	4	4
d. Leishmaniasis	1 628	991	637	78	460	302	129	17	4	1	52	303	187	80	12	3	2
10. Leprosy	**46**	**24**	**22**	**1**	**4**	**2**	**4**	**7**	**4**	**1**	**7**	**1**	**3**	**3**	**4**	**3**	-
11. Dengue	**743**	**341**	**403**	**69**	**262**	**4**	**3**	**2**	-	-	**82**	**311**	**5**	**3**	**2**	-	-
12. Japanese encephalitis	**163**	**85**	**77**	**45**	**30**	**4**	**4**	**1**	-	-	**45**	**24**	**4**	**2**	**1**	-	-
13. Trachoma	-	-	-	-	-	-	-	-	-	-	-	-	-	-	-	-	-
14. Intestinal nematode infections	**753**	**386**	**367**	-	**341**	**21**	**12**	**7**	**2**	**2**	**1**	**322**	**20**	**12**	**7**	**2**	**2**
a. Ascariasis	406	209	198	-	202	3	2	1	-	-	-	192	3	2	1	-	-
b. Trichuriasis	269	138	130	-	138	-	-	-	-	-	-	130	-	-	-	-	-
c. Ancylostomiasis, necatoriasis	78	39	39	-	-	18	10	7	2	2	-	-	17	10	7	2	2
15. Other infectious and parasitic	**14 299**	**7 351**	**6 948**	**4 574**	**1 100**	**472**	**490**	**353**	**216**	**147**	**4 299**	**1 241**	**439**	**322**	**254**	**203**	**191**

Annex Table 7i, continued. YLLs by age, sex and cause (thousands): World, 1990

Cause	Total	Male	Female	Males							Females						
				0-4	5-14	15-29	30-44	45-59	60-69	70+	0-4	5-14	15-29	30-44	45-59	60-69	70+
B. Respiratory infections	**110 992**	**56 587**	**54 404**	**46 033**	**4 941**	**1 093**	**854**	**794**	**1 460**	**1 412**	**43 288**	**5 613**	**1 254**	**750**	**709**	**1 139**	**1 651**
1. Lower respiratory infections	108 601	55 547	53 054	45 147	4 852	1 073	844	786	1 446	1 399	42 106	5 512	1 230	742	701	1 127	1 635
2. Upper respiratory infections	1 114	571	543	466	50	12	9	8	14	13	431	57	13	8	7	11	16
3. Otitis media	952	469	483	420	39	8	1	-	-	-	427	45	10	1	-	-	-
C. Maternal conditions	**13 299**	**-**	**13 299**								**-**	**382**	**7 379**	**5 367**	**171**	**-**	**-**
1. Maternal haemorrhage	3 327	-	3 327								-	92	1 873	1 317	45	-	-
2. Maternal sepsis	1 976	-	1 976								-	61	1 070	821	24	-	-
3. Hypertensive disorders*	1 656	-	1 656								-	46	913	676	21	-	-
4. Obstructed labour	1 004	-	1 004								-	31	545	416	12	-	-
5. Abortion	1 794	-	1 794								-	52	997	725	20	-	-
6. Other maternal	3 541	-	3 541								-	101	1 981	1 411	48	-	-
D. Perinatal conditions*	**82 681**	**42 626**	**40 055**	**42 623**	**2**	**1**	**-**	**-**	**-**	**-**	**40 053**	**1**	**-**	**-**	**-**	**-**	**-**
1. Low birth weight	35 092	17 965	17 126	17 965	-	-	-	-	-	-	17 126	-	-	-	-	-	-
2. Birth asphyxia and birth trauma	26 049	13 365	12 684	13 364	1	-	-	-	-	-	12 684	-	-	-	-	-	-
3. Other perinatal	21 542	11 297	10 245	11 295	1	1	-	-	-	-	10 243	1	-	-	-	-	-
E. Nutritional deficiencies	**18 282**	**8 709**	**9 573**	**6 799**	**1 064**	**342**	**172**	**131**	**101**	**101**	**7 138**	**1 195**	**511**	**316**	**166**	**108**	**139**
1. Protein-energy malnutrition	11 080	5 329	5 750	4 913	139	64	57	53	50	53	5 212	223	101	61	44	43	67
2. Iodine deficiency	795	404	391	302	72	27	3	-	-	-	293	70	25	3	-	-	-
3. Vitamin A deficiency	3 722	1 882	1 840	1 180	657	45	-	-	-	-	1 140	655	45	-	-	-	-
4. Iron-deficiency anaemia	2 627	1 064	1 563	389	194	204	108	74	49	46	480	245	339	249	119	63	68
II. Noncommunicable diseases	**283 395**	**152 937**	**130 458**	**19 269**	**12 451**	**12 308**	**21 085**	**38 075**	**30 155**	**19 593**	**18 597**	**11 922**	**11 625**	**14 158**	**26 713**	**23 826**	**23 618**
A. Malignant neoplasms	**64 837**	**36 083**	**28 753**	**927**	**2 340**	**2 659**	**5 647**	**12 306**	**8 602**	**3 602**	**903**	**1 739**	**2 656**	**4 996**	**9 317**	**6 091**	**3 050**
1. Mouth and oropharynx cancers	3 247	2 080	1 167	19	40	171	413	769	490	178	17	41	141	197	381	271	117
2. Oesophagus cancer	3 375	2 280	1 095	-	1	70	274	1 002	687	246	-	2	67	77	423	374	151
3. Stomach cancer	6 984	4 382	2 602	-	14	154	544	1 853	1 313	500	1	10	172	441	875	715	388
4. Colon and rectum cancers	3 926	2 063	1 863	2	18	161	327	645	595	314	5	19	94	256	567	562	360
5. Liver cancer	6 333	4 712	1 621	24	67	352	1 379	1 892	782	215	21	54	106	329	586	366	159
6. Pancreas cancer	1 483	877	606	-	-	41	106	345	268	117	2	2	19	47	192	212	131
7. Trachea, bronchus, lung cancers	8 303	6 268	2 035	-	-	170	500	2 677	2 121	754	5	11	64	190	770	687	308
8. Melanoma and other skin cancers	508	272	237	-	-	24	72	98	49	25	1	2	21	54	78	49	32
9. Breast cancer	3 785	-	3 785								-	7	303	926	1 562	685	298
10. Cervix uteri cancer	2 661	-	2 661								-	2	299	564	1 220	411	163
11. Corpus uteri cancer	576	-	576								-	4	26	67	235	161	81
12. Ovary cancer	1 309	-	1 309								23	50	158	284	445	250	99
13. Prostate cancer	1 055	1 055	-	-	-	9	16	194	447	384							
14. Bladder cancer	976	728	249	-	-	30	57	236	253	144	2	3	12	22	69	81	60
15. Lymphomas, multiple myeloma	2 953	1 841	1 112	129	417	274	327	344	243	107	78	222	125	165	223	189	110
16. Leukaemia	4 422	2 394	2 028	301	724	473	414	253	152	77	295	536	399	352	227	139	79
17. Other cancers	12 941	7 132	5 809	429	1 016	729	1 218	1 997	1 203	541	450	773	648	1 024	1 463	936	514
B. Other neoplasms	**1 650**	**868**	**782**	**112**	**211**	**134**	**129**	**146**	**88**	**47**	**103**	**182**	**121**	**117**	**120**	**85**	**53**

Annex Table 7i, continued. YLLs by age, sex and cause (thousands): World, 1990

Cause	Total	Male	Female	Males							Females						
				0-4	5-14	15-29	30-44	45-59	60-69	70+	0-4	5-14	15-29	30-44	45-59	60-69	70+
C. Diabetes mellitus	5 769	2 650	3 119	146	358	164	426	713	548	295	145	348	231	296	799	810	490
D. Endocrine disorders	2 363	1 130	1 233	413	178	133	143	121	81	61	376	241	166	127	137	86	100
E. Neuro-psychiatric conditions	10 424	6 027	4 397	847	965	1 355	1 255	797	441	368	800	808	882	588	436	381	501
2. Bipolar disorder	116	51	65		1	8	14	12	8	8			8	7	11	11	26
3. Schizophrenia	615	384	230			111	139	71	34	30			52	58	47	34	40
4. Epilepsy	1 641	943	698	76	175	310	242	99	30	12	69	130	284	132	51	23	10
5. Alcohol use	890	761	130			61	347	265	73	15			12	44	50	20	4
6. Dementia*	1 435	656	780	93	54	66	57	105	120	160	124	46	56	49	97	138	269
7. Parkinson disease	241	133	108			1	1	11	43	77				1	8	32	66
8. Multiple sclerosis	352	150	202			16	56	52	21	5			15	71	75	32	9
9. Drug use	299	248	51		3	155	84	5	1			1	32	16	1		
13. Other neuro-psychiatric	4 835	2 702	2 133	677	732	628	314	178	111	61	606	630	425	210	96	89	77
F. Sense organ diseases	272	142	130	39	5	19	5	37	29	8	26	11	12	16	30	27	7
1. Glaucoma	75	46	30	7		13		11	11	3	9				9	9	3
2. Cataracts	72	44	28	14				16	11	2	2			5	12	7	2
G. Cardiovascular diseases	116 325	60 921	55 404	3 649	4 255	4 241	7 648	15 885	14 258	10 985	3 420	4 474	4 253	4 886	10 930	12 209	15 231
1. Rheumatic heart disease	5 527	2 347	3 180	5	313	765	500	462	197	106	32	447	829	663	716	319	174
2. Ischaemic heart disease	41 595	23 093	18 501			480	2 980	7 558	6 890	5 185	140		345	1 549	4 137	5 410	6 920
3. Cerebrovascular disease	32 115	16 098	16 017	475	899	910	1 822	4 312	4 304	3 376	441	774	737	1 286	3 618	4 174	4 986
4. Inflammatory heart diseases	8 347	4 236	4 111	703	856	732	713	726	288	219	839	948	691	497	560	271	305
5. Other cardiovascular	28 741	15 146	13 595	2 466	2 188	1 354	1 634	2 827	2 579	2 100	1 967	2 305	1 650	892	1 900	2 034	2 846
H. Respiratory diseases	24 755	13 488	11 266	2 227	930	632	1 046	2 558	3 344	2 751	2 350	951	574	726	1 773	2 198	2 696
1. COPD*	14 444	7 948	6 496	575	146	160	380	1 726	2 690	2 270	797	169	102	290	1 172	1 772	2 218
2. Asthma	1 665	910	755	41	145	142	190	177	127	87	26	86	102	148	173	125	95
3. Other respiratory	8 646	4 631	4 016	1 611	639	329	476	655	527	394	1 527	695	394	288	428	300	383
I. Digestive diseases	26 050	15 890	10 159	2 008	1 288	1 568	3 695	4 443	2 007	880	2 031	1 211	1 241	1 396	2 113	1 256	912
1. Peptic ulcer	1 789	1 134	655	22	25	142	259	357	199	129	26	27	96	99	168	112	127
2. Cirrhosis of the liver	10 549	7 281	3 268	155	184	627	2 156	2 750	1 092	318	114	233	382	627	1 104	577	231
3. Appendicitis	1 676	983	693	27	388	344	176	33	12		27	314	213	102	24	10	3
4. Other digestive	12 043	6 497	5 547	1 804	692	455	1 105	1 305	705	431	1 865	637	550	568	817	558	552
J. Genito-urinary diseases	9 875	5 195	4 680	521	979	787	855	908	643	503	406	998	749	709	826	555	436
1. Nephritis and nephrosis	7 837	4 061	3 776	423	849	678	667	680	447	317	363	907	593	566	620	413	314
2. Benign prostatic hypertrophy	162	162		7		1	9	9	59	77							
3. Other genito-urinary	1 877	973	904	90	130	108	179	219	136	110	43	91	155	143	206	142	122
K. Skin diseases	635	336	299	165	48	23	24	32	19	26	127	15	59	21	25	20	32
L. Musculo-skeletal diseases	970	360	610	20	61	53	39	55	74	58	25	53	125	118	111	81	99
1. Rheumatoid arthritis	118	39	79	1	3	3	4	7	12	8	1	1	6	8	24	21	18
3. Other musculo-skeletal	850	320	530	19	58	49	34	48	61	49	24	51	119	110	86	59	80

Annex Table 7i, continued. YLLs by age, sex and cause (thousands): World, 1990

Cause	Total	Male	Female	Males 0-4	5-14	15-29	30-44	45-59	60-69	70+	Females 0-4	5-14	15-29	30-44	45-59	60-69	70+
M. Congenital anomalies	19 414	9 831	9 582	8 192	828	536	171	75	21	8	7 881	877	533	161	94	27	10
1. Abdominal wall defect	174	94	80	94	-	-	-	-	-	-	80	-	-	-	-	-	-
2. Anencephaly	4 993	1 945	3 048	1 945	-	-	-	-	-	-	3 048	-	-	-	-	-	-
3. Anorectal atresia	61	34	27	34	-	-	-	-	-	-	27	-	-	-	-	-	-
4. Cleft lip	171	102	68	102	-	-	-	-	-	-	68	-	-	-	-	-	-
5. Cleft palate	137	68	68	68	-	-	-	-	-	-	68	-	-	-	-	-	-
6. Oesophageal atresia	103	57	45	57	-	-	-	-	-	-	45	-	-	-	-	-	-
7. Renal agenesis	394	199	194	199	-	-	-	-	-	-	194	-	-	-	-	-	-
8. Down syndrome	1 855	1 009	845	568	189	179	59	12	2	1	417	189	169	53	14	2	1
9. Congenital heart anomalies	6 654	3 655	2 999	2 870	386	247	78	53	16	6	2 179	392	254	80	67	19	8
10. Spina bifida	1 995	1 054	942	941	98	9	3	1	-	-	780	118	26	11	5	1	-
11. Other congenital	2 878	1 614	1 265	1 313	156	102	31	8	3	1	972	179	83	16	8	5	2
N. Oral conditions	57	15	42	2	5	5	2	1	-	-	2	14	23	1	1	-	-
III. Injuries	132 519	87 125	45 394	12 836	14 628	33 692	17 282	6 351	1 664	673	10 727	8 912	15 019	6 197	2 781	1 075	683
A. Unintentional injuries	84 536	56 474	28 062	10 343	12 147	18 295	10 113	4 058	1 054	464	8 090	7 369	6 795	3 031	1 613	658	507
1. Road traffic accidents	26 162	19 184	6 978	1 725	3 564	7 697	4 231	1 479	368	120	1 099	2 002	2 043	968	592	198	77
2. Poisonings	6 090	3 620	2 470	968	456	804	817	456	91	28	660	373	821	368	163	59	26
3. Falls	4 731	3 197	1 533	451	615	865	611	379	153	122	453	292	181	140	141	110	217
4. Fires	7 295	3 015	4 280	1 058	521	741	436	186	40	33	926	932	1 579	570	165	66	43
5. Drownings	15 691	10 457	5 234	2 920	4 004	2 303	834	288	74	34	2 106	1 969	704	249	124	48	33
6. Other unintentional	24 566	17 000	7 566	3 221	2 987	5 885	3 184	1 270	327	126	2 847	1 802	1 467	734	429	176	111
B. Intentional injuries	47 983	30 651	17 332	2 493	2 481	15 397	7 169	2 292	610	208	2 637	1 543	8 225	3 166	1 168	417	176
1. Self-inflicted injuries	17 231	9 698	7 533	-	675	4 285	2 810	1 339	419	169	-	373	4 400	1 581	756	277	145
2. Violence	15 540	12 174	3 365	788	675	6 979	2 851	727	124	30	922	413	1 108	579	255	68	21
3. War	15 213	8 778	6 434	1 705	1 131	4 133	1 508	226	66	9	1 715	757	2 717	1 007	157	71	10

Notes:

Causes responsible for no deaths have been omitted from this table.

A dash (-) symbol indicates fewer than 500 YLLs.

*IA6 is Bacterial meningitis and meningococcaemia; IC3 is Hypertensive disorders of pregnancy; ID is Conditions arising during the perinatal period; IIE6 is Dementia and other degenerative and hereditary CNS disorders; IIH1 is Chronic obstructive pulmonary disease.

Annex Table 8a. YLDs by age, sex and cause (thousands): Established Market Economies, 1990

Cause	Total	Male	Female	Males					Females				
				0-4	5-14	15-44	45-59	60+	0-4	5-14	15-44	45-59	60+
Population (millions)	*798*	*390*	*407*	*26*	*53*	*184*	*66*	*61*	*25*	*51*	*179*	*68*	*85*
All causes	**49 120**	**24 911**	**24 209**	**1 240**	**941**	**13 752**	**4 432**	**4 546**	**1 110**	**719**	**12 291**	**4 631**	**5 459**
I. Communicable, maternal, perinatal and nutritional conditions													
A. Infectious and parasitic diseases	2 682	946	1 736	291	124	407	58	67	276	121	1 136	113	90
1. Tuberculosis	1 255	516	739	93	36	330	38	19	86	37	558	33	25
1. Tuberculosis	**11**	**8**	**3**	–	–	4	2	2			2	1	
2. STDs excluding HIV	**397**	**22**	**375**			22					370	2	1
a. Syphilis	2	1	1			1					1		
b. Chlamydia	348	14	335			13					330		
c. Gonorrhoea	44	8	36			8					36		
3. HIV	**317**	**265**	**52**	1		243	20	2	1		49	2	
4. Diarrhoeal diseases	**207**	**104**	**103**	38	9	40	10	6	36	9	39	10	8
5. Childhood-cluster diseases	**31**	**17**	**14**	13	4				10	4			
a. Pertussis	24	12	12	9	3				9	3			
b. Poliomyelitis													
c. Diphtheria	–												
d. Measles	7	5	2	4	1				1	1			
e. Tetanus	–												
6. Bacterial meningitis*	**91**	**46**	**45**	34	7	3	1	1	33	7	3	1	1
7. Hepatitis B and hepatitis C	**6**	**4**	**2**			3	1				1	1	
8. Malaria	–	–	–	–	–	–	–	–	–	–	–	–	–
9. Tropical-cluster diseases	1	1	–	–	–	–	–	–	–	–	–	–	–
a. Trypanosomiasis	–	–	–	–	–	–	–	–	–	–	–	–	–
b. Chagas disease	–	–	–	–	–	–	–	–	–	–	–	–	–
c. Schistosomiasis	–	–	–	–	–	–	–	–	–	–	–	–	–
d. Leishmaniasis	1	1	–	–	–	–	–	–	–	–	–	–	–
e. Lymphatic filariasis	–	–	–	–	–	–	–	–	–	–	–	–	–
f. Onchocerciasis	–	–	–	–	–	–	–	–	–	–	–	–	–
10. Leprosy	1	1	–	–	–	–	–	–	–	–	–	–	–
11. Dengue	–	–	–	–	–	–	–	–	–	–	–	–	–
12. Japanese encephalitis	–	–	–	–	–	–	–	–	–	–	–	–	–
13. Trachoma	–	–	–	–	–	–	–	–	–	–	–	–	–
14. Intestinal nematode infections	–	–	–	–	–	–	–	–	–	–	–	–	–
a. Ascariasis	–	–	–	–	–	–	–	–	–	–	–	–	–
b. Trichuriasis	–	–	–	–	–	–	–	–	–	–	–	–	–
c. Ancylostomiasis and necatoriasis	–	–	–	–	–	–	–	–	–	–	–	–	–

Annex Table 8a, continued. YLDs by age, sex and cause (thousands): Established Market Economies, 1990

Cause	Total	Male	Female	Males 0-4	5-14	15-44	45-59	60+	Females 0-4	5-14	15-44	45-59	60+
B. Respiratory infections	154	76	77	10	40	17	4	6	9	38	18	4	8
1. Lower respiratory infections	45	22	23	2	5	9	2	4	2	5	9	2	6
2. Upper respiratory infections	29	14	15			8	2	2			9	2	2
3. Otitis media	79	41	39	7	33				7	32			
C. Maternal conditions	307	–	307								306		
1. Maternal haemorrhage	16	–	16								16		
2. Maternal sepsis	32	–	32								32		
3. Hypertensive disorders of pregnancy	3	–	3								3		
4. Obstructed labour	230	–	230								230		
5. Abortion	9	–	9								9		
D. Perinatal conditions*	234	119	115	119					115				
E. Nutritional deficiencies	732	235	498	69	48	60	15	42	66	46	254	75	57
1. Protein-energy malnutrition	64	33	31	33					31				
2. Iodine deficiency	21	10	11	10					10				
3. Vitamin A deficiency	–	–	–										
4. Iron-deficiency anaemia	643	191	453	26	48	59	15	42	24	45	251	75	57
II. Noncommunicable diseases	*42 584*	*21 370*	*21 214*	*814*	*581*	*11 545*	*4 075*	*4 354*	*742*	*479*	*10 465*	*4 329*	*5 200*
A. Malignant neoplasms	1 858	1 087	771	2	4	91	224	767	1	4	141	207	417
1. Mouth and oropharynx cancers	50	39	11			9	15	15			3	3	5
2. Oesophagus cancer	23	17	6			1	6	10				1	5
3. Stomach cancer	129	88	41			7	19	62			6	10	25
4. Colon and rectum cancers	330	175	154			11	41	124			10	31	113
5. Liver cancer	15	12	3			1	5	5				1	2
6. Pancreas cancer	43	26	18			2	5	19			1	6	10
7. Trachea, bronchus, lung cancers	216	146	70			8	40	98			4	20	46
8. Melanoma and other skin cancers	30	17	14			6	4	7			7	3	4
9. Breast cancer	193	–	193								50	61	82
10. Cervix uteri cancer	17	–	17								8	4	4
11. Corpus uteri cancer	22	–	22								6	16	
12. Ovary cancer	30	–	30								9	9	11
13. Prostate cancer	188	188	–			1	18	169					
14. Bladder cancer	135	121	15			3	13	105			1	2	11
15. Lymphomas and multiple myeloma	59	33	25			11	8	14			6	5	13
16. Leukaemia	33	19	14	1	1	5	4	9	1	1	3	2	7
C. Diabetes mellitus	1 547	705	842	2	3	198	266	237	2	4	202	295	339
D. Endocrine disorders	856	334	522	66	45	120	47	56	65	34	192	139	91

Annex Table 8a, continued. YLDs by age, sex and cause (thousands): Established Market Economies, 1990

Cause	Total	Male	Female	Males 0-4	Males 5-14	Males 15-44	Males 45-59	Males 60+	Females 0-4	Females 5-14	Females 15-44	Females 45-59	Females 60+
E. Neuro-psychiatric conditions	**23 183**	**11 959**	**11 223**	**87**	**288**	**9 193**	**1 331**	**1 060**	**76**	**244**	**7 647**	**1 415**	**1 841**
1. Unipolar major depression	6 684	2 331	4 353	-	-	1 830	381	121	-	-	3 359	706	287
2. Bipolar disorder	1 705	858	847	-	-	770	63	26	-	-	749	64	34
3. Schizophrenia	2 186	1 137	1 049	-	-	1 137	-	-	-	-	1 049	-	-
4. Epilepsy	375	186	188	5	45	96	29	11	6	48	85	31	19
5. Alcohol use	4 467	3 779	689	-	-	3 297	396	86	-	-	596	67	26
6. Dementia*	2 429	924	1 506	21	10	26	205	661	21	9	26	227	1 222
7. Parkinson disease	349	149	199	-	-	-	62	87	-	-	-	69	130
8. Multiple sclerosis	166	71	95	-	-	69	3	-	-	-	91	4	-
9. Drug use	1 413	1 060	353	4	84	939	31	5	6	28	313	10	2
10. Post-traumatic stress disorder	269	102	168	-	16	71	9	2	-	26	117	15	4
11. Obsessive-compulsive disorders	1 454	620	834	-	53	502	41	25	-	66	650	74	44
12. Panic disorder	688	228	460	-	18	167	42	-	-	18	356	69	18
F. Sense organ diseases	**107**	**49**	**58**	**-**	**-**	**4**	**20**	**24**	**-**	**-**	**2**	**22**	**33**
1. Glaucoma	71	31	39	-	-	2	17	12	-	-	1	19	20
2. Cataracts	33	16	17	-	-	1	3	11	-	-	1	3	13
G. Cardiovascular diseases	**3 051**	**1 714**	**1 337**	**2**	**3**	**387**	**444**	**878**	**2**	**2**	**289**	**290**	**754**
1. Rheumatic heart disease	21	7	14	-	-	1	2	4	-	1	1	3	9
2. Ischaemic heart disease	764	521	243	-	-	39	164	318	-	-	12	47	184
3. Cerebrovascular disease	1 553	778	776	-	-	202	196	379	-	-	167	192	417
4. Inflammatory heart diseases	180	98	82	1	2	54	20	21	1	1	40	13	27
H. Respiratory diseases	**3 006**	**1 702**	**1 304**	**83**	**125**	**512**	**386**	**596**	**59**	**80**	**473**	**297**	**395**
1. COPD*	1 162	750	411	-	-	93	212	445	-	-	49	128	235
2. Asthma	1 045	560	485	46	112	295	74	34	28	73	276	71	36
I. Digestive diseases	**2 015**	**1 007**	**1 008**	**42**	**14**	**325**	**382**	**243**	**31**	**13**	**293**	**308**	**363**
1. Peptic ulcer	80	48	32	-	1	28	16	4	-	-	18	11	3
2. Cirrhosis of the liver	346	238	108	-	-	60	126	53	-	-	22	46	40
3. Appendicitis	22	13	9	-	2	9	1	1	-	2	6	1	1
J. Genito-urinary diseases	**513**	**309**	**204**	**8**	**1**	**35**	**126**	**139**	**8**	**3**	**52**	**52**	**88**
1. Nephritis and nephrosis	38	22	16	6	1	11	1	4	5	2	3	1	4
2. Benign prostatic hypertrophy	193	193	-	6	-	-	99	93	-	-	-	-	-
L. Musculo-skeletal diseases	**3 932**	**1 317**	**2 615**	**1**	**2**	**406**	**684**	**224**	**1**	**9**	**842**	**1 090**	**673**
1. Rheumatoid arthritis	887	205	682	-	-	57	85	63	-	4	329	153	196
2. Osteoarthritis	2 701	1 044	1 657	-	-	323	578	144	-	-	371	865	420

508

Annex Table 8a, continued. YLDs by age, sex and cause (thousands): Established Market Economies, 1990

Cause	Total	Male	Female	Males 0-4	Males 5-14	Males 15-44	Males 45-59	Males 60+	Females 0-4	Females 5-14	Females 15-44	Females 45-59	Females 60+
M. Congenital anomalies	**962**	**493**	**469**	**493**	–	–	–	–	**469**	–	–	–	–
1. Abdominal wall defect	–	–	–	–	–	–	–	–	–	–	–	–	–
2. Anencephaly	–	–	–	–	–	–	–	–	–	–	–	–	–
3. Anorectal atresia	–	–	–	–	–	–	–	–	–	–	–	–	–
4. Cleft lip	8	5	3	5	–	–	–	–	3	–	–	–	–
5. Cleft palate	7	3	4	3	–	–	–	–	4	–	–	–	–
6. Oesophageal atresia	–	–	–	–	–	–	–	–	–	–	–	–	–
7. Renal agenesis	214	121	92	121	–	–	–	–	92	–	–	–	–
8. Down syndrome	645	328	317	328	–	–	–	–	317	–	–	–	–
9. Congenital heart anomalies	88	35	53	35	–	–	–	–	53	–	–	–	–
10. Spina bifida	–	–	–	–	–	–	–	–	–	–	–	–	–
N. Oral conditions	**867**	**416**	**451**	**13**	**69**	**180**	**80**	**73**	**12**	**66**	**177**	**87**	**109**
1. Dental caries	405	202	203	13	69	88	16	17	12	66	85	16	23
2. Periodontal disease	35	18	18	–	–	16	1	1	–	–	15	1	1
3. Edentulism	423	195	229	–	–	76	63	56	–	–	76	69	84
III. Injuries	**3 854**	**2 595**	**1 259**	**136**	**236**	**1 800**	**299**	**124**	**92**	**119**	**690**	**189**	**169**
A. Unintentional injuries	**3 474**	**2 351**	**1 123**	**131**	**231**	**1 586**	**280**	**122**	**88**	**116**	**579**	**173**	**167**
1. Road traffic accidents	1 349	912	437	9	81	726	77	19	7	47	335	34	14
2. Poisonings	10	7	3	2	1	4	–	–	1	–	1	–	–
3. Falls	916	525	391	50	79	300	69	28	31	32	141	99	88
4. Fires	78	46	32	7	23	13	3	1	5	19	6	1	1
5. Drownings	–	–	–	–	–	–	–	–	–	–	–	–	–
6. Other unintentional	1 121	861	260	63	48	543	132	75	43	17	96	39	65
B. Intentional injuries	**381**	**244**	**136**	**4**	**5**	**215**	**19**	**2**	**4**	**4**	**111**	**16**	**2**
1. Self-inflicted injuries	166	81	85	–	–	69	12	1	–	–	70	13	1
2. Violence	214	163	51	4	5	146	7	1	4	4	40	3	–
3. War	1	–	–	–	–	–	–	–	–	–	–	–	–

Notes:

A dash (–) symbol indicates fewer than 500 YLDs.

*IA6 is Bacterial meningitis and meningococcaemia; ID is Conditions arising during the perinatal period;
IIE6 is Dementia and other degenerative and hereditary CNS disorders; IIH1 is Chronic obstructive pulmonary disease.

Annex Table 8b. YLDs by age, sex and cause (thousands): Formerly Socialist Economies of Europe, 1990

Cause	Total	Male	Female	Males					Females				
				0-4	5-14	15-44	45-59	60+	0-4	5-14	15-44	45-59	60+
Population (millions)	346	165	181	14	27	76	27	21	13	26	75	30	36
All causes	26 269	13 331	12 938	863	637	7 628	2 587	1 616	779	471	6 711	2 603	2 373
I. Communicable, maternal, perinatal and nutritional conditions	2 061	548	1 512	258	117	127	21	25	250	115	1 052	53	42
A. Infectious and parasitic diseases	781	225	556	85	29	91	12	7	80	29	419	14	13
1. Tuberculosis	27	19	7	-	-	13	5	2	-	1	5	1	1
2. STDs excluding HIV	376	48	327	5	1	42	-	-	5	4	316	1	-
a. Syphilis	2	1	1	-	-	1	-	-	-	-	-	1	-
b. Chlamydia	295	20	275	2	-	17	-	-	2	4	268	-	-
c. Gonorrhoea	76	26	50	3	-	23	-	-	3	1	46	-	-
3. HIV	10	9	1	-	-	8	-	-	-	-	1	-	-
4. Diarrhoeal diseases	107	53	54	25	5	17	4	2	24	5	16	5	4
5. Childhood-cluster diseases	26	13	12	10	3	-	-	-	9	3	-	-	-
a. Pertussis	24	12	12	9	3	-	-	-	9	3	-	-	-
b. Poliomyelitis	-	-	-	-	-	-	-	-	-	-	-	-	-
c. Diphtheria	-	-	-	-	-	-	-	-	-	-	-	-	-
d. Measles	2	1	1	1	-	-	-	-	1	-	-	-	-
e. Tetanus	2	2	-	1	-	1	-	-	-	-	-	-	-
6. Bacterial meningitis*	87	43	44	29	6	6	1	1	28	6	7	2	2
7. Hepatitis B and hepatitis C	2	1	1	-	-	1	-	-	-	-	1	-	-
8. Malaria	-	-	-	-	-	-	-	-	-	-	-	-	-
9. Tropical-cluster diseases	-	-	-	-	-	-	-	-	-	-	-	-	-
a. Trypanosomiasis	-	-	-	-	-	-	-	-	-	-	-	-	-
b. Chagas disease	-	-	-	-	-	-	-	-	-	-	-	-	-
c. Schistosomiasis	-	-	-	-	-	-	-	-	-	-	-	-	-
d. Leishmaniasis	-	-	-	-	-	-	-	-	-	-	-	-	-
e. Lymphatic filariasis	-	-	-	-	-	-	-	-	-	-	-	-	-
f. Onchocerciasis	-	-	-	-	-	-	-	-	-	-	-	-	-
10. Leprosy	-	-	-	-	-	-	-	-	-	-	-	-	-
11. Dengue	-	-	-	-	-	-	-	-	-	-	-	-	-
12. Japanese encephalitis	-	-	-	-	-	-	-	-	-	-	-	-	-
13. Trachoma	-	-	-	-	-	-	-	-	-	-	-	-	-
14. Intestinal nematode infections	2	-	2	-	-	-	-	-	-	-	-	-	-
a. Ascariasis	-	-	-	-	-	-	-	-	-	-	-	-	-
b. Trichuriasis	2	-	2	-	-	-	-	-	-	-	1	-	-
c. Ancylostomiasis and necatoriasis	-	-	-	-	-	-	-	-	-	-	-	-	-

Annex Table 8b, continued. YLDs by age, sex and cause (thousands): Formerly Socialist Economies of Europe, 1990

Cause	Total	Male	Female	Males 0-4	Males 5-14	Males 15-44	Males 45-59	Males 60+	Females 0-4	Females 5-14	Females 15-44	Females 45-59	Females 60+
B. Respiratory infections	110	55	55	13	28	9	2	2	13	27	10	3	3
1. Lower respiratory infections	57	28	28	9	10	6	2	1	9	9	6	2	2
2. Upper respiratory infections	12	6	7	-	1	3	1	1	-	1	4	1	1
3. Otitis media	41	21	20	4	17	-	-	-	4	16	-	-	-
C. Maternal conditions	502		502								502		
1. Maternal haemorrhage	8		8								8		
2. Maternal sepsis	104		104								104		
3. Hypertensive disorders of pregnancy	2		2								2		
4. Obstructed labour	155		155								155		
5. Abortion	129		129								129		
D. Perinatal conditions*	134	68	66	68					66				
E. Nutritional deficiencies	533	201	332	92	61	26	7	15	90	59	122	36	26
1. Protein-energy malnutrition	100	51	49	51					49				
2. Iodine deficiency	21	9	11	9					10		1		
3. Vitamin A deficiency	-	-	-										
4. Iron-deficiency anaemia	375	130	245	29	56	25	6	15	28	54	105	33	25
II. Noncommunicable diseases	*20 874*	*10 307*	*10 567*	*421*	*295*	*5 807*	*2 240*	*1 545*	*395*	*256*	*5 225*	*2 418*	*2 273*
A. Malignant neoplasms	652	378	274	1	3	53	138	184	1	2	60	96	115
1. Mouth and oropharynx cancers	31	26	5			7	12	6				1	1
2. Oesophagus cancer	6	5	1			1	2	2					1
3. Stomach cancer	98	65	33			8	25	33			5	11	17
4. Colon and rectum cancers	103	51	52			5	16	30			5	15	32
5. Liver cancer	7	5	3			1	2	2			1	1	2
6. Pancreas cancer	16	9	7			1	3	5			2	3	2
7. Trachea, bronchus, lung cancers	102	85	16			8	40	37			3	5	9
8. Melanoma and other skin cancers	12	5	7			2	2	2				2	2
9. Breast cancer	53	-	53								15	21	18
10. Cervix uteri cancer	14	-	14								6	4	4
11. Corpus uteri cancer	15		15								4	11	
12. Ovary cancer	13		13								5	5	3
13. Prostate cancer	22	22	-				4	18					
14. Bladder cancer	28	24	4			1	6	17				1	3
15. Lymphomas and multiple myeloma	14	8	6			3	2	2			2		2
16. Leukaemia	12	7	5			2	2	2		1	1	1	2
C. Diabetes mellitus	399	166	232	-	1	49	64	53	-	1	50	76	105
D. Endocrine disorders	175	66	109	12	6	37	8	2	13	6	55	27	9

Annex Table 8b, continued. YLDs by age, sex and cause (thousands): Formerly Socialist Economies of Europe, 1990

Cause	Total	Male	Female	Males 0-4	5-14	15-44	45-59	60+	Females 0-4	5-14	15-44	45-59	60+
E. Neuro-psychiatric conditions	**9 886**	**5 005**	**4 881**	**68**	**190**	**3 874**	**549**	**324**	**65**	**156**	**3 328**	**637**	**696**
1. Unipolar major depression	3 095	1 056	2 039	-	-	834	172	50	-	-	1 551	345	143
2. Bipolar disorder	800	398	402	-	-	359	29	10	-	-	353	32	17
3. Schizophrenia	814	420	394	-	-	420	-	-	-	-	394	-	-
4. Epilepsy	249	153	95	5	49	76	17	6	6	37	31	14	8
5. Alcohol use	1 645	1 452	193	-	-	1 268	155	29	-	-	180	9	4
6. Dementia*	835	286	549	11	5	10	75	185	11	5	11	97	426
7. Parkinson disease	97	37	60	-	-	-	17	21	-	-	-	21	39
8. Multiple sclerosis	67	28	39	-	-	27	1	-	-	-	37	2	-
9. Drug use	530	424	106	-	34	376	13	2	-	8	94	3	-
10. Post-traumatic stress disorder	118	44	74	2	8	29	4	1	3	13	49	6	2
11. Obsessive-compulsive disorders	644	271	373	-	28	217	17	9	-	36	283	34	20
12. Panic disorder	308	101	207	-	10	73	18	-	-	10	157	32	8
F. Sense organ diseases	**64**	**26**	**38**	-	-	**1**	**7**	**17**	-	-	**2**	**13**	**22**
1. Glaucoma	29	10	20	-	-	-	4	6	-	-	1	10	8
2. Cataracts	34	16	18	-	-	1	3	12	-	-	1	3	14
G. Cardiovascular diseases	**1 861**	**1 041**	**820**	**1**	**2**	**205**	**368**	**465**	**1**	**1**	**174**	**199**	**444**
1. Rheumatic heart disease	38	17	21	-	-	7	9	1	-	1	5	13	3
2. Ischaemic heart disease	708	485	223	-	-	50	216	220	-	-	11	54	158
3. Cerebrovascular disease	790	349	441	-	-	89	97	163	-	-	118	116	207
4. Inflammatory heart diseases	100	54	46	-	1	30	13	10	-	1	21	9	16
H. Respiratory diseases	**1 866**	**1 090**	**776**	**30**	**49**	**344**	**447**	**221**	**21**	**33**	**255**	**211**	**256**
1. COPD*	577	400	177	-	-	103	216	80	-	-	49	41	87
2. Asthma	422	222	200	20	48	112	30	12	12	32	108	32	16
I. Digestive diseases	**1 450**	**734**	**716**	**41**	**9**	**377**	**226**	**81**	**32**	**7**	**253**	**244**	**181**
1. Peptic ulcer	60	36	25	-	1	21	12	2	-	1	13	8	2
2. Cirrhosis of the liver	157	104	54	-	-	26	58	20	-	-	10	26	18
3. Appendicitis	10	6	4	1	1	4	-	-	1	1	3	-	-
J. Genito-urinary diseases	**537**	**227**	**310**	**3**	**3**	**72**	**91**	**57**	**3**	**5**	**115**	**122**	**66**
1. Nephritis and nephrosis	28	14	14	1	1	10	1	-	1	3	8	1	-
2. Benign prostatic hypertrophy	85	85	-	-	-	-	50	35	-	-	-	-	-
L. Musculo-skeletal diseases	**2 666**	**987**	**1 679**	**1**	**3**	**627**	**250**	**106**	**1**	**6**	**716**	**648**	**308**
1. Rheumatoid arthritis	484	114	370	-	-	68	28	18	-	3	218	95	54
2. Osteoarthritis	1 980	826	1 154	-	-	528	212	85	-	-	411	503	239

Annex Table 8b, continued. YLDs by age, sex and cause (thousands): Formerly Socialist Economies of Europe, 1990

Cause	Total	Male	Female	Males 0-4	5-14	15-44	45-59	60+	Females 0-4	5-14	15-44	45-59	60+
M. Congenital anomalies	474	238	236	238	-	-	-	-	236	-	-	-	-
1. Abdominal wall defect	-	-	-	-	-	-	-	-	-	-	-	-	-
2. Anencephaly	-	-	-	-	-	-	-	-	-	-	-	-	-
3. Anorectal atresia	-	-	-	-	-	-	-	-	-	-	-	-	-
4. Cleft lip	5	3	2	3	-	-	-	-	2	-	-	-	-
5. Cleft palate	4	2	2	2	-	-	-	-	2	-	-	-	-
6. Oesophageal atresia	-	-	-	-	-	-	-	-	-	-	-	-	-
7. Renal agenesis	76	43	33	43	-	-	-	-	33	-	-	-	-
8. Down syndrome	332	169	164	169	-	-	-	-	164	-	-	-	-
9. Congenital heart anomalies	57	23	35	23	-	-	-	-	35	-	-	-	-
10. Spina bifida	-	-	-	-	-	-	-	-	-	-	-	-	-
N. Oral conditions	480	219	262	16	21	96	60	25	15	31	100	72	44
1. Dental caries	243	112	130	16	21	45	19	10	15	31	45	21	18
2. Periodontal disease	17	7	10	-	-	5	1	1	-	-	8	1	1
3. Edentulism	221	99	122	-	-	46	40	13	-	-	47	49	25
III. Injuries	*3 334*	*2 475*	*859*	*184*	*224*	*1 695*	*326*	*47*	*135*	*100*	*434*	*133*	*57*
A. Unintentional injuries	2 810	2 145	664	167	213	1 419	302	45	119	86	287	117	55
1. Road traffic accidents	666	534	132	5	55	409	58	7	3	29	75	19	6
2. Poisonings	40	26	15	15	3	6	1	-	11	2	1	-	-
3. Falls	759	505	254	51	76	314	54	10	37	29	109	52	27
4. Fires	46	31	16	5	11	12	3	-	4	7	3	1	-
5. Drownings	-	-	-	-	-	-	-	-	-	-	-	-	-
6. Other unintentional	1 298	1 049	248	90	69	678	185	27	65	19	98	44	21
B. Intentional injuries	524	330	194	17	11	276	24	2	15	14	147	16	2
1. Self-inflicted injuries	107	64	43	-	-	53	11	-	-	-	34	8	1
2. Violence	149	114	35	3	2	100	8	1	1	2	27	4	1
3. War	269	152	117	14	9	124	5	1	14	12	86	4	1

Notes:
A dash (-) symbol indicates fewer than 500 YLDs.
A dash (-) symbol indicates fewer than 500 YLDs.
*IA6 is Bacterial meningitis and meningococcaemia; ID is Conditions arising during the perinatal period;
*IIA6 is Bacterial meningitis and meningococcaemia; ID is Conditions arising during the perinatal period;
IIH1 is Chronic obstructive pulmonary disease.
IIE6 is Dementia and other degenerative and hereditary CNS disorders; IIH1 is Chronic obstructive pulmonary disease.

Annex Table 8c. YLDs by age, sex and cause (thousands): India, 1990

Cause	Total	Male	Female	Males					Females				
				0-4	5-14	15-44	45-59	60+	0-4	5-14	15-44	45-59	60+
Population (millions)	*850*	*439*	*410*	*60*	*102*	*201*	*48*	*30*	*57*	*95*	*183*	*46*	*29*
All causes	**87 680**	**42 624**	**45 056**	**10 086**	**8 921**	**15 506**	**5 004**	**3 108**	**9 625**	**6 371**	**21 457**	**4 653**	**2 949**
I. Communicable, maternal, perinatal and nutritional conditions	**29 434**	**12 405**	**17 029**	**5 618**	**2 084**	**3 923**	**471**	**309**	**5 197**	**1 644**	**9 384**	**572**	**230**
A. Infectious and parasitic diseases	**12 502**	**6 290**	**6 212**	**1 656**	**1 273**	**2 898**	**297**	**166**	**1 424**	**885**	**3 558**	**253**	**92**
1. Tuberculosis	**1 199**	**725**	**474**	**14**	**50**	**409**	**140**	**112**	**11**	**38**	**336**	**57**	**32**
2. STDs excluding HIV	**3 647**	**1 080**	**2 567**	**282**	**13**	**780**	**4**	**1**	**270**	**43**	**2 247**	**5**	**1**
a. Syphilis	239	112	127	7	1	103	1	-	7	1	118	1	-
b. Chlamydia	2 014	311	1 703	67	5	239	1	-	64	31	1 604	3	1
c. Gonorrhoea	1 394	657	738	209	7	438	2	-	200	10	526	1	-
3. HIV	**219**	**141**	**77**	-	-	**135**	**5**	**1**	-	-	**76**	**1**	-
4. Diarrhoeal diseases	**923**	**476**	**446**	**217**	**108**	**130**	**15**	**6**	**205**	**101**	**119**	**14**	**6**
5. Childhood-cluster diseases	**1 272**	**714**	**559**	**653**	**44**	**15**	**1**	-	**505**	**42**	**11**	**1**	-
a. Pertussis	306	157	150	119	38	-	-	-	114	36	-	-	-
b. Poliomyelitis	951	549	402	531	3	14	1	-	389	2	10	1	-
c. Diphtheria	10	6	4	3	3	-	-	-	1	3	-	-	-
d. Measles	4	2	2	-	1	1	-	-	-	1	1	-	-
e. Tetanus													
6. Bacterial meningitis*	**325**	**167**	**158**	**126**	**21**	**17**	**3**	-	**120**	**20**	**15**	**3**	-
7. Hepatitis B and hepatitis C	**9**	**5**	**4**	-	-	**2**	**1**	**1**	-	-	**2**	**1**	**1**
8. Malaria	**425**	**220**	**205**	**41**	**84**	**77**	**13**	**5**	**39**	**79**	**70**	**13**	**5**
9. Tropical-cluster diseases	**2 022**	**1 491**	**531**	**64**	**494**	**868**	**60**	**5**	**30**	**174**	**229**	**91**	**6**
a. Trypanosomiasis													
b. Chagas disease													
c. Schistosomiasis													
d. Leishmaniasis	251	151	100	9	55	85	2	-	6	36	56	2	-
e. Lymphatic filariasis	1 770	1 339	431	56	439	782	58	4	24	138	173	90	5
f. Onchocerciasis													
10. Leprosy	**173**	**89**	**84**	**2**	**33**	**48**	**6**	-	**2**	**31**	**44**	**6**	-
11. Dengue	**3**	**1**	**2**	-	**1**	-	-	-	-	**1**	-	-	-
12. Japanese encephalitis	**51**	**26**	**25**	**15**	**10**	**2**	-	-	**14**	**9**	**2**	-	-
13. Trachoma	**26**	**7**	**19**	-	-	**2**	**3**	**3**	-	-	**4**	**6**	**8**
14. Intestinal nematode infections	**688**	**356**	**332**	**3**	**171**	**148**	**25**	**10**	**2**	**161**	**135**	**24**	**10**
a. Ascariasis	148	76	72	2	74	-	-	-	2	69	-	-	-
b. Trichuriasis	104	54	50	-	54	-	-	-	-	50	-	-	-
c. Ancylostomiasis and necatoriasis	436	226	209	-	44	148	25	10	-	41	135	24	10

Annex Table 8c, continued. YLDs by age, sex and cause (thousands): India, 1990

Cause	Total	Male	Female	Males					Females				
				0-4	5-14	15-44	45-59	60+	0-4	5-14	15-44	45-59	60+
B. Respiratory infections	**1 199**	**617**	**582**	**414**	**152**	**34**	**5**	**12**	**393**	**142**	**30**	**5**	**12**
1. Lower respiratory infections	929	477	452	387	52	23	4	11	368	49	21	4	11
2. Upper respiratory infections	37	20	17	2	4	12	1	1	1	4	9	2	1
3. Otitis media	233	120	113	25	95	-	-	-	24	89	-	-	-
C. Maternal conditions	**4 081**	**-**	**4 081**	**-**	**-**	**-**	**-**	**-**	**-**	**-**	**4 077**	**4**	**-**
1. Maternal haemorrhage	47		47								47		
2. Maternal sepsis	725		725								725		
3. Hypertensive disorders of pregnancy	14		14								14		
4. Obstructed labour	1 236		1 236								1 236		
5. Abortion	1 106		1 106								1 106		
D. Perinatal conditions*	**3 102**	**1 589**	**1 513**	**1 589**					**1 513**				
E. Nutritional deficiencies	**8 550**	**3 909**	**4 641**	**1 960**	**659**	**990**	**169**	**131**	**1 867**	**617**	**1 720**	**310**	**126**
1. Protein-energy malnutrition	3 005	1 538	1 467	1 538	-	-	-	-	1 467	-	-	-	-
2. Iodine deficiency	175	89	86	88	1	-	-	-	83	1	2	-	-
3. Vitamin A deficiency	21	11	10	11	-	-	-	-	10	-	-	-	-
4. Iron-deficiency anaemia	5 349	2 271	3 077	323	658	990	169	131	307	616	1 718	310	126
II. Noncommunicable diseases	**38 280**	**18 797**	**19 483**	**2 225**	**789**	**9 056**	**4 022**	**2 704**	**2 273**	**778**	**10 195**	**3 616**	**2 622**
A. Malignant neoplasms	**525**	**246**	**279**	**1**	**5**	**63**	**85**	**93**	**1**	**3**	**97**	**115**	**63**
1. Mouth and oropharynx cancers	145	80	65	-	-	22	30	27	-	1	23	27	13
2. Oesophagus cancer	39	14	25	-	-	2	5	6	-	-	8	11	7
3. Stomach cancer	43	28	15	-	-	5	11	12	-	-	4	7	4
4. Colon and rectum cancers	26	14	12	-	-	4	4	6	-	-	2	5	5
5. Liver cancer	5	3	1	-	-	1	1	1	-	-	-	-	1
6. Pancreas cancer	5	2	2	-	-	-	1	1	-	-	-	1	1
7. Trachea, bronchus, lung cancers	18	15	3	-	-	2	6	7	-	-	-	1	1
8. Melanoma and other skin cancers	1	-	1	-	-	-	-	-	-	-	-	-	1
9. Breast cancer	38	-	38	-	-	-	-	-	-	-	14	16	8
10. Cervix uteri cancer	45	-	45	-	-	-	-	-	-	-	14	23	8
11. Corpus uteri cancer	3	-	3	-	-	-	-	-	-	-	1	2	-
12. Ovary cancer	10	-	10	-	-	-	-	-	-	-	5	3	2
13. Prostate cancer	9	9	-	-	-	-	1	8	-	-	-	-	-
14. Bladder cancer	5	5	-	-	-	-	1	3	-	-	-	1	-
15. Lymphomas and multiple myeloma	11	7	4	-	-	3	2	2	-	-	1	1	1
16. Leukaemia	10	6	4	-	1	2	1	2	-	1	2	1	1
C. Diabetes mellitus	**866**	**440**	**426**	**-**	**-**	**146**	**182**	**112**	**-**	**-**	**135**	**182**	**109**
D. Endocrine disorders	**56**	**29**	**27**	**12**	**2**	**8**	**5**	**1**	**9**	**-**	**7**	**6**	**4**

Annex Table 8c, continued. YLDs by age, sex and cause (thousands): India, 1990

Cause	Total	Male	Female	Males					Females				
				0-4	5-14	15-44	45-59	60+	0-4	5-14	15-44	45-59	60+
E. Neuro-psychiatric conditions	**18 334**	**8 332**	**10 002**	**250**	**317**	**6 576**	**751**	**438**	**299**	**429**	**7 803**	**944**	**527**
1. Unipolar major depression	8 063	2 961	5 102	-	-	2 528	350	83	-	-	4 346	612	144
2. Bipolar disorder	2 285	1 190	1 094	-	-	1 113	60	17	-	-	1 021	57	16
3. Schizophrenia	1 600	862	738	-	-	862	-	-	-	-	738	-	-
4. Epilepsy	668	342	326	21	95	196	18	11	24	166	120	6	10
5. Alcohol use	825	753	72	-	-	710	38	5	-	-	69	3	-
6. Dementia*	803	399	404	45	17	26	99	213	42	16	24	101	221
7. Parkinson disease	104	47	57	-	-	-	24	23	-	-	-	29	28
8. Multiple sclerosis	165	74	91	-	-	72	2	-	-	-	88	2	1
9. Drug use	71	64	7	-	-	56	6	2	-	-	6	1	-
10. Post-traumatic stress disorder	316	123	193	8	31	77	6	1	13	48	120	10	2
11. Obsessive-compulsive disorders	1 640	731	908	-	106	581	31	13	-	132	706	53	17
12. Panic disorder	738	239	498	-	4	202	34	-	-	36	403	52	7
F. Sense organ diseases	**3 013**	**1 488**	**1 525**	**5**	**1**	**145**	**721**	**617**	**4**	**1**	**124**	**663**	**734**
1. Glaucoma	573	329	243	-	-	34	228	67	-	-	12	162	69
2. Cataracts	2 439	1 158	1 281	4	1	111	493	549	4	1	112	501	665
G. Cardiovascular diseases	**3 145**	**1 834**	**1 311**	**15**	**23**	**503**	**597**	**695**	**8**	**34**	**420**	**391**	**458**
1. Rheumatic heart disease	152	63	89	-	4	34	21	4	-	6	47	31	6
2. Ischaemic heart disease	1 281	820	460	-	-	49	330	442	-	-	37	163	261
3. Cerebrovascular disease	651	327	324	-	-	100	104	124	-	-	123	96	105
4. Inflammatory heart diseases	420	232	187	6	8	156	40	23	3	6	116	33	23
H. Respiratory diseases	**4 408**	**2 237**	**2 170**	**330**	**296**	**634**	**579**	**398**	**334**	**205**	**721**	**565**	**345**
1. COPD*	1 257	707	549	-	-	213	311	183	-	-	207	240	103
2. Asthma	1 251	693	559	104	221	305	48	15	70	153	279	46	11
I. Digestive diseases	**2 102**	**1 270**	**832**	**144**	**29**	**509**	**483**	**106**	**148**	**5**	**328**	**265**	**86**
1. Peptic ulcer	338	231	107	-	6	150	64	11	-	3	68	31	5
2. Cirrhosis of the liver	551	391	159	16	-	140	189	46	20	-	52	68	19
3. Appendicitis	11	6	4	-	2	4	-	-	-	1	3	-	-
J. Genito-urinary diseases	**423**	**342**	**81**	**18**	**33**	**15**	**245**	**31**	**10**	**28**	**28**	**10**	**6**
1. Nephritis and nephrosis	107	50	57	7	30	8	3	1	7	28	19	2	1
2. Benign prostatic hypertrophy	264	264	-	-	-	-	237	27	-	-	-	-	-
L. Musculo-skeletal diseases	**1 393**	**558**	**835**	**1**	**2**	**235**	**236**	**85**	**1**	**4**	**325**	**342**	**162**
1. Rheumatoid arthritis	160	45	115	-	-	35	8	2	-	3	68	34	11
2. Osteoarthritis	1 218	504	714	-	-	197	226	81	-	-	256	308	150

Annex Table 8c, continued. YLDs by age, sex and cause (thousands): India, 1990

Cause	Total	Male	Female	Males 0-4	5-14	15-44	45-59	60+	Females 0-4	5-14	15-44	45-59	60+
M. Congenital anomalies	2 780	1 381	1 399	1 381	-	-	-	-	1 399	-	-	-	-
1. Abdominal wall defect	-	-	-	-	-	-	-	-	-	-	-	-	-
2. Anencephaly	-	-	-	-	-	-	-	-	-	-	-	-	-
3. Anorectal atresia	-	-	-	-	-	-	-	-	-	-	-	-	-
4. Cleft lip	42	25	17	25	-	-	-	-	17	-	-	-	-
5. Cleft palate	45	21	24	21	-	-	-	-	24	-	-	-	-
6. Oesophageal atresia	-	-	-	-	-	-	-	-	-	-	-	-	-
7. Renal agenesis	-	-	-	-	-	-	-	-	-	-	-	-	-
8. Down syndrome	580	330	250	330	-	-	-	-	250	-	-	-	-
9. Congenital heart anomalies	1 458	745	712	745	-	-	-	-	712	-	-	-	-
10. Spina bifida	655	260	395	260	-	-	-	-	395	-	-	-	-
N. Oral conditions	1 045	531	513	42	71	175	121	123	40	67	166	120	121
1. Dental caries	672	347	325	41	71	143	52	39	39	66	131	51	38
2. Periodontal disease	71	37	34	-	-	30	5	2	-	-	28	5	2
3. Edentulism	289	145	145	-	-	-	64	81	-	-	-	64	81
III. Injuries	*19 966*	*11 423*	*8 544*	*2 242*	*6 047*	*2 528*	*511*	*94*	*2 154*	*3 949*	*1 878*	*465*	*97*
A. Unintentional injuries	19 595	11 210	8 385	2 212	6 035	2 381	492	91	2 116	3 938	1 792	445	94
1. Road traffic accidents	1 375	957	418	77	320	488	63	9	23	233	115	37	9
2. Poisonings	85	20	66	12	7	1	-	-	8	5	1	48	3
3. Falls	9 046	5 549	3 496	895	4 056	508	77	13	1 047	1 774	493	167	16
4. Fires	2 115	593	1 523	129	315	129	18	1	112	969	420	19	2
5. Drownings	1	1	-	-	-	1	-	-	-	-	-	-	-
6. Other unintentional	6 972	4 090	2 882	1 097	1 337	1 254	334	68	927	957	762	174	63
B. Intentional injuries	372	213	159	31	13	147	19	3	38	11	86	21	3
1. Self-inflicted injuries	166	81	85	-	-	69	12	1	-	-	70	13	1
2. Violence	182	108	74	31	13	55	8	2	38	11	16	7	2
3. War	23	23	-	-	-	23	-	-	-	-	-	-	-

Notes:
A dash (-) symbol indicates fewer than 500 YLDs.
*IA6 is Bacterial meningitis and meningococcaemia; ID is Conditions arising during the perinatal period;
IIE6 is Dementia and other degenerative and hereditary CNS disorders; IIH1 is Chronic obstructive pulmonary disease.

Annex Table 8d. YLDs by age, sex and cause (thousands): China, 1990

Cause	Total	Male	Female	Males 0-4	Males 5-14	Males 15-44	Males 45-59	Males 60+	Females 0-4	Females 5-14	Females 15-44	Females 45-59	Females 60+
Population (millions)	*1 134*	*585*	*548*	*60*	*97*	*306*	*73*	*49*	*58*	*90*	*284*	*64*	*52*
All causes	*90 524*	*45 158*	*45 367*	*7 455*	*3 194*	*22 488*	*6 549*	*5 472*	*7 447*	*2 692*	*23 827*	*6 181*	*5 220*
I. Communicable, maternal, perinatal and nutritional conditions	*17 118*	*8 247*	*8 871*	*2 405*	*1 548*	*3 265*	*657*	*371*	*2 325*	*1 439*	*4 071*	*633*	*402*
A. Infectious and parasitic diseases	*5 827*	*3 082*	*2 745*	*628*	*831*	*1 150*	*296*	*177*	*609*	*770*	*929*	*236*	*202*
1. Tuberculosis	673	426	247	4	7	231	111	75	8	18	150	45	26
2. STDs excluding HIV	97	19	78	2	-	17	-	-	2	1	76	-	-
a. Syphilis	67	7	60	-	-	7	-	-	1	-	59	-	-
b. Chlamydia	30	12	18	1	-	10	-	-	1	1	17	-	-
c. Gonorrhoea	-	-	-	-	-	-	-	-	-	-	-	-	-
3. HIV	3	3	-	-	-	3	-	-	-	-	-	-	-
4. Diarrhoeal diseases	1 573	794	779	112	103	464	79	36	145	96	431	70	37
5. Childhood-cluster diseases	490	268	222	229	28	11	1	-	187	27	8	-	-
a. Pertussis	202	103	99	79	25	-	-	-	75	24	-	-	-
b. Poliomyelitis	280	160	120	148	1	11	1	-	110	1	8	-	-
c. Diphtheria	8	5	3	3	2	-	-	-	1	2	-	-	-
d. Measles	-	-	-	-	-	-	-	-	-	-	-	-	-
e. Tetanus	-	-	-	-	-	-	-	-	-	-	-	-	-
6. Bacterial meningitis*	353	180	173	129	19	24	5	3	125	18	23	5	3
7. Hepatitis B and hepatitis C	19	13	6	-	-	6	4	2	-	-	2	1	2
8. Malaria	50	26	24	4	8	11	2	1	4	7	10	2	1
9. Tropical-cluster diseases	225	188	37	6	23	151	7	2	1	4	30	1	-
a. Trypanosomiasis	-	-	-	-	-	-	-	-	-	-	-	-	-
b. Chagas disease	-	-	-	-	-	-	-	-	-	-	-	-	-
c. Schistosomiasis	11	7	4	-	1	4	1	1	1	1	3	1	-
d. Leishmaniasis	-	-	-	-	-	-	-	-	-	-	-	-	-
e. Lymphatic filariasis	214	181	33	6	22	146	6	1	1	4	28	-	-
f. Onchocerciasis	-	-	-	-	-	-	-	-	-	-	-	-	-
10. Leprosy	6	3	3	-	-	2	1	-	-	1	2	-	-
11. Dengue	-	-	-	-	-	-	-	-	-	-	-	-	-
12. Japanese encephalitis	395	202	193	113	73	15	1	-	109	68	14	-	-
13. Trachoma	347	98	249	-	-	22	34	42	-	-	57	79	113
14. Intestinal nematode infections	1 137	587	550	9	531	38	6	3	9	498	35	6	3
a. Ascariasis	497	256	241	9	246	1	-	-	9	231	1	-	-
b. Trichuriasis	527	272	255	-	271	1	-	-	-	254	1	-	-
c. Ancylostomiasis and necatoriasis	113	59	55	-	14	36	6	3	-	13	33	6	3

Annex Table 8d, continued. YLDs by age, sex and cause (thousands): China, 1990

Cause	Total	Male	Female	Males					Females				
				0-4	5-14	15-44	45-59	60+	0-4	5-14	15-44	45-59	60+
B. Respiratory infections	**1 225**	**626**	**599**	**423**	**143**	**46**	**8**	**6**	**409**	**134**	**42**	**7**	**7**
1. Lower respiratory infections	965	492	473	397	50	35	6	5	384	46	32	5	5
2. Upper respiratory infections	34	18	16	1	3	11	2	1	1	3	10	2	1
3. Otitis media	226	116	109	25	91				25	85			
C. Maternal conditions	**1 708**		**1 708**								**1 696**	**12**	
1. Maternal haemorrhage	39		39								39		
2. Maternal sepsis	430		430								430		
3. Hypertensive disorders of pregnancy	15		15								15		
4. Obstructed labour	566		566								566		
5. Abortion													
D. Perinatal conditions*	**977**	**498**	**479**	**498**					**479**				
E. Nutritional deficiencies	**7 381**	**4 042**	**3 340**	**857**	**574**	**2 070**	**354**	**187**	**829**	**535**	**1 404**	**378**	**194**
1. Protein-energy malnutrition	1 013	514	499	514					499	1	3		
2. Iodine deficiency	218	110	108	109	1				104				
3. Vitamin A deficiency	11	6	5	6					5				
4. Iron-deficiency anaemia	6 140	3 412	2 728	229	573	2 069	354	187	221	534	1 401	378	194
II. Noncommunicable diseases	***60 539***	***29 423***	***31 115***	***3 226***	***806***	***15 013***	***5 403***	***4 976***	***3 163***	***671***	***17 340***	***5 239***	***4 702***
A. Malignant neoplasms	**1 127**	**714**	**413**	**2**	**10**	**167**	**216**	**320**	**3**	**7**	**135**	**131**	**137**
1. Mouth and oropharynx cancers	78	52	26			29	11	11			14	7	5
2. Oesophagus cancer	79	67	12		1	7	21	39			6	3	3
3. Stomach cancer	299	207	92			21	68	118			22	30	40
4. Colon and rectum cancers	118	67	51			17	19	31		1	11	16	23
5. Liver cancer	133	106	27		1	38	44	24		1	6	10	10
6. Pancreas cancer	15	10	5			2	2	6			1	2	2
7. Trachea, bronchus, lung cancers	140	92	47			13	26	53			8	16	23
8. Melanoma and other skin cancers	1												
9. Breast cancer	34		34								15	11	8
10. Cervix uteri cancer	19		19								6	7	6
11. Corpus uteri cancer	11		11								3	8	
12. Ovary cancer	12		12								7	3	2
13. Prostate cancer	5	5						4					
14. Bladder cancer	22	18	3			2	3	13			2		1
15. Lymphomas and multiple myeloma	15	10	5			4	3	3			2	2	1
16. Leukaemia	48	25	23	1	4	13	4	2	1	2	13	3	3
C. Diabetes mellitus	**459**	**236**	**223**			**72**	**92**	**71**			**64**	**87**	**72**
D. Endocrine disorders	**348**	**89**	**259**	**13**	**7**	**36**	**22**	**11**	**82**	**12**	**131**	**19**	**14**

Annex Table 8d, continued. YLDs by age, sex and cause (thousands): China, 1990

Cause	Total	Male	Female	Males					Females				
				0-4	5-14	15-44	45-59	60+	0-4	5-14	15-44	45-59	60+
E. Neuro-psychiatric conditions	**27 824**	**12 657**	**15 167**	**166**	**314**	**10 506**	**1 066**	**605**	**137**	**327**	**12 536**	**1 351**	**816**
1. Unipolar major depression	12 975	4 749	8 226			4 050	558	142			7 072	895	260
2. Bipolar disorder	3 693	1 917	1 776			1 790	96	30			1 662	85	30
3. Schizophrenia	2 347	1 252	1 094			1 252					1 094		
4. Epilepsy	621	316	305	11	76	184	33	12	11	87	178	19	9
5. Alcohol use	1 453	1 350	103			1 263	76	11			100	3	
6. Dementia*	1 298	616	682	48	16	40	154	359	47	15	38	146	436
7. Parkinson disease	74	37	37				19	18				17	20
8. Multiple sclerosis	257	114	143			111	3				139	3	1
9. Drug use	177	159	18		13	141	5			1	16	1	
10. Post-traumatic stress disorder	429	167	262	8	29	118	10	2	13	46	186	14	3
11. Obsessive-compulsive disorders	2 381	1 057	1 324		101	887	47	22		126	1 093	74	30
12. Panic disorder	1 141	396	745		35	308	52			35	626	72	12
F. Sense organ diseases	**1 821**	**706**	**1 115**	**15**		**70**	**276**	**344**	**16**	**7**	**151**	**499**	**442**
1. Glaucoma	731	215	516			23	124	68			70	339	107
2. Cataracts	963	453	510	2		42	139	270	3		41	141	324
G. Cardiovascular diseases	**3 184**	**1 783**	**1 401**	**8**	**10**	**648**	**467**	**650**	**5**	**9**	**646**	**341**	**400**
1. Rheumatic heart disease	288	125	163		4	54	27	39		5	63	46	50
2. Ischaemic heart disease	739	465	274			67	151	247			52	84	138
3. Cerebrovascular disease	1 716	976	740			382	255	339			373	181	186
4. Inflammatory heart diseases	359	198	162	4	4	137	32	21	3	3	108	25	23
H. Respiratory diseases	**12 710**	**7 028**	**5 682**	**489**	**328**	**2 416**	**1 699**	**2 096**	**321**	**212**	**1 922**	**1 299**	**1 928**
1. COPD*	9 341	5 129	4 212			1 594	1 548	1 987			1 207	1 182	1 823
2. Asthma	2 373	1 324	1 048	164	314	700	111	36	103	202	622	92	29
I. Digestive diseases	**4 643**	**2 375**	**2 268**	**898**	**43**	**556**	**593**	**285**	**943**	**27**	**569**	**477**	**252**
1. Peptic ulcer	174	114	60		2	73	33	6		1	39	16	3
2. Cirrhosis of the liver	625	428	197	18		159	170	81	7		48	84	58
3. Appendicitis	15	9	6		2	7				1	4		
J. Genito-urinary diseases	**765**	**570**	**195**	**21**	**12**	**65**	**400**	**71**	**12**	**9**	**83**	**58**	**32**
1. Nephritis and nephrosis	130	71	59	8	12	45	3	2	12	9	35	2	1
2. Benign prostatic hypertrophy	404	404					361	42					
L. Musculo-skeletal diseases	**3 217**	**1 074**	**2 143**		**13**	**291**	**397**	**372**	**13**	**11**	**848**	**821**	**449**
1. Rheumatoid arthritis	649	211	438			83	96	32		5	170	172	91
2. Osteoarthritis	2 153	735	1 418			169	277	289			515	590	313

Annex Table 8d, continued. YLDs by age, sex and cause (thousands): China, 1990

Cause	Total	Male	Female	Males 0-4	Males 5-14	Males 15-44	Males 45-59	Males 60+	Females 0-4	Females 5-14	Females 15-44	Females 45-59	Females 60+
M. Congenital anomalies	2 706	1 338	1 368	1 338	-	-	-	-	1 368	-	-	-	-
1. Abdominal wall defect	-	-	-	-	-	-	-	-	-	-	-	-	-
2. Anencephaly	-	-	-	-	-	-	-	-	-	-	-	-	-
3. Anorectal atresia	57	29	29	29	-	-	-	-	29	-	-	-	-
4. Cleft lip	7	3	4	3	-	-	-	-	4	-	-	-	-
5. Cleft palate	-	-	-	-	-	-	-	-	-	-	-	-	-
6. Oesophageal atresia	-	-	-	-	-	-	-	-	-	-	-	-	-
7. Renal agenesis	564	313	251	313	-	-	-	-	251	-	-	-	-
8. Down syndrome	1 614	814	800	814	-	-	-	-	800	-	-	-	-
9. Congenital heart anomalies	464	179	285	179	-	-	-	-	285	-	-	-	-
10. Spina bifida	-	-	-	-	-	-	-	-	-	-	-	-	-
N. Oral conditions	999	497	503	188	34	62	99	113	181	33	73	91	124
1. Dental caries	583	299	284	188	34	44	23	11	180	31	41	20	11
2. Periodontal disease	33	17	16	-	-	15	1	1	-	-	14	1	1
3. Edentulism	358	176	182	-	-	-	74	102	-	-	-	69	112
III. Injuries	*12 867*	*7 487*	*5 380*	*1 823*	*840*	*4 210*	*490*	*125*	*1 959*	*582*	*2 415*	*308*	*116*
A. Unintentional injuries	11 688	7 176	4 513	1 794	831	3 961	468	122	1 904	569	1 668	260	111
1. Road traffic accidents	1 082	760	322	21	114	542	71	12	16	107	158	35	6
2. Poisonings	108	73	35	59	9	4	1	-	18	12	5	-	-
3. Falls	3 578	2 047	1 531	523	305	1 102	98	19	669	201	511	102	47
4. Fires	235	122	113	35	49	33	3	2	24	71	12	3	2
5. Drownings	2	1	1	-	-	-	-	-	-	-	-	-	-
6. Other unintentional	6 685	4 174	2 511	1 156	354	2 280	295	88	1 176	178	982	119	57
B. Intentional injuries	1 179	311	868	30	9	249	21	3	55	13	747	48	5
1. Self-inflicted injuries	937	169	769	-	-	149	18	2	-	1	719	46	3
2. Violence	234	135	99	30	9	92	4	1	55	12	28	2	1
3. War	7	7	-	-	-	7	-	-	-	-	-	-	-

Notes:
A dash (-) symbol indicates fewer than 500 YLDs.
*IA6 is Bacterial meningitis and meningococcaemia; ID is Conditions arising during the perinatal period;
IIE6 is Dementia and other degenerative and hereditary CNS disorders; IIH1 is Chronic obstructive pulmonary disease.

Annex Table 8e. YLDs by age, sex and cause (thousands): Other Asia and Islands, 1990

Cause	Total	Male	Female	Males					Females				
				0–4	5–14	15–44	45–59	60+	0–4	5–14	15–44	45–59	60+
Population (millions)	*683*	*343*	*340*	*44*	*84*	*161*	*34*	*20*	*42*	*80*	*160*	*35*	*23*
All causes	**63 080**	**31 168**	**31 912**	**6 145**	**3 868**	**15 314**	**3 741**	**2 100**	**5 654**	**2 820**	**17 548**	**3 683**	**2 207**
I. Communicable, maternal, perinatal and nutritional conditions	***17 977***	***6 967***	***11 010***	***2 749***	***1 311***	***2 399***	***341***	***167***	***2 592***	***1 211***	***6 640***	***393***	***174***
A. Infectious and parasitic diseases	**7 976**	**3 563**	**4 413**	**807**	**870**	**1 577**	**216**	**93**	**711**	**789**	**2 622**	**199**	**92**
1. Tuberculosis	1 040	587	453	1	31	369	120	65	1	24	286	93	50
2. STDs excluding HIV	2 767	781	1 986	200	10	568	2	-	200	33	1 749	4	1
a. Syphilis	160	72	88	4	1	66	1	-	4	1	82	1	-
b. Chlamydia	1 530	220	1 310	45	3	171	1	-	46	23	1 238	2	-
c. Gonorrhoea	1 077	489	589	151	5	331	1	-	151	8	429	1	-
3. HIV	109	71	39	-	-	68	2	1	-	-	38	-	-
4. Diarrhoeal diseases	613	285	328	141	60	70	11	4	101	57	138	22	9
5. Childhood-cluster diseases	481	264	217	228	26	9	1	-	185	25	7	-	-
a. Pertussis	175	89	86	68	21	-	-	-	65	21	-	-	-
b. Poliomyelitis	296	169	127	158	2	9	-	-	119	1	7	-	-
c. Diphtheria	8	5	3	3	2	-	-	-	1	2	-	-	-
d. Measles	2	1	1	-	1	-	-	-	-	1	-	-	-
e. Tetanus	-	-	-	-	-	-	-	-	-	-	-	-	-
6. Bacterial meningitis*	241	122	119	92	16	11	2	1	89	15	11	3	1
7. Hepatitis B and hepatitis C	10	6	5	-	-	2	1	1	-	-	2	1	1
8. Malaria	252	127	124	28	49	42	6	2	27	46	42	7	3
9. Tropical-cluster diseases	530	373	157	10	80	244	35	3	8	22	96	29	2
a. Trypanosomiasis	-	-	-	-	-	-	-	-	-	-	-	-	-
b. Chagas disease	-	-	-	-	-	-	-	-	-	-	-	-	-
c. Schistosomiasis	6	3	2	-	1	2	-	-	-	1	1	-	-
d. Leishmaniasis	18	11	7	-	2	8	-	-	-	1	5	-	-
e. Lymphatic filariasis	507	359	147	10	77	235	35	3	7	19	90	29	2
f. Onchocerciasis	-	-	-	-	-	-	-	-	-	-	-	-	-
10. Leprosy	65	33	33	1	13	16	2	-	1	13	17	2	-
11. Dengue	3	1	1	-	1	-	-	-	-	1	-	-	-
12. Japanese encephalitis	136	69	67	39	25	5	-	-	37	24	5	-	-
13. Trachoma	47	13	35	-	-	3	4	5	-	-	9	12	14
14. Intestinal nematode infections	1 288	654	634	6	504	119	18	7	6	485	118	18	8
a. Ascariasis	378	192	185	6	186	-	-	-	6	179	-	-	-
b. Trichuriasis	556	284	273	-	283	-	-	-	-	272	-	-	-
c. Ancylostomiasis and necatoriasis	354	178	176	-	35	118	18	7	-	34	117	18	8

Annex Table 8e, continued. YLDs by age, sex and cause (thousands): Other Asia and Islands, 1990

Cause	Total	Male	Female	Males					Females				
				0-4	5-14	15-44	45-59	60+	0-4	5-14	15-44	45-59	60+
B. Respiratory infections	**909**	**463**	**446**	**303**	**125**	**27**	**4**	**4**	**292**	**120**	**26**	**4**	**4**
1. Lower respiratory infections	689	351	339	284	43	18	3	3	273	41	18	3	4
2. Upper respiratory infections	30	16	15	1	4	9	1	1	1	3	8	1	1
3. Otitis media	190	97	93	18	79	-	-	-	18	75	-	-	-
C. Maternal conditions	**2 542**	–	**2 542**								**2 539**	**3**	
1. Maternal haemorrhage	30		30								30		
2. Maternal sepsis	471		471								471		
3. Hypertensive disorders of pregnancy	10		10								10		
4. Obstructed labour	790		790								790		
5. Abortion	576		576								576		
D. Perinatal conditions*	**1 061**	**537**	**524**	**537**					**524**				
E. Nutritional deficiencies	**5 489**	**2 404**	**3 085**	**1 102**	**316**	**795**	**121**	**70**	**1 066**	**302**	**1 453**	**186**	**77**
1. Protein-energy malnutrition	1 633	830	803	830					803	1	2		
2. Iodine deficiency	81	40	41	39					39				
3. Vitamin A deficiency	19	10	9	10					9				
4. Iron-deficiency anaemia	3 756	1 524	2 231	223	315	794	121	70	216	301	1 451	186	77
II. Noncommunicable diseases	**35 368**	**17 694**	**17 675**	**2 056**	**1 031**	**9 623**	**3 086**	**1 898**	**1 854**	**823**	**9 826**	**3 165**	**2 007**
A. Malignant neoplasms	**593**	**307**	**286**	**3**	**17**	**69**	**78**	**140**	**3**	**14**	**99**	**76**	**94**
1. Mouth and oropharynx cancers	105	64	42		2	21	11	30		2	16	6	17
2. Oesophagus cancer	26	8	18			1	3	4			6	3	9
3. Stomach cancer	55	38	17			6	14	17			4	7	7
4. Colon and rectum cancers	50	27	23			6	5	15			5	5	13
5. Liver cancer	28	22	6			5	11	6			1	2	2
6. Pancreas cancer	5	3	2				1	2			1		1
7. Trachea, bronchus, lung cancers	45	35	10			4	11	20			1	3	7
8. Melanoma and other skin cancers	2	1	1										
9. Breast cancer	34	–	34								13	13	8
10. Cervix uteri cancer	33	–	33								12	14	6
11. Corpus uteri cancer	4	–	4								1	3	
12. Ovary cancer	12	–	12								7	2	2
13. Prostate cancer	12	12	–				2	10					
14. Bladder cancer	12	9	2			1	2	6					2
15. Lymphomas and multiple myeloma	16	10	6			3	1	3			2	1	2
16. Leukaemia	20	11	9	1	5	3	1	2	1	3	2	1	1
C. Diabetes mellitus	**643**	**310**	**333**			**116**	**125**	**70**			**117**	**134**	**82**
D. Endocrine disorders	**260**	**117**	**143**	**63**	**18**	**18**	**11**	**7**	**53**	**9**	**41**	**24**	**16**

Annex Table 8e, continued. YLDs by age, sex and cause (thousands): Other Asia and Islands, 1990

Cause	Total	Male	Female	Males					Females				
				0-4	5-14	15-44	45-59	60+	0-4	5-14	15-44	45-59	60+
E. Neuro-psychiatric conditions	**18 003**	**8 886**	**9 117**	**130**	**404**	**7 445**	**619**	**289**	**130**	**392**	**7 396**	**793**	**405**
1. Unipolar major depression	6 701	2 335	4 366	-	-	2 026	252	57	-	-	3 787	467	112
2. Bipolar disorder	1 888	947	942	-	-	892	43	12	-	-	885	44	13
3. Schizophrenia	2 201	1 140	1 061	-	-	1 140	-	-	-	-	1 061	-	-
4. Epilepsy	657	324	333	7	127	156	26	8	9	146	152	18	7
5. Alcohol use	1 825	1 688	137	-	-	1 610	67	11	-	-	134	3	-
6. Dementia*	702	315	387	32	15	22	94	152	32	14	22	103	216
7. Parkinson disease	75	40	35	-	-	-	21	19	-	-	-	18	17
8. Multiple sclerosis	137	59	79	-	-	57	1	4	-	-	77	2	-
9. Drug use	885	796	88	6	63	706	24	1	-	7	78	3	-
10. Post-traumatic stress disorder	262	99	164	-	25	62	5	-	10	41	105	8	1
11. Obsessive-compulsive disorders	1 365	585	780	-	88	466	22	9	-	112	615	40	13
12. Panic disorder	644	217	427	-	31	162	24	-	-	31	351	39	5
F. Sense organ diseases	**1 675**	**707**	**968**	**4**	**2**	**67**	**336**	**297**	**4**	**-**	**94**	**499**	**371**
1. Glaucoma	524	156	369	-	-	14	103	38	-	-	42	264	63
2. Cataracts	1 142	545	597	2	-	52	233	258	2	-	52	235	308
G. Cardiovascular diseases	**1 852**	**999**	**853**	**43**	**41**	**449**	**213**	**252**	**42**	**19**	**436**	**169**	**187**
1. Rheumatic heart disease	21	9	12	-	1	3	1	4	-	1	4	2	5
2. Ischaemic heart disease	462	288	175	-	-	54	96	137	-	-	41	52	82
3. Cerebrovascular disease	582	289	294	-	-	137	71	82	-	-	140	81	72
4. Inflammatory heart diseases	302	167	134	14	17	100	22	14	15	7	79	18	15
H. Respiratory diseases	**2 968**	**1 645**	**1 323**	**455**	**311**	**453**	**218**	**208**	**370**	**204**	**450**	**136**	**164**
1. COPD*	578	359	219	-	-	135	113	111	-	-	94	50	74
2. Asthma	1 214	678	536	117	247	268	36	10	75	163	255	35	8
I. Digestive diseases	**3 684**	**1 958**	**1 726**	**418**	**125**	**443**	**664**	**309**	**358**	**80**	**408**	**567**	**312**
1. Peptic ulcer	104	66	38	-	2	44	17	3	-	1	25	10	2
2. Cirrhosis of the liver	445	332	113	12	-	108	170	42	8	1	24	55	27
3. Appendicitis	8	5	3	-	1	3	-	-	-	1	2	-	-
J. Genito-urinary diseases	**508**	**335**	**173**	**18**	**32**	**37**	**209**	**39**	**8**	**26**	**58**	**47**	**34**
1. Nephritis and nephrosis	93	50	173	7	21	18	2	1	8	20	10	3	1
2. Benign prostatic hypertrophy	198	198	-	-	-	-	181	17	-	-	-	-	-
L. Musculo-skeletal diseases	**1 948**	**827**	**1 121**	**11**	**9**	**229**	**426**	**152**	**11**	**11**	**393**	**521**	**184**
1. Rheumatoid arthritis	182	48	134	-	-	3	16	29	-	2	49	26	57
2. Osteoarthritis	1 592	722	869	-	-	212	397	113	-	-	293	470	107

Annex Table 8e, continued. YLDs by age, sex and cause (thousands): Other Asia and Islands, 1990

Cause	Total	Male	Female	Males 0-4	5-14	15-44	45-59	60+	Females 0-4	5-14	15-44	45-59	60+
M. Congenital anomalies	**1 638**	**831**	**807**	**831**					**807**				
1. Abdominal wall defect	-	-	-	-	-	-	-	-	-	-	-	-	-
2. Anencephaly	-	-	-	-	-	-	-	-	-	-	-	-	-
3. Anorectal atresia	-	-	-	-	-	-	-	-	-	-	-	-	-
4. Cleft lip	35	20	14	20	-	-	-	-	14	-	-	-	-
5. Cleft palate	38	18	21	18	-	-	-	-	21	-	-	-	-
6. Oesophageal atresia	-	-	-	-	-	-	-	-	-	-	-	-	-
7. Renal agenesis	-	-	-	-	-	-	-	-	-	-	-	-	-
8. Down syndrome	363	204	159	204	-	-	-	-	159	-	-	-	-
9. Congenital heart anomalies	1 047	530	517	530	-	-	-	-	517	-	-	-	-
10. Spina bifida	155	60	95	60	-	-	-	-	95	-	-	-	-
N. Oral conditions	**1 273**	**619**	**654**	**31**	**44**	**265**	**155**	**124**	**29**	**43**	**272**	**165**	**144**
1. Dental caries	530	265	265	30	44	115	54	22	29	42	114	55	25
2. Periodontal disease	33	17	17	-	-	13	2	1	-	-	13	2	1
3. Edentulism	699	336	363	-	-	136	99	101	-	-	137	107	118
III. Injuries	***9 734***	***6 507***	***3 227***	***1 340***	***1 526***	***3 292***	***314***	***35***	***1 208***	***786***	***1 081***	***125***	***26***
A. Unintentional injuries	**9 222**	**6 233**	**2 989**	**1 327**	**1 506**	**3 066**	**300**	**33**	**1 194**	**769**	**883**	**118**	**25**
1. Road traffic accidents	980	698	282	56	206	396	36	5	52	111	102	15	3
2. Poisonings	52	27	26	15	9	2	-	-	14	10	2	-	-
3. Falls	3 221	2 040	1 181	710	558	709	57	5	549	263	326	39	5
4. Fires	204	89	115	3	63	20	2	-	33	72	10	1	-
5. Drownings	1	1	-	-	-	-	-	-	-	-	-	-	-
6. Other unintentional	4 764	3 379	1 385	542	670	1 939	205	23	547	314	444	62	17
B. Intentional injuries	**512**	**274**	**238**	**13**	**20**	**226**	**14**	**2**	**14**	**17**	**198**	**7**	**1**
1. Self-inflicted injuries	192	54	138	-	-	50	4	-	-	1	133	4	-
2. Violence	179	138	41	6	15	109	7	1	7	10	23	1	-
3. War	141	83	59	7	5	67	3	-	8	6	43	2	-

Notes:
A dash (-) symbol indicates fewer than 500 YLDs.
¹IA6 is Bacterial meningitis and meningococcaemia; ID is Conditions arising during the perinatal period;
IIH1 is Chronic obstructive pulmonary disease.
IIE6 is Dementia and other degenerative and hereditary CNS disorders;

Annex Table 8f. YLDs by age, sex and cause (thousands): Sub-Saharan Africa, 1990

Cause	Total	Male	Female	Males					Females				
				0-4	5-14	15-44	45-59	60+	0-4	5-14	15-44	45-59	60+
Population (millions)	*510*	*252*	*258*	*47*	*70*	*104*	*20*	*11*	*47*	*70*	*106*	*22*	*13*
All causes	**68 403**	**33 869**	**34 535**	**8 859**	**5 011**	**15 492**	**3 075**	**1 432**	**8 557**	**4 297**	**16 946**	**2 982**	**1 753**
I. Communicable, maternal, perinatal and nutritional conditions	*26 882*	*11 192*	*15 690*	*5 100*	*1 703*	*3 755*	*472*	*162*	*5 044*	*1 363*	*8 584*	*483*	*217*
A. Infectious and parasitic diseases	**15 351**	**7 526**	**7 824**	**2 385**	**1 246**	**3 355**	**416**	**124**	**2 303**	**891**	**4 056**	**403**	**172**
1. Tuberculosis	750	389	361	11	52	264	46	15	11	63	231	42	14
2. STDs excluding HIV	3 595	1 070	2 525	365	15	687	3	-	390	50	2 080	4	1
a. Syphilis	277	124	154	13	2	108	1	-	13	2	138	1	-
b. Chlamydia	1 653	224	1 429	65	4	154	1	-	70	33	1 324	2	-
c. Gonorrhoea	1 665	722	943	287	9	424	2	-	308	15	619	1	-
3. HIV	1 350	674	676	5	3	644	18	3	5	7	647	15	1
4. Diarrhoeal diseases	733	377	356	184	112	68	9	3	161	112	69	10	4
5. Childhood-cluster diseases	885	474	411	405	62	6	-	-	346	60	5	-	-
a. Pertussis	436	221	215	166	55	-	-	-	162	53	-	-	-
b. Poliomyelitis	427	240	187	232	2	5	-	-	181	1	4	-	-
c. Diphtheria													
d. Measles	20	12	8	7	5	-	-	-	3	5	-	-	-
e. Tetanus	2	1	1	-	-	-	-	-	-	-	-	-	-
6. Bacterial meningitis*	240	119	121	95	14	8	1	1	96	14	9	2	1
7. Hepatitis B and hepatitis C	8	5	4	-	-	2	1	-	-	-	2	1	-
8. Malaria	2 704	1 367	1 336	1 171	75	102	14	5	1 148	74	95	14	6
9. Tropical-cluster diseases	3 775	2 488	1 287	66	751	1 357	260	54	70	359	632	191	36
a. Trypanosomiasis	121	65	57	2	17	35	10	1	4	15	32	6	1
b. Chagas disease													
c. Schistosomiasis	1 175	695	480	24	261	348	47	14	16	176	245	33	10
d. Leishmaniasis	111	74	38	3	37	34	-	-	1	19	17	-	-
e. Lymphatic filariasis	1 486	1 151	335	30	352	695	71	3	42	81	150	57	5
f. Onchocerciasis	881	503	378	7	84	245	132	35	6	68	188	95	21
10. Leprosy	39	19	20	1	7	10	1	-	1	8	10	1	-
11. Dengue													
12. Japanese encephalitis													
13. Trachoma	355	92	262	-	-	26	33	33	-	-	69	94	98
14. Intestinal nematode infections	437	217	221	1	99	98	14	5	1	99	100	15	5
a. Ascariasis	70	35	35	1	34	-	-	-	1	34	-	-	-
b. Trichuriasis	79	39	39	-	39	-	-	-	-	39	-	-	-
c. Ancylostomiasis and necatoriasis	288	142	146	-	26	98	14	5	-	26	100	15	5

Annex Table 8f, continued. YLDs by age, sex and cause (thousands): Sub-Saharan Africa, 1990

Cause	Total	Male	Female	Males					Females				
				0-4	5-14	15-44	45-59	60+	0-4	5-14	15-44	45-59	60+
B. Respiratory infections	**878**	**437**	**441**	**309**	**105**	**16**	**2**	**4**	**312**	**104**	**17**	**2**	**5**
1. Lower respiratory infections	688	342	346	289	36	12	2	4	292	36	12	2	5
2. Upper respiratory infections	21	10	11	1	4	4	1	-	1	4	5	1	-
3. Otitis media	168	84	84	19	65	-	-	-	19	65	-	-	-
C. Maternal conditions	**3 983**		**3 983**							**17**	**3 966**	**1**	
1. Maternal haemorrhage	45		45								45		
2. Maternal sepsis	923		923								923		
3. Hypertensive disorders of pregnancy	14		14								14		
4. Obstructed labour	1 221		1 221								1 221		
5. Abortion	928		928								928		
D. Perinatal conditions*	**2 163**	**1 075**	**1 088**	**1 075**					**1 088**				
E. Nutritional deficiencies	**4 507**	**2 154**	**2 354**	**1 331**	**352**	**384**	**54**	**33**	**1 340**	**350**	**546**	**77**	**40**
1. Protein-energy malnutrition	2 140	1 066	1 074	1 066					1 074				
2. Iodine deficiency	72	33	39	31	1	1	-	-	32	2	4	1	-
3. Vitamin A deficiency	36	18	18	18					18				
4. Iron-deficiency anaemia	2 260	1 036	1 223	216	350	383	54	33	217	348	542	76	40
II. Noncommunicable diseases	**27 215**	**13 245**	**13 970**	**2 576**	**850**	**6 312**	**2 287**	**1 220**	**2 507**	**877**	**6 709**	**2 378**	**1 498**
A. Malignant neoplasms	**351**	**177**	**174**	**1**	**9**	**40**	**50**	**77**	**1**	**12**	**57**	**53**	**51**
1. Mouth and oropharynx cancers	38	21	16			7	4	10		2	6	2	6
2. Oesophagus cancer	15	9	6			2	4	3			2	1	3
3. Stomach cancer	31	18	12			3	8	8			3	6	4
4. Colon and rectum cancers	17	9	8			2	2	5			2	2	5
5. Liver cancer	24	18	6			7	7	3			2	2	2
6. Pancreas cancer	4	2	2			-	1	1			1	-	1
7. Trachea, bronchus, lung cancers	9	7	2			1	2	3			-	1	-
8. Melanoma and other skin cancers	5	2	3			-	1	1			-	1	2
9. Breast cancer	19	-	19								6	7	5
10. Cervix uteri cancer	30	-	30								10	12	8
11. Corpus uteri cancer	3		3								1	2	-
12. Ovary cancer	7		7								3	2	1
13. Prostate cancer	26	26	-			1	5	20					
14. Bladder cancer	13	9	4			1	3	5			1	2	2
15. Lymphomas and multiple myeloma	17	10	7			2	1	2		3	2	1	1
16. Leukaemia	5	2	3			1	-	1		1	1	-	1
C. Diabetes mellitus	**190**	**89**	**101**	**-**	**13**	**31**	**37**	**21**	**-**	**25**	**33**	**42**	**26**
D. Endocrine disorders	**631**	**289**	**343**	**131**		**63**	**61**	**19**	**83**		**92**	**83**	**59**

Annex Table 8f, continued. YLDs by age, sex and cause (thousands): Sub-Saharan Africa, 1990

Cause	Total	Male	Female	Males 0-4	5-14	15-44	45-59	60+	Females 0-4	5-14	15-44	45-59	60+
E. Neuro-psychiatric conditions	11 147	5 296	5 851	127	261	4 444	355	110	152	286	4 726	471	216
1. Unipolar major depression	4 552	1 550	3 003	-	-	1 362	156	32	-	-	2 626	308	68
2. Bipolar disorder	1 303	641	661	-	-	608	27	7	-	-	623	30	8
3. Schizophrenia	434	223	211	-	-	223	-	-	-	-	211	-	-
4. Epilepsy	380	186	193	15	73	82	11	4	18	77	85	9	5
5. Alcohol use	1 695	1 374	321	-	-	1 306	62	5	-	-	310	9	2
6. Dementia*	264	77	187	11	4	5	20	36	32	15	18	23	99
7. Parkinson disease	37	19	18	-	-	-	10	8	-	-	-	9	8
8. Multiple sclerosis	87	36	50	-	-	36	1	-	-	-	49	1	-
9. Drug use	355	319	35	-	25	283	9	2	-	3	31	1	-
10. Post-traumatic stress disorder	192	71	121	6	21	40	3	-	10	36	70	5	-
11. Obsessive-compulsive disorders	933	393	540	-	73	301	13	5	-	97	410	26	8
12. Panic disorder	438	146	292	-	26	105	15	-	-	27	237	25	3
F. Sense organ diseases	1 950	903	1 047	7	1	76	453	367	7	1	80	510	449
1. Glaucoma	389	155	234	-	-	1	75	79	-	-	2	120	112
2. Cataracts	1 558	746	811	7	1	72	378	288	7	1	76	390	337
G. Cardiovascular diseases	1 084	535	550	18	23	245	130	119	14	33	236	150	117
1. Rheumatic heart disease	59	23	36	-	8	14	1	-	-	13	21	2	-
2. Ischaemic heart disease	272	145	126	-	-	37	59	49	-	-	35	49	43
3. Cerebrovascular disease	351	164	187	-	-	77	37	50	-	-	66	71	49
4. Inflammatory heart diseases	260	131	129	8	7	80	21	15	12	7	67	19	23
H. Respiratory diseases	4 533	2 375	2 159	634	292	744	467	237	620	254	668	408	209
1. COPD*	740	474	266	-	-	242	145	87	-	-	119	93	53
2. Asthma	1 207	599	608	114	222	226	30	8	94	189	279	38	9
I. Digestive diseases	2 488	1 278	1 209	280	93	381	373	151	280	133	364	253	180
1. Peptic ulcer	109	58	51	-	2	38	15	2	-	2	33	13	2
2. Cirrhosis of the liver	126	86	40	-	8	32	34	13	-	4	14	14	8
3. Appendicitis	6	4	2	-	1	2	-	-	-	1	1	-	-
J. Genito-urinary diseases	626	394	232	52	76	35	206	26	24	56	64	59	28
1. Nephritis and nephrosis	166	90	76	24	56	7	2	-	20	44	9	3	1
2. Benign prostatic hypertrophy	174	174	-	-	-	-	168	6	-	-	-	-	-
L. Musculo-skeletal diseases	1 038	345	692	-	-	179	115	51	-	-	281	305	104
1. Rheumatoid arthritis	85	23	62	-	-	15	6	2	-	-	38	16	5
2. Osteoarthritis	939	318	621	-	-	161	108	48	-	-	237	286	98

Annex Table 8f, continued. YLDs by age, sex and cause (thousands): Sub-Saharan Africa, 1990

Cause	Total	Male	Female	Males					Females				
				0-4	5-14	15-44	45-59	60+	0-4	5-14	15-44	45-59	60+
M. Congenital anomalies	**2 137**	**1 042**	**1 095**	**1 042**	–	–	–	–	**1 095**	–	–	–	–
1. Abdominal wall defect	–	–	–	–	–	–	–	–	–	–	–	–	–
2. Anencephaly	–	–	–	–	–	–	–	–	–	–	–	–	–
3. Anorectal atresia	–	–	–	–	–	–	–	–	–	–	–	–	–
4. Cleft lip	50	28	22	28	–	–	–	–	22	–	–	–	–
5. Cleft palate	57	25	32	25	–	–	–	–	32	–	–	–	–
6. Oesophageal atresia	–	–	–	–	–	–	–	–	–	–	–	–	–
7. Renal agenesis	480	262	219	262	–	–	–	–	219	–	–	–	–
8. Down syndrome	1 188	591	597	591	–	–	–	–	597	–	–	–	–
9. Congenital heart anomalies	362	136	226	136	–	–	–	–	226	–	–	–	–
10. Spina bifida	–	–	–	–	–	–	–	–	–	–	–	–	–
N. Oral conditions	**387**	**187**	**200**	**47**	**49**	**47**	**11**	**33**	**47**	**50**	**51**	**12**	**41**
1. Dental caries	286	142	144	46	49	35	10	3	46	48	35	10	4
2. Periodontal disease	27	13	14	–	–	12	1	–	–	–	12	1	–
3. Edentulism	65	29	36	–	–	–	–	29	–	–	–	–	36
III. Injuries	***14 306***	***9 431***	***4 875***	***1 183***	***2 458***	***5 425***	***316***	***50***	***1 006***	***2 058***	***1 652***	***121***	***38***
A. Unintentional injuries	**11 132**	**7 460**	**3 671**	**1 041**	**2 329**	**3 795**	**255**	**41**	**868**	**1 923**	**766**	**84**	**30**
1. Road traffic accidents	1 061	752	309	31	359	331	28	4	22	187	90	9	1
2. Poisonings	24	15	10	10	4	–	–	–	7	2	–	–	–
3. Falls	1 710	955	755	192	564	172	21	6	212	354	152	23	14
4. Fires	1 498	682	815	170	427	79	6	1	149	601	60	4	1
5. Drownings	1	1	–	–	–	–	–	–	–	–	–	–	–
6. Other unintentional	6 838	5 056	1 782	637	974	3 213	200	31	477	780	464	48	13
B. Intentional injuries	**3 175**	**1 971**	**1 203**	**142**	**129**	**1 630**	**61**	**9**	**138**	**135**	**886**	**37**	**8**
1. Self-inflicted injuries	33	18	15	–	–	17	1	–	–	–	14	1	–
2. Violence	568	483	85	15	43	411	11	2	8	19	55	2	1
3. War	2 574	1 470	1 104	127	86	1 202	49	7	130	116	817	34	7

Notes:
A dash (-) symbol indicates fewer than 500 YLDs.
*IA6 is Bacterial meningitis and meningococcaemia; ID is Conditions arising during the perinatal period;
*IIE6 is Dementia and other degenerative and hereditary CNS disorders; IIH1 is Chronic obstructive pulmonary disease.

Annex Table 8g. YLDs by age, sex and cause (thousands): Latin America and the Caribbean, 1990

Cause	Total	Male	Female	Males					Females				
				0-4	5-14	15-44	45-59	60+	0-4	5-14	15-44	45-59	60+
Population (millions)	444	222	223	29	52	104	22	14	28	51	104	23	17
All causes	42 045	21 633	20 412	3 161	2 844	11 778	2 519	1 331	2 963	2 167	11 502	2 333	1 447
I. Communicable, maternal, perinatal and nutritional conditions	8 005	2 896	5 109	1 083	702	979	90	41	1 192	688	3 088	100	42
A. Infectious and parasitic diseases	4 087	1 802	2 285	375	500	835	68	24	348	489	1 369	57	22
1. Tuberculosis	179	98	81	2	11	61	15	9	2	14	51	9	6
2. STDs excluding HIV	856	151	706	24	2	124	1	–	24	12	668	1	–
a. Syphilis	34	15	19	1	–	14	1	–	1	–	17	1	–
b. Chlamydia	559	48	511	6	1	42	–	–	6	9	495	–	–
c. Gonorrhoea	263	87	176	17	1	68	–	–	17	3	156	–	–
3. HIV	300	234	66	–	–	224	9	1	–	–	62	3	–
4. Diarrhoeal diseases	567	286	281	93	111	68	10	4	89	108	68	11	5
5. Childhood-cluster diseases	301	164	138	142	18	3	–	–	118	18	2	–	–
a. Pertussis	138	70	68	54	16	–	–	–	52	16	–	–	–
b. Poliomyelitis	158	90	68	87	1	2	–	–	65	–	2	–	–
c. Diphtheria													
d. Measles	5	3	2	2	1	–	–	–	1	1	–	–	–
e. Tetanus				2	1	–	–	–	1	1	–	–	–
6. Bacterial meningitis*	157	79	78	58	10	8	2	1	57	10	9	2	1
7. Hepatitis B and hepatitis C	3	1	1	–	–	–	–	1	–	–	1	–	–
8. Malaria	64	32	32	7	12	12	2	1	6	11	12	2	1
9. Tropical-cluster diseases	448	236	212	2	15	203	14	2	2	11	187	11	1
a. Trypanosomiasis	341	172	169	–	–	163	8	1	1	–	161	7	1
b. Chagas disease	69	35	34	–	8	22	3	1	1	10	20	3	1
c. Schistosomiasis	28	22	6	1	4	14	1	1	1	1	4	1	–
d. Leishmaniasis	8	6	2	1	2	3	1	–	–	–	1	–	–
e. Lymphatic filariasis	3	2	1	–	–	1	–	–	–	–	1	–	–
f. Onchocerciasis	3	2	1	–	–	1	–	–	–	–	1	–	–
10. Leprosy	45	22	23	1	9	11	2	1	1	9	11	2	1
11. Dengue													
12. Japanese encephalitis													
13. Trachoma													
14. Intestinal nematode infections	560	282	278	3	229	41	6	3	3	225	41	6	3
a. Ascariasis	182	92	90	3	89	–	–	–	3	87	–	–	–
b. Trichuriasis	253	128	125	–	127	–	–	–	–	125	–	–	–
c. Ancylostomiasis and necatoriasis	125	62	63	–	13	40	–	3	–	13	40	–	3

Annex Table 8g, continued. YLDs by age, sex and cause (thousands): Latin America and the Caribbean, 1990

				Males					Females				
Cause	Total	Male	Female	0-4	5-14	15-44	45-59	60+	0-4	5-14	15-44	45-59	60+
B. Respiratory infections	**433**	**141**	**292**	**43**	**77**	**16**	**2**	**2**	**195**	**75**	**16**	**3**	**2**
1. Lower respiratory infections	297	72	225	31	27	12	2	2	183	26	12	2	2
2. Upper respiratory infections	16	8	8			4				1	4	1	
3. Otitis media	120	61	59	12	49				12	48			
C. Maternal conditions	**1 123**	**–**	**1 123**								**1 122**		
1. Maternal haemorrhage	20	–	20								20		
2. Maternal sepsis	245	–	245								245		
3. Hypertensive disorders of pregnancy	7	–	7								7		
4. Obstructed labour	366	–	366								366		
5. Abortion	314	–	314								314		
D. Perinatal conditions*	**660**	**334**	**326**	**334**					**326**				
E. Nutritional deficiencies	**1 702**	**619**	**1 083**	**331**	**125**	**128**	**20**	**15**	**322**	**122**	**581**	**40**	**18**
1. Protein-energy malnutrition	361	183	178	183					178				
2. Iodine deficiency	47	22	25	20	1	1			20	1	3		
3. Vitamin A deficiency	6	3	3	3					3				
4. Iron-deficiency anaemia	1 283	409	874	124	124	127	19	15	120	121	577	39	18
II. Noncommunicable diseases	**28 303**	**14 654**	**13 649**	**1 534**	**1 049**	**8 654**	**2 189**	**1 229**	**1 397**	**1 012**	**7 727**	**2 147**	**1 365**
A. Malignant neoplasms	**346**	**161**	**185**	**1**	**7**	**26**	**41**	**86**	**1**	**6**	**64**	**60**	**54**
1. Mouth and oropharynx cancers	19	14	5			4	5	4			1	2	2
2. Oesophagus cancer	6	4	3				1	2			1	1	1
3. Stomach cancer	35	23	12			3	7	13			2	4	6
4. Colon and rectum cancers	31	15	16			3	4	8			2	4	9
5. Liver cancer	2	1	1					1					1
6. Pancreas cancer	4	2	2				1	1				1	
7. Trachea, bronchus, lung cancers	22	16	6			2	5	9			1	2	3
8. Melanoma and other skin cancers	4	1	2								1	1	
9. Breast cancer	38	–	38								13	14	11
10. Cervix uteri cancer	27	–	27								13	9	5
11. Corpus uteri cancer	8	–	8								2	6	
12. Ovary cancer	6	–	6								3	1	1
13. Prostate cancer	22	22	–				3	19					
14. Bladder cancer	11	9	2			1	2	6				1	1
15. Lymphomas and multiple myeloma	12	7	5		1	3	1	1		1	2	1	2
16. Leukaemia	9	5	4		2	2	1	1		2	1		1
C. Diabetes mellitus	**564**	**269**	**294**			**97**	**102**	**70**			**100**	**117**	**77**
D. Endocrine disorders	**873**	**409**	**464**	**195**	**54**	**99**	**38**	**23**	**159**	**48**	**157**	**64**	**36**

Annex Table 8g, continued. YLDs by age, sex and cause (thousands): Latin America and the Caribbean, 1990

Cause	Total	Male	Female	Males					Females				
				0-4	5-14	15-44	45-59	60+	0-4	5-14	15-44	45-59	60+
E. Neuro-psychiatric conditions	**14 565**	**8 114**	**6 451**	**138**	**389**	**6 767**	**568**	**253**	**127**	**383**	**5 130**	**508**	**303**
1. Unipolar major depression	4 183	1 448	2 735	-	-	1 255	156	36	-	-	2 363	296	75
2. Bipolar disorder	1 168	583	584	-	-	549	27	8	-	-	548	28	9
3. Schizophrenia	1 231	635	597	-	-	635	-	-	-	-	597	-	-
4. Epilepsy	500	273	227	4	85	151	24	7	6	87	119	10	6
5. Alcohol use	3 612	3 316	296	-	-	3 023	232	60	-	-	285	8	3
6. Dementia*	516	214	302	22	9	15	51	118	22	9	15	73	183
7. Parkinson disease	27	14	12	-	-	-	7	7	-	-	-	6	6
8. Multiple sclerosis	91	39	52	-	-	38	1	-	-	-	51	1	-
9. Drug use	1 061	690	371	-	55	611	20	3	-	29	329	11	2
10. Post-traumatic stress disorder	169	63	106	4	16	40	3	1	6	26	68	5	1
11. Obsessive-compulsive disorders	852	363	489	-	52	290	14	6	-	68	386	26	9
12. Panic disorder	388	130	259	-	18	97	15	-	-	18	213	24	4
F. Sense organ diseases	**571**	**262**	**309**	**14**	**3**	**18**	**67**	**159**	**10**	**5**	**20**	**82**	**192**
1. Glaucoma	83	30	53	-	-	1	15	14	-	-	2	30	20
2. Cataracts	453	214	240	3	-	14	51	145	3	1	14	51	171
G. Cardiovascular diseases	**990**	**569**	**421**	**6**	**8**	**205**	**161**	**190**	**5**	**7**	**170**	**107**	**132**
1. Rheumatic heart disease	19	7	13	-	2	3	1	1	-	2	7	2	1
2. Ischaemic heart disease	323	202	121	-	-	32	82	88	-	-	28	43	50
3. Cerebrovascular disease	377	207	170	-	-	89	50	68	-	-	70	43	57
4. Inflammatory heart diseases	122	67	56	2	3	46	10	6	2	2	38	8	6
H. Respiratory diseases	**2 570**	**1 294**	**1 275**	**345**	**187**	**406**	**208**	**148**	**301**	**164**	**514**	**176**	**120**
1. COPD*	527	298	230	-	-	118	99	81	-	-	112	64	53
2. Asthma	817	423	395	62	135	190	27	8	50	117	183	33	13
I. Digestive diseases	**1 793**	**916**	**878**	**148**	**67**	**316**	**277**	**107**	**113**	**54**	**361**	**220**	**130**
1. Peptic ulcer	49	31	19	-	1	20	8	1	-	-	12	5	-
2. Cirrhosis of the liver	228	167	61	3	-	69	78	17	3	-	21	26	11
3. Appendicitis	8	5	3	-	1	3	-	-	-	1	2	-	-
J. Genito-urinary diseases	**533**	**288**	**245**	**29**	**34**	**23**	**176**	**26**	**29**	**47**	**111**	**35**	**22**
1. Nephritis and nephrosis	97	39	57	10	25	2	2	1	13	34	8	1	1
2. Benign prostatic hypertrophy	165	165	-	-	-	-	157	8	-	-	-	-	-
L. Musculo-skeletal diseases	**2 911**	**1 119**	**1 792**	**5**	**17**	**473**	**499**	**124**	**3**	**27**	**814**	**707**	**241**
1. Rheumatoid arthritis	556	114	442	-	-	69	34	11	-	5	310	94	32
2. Osteoarthritis	2 093	951	1 142	-	-	387	456	107	-	-	366	580	195

Annex Table 8g, continued. YLDs by age, sex and cause (thousands): Latin America and the Caribbean, 1990

Cause	Total	Male	Female	Males					Females				
				0-4	5-14	15-44	45-59	60+	0-4	5-14	15-44	45-59	60+
M. Congenital anomalies	**1 177**	**589**	**588**	**589**	–	–	–	–	**588**	–	–	–	–
1. Abdominal wall defect	–	–	–	–	–	–	–	–	–	–	–	–	–
2. Anencephaly	–	–	–	–	–	–	–	–	–	–	–	–	–
3. Anorectal atresia	–	–	–	–	–	–	–	–	–	–	–	–	–
4. Cleft lip	19	11	8	11	–	–	–	–	8	–	–	–	–
5. Cleft palate	14	6	7	6	–	–	–	–	7	–	–	–	–
6. Oesophageal atresia	–	–	–	–	–	–	–	–	–	–	–	–	–
7. Renal agenesis	–	–	–	–	–	–	–	–	–	–	–	–	–
8. Down syndrome	247	139	108	139	–	–	–	–	108	–	–	–	–
9. Congenital heart anomalies	712	361	351	361	–	–	–	–	351	–	–	–	–
10. Spina bifida	185	72	113	72	–	–	–	–	113	–	–	–	–
N. Oral conditions	**1 004**	**501**	**503**	**36**	**236**	**178**	**21**	**30**	**35**	**230**	**178**	**22**	**37**
1. Dental caries	902	455	448	36	235	174	7	3	34	229	173	7	4
2. Periodontal disease	18	9	9	–	–	3	4	2	–	–	3	4	2
3. Edentulism	77	35	42	–	–	–	10	26	–	–	–	11	31
III. Injuries	***5 736***	***4 083***	***1 654***	***544***	***1 093***	***2 145***	***240***	***61***	***374***	***467***	***687***	***86***	***40***
A. Unintentional injuries	***5 170***	***3 671***	***1 499***	**529**	**1 061**	**1 798**	**225**	**58**	**360**	**448**	**570**	**81**	**39**
1. Road traffic accidents	1 061	765	296	18	242	449	49	7	14	123	141	16	3
2. Poisonings	18	10	8	7	2	3	–	–	5	2	3	–	–
3. Falls	1 347	978	369	182	437	314	30	14	84	137	108	25	15
4. Fires	129	68	61	13	43	11	1	–	12	42	6	1	–
5. Drownings	–	–	–	–	–	–	–	–	–	–	–	–	–
6. Other unintentional	2 616	1 850	766	308	337	1 024	145	37	245	145	315	40	21
B. Intentional injuries	***566***	***412***	***154***	**15**	**32**	**347**	**15**	**3**	**14**	**18**	**116**	**5**	**1**
1. Self-inflicted injuries	53	20	33	–	–	18	2	–	–	–	31	2	–
2. Violence	347	297	50	7	26	252	10	2	5	11	33	1	–
3. War	166	95	71	8	5	77	3	–	9	7	53	2	–

Notes:
A dash (–) symbol indicates fewer than 500 YLDs.
*IA6 is Bacterial meningitis and meningococcaemia; ID is Conditions arising during the perinatal period;
IIE6 is Dementia and other degenerative and hereditary CNS disorders; IIH1 is Chronic obstructive pulmonary disease.

Annex Table 8h. YLDs by age, sex and cause (thousands): Middle Eastern Crescent, 1990

Cause	Total	Male	Female	Males 0-4	5-14	15-44	45-59	60+	Females 0-4	5-14	15-44	45-59	60+
Population (millions)	*503*	*256*	*247*	*41*	*65*	*114*	*22*	*14*	*40*	*62*	*107*	*22*	*15*
All causes	**45 615**	**22 402**	**23 213**	**6 454**	**2 632**	**9 577**	**2 365**	**1 374**	**6 146**	**1 821**	**11 651**	**2 216**	**1 380**
I. Communicable, maternal, perinatal and nutritional conditions	***11 213***	***4 098***	***7 115***	***2 632***	***593***	***686***	***116***	***71***	***2 500***	***554***	***3 773***	***169***	***119***
A. Infectious and parasitic diseases	**2 936**	**1 397**	**1 539**	**602**	**248**	**422**	**79**	**47**	**523**	**225**	**595**	**104**	**92**
1. Tuberculosis	**243**	**156**	**87**	**4**	**12**	**108**	**23**	**9**	**3**	**7**	**57**	**13**	**7**
2. STDs excluding HIV	**364**	**73**	**291**	**13**	**1**	**59**	-	-	**13**	**6**	**272**	**1**	-
a. Syphilis	28	13	15	2	-	11			2	-	13		
b. Chlamydia	240	27	213	3	-	23			3	4	205		
c. Gonorrhoea	97	33	63	8	-	25			8	1	54		
3. HIV	**31**	**27**	**4**	-	-	**25**	**2**	-	-	-	**4**		
4. Diarrhoeal diseases	**477**	**250**	**227**	**133**	**58**	**49**	**7**	**3**	**115**	**55**	**46**	**7**	**3**
5. Childhood-cluster diseases	**582**	**319**	**263**	**282**	**31**	**6**	-	-	**229**	**29**	**4**	-	-
a. Pertussis	221	113	108	86	27				83	26	4		
b. Poliomyelitis	350	200	150	192	1	6			145	1	4		
c. Diphtheria				-									
d. Measles	10	6	4	3	3				1	3			
e. Tetanus	1	1	-										
6. Bacterial meningitis*	**215**	**109**	**106**	**84**	**13**	**9**	**2**	**1**	**82**	**12**	**9**	**2**	**1**
7. Hepatitis B and hepatitis C	**7**	**4**	**3**	-	-	**2**	**1**	**1**	-	-	**1**	-	**1**
8. Malaria	**174**	**89**	**85**	**16**	**36**	**30**	**4**	**2**	**16**	**34**	**29**	**4**	**2**
9. Tropical-cluster diseases	**170**	**102**	**68**	**6**	**36**	**51**	**7**	**2**	**4**	**23**	**34**	**4**	**1**
a. Trypanosomiasis													
b. Chagas disease													
c. Schistosomiasis	103	60	43	1	18	35	5	1	1	11	26	4	1
d. Leishmaniasis	54	33	22	5	17	9	1		3	11	6		
e. Lymphatic filariasis	12	9	3	-	1	7	1		-	-	2		
f. Onchocerciasis													
10. Leprosy	**9**	**5**	**5**	-	**2**	**2**	-	-	-	**2**	**2**	-	-
11. Dengue	-	-	-										
12. Japanese encephalitis	-	-	-										
13. Trachoma	**249**	**68**	**181**	-	**43**	**19**	**23**	**26**	-	**41**	**45**	**63**	**73**
14. Intestinal nematode infections	**160**	**82**	**78**	**1**	**43**	**31**	**4**	**2**	**1**	**41**	**29**	**4**	**2**
a. Ascariasis	69	35	34	1	34				1	32			
b. Trichuriasis	1	1	1	1	1				1				
c. Ancylostomiasis and necatoriasis	90	46	44	-	9	31	4	2	-	8	29	4	2

Annex Table 8h, continued. YLDs by age, sex and cause (thousands): Middle Eastern Crescent, 1990

Cause	Total	Male	Female	Males					Females				
				0-4	5-14	15-44	45-59	60+	0-4	5-14	15-44	45-59	60+
B. Respiratory infections	**797**	**405**	**392**	**286**	**97**	**18**	**2**	**2**	**278**	**92**	**18**	**2**	**2**
1. Lower respiratory infections	626	318	308	268	33	13	2	2	260	32	12	2	2
2. Upper respiratory infections	18	9	9	1	2	5	1	-	1	2	5	1	-
3. Otitis media	153	78	75	17	61	-	-	-	17	58	-	-	-
C. Maternal conditions	**2 282**	**-**	**2 282**	**-**	**-**	**-**	**-**	**-**	**-**	**-**	**2 276**	**6**	**-**
1. Maternal haemorrhage	32	-	32	-	-	-	-	-	-	-	32	-	-
2. Maternal sepsis	547	-	547	-	-	-	-	-	-	-	547	-	-
3. Hypertensive disorders of pregnancy	11	-	11	-	-	-	-	-	-	-	11	-	-
4. Obstructed labour	893	-	893	-	-	-	-	-	-	-	893	-	-
5. Abortion	243	-	243	-	-	-	-	-	-	-	243	-	-
D. Perinatal conditions*	**1 299**	**658**	**642**	**658**	**-**	**-**	**-**	**-**	**642**	**-**	**-**	**-**	**-**
E. Nutritional deficiencies	**3 898**	**1 639**	**2 260**	**1 088**	**248**	**247**	**35**	**22**	**1 059**	**237**	**884**	**56**	**25**
1. Protein-energy malnutrition	1 562	791	771	791	-	-	-	-	771	-	-	-	-
2. Iodine deficiency	132	62	70	57	2	2	-	-	56	4	9	1	-
3. Vitamin A deficiency	23	12	11	12	-	-	-	-	11	-	-	-	-
4. Iron-deficiency anaemia	2 181	773	1 407	227	245	244	35	22	221	233	875	55	24
II. Noncommunicable diseases	***28 073***	***14 199***	***13 874***	***2 973***	***1 070***	***6 781***	***2 096***	***1 279***	***2 914***	***749***	***6 993***	***1 976***	***1 242***
A. Malignant neoplasms	**225**	**118**	**107**	**1**	**8**	**33**	**34**	**43**	**1**	**8**	**41**	**30**	**27**
1. Mouth and oropharynx cancers	30	19	11	-	1	9	4	6	-	1	5	2	3
2. Oesophagus cancer	8	3	5	-	-	1	-	1	-	-	1	1	2
3. Stomach cancer	21	14	8	-	-	3	5	5	-	-	3	2	3
4. Colon and rectum cancers	17	9	8	-	-	3	2	4	-	-	3	2	3
5. Liver cancer	3	2	1	-	-	2	1	1	-	-	1	-	-
6. Pancreas cancer	3	2	1	-	-	-	1	1	-	-	-	-	1
7. Trachea, bronchus, lung cancers	16	14	3	-	-	3	6	6	-	-	1	1	1
8. Melanoma and other skin cancers	2	1	1	-	-	-	-	1	-	-	-	-	1
9. Breast cancer	16	-	16	-	-	-	-	-	-	-	7	6	3
10. Cervix uteri cancer	8	-	8	-	-	-	-	-	-	-	7	3	2
11. Corpus uteri cancer	2	-	2	-	-	-	-	-	-	-	1	1	-
12. Ovary cancer	4	-	4	-	-	-	-	-	-	-	3	1	-
13. Prostate cancer	5	5	-	-	-	-	1	3	-	-	-	-	-
14. Bladder cancer	12	10	2	-	-	2	3	5	-	-	-	1	1
15. Lymphomas and multiple myeloma	7	5	2	-	1	2	1	1	-	1	-	1	1
16. Leukaemia	9	5	4	-	2	2	-	1	-	2	1	-	1
C. Diabetes mellitus	**664**	**331**	**334**	**-**	**1**	**131**	**133**	**67**	**-**	**1**	**125**	**134**	**74**
D. Endocrine disorders	**525**	**264**	**261**	**129**	**37**	**59**	**28**	**11**	**121**	**39**	**67**	**23**	**11**

Annex Table 8h, continued. YLDs by age, sex and cause (thousands): Middle Eastern Crescent, 1990

Cause	Total	Male	Female	Males					Females				
				0-4	5-14	15-44	45-59	60+	0-4	5-14	15-44	45-59	60+
E. Neuro-psychiatric conditions	11 584	5 579	6 005	303	389	4 437	325	125	242	313	4 850	429	171
1. Unipolar major depression	4 556	1 639	2 917	-	-	1 437	164	38	-	-	2 546	296	75
2. Bipolar disorder	1 300	668	631	-	-	632	28	8	-	-	595	28	9
3. Schizophrenia	1 371	728	643	-	-	728	-	-	-	-	643	-	-
4. Epilepsy	259	129	130	10	56	53	7	3	9	80	33	6	2
5. Alcohol use	248	224	25	-	-	213	9	2	-	-	24	1	-
6. Dementia*	218	107	110	31	9	12	17	38	31	8	13	10	49
7. Parkinson disease	47	25	22	-	-	-	13	12	-	-	-	11	11
8. Multiple sclerosis	95	42	53	-	-	41	-	-	-	-	52	1	-
9. Drug use	884	796	88	-	63	705	24	4	-	7	78	3	-
10. Post-traumatic stress disorder	189	73	116	6	20	44	3	-	9	32	70	5	-
11. Obsessive-compulsive disorders	944	415	529	-	68	327	14	6	-	85	409	25	9
12. Panic disorder	422	147	275	-	23	109	15	-	-	23	225	24	4
F. Sense organ diseases	926	428	498	2	-	35	190	200	3	-	36	216	242
1. Glaucoma	103	39	64	-	-	1	26	13	-	-	2	45	17
2. Cataracts	816	386	430	2	-	32	164	187	2	-	33	170	224
G. Cardiovascular diseases	1 743	972	771	54	37	342	255	284	49	35	311	173	203
1. Rheumatic heart disease	65	27	38	-	9	17	1	-	-	12	23	2	-
2. Ischaemic heart disease	556	350	206	-	-	63	134	153	-	-	39	69	98
3. Cerebrovascular disease	387	199	188	-	-	96	46	57	-	-	89	48	51
4. Inflammatory heart diseases	231	126	106	14	7	74	18	13	15	4	60	14	12
H. Respiratory diseases	3 555	1 881	1 673	726	289	485	176	206	682	151	469	222	149
1. COPD*	512	240	271	-	-	121	10	109	-	-	130	87	54
2. Asthma	781	526	255	110	194	192	24	7	37	73	123	17	5
I. Digestive diseases	3 248	1 709	1 538	762	111	390	323	124	859	49	279	238	113
1. Peptic ulcer	62	40	22	-	1	27	10	2	-	1	15	6	1
2. Cirrhosis of the liver	155	88	67	4	3	25	40	16	3	14	9	27	14
3. Appendicitis	8	5	3	-	1	3	-	-	-	1	2	-	-
J. Genito-urinary diseases	1 527	920	608	57	69	316	372	105	46	42	266	174	81
1. Nephritis and nephrosis	111	54	57	12	29	11	1	1	12	28	16	1	-
2. Benign prostatic hypertrophy	174	174	-	-	-	-	164	10	-	-	-	-	-
L. Musculo-skeletal diseases	836	371	465	7	5	214	107	38	6	4	201	170	85
1. Rheumatoid arthritis	165	100	66	-	-	96	3	1	-	2	37	20	7
2. Osteoarthritis	600	241	359	-	-	106	100	35	-	-	142	142	75

Annex Table 8h, continued. YLDs by age, sex and cause (thousands): Middle Eastern Crescent, 1990

Cause	Total	Male	Female	Males					Females				
				0-4	5-14	15-44	45-59	60+	0-4	5-14	15-44	45-59	60+
M. Congenital anomalies	**1 633**	**827**	**806**	**827**	–	–	–	–	**806**	–	–	–	–
1. Abdominal wall defect	–	–	–	–	–	–	–	–	–	–	–	–	–
2. Anencephaly	–	–	–	–	–	–	–	–	–	–	–	–	–
3. Anorectal atresia	–	–	–	–	–	–	–	–	–	–	–	–	–
4. Cleft lip	26	15	11	15	–	–	–	–	11	–	–	–	–
5. Cleft palate	27	12	15	12	–	–	–	–	15	–	–	–	–
6. Oesophageal atresia	–	–	–	–	–	–	–	–	–	–	–	–	–
7. Renal agenesis	367	205	161	205	–	–	–	–	161	–	–	–	–
8. Down syndrome	1 057	534	523	534	–	–	–	–	523	–	–	–	–
9. Congenital heart anomalies	156	60	96	60	–	–	–	–	96	–	–	–	–
10. Spina bifida	–	–	–	–	–	–	–	–	–	–	–	–	–
N. Oral conditions	**1 374**	**689**	**686**	**86**	**102**	**298**	**138**	**65**	**83**	**97**	**287**	**142**	**76**
1. Dental caries	692	352	340	85	102	108	35	21	82	97	102	35	24
2. Periodontal disease	20	10	10	–	–	10	–	–	–	–	9	–	–
3. Edentulism	655	325	330	–	–	179	102	44	–	–	171	107	52
III. Injuries	***6 329***	***4 105***	***2 224***	***848***	***969***	***2 110***	***153***	***24***	***732***	***518***	***884***	***71***	***19***
A. Unintentional injuries	**4 562**	**3 090**	**1 472**	**763**	**912**	**1 277**	**118**	**20**	**647**	**442**	**322**	**47**	**14**
1. Road traffic accidents	582	456	126	12	133	287	21	2	11	63	45	6	1
2. Poisonings	27	14	13	12	2	1	–	–	11	2	–	–	–
3. Falls	1 373	876	497	281	377	202	14	2	239	159	82	14	2
4. Fires	275	131	145	29	80	20	2	–	30	83	29	2	–
5. Drownings	–	–	–	–	–	–	–	–	–	–	–	–	–
6. Other unintentional	2 304	1 613	691	429	320	768	81	15	356	135	165	25	10
B. Intentional injuries	**1 767**	**1 014**	**753**	**85**	**57**	**833**	**35**	**5**	**85**	**76**	**562**	**25**	**5**
1. Self-inflicted injuries	82	34	48	–	1	30	3	–	–	2	43	3	–
2. Violence	60	51	9	2	2	46	1	–	1	1	6	–	–
3. War	1 625	929	696	83	54	757	31	4	84	73	513	22	5

Notes:
A dash (-) symbol indicates fewer than 500 YLDs.
*IA6 is Bacterial meningitis and meningococcaemia; ID is Conditions arising during the perinatal period;
IIE6 is Dementia and other degenerative and hereditary CNS disorders; IIH1 is Chronic obstructive pulmonary disease.

Annex Table 8i. YLDs by age, sex and cause (thousands): World, 1990

Cause	Total	Male	Female	Males					Females				
				0-4	5-14	15-44	45-59	60+	0-4	5-14	15-44	45-59	60+
Population (millions)	5 267	2 654	2 614	321	551	1 250	312	219	309	526	1 199	311	269
All causes	472 736	235 096	237 641	44 262	28 047	111 536	30 272	20 979	42 283	21 358	121 931	29 281	22 787
I. Communicable, maternal, perinatal and nutritional conditions	115 372	47 300	68 072	20 137	8 182	15 541	2 226	1 213	19 377	7 134	37 729	2 516	1 316
A. Infectious and parasitic diseases	50 715	24 400	26 315	6 630	5 034	10 659	1 420	657	6 084	4 116	14 106	1 300	709
1. Tuberculosis	4 122	2 407	1 714	35	163	1 460	461	289	36	165	1 119	260	135
2. STDs excluding HIV	12 100	3 244	8 856	891	41	2 299	11	2	904	152	7 778	18	4
a. Syphilis	743	339	405	27	4	305	2	-	26	5	370	3	-
b. Chlamydia	6 706	871	5 834	188	13	666	3	1	190	109	5 522	11	2
c. Gonorrhoea	4 646	2 033	2 614	676	23	1 327	6	1	688	39	1 883	3	1
3. HIV	2 340	1 423	917	6	4	1 349	56	7	6	8	879	21	2
4. Diarrhoeal diseases	5 199	2 626	2 573	943	567	906	145	66	878	543	926	149	77
5. Childhood-cluster diseases	4 068	2 232	1 836	1 963	217	49	3	-	1 588	208	37	2	-
a. Pertussis	1 525	777	749	589	188	-	-	-	568	180	-	-	-
b. Poliomyelitis	2 462	1 408	1 055	1 348	11	46	2	-	1 010	8	35	2	-
c. Diphtheria	1	1	1	-	-	-	-	-	-	-	-	-	-
d. Measles	70	43	27	25	18	-	-	-	10	18	2	-	-
e. Tetanus	9	4	5	-	1	2	-	-	-	2	2	-	-
6. Bacterial meningitis*	1 710	865	845	647	106	88	17	8	630	102	85	18	10
7. Hepatitis B and hepatitis C	64	38	26	1	2	16	11	9	1	2	11	4	8
8. Malaria	3 669	1 862	1 807	1 267	263	274	42	16	1 239	252	257	41	18
9. Tropical-cluster diseases	7 171	4 878	2 293	155	1 399	2 875	382	67	115	594	1 208	329	48
a. Trypanosomiasis	121	65	57	2	17	35	10	1	4	15	32	6	1
b. Chagas disease	341	172	169	-	-	163	8	1	-	-	161	7	-
c. Schistosomiasis	1 364	800	563	26	289	412	56	17	18	198	295	40	12
d. Leishmaniasis	464	290	173	18	116	151	4	2	11	69	89	3	1
e. Lymphatic filariasis	3 997	3 046	952	101	893	1 868	171	11	75	243	443	177	12
f. Onchocerciasis	884	505	379	7	84	246	132	35	6	69	189	95	21
10. Leprosy	338	172	167	5	65	89	12	-	5	63	86	13	-
11. Dengue	6	3	3	-	2	-	-	-	-	3	-	-	-
12. Japanese encephalitis	582	297	285	166	107	22	2	1	161	101	21	2	1
13. Trachoma	1 024	279	745	-	-	72	98	109	-	-	184	256	305
14. Intestinal nematode infections	4 271	2 176	2 095	23	1 576	474	73	29	23	1 509	459	73	30
a. Ascariasis	1 344	687	657	23	661	2	-	-	22	633	2	-	-
b. Trichuriasis	1 519	776	743	1	775	1	-	-	1	741	1	-	-
c. Ancylostomiasis and necatoriasis	1 406	713	693	-	140	471	73	29	-	135	455	73	30

Annex Table 8i, continued. YLDs by age, sex and cause (thousands): World, 1990

Cause	Total	Male	Female	Males 0-4	5-14	15-44	45-59	60+	Females 0-4	5-14	15-44	45-59	60+
B. Respiratory infections	**5 705**	**2 820**	**2 884**	**1 801**	**766**	**184**	**31**	**39**	**1 901**	**732**	**177**	**31**	**44**
1. Lower respiratory infections	4 297	2 103	2 194	1 666	255	127	21	33	1 771	243	121	21	37
2. Upper respiratory infections	197	99	98	6	21	57	9	6	6	20	55	10	7
3. Otitis media	1 211	618	592	128	490	–	–	–	124	468	–	–	–
C. Maternal conditions	**16 528**		**16 528**							**18**	**16 484**	**26**	–
1. Maternal haemorrhage	237		237								237		
2. Maternal sepsis	3 476		3 476								3 476		
3. Hypertensive disorders of pregnancy	75		75								75		
4. Obstructed labour	5 457		5 457								5 457		
5. Abortion	3 304		3 304								3 304		
D. Perinatal conditions*	**9 631**	**4 878**	**4 753**	**4 878**					**4 753**				
E. Nutritional deficiencies	**32 792**	**15 201**	**17 592**	**6 828**	**2 382**	**4 699**	**775**	**517**	**6 639**	**2 269**	**6 963**	**1 158**	**563**
1. Protein-energy malnutrition	9 878	5 006	4 871	5 006	6	6	1	–	4 871	10	23	4	1
2. Iodine deficiency	766	375	391	363					353				
3. Vitamin A deficiency	116	59	57	59					57				
4. Iron-deficiency anaemia	21 987	9 748	12 239	1 396	2 370	4 691	774	516	1 353	2 253	6 920	1 152	561
II. Noncommunicable diseases	***281 237***	***139 689***	***141 548***	***15 824***	***6 472***	***72 789***	***25 398***	***19 206***	***15 245***	***5 645***	***74 480***	***25 267***	***20 910***
A. Malignant neoplasms	**5 677**	**3 189**	**2 488**	**13**	**61**	**541**	**865**	**1 709**	**13**	**55**	**693**	**768**	**959**
1. Mouth and oropharynx cancers	496	316	180		4	108	93	111		6	70	51	54
2. Oesophagus cancer	203	127	76			14	44	69			25	22	30
3. Stomach cancer	711	481	230		1	56	157	267			47	77	106
4. Colon and rectum cancers	691	366	325		1	49	94	222		1	40	79	205
5. Liver cancer	217	170	47		2	53	72	43			10	17	19
6. Pancreas cancer	94	56	38			7	14	35			5	16	17
7. Trachea, bronchus, lung cancers	568	410	158			41	136	233			19	48	91
8. Melanoma and other skin cancers	57	28	29			9	8	11			12	8	10
9. Breast cancer	425		425								133	149	143
10. Cervix uteri cancer	193		193								74	76	44
11. Corpus uteri cancer	68		68								19	49	
12. Ovary cancer	95		95								43	27	24
13. Prostate cancer	290	290					35	252					
14. Bladder cancer	239	205	34			10	34	160			4	8	22
15. Lymphomas and multiple myeloma	151	91	60		11	31	20	28		6	17	12	24
16. Leukaemia	146	80	66	4	16	29	13	18	4	13	25	10	15
C. Diabetes mellitus	**5 333**	**2 548**	**2 786**	**2**	**6**	**840**	**1 001**	**699**	**2**	**7**	**827**	**1 066**	**885**
D. Endocrine disorders	**3 724**	**1 597**	**2 127**	**621**	**182**	**440**	**222**	**131**	**585**	**172**	**742**	**386**	**241**

Annex Table 8i, continued. YLDs by age, sex and cause (thousands): World, 1990

Cause	Total	Male	Female	Males 0-4	5-14	15-44	45-59	60+	Females 0-4	5-14	15-44	45-59	60+
E. Neuro-psychiatric conditions	**134 526**	**65 828**	**68 697**	**1 269**	**2 551**	**53 241**	**5 564**	**3 204**	**1 228**	**2 532**	**53 415**	**6 548**	**4 975**
1. Unipolar major depression	50 810	18 070	32 740			15 321	2 189	559			27 651	3 925	1 165
2. Bipolar disorder	14 141	7 203	6 938			6 713	373	117			6 436	367	134
3. Schizophrenia	12 183	6 397	5 786			6 397					5 786		
4. Epilepsy	3 709	1 910	1 798	79	606	995	166	64	89	728	803	113	65
5. Alcohol use	15 770	13 935	1 836			12 689	1 036	209			1 696	103	36
6. Dementia*	7 064	2 938	4 126	221	84	156	715	1 762	237	91	168	779	2 851
7. Parkinson disease	809	369	440				173	196				180	260
8. Multiple sclerosis	1 065	464	602			451	11	1			585	17	
9. Drug use	5 375	4 308	1 067		342	3 818	127	21		85	946	32	5
10. Post-traumatic stress disorder	1 945	741	1 204	43	165	482	42	8	70	267	785	67	14
11. Obsessive-compulsive disorders	10 213	4 435	5 778		569	3 571	200	95		722	4 552	352	152
12. Panic disorder	4 766	1 603	3 163		163	1 223	215	1		197	2 568	338	61
F. Sense organ diseases	**10 126**	**4 569**	**5 558**	**49**	**8**	**415**	**2 071**	**2 025**	**45**	**14**	**509**	**2 504**	**2 485**
1. Glaucoma	2 503	965	1 538			76	592	296			132	990	416
2. Cataracts	7 439	3 534	3 905	21	3	324	1 464	1 721	22	3	329	1 493	2 058
G. Cardiovascular diseases	**16 911**	**9 447**	**7 463**	**147**	**148**	**2 983**	**2 636**	**3 534**	**125**	**141**	**2 683**	**1 820**	**2 694**
1. Rheumatic heart disease	664	278	386		28	133	63	53		39	171	101	75
2. Ischaemic heart disease	5 105	3 277	1 828			391	1 233	1 653			254	561	1 013
3. Cerebrovascular disease	6 408	3 288	3 120			1 171	855	1 262	51		1 147	829	1 144
4. Inflammatory heart diseases	1 974	1 073	901	48	49	678	175	123		36	530	140	145
H. Respiratory diseases	**35 616**	**19 253**	**16 363**	**3 092**	**1 877**	**5 994**	**4 180**	**4 110**	**2 709**	**1 304**	**5 472**	**3 314**	**3 564**
1. COPD*	14 692	8 357	6 335			2 620	2 655	3 083			1 967	1 885	2 483
2. Asthma	9 111	5 025	4 086	736	1 493	2 288	380	129	469	1 001	2 125	364	126
I. Digestive diseases	**21 422**	**11 247**	**10 175**	**2 733**	**492**	**3 297**	**3 321**	**1 405**	**2 764**	**368**	**2 855**	**2 571**	**1 617**
1. Peptic ulcer	977	624	353		15	403	175	30	1	8	223	101	20
2. Cirrhosis of the liver	2 633	1 834	799	54	11	617	865	287	41	18	198	346	195
3. Appendicitis	88	52	36		12	35	3	1		9	23	2	1
J. Genito-urinary diseases	**5 433**	**3 384**	**2 049**	**206**	**260**	**599**	**1 825**	**494**	**139**	**217**	**777**	**558**	**357**
1. Nephritis and nephrosis	770	391	379	75	176	112	17	10	79	168	108	15	10
2. Benign prostatic hypertrophy	1 656	1 656					1 417	239					
L. Musculo-skeletal diseases	**17 941**	**6 599**	**11 342**	**26**	**53**	**2 654**	**2 714**	**1 153**	**36**	**74**	**4 420**	**4 604**	**2 207**
1. Rheumatoid arthritis	3 168	859	2 309			426	275	158		26	1 218	611	454
2. Osteoarthritis	13 275	5 341	7 934			2 083	2 354	903			2 591	3 745	1 598

Annex Table 8i, continued. YLDs by age, sex and cause (thousands): World, 1990

Cause	Total	Male	Female	Males					Females				
				0-4	5-14	15-44	45-59	60+	0-4	5-14	15-44	45-59	60+
M. Congenital anomalies	**13 507**	**6 740**	**6 767**	**6 740**	-	-	-	-	**6 767**	-	-	-	-
1. Abdominal wall defect	-	-	-	-	-	-	-	-	-	-	-	-	-
2. Anencephaly	-	-	-	-	-	-	-	-	-	-	-	-	-
3. Anorectal atresia	-	-	-	-	-	-	-	-	-	-	-	-	-
4. Cleft lip	241	135	106	135					106				
5. Cleft palate	200	91	108	91					108				
6. Oesophageal atresia	-	-	-	-					-				
7. Renal agenesis													
8. Down syndrome	2 891	1 617	1 274	1 617					1 274				
9. Congenital heart anomalies	8 053	4 071	3 982	4 071					3 982				
10. Spina bifida	2 122	824	1 297	824					1 297				
N. Oral conditions	**7 430**	**3 659**	**3 771**	**459**	**628**	**1 301**	**685**	**586**	**442**	**618**	**1 305**	**711**	**695**
1. Dental caries	4 313	2 174	2 139	455	625	751	216	127	439	610	726	217	147
2. Periodontal disease	255	128	127	-	-	104	16	7	-	-	103	16	8
3. Edentulism	2 787	1 339	1 448	-	-	437	451	451	-	-	432	476	539
III. Injuries	***76 128***	***48 107***	***28 021***	***8 301***	***13 393***	***23 205***	***2 648***	***560***	***7 660***	***8 579***	***9 722***	***1 499***	***561***
A. Unintentional injuries	**67 652**	**43 336**	**24 316**	**7 964**	**13 118**	**19 282**	**2 440**	**532**	**7 297**	**8 292**	**6 868**	**1 324**	**535**
1. Road traffic accidents	8 154	5 834	2 321	230	1 509	3 627	404	64	147	900	1 061	171	43
2. Poisonings	365	191	174	133	36	19	2	1	76	35	11	49	4
3. Falls	21 949	13 474	8 475	2 884	6 453	3 621	419	97	2 868	2 948	1 923	521	214
4. Fires	4 580	1 761	2 819	392	1 010	316	38	5	369	1 864	547	32	7
5. Drownings	6	4	2	1	1	1	-	-	1	-	-	-	-
6. Other unintentional	32 598	22 073	10 525	4 324	4 109	11 699	1 577	365	3 835	2 545	3 327	551	268
B. Intentional injuries	**8 475**	**4 770**	**3 705**	**337**	**275**	**3 923**	**208**	**28**	**363**	**287**	**2 854**	**175**	**26**
1. Self-inflicted injuries	1 736	522	1 214	-	2	455	61	4	-	3	1 114	91	6
2. Violence	1 932	1 488	444	97	114	1 210	56	11	119	69	228	21	7
3. War	4 807	2 760	2 047	239	159	2 258	91	13	244	215	1 512	63	13

Notes:
A dash (-) symbol indicates fewer than 500 YLDs.
*IA6 is Bacterial meningitis and meningococcaemia; ID is Conditions arising during the perinatal period;
IIE6 is Dementia and other degenerative and hereditary CNS disorders; IIH1 is Chronic obstructive pulmonary disease.

Annex Table 9a. DALYs by age, sex and cause (thousands): Established Market Economies, 1990

Cause	Total	Male	Female	Males					Females				
				0-4	5-14	15-44	45-59	60+	0-4	5-14	15-44	45-59	60+
Population (millions)	798	390	407	26	53	184	66	61	25	51	179	68	85
All causes	98 794	54 715	44 080	3 250	1 457	22 039	11 253	16 716	2 625	1 051	15 724	8 360	16 320
I. Communicable, maternal, perinatal and nutritional conditions	7 049	3 664	3 386	1 316	149	1 245	331	623	1 021	145	1 371	208	641
A. Infectious and parasitic diseases	2 750	1 642	1 108	164	46	1 071	221	139	139	48	709	77	134
1. Tuberculosis	118	85	33	-	-	22	25	36	-	-	8	7	17
2. STDs excluding HIV	404	25	379	1	-	23	1	1	-	3	371	7	2
a. Syphilis	6	4	2	1	-	2	1	1	-	-	1	2	-
b. Chlamydia	349	14	336	-	-	13	-	-	-	4	330	1	-
c. Gonorrhoea	44	8	37	-	-	8	-	-	-	-	36	-	-
3. HIV	1 267	1 077	191	17	3	899	144	13	13	3	156	16	3
4. Diarrhoeal diseases	230	117	113	45	10	42	11	9	41	9	39	11	12
5. Childhood-cluster diseases	41	22	19	15	5	1	1	1	12	5	1	1	1
a. Pertussis	25	13	12	10	3	-	-	-	10	3	-	-	-
b. Poliomyelitis	3	2	1	-	-	1	-	1	-	-	-	-	1
c. Diphtheria	-	-	-	-	-	-	-	-	-	-	-	-	-
d. Measles	11	7	4	5	2	-	-	-	2	2	-	-	-
e. Tetanus	1	1	1	-	-	-	-	-	-	-	-	-	-
6. Bacterial meningitis*	181	97	84	62	10	15	5	5	53	11	11	4	5
7. Hepatitis B and hepatitis C	54	34	21	1	1	15	9	7	1	-	9	5	6
8. Malaria	2	1	1	-	-	1	-	-	-	-	-	-	-
9. Tropical-cluster diseases	2	1	1	-	-	1	-	-	-	-	-	-	-
a. Trypanosomiasis	-	-	-	-	-	-	-	-	-	-	-	-	-
b. Chagas disease	-	-	-	-	-	-	-	-	-	-	-	-	-
c. Schistosomiasis	-	-	-	-	-	-	-	-	-	-	-	-	-
d. Leishmaniasis	1	1	1	-	-	1	-	-	-	-	-	-	-
e. Lymphatic filariasis	-	-	-	-	-	-	-	-	-	-	-	-	-
f. Onchocerciasis	-	-	-	-	-	-	-	-	-	-	-	-	-
10. Leprosy	1	1	1	-	-	1	-	-	-	-	-	-	-
11. Dengue	-	-	-	-	-	-	-	-	-	-	-	-	-
12. Japanese encephalitis	-	-	-	-	-	-	-	-	-	-	-	-	-
13. Trachoma	-	-	-	-	-	-	-	-	-	-	-	-	-
14. Intestinal nematode infections	-	-	-	-	-	-	-	-	-	-	-	-	-
a. Ascariasis	-	-	-	-	-	-	-	-	-	-	-	-	-
b. Trichuriasis	-	-	-	-	-	-	-	-	-	-	-	-	-
c. Ancylostomiasis and necatoriasis	-	-	-	-	-	-	-	-	-	-	-	-	-

Annex Table 9a, continued. DALYs by age, sex and cause (thousands): Established Market Economies, 1990

Cause	Total	Male	Female	Males 0-4	Males 5-14	Males 15-44	Males 45-59	Males 60+	Females 0-4	Females 5-14	Females 15-44	Females 45-59	Females 60+
B. Respiratory infections	**1 346**	**720**	**626**	**74**	**50**	**95**	**85**	**416**	**53**	**47**	**64**	**49**	**414**
1. Lower respiratory infections	1 208	648	559	57	14	84	82	411	40	13	54	46	408
2. Upper respiratory infections	55	29	26	8	3	10	3	4	5	2	10	3	6
3. Otitis media	84	43	41	9	33	-	-	-	8	32	-	-	-
C. Maternal conditions	**330**	**-**	**330**	**-**	**-**	**-**	**-**	**-**	**-**	**-**	**329**	**-**	**-**
1. Maternal haemorrhage	19		19								19		
2. Maternal sepsis	34		34								34		
3. Hypertensive disorders of pregnancy	14		14								14		
4. Obstructed labour	230		230								230		
5. Abortion	12		12								12		
D. Perinatal conditions*	**1 767**	**1 007**	**761**	**1 005**	**1**	**1**	**-**	**-**	**760**	**-**	**-**	**-**	**-**
E. Nutritional deficiencies	**856**	**295**	**561**	**73**	**51**	**79**	**25**	**67**	**69**	**49**	**268**	**82**	**92**
1. Protein-energy malnutrition	88	43	45	33	-	2	2	7	32	-	1	1	11
2. Iodine deficiency	21	10	11	10	-	-	-	-	10	-	-	-	-
3. Vitamin A deficiency													
4. Iron-deficiency anaemia	737	237	500	30	51	76	21	60	27	49	263	80	81
II. Noncommunicable diseases	***79 987***	***42 557***	***37 430***	***1 600***	***806***	***14 735***	***9 872***	***15 544***	***1 377***	***656***	***12 517***	***7 684***	***15 196***
A. Malignant neoplasms	**14 843**	**8 333**	**6 510**	**41**	**87**	**1 079**	**2 604**	**4 523**	**33**	**66**	**1 149**	**2 026**	**3 236**
1. Mouth and oropharynx cancers	362	289	74	-	-	49	137	102	-	-	13	26	34
2. Oesophagus cancer	346	279	67			23	121	136			5	20	43
3. Stomach cancer	1 061	668	392			73	217	378			68	106	218
4. Colon and rectum cancers	1 626	863	763		1	81	262	520		1	71	204	487
5. Liver cancer	321	248	73		1	23	106	116		1	7	20	45
6. Pancreas cancer	596	337	259			31	116	189			18	72	169
7. Trachea, bronchus, lung cancers	2 987	2 183	804			148	769	1 264			69	273	461
8. Melanoma and other skin cancers	248	147	101			54	46	47			39	29	33
9. Breast cancer	1 421	-	1 421								332	558	531
10. Cervix uteri cancer	192	-	192								80	62	51
11. Corpus uteri cancer	185	-	185								25	66	94
12. Ovary cancer	375	-	375								63	145	166
13. Prostate cancer	574	574	-			4	61	508					
14. Bladder cancer	370	296	74			8	53	234			4	13	58
15. Lymphomas and multiple myeloma	701	408	293	2	10	126	113	158	1	4	66	72	149
16. Leukaemia	602	346	256	13	35	124	67	107	11	24	83	51	86
C. Diabetes mellitus	**2 357**	**1 087**	**1 270**	**3**	**4**	**265**	**373**	**443**	**2**	**5**	**244**	**373**	**645**
D. Endocrine disorders	**1 257**	**535**	**721**	**103**	**63**	**175**	**70**	**125**	**97**	**47**	**235**	**175**	**167**

Annex Table 9a, continued. DALYs by age, sex and cause (thousands): Established Market Economies, 1990

Cause	Total	Male	Female	Males 0-4	Males 5-14	Males 15-44	Males 45-59	Males 60+	Females 0-4	Females 5-14	Females 15-44	Females 45-59	Females 60+
E. Neuro-psychiatric conditions	**24 747**	**12 892**	**11 855**	**141**	**324**	**9 588**	**1 510**	**1 328**	**118**	**272**	**7 803**	**1 511**	**2 151**
1. Unipolar major depression	6 684	2 331	4 353	-	-	1 830	381	121	-	-	3 359	706	287
2. Bipolar disorder	1 709	860	849	-	-	770	63	26	-	-	750	64	35
3. Schizophrenia	2 249	1 173	1 076	-	-	1 147	10	17	-	-	1 051	4	21
4. Epilepsy	505	270	236	9	50	151	43	18	9	51	114	38	24
5. Alcohol use	4 690	3 955	736	-	-	3 370	470	115	-	-	615	86	34
6. Dementia*	2 866	1 124	1 743	40	17	51	237	778	39	14	42	252	1 396
7. Parkinson disease	447	202	245	-	-	1	65	137	-	-	-	71	173
8. Multiple sclerosis	236	99	136	-	-	79	13	7	-	-	105	21	11
9. Drug use	1 522	1 149	372	-	85	1 027	33	5	-	28	331	11	2
10. Post-traumatic stress disorder	269	102	168	4	16	71	9	2	6	26	117	15	4
11. Obsessive-compulsive disorders	1 454	620	834	-	53	502	41	25	-	66	650	74	44
12. Panic disorder	688	228	460	-	18	167	42	-	-	18	356	69	18
F. Sense organ diseases	**109**	**50**	**59**	**1**	**-**	**4**	**20**	**24**	**1**	**-**	**2**	**22**	**34**
1. Glaucoma	71	32	39	-	-	2	17	13	-	-	1	19	20
2. Cataracts	33	16	18	-	-	1	3	11	-	-	1	3	13
G. Cardiovascular diseases	**18 339**	**10 409**	**7 930**	**62**	**28**	**1 430**	**2 714**	**6 176**	**50**	**22**	**723**	**1 170**	**5 965**
1. Rheumatic heart disease	163	58	105	-	-	14	17	26	-	-	15	28	61
2. Ischaemic heart disease	8 876	5 418	3 459	-	-	490	1 589	3 339	-	-	133	484	2 841
3. Cerebrovascular disease	4 977	2 423	2 554	9	6	395	552	1 460	7	5	305	427	1 810
4. Inflammatory heart diseases	684	412	272	12	6	169	111	114	14	5	84	52	116
H. Respiratory diseases	**4 773**	**2 798**	**1 975**	**112**	**139**	**620**	**572**	**1 356**	**78**	**88**	**547**	**413**	**849**
1. COPD*	2 284	1 475	809	5	2	112	328	1 029	3	1	59	198	549
2. Asthma	1 236	657	579	48	119	329	94	67	30	77	307	92	73
I. Digestive diseases	**4 307**	**2 456**	**1 850**	**67**	**21**	**687**	**909**	**772**	**47**	**18**	**443**	**524**	**819**
1. Peptic ulcer	239	145	94	1	1	43	42	58	1	1	23	20	50
2. Cirrhosis of the liver	1 584	1 105	479	1	1	300	506	298	1	2	110	187	180
3. Appendicitis	36	21	15	-	3	11	3	4	-	3	7	2	4
J. Genito-urinary diseases	**1 105**	**617**	**488**	**20**	**3**	**81**	**183**	**330**	**16**	**5**	**83**	**96**	**288**
1. Nephritis and nephrosis	446	241	204	16	2	46	45	133	12	3	23	31	135
2. Benign prostatic hypertrophy	205	205	-	-	-	-	100	105	-	-	-	-	-
L. Musculo-skeletal diseases	**4 125**	**1 375**	**2 750**	**2**	**-**	**418**	**697**	**254**	**2**	**11**	**876**	**1 116**	**745**
1. Rheumatoid arthritis	935	217	718	-	3	58	88	71	-	4	331	160	222
2. Osteoarthritis	2 701	1 044	1 657	-	-	323	578	144	-	-	371	865	420

Annex Table 9a, continued. DALYs by age, sex and cause (thousands): Established Market Economies, 1990

Cause	Total	Male	Female	Males					Females				
				0-4	5-14	15-44	45-59	60+	0-4	5-14	15-44	45-59	60+
M. Congenital anomalies	**2 133**	**1 136**	**997**	**1 015**	**31**	**68**	**12**	**8**	**899**	**28**	**48**	**12**	**10**
1. Abdominal wall defect	15	5	10	5	-	-	-	-	10	-	-	-	-
2. Anencephaly	87	35	52	35	-	-	-	-	52	-	-	-	-
3. Anorectal atresia	3	1	2	1	-	-	-	-	2	-	-	-	-
4. Cleft lip	24	13	12	13	-	-	-	-	12	-	-	-	-
5. Cleft palate	21	9	13	9	-	-	-	-	13	-	-	-	-
6. Oesophageal atresia	8	3	4	3	-	-	-	-	4	-	-	-	-
7. Renal agenesis	62	32	30	32	-	-	-	-	30	-	-	-	-
8. Down syndrome	284	160	123	147	3	3	5	3	112	2	2	5	2
9. Congenital heart anomalies	1 096	581	515	517	15	38	6	4	466	13	25	6	5
10. Spina bifida	148	63	85	56	3	3	-	-	78	2	3	1	-
N. Oral conditions	**870**	**417**	**452**	**13**	**69**	**181**	**81**	**74**	**13**	**66**	**177**	**87**	**109**
1. Dental caries	405	202	203	13	69	88	16	17	12	66	85	16	23
2. Periodontal disease	35	18	18	-	-	16	1	1	-	-	15	1	1
3. Edentulism	423	195	229	-	-	76	63	56	-	-	76	69	84
III. Injuries	***11 758***	***8 494***	***3 264***	***334***	***502***	***6 059***	***1 050***	***549***	***227***	***250***	***1 836***	***467***	***483***
A. Unintentional injuries	**8 608**	**6 164**	**2 444**	**311**	**468**	**4 251**	**721**	**414**	**205**	**230**	**1 278**	**322**	**409**
1. Road traffic accidents	4 310	3 112	1 197	55	206	2 466	269	116	41	120	850	112	74
2. Poisonings	276	206	70	5	4	168	21	7	4	2	48	10	6
3. Falls	1 350	804	547	57	86	420	131	109	36	35	163	115	198
4. Fires	261	162	99	29	37	67	18	12	22	30	28	9	10
5. Drownings	276	222	54	36	35	119	20	12	18	8	16	5	6
6. Other unintentional	2 135	1 657	478	129	100	1 010	261	157	85	34	172	70	115
B. Intentional injuries	**3 150**	**2 331**	**819**	**23**	**34**	**1 808**	**330**	**135**	**22**	**20**	**558**	**146**	**73**
1. Self-inflicted injuries	2 155	1 573	582	-	13	1 157	279	124	-	4	383	128	67
2. Violence	993	756	237	23	21	650	50	11	22	16	175	17	7
3. War	2	1	-	-	-	1	-	-	-	-	-	-	-

Notes:

A dash (-) symbol indicates fewer than 500 DALYs.

[a]IA6 is Bacterial meningitis and meningococcaemia; ID is Conditions arising during the perinatal period;
IIE6 is Dementia and other degenerative and hereditary CNS disorders; IIH1 is Chronic obstructive pulmonary disease.

Annex Table 9b. DALYs by age, sex and cause (thousands): Formerly Socialist Economies of Europe, 1990

Cause	Total	Male	Female	Males 0-4	5-14	15-44	45-59	60+	Females 0-4	5-14	15-44	45-59	60+
Population (millions)	*346*	*165*	*181*	*14*	*27*	*76*	*27*	*21*	*13*	*26*	*75*	*30*	*36*
All causes	**62 200**	**35 664**	**26 536**	**3 079**	**1 261**	**14 904**	**8 790**	**7 630**	**2 395**	**828**	**9 040**	**5 367**	**8 905**
I. Communicable, maternal, perinatal and nutritional conditions	**5 451**	**2 567**	**2 884**	**1 540**	**153**	**414**	**230**	**229**	**1 144**	**145**	**1 206**	**106**	**283**
A. Infectious and parasitic diseases	1 659	821	838	278	42	287	143	71	227	40	468	40	63
1. Tuberculosis	378	324	54	2	–	167	114	41	1	1	24	14	13
2. STDs excluding HIV	382	52	329	5	1	44	1	–	5	4	318	2	1
a. Syphilis	3	2	1	–	–	1	–	–	–	–	1	–	–
b. Chlamydia	296	20	276	2	–	17	–	–	2	4	269	1	–
c. Gonorrhoea	77	26	51	3	–	23	–	–	3	1	47	–	–
3. HIV	41	25	16	10	2	13	1	–	10	2	3	–	–
4. Diarrhoeal diseases	235	123	113	91	6	18	5	3	80	6	17	5	5
5. Childhood-cluster diseases	39	21	18	14	4	2	1	–	12	4	1	1	1
a. Pertussis	24	12	12	9	3	–	–	–	9	3	–	–	–
b. Poliomyelitis	1	1	–	1	–	–	–	–	–	–	–	–	–
c. Diphtheria	1	–	1	–	–	–	–	–	1	–	–	–	–
d. Measles	11	7	5	4	1	1	1	–	2	1	1	–	–
e. Tetanus	2	1	1	–	–	1	–	–	–	–	–	1	1
6. Bacterial meningitis*	228	129	98	82	9	21	10	8	64	8	14	6	7
7. Hepatitis B and hepatitis C	37	20	17	7	2	6	2	2	6	1	7	2	2
8. Malaria	–	–	–	–	–	–	–	–	–	–	–	–	–
9. Tropical-cluster diseases	–	–	–	–	–	–	–	–	–	–	–	–	–
a. Trypanosomiasis	–	–	–	–	–	–	–	–	–	–	–	–	–
b. Chagas disease	–	–	–	–	–	–	–	–	–	–	–	–	–
c. Schistosomiasis	–	–	–	–	–	–	–	–	–	–	–	–	–
d. Leishmaniasis	–	–	–	–	–	–	–	–	–	–	–	–	–
e. Lymphatic filariasis	–	–	–	–	–	–	–	–	–	–	–	–	–
f. Onchocerciasis	–	–	–	–	–	–	–	–	–	–	–	–	–
10. Leprosy	–	–	–	–	–	–	–	–	–	–	–	–	–
11. Dengue	–	–	–	–	–	–	–	–	–	–	–	–	–
12. Japanese encephalitis	–	–	–	–	–	–	–	–	–	–	–	–	–
13. Trachoma	–	–	–	–	–	–	–	–	–	–	–	–	–
14. Intestinal nematode infections	2	–	2	–	–	–	–	–	–	–	2	–	–
a. Ascariasis	2	–	2	–	–	–	–	–	–	–	2	–	–
b. Trichuriasis	–	–	–	–	–	–	–	–	–	–	–	–	–
c. Ancylostomiasis and necatoriasis	–	–	–	–	–	–	–	–	–	–	–	–	–

Annex Table 9b, continued. DALYs by age, sex and cause (thousands): Formerly Socialist Economies of Europe, 1990

Cause	Total	Male	Female	Males					Females				
				0-4	5-14	15-44	45-59	60+	0-4	5-14	15-44	45-59	60+
B. Respiratory infections	1 256	698	558	351	47	92	74	134	271	44	44	24	175
1. Lower respiratory infections	1 184	661	523	339	28	88	73	133	261	26	40	23	174
2. Upper respiratory infections	24	12	12	5	1	4	1	1	4	-	4	1	2
3. Otitis media	48	25	23	8	17	-	-	-	6	17	-	-	-
C. Maternal conditions	565	-	565	-	-	-	-	-	-	-	565	-	-
1. Maternal haemorrhage	14	-	14	-	-	-	-	-	-	-	14	-	-
2. Maternal sepsis	108	-	108	-	-	-	-	-	-	-	108	-	-
3. Hypertensive disorders of pregnancy	10	-	10	-	-	-	-	-	-	-	10	-	-
4. Obstructed labour	155	-	155	-	-	-	-	-	-	-	155	-	-
5. Abortion	158	-	158	-	-	-	-	-	-	-	158	-	-
D. Perinatal conditions*	1 353	806	547	806	-	-	-	-	547	-	-	-	-
E. Nutritional deficiencies	618	241	376	105	64	35	13	24	100	62	129	41	45
1. Protein-energy malnutrition	111	55	55	51	-	1	1	2	50	-	1	1	4
2. Iodine deficiency	21	9	11	9	-	-	-	-	10	-	-	-	-
3. Vitamin A deficiency	-	-	-	-	-	-	-	-	-	-	-	-	-
4. Iron-deficiency anaemia	411	147	265	31	57	29	9	20	30	55	109	36	35
II. Noncommunicable diseases	45 145	24 156	20 989	1 038	487	8 369	7 186	7 075	873	403	6 498	4 845	8 371
A. Malignant neoplasms	7 253	4 288	2 965	44	78	719	1 865	1 582	33	52	619	1 058	1 203
1. Mouth and oropharynx cancers	233	202	31		1	42	110	49			8	11	13
2. Oesophagus cancer	115	98	16			13	55	31			2	6	8
3. Stomach cancer	1 023	648	374			95	295	258			59	127	189
4. Colon and rectum cancers	673	333	340			48	124	160			42	113	185
5. Liver cancer	189	112	78	1		15	46	48	1	1	8	24	44
6. Pancreas cancer	275	168	107			25	76	67			11	36	60
7. Trachea, bronchus, lung cancers	1 600	1 360	240		1	139	713	506		1	35	94	110
8. Melanoma and other skin cancers	102	52	50			20	17	14			19	14	17
9. Breast cancer	509	-	509								130	227	152
10. Cervix uteri cancer	186	-	186								61	65	59
11. Corpus uteri cancer	134	-	134								22	57	55
12. Ovary cancer	189	-	189								43	84	62
13. Prostate cancer	108	108	-				23	81					
14. Bladder cancer	149	119	29			4	41	71			3	8	18
15. Lymphomas and multiple myeloma	248	152	96	5	15	62	42	28	3	6	37	24	27
16. Leukaemia	298	170	128	14	30	59	35	32	11	20	41	27	29
C. Diabetes mellitus	665	281	384	1	2	83	100	96	1	2	75	114	192
D. Endocrine disorders	246	101	145	23	9	50	14	6	21	9	66	34	15

Annex Table 9b, continued. DALYs by age, sex and cause (thousands): Formerly Socialist Economies of Europe, 1990

Cause	Total	Male	Female	Males					Females				
				0-4	5-14	15-44	45-59	60+	0-4	5-14	15-44	45-59	60+
E. Neuro-psychiatric conditions	**10 704**	**5 480**	**5 223**	**124**	**241**	**4 066**	**643**	**406**	**107**	**193**	**3 430**	**684**	**809**
1. Unipolar major depression	3 095	1 056	2 039	-	-	834	172	50	-	-	1 551	345	143
2. Bipolar disorder	834	411	422	-	-	364	32	15	-	-	356	35	31
3. Schizophrenia	857	446	410	-	-	432	9	6	-	-	399	4	7
4. Epilepsy	379	234	145	9	58	126	29	12	9	42	61	21	12
5. Alcohol use	1 756	1 545	211	-	-	1 306	192	46	-	-	185	16	9
6. Dementia*	950	336	613	21	11	20	81	203	19	9	18	102	465
7. Parkinson disease	127	50	77	-	-	-	18	31	-	-	-	22	55
8. Multiple sclerosis	121	51	70	-	-	38	7	5	-	-	52	10	8
9. Drug use	532	425	106	-	34	377	13	2	-	8	94	3	1
10. Post-traumatic stress disorder	118	44	73	2	8	29	4	1	3	13	49	6	2
11. Obsessive-compulsive disorders	644	271	373	-	28	217	17	9	-	36	283	34	20
12. Panic disorder	308	101	207	-	10	73	18	-	-	10	157	32	8
F. Sense organ diseases	**64**	**25**	**38**	-	-	**1**	**7**	**17**	-	-	**2**	**13**	**22**
1. Glaucoma	29	10	20	-	-	1	4	6	-	-	1	10	8
2. Cataracts	34	16	18	-	-	1	3	12	-	-	1	3	14
G. Cardiovascular diseases	**14 449**	**7 945**	**6 505**	**25**	**15**	**1 374**	**2 764**	**3 766**	**23**	**12**	**499**	**1 243**	**4 729**
1. Rheumatic heart disease	383	176	206	-	2	74	76	24	-	2	48	103	54
2. Ischaemic heart disease	7 074	4 264	2 810	-	-	670	1 672	1 921	-	-	120	516	2 174
3. Cerebrovascular disease	4 447	2 045	2 402	4	3	292	637	1 110	3	3	215	499	1 683
4. Inflammatory heart diseases	466	283	183	5	4	127	87	60	7	3	51	46	77
H. Respiratory diseases	**2 958**	**1 828**	**1 130**	**40**	**53**	**423**	**706**	**606**	**28**	**37**	**295**	**287**	**483**
1. COPD*	1 081	747	333	-	1	127	339	281	1	-	59	72	202
2. Asthma	497	258	239	21	50	125	38	24	13	33	119	41	32
I. Digestive diseases	**2 752**	**1 578**	**1 174**	**77**	**15**	**636**	**553**	**297**	**55**	**13**	**343**	**390**	**374**
1. Peptic ulcer	203	146	57	-	1	53	57	35	-	-	19	18	20
2. Cirrhosis of the liver	761	508	253	2	1	140	239	125	2	2	51	106	93
3. Appendicitis	18	10	8	-	2	5	1	2	-	1	4	1	2
J. Genito-urinary diseases	**988**	**475**	**514**	**8**	**8**	**155**	**161**	**142**	**5**	**9**	**174**	**187**	**138**
1. Nephritis and nephrosis	276	154	122	3	5	73	44	30	3	6	47	33	31
2. Benign prostatic hypertrophy	112	112	-	-	-	-	52	60	-	-	-	-	-
L. Musculo-skeletal diseases	**2 736**	**1 011**	**1 725**	**2**	**5**	**638**	**256**	**110**	**2**	**9**	**733**	**662**	**320**
1. Rheumatoid arthritis	490	116	375	-	-	68	29	19	-	3	218	97	57
2. Osteoarthritis	1 980	826	1 154	-	-	528	212	85	-	-	411	503	239

Annex Table 9b, continued. DALYs by age, sex and cause (thousands): Formerly Socialist Economies of Europe, 1990

Cause	Total	Male	Female	Males					Females				
				0-4	5-14	15-44	45-59	60+	0-4	5-14	15-44	45-59	60+
M. Congenital anomalies	**1 347**	**725**	**622**	**662**	**26**	**32**	**4**	**1**	**569**	**25**	**22**	**4**	**1**
1. Abdominal wall defect	9	3	6	3	-	-	-	-	6	-	-	-	-
2. Anencephaly	26	10	16	10	-	-	-	-	16	-	-	-	-
3. Anorectal atresia	1	1	1	1	-	-	-	-	1	-	-	-	-
4. Cleft lip	16	10	6	10	-	-	-	-	6	-	-	-	-
5. Cleft palate	13	6	6	6	-	-	-	-	6	-	-	-	-
6. Oesophageal atresia	4	2	2	2	-	-	-	-	2	-	-	-	-
7. Renal agenesis	15	7	7	7	-	-	-	-	7	-	-	-	-
8. Down syndrome	109	62	47	55	3	1	-	-	42	1	1	-	-
9. Congenital heart anomalies	680	364	317	330	10	22	2	1	295	9	11	3	1
10. Spina bifida	134	59	74	54	3	1	1	-	70	3	1	2	-
N. Oral conditions	**481**	**219**	**262**	**16**	**21**	**96**	**60**	**25**	**15**	**31**	**100**	**72**	**44**
1. Dental caries	243	112	130	16	21	45	19	10	15	31	45	21	18
2. Periodontal disease	17	7	10	-	-	5	1	1	-	-	8	1	1
3. Edentulism	221	99	122	-	-	46	40	13	-	-	47	49	25
III. Injuries	***11 604***	***8 941***	***2 663***	***501***	***621***	***6 120***	***1 373***	***325***	***378***	***280***	***1 337***	***417***	***251***
A. Unintentional injuries	**7 994**	**6 334**	**1 660**	**379**	**517**	**4 209**	**1 002**	**228**	**257**	**211**	**715**	**291**	**187**
1. Road traffic accidents	2 754	2 240	514	39	164	1 701	270	66	24	84	287	77	43
2. Poisonings	905	706	199	47	17	412	195	35	34	12	78	53	21
3. Falls	1 098	761	337	61	90	459	109	42	43	34	130	64	66
4. Fires	191	133	57	20	18	65	23	7	17	12	15	7	7
5. Drownings	601	511	90	36	94	316	54	11	16	31	30	8	5
6. Other unintentional	2 445	1 983	462	175	135	1 256	351	67	124	37	175	81	45
B. Intentional injuries	**3 609**	**2 607**	**1 003**	**123**	**104**	**1 911**	**371**	**98**	**121**	**69**	**622**	**126**	**64**
1. Self-inflicted injuries	1 613	1 294	319	-	19	915	280	79	-	4	186	82	47
2. Violence	847	652	195	10	10	546	73	13	8	9	135	32	11
3. War	1 149	661	488	113	75	450	18	5	113	56	301	13	5

Notes:
A dash (-) symbol indicates fewer than 500 DALYs.
*IA6 is Bacterial meningitis and meningococcaemia; ID is Conditions arising during the perinatal period;
IIE6 is Dementia and other degenerative and hereditary CNS disorders; IIH1 is Chronic obstructive pulmonary disease.

Annex Table 9c. DALYs by age, sex and cause (thousands): India, 1990

Cause	Total	Male	Female	Males 0-4	Males 5-14	Males 15-44	Males 45-59	Males 60+	Females 0-4	Females 5-14	Females 15-44	Females 45-59	Females 60+
Population (millions)	850	439	410	60	102	201	48	30	57	95	183	46	29
All causes	287 739	142 190	145 549	63 464	18 512	32 273	14 927	13 015	65 844	17 427	38 298	12 131	11 848
I. Communicable, maternal, perinatal and nutritional conditions	162 354	76 534	85 820	52 685	6 901	10 705	3 487	2 756	55 589	8 080	17 514	2 674	1 963
A. Infectious and parasitic diseases	83 146	42 483	40 663	24 304	4 620	8 821	3 012	1 726	25 214	4 821	7 613	1 970	1 046
1. Tuberculosis	13 763	8 747	5 016	502	396	4 259	2 407	1 184	387	308	2 475	1 362	484
2. STDs excluding HIV	5 566	1 871	3 695	1 012	13	804	19	24	1 066	51	2 521	27	30
a. Syphilis	1 898	903	995	736	1	126	16	24	802	1	143	19	30
b. Chlamydia	2 187	311	1 876	67	5	239	1	-	64	37	1 770	5	1
c. Gonorrhoea	1 480	656	824	209	7	438	2	-	200	13	609	2	-
3. HIV	236	152	83	5	1	140	5	1	5	1	77	1	-
4. Diarrhoeal diseases	29 480	14 060	15 420	12 067	953	651	158	231	13 069	1 311	648	159	233
5. Childhood-cluster diseases	18 328	9 150	9 178	7 682	996	396	54	21	7 556	1 150	395	56	21
a. Pertussis	3 013	1 507	1 506	1 349	157	-	-	-	1 347	159	-	-	-
b. Poliomyelitis	1 322	758	564	739	4	15	1	-	549	9	11	1	-
c. Diphtheria	151	75	76	65	9	1	-	-	66	9	1	-	-
d. Measles	7 066	3 507	3 559	2 973	528	6	1	-	3 007	546	5	-	-
e. Tetanus	6 777	3 302	3 474	2 557	299	374	52	20	2 588	433	378	55	21
6. Bacterial meningitis*	1 506	767	739	537	27	145	38	20	530	26	123	38	21
7. Hepatitis B and hepatitis C	355	195	160	44	28	70	34	19	37	29	60	17	18
8. Malaria	1 195	614	581	144	201	225	33	11	129	219	193	30	10
9. Tropical-cluster diseases	3 145	2 166	980	111	786	1 187	72	9	63	385	423	100	9
a. Trypanosomiasis	-	-	-	-	-	-	-	-	-	-	-	-	-
b. Chagas disease	-	-	-	-	-	-	-	-	-	-	-	-	-
c. Schistosomiasis	-	-	-	-	-	-	-	-	-	-	-	-	-
d. Leishmaniasis	1 375	826	549	56	347	405	14	5	39	247	250	10	4
e. Lymphatic filariasis	1 770	1 339	431	56	439	782	58	4	24	138	173	90	5
f. Onchocerciasis	-	-	-	-	-	-	-	-	-	-	-	-	-
10. Leprosy	186	95	90	2	33	50	8	2	3	32	46	7	2
11. Dengue	444	200	244	40	155	4	1	-	48	190	5	1	-
12. Japanese encephalitis	85	42	42	23	15	3	-	3	23	16	3	-	-
13. Trachoma	26	7	19	-	-	2	3	3	-	-	4	7	8
14. Intestinal nematode infections	788	407	381	3	207	158	27	12	2	198	144	26	11
a. Ascariasis	200	102	98	2	99	1	-	-	2	95	1	-	-
b. Trichuriasis	126	65	62	-	65	-	-	-	-	61	-	-	-
c. Ancylostomiasis and necatoriasis	462	240	222	-	44	158	27	12	-	41	143	26	11

Annex Table 9c, continued. DALYs by age, sex and cause (thousands): India, 1990

Cause	Total	Male	Female	Males					Females				
				0-4	5-14	15-44	45-59	60+	0-4	5-14	15-44	45-59	60+
B. Respiratory infections	**34 251**	**16 059**	**18 192**	**12 819**	**1 374**	**738**	**275**	**854**	**14 203**	**2 323**	**639**	**284**	**743**
1. Lower respiratory infections	32 940	15 592	17 349	12 507	1 252	716	270	845	13 523	2 190	621	280	735
2. Upper respiratory infections	358	171	187	123	17	19	4	9	133	26	16	4	8
3. Otitis media	629	296	332	189	105	3	-	-	223	107	3	-	-
C. Maternal conditions	**7 409**		**7 409**								**7 349**	**61**	**-**
1. Maternal haemorrhage	846		846								833	14	-
2. Maternal sepsis	1 256		1 256								1 247	9	-
3. Hypertensive disorders of pregnancy	414		414								407	7	-
4. Obstructed labour	1 503		1 503								1 499	5	-
5. Abortion	1 600		1 600								1 592	8	-
D. Perinatal conditions*	**25 363**	**12 463**	**12 900**	**12 463**					**12 900**				
E. Nutritional deficiencies	**12 185**	**5 530**	**6 655**	**3 100**	**907**	**1 147**	**201**	**175**	**3 272**	**937**	**1 914**	**359**	**173**
1. Protein-energy malnutrition	5 076	2 414	2 661	2 298	38	45	11	22	2 494	108	28	9	23
2. Iodine deficiency	378	192	187	163	21	8	-	-	157	21	8	-	-
3. Vitamin A deficiency	746	373	372	230	133	11	-	-	228	135	9	-	-
4. Iron-deficiency anaemia	5 985	2 550	3 435	409	715	1 083	190	154	393	673	1 869	350	150
II. Noncommunicable diseases	**83 437**	**42 071**	**41 366**	**6 106**	**2 605**	**13 575**	**9 906**	**9 880**	**6 243**	**2 806**	**14 479**	**8 323**	**9 514**
A. Malignant neoplasms	**7 158**	**3 331**	**3 827**	**132**	**211**	**889**	**1 232**	**867**	**64**	**111**	**1 266**	**1 576**	**810**
1. Mouth and oropharynx cancers	1 100	613	487	2	4	142	276	187	2	5	136	230	115
2. Oesophagus cancer	593	284	309			52	136	97			69	144	95
3. Stomach cancer	557	340	217		1	80	160	100			65	93	59
4. Colon and rectum cancers	266	140	126		1	51	47	41			32	52	42
5. Liver cancer	149	102	47	1	2	26	45	27	1	1	12	19	14
6. Pancreas cancer	88	51	37			12	24	15			11	15	12
7. Trachea, bronchus, lung cancers	387	318	68		1	57	156	105			15	28	24
8. Melanoma and other skin cancers	16	7	8			2	3	1			3	4	2
9. Breast cancer	562	-	562								227	239	96
10. Cervix uteri cancer	761	-	761								227	410	124
11. Corpus uteri cancer	38	-	38								5	19	13
12. Ovary cancer	183	-	183							1	86	55	39
13. Prostate cancer	76	76	-			2	16	57					
14. Bladder cancer	67	52	15			7	19	24			3	5	6
15. Lymphomas and multiple myeloma	312	214	98	22	38	84	46	24	4	8	35	26	24
16. Leukaemia	379	221	158	40	68	77	24	12	20	40	65	23	10
C. Diabetes mellitus	**2 257**	**1 103**	**1 154**	**70**	**163**	**267**	**330**	**274**	**70**	**158**	**252**	**349**	**325**
D. Endocrine disorders	**105**	**57**	**48**	**24**	**6**	**15**	**9**	**2**	**18**	**2**	**13**	**9**	**6**

Annex Table 9c, continued. DALYs by age, sex and cause (thousands): India, 1990

Cause	Total	Male	Female	Males 0-4	5-14	15-44	45-59	60+	Females 0-4	5-14	15-44	45-59	60+
E. Neuro-psychiatric conditions	**20 161**	**9 338**	**10 823**	**439**	**500**	**6 914**	**891**	**595**	**543**	**572**	**8 055**	**993**	**661**
1. Unipolar major depression	8 063	2 961	5 102	-	-	2 528	350	83	-	-	4 346	612	144
2. Bipolar disorder	2 305	1 200	1 105	-	-	1 117	62	21	-	-	1 023	59	22
3. Schizophrenia	1 650	892	758	-	-	875	10	7	-	-	744	4	9
4. Epilepsy	975	510	465	38	128	283	39	22	44	189	201	14	17
5. Alcohol use	915	838	77	-	-	758	67	13	-	-	71	4	2
6. Dementia*	1 002	490	512	55	21	46	115	253	65	23	43	114	265
7. Parkinson disease	137	69	68	-	-	-	26	42	-	-	-	30	38
8. Multiple sclerosis	215	96	119	-	-	83	10	4	-	-	102	12	5
9. Drug use	78	70	8	-	6	62	2	-	-	1	7	-	-
10. Post-traumatic stress disorder	316	123	193	8	31	77	6	1	13	48	120	10	2
11. Obsessive-compulsive disorders	1 640	731	908	-	106	581	31	13	-	132	706	53	17
12. Panic disorder	738	239	498	-	4	202	34	-	-	36	403	52	7
F. Sense organ diseases	**3 014**	**1 490**	**1 525**	**6**	**1**	**145**	**721**	**617**	**4**	**1**	**124**	**663**	**734**
1. Glaucoma	573	329	243	-	-	34	228	67	-	-	12	162	69
2. Cataracts	2 439	1 158	1 281	4	1	111	493	549	4	1	112	501	665
G. Cardiovascular diseases	**23 447**	**12 251**	**11 197**	**550**	**397**	**2 023**	**3 665**	**5 616**	**614**	**612**	**1 848**	**2 582**	**5 542**
1. Rheumatic heart disease	1 504	613	890	1	46	343	170	52	2	69	480	258	82
2. Ischaemic heart disease	10 131	5 603	4 528	-	-	384	1 985	3 234	-	-	294	1 210	3 024
3. Cerebrovascular disease	4 235	2 129	2 106	109	63	237	582	1 138	116	76	307	408	1 201
4. Inflammatory heart diseases	1 820	899	921	100	95	386	197	121	135	155	328	173	131
H. Respiratory diseases	**7 615**	**3 874**	**3 740**	**609**	**547**	**830**	**904**	**984**	**665**	**474**	**983**	**865**	**753**
1. COPD*	2 494	1 391	1 103	64	40	254	477	555	84	48	250	380	342
2. Asthma	1 508	830	678	112	249	343	77	48	75	173	314	75	42
I. Digestive diseases	**6 335**	**3 974**	**2 361**	**314**	**185**	**1 654**	**1 360**	**461**	**335**	**149**	**975**	**643**	**259**
1. Peptic ulcer	926	585	341	4	11	297	188	86	7	16	174	98	46
2. Cirrhosis of the liver	2 867	1 968	900	58	37	795	798	280	76	73	342	295	113
3. Appendicitis	381	219	162	8	65	136	8	3	8	54	92	6	2
J. Genito-urinary diseases	**2 085**	**1 161**	**924**	**94**	**276**	**168**	**391**	**232**	**48**	**401**	**229**	**126**	**120**
1. Nephritis and nephrosis	1 660	778	882	74	266	154	145	139	44	398	214	114	111
2. Benign prostatic hypertrophy	326	326	-	-	-	-	238	87	-	-	-	-	-
L. Musculo-skeletal diseases	**1 434**	**579**	**855**	**3**	**9**	**240**	**238**	**90**	**2**	**7**	**330**	**351**	**164**
1. Rheumatoid arthritis	182	54	128	1	1	37	8	7	-	3	71	42	13
2. Osteoarthritis	1 218	504	714	-	-	197	226	81	-	-	256	308	150

Annex Table 9c, continued. DALYs by age, sex and cause (thousands): India, 1990

Cause	Total	Male	Female	Males					Females				
				0-4	5-14	15-44	45-59	60+	0-4	5-14	15-44	45-59	60+
M. Congenital anomalies	8 400	4 163	4 237	3 775	203	159	19	7	3 798	243	160	27	10
1. Abdominal wall defect	43	23	19	23	-	-	-	-	19	-	-	-	-
2. Anencephaly	1 552	612	940	612	-	-	-	-	940	-	-	-	-
3. Anorectal atresia	22	12	10	12	-	-	-	-	10	-	-	-	-
4. Cleft lip	80	48	32	48	-	-	-	-	32	-	-	-	-
5. Cleft palate	75	37	38	37	-	-	-	-	38	-	-	-	-
6. Oesophageal atresia	29	16	13	16	-	-	-	-	13	-	-	-	-
7. Renal agenesis	82	41	40	41	-	-	-	-	40	-	-	-	-
8. Down syndrome	1 108	629	478	495	57	76	-	-	360	55	63	-	-
9. Congenital heart anomalies	3 297	1 715	1 582	1 539	97	57	17	6	1 376	116	60	22	8
10. Spina bifida	1 367	640	728	620	18	1	-	-	689	23	13	2	1
N. Oral conditions	1 057	534	523	42	72	176	121	123	40	70	172	120	121
1. Dental caries	672	347	325	41	71	143	52	39	39	66	131	51	38
2. Periodontal disease	71	37	34	-	-	30	5	2	-	-	28	5	2
3. Edentulism	289	145	145	-	-	-	64	81	-	-	-	64	81
III. Injuries	*41 947*	*23 584*	*18 363*	*4 672*	*9 006*	*7 993*	*1 534*	*379*	*4 012*	*6 541*	*6 305*	*1 134*	*371*
A. Unintentional injuries	37 515	21 167	16 348	4 450	8 826	6 342	1 230	319	3 730	6 373	4 979	937	329
1. Road traffic accidents	5 992	4 292	1 700	632	1 027	2 231	322	79	186	744	516	188	66
2. Poisonings	966	469	496	170	107	163	24	6	119	81	215	76	5
3. Falls	10 182	6 288	3 894	1 013	4 360	716	150	49	1 174	1 906	574	198	42
4. Fires	5 647	1 595	4 052	431	463	580	103	18	378	1 437	2 070	119	49
5. Drownings	2 712	1 457	1 255	359	613	419	49	17	302	592	287	53	22
6. Other unintentional	12 017	7 065	4 951	1 845	2 255	2 233	582	150	1 572	1 613	1 317	304	145
B. Intentional injuries	4 432	2 417	2 015	222	180	1 651	304	60	281	168	1 325	198	42
1. Self-inflicted injuries	2 803	1 406	1 397	-	106	1 077	195	28	-	105	1 187	96	9
2. Violence	1 510	893	618	222	74	456	109	32	281	64	138	102	33
3. War	119	119	-	-	-	119	-	-	-	-	-	-	-

Notes:
A dash (–) symbol indicates fewer than 500 DALYs.
*IA6 is Bacterial meningitis and meningococcaemia; ID is Conditions arising during the perinatal period;
IIE6 is Dementia and other degenerative and hereditary CNS disorders; IIH1 is Chronic obstructive pulmonary disease.

Annex Table 9d. DALYs by age, sex and cause (thousands): China, 1990

Cause	Total	Male	Female	Males					Females				
				0-4	5-14	15-44	45-59	60+	0-4	5-14	15-44	45-59	60+
Population (millions)	1 134	585	548	60	97	306	73	49	58	90	284	64	52
All causes	208 407	108 652	99 755	24 406	6 416	40 202	17 526	20 101	26 519	5 062	37 327	13 324	17 523
I. Communicable, maternal, perinatal and nutritional conditions	50 446	23 938	26 508	13 874	2 132	4 763	1 701	1 468	15 786	2 080	6 201	1 199	1 243
A. Infectious and parasitic diseases	15 622	8 390	7 232	2 666	1 157	2 403	1 247	918	2 821	1 108	1 885	716	701
1. Tuberculosis	4 155	2 449	1 706	94	27	900	798	630	107	86	753	410	350
2. STDs excluding HIV	107	23	84	2	-	19	1	1	2	1	79	1	1
a. Syphilis	7	4	2	1	-	2	1	1	1	-	1	-	1
b. Chlamydia	69	7	62	-	-	7	1	-	-	1	61	1	-
c. Gonorrhoea	31	12	19	1	-	10	-	-	1	-	18	-	-
3. HIV	3	3	-	-	-	3	-	-	-	-	-	-	-
4. Diarrhoeal diseases	3 685	1 772	1 913	847	156	550	104	114	1 098	142	483	89	102
5. Childhood-cluster diseases	2 254	1 190	1 064	1 029	103	51	6	2	944	88	28	3	1
a. Pertussis	774	398	377	351	47	-	-	-	332	45	-	-	-
b. Poliomyelitis	365	209	156	195	2	12	1	-	146	1	9	-	-
c. Diphtheria	7	3	3	3	-	-	-	-	3	-	-	-	-
d. Measles	517	264	253	219	34	9	1	-	211	33	8	1	-
e. Tetanus	590	315	275	261	19	29	4	1	253	9	11	1	1
6. Bacterial meningitis*	1 281	656	626	359	23	186	52	35	348	21	170	49	38
7. Hepatitis B and hepatitis C	626	428	197	62	12	212	111	31	52	11	72	23	40
8. Malaria	58	30	28	4	9	14	2	1	4	8	13	2	1
9. Tropical-cluster diseases	243	199	43	6	24	155	10	4	2	5	32	3	2
a. Trypanosomiasis	-	-	-	-	-	-	-	-	-	-	-	-	-
b. Chagas disease	-	-	-	-	-	-	-	-	-	-	-	-	-
c. Schistosomiasis	27	17	9	-	-	9	5	3	-	1	4	3	2
d. Leishmaniasis	1	1	-	-	1	-	-	-	-	-	-	-	-
e. Lymphatic filariasis	214	181	33	6	22	146	6	1	1	4	28	1	-
f. Onchocerciasis	-	-	-	-	-	-	-	-	-	-	-	-	-
10. Leprosy	7	3	3	-	1	2	-	-	-	1	2	-	-
11. Dengue	29	14	15	3	10	-	-	-	1	12	2	-	-
12. Japanese encephalitis	479	245	234	135	88	19	2	1	134	80	18	2	1
13. Trachoma	347	98	249	-	-	22	34	42	-	-	57	79	113
14. Intestinal nematode infections	1 383	714	668	9	652	43	7	3	9	610	40	6	3
a. Ascariasis	646	333	312	9	319	4	1	-	9	299	4	-	-
b. Trichuriasis	617	319	298	-	318	1	-	-	-	298	-	-	-
c. Ancylostomiasis and necatoriasis	119	62	58	-	14	38	7	3	-	13	36	6	3

Annex Table 9d, continued. DALYs by age, sex and cause (thousands): China, 1990

Cause	Total	Male	Female	Males 0-4	Males 5-14	Males 15-44	Males 45-59	Males 60+	Females 0-4	Females 5-14	Females 15-44	Females 45-59	Females 60+
B. Respiratory infections	**12 378**	**5 755**	**6 623**	**4 844**	**303**	**196**	**87**	**325**	**5 780**	**297**	**195**	**51**	**300**
1. Lower respiratory infections	11 924	5 533	6 392	4 738	206	183	85	321	5 658	207	183	49	296
2. Upper respiratory infections	145	69	77	45	4	13	3	4	54	4	12	2	4
3. Otitis media	308	154	155	61	92	1	–	–	68	86	1	–	–
C. Maternal conditions	**2 621**		**2 621**								**2 581**	**40**	
1. Maternal haemorrhage	396		396								385	11	
2. Maternal sepsis	473		473								472	1	
3. Hypertensive disorders of pregnancy	88		88								86	2	
4. Obstructed labour	578		578								578	–	
5. Abortion	76		76								74	2	
D. Perinatal conditions*	**10 279**	**4 953**	**5 326**	**4 953**					**5 326**				
E. Nutritional deficiencies	**9 547**	**4 840**	**4 707**	**1 411**	**672**	**2 165**	**367**	**225**	**1 860**	**675**	**1 539**	**392**	**242**
1. Protein-energy malnutrition	2 024	838	1 187	799	3	11	5	20	1 153	3	12	3	17
2. Iodine deficiency	491	251	240	214	22	15	–	–	204	21	15	1	–
3. Vitamin A deficiency	340	174	165	115	52	8	–	–	111	48	7	–	–
4. Iron-deficiency anaemia	6 691	3 576	3 115	284	595	2 131	361	204	393	603	1 505	389	225
II. Noncommunicable diseases	***121 248***	***63 381***	***57 867***	***6 179***	***1 886***	***23 348***	***14 140***	***17 828***	***6 385***	***1 391***	***23 457***	***11 046***	***15 588***
A. Malignant neoplasms	**18 076**	**11 292**	**6 785**	**177**	**384**	**3 237**	**3 863**	**3 630**	**230**	**194**	**2 120**	**2 128**	**2 113**
1. Mouth and oropharynx cancers	587	399	188	7	9	191	109	83	–	1	88	59	41
2. Oesophagus cancer	1 773	1 237	535	–	–	183	480	574	–	–	47	184	305
3. Stomach cancer	3 350	2 157	1 193	–	8	282	877	989	–	8	323	369	492
4. Colon and rectum cancers	1 029	577	452	–	8	200	175	194	–	9	125	153	165
5. Liver cancer	3 986	3 010	976	7	24	1 203	1 169	606	7	23	295	362	288
6. Pancreas cancer	298	192	107	–	–	42	62	87	1	–	12	30	64
7. Trachea, bronchus, lung cancers	2 085	1 449	636	–	–	157	541	729	–	–	81	255	301
8. Melanoma and other skin cancers	14	8	6	7	15	3	2	3	–	–	2	2	2
9. Breast cancer	392		392						–	–	178	138	76
10. Cervix uteri cancer	272		272						–	–	83	109	80
11. Corpus uteri cancer	91		91						–	–	22	53	16
12. Ovary cancer	176		176						5	7	87	51	27
13. Prostate cancer	37	37		–	–	3	5	30					
14. Bladder cancer	170	136	34	–	–	19	33	83	–	–	3	7	23
15. Lymphomas and multiple myeloma	349	243	106	–	32	104	54	54	–	–	39	45	22
16. Leukaemia	1 613	853	760	99	193	429	94	39	106	100	423	86	45
C. Diabetes mellitus	**1 094**	**531**	**563**	**8**	**14**	**164**	**177**	**168**	**8**	**13**	**143**	**184**	**215**
D. Endocrine disorders	**576**	**157**	**419**	**20**	**14**	**62**	**35**	**25**	**135**	**30**	**195**	**28**	**31**

Annex Table 9d, continued. DALYs by age, sex and cause (thousands): China, 1990

Cause	Total	Male	Female	Males					Females				
				0-4	5-14	15-44	45-59	60+	0-4	5-14	15-44	45-59	60+
E. Neuro-psychiatric conditions	**29 516**	**13 665**	**15 850**	**243**	**384**	**11 200**	**1 145**	**692**	**198**	**361**	**12 931**	**1 427**	**933**
1. Unipolar major depression	12 975	4 749	8 226	-	-	4 050	558	142	-	-	7 072	895	260
2. Bipolar disorder	3 713	1 925	1 788	-	-	1 795	98	32	-	-	1 665	87	36
3. Schizophrenia	2 644	1 450	1 193	-	88	1 426	11	14	-	-	1 168	15	10
4. Epilepsy	923	490	433	18	-	322	44	17	16	92	281	29	15
5. Alcohol use	1 549	1 438	111	-	-	1 331	92	15	-	-	105	5	1
6. Dementia*	1 526	723	803	63	25	68	172	395	62	19	62	165	495
7. Parkinson disease	97	49	48	-	-	-	20	29	-	-	-	18	29
8. Multiple sclerosis	334	148	186	-	-	128	14	6	-	-	159	19	8
9. Drug use	189	170	19	-	13	151	5	1	-	1	17	1	-
10. Post-traumatic stress disorder	429	167	262	8	29	118	10	2	13	46	186	14	3
11. Obsessive-compulsive disorders	2 381	1 057	1 324	-	101	887	47	22	-	126	1 093	74	30
12. Panic disorder	1 141	395	745	-	35	308	52	-	-	35	626	72	12
F. Sense organ diseases	**2 051**	**823**	**1 228**	**44**	-	**88**	**312**	**380**	**34**	**16**	**175**	**529**	**474**
1. Glaucoma	805	260	545	7	-	36	135	82	9	-	70	348	119
2. Cataracts	1 032	497	535	17	-	42	155	283	3	-	46	153	333
G. Cardiovascular diseases	**22 882**	**12 199**	**10 683**	**334**	**158**	**2 727**	**3 285**	**5 696**	**246**	**92**	**2 541**	**2 553**	**5 251**
1. Rheumatic heart disease	2 361	1 016	1 346	-	28	548	215	225	26	30	618	346	326
2. Ischaemic heart disease	6 004	3 271	2 733	-	-	614	926	1 731	-	-	445	655	1 634
3. Cerebrovascular disease	10 821	5 918	4 904	78	62	1 055	1 691	3 032	60	24	878	1 281	2 659
4. Inflammatory heart diseases	1 300	679	621	59	28	361	133	98	52	20	334	116	101
H. Respiratory diseases	**22 265**	**12 068**	**10 197**	**819**	**376**	**2 840**	**2 685**	**5 347**	**791**	**240**	**2 222**	**2 030**	**4 914**
1. COPD*	17 810	9 553	8 256	141	7	1 863	2 460	5 082	325	5	1 405	1 857	4 664
2. Asthma	2 755	1 538	1 218	173	340	768	160	97	109	211	677	135	85
I. Digestive diseases	**10 252**	**5 699**	**4 554**	**1 456**	**169**	**1 668**	**1 432**	**973**	**1 573**	**129**	**1 147**	**943**	**762**
1. Peptic ulcer	461	284	177	10	6	121	76	72	11	4	65	40	56
2. Cirrhosis of the liver	3 080	2 121	959	74	23	865	718	440	24	24	277	349	286
3. Appendicitis	359	213	147	5	56	140	8	3	5	43	91	6	2
J. Genito-urinary diseases	**2 499**	**1 563**	**936**	**76**	**75**	**573**	**566**	**272**	**73**	**51**	**442**	**186**	**185**
1. Nephritis and nephrosis	1 662	948	714	51	75	530	145	147	73	51	369	104	117
2. Benign prostatic hypertrophy	442	442	-	7	-	8	364	63	-	-	-	-	-
L. Musculo-skeletal diseases	**3 537**	**1 206**	**2 331**	-	**29**	**320**	**414**	**443**	**22**	**20**	**933**	**850**	**506**
1. Rheumatoid arthritis	665	217	448	-	1	84	96	35	-	6	174	173	94
2. Osteoarthritis	2 153	735	1 418	-	-	169	277	289	-	-	515	590	313

Annex Table 9d, continued. DALYs by age, sex and cause (thousands): China, 1990

Cause	Total	Male	Female	Males 0-4	5-14	15-44	45-59	60+	Females 0-4	5-14	15-44	45-59	60+
M. Congenital anomalies	6 242	3 050	3 193	2 675	172	198	5	-	2 761	173	253	6	-
1. Abdominal wall defect	23	13	10	13	-	-	-	-	10	-	-	-	-
2. Anencephaly	1 314	506	808	506	-	-	-	-	808	-	-	-	-
3. Anorectal atresia	5	3	2	3	-	-	-	-	2	-	-	-	-
4. Cleft lip	82	44	38	44	-	-	-	-	38	-	-	-	-
5. Cleft palate	26	13	13	13	-	-	-	-	13	-	-	-	-
6. Oesophageal atresia	4	2	2	2	-	-	-	-	2	-	-	-	-
7. Renal agenesis	18	9	9	9	-	-	-	-	9	-	-	-	-
8. Down syndrome	976	502	474	405	36	58	2	-	343	43	84	3	-
9. Congenital heart anomalies	2 603	1 366	1 237	1 190	76	98	2	-	1 030	64	140	2	-
10. Spina bifida	883	412	471	376	34	2	-	-	429	39	3	-	-
N. Oral conditions	1 015	500	514	189	35	65	99	113	182	35	82	91	124
1. Dental caries	583	299	284	188	34	44	23	11	180	31	41	20	11
2. Periodontal disease	33	17	16	-	-	15	1	1	-	-	14	1	-
3. Edentulism	358	176	182	-	-	-	74	102	-	-	-	69	112
III. Injuries	*36 712*	*21 333*	*15 379*	*4 353*	*2 399*	*12 091*	*1 685*	*806*	*4 348*	*1 591*	*7 670*	*1 079*	*692*
A. Unintentional injuries	26 970	17 091	9 879	4 164	2 263	8 936	1 223	505	3 997	1 463	3 403	605	411
1. Road traffic accidents	4 276	3 025	1 251	152	332	2 118	314	109	111	314	624	152	49
2. Poisonings	1 544	862	682	226	67	389	133	47	70	94	445	36	38
3. Falls	4 485	2 592	1 894	603	340	1 393	164	92	791	230	569	153	151
4. Fires	680	386	294	122	73	151	19	20	86	106	58	19	25
5. Drownings	4 425	2 772	1 653	1 019	819	830	66	39	865	402	318	33	36
6. Other unintentional	11 559	7 454	4 105	2 042	632	4 055	528	198	2 074	317	1 390	212	112
B. Intentional injuries	9 742	4 242	5 500	189	135	3 154	462	301	351	127	4 266	475	281
1. Self-inflicted injuries	8 078	3 232	4 846	-	90	2 439	419	284	-	66	4 069	447	265
2. Violence	1 638	984	654	189	45	690	43	17	351	62	198	27	16
3. War	26	26	-	-	-	26	-	-	-	-	-	-	-

Notes:

A dash (-) symbol indicates fewer than 500 DALYs.

*IA6 is Bacterial meningitis and meningococcaemia; ID is Conditions arising during the perinatal period;
IIE6 is Dementia and other degenerative and hereditary CNS disorders; IIH1 is Chronic obstructive pulmonary disease.

Annex Table 9e. DALYs by age, sex and cause (thousands): Other Asia and Islands, 1990

Cause	Total	Male	Female	Males					Females				
				0-4	5-14	15-44	45-59	60+	0-4	5-14	15-44	45-59	60+
Population (millions)	683	343	340	44	84	161	34	20	42	80	160	35	23
All causes	177 671	94 900	82 771	36 552	12 482	28 324	9 667	7 875	30 097	9 265	27 519	8 042	7 848
I. Communicable, maternal, perinatal and nutritional conditions	79 341	39 634	39 707	27 969	4 390	4 711	1 375	1 189	22 616	3 907	10 572	1 483	1 129
A. Infectious and parasitic diseases	39 588	20 569	19 019	12 495	2 733	3 506	1 137	698	10 068	2 425	4 701	1 129	696
1. Tuberculosis	5 501	2 806	2 695	39	103	1 325	809	529	14	102	1 253	797	529
2. STDs excluding HIV	4 011	1 397	2 614	778	10	581	12	16	611	38	1 927	19	19
a. Syphilis	1 232	688	545	582	1	79	10	15	415	1	97	13	19
b. Chlamydia	1 642	220	1 422	45	3	171	1	-	46	27	1 346	4	-
c. Gonorrhoea	1 136	489	648	151	5	331	1	-	151	10	485	2	-
3. HIV	118	76	42	3	-	69	3	1	3	1	39	-	-
4. Diarrhoeal diseases	13 711	7 720	5 990	6 961	533	140	44	42	5 242	407	240	62	40
5. Childhood-cluster diseases	8 084	4 214	3 869	3 499	514	169	24	9	3 151	506	178	26	9
a. Pertussis	1 313	688	625	616	72	-	-	-	560	64	-	-	-
b. Poliomyelitis	407	234	173	219	3	11	1	-	162	2	9	1	-
c. Diphtheria	81	43	38	37	5	1	-	-	34	4	1	-	-
d. Measles	3 907	2 048	1 858	1 749	294	4	1	-	1 595	259	4	-	-
e. Tetanus	2 377	1 202	1 175	877	140	153	23	8	801	176	165	25	8
6. Bacterial meningitis*	847	433	414	289	21	80	28	15	269	19	81	31	14
7. Hepatitis B and hepatitis C	378	216	162	52	31	70	40	23	39	27	59	19	18
8. Malaria	2 529	1 331	1 198	211	480	547	71	20	194	423	486	76	19
9. Tropical-cluster diseases	596	414	182	12	91	268	38	4	9	28	110	31	3
a. Trypanosomiasis	-	-	-	-	-	-	-	-	-	-	-	-	-
b. Chagas disease	-	-	-	-	-	-	-	-	-	-	-	-	-
c. Schistosomiasis	12	7	5	-	1	3	2	1	-	1	2	1	-
d. Leishmaniasis	77	47	29	2	13	30	2	1	1	8	19	1	-
e. Lymphatic filariasis	507	359	147	10	77	235	35	3	7	19	90	29	2
f. Onchocerciasis	-	-	-	-	-	-	-	-	-	-	-	-	-
10. Leprosy	82	41	41	1	15	18	5	1	7	13	18	3	-
11. Dengue	255	120	135	25	92	2	1	-	29	102	3	1	-
12. Japanese encephalitis	180	95	86	53	34	7	1	-	48	30	6	1	-
13. Trachoma	47	13	35	-	-	3	4	5	-	-	9	12	14
14. Intestinal nematode infections	1 527	781	746	6	621	126	20	8	6	587	124	20	9
a. Ascariasis	494	254	240	6	247	1	-	-	6	233	1	-	-
b. Trichuriasis	660	339	321	-	338	-	-	-	-	320	-	-	-
c. Ancylostomiasis and necatoriasis	372	187	185	-	35	125	19	8	-	34	123	20	8

Annex Table 9e, continued. DALYs by age, sex and cause (thousands): Other Asia and Islands, 1990

Cause	Total	Male	Female	Males 0-4	5-14	15-44	45-59	60+	Females 0-4	5-14	15-44	45-59	60+
B. Respiratory infections	**15 515**	**8 664**	**6 850**	**6 668**	**1 168**	**329**	**96**	**403**	**5 089**	**1 030**	**292**	**103**	**337**
1. Lower respiratory infections	15 041	8 409	6 632	6 534	1 067	315	94	398	4 984	935	279	101	333
2. Upper respiratory infections	176	98	79	65	14	12	2	5	49	13	11	2	4
3. Otitis media	298	158	140	69	87	2	–	–	56	82	1	–	–
C. Maternal conditions	**4 040**	–	**4 040**						–	–	**4 004**	**36**	–
1. Maternal haemorrhage	389		389								381	8	
2. Maternal sepsis	710		710								705	5	
3. Hypertensive disorders of pregnancy	189		189								185	4	
4. Obstructed labour	910		910								907	3	
5. Abortion	775		775								771	4	
D. Perinatal conditions*	**12 293**	**6 760**	**5 533**	**6 760**					**5 533**				
E. Nutritional deficiencies	**7 906**	**3 641**	**4 265**	**2 045**	**490**	**876**	**142**	**88**	**1 927**	**452**	**1 576**	**215**	**96**
1. Protein-energy malnutrition	2 945	1 517	1 428	1 486	14	6	5	6	1 400	11	9	4	5
2. Iodine deficiency	174	88	86	74	10	3	–	–	72	10	4	–	–
3. Vitamin A deficiency	636	336	301	203	124	9	–	–	185	108	7	–	–
4. Iron-deficiency anaemia	4 150	1 700	2 450	283	341	858	136	82	270	323	1 556	210	91
II. Noncommunicable diseases	**72 740**	**38 024**	**34 716**	**5 412**	**4 393**	**14 431**	**7 324**	**6 465**	**4 743**	**3 504**	**13 682**	**6 207**	**6 580**
A. Malignant neoplasms	**8 978**	**4 795**	**4 183**	**247**	**676**	**1 068**	**1 418**	**1 386**	**251**	**455**	**1 243**	**1 150**	**1 084**
1. Mouth and oropharynx cancers	800	477	323	7	20	134	105	212	8	16	98	55	146
2. Oesophagus cancer	248	157	91	–	–	20	74	63	–	–	18	32	41
3. Stomach cancer	670	429	241	1	2	90	192	145	–	1	59	88	93
4. Colon and rectum cancers	455	232	223	2	6	66	50	106	–	5	57	49	109
5. Liver cancer	870	653	217	9	24	178	308	133	7	13	47	76	74
6. Pancreas cancer	103	64	40	–	–	14	25	24	1	1	5	15	18
7. Trachea, bronchus, lung cancers	887	661	226	–	8	87	295	268	3	5	33	81	105
8. Melanoma and other skin cancers	30	13	17	–	1	4	5	3	–	3	5	5	6
9. Breast cancer	444	–	444	–	–	–	–	–	2	3	178	181	80
10. Cervix uteri cancer	504	–	504						–	1	171	239	92
11. Corpus uteri cancer	51		51						–	–	9	22	16
12. Ovary cancer	201		201						10	17	100	47	26
13. Prostate cancer	103	103	–	1	3	2	20	77					
14. Bladder cancer	106	77	30	–	–	9	27	41	–	1	4	7	18
15. Lymphomas and multiple myeloma	415	266	149	32	84	75	31	44	16	28	44	19	44
16. Leukaemia	824	454	370	86	228	98	17	24	91	160	77	17	26
C. Diabetes mellitus	**1 307**	**613**	**695**	**10**	**28**	**196**	**219**	**160**	**10**	**27**	**190**	**240**	**227**
D. Endocrine disorders	**465**	**226**	**238**	**112**	**50**	**33**	**18**	**13**	**89**	**26**	**63**	**32**	**28**

Annex Table 9e, continued. DALYs by age, sex and cause (thousands): Other Asia and Islands, 1990

Cause	Total	Male	Female	Males 0-4	Males 5-14	Males 15-44	Males 45-59	Males 60+	Females 0-4	Females 5-14	Females 15-44	Females 45-59	Females 60+
E. Neuro-psychiatric conditions	**19 206**	**9 605**	**9 601**	**213**	**533**	**7 765**	**725**	**369**	**209**	**504**	**7 548**	**848**	**492**
1. Unipolar major depression	6 701	2 335	4 366	-	-	2 026	252	57	-	-	3 787	467	112
2. Bipolar disorder	1 902	953	948	-	-	895	45	14	-	-	887	45	16
3. Schizophrenia	2 261	1 177	1 085	-	-	1 156	12	8	-	-	1 067	6	12
4. Epilepsy	867	449	418	16	153	225	42	13	18	166	198	25	11
5. Alcohol use	1 916	1 771	145	-	-	1 653	99	19	-	-	137	6	2
6. Dementia*	861	383	477	40	19	37	107	181	49	21	36	116	256
7. Parkinson disease	97	53	44	-	-	-	22	31	-	-	-	18	25
8. Multiple sclerosis	171	73	98	-	-	65	6	2	-	-	85	9	3
9. Drug use	932	839	93	-	64	746	24	4	-	7	82	3	3
10. Post-traumatic stress disorder	262	99	164	6	25	62	5	1	10	41	105	8	1
11. Obsessive-compulsive disorders	1 365	585	780	-	88	466	22	9	-	112	615	40	13
12. Panic disorder	644	217	427	-	31	162	24	-	-	31	351	39	5
F. Sense organ diseases	**1 686**	**714**	**972**	**6**	**6**	**68**	**336**	**297**	**7**	**-**	**94**	**499**	**371**
1. Glaucoma	524	156	369	-	-	14	103	38	-	-	42	264	63
2. Cataracts	1 144	545	599	2	-	52	233	258	4	-	52	235	308
G. Cardiovascular diseases	**17 952**	**9 446**	**8 507**	**1 083**	**1 669**	**2 550**	**1 729**	**2 415**	**985**	**1 401**	**2 060**	**1 342**	**2 720**
1. Rheumatic heart disease	147	62	85	-	9	23	11	18	-	13	32	15	24
2. Ischaemic heart disease	3 958	2 118	1 840	-	-	446	627	1 045	-	-	301	431	1 109
3. Cerebrovascular disease	4 478	2 307	2 171	135	312	588	506	766	123	237	437	451	923
4. Inflammatory heart diseases	2 245	1 195	1 050	211	378	427	115	64	233	330	325	89	73
H. Respiratory diseases	**4 839**	**2 709**	**2 130**	**797**	**479**	**586**	**352**	**496**	**641**	**328**	**569**	**213**	**378**
1. COPD*	1 237	745	493	79	27	162	182	295	69	22	115	86	201
2. Asthma	1 473	820	653	122	274	329	61	36	77	180	301	59	36
I. Digestive diseases	**8 346**	**4 928**	**3 418**	**773**	**482**	**1 288**	**1 545**	**840**	**627**	**355**	**800**	**946**	**690**
1. Peptic ulcer	341	214	126	6	13	79	63	53	5	9	42	30	40
2. Cirrhosis of the liver	2 292	1 678	614	46	46	586	715	285	31	42	155	230	155
3. Appendicitis	313	181	132	4	83	87	5	2	66	57	4	4	1
J. Genito-urinary diseases	**1 878**	**1 017**	**861**	**67**	**209**	**235**	**331**	**175**	**45**	**152**	**270**	**181**	**213**
1. Nephritis and nephrosis	1 305	653	652	49	179	198	109	118	45	132	197	122	156
2. Benign prostatic hypertrophy	200	200	-	-	-	-	181	19	-	-	-	-	-
L. Musculo-skeletal diseases	**2 089**	**884**	**1 205**	**19**	**27**	**242**	**434**	**162**	**18**	**31**	**422**	**533**	**201**
1. Rheumatoid arthritis	191	52	139	-	-	4	17	30	-	2	51	28	59
2. Osteoarthritis	1 592	722	869	-	-	212	397	113	-	-	293	470	107

Annex Table 9e, continued. DALYs by age, sex and cause (thousands): Other Asia and Islands, 1990

Cause	Total	Male	Female	Males 0-4	5-14	15-44	45-59	60+	Females 0-4	5-14	15-44	45-59	60+
M. Congenital anomalies	4 116	2 170	1 946	1 967	114	75	10	4	1 764	108	58	12	4
1. Abdominal wall defect	24	14	9	14	-	-	-	-	9	-	-	-	-
2. Anencephaly	658	257	401	257	-	-	-	-	401	-	-	-	-
3. Anorectal atresia	8	5	3	5	-	-	-	-	3	-	-	-	-
4. Cleft lip	60	37	23	37	-	-	-	-	23	-	-	-	-
5. Cleft palate	58	29	29	29	-	-	-	-	29	-	-	-	-
6. Oesophageal atresia	16	10	6	10	-	-	-	-	6	-	-	-	-
7. Renal agenesis	58	30	29	30	-	-	-	-	29	-	-	-	-
8. Down syndrome	573	337	236	290	21	26	-	-	204	16	15	-	-
9. Congenital heart anomalies	1 984	1 093	891	989	54	37	9	3	802	48	29	10	4
10. Spina bifida	353	166	187	149	16	1	-	-	159	22	5	1	-
N. Oral conditions	1 281	621	660	31	45	266	155	124	30	45	276	165	144
1. Dental caries	530	265	265	30	44	115	54	22	29	42	114	55	25
2. Periodontal disease	33	17	17	-	-	13	2	1	-	-	13	2	1
3. Edentulism	699	336	363	-	-	136	99	101	-	-	137	107	118
III. Injuries	*25 590*	*17 242*	*8 348*	*3 171*	*3 699*	*9 182*	*969*	*221*	*2 738*	*1 854*	*3 265*	*352*	*139*
A. Unintentional injuries	21 545	14 656	6 889	3 068	3 496	7 162	764	166	2 627	1 724	2 140	284	113
1. Road traffic accidents	4 720	3 320	1 400	485	716	1 876	192	52	446	366	475	78	35
2. Poisonings	1 036	538	498	82	104	294	44	14	75	109	280	23	12
3. Falls	4 100	2 678	1 422	845	651	1 043	117	22	652	304	396	56	15
4. Fires	510	257	253	70	91	84	9	3	102	102	43	4	3
5. Drownings	2 775	1 916	859	647	769	452	35	12	406	300	134	12	7
6. Other unintentional	8 403	5 948	2 456	940	1 164	3 414	367	63	946	544	812	112	42
B. Intentional injuries	4 045	2 586	1 460	103	203	2 020	205	55	111	130	1 125	68	26
1. Self-inflicted injuries	1 918	1 047	871	-	72	846	94	35	-	44	765	43	19
2. Violence	1 534	1 197	337	45	93	942	101	17	52	57	206	18	5
3. War	593	341	252	58	39	232	9	3	59	29	154	7	3

Notes:
A dash (-) symbol indicates fewer than 500 DALYs.
*IA6 is Bacterial meningitis and meningococcaemia; ID is Conditions arising during the perinatal period;
IIE6 is Dementia and other degenerative and hereditary CNS disorders; IIH1 is Chronic obstructive pulmonary disease.

Annex Table 9f. DALYs by age, sex and cause (thousands): Sub-Saharan Africa, 1990

Cause	Total	Male	Female	Males 0-4	5-14	15-44	45-59	60+	Females 0-4	5-14	15-44	45-59	60+
Population (millions)	510	252	258	47	70	104	20	11	47	70	106	22	13
All causes	295 294	154 602	140 692	82 566	19 439	39 356	8 197	5 045	72 243	17 638	37 281	7 513	6 017
I. Communicable, maternal, perinatal and nutritional conditions	194 577	95 783	98 794	73 326	9 295	10 417	1 752	993	63 895	9 384	22 583	1 727	1 205
A. Infectious and parasitic diseases	125 495	64 605	60 890	45 979	6 887	9 589	1 596	555	39 613	6 832	12 284	1 522	639
1. Tuberculosis	10 184	4 773	5 410	629	450	2 773	706	217	688	650	3 178	675	220
2. STDs excluding HIV	6 191	2 253	3 938	1 487	15	705	19	27	1 459	58	2 351	31	39
a. Syphilis	2 620	1 306	1 314	1 134	2	127	17	26	1 082	2	168	23	38
b. Chlamydia	1 801	224	1 577	65	4	154	1	-	70	37	1 464	5	-
c. Gonorrhoea	1 769	722	1 048	287	9	424	2	-	308	19	718	3	-
3. HIV	8 370	3 904	4 467	1 090	167	2 474	146	27	1 037	176	3 126	110	17
4. Diarrhoeal diseases	32 126	17 272	14 854	15 383	1 403	332	70	84	12 540	1 486	632	91	105
5. Childhood-cluster diseases	30 445	15 814	14 630	13 526	2 085	162	29	11	12 301	2 100	192	27	11
a. Pertussis	5 529	2 888	2 641	2 587	301	-	-	-	2 347	294	-	-	-
b. Poliomyelitis	588	335	255	323	-	7	-	-	247	-	6	-	-
c. Diphtheria	64	33	30	29	4	-	-	-	26	4	1	-	-
d. Measles	19 943	10 351	9 592	8 731	1 618	2	-	-	7 982	1 606	3	-	-
e. Tetanus	4 321	2 210	2 111	1 857	160	152	29	11	1 699	193	182	26	11
6. Bacterial meningitis*	996	495	501	392	18	59	18	8	376	18	76	21	11
7. Hepatitis B and hepatitis C	309	164	145	39	26	49	32	18	30	25	57	16	18
8. Malaria	27 089	14 432	12 657	12 225	1 150	901	125	32	10 150	1 177	1 147	141	42
9. Tropical-cluster diseases	5 556	3 404	2 152	92	1 133	1 761	350	68	106	690	1 058	253	46
a. Trypanosomiasis	1 467	708	759	18	260	331	88	12	35	271	382	62	9
b. Chagas disease	-	-	-	-	-	-	-	-	-	-	-	-	-
c. Schistosomiasis	1 255	742	513	25	273	371	56	18	17	184	264	37	11
d. Leishmaniasis	467	300	167	12	165	118	5	-	6	85	74	3	-
e. Lymphatic filariasis	1 486	1 151	335	30	352	695	71	3	42	81	150	57	5
f. Onchocerciasis	881	503	378	7	84	245	132	35	6	68	188	95	21
10. Leprosy	46	23	22	1	9	12	2	-	1	8	12	2	-
11. Dengue	21	9	11	2	7	-	-	-	2	9	-	-	-
12. Japanese encephalitis	-	-	-	-	-	-	-	-	-	-	-	-	-
13. Trachoma	355	92	262	-	-	26	33	33	-	-	69	94	98
14. Intestinal nematode infections	495	244	251	1	119	103	15	5	1	120	107	16	6
a. Ascariasis	95	47	48	1	46	-	-	-	1	46	-	-	-
b. Trichuriasis	95	48	48	1	48	-	-	-	-	48	-	-	-
c. Ancylostomiasis and necatoriasis	304	149	155	-	26	103	15	5	-	26	107	16	6

Annex Table 9f, continued. DALYs by age, sex and cause (thousands): Sub-Saharan Africa, 1990

Cause	Total	Male	Female	Males					Females				
				0-4	5-14	15-44	45-59	60+	0-4	5-14	15-44	45-59	60+
B. Respiratory infections	**30 941**	**16 755**	**14 186**	**14 126**	**1 773**	**384**	**86**	**386**	**11 565**	**1 518**	**500**	**99**	**503**
1. Lower respiratory infections	30 221	16 371	13 850	13 858	1 674	373	85	381	11 343	1 424	488	97	498
2. Upper respiratory infections	322	174	148	139	20	8	1	4	114	18	9	2	5
3. Otitis media	398	210	188	130	79	2	-	-	109	76	3	-	-
C. Maternal conditions	**9 513**		**9 513**						-	**391**	**9 115**	**7**	-
1. Maternal haemorrhage	1 372		1 372							90	1 280	1	
2. Maternal sepsis	1 806		1 806							60	1 745	1	
3. Hypertensive disorders of pregnancy	679		679							45	633	1	
4. Obstructed labour	1 665		1 664							30	1 634	1	
5. Abortion	1 674		1 674							51	1 623		
D. Perinatal conditions [a]	**19 314**	**9 855**	**9 459**	**9 855**						**9 459**				
E. Nutritional deficiencies	**9 314**	**4 567**	**4 747**	**3 366**	**635**	**444**	**70**	**53**	**3 258**	**643**	**683**	**99**	**63**
1. Protein-energy malnutrition	5 424	2 737	2 687	2 653	38	23	9	14	2 569	42	52	9	15
2. Iodine deficiency	129	61	68	52	7	2	-	-	53	8	6	1	-
3. Vitamin A deficiency	1 196	605	590	387	209	9	-	-	365	213	12	-	-
4. Iron-deficiency anaemia	2 565	1 164	1 401	274	380	410	61	39	271	379	613	90	48
II. Noncommunicable diseases	***55 380***	***27 757***	***27 623***	***4 722***	***3 249***	***10 628***	***5 363***	***3 795***	***4 734***	***3 689***	***9 149***	***5 402***	***4 649***
A. Malignant neoplasms	**6 217**	**3 356**	**2 862**	**128**	**403**	**946**	**1 047**	**832**	**155**	**444**	**618**	**947**	**698**
1. Mouth and oropharynx cancers	280	161	119	1	4	47	39	70	5	17	26	21	51
2. Oesophagus cancer	282	210	72			44	112	54			12	29	30
3. Stomach cancer	393	229	164		1	49	109	69	1		28	85	51
4. Colon and rectum cancers	168	91	77			30	23	37		1	17	18	41
5. Liver cancer	865	658	207	3	10	314	248	83	4	12	60	77	54
6. Pancreas cancer	86	49	37			12	24	12			8	19	11
7. Trachea, bronchus, lung cancers	225	170	55			30	86	53			8	28	19
8. Melanoma and other skin cancers	94	40	54			8	20	11		1	6	22	24
9. Breast cancer	238	-	238						1	2	65	110	60
10. Cervix uteri cancer	434	-	434						-	1	101	211	122
11. Corpus uteri cancer	40		40								5	18	16
12. Ovary cancer	117		117						4	14	32	44	24
13. Prostate cancer	265	265				6	72	187					
14. Bladder cancer	155	99	56			18	40	40			12	22	21
15. Lymphomas and multiple myeloma	596	352	245	45	162	72	35	37	39	128	33	21	24
16. Leukaemia	196	83	114	8	29	26	7	12	17	56	17	13	11
C. Diabetes mellitus	**523**	**243**	**280**	**13**	**52**	**56**	**69**	**52**	**16**	**54**	**46**	**83**	**82**
D. Endocrine disorders	**1 070**	**507**	**564**	**198**	**44**	**134**	**95**	**36**	**124**	**86**	**139**	**119**	**95**

Annex Table 9f, continued. DALYs by age, sex and cause (thousands): Sub-Saharan Africa, 1990

Cause	Total	Male	Female	Males					Females				
				0-4	5-14	15-44	45-59	60+	0-4	5-14	15-44	45-59	60+
E. Neuro-psychiatric conditions	**11 957**	**5 789**	**6 168**	**185**	**374**	**4 663**	**414**	**153**	**216**	**389**	**4 789**	**511**	**262**
1. Unipolar major depression	4 552	1 550	3 003	-	-	1 362	156	32	-	-	2 626	308	68
2. Bipolar disorder	1 311	646	665	-	-	610	28	8	-	-	624	31	10
3. Schizophrenia	452	235	217	-	-	230	3	2	-	-	212	2	3
4. Epilepsy	521	278	243	22	96	133	21	7	25	95	104	12	7
5. Alcohol use	1 766	1 426	340	-	-	1 332	82	12	-	-	315	19	6
6. Dementia*	350	115	235	16	-	14	27	51	43	20	23	31	118
7. Parkinson disease	49	26	23	-	-	-	11	15	-	-	-	10	13
8. Multiple sclerosis	108	46	62	-	-	41	4	1	-	-	53	7	2
9. Drug use	374	338	37	-	25	301	10	2	-	3	32	1	-
10. Post-traumatic stress disorder	192	71	121	-	21	40	-	-	10	36	70	5	1
11. Obsessive-compulsive disorders	933	393	540	-	73	301	13	5	-	97	410	26	8
12. Panic disorder	438	146	292	-	26	105	15	-	-	27	237	25	3
F. Sense organ diseases	**1 953**	**905**	**1 048**	**7**	**1**	**78**	**453**	**367**	**7**	**1**	**81**	**510**	**449**
1. Glaucoma	389	155	234	-	-	1	75	79	-	-	2	120	112
2. Cataracts	1 558	746	811	7	1	72	378	288	7	1	76	390	337
G. Cardiovascular diseases	**11 612**	**5 308**	**6 303**	**407**	**739**	**1 775**	**1 237**	**1 150**	**470**	**1 067**	**1 277**	**1 555**	**1 934**
1. Rheumatic heart disease	666	302	364	1	126	161	11	3	2	194	144	19	5
2. Ischaemic heart disease	2 367	1 094	1 273	-	-	327	386	382	140	-	167	410	555
3. Cerebrovascular disease	4 595	2 064	2 531	65	232	704	517	546	74	232	440	758	1 027
4. Inflammatory heart diseases	1 450	644	806	108	123	228	107	77	177	216	190	99	125
H. Respiratory diseases	**7 618**	**4 172**	**3 445**	**989**	**517**	**1 212**	**836**	**618**	**972**	**470**	**868**	**664**	**471**
1. COPD*	1 826	1 125	701	82	36	346	333	329	89	39	153	212	208
2. Asthma	1 426	733	693	124	248	285	49	26	99	204	309	55	26
I. Digestive diseases	**5 416**	**3 009**	**2 407**	**429**	**448**	**1 088**	**705**	**339**	**425**	**580**	**637**	**426**	**339**
1. Peptic ulcer	297	189	108	-	2	119	49	18	-	2	50	35	21
2. Cirrhosis of the liver	646	455	191	-	38	200	147	70	-	20	66	63	42
3. Appendicitis	446	269	178	6	138	117	6	1	7	117	47	5	1
J. Genito-urinary diseases	**2 524**	**1 434**	**1 090**	**247**	**406**	**315**	**324**	**141**	**181**	**334**	**233**	**207**	**135**
1. Nephritis and nephrosis	1 834	1 003	831	205	343	257	101	97	174	291	149	126	91
2. Benign prostatic hypertrophy	176	176	-	-	-	-	168	8	-	-	-	-	-
L. Musculo-skeletal diseases	**1 049**	**351**	**698**	-	-	**181**	**117**	**53**	-	**2**	**283**	**307**	**106**
1. Rheumatoid arthritis	88	25	63	-	-	15	7	3	-	2	38	18	5
2. Osteoarthritis	939	318	621	-	-	161	108	48	-	-	237	286	98

Annex Table 9f, continued. DALYs by age, sex and cause (thousands): Sub-Saharan Africa, 1990

Cause	Total	Male	Female	Males					Females				
				0-4	5-14	15-44	45-59	60+	0-4	5-14	15-44	45-59	60+
M. Congenital anomalies	3 936	1 907	2 029	1 715	107	72	10	4	1 848	122	38	15	5
1. Abdominal wall defect	14	7	7	7	-	-	-	-	7	-	-	-	-
2. Anencephaly	410	154	255	154	-	-	-	-	255	-	-	-	-
3. Anorectal atresia	7	4	4	4	-	-	-	-	4	-	-	-	-
4. Cleft lip	62	35	27	35	-	-	-	-	27	-	-	-	-
5. Cleft palate	67	30	37	30	-	-	-	-	37	-	-	-	-
6. Oesophageal atresia	10	5	5	5	-	-	-	-	5	-	-	-	-
7. Renal agenesis	70	35	35	35	-	-	-	-	35	-	-	-	-
8. Down syndrome	686	376	309	312	29	35	-	-	260	29	20	-	-
9. Congenital heart anomalies	1 848	919	928	832	49	26	8	-	834	60	18	12	4
10. Spina bifida	524	215	309	208	6	-	-	-	297	8	3	1	-
N. Oral conditions	396	189	206	47	51	48	11	33	47	54	53	12	41
1. Dental caries	286	142	144	46	49	35	10	3	46	48	35	10	4
2. Periodontal disease	27	13	14	-	-	12	1	-	-	-	12	1	-
3. Edentulism	65	29	36	-	-	-	-	29	-	-	-	-	36
III. Injuries	*45 337*	*31 062*	*14 275*	*4 517*	*6 895*	*18 312*	*1 082*	*256*	*3 613*	*4 565*	*5 549*	*384*	*163*
A. Unintentional injuries	27 591	18 898	8 692	3 318	5 818	8 933	667	163	2 480	3 904	2 002	210	97
1. Road traffic accidents	5 729	4 139	1 590	357	1 487	2 054	192	49	249	711	557	59	14
2. Poisonings	1 231	726	505	481	154	72	14	5	356	77	66	4	2
3. Falls	2 126	1 246	880	222	630	332	43	18	245	393	183	28	30
4. Fires	3 557	1 741	1 816	625	663	403	37	14	541	919	311	28	17
5. Drownings	3 125	2 263	862	535	1 249	443	27	8	274	501	78	7	3
6. Other unintentional	11 823	8 784	3 039	1 098	1 635	5 627	354	69	814	1 302	808	85	30
B. Intentional injuries	17 746	12 164	5 582	1 200	1 077	9 379	415	93	1 133	661	3 547	174	66
1. Self-inflicted injuries	472	379	93	-	52	300	21	6	-	-	85	7	1
2. Violence	6 576	5 657	918	154	333	4 908	222	40	78	139	639	48	14
3. War	10 698	6 128	4 571	1 045	693	4 171	171	47	1 055	522	2 823	119	51

Notes:
A dash (-) symbol indicates fewer than 500 DALYs.
*IA6 is Bacterial meningitis and meningococcaemia; ID is Conditions arising during the perinatal period;
IIE6 is Dementia and other degenerative and hereditary CNS disorders; IIH1 is Chronic obstructive pulmonary disease.

Annex Table 9g. DALYs by age, sex and cause (thousands): Latin America and the Caribbean, 1990

Cause	Total	Male	Female	Males					Females				
				0-4	5-14	15-44	45-59	60+	0-4	5-14	15-44	45-59	60+
Population (millions)	444	222	223	29	52	104	22	14	28	51	104	23	17
All causes	98 285	53 718	44 567	16 731	5 580	20 992	5 890	4 525	13 286	4 225	17 592	4 968	4 496
I. Communicable, maternal, perinatal and nutritional conditions	34 731	17 492	17 239	12 528	1 418	2 643	522	381	9 670	1 523	5 240	447	359
A. Infectious and parasitic diseases	17 311	9 106	8 206	5 242	966	2 284	394	220	4 116	1 020	2 577	307	186
1. Tuberculosis	1 778	953	826	52	65	571	161	103	41	98	521	102	64
2. STDs excluding HIV	1 220	332	888	198	2	127	3	3	169	13	699	4	4
a. Syphilis	370	197	173	176	-	16	2	3	146	-	21	3	4
b. Chlamydia	579	48	530	6	1	42	-	-	6	9	514	1	-
c. Gonorrhoea	272	87	185	17	1	68	-	-	17	3	165	-	-
3. HIV	1 090	857	233	36	4	761	47	9	34	4	186	8	2
4. Diarrhoeal diseases	5 371	3 028	2 343	2 660	199	112	31	27	1 897	214	165	35	32
5. Childhood-cluster diseases	3 377	1 777	1 600	1 618	144	11	3	1	1 429	149	18	3	1
a. Pertussis	718	375	343	341	34	-	-	-	307	35	-	-	-
b. Poliomyelitis	209	120	89	117	1	3	-	-	86	-	2	-	-
c. Diphtheria	16	8	8	5	-	-	-	-	4	-	1	-	-
d. Measles	1 763	919	844	823	93	2	-	-	735	103	6	-	-
e. Tetanus	672	356	316	333	14	6	2	1	297	6	9	3	1
6. Bacterial meningitis*	501	250	252	162	12	50	15	10	150	12	61	17	12
7. Hepatitis B and hepatitis C	121	51	69	19	15	12	3	2	14	17	32	5	2
8. Malaria	457	221	236	39	60	105	13	4	36	66	116	14	5
9. Tropical-cluster diseases	780	384	397	9	24	266	61	23	6	17	287	63	23
a. Trypanosomiasis	-	-	-	-	-	-	-	-	-	-	-	-	-
b. Chagas disease	641	301	340	1	3	220	55	22	1	1	258	58	22
c. Schistosomiasis	79	40	38	1	9	25	4	-	1	10	22	4	1
d. Leishmaniasis	50	35	15	7	10	16	1	-	4	6	5	-	-
e. Lymphatic filariasis	8	6	2	-	2	3	1	-	-	-	1	1	-
f. Onchocerciasis	3	2	1	-	-	1	1	-	-	-	1	-	-
10. Leprosy	52	26	26	1	9	12	3	1	1	9	12	3	1
11. Dengue	1	-	-	-	-	-	-	-	-	-	-	-	-
12. Japanese encephalitis	-	-	-	-	-	-	-	-	-	-	-	-	-
13. Trachoma	-	-	-	-	-	-	-	-	-	-	-	-	-
14. Intestinal nematode infections	644	321	323	3	265	44	7	3	3	265	44	7	3
a. Ascariasis	224	112	113	3	108	1	-	-	3	109	1	-	-
b. Trichuriasis	288	144	144	3	144	-	-	-	3	143	-	-	-
c. Ancylostomiasis and necatoriasis	132	66	66	-	13	43	7	3	-	13	43	7	3

Annex Table 9g, continued. DALYs by age, sex and cause (thousands): Latin America and the Caribbean, 1990

Cause	Total	Male	Female	Males					Females				
				0-4	5-14	15-44	45-59	60+	0-4	5-14	15-44	45-59	60+
B. Respiratory infections	**4 856**	**2 587**	**2 269**	**2 008**	**222**	**168**	**80**	**108**	**1 595**	**246**	**253**	**67**	**109**
1. Lower respiratory infections	4 668	2 491	2 177	1 975	170	162	79	106	1 567	193	244	65	108
2. Upper respiratory infections	60	32	28	20	3	6	1	1	14	4	7	1	1
3. Otitis media	128	63	65	13	49	1	-	-	13	49	2	-	-
C. Maternal conditions	**1 703**	-	**1 703**	-	-	-	-	-	-	**6**	**1 695**	**2**	-
1. Maternal haemorrhage	161	-	161	-	-	-	-	-	-	1	159	-	-
2. Maternal sepsis	293	-	293	-	-	-	-	-	-	1	293	-	-
3. Hypertensive disorders of pregnancy	99	-	99	-	-	-	-	-	-	1	98	-	-
4. Obstructed labour	414	-	414	-	-	-	-	-	-	1	414	-	-
5. Abortion	445	-	445	-	-	-	-	-	-	1	444	-	-
D. Perinatal conditions*	**7 253**	**4 194**	**3 059**	**4 193**	**1**	-	-	-	**3 058**	**1**	-	-	-
E. Nutritional deficiencies	**3 607**	**1 605**	**2 002**	**1 085**	**229**	**190**	**48**	**53**	**901**	**251**	**714**	**71**	**64**
1. Protein-energy malnutrition	1 671	899	772	789	39	28	17	26	628	52	47	15	30
2. Iodine deficiency	93	45	48	39	4	2	-	-	38	5	5	-	-
3. Vitamin A deficiency	184	93	90	65	25	3	-	-	59	28	3	-	-
4. Iron-deficiency anaemia	1 640	561	1 079	187	161	156	30	27	169	164	657	55	34
II. Noncommunicable diseases	***47 401***	***24 328***	***23 074***	***3 027***	***1 879***	***10 908***	***4 598***	***3 916***	***2 754***	***1 674***	***10 326***	***4 303***	***4 018***
A. Malignant neoplasms	**4 408**	**1 985**	**2 422**	**77**	**254**	**410**	**575**	**669**	**70**	**187**	**788**	**763**	**614**
1. Mouth and oropharynx cancers	155	114	41	1	2	29	52	30	-	1	9	14	16
2. Oesophagus cancer	98	70	28	-	-	8	34	27	-	-	3	9	15
3. Stomach cancer	371	227	144	-	-	42	86	99	-	-	29	46	69
4. Colon and rectum cancers	240	112	128	-	1	28	39	44	-	-	24	40	62
5. Liver cancer	56	29	27	1	2	7	10	10	-	1	4	9	13
6. Pancreas cancer	74	38	35	-	-	6	15	16	-	-	4	12	19
7. Trachea, bronchus, lung cancers	336	245	91	-	1	37	105	102	-	-	17	33	40
8. Melanoma and other skin cancers	43	20	23	-	1	9	7	4	-	-	9	7	5
9. Breast cancer	428	-	428	-	-	-	-	-	-	-	155	176	97
10. Cervix uteri cancer	377	-	377	-	-	-	-	-	-	-	166	145	66
11. Corpus uteri cancer	79	-	79	-	-	-	-	-	-	-	16	38	24
12. Ovary cancer	90	-	90	-	-	-	-	-	2	5	39	25	19
13. Prostate cancer	142	142	-	-	-	4	21	116	-	-	-	-	-
14. Bladder cancer	77	58	19	-	1	7	19	31	-	-	3	5	11
15. Lymphomas and multiple myeloma	279	165	115	14	43	59	28	20	9	27	33	21	24
16. Leukaemia	311	174	138	24	76	51	12	10	20	60	35	12	11
C. Diabetes mellitus	**1 436**	**630**	**806**	**12**	**28**	**176**	**217**	**197**	**11**	**24**	**198**	**281**	**292**
D. Endocrine disorders	**1 384**	**672**	**712**	**326**	**87**	**155**	**58**	**46**	**262**	**73**	**220**	**90**	**66**

Annex Table 9g, continued. DALYs by age, sex and cause (thousands): Latin America and the Caribbean, 1990

Cause	Total	Male	Female	Males 0-4	5-14	15-44	45-59	60+	Females 0-4	5-14	15-44	45-59	60+
E. Neuro-psychiatric conditions	**15 604**	**8 724**	**6 880**	**240**	**523**	**7 003**	**660**	**298**	**215**	**487**	**5 301**	**544**	**333**
1. Unipolar major depression	4 183	1 448	2 735	-	-	1 255	156	36	-	-	2 363	296	75
2. Bipolar disorder	1 175	587	588	-	-	551	27	8	-	-	550	28	10
3. Schizophrenia	1 270	659	611	-	-	645	9	5	-	-	601	4	6
4. Epilepsy	662	355	308	14	109	191	31	10	13	103	169	14	8
5. Alcohol use	3 807	3 488	319	-	-	3 126	287	76	-	-	299	15	5
6. Dementia*	637	275	362	42	26	23	57	127	43	20	27	78	194
7. Parkinson disease	34	19	16	-	-	-	8	11	-	-	-	7	9
8. Multiple sclerosis	115	49	66	-	-	43	4	2	-	-	57	7	2
9. Drug use	1 115	725	391	-	55	645	21	4	-	30	348	11	2
10. Post-traumatic stress disorder	169	63	106	4	16	40	3	1	6	26	68	5	1
11. Obsessive-compulsive disorders	852	363	489	-	52	290	14	6	-	68	386	26	9
12. Panic disorder	388	130	259	-	18	97	15	-	-	18	213	24	4
F. Sense organ diseases	**592**	**273**	**319**	**22**	**5**	**20**	**68**	**159**	**15**	**7**	**22**	**82**	**192**
1. Glaucoma	83	30	53	-	-	1	15	14	-	-	2	30	20
2. Cataracts	453	214	240	3	-	14	51	145	3	1	14	51	171
G. Cardiovascular diseases	**7 809**	**4 071**	**3 738**	**136**	**125**	**988**	**1 246**	**1 576**	**117**	**111**	**1 027**	**959**	**1 524**
1. Rheumatic heart disease	182	59	123	1	15	28	10	5	1	21	66	24	11
2. Ischaemic heart disease	2 958	1 636	1 322	-	-	304	588	744	-	-	250	388	684
3. Cerebrovascular disease	2 489	1 251	1 238	11	22	327	393	498	9	20	354	346	508
4. Inflammatory heart diseases	499	252	247	26	27	117	49	32	27	24	120	42	33
H. Respiratory diseases	**3 955**	**2 032**	**1 924**	**599**	**240**	**515**	**323**	**356**	**524**	**205**	**650**	**271**	**275**
1. COPD*	1 031	579	452	58	8	142	157	214	56	7	136	108	145
2. Asthma	967	499	468	65	148	220	41	24	53	126	207	50	32
I. Digestive diseases	**3 711**	**2 122**	**1 589**	**257**	**131**	**773**	**644**	**317**	**194**	**99**	**609**	**394**	**294**
1. Peptic ulcer	157	97	60	1	3	42	28	23	2	2	23	15	18
2. Cirrhosis of the liver	1 132	827	305	13	10	365	325	114	10	9	116	110	60
3. Appendicitis	57	33	24	1	13	17	1	1	1	9	12	1	-
J. Genito-urinary diseases	**1 209**	**596**	**612**	**77**	**73**	**105**	**234**	**108**	**67**	**86**	**262**	**102**	**95**
1. Nephritis and nephrosis	617	283	334	44	59	73	50	58	41	67	117	54	56
2. Benign prostatic hypertrophy	174	174	-	-	-	-	158	16	-	-	-	-	-
L. Musculo-skeletal diseases	**3 052**	**1 158**	**1 894**	**8**	**29**	**484**	**505**	**132**	**5**	**38**	**872**	**723**	**257**
1. Rheumatoid arthritis	567	117	450	-	-	69	34	13	-	6	312	96	36
2. Osteoarthritis	2 095	952	1 144	-	-	387	456	108	-	-	367	581	196

Annex Table 9g, continued. DALYs by age, sex and cause (thousands): Latin America and the Caribbean, 1990

Cause	Total	Male	Female	Males					Females				
				0-4	5-14	15-44	45-59	60+	0-4	5-14	15-44	45-59	60+
M. Congenital anomalies	**2 609**	**1 299**	**1 310**	**1 193**	**73**	**28**	**3**	**2**	**1 193**	**63**	**46**	**5**	**2**
1. Abdominal wall defect	17	8	8	8	-	-	-	-	8	-	-	-	-
2. Anencephaly	288	113	175	113	-	-	-	-	175	-	-	-	-
3. Anorectal atresia	5	3	3	3	-	-	-	-	3	-	-	-	-
4. Cleft lip	40	23	17	23	-	-	-	-	17	-	-	-	-
5. Cleft palate	31	14	16	14	-	-	-	-	16	-	-	-	-
6. Oesophageal atresia	11	6	6	6	-	-	-	-	6	-	-	-	-
7. Renal agenesis	31	16	15	16	-	-	-	-	15	-	-	-	-
8. Down syndrome	381	210	171	187	14	7	2	-	147	12	10	3	-
9. Congenital heart anomalies	1 202	621	581	571	33	14	1	2	526	26	25	2	2
10. Spina bifida	398	178	220	163	12	3	-	-	203	12	4	-	-
N. Oral conditions	**1 007**	**502**	**504**	**36**	**236**	**178**	**21**	**31**	**35**	**231**	**178**	**23**	**37**
1. Dental caries	902	455	448	36	235	174	7	3	34	229	173	7	4
2. Periodontal disease	18	9	10	-	-	4	4	2	-	-	4	4	2
3. Edentulism	77	35	42	-	-	-	10	26	-	-	-	11	31
III. Injuries	***16 153***	***11 899***	***4 254***	***1 176***	***2 283***	***7 441***	***770***	***228***	***862***	***1 029***	***2 026***	***218***	***119***
A. Unintentional injuries	**11 699**	**8 369**	**3 330**	**1 065**	**2 085**	**4 474**	**564**	**182**	**762**	**926**	**1 359**	**177**	**105**
1. Road traffic accidents	3 991	2 892	1 099	131	700	1 790	213	58	98	354	556	66	25
2. Poisonings	150	87	63	29	17	35	5	2	21	15	24	2	1
3. Falls	1 659	1 211	449	204	478	440	56	33	98	157	130	31	33
4. Fires	317	174	144	48	65	51	7	3	44	64	29	4	2
5. Drownings	884	684	200	99	217	338	24	6	63	76	56	4	1
6. Other unintentional	4 698	3 322	1 376	554	609	1 820	259	80	438	261	564	71	43
B. Intentional injuries	**4 453**	**3 530**	**924**	**111**	**198**	**2 968**	**206**	**46**	**100**	**102**	**667**	**41**	**14**
1. Self-inflicted injuries	593	383	209	-	17	307	43	17	-	13	175	15	5
2. Violence	3 172	2 751	421	44	136	2 392	152	27	32	55	310	18	5
3. War	689	395	293	67	45	269	11	3	68	34	181	8	3

Notes:
A dash (-) symbol indicates fewer than 500 DALYs.
*IA6 is Bacterial meningitis and meningococcaemia; ID is Conditions arising during the perinatal period;
IIE6 is Dementia and other degenerative and hereditary CNS disorders; IIH1 is Chronic obstructive pulmonary disease.

Annex Table 9h. DALYs by age, sex and cause (thousands): Middle Eastern Crescent, 1990

Cause	Total	Male	Female	Males					Females				
				0-4	5-14	15-44	45-59	60+	0-4	5-14	15-44	45-59	60+
Population (millions)	503	256	247	41	65	114	22	14	40	62	107	22	15
All causes	150 849	77 592	73 257	38 740	8 561	19 063	6 123	5 105	36 994	7 118	19 210	4 900	5 035
I. Communicable, maternal, perinatal and nutritional conditions	72 010	34 563	37 446	29 319	2 326	1 893	503	522	28 052	2 291	6 104	501	497
A. Infectious and parasitic diseases	30 479	15 737	14 742	12 466	1 159	1 487	420	206	11 805	1 052	1 353	321	210
1. Tuberculosis	2 549	1 604	945	176	113	920	277	119	110	71	524	158	82
2. STDs excluding HIV	804	292	511	226	1	61	2	2	218	6	282	3	3
a. Syphilis	459	232	227	215	–	13	2	2	207	–	15	2	3
b. Chlamydia	246	27	219	–	–	23	–	–	3	5	210	–	–
c. Gonorrhoea	99	33	66	8	–	25	–	–	8	1	56	–	–
3. HIV	47	39	7	2	–	34	3	–	2	–	6	–	–
4. Diarrhoeal diseases	14 795	7 549	7 245	7 108	334	79	16	11	6 774	337	106	17	11
5. Childhood-cluster diseases	8 605	4 403	4 203	3 960	411	23	6	2	3 759	377	54	11	2
a. Pertussis	2 007	1 025	983	925	99	–	–	–	886	97	–	–	–
b. Poliomyelitis	477	273	205	264	2	6	–	–	198	1	5	–	–
c. Diphtheria	42	21	20	19	2	–	–	–	18	2	–	–	–
d. Measles	3 302	1 676	1 626	1 445	230	1	–	–	1 394	228	3	–	–
e. Tetanus	2 777	1 408	1 369	1 307	77	16	6	2	1 263	48	46	10	2
6. Bacterial meningitis*	701	356	345	254	16	58	18	10	247	16	54	18	10
7. Hepatitis B and hepatitis C	255	141	115	37	21	41	27	15	29	20	40	13	13
8. Malaria	378	191	187	38	75	66	9	3	36	72	65	10	3
9. Tropical-cluster diseases	279	171	107	21	65	69	12	4	14	38	46	7	2
a. Trypanosomiasis	–	–	–	–	–	–	–	–	–	–	–	–	–
b. Chagas disease	–	–	–	–	–	–	–	–	–	–	–	–	–
c. Schistosomiasis	146	91	56	2	25	50	10	4	1	11	36	6	2
d. Leishmaniasis	120	72	48	19	40	12	1	–	13	27	8	–	–
e. Lymphatic filariasis	12	9	3	–	–	7	1	–	–	–	2	–	–
f. Onchocerciasis	–	–	–	–	–	–	–	–	–	–	–	–	–
10. Leprosy	11	6	4	1	2	2	1	–	1	2	3	–	–
11. Dengue	–	–	–	–	–	–	–	–	–	–	–	–	–
12. Japanese encephalitis	–	–	–	–	–	–	–	–	–	–	–	–	–
13. Trachoma	249	68	181	–	–	19	23	26	–	–	45	63	73
14. Intestinal nematode infections	185	95	91	1	53	33	5	2	1	51	31	5	2
a. Ascariasis	90	46	44	1	44	1	–	–	1	43	–	–	–
b. Trichuriasis	1	1	0	–	1	–	–	–	–	–	–	–	–
c. Ancylostomiasis and necatoriasis	94	48	46	–	8	33	5	2	–	8	31	5	2

Annex Table 9h, continued. DALYs by age, sex and cause (thousands): Middle Eastern Crescent, 1990

Cause	Total	Male	Female	Males					Females				
				0–4	5–14	15–44	45–59	60+	0–4	5–14	15–44	45–59	60+
B. Respiratory infections	**16 152**	**8 169**	**7 983**	**6 944**	**770**	**129**	**41**	**285**	**6 634**	**841**	**193**	**64**	**252**
1. Lower respiratory infections	15 711	7 945	7 765	6 807	695	122	40	282	6 502	767	184	62	249
2. Upper respiratory infections	171	86	85	67	9	6	1	3	64	9	7	1	3
3. Otitis media	270	138	133	71	67	1	–	–	68	64	1	–	–
C. Maternal conditions	**3 646**	**–**	**3 646**	–	–	–	–	–	–	2	**3 592**	**51**	–
1. Maternal haemorrhage	367	–	367	–	–	–	–	–	–	1	356	11	–
2. Maternal sepsis	772	–	771	–	–	–	–	–	–	–	764	7	–
3. Hypertensive disorders of pregnancy	236	–	236	–	–	–	–	–	–	–	228	7	–
4. Obstructed labour	1 006	–	1 005	–	–	–	–	–	–	–	1 002	4	–
5. Abortion	356	–	356	–	–	–	–	–	–	–	352	4	–
D. Perinatal conditions*	**14 691**	**7 466**	**7 224**	**7 466**	–	–	–	–	**7 224**	–	–	–	–
E. Nutritional deficiencies	**7 042**	**3 190**	**3 852**	**2 442**	**398**	**277**	**42**	**32**	**2 389**	**396**	**967**	**65**	**35**
1. Protein-energy malnutrition	3 617	1 832	1 786	1 809	7	6	3	7	1 758	7	12	2	6
2. Iodine deficiency	255	123	131	105	13	5	–	–	103	15	12	1	–
3. Vitamin A deficiency	736	358	378	240	113	6	–	–	248	123	7	–	–
4. Iron-deficiency anaemia	2 433	877	1 557	288	264	260	39	25	280	251	936	61	28
II. Noncommunicable diseases	**59 293**	**30 352**	**28 941**	**7 010**	**3 618**	**10 189**	**5 085**	**4 450**	**6 732**	**3 446**	**10 156**	**4 171**	**4 437**
A. Malignant neoplasms	**3 580**	**1 892**	**1 688**	**94**	**308**	**500**	**566**	**423**	**81**	**285**	**543**	**437**	**343**
1. Mouth and oropharynx cancers	226	142	84	1	5	57	34	45	1	6	31	18	28
2. Oesophagus cancer	124	71	53	–	1	16	35	19	–	2	14	21	17
3. Stomach cancer	269	164	105	1	2	44	74	43	–	1	28	37	38
4. Colon and rectum cancers	161	82	79	1	1	31	20	28	1	3	23	16	36
5. Liver cancer	113	70	43	1	4	18	30	16	1	4	10	15	13
6. Pancreas cancer	58	35	22	–	–	10	17	9	1	–	4	10	9
7. Trachea, bronchus, lung cancers	365	292	73	–	5	57	148	80	1	5	15	27	25
8. Melanoma and other skin cancers	19	11	8	–	–	4	5	2	–	4	4	2	1
9. Breast cancer	216	–	216	–	–	–	–	–	1	2	96	82	35
10. Cervix uteri cancer	129	–	129	–	–	–	–	–	–	1	49	56	23
11. Corpus uteri cancer	27	–	27	–	–	–	–	–	–	–	6	12	9
12. Ovary cancer	72	–	72	–	–	–	–	–	1	6	35	21	9
13. Prostate cancer	41	41	–	–	–	3	11	26	–	–	–	–	–
14. Bladder cancer	122	96	25	–	2	23	38	32	–	1	6	9	9
15. Lymphomas and multiple myeloma	203	132	70	11	44	50	14	13	7	28	20	6	9
16. Leukaemia	343	174	169	20	81	52	10	11	22	90	35	8	13
C. Diabetes mellitus	**1 463**	**709**	**754**	**31**	**73**	**222**	**230**	**153**	**29**	**71**	**205**	**241**	**206**
D. Endocrine disorders	**985**	**472**	**513**	**229**	**87**	**93**	**44**	**20**	**215**	**140**	**104**	**34**	**19**

Annex Table 9h, continued. DALYs by age, sex and cause (thousands): Middle Eastern Crescent, 1990

Cause	Total	Male	Female	Males 0-4	Males 5-14	Males 15-44	Males 45-59	Males 60+	Females 0-4	Females 5-14	Females 15-44	Females 45-59	Females 60+
E. Neuro-psychiatric conditions	**13 056**	**6 362**	**6 694**	**530**	**638**	**4 652**	**373**	**170**	**420**	**562**	**5 029**	**468**	**215**
1. Unipolar major depression	4 556	1 639	2 917	-	-	1 437	164	38	-	-	2 546	296	75
2. Bipolar disorder	1 309	673	636	-	-	634	29	9	-	-	597	29	10
3. Schizophrenia	1 416	748	667	-	-	736	7	5	-	-	653	9	6
4. Epilepsy	517	267	251	30	100	115	16	6	24	120	91	12	4
5. Alcohol use	260	235	26	-	-	219	13	3	-	-	24	1	1
6. Dementia*	309	147	161	37	11	21	24	54	43	12	21	17	68
7. Parkinson disease	62	34	28	-	-	-	13	20	-	-	-	11	16
8. Multiple sclerosis	118	52	66	-	-	46	4	1	-	-	58	6	2
9. Drug use	933	840	93	-	64	748	24	4	-	7	83	3	-
10. Post-traumatic stress disorder	189	73	116	6	20	44	3	-	9	32	70	5	1
11. Obsessive-compulsive disorders	944	415	529	-	68	327	14	6	-	85	409	25	9
12. Panic disorder	422	147	275	-	23	109	15	-	-	23	225	24	4
F. Sense organ diseases	**930**	**430**	**500**	**3**	**-**	**36**	**191**	**201**	**4**	**1**	**37**	**216**	**242**
1. Glaucoma	103	39	64	-	-	1	26	13	-	-	2	45	17
2. Cataracts	816	386	430	2	-	32	164	187	2	-	33	170	224
G. Cardiovascular diseases	**16 745**	**8 740**	**8 005**	**1 200**	**1 271**	**2 005**	**1 881**	**2 383**	**1 041**	**1 300**	**1 847**	**1 346**	**2 471**
1. Rheumatic heart disease	786	339	447	1	114	205	15	3	2	156	260	23	6
2. Ischaemic heart disease	5 331	2 967	2 364	-	-	616	1 018	1 333	-	-	438	605	1 321
3. Cerebrovascular disease	2 481	1 251	1 230	64	199	307	290	392	50	177	234	275	494
4. Inflammatory heart diseases	1 858	946	912	230	243	308	102	64	246	230	287	83	66
H. Respiratory diseases	**6 347**	**3 259**	**3 088**	**1 356**	**456**	**645**	**360**	**443**	**1 358**	**413**	**639**	**343**	**335**
1. COPD*	1 373	690	683	145	26	154	104	260	171	47	158	144	164
2. Asthma	913	601	313	113	210	221	37	20	39	83	142	29	19
I. Digestive diseases	**6 353**	**3 371**	**2 981**	**1 367**	**328**	**767**	**616**	**293**	**1 539**	**237**	**538**	**420**	**248**
1. Peptic ulcer	142	98	45	1	5	50	29	14	1	2	22	12	7
2. Cirrhosis of the liver	821	453	367	15	39	149	165	86	11	81	92	110	74
3. Appendicitis	152	88	64	3	40	43	2	1	3	32	27	2	1
J. Genito-urinary diseases	**3 021**	**1 716**	**1 304**	**137**	**189**	**609**	**543**	**239**	**109**	**177**	**543**	**300**	**175**
1. Nephritis and nephrosis	808	391	417	57	96	128	58	52	49	127	152	50	39
2. Benign prostatic hypertrophy	183	183	-	-	-	1	165	17	-	-	-	-	-
L. Musculo-skeletal diseases	**888**	**396**	**493**	**13**	**12**	**222**	**109**	**40**	**10**	**8**	**214**	**173**	**87**
1. Rheumatoid arthritis	167	100	66	-	-	96	3	1	-	2	37	20	7
2. Osteoarthritis	600	241	359	-	-	106	100	35	-	-	142	142	75

Annex Table 9h, continued. DALYs by age, sex and cause (thousands): Middle Eastern Crescent, 1990

Cause	Total	Male	Female	Males					Females				
				0-4	5-14	15-44	45-59	60+	0-4	5-14	15-44	45-59	60+
M. Congenital anomalies	**4 137**	**2 121**	**2 016**	**1 930**	**102**	**75**	**10**	**3**	**1 814**	**116**	**68**	**13**	**5**
1. Abdominal wall defect	30	19	10	19	-	-	-	-	10	-	-	-	-
2. Anencephaly	659	258	401	258	-	-	-	-	401	-	-	-	-
3. Anorectal atresia	10	6	3	6	-	-	-	-	3	-	-	-	-
4. Cleft lip	48	28	20	28	-	-	-	-	20	-	-	-	-
5. Cleft palate	45	21	24	21	-	-	-	-	24	-	-	-	-
6. Oesophageal atresia	20	13	7	13	-	-	-	-	7	-	-	-	-
7. Renal agenesis	59	30	29	30	-	-	-	-	29	-	-	-	-
8. Down syndrome	630	350	280	293	25	31	-	-	223	31	27	-	-
9. Congenital heart anomalies	1 997	1 068	929	974	51	32	8	3	832	55	27	11	4
10. Spina bifida	310	146	164	139	6	1	-	-	152	7	4	1	-
N. Oral conditions	**1 381**	**691**	**690**	**86**	**103**	**299**	**138**	**65**	**83**	**99**	**290**	**143**	**76**
1. Dental caries	692	352	340	85	102	108	35	21	82	97	102	35	24
2. Periodontal disease	20	10	10	-	-	10	-	-	-	-	9	-	-
3. Edentulism	655	325	330	-	-	179	102	44	-	-	171	107	52
III. Injuries	***19 546***	***12 676***	***6 870***	***2 411***	***2 617***	***6 981***	***535***	***133***	***2 210***	***1 381***	***2 950***	***228***	***100***
A. Unintentional injuries	**10 266**	**7 130**	**3 135**	**1 552**	**1 792**	**3 383**	**328**	**75**	**1 329**	**829**	**817**	**112**	**49**
1. Road traffic accidents	2 545	1 997	548	104	441	1 317	111	23	91	207	207	31	12
2. Poisonings	348	218	130	61	23	107	22	4	57	18	44	8	3
3. Falls	1 680	1 093	587	331	433	294	28	7	282	182	99	17	6
4. Fires	711	327	384	104	120	91	9	2	106	125	141	8	4
5. Drownings	898	636	262	191	210	220	12	3	164	58	36	3	1
6. Other unintentional	4 084	2 860	1 224	761	565	1 353	145	35	628	238	291	45	22
B. Intentional injuries	**9 280**	**5 546**	**3 734**	**859**	**825**	**3 597**	**207**	**58**	**881**	**552**	**2 134**	**116**	**52**
1. Self-inflicted injuries	1 335	906	429	-	308	510	68	20	-	140	246	27	16
2. Violence	1 201	772	429	198	78	456	32	8	216	82	113	14	4
3. War	6 744	3 868	2 876	661	439	2 631	107	29	665	330	1 775	75	32

Notes:
A dash (-) symbol indicates fewer than 500 DALYs.
*IA6 is Bacterial meningitis and meningococcaemia; ID is Conditions arising during the perinatal period;
IIE6 is Dementia and other degenerative and hereditary CNS disorders; IIH1 is Chronic obstructive pulmonary disease.

Annex Table 9i. DALYs by age, sex and cause (thousands): World, 1990

Cause	Total	Male	Female	Males 0-4	Males 5-14	Males 15-44	Males 45-59	Males 60+	Females 0-4	Females 5-14	Females 15-44	Females 45-59	Females 60+
Population (millions)	*5 267*	*2 654*	*2 614*	*309*	*551*	*1 250*	*312*	*219*	*309*	*526*	*1 199*	*311*	*269*
All causes	*1 379 238*	*722 032*	*657 206*	*268 786*	*73 708*	*217 153*	*82 373*	*80 012*	*250 003*	*62 615*	*201 991*	*64 604*	*77 993*
I. Communicable, maternal, perinatal and nutritional conditions	*605 959*	*294 175*	*311 784*	*212 557*	*26 764*	*36 792*	*9 901*	*8 162*	*197 774*	*27 555*	*70 790*	*8 344*	*7 320*
A. Infectious and parasitic diseases	*316 050*	*163 353*	*152 697*	*103 594*	*17 608*	*29 448*	*8 169*	*4 533*	*94 002*	*17 346*	*31 590*	*6 083*	*3 676*
1. Tuberculosis	38 426	21 741	16 685	1 494	1 155	10 937	5 297	2 858	1 350	1 315	8 736	3 525	1 759
2. STDs excluding HIV	18 684	6 246	12 439	3 710	41	2 363	58	74	3 530	174	8 548	88	99
a. Syphilis	6 596	3 337	3 259	2 845	4	366	49	72	2 652	5	447	61	94
b. Chlamydia	7 169	871	6 298	188	13	666	3	1	190	123	5 964	18	2
c. Gonorrhoea	4 909	2 033	2 876	676	23	1 327	6	1	688	47	2 133	8	1
3. HIV	11 172	6 132	5 040	1 163	177	4 392	348	52	1 103	186	3 593	135	22
4. Diarrhoeal diseases	99 633	51 642	47 991	45 163	3 593	1 924	439	522	40 740	3 912	2 330	469	540
5. Childhood-cluster diseases	71 173	36 591	34 581	31 343	4 262	815	123	47	29 165	4 377	865	128	46
a. Pertussis	13 403	6 904	6 499	6 187	717	–	–	–	5 799	700	–	–	–
b. Poliomyelitis	3 371	1 929	1 442	1 857	14	55	3	1	1 388	10	41	3	1
c. Diphtheria	361	184	177	159	22	3	–	1	150	23	3	–	–
d. Measles	36 520	18 780	17 741	15 948	2 800	26	3	–	14 928	2 779	30	3	–
e. Tetanus	17 517	8 794	8 722	7 192	709	731	116	46	6 900	865	791	122	44
6. Bacterial meningitis*	6 242	3 183	3 058	2 137	136	615	185	111	2 037	132	589	182	119
7. Hepatitis B and hepatitis C	2 136	1 249	887	262	135	476	259	117	207	130	335	99	116
8. Malaria	31 706	16 819	14 888	12 661	1 975	1 858	254	71	10 549	1 966	2 020	272	80
9. Tropical-cluster diseases	10 600	6 739	3 861	251	2 124	3 707	544	113	199	1 163	1 956	457	85
a. Trypanosomiasis	1 467	708	759	18	260	331	88	12	35	271	382	62	9
b. Chagas disease	641	301	340	1	3	220	55	22	1	1	258	58	22
c. Schistosomiasis	1 519	898	622	28	308	458	77	27	19	207	328	51	17
d. Leishmaniasis	2 092	1 282	810	96	576	583	21	6	63	372	356	15	4
e. Lymphatic filariasis	3 997	3 046	952	101	893	1 868	171	11	75	243	443	177	12
f. Onchocerciasis	884	505	379	7	84	246	132	35	6	69	189	95	21
10. Leprosy	384	195	189	6	69	96	19	5	12	64	93	16	4
11. Dengue	750	344	406	69	265	7	2	–	82	313	8	2	–
12. Japanese encephalitis	744	382	362	211	137	30	3	1	206	126	27	3	1
13. Trachoma	1 024	279	745	–	–	72	98	109	–	–	184	256	305
14. Intestinal nematode infections	5 024	2 562	2 462	24	1 918	507	80	33	23	1 832	491	81	35
a. Ascariasis	1 750	895	855	23	864	7	1	–	22	825	7	–	–
b. Trichuriasis	1 788	915	873	1	913	1	–	–	1	871	1	–	–
c. Ancylostomiasis and necatoriasis	1 484	752	732	–	141	499	79	33	–	136	482	80	34

Annex Table 9i, continued. DALYs by age, sex and cause (thousands): World, 1990

				Males					Females				
Cause	Total	Male	Female	0-4	5-14	15-44	45-59	60+	0-4	5-14	15-44	45-59	60+
B. Respiratory infections	**116 696**	**59 408**	**57 288**	**47 834**	**5 708**	**2 130**	**824**	**2 911**	**45 190**	**6 345**	**2 180**	**740**	**2 834**
1. Lower respiratory infections	112 898	57 650	55 248	46 813	5 108	2 044	807	2 878	43 877	5 755	2 093	722	2 800
2. Upper respiratory infections	1 311	670	641	472	71	78	17	32	437	77	76	17	34
3. Otitis media	2 163	1 087	1 075	549	529	9	-	-	551	513	11	-	-
C. Maternal conditions	**29 827**		**29 827**							**400**	**29 231**	**197**	
1. Maternal haemorrhage	3 564		3 564							92	3 427	45	
2. Maternal sepsis	5 452		5 452							61	5 367	24	
3. Hypertensive disorders of pregnancy	1 731		1 731							46	1 663	21	
4. Obstructed labour	6 462		6 462							31	6 419	12	
5. Abortion	5 097		5 097							52	5 025	20	
D. Perinatal conditions*	**92 313**	**47 504**	**44 808**	**47 501**	**2**	**1**			**44 806**	**1**	**1**		
E. Nutritional deficiencies	**51 074**	**23 910**	**27 164**	**13 626**	**3 446**	**5 213**	**907**	**718**	**13 776**	**3 464**	**7 789**	**1 324**	**810**
1. Protein-energy malnutrition	20 957	10 336	10 621	9 919	139	122	53	103	10 083	223	162	44	110
2. Iodine deficiency	1 562	779	782	665	78	36	1	-	646	80	50	4	1
3. Vitamin A deficiency	3 838	1 941	1 897	1 239	657	45	-	-	1 197	655	45	-	-
4. Iron-deficiency anaemia	24 613	10 812	13 802	1 786	2 564	5 003	847	611	1 833	2 498	7 508	1 272	691
II. Noncommunicable diseases	***564 632***	***292 626***	***272 006***	***35 094***	***18 924***	***106 183***	***63 473***	***68 953***	***33 842***	***17 568***	***100 263***	***51 980***	***68 354***
A. Malignant neoplasms	**70 513**	**39 272**	**31 241**	**940**	**2 402**	**8 847**	**13 171**	**13 913**	**916**	**1 794**	**8 346**	**10 085**	**10 101**
1. Mouth and oropharynx cancers	3 743	2 396	1 347	19	44	692	862	778	17	47	409	432	442
2. Oesophagus cancer	3 578	2 407	1 171	-	1	358	1 047	1 001	-	2	169	445	555
3. Stomach cancer	7 694	4 862	2 832	2	15	755	2 010	2 080	1	10	660	952	1 208
4. Colon and rectum cancers	4 617	2 429	2 188	4	19	537	739	1 130	5	20	390	646	1 127
5. Liver cancer	6 550	4 882	1 668	25	69	1 784	1 964	1 040	22	55	444	603	544
6. Pancreas cancer	1 577	933	644	13	-	153	359	421	2	3	71	208	360
7. Trachea, bronchus, lung cancers	8 871	6 678	2 194	1	31	712	2 813	3 108	5	11	273	818	1 086
8. Melanoma and other skin cancers	565	299	266	-	3	104	106	85	1	2	87	85	90
9. Breast cancer	4 210		4 210						3	8	1 362	1 711	1 126
10. Cervix uteri cancer	2 854		2 854						1	2	937	1 296	617
11. Corpus uteri cancer	644		644						-	4	111	284	242
12. Ovary cancer	1 403		1 403						23	52	485	471	371
13. Prostate cancer	1 345	1 345	-			28	229	1 083					
14. Bladder cancer	1 215	932	283	2	5	97	270	557	-	3	38	77	163
15. Lymphomas and multiple myeloma	3 104	1 932	1 172	131	428	632	363	377	79	228	307	235	323
16. Leukaemia	4 567	2 474	2 093	305	740	916	266	248	299	549	776	237	233
C. Diabetes mellitus	**11 103**	**5 198**	**5 905**	**148**	**363**	**1 430**	**1 714**	**1 542**	**147**	**355**	**1 353**	**1 865**	**2 184**
D. Endocrine disorders	**6 087**	**2 726**	**3 361**	**1 034**	**360**	**717**	**343**	**273**	**962**	**413**	**1 035**	**523**	**428**

Annex Table 9i, continued. DALYs by age, sex and cause (thousands): World, 1990

Cause	Total	Male	Female	Males					Females				
				0-4	5-14	15-44	45-59	60+	0-4	5-14	15-44	45-59	60+
E. Neuro-psychiatric conditions	**144 950**	**71 855**	**73 095**	**2 116**	**3 516**	**55 850**	**6 361**	**4 012**	**2 028**	**3 340**	**54 886**	**6 984**	**5 856**
1. Unipolar major depression	50 810	18 070	32 740	-	1	15 321	2 189	559	-	1	27 651	3 925	1 165
2. Bipolar disorder	14 257	7 254	7 003	-	1	6 736	385	132	-	-	6 453	378	172
3. Schizophrenia	12 798	6 781	6 017	-	-	6 646	71	64	-	1	5 896	47	73
4. Epilepsy	5 350	2 853	2 496	155	781	1 547	264	106	157	858	1 219	164	98
5. Alcohol use	16 661	14 696	1 965	-	-	13 096	1 301	298	-	-	1 752	153	60
6. Dementia*	8 500	3 594	4 906	314	138	279	820	2 042	362	138	272	876	3 258
7. Parkinson disease	1 050	502	548	-	-	1	184	316	-	-	1	188	358
8. Multiple sclerosis	1 417	614	804	-	-	523	63	27	-	-	670	92	41
9. Drug use	5 675	4 556	1 118	-	345	4 057	132	22	-	86	994	33	6
10. Post-traumatic stress disorder	1 945	741	1 204	43	165	482	42	8	70	267	785	67	14
11. Obsessive-compulsive disorders	10 213	4 435	5 778	-	569	3 571	200	95	-	722	4 552	352	152
12. Panic disorder	4 766	1 603	3 163	-	163	1 223	215	1	-	197	2 568	338	61
F. Sense organ diseases	**10 398**	**4 710**	**5 688**	**88**	**13**	**439**	**2 108**	**2 062**	**71**	**26**	**537**	**2 535**	**2 519**
1. Glaucoma	2 578	1 010	1 567	7	-	90	603	311	9	-	132	998	428
2. Cataracts	7 510	3 578	3 933	35	3	324	1 481	1 735	24	3	334	1 505	2 066
G. Cardiovascular diseases	**133 236**	**70 368**	**62 867**	**3 796**	**4 403**	**14 872**	**18 521**	**28 777**	**3 545**	**4 615**	**11 822**	**12 750**	**30 135**
1. Rheumatic heart disease	6 191	2 625	3 566	5	341	1 397	525	357	33	486	1 662	817	568
2. Ischaemic heart disease	46 699	26 370	20 329	-	-	3 851	8 791	13 728	140	-	2 148	4 698	13 343
3. Cerebrovascular disease	38 523	19 387	19 136	475	899	3 903	5 168	8 942	441	774	3 170	4 446	10 304
4. Inflammatory heart diseases	10 322	5 309	5 013	751	905	2 123	901	629	891	983	1 718	700	721
H. Respiratory diseases	**60 370**	**32 741**	**27 629**	**5 320**	**2 807**	**7 671**	**6 738**	**10 205**	**5 058**	**2 255**	**6 772**	**5 086**	**8 458**
1. COPD*	29 136	16 305	12 831	575	146	3 160	4 381	8 043	797	169	2 335	3 057	6 473
2. Asthma	10 775	5 935	4 840	778	1 638	2 620	557	343	495	1 087	2 376	536	346
I. Digestive diseases	**47 472**	**27 138**	**20 334**	**4 741**	**1 780**	**8 561**	**7 764**	**4 292**	**4 795**	**1 579**	**5 491**	**4 684**	**3 784**
1. Peptic ulcer	2 766	1 758	1 007	23	40	804	531	359	26	35	418	269	258
2. Cirrhosis of the liver	13 182	9 116	4 067	209	195	3 400	3 614	1 697	155	251	1 208	1 450	1 003
3. Appendicitis	1 763	1 034	729	28	400	555	36	16	28	323	338	26	14
J. Genito-urinary diseases	**15 308**	**8 580**	**6 728**	**726**	**1 239**	**2 241**	**2 733**	**1 640**	**545**	**1 215**	**2 235**	**1 384**	**1 349**
1. Nephritis and nephrosis	8 607	4 452	4 155	499	1 025	1 457	697	774	441	1 075	1 268	635	737
2. Benign prostatic hypertrophy	1 818	1 818	-	7	1	9	1 426	375	-	-	-	-	-
L. Musculo-skeletal diseases	**18 910**	**6 959**	**11 952**	**46**	**114**	**2 745**	**2 769**	**1 284**	**61**	**126**	**4 663**	**4 715**	**2 387**
1. Rheumatoid arthritis	3 286	898	2 388	1	3	433	283	179	1	27	1 232	635	493
2. Osteoarthritis	13 278	5 342	7 935	-	-	2 083	2 354	904	-	-	2 591	3 745	1 599

Annex Table 9i, continued. DALYs by age, sex and cause (thousands): World, 1990

Cause	Total	Male	Female	Males 0-4	Males 5-14	Males 15-44	Males 45-59	Males 60+	Females 0-4	Females 5-14	Females 15-44	Females 45-59	Females 60+
M. Congenital anomalies	32 921	16 571	16 350	14 932	828	707	75	29	14 648	877	693	94	37
1. Abdominal wall defect	174	94	80	94	-	-	-	-	80	-	-	-	-
2. Anencephaly	4 993	1 945	3 048	1 945	-	-	-	-	3 048	-	-	-	-
3. Anorectal atresia	61	34	27	34	-	-	-	-	27	-	-	-	-
4. Cleft lip	412	238	174	238	-	-	-	-	174	-	-	-	-
5. Cleft palate	336	159	177	159	-	-	-	-	177	-	-	-	-
6. Oesophageal atresia	103	57	45	57	-	-	-	-	45	-	-	-	-
7. Renal agenesis	394	199	194	199	-	-	-	-	194	-	-	-	-
8. Down syndrome	4 746	2 626	2 119	2 185	189	238	12	3	1 691	189	223	14	2
9. Congenital heart anomalies	14 707	7 727	6 981	6 942	386	324	53	21	6 161	392	334	67	27
10. Spina bifida	4 117	1 878	2 239	1 766	98	13	1	-	2 077	118	37	5	2
N. Oral conditions	7 487	3 674	3 813	462	633	1 308	685	586	445	631	1 329	712	696
1. Dental caries	4 313	2 174	2 139	455	625	751	216	127	439	610	726	217	147
2. Periodontal disease	255	128	127	-	-	104	16	7	-	-	103	16	8
3. Edentulism	2 787	1 339	1 448	-	-	437	451	451	-	-	432	476	539
III. Injuries	*208 647*	*135 231*	*73 415*	*21 136*	*28 021*	*74 179*	*8 999*	*2 897*	*18 387*	*17 491*	*30 938*	*4 280*	*2 319*
A. Unintentional injuries	152 188	99 810	52 378	18 307	25 265	47 690	6 498	2 051	15 387	15 661	16 693	2 937	1 700
1. Road traffic accidents	34 317	25 018	9 299	1 956	5 073	15 554	1 883	552	1 246	2 901	4 072	762	318
2. Poisonings	6 455	3 811	2 644	1 101	492	1 639	458	120	736	408	1 200	211	89
3. Falls	26 680	16 672	10 008	3 335	7 068	5 098	798	373	3 321	3 240	2 244	662	541
4. Fires	11 875	4 776	7 100	1 449	1 530	1 493	224	79	1 295	2 796	2 695	197	116
5. Drownings	15 697	10 461	5 236	2 921	4 006	3 138	288	108	2 107	1 970	954	124	81
6. Other unintentional	57 164	39 073	18 091	7 544	7 096	20 768	2 847	819	6 681	4 347	5 528	980	555
B. Intentional injuries	56 459	35 421	21 037	2 829	2 756	26 489	2 500	846	3 000	1 830	14 245	1 343	619
1. Self-inflicted injuries	18 967	10 220	8 747	-	677	7 550	1 400	593	-	376	7 095	847	429
2. Violence	17 472	13 662	3 810	885	789	11 040	783	165	1 041	482	1 915	276	95
3. War	20 019	11 538	8 481	1 945	1 290	7 899	317	88	1 959	972	5 235	221	95

Notes:
A dash (-) symbol indicates fewer than 500 DALYs.
*IA6 is Bacterial meningitis and meningococcaemia; ID is Conditions arising during the perinatal period;
IIE6 is Dementia and other degenerative and hereditary CNS disorders; IIH1 is Chronic obstructive pulmonary disease.

Annex Table 10a. DALYs [0,0] by age, sex and cause (thousands): Established Market Economies, 1990

Cause	Total	Male	Female	Males					Females				
				0-4	5-14	15-44	45-59	60+	0-4	5-14	15-44	45-59	60+
Population (millions)	798	390	407	26	53	184	66	61	25	51	179	68	85
All causes	161 524	87 426	74 098	6 119	1 999	27 030	18 232	34 046	4 924	1 409	17 923	13 826	36 015
I. Communicable, maternal, perinatal and nutritional conditions	12 823	6 913	5 911	3 087	171	1 755	564	1 336	2 473	169	1 495	297	1 476
A. Infectious and parasitic diseases	4 163	2 649	1 514	388	62	1 534	379	287	345	65	689	120	296
1. Tuberculosis	224	157	66	1	–	35	45	76	1	–	13	14	39
2. STDs excluding HIV	289	21	268	2	–	16	1	1	1	2	257	3	4
a. Syphilis	11	7	4	2	–	2	1	1	1	–	1	–	1
b. Chlamydia	241	9	232	–	–	9	1	–	1	3	227	1	1
c. Gonorrhoea	30	5	25	–	–	5	–	–	–	–	25	–	–
3. HIV	1 955	1 650	305	41	–	1 325	252	26	31	6	232	30	6
4. Diarrhoeal diseases	361	184	177	118	5	30	11	16	108	9	26	11	22
5. Childhood-cluster diseases	94	47	47	35	9	2	1	2	35	9	1	1	2
a. Pertussis	54	27	27	35	7	2	1	2	35	8	1	1	2
b. Poliomyelitis	6	3	3	22	5	–	–	–	22	5	–	–	–
c. Diphtheria				–	–	1	1	1	–	–	–	–	–
d. Measles	30	15	15	12	2	1	–	–	12	3	–	–	–
e. Tetanus	3	1	1	–	–	1	–	–	–	–	–	–	–
6. Bacterial meningitis*	377	198	179	135	18	26	10	10	121	20	19	7	12
7. Hepatitis B and hepatitis C	98	59	39	2	1	25	16	14	2	1	15	9	12
8. Malaria	3	2	1	–	–	1	–	–	–	–	1	–	–
9. Tropical-cluster diseases	2	1	1	–	–	1	–	–	–	–	1	–	–
a. Trypanosomiasis				–	–	–	–	–	–	–	–	–	–
b. Chagas disease													
c. Schistosomiasis													
d. Leishmaniasis	2	2	1	–	–	1	–	–	–	–	1	–	–
e. Lymphatic filariasis													
f. Onchocerciasis													
10. Leprosy	2	1	1	–	–	1	1	–	–	–	–	1	–
11. Dengue				–	–	–	–	–	–	–	–	–	–
12. Japanese encephalitis													
13. Trachoma													
14. Intestinal nematode infections				–	–	–	–	–	–	–	–	–	–
a. Ascariasis													
b. Trichuriasis													
c. Ancylostomiasis and necatoriasis													

Annex Table 10a, continued. DALYs [0.0] by age, sex and cause (thousands): Established Market Economies, 1990

Cause	Total	Male	Female	Males					Females				
				0-4	5-14	15-44	45-59	60+	0-4	5-14	15-44	45-59	60+
B. Respiratory infections	**2 847**	**1 467**	**1 380**	**178**	**59**	**146**	**154**	**930**	**131**	**56**	**95**	**91**	**1 007**
1. Lower respiratory infections	2 649	1 363	1 285	136	21	136	149	921	98	20	87	87	993
2. Upper respiratory infections	84	45	39	20	3	9	4	9	12	3	8	4	13
3. Otitis media	114	58	56	22	35	1	-	1	20	34	-	-	1
C. Maternal conditions	**512**		**512**								**511**	**1**	
1. Maternal haemorrhage	33		33								33		
2. Maternal sepsis	30		30								30		
3. Hypertensive disorders of pregnancy	25		25								25		
4. Obstructed labour	389		389								389		
5. Abortion	13		13								13		
D. Perinatal conditions*	**4 215**	**2 368**	**1 847**	**2 365**	**2**	**1**			**1 845**	**1**	**1**		
E. Nutritional deficiencies	**1 086**	**429**	**658**	**155**	**49**	**73**	**32**	**119**	**152**	**47**	**199**	**86**	**174**
1. Protein-energy malnutrition	196	94	103	72	-	3	4	15	72	-	2	2	26
2. Iodine deficiency	36	18	19	18					18				
3. Vitamin A deficiency	-	-	-										
4. Iron-deficiency anaemia	837	309	528	64	48	69	26	102	62	46	193	83	145
II. Noncommunicable diseases	***128 355***	***66 153***	***62 202***	***2 284***	***942***	***15 496***	***15 838***	***31 592***	***1 920***	***775***	***13 335***	***12 679***	***33 494***
A. Malignant neoplasms	**28 847**	**15 813**	**13 034**	**97**	**159**	**1 775**	**4 624**	**9 158**	**81**	**124**	**1 934**	**3 792**	**7 103**
1. Mouth and oropharynx cancers	665	521	144	-	1	77	241	203	-	1	21	48	74
2. Oesophagus cancer	672	532	140			38	218	275			8	37	95
3. Stomach cancer	2 078	1 274	804			120	386	768			118	198	487
4. Colon and rectum cancers	3 167	1 623	1 544	-	1	130	450	1 041	-	1	118	373	1 053
5. Liver cancer	625	472	153	4	1	39	192	236	2	1	13	39	99
6. Pancreas cancer	1 197	650	547	-	-	53	211	387	-	-	31	135	380
7. Trachea, bronchus, lung cancers	5 864	4 221	1 643	1	1	249	1 386	2 583	1	1	121	518	1 002
8. Melanoma and other skin cancers	455	265	190	-	-	87	82	96	-	-	63	54	72
9. Breast cancer	2 739		2 739						-	-	551	1 041	1 147
10. Cervix uteri cancer	365		365						-	-	136	117	112
11. Corpus uteri cancer	366		366						-	-	39	115	212
12. Ovary cancer	748		748						-	1	105	277	365
13. Prostate cancer	1 130	1 130		-	-	6	99	1 025					
14. Bladder cancer	711	554	157	1		11	89	453	-		6	22	128
15. Lymphomas and multiple myeloma	1 351	757	593	5	17	206	202	327	3	7	113	138	332
16. Leukaemia	1 162	649	514	30	64	209	120	225	28	46	147	99	194
C. Diabetes mellitus	**4 043**	**1 766**	**2 277**	**5**	**6**	**362**	**557**	**836**	**5**	**9**	**354**	**592**	**1 317**
D. Endocrine disorders	**1 959**	**811**	**1 148**	**160**	**73**	**227**	**109**	**242**	**154**	**56**	**295**	**293**	**351**

Annex Table 10a, continued. DALYs [0,0] by age, sex and cause (thousands): Established Market Economies, 1990

Cause	Total	Male	Female	Males 0-4	5-14	15-44	45-59	60+	Females 0-4	5-14	15-44	45-59	60+
E. Neuro-psychiatric conditions	26 675	13 151	13 524	234	326	8 137	1 815	2 640	200	273	6 749	1 821	4 480
1. Unipolar major depression	5 161	1 780	3 381			1 253	361	166			2 304	671	406
2. Bipolar disorder	1 260	629	631			529	61	38			516	63	53
3. Schizophrenia	3 627	1 826	1 801			1 771	18	37			1 742	7	52
4. Epilepsy	615	332	283	16	48	174	61	33	16	48	123	52	45
5. Alcohol use	3 699	3 094	605			2 380	523	192			442	103	59
6. Dementia*	5 955	2 231	3 724	72	26	75	378	1 679	70		62	427	3 143
7. Parkinson disease	893	388	506			1	105	282		21		128	377
8. Multiple sclerosis	363	147	216			110	23	13			153	39	23
9. Drug use	1 190	905	285	1	76	788	32	8		26	245	11	3
10. Post-traumatic stress disorder	220	83	137	7	14	50	9	3	11	23	82	15	7
11. Obsessive-compulsive disorders	1 116	468	647		46	345	40	37		59	447	72	70
12. Panic disorder	520	170	350		16	113	41			16	241	66	27
F. Sense organ diseases	168	73	96	1		5	27	40	1		3	33	59
1. Glaucoma	115	48	68			3	23	22			1	29	37
2. Cataracts	46	21	25	1		1	3	17			1	3	21
G. Cardiovascular diseases	37 313	20 051	17 262	145	49	2 195	4 707	12 955	122	40	1 106	2 113	13 882
1. Rheumatic heart disease	323	108	215	1	1	23	30	53	1	1	25	52	136
2. Ischaemic heart disease	18 375	10 592	7 783			811	2 790	6 991			230	905	6 649
3. Cerebrovascular disease	9 985	4 591	5 394	23	12	563	920	3 073	17	9	457	737	4 174
4. Inflammatory heart diseases	1 197	698	499	29	11	237	188	233	34	9	108	89	258
H. Respiratory diseases	7 617	4 443	3 174	186	134	648	822	2 653	130	85	564	620	1 774
1. COPD*	4 162	2 639	1 523	12	3	135	475	2 014	7	2	73	297	1 144
2. Asthma	1 362	713	649	82	110	279	115	126	51	71	264	117	146
I. Digestive diseases	7 431	4 095	3 337	106	25	954	1 474	1 535	76	22	590	890	1 760
1. Peptic ulcer	412	239	172	1	1	47	66	125	1	1	23	30	118
2. Cirrhosis of the liver	2 808	1 910	898	3	1	465	849	593	2	1	179	331	385
3. Appendicitis	44	26	18	1	4	9	4	8		2	6	2	8
J. Genito-urinary diseases	2 015	1 049	966	38	4	115	248	644	30	7	114	168	648
1. Nephritis and nephrosis	920	476	444	32	3	69	83	290	24	4	38	60	318
2. Benign prostatic hypertrophy	275	275					107	168					
L. Musculo-skeletal diseases	6 758	2 201	4 557	4	4	595	1 114	484	3	12	1 107	1 924	1 511
1. Rheumatoid arthritis	1 130	271	859			46	102	123		4	261	189	406
2. Osteoarthritis	4 846	1 748	3 099			500	965	282			628	1 584	887

Annex Table 10a, continued. DALYs [0,0] by age, sex and cause (thousands): Established Market Economies, 1990

Cause	Total	Male	Female	Males 0-4	5-14	15-44	45-59	60+	Females 0-4	5-14	15-44	45-59	60+
M. Congenital anomalies	**2 707**	**1 463**	**1 244**	**1 246**	**59**	**117**	**23**	**18**	**1 058**	**54**	**87**	**24**	**22**
1. Abdominal wall defect	37	12	25	12	-	-	-	-	25	-	-	-	-
2. Anencephaly	212	84	128	84	-	-	-	-	128	-	-	-	-
3. Anorectal atresia	7	3	4	3	-	-	-	-	4	-	-	-	-
4. Cleft lip	40	19	21	19	-	-	-	-	21	-	-	-	-
5. Cleft palate	34	13	21	13	-	-	-	-	21	-	-	-	-
6. Oesophageal atresia	19	8	11	8	-	-	-	-	11	-	-	-	-
7. Renal agenesis	150	76	74	76	-	-	-	-	74	-	-	-	-
8. Down syndrome	156	86	70	62	5	5	9	6	48	4	4	10	4
9. Congenital heart anomalies	1 025	564	461	450	29	66	12	8	369	26	45	12	10
10. Spina bifida	138	63	75	50	6	6	-	-	63	5	6	1	1
N. Oral conditions	**1 175**	**536**	**639**	**29**	**62**	**188**	**123**	**133**	**28**	**59**	**196**	**145**	**211**
1. Dental caries	379	188	191	29	62	57	15	24	27	59	56	16	33
2. Periodontal disease	27	13	13	-	-	11	1	1	-	-	11	1	2
3. Edentulism	759	330	428	-	-	118	105	107	-	-	129	126	173
III. Injuries	***20 346***	***14 361***	***5 985***	***749***	***886***	***9 779***	***1 830***	***1 117***	***532***	***465***	***3 093***	***850***	***1 045***
A. Unintentional injuries	**14 771**	**10 307**	**4 464**	**695**	**823**	**6 727**	**1 226**	**836**	**479**	**427**	**2 110**	**567**	**882**
1. Road traffic accidents	7 251	5 144	2 107	129	367	3 948	465	236	99	225	1 416	207	161
2. Poisonings	492	359	133	13	6	286	39	15	9	4	85	20	14
3. Falls	2 284	1 292	992	117	140	598	213	225	78	61	242	186	425
4. Fires	496	299	196	66	65	112	32	24	53	56	50	16	22
5. Drownings	533	418	114	85	66	204	38	25	44	16	30	10	14
6. Other unintentional	3 716	2 794	921	286	178	1 580	440	310	196	65	288	128	246
B. Intentional injuries	**5 575**	**4 054**	**1 521**	**53**	**64**	**3 052**	**604**	**281**	**53**	**39**	**984**	**283**	**163**
1. Self-inflicted injuries	3 857	2 773	1 084	-	25	1 977	513	257	-	8	678	250	148
2. Violence	1 713	1 278	436	53	38	1 073	90	23	53	30	305	33	15
3. War	3	3	-	-	-	1	-	1	-	-	-	-	-

Notes:
A dash (-) symbol indicates fewer than 500 DALYs.

*IA6 is Bacterial meningitis and meningococcaemia; ID is Conditions arising during the perinatal period;
*IIH1 is Chronic obstructive pulmonary disease.
IIE6 is Dementia and other degenerative and hereditary CNS disorders;

Annex Table 10b. DALYs [0,0] by age, sex and cause (thousands): Formerly Socialist Economies of Europe, 1990

Cause	Total	Male	Female	Males					Females				
				0-4	5-14	15-44	45-59	60+	0-4	5-14	15-44	45-59	60+
Population (millions)	*346*	*165*	*181*	*14*	*27*	*76*	*27*	*21*	*13*	*26*	*75*	*30*	*36*
All causes	*103 250*	*57 930*	*45 320*	*6 368*	*1 879*	*19 942*	*14 538*	*15 202*	*5 004*	*1 193*	*10 752*	*8 992*	*19 379*
I. Communicable, maternal, perinatal and nutritional conditions	*10 150*	*5 215*	*4 935*	*3 567*	*181*	*586*	*407*	*474*	*2 740*	*172*	*1 228*	*156*	*638*
A. Infectious and parasitic diseases	2 686	1 495	1 191	638	58	404	254	141	539	54	397	66	135
1. Tuberculosis	666	567	99	5	1	275	206	81	3	2	39	26	29
2. STDs excluding HIV	273	42	231	5	1	32	2	1	5	3	219	2	1
a. Syphilis	4	3	2	–	–	1	–	–	–	–	1	–	–
b. Chlamydia	206	14	192	2	–	12	–	–	2	3	185	–	–
c. Gonorrhoea	54	18	36	3	–	15	–	–	3	–	32	–	–
3. HIV	76	43	34	24	3	14	1	–	25	–	5	1	–
4. Diarrhoeal diseases	485	253	233	223	7	13	6	4	201	6	13	5	7
5. Childhood-cluster diseases	83	41	42	30	6	3	2	1	31	6	1	1	1
a. Pertussis	50	24	26	19	4	–	–	–	21	5	–	–	–
b. Poliomyelitis	1	1	–	–	–	–	–	–	–	–	–	–	–
c. Diphtheria	2	1	1	1	–	–	–	–	1	–	–	–	–
d. Measles	26	14	12	9	–	2	–	–	9	–	1	–	–
e. Tetanus	4	2	2	–	–	–	–	–	–	–	–	–	–
6. Bacterial meningitis*	472	262	210	180	15	34	17	16	147	15	23	10	14
7. Hepatitis B and hepatitis C	73	39	34	17	3	10	4	4	14	2	12	3	3
8. Malaria	–	–	–	–	–	–	–	–	–	–	–	–	–
9. Tropical-cluster diseases	–	–	–	–	–	–	–	–	–	–	–	–	–
a. Trypanosomiasis	–	–	–	–	–	–	–	–	–	–	–	–	–
b. Chagas disease	–	–	–	–	–	–	–	–	–	–	–	–	–
c. Schistosomiasis	–	–	–	–	–	–	–	–	–	–	–	–	–
d. Leishmaniasis	–	–	–	–	–	–	–	–	–	–	–	–	–
e. Lymphatic filariasis	–	–	–	–	–	–	–	–	–	–	–	–	–
f. Onchocerciasis	–	–	–	–	–	–	–	–	–	–	–	–	–
10. Leprosy	–	–	–	–	–	–	–	–	–	–	–	–	–
11. Dengue	–	–	–	–	–	–	–	–	–	–	–	–	–
12. Japanese encephalitis	–	–	–	–	–	–	–	–	–	–	–	–	–
13. Trachoma	–	–	–	–	–	–	–	–	–	–	–	–	–
14. Intestinal nematode infections	2	–	2	–	–	–	–	–	–	–	2	–	–
a. Ascariasis	2	–	2	–	–	–	–	–	–	–	2	–	–
b. Trichuriasis	–	–	–	–	–	–	–	–	–	–	–	–	–
c. Ancylostomiasis and necatoriasis	–	–	–	–	–	–	–	–	–	–	–	–	–

Annex Table 10b, continued. DALYs [0,0] by age, sex and cause (thousands): Formerly Socialist Economies of Europe, 1990

Cause	Total	Male	Female	Males 0-4	5-14	15-44	45-59	60+	Females 0-4	5-14	15-44	45-59	60+
B. Respiratory infections	**2 727**	**1 471**	**1 256**	**833**	**62**	**149**	**135**	**291**	**665**	**59**	**68**	**45**	**419**
1. Lower respiratory infections	2 620	1 415	1 204	804	44	145	133	289	640	41	65	44	415
2. Upper respiratory infections	37	19	18	11	1	3	1	2	10	17	3	1	3
3. Otitis media	70	36	33	18	18	1	-	-	15	17	-	-	-
C. Maternal conditions	**664**		**664**								**664**		
1. Maternal haemorrhage	23		23								23		
2. Maternal sepsis	95		95								95		
3. Hypertensive disorders of pregnancy	18		18								18		
4. Obstructed labour	249		249								249		
5. Abortion	156		156								156		
D. Perinatal conditions*	**3 202**	**1 882**	**1 320**	**1 882**					**1 320**				
E. Nutritional deficiencies	**871**	**368**	**503**	**214**	**61**	**33**	**18**	**42**	**216**	**58**	**99**	**45**	**84**
1. Protein-energy malnutrition	234	112	122	104	-	1	2	5	109	-	1	1	11
2. Iodine deficiency	35	16	19	16					18				
3. Vitamin A deficiency													
4. Iron-deficiency anaemia	477	185	292	65	53	25	11	32	65	51	79	37	61
II. Noncommunicable diseases	**73 232**	**37 785**	**35 447**	**1 696**	**622**	**9 638**	**11 747**	**14 081**	**1 384**	**510**	**7 273**	**8 077**	**18 202**
A. Malignant neoplasms	**13 716**	**7 893**	**5 824**	**104**	**145**	**1 184**	**3 325**	**3 136**	**80**	**98**	**1 059**	**1 989**	**2 598**
1. Mouth and oropharynx cancers	417	356	60	1	1	65	193	97	-	1	12	20	27
2. Oesophagus cancer	214	181	33	-	-	21	98	61	-	-	4	11	18
3. Stomach cancer	1 943	1 192	751	-	-	156	523	512	-	-	102	238	410
4. Colon and rectum cancers	1 283	610	673	1	1	78	216	315	1	-	70	208	393
5. Liver cancer	372	210	161	2	1	25	84	97	2	-	15	47	97
6. Pancreas cancer	531	313	218	-	-	42	137	134	-	1	18	68	132
7. Trachea, bronchus, lung cancers	2 996	2 517	480	-	-	231	1 280	1 002	-	1	62	180	237
8. Melanoma and other skin cancers	187	92	95	2	2	32	31	28	1	-	32	25	36
9. Breast cancer	971		971						-	-	221	427	323
10. Cervix uteri cancer	358		358						-	-	105	124	128
11. Corpus uteri cancer	259		259								35	102	121
12. Ovary cancer	367		367								73	160	132
13. Prostate cancer	207	207				6	39	162					
14. Bladder cancer	282	222	60	2	2	9	70	139	-	-	5	15	40
15. Lymphomas and multiple myeloma	460	274	186	12	27	103	75	57	7	11	64	46	58
16. Leukaemia	568	316	252	34	56	100	63	64	26	38	73	52	63
C. Diabetes mellitus	**1 079**	**432**	**646**	**1**	**2**	**112**	**144**	**173**	**2**	**4**	**103**	**174**	**364**
D. Endocrine disorders	**362**	**145**	**217**	**38**	**11**	**65**	**21**	**11**	**36**	**11**	**85**	**55**	**30**

Annex Table 10b, continued. DALYs [0,0] by age, sex and cause (thousands): Formerly Socialist Economies of Europe, 1990

Cause	Total	Male	Female	Males 0-4	Males 5-14	Males 15-44	Males 45-59	Males 60+	Females 0-4	Females 5-14	Females 15-44	Females 45-59	Females 60+
E. Neuro-psychiatric conditions	**11 138**	**5 387**	**5 751**	**215**	**264**	**3 392**	**758**	**758**	**183**	**211**	**2 943**	**805**	**1 608**
1. Unipolar major depression	2 391	801	1 590	-	-	571	163	67	-	-	1 063	328	199
2. Bipolar disorder	659	314	345	-	-	256	34	24	-	-	249	37	59
3. Schizophrenia	1 287	633	653	-	-	605	16	12	-	-	628	8	17
4. Epilepsy	470	284	185	19	60	146	39	21	15	43	77	28	23
5. Alcohol use	1 404	1 230	174	-	-	932	219	79	-	-	133	23	17
6. Dementia*	1 880	621	1 259	37	17	29	121	417	34	14	27	165	1 019
7. Parkinson disease	243	89	153	-	-	-	28	61	-	-	-	38	115
8. Multiple sclerosis	191	76	115	-	-	53	13	10	-	-	77	20	18
9. Drug use	378	302	76	-	30	257	12	3	-	7	64	3	1
10. Post-traumatic stress disorder	97	36	61	4	7	21	4	1	6	12	34	6	3
11. Obsessive-compulsive disorders	494	204	291	-	25	149	17	13	-	32	194	33	31
12. Panic disorder	233	75	158	-	8	49	17	-	-	9	106	31	12
F. Sense organ diseases	**92**	**36**	**56**	**1**	-	**1**	**8**	**26**	**1**	-	**2**	**18**	**36**
1. Glaucoma	45	14	31	-	-	-	5	9	-	-	1	15	15
2. Cataracts	46	21	25	1	-	1	3	17	1	-	1	3	21
G. Cardiovascular diseases	**28 624**	**14 747**	**13 877**	**58**	**26**	**2 181**	**4 796**	**7 686**	**55**	**21**	**764**	**2 277**	**10 760**
1. Rheumatic heart disease	696	306	390	-	4	121	133	48	-	3	82	191	114
2. Ischaemic heart disease	14 038	7 907	6 131	-	-	1 105	2 896	3 907	-	-	206	961	4 964
3. Cerebrovascular disease	8 833	3 818	5 015	9	6	430	1 105	2 268	7	5	304	895	3 803
4. Inflammatory heart diseases	818	478	340	12	6	188	150	122	16	5	70	81	169
H. Respiratory diseases	**4 635**	**2 797**	**1 839**	**67**	**50**	**483**	**1 028**	**1 169**	**47**	**35**	**327**	**446**	**983**
1. COPD*	1 791	1 190	602	1	1	151	487	549	1	1	73	111	415
2. Asthma	549	279	270	35	47	107	47	43	22	31	102	52	63
I. Digestive diseases	**4 446**	**2 474**	**1 972**	**130**	**19**	**867**	**883**	**575**	**93**	**17**	**455**	**646**	**761**
1. Peptic ulcer	332	239	93	-	-	71	95	71	-	-	20	28	45
2. Cirrhosis of the liver	1 345	872	473	5	1	218	401	245	4	3	82	188	196
3. Appendicitis	23	13	11	1	2	5	2	3	-	2	4	2	3
J. Genito-urinary diseases	**1 609**	**753**	**856**	**14**	**12**	**224**	**235**	**268**	**10**	**12**	**241**	**314**	**278**
1. Nephritis and nephrosis	497	272	226	6	8	115	81	62	6	9	77	65	69
2. Benign prostatic hypertrophy	164	164	-	-	-	-	57	107	-	-	-	-	-
L. Musculo-skeletal diseases	**4 122**	**1 440**	**2 682**	**4**	**6**	**850**	**381**	**200**	**3**	**10**	**964**	**1 082**	**625**
1. Rheumatoid arthritis	499	116	382	-	-	53	32	31	-	3	171	111	98
2. Osteoarthritis	3 236	1 226	2 010	-	-	743	325	158	-	-	660	870	480

Annex Table 10b, continued. DALYs [0,0] by age, sex and cause (thousands): Formerly Socialist Economies of Europe, 1990

Cause	Total	Male	Female	Males					Females				
				0-4	5-14	15-44	45-59	60+	0-4	5-14	15-44	45-59	60+
M. Congenital anomalies	2 032	1 116	916	1 003	49	54	8	2	816	49	39	9	3
1. Abdominal wall defect	21	7	15	7	-	-	-	-	15	-	-	-	-
2. Anencephaly	63	24	39	24	-	-	-	-	39	-	-	-	-
3. Anorectal atresia	3	2	2	2	-	-	-	-	2	-	-	-	-
4. Cleft lip	27	16	11	16	-	-	-	-	11	-	-	-	-
5. Cleft palate	21	11	11	11	-	-	-	-	11	-	-	-	-
6. Oesophageal atresia	10	5	5	5	-	-	-	-	5	-	-	-	-
7. Renal agenesis	36	18	18	18	-	-	-	-	18	-	-	-	-
8. Down syndrome	73	42	31	28	6	2	4	1	22	2	2	5	1
9. Congenital heart anomalies	803	442	361	381	19	37	3	1	321	17	19	3	2
10. Spina bifida	179	84	95	75	6	2	-	-	86	6	2	-	-
N. Oral conditions	634	276	358	37	19	100	81	40	35	28	111	107	77
1. Dental caries	258	119	139	37	19	30	19	15	35	28	29	21	26
2. Periodontal disease	15	7	8	-	-	5	1	1	-	-	5	-	1
3. Edentulism	361	150	211	-	-	65	61	24	-	-	76	85	50
III. Injuries	*19 869*	*14 930*	*4 939*	*1 105*	*1 076*	*9 718*	*2 385*	*647*	*879*	*512*	*2 251*	*759*	*538*
A. Unintentional injuries	13 454	10 403	3 051	823	884	6 538	1 709	448	590	381	1 168	515	397
1. Road traffic accidents	4 607	3 676	931	91	287	2 700	466	132	56	155	484	143	93
2. Poisonings	1 673	1 275	398	116	29	702	359	69	87	22	140	104	45
3. Falls	1 678	1 117	561	119	132	611	172	84	92	54	180	96	140
4. Fires	355	239	116	46	31	108	41	14	39	22	26	13	16
5. Drownings	1 106	927	179	85	176	543	100	23	38	60	54	17	11
6. Other unintentional	4 035	3 169	866	368	230	1 874	571	127	278	68	284	144	93
B. Intentional injuries	6 415	4 527	1 888	282	192	3 179	676	198	289	131	1 083	244	141
1. Self-inflicted injuries	2 862	2 264	598	-	36	1 554	512	162	-	8	326	159	105
2. Violence	1 447	1 091	356	22	18	893	132	27	18	16	235	61	25
3. War	2 106	1 171	934	260	138	732	32	10	271	107	521	24	11

Notes:
A dash (-) symbol indicates fewer than 500 DALYs.
*IA6 is Bacterial meningitis and meningococcaemia; ID is Conditions arising during the perinatal period;
IIH1 is Chronic obstructive pulmonary disease.
IIE6 is Dementia and other degenerative and hereditary CNS disorders; IIH1 is Chronic obstructive pulmonary disease.

Annex Table 10c. DALYs [0,0] by age, sex and cause (thousands): India, 1990

Cause	Total	Male	Female	Males 0-4	5-14	15-44	45-59	60+	Females 0-4	5-14	15-44	45-59	60+
Population (millions)	850	439	410	60	102	201	48	30	57	95	183	46	29
All causes	539 143	266 004	273 139	143 381	30 122	42 989	24 181	25 332	149 887	130 998	49 040	20 115	24 334
I. Communicable, maternal, perinatal and nutritional conditions	337 903	161 303	176 600	123 282	11 375	15 076	6 056	5 515	130 998	29 763	22 613	4 742	4 171
A. Infectious and parasitic diseases	171 220	86 885	84 335	57 278	7 902	12 900	5 334	3 470	59 819	8 608	9 983	3 681	2 244
1. Tuberculosis	24 704	15 497	9 207	1 196	688	6 919	4 314	2 380	925	549	4 074	2 615	1 045
2. STDs excluding HIV	7 166	2 740	4 426	2 061	10	587	32	51	2 213	47	2 051	48	67
a. Syphilis	4 174	1 984	2 190	1 776	1	127	29	50	1 941	1	144	37	66
b. Chlamydia	1 742	236	1 506	70	3	161	1	-	67	33	1 398	8	1
c. Gonorrhoea	1 251	521	730	215	5	298	2	1	205	13	509	3	-
3. HIV	206	133	73	11	1	112	6	2	12	2	59	1	-
4. Diarrhoeal diseases	68 014	32 332	35 682	28 925	1 671	985	278	474	31 441	2 405	1 029	297	510
5. Childhood-cluster diseases	41 687	20 726	20 962	18 069	1 838	677	99	42	17 921	2 180	704	110	46
a. Pertussis	6 922	3 450	3 472	3 171	279	-	-	-	3 183	290	-	-	-
b. Poliomyelitis	2 682	1 532	1 151	1 503	7	21	1	-	1 129	5	16	1	-
c. Diphtheria	351	175	176	157	16	2	-	-	158	17	2	-	-
d. Measles	16 401	8 113	8 288	7 120	981	10	1	-	7 235	1 042	9	1	-
e. Tetanus	15 331	7 456	7 875	6 118	556	644	96	42	6 217	827	678	107	46
6. Bacterial meningitis*	3 192	1 609	1 584	1 210	44	245	69	41	1 204	43	217	74	46
7. Hepatitis B and hepatitis C	696	376	320	106	52	118	61	38	89	54	106	32	38
8. Malaria	1 981	1 007	974	338	292	307	50	20	304	338	268	45	18
9. Tropical-cluster diseases	4 984	3 372	1 613	228	1 289	1 724	114	16	135	658	641	162	17
a. Trypanosomiasis	-	-	-	-	-	-	-	-	-	-	-	-	-
b. Chagas disease	-	-	-	-	-	-	-	-	-	-	-	-	-
c. Schistosomiasis	-	-	-	-	-	-	-	-	-	-	-	-	-
d. Leishmaniasis	2 300	1 363	937	129	593	609	23	9	91	434	386	18	7
e. Lymphatic filariasis	2 684	2 008	676	99	697	1 115	90	7	44	224	255	144	10
f. Onchocerciasis	-	-	-	-	-	-	-	-	-	-	-	-	-
10. Leprosy	288	146	142	4	52	72	13	5	7	52	68	12	4
11. Dengue	879	391	488	95	287	7	2	-	114	362	8	3	-
12. Japanese encephalitis	160	78	81	47	25	5	1	-	48	27	5	1	-
13. Trachoma	36	10	26	-	-	2	3	5	-	-	5	9	12
14. Intestinal nematode infections	956	488	469	4	319	118	28	18	4	312	108	28	18
a. Ascariasis	328	165	162	4	160	1	-	-	4	157	1	-	-
b. Trichuriasis	180	91	89	-	91	-	-	-	-	89	-	-	-
c. Ancylostomiasis and necatoriasis	448	231	217	-	68	117	28	18	-	66	107	27	17

Annex Table 10c, continued. DALYs [0,0] by age, sex and cause (thousands): India, 1990

Cause	Total	Male	Female	Males 0-4	5-14	15-44	45-59	60+	Females 0-4	5-14	15-44	45-59	60+
B. Respiratory infections	**77 990**	**36 421**	**41 569**	**30 497**	**2 425**	**1 235**	**501**	**1 763**	**33 957**	**4 309**	**1 113**	**552**	**1 638**
1. Lower respiratory infections	75 207	35 486	39 721	29 753	2 283	1 210	495	1 744	32 325	4 139	1 091	545	1 620
2. Upper respiratory infections	772	365	407	294	27	20	6	19	320	45	17	7	17
3. Otitis media	1 233	570	663	450	115	5	–	–	533	125	5	–	–
C. Maternal conditions	**10 117**	–	**10 117**	–	–	–	–	–	–	–	**10 001**	**115**	–
1. Maternal haemorrhage	1 499		1 499								1 473	27	
2. Maternal sepsis	1 571		1 571								1 553	18	
3. Hypertensive disorders of pregnancy	739		739								726	13	
4. Obstructed labour	2 202		2 202								2 193	9	
5. Abortion	1 787		1 787								1 771	17	
D. Perinatal conditions*	**59 273**	**29 026**	**30 247**	**29 026**					**30 247**				
E. Nutritional deficiencies	**19 304**	**8 972**	**10 332**	**6 480**	**1 048**	**941**	**221**	**282**	**6 976**	**1 159**	**1 515**	**393**	**289**
1. Protein-energy malnutrition	10 574	4 965	5 608	4 751	72	78	20	45	5 284	206	49	17	51
2. Iodine deficiency	760	384	376	333	38	13	–	–	323	40	12	–	–
3. Vitamin A deficiency	1 626	809	816	543	248	18	–	–	543	257	16	–	–
4. Iron-deficiency anaemia	6 345	2 813	3 532	854	689	832	200	237	826	656	1 437	376	238
II. Noncommunicable diseases	**128 077**	**64 185**	**63 893**	**10 305**	**4 077**	**15 222**	**15 510**	**19 070**	**10 559**	**4 564**	**15 966**	**13 408**	**19 396**
A. Malignant neoplasms	**13 355**	**6 114**	**7 242**	**315**	**389**	**1 469**	**2 200**	**1 742**	**154**	**208**	**2 171**	**2 983**	**1 726**
1. Mouth and oropharynx cancers	1 992	1 093	900	6	8	223	485	372	5	8	219	426	242
2. Oesophagus cancer	1 120	528	592	–	–	87	245	196	–	–	115	272	204
3. Stomach cancer	1 032	618	414	1	1	132	285	199	1	1	113	176	126
4. Colon and rectum cancers	492	250	242	–	–	84	82	82	–	–	54	97	88
5. Liver cancer	282	189	94	3	4	43	82	55	2	3	22	37	30
6. Pancreas cancer	166	94	72	–	–	20	43	31	–	–	18	28	26
7. Trachea, bronchus, lung cancers	726	591	135	1	1	95	282	212	1	1	27	54	52
8. Melanoma and other skin cancers	29	14	16	–	–	4	6	2	–	–	5	7	4
9. Breast cancer	1 050	–	1 050						–	–	392	453	204
10. Cervix uteri cancer	1 438	–	1 438								393	782	263
11. Corpus uteri cancer	74	–	74								9	35	29
12. Ovary cancer	343	–	343						2	3	149	105	84
13. Prostate cancer	150	150	–				28	117					
14. Bladder cancer	127	97	30			12	35	49	1		5	10	14
15. Lymphomas and multiple myeloma	585	396	190	52	69	142	83	49	10	15	62	51	51
16. Leukaemia	723	419	305	96	126	130	43	23	49	75	116	44	22
C. Diabetes mellitus	**3 880**	**1 845**	**2 035**	**168**	**303**	**369**	**499**	**506**	**168**	**302**	**363**	**560**	**643**
D. Endocrine disorders	**161**	**87**	**75**	**40**	**10**	**20**	**13**	**4**	**29**	**4**	**18**	**13**	**11**

Annex Table 10c, continued. DALYs [0,0] by age, sex and cause (thousands): India, 1990

Cause	Total	Male	Female	Males					Females				
				0-4	5-14	15-44	45-59	60+	0-4	5-14	15-44	45-59	60+
E. Neuro-psychiatric conditions	19 666	9 323	10 343	741	622	5 817	1 065	1 077	929	655	6 494	1 075	1 190
1. Unipolar major depression	5 929	2 174	3 755	-	-	1 732	332	111	-	-	2 980	582	194
2. Bipolar disorder	1 672	868	804			773	63	32			709	58	37
3. Schizophrenia	2 368	1 269	1 099	85	143	1 236	18	15	95	188	1 070	8	21
4. Epilepsy	1 215	623	592	-	-	300	57	39	-	-	256	21	31
5. Alcohol use	740	679	60	-	-	567	90	23	-	-	51	6	3
6. Dementia*	1 784	856	928	80	29	64	175	508	107	33	64	179	545
7. Parkinson disease	242	124	117	-	-	-	41	83	-	-	-	45	73
8. Multiple sclerosis	304	134	170	-	-	109	17	7	-	-	137	23	10
9. Drug use	62	56	6	-	6	48	2	1	-	1	5	-	-
10. Post-traumatic stress disorder	268	104	164	16	27	54	6	2	25	42	84	10	2
11. Obsessive-compulsive disorders	1 221	542	679	-	94	399	30	20	-	117	485	52	25
12. Panic disorder	536	172	364	-	3	136	32	-	-	32	273	49	10
F. Sense organ diseases	3 719	1 813	1 905	10	1	114	778	910	7	1	91	711	1 096
1. Glaucoma	786	441	345	-	-	38	295	108	-	-	14	217	113
2. Cataracts	2 929	1 369	1 560	7	1	76	483	801	7	1	77	493	982
G. Cardiovascular diseases	44 669	22 509	22 160	1 307	717	3 013	6 257	11 214	1 470	1 135	2 903	4 704	11 948
1. Rheumatic heart disease	2 638	1 044	1 594	3	82	558	298	103	4	126	814	478	172
2. Ischaemic heart disease	19 604	10 398	9 206	-	-	614	3 369	6 414	-	-	492	2 211	6 503
3. Cerebrovascular disease	8 200	4 012	4 189	261	116	330	999	2 304	278	145	447	724	2 595
4. Inflammatory heart diseases	3 126	1 477	1 649	236	170	506	329	237	323	285	460	307	274
H. Respiratory diseases	11 560	5 828	5 732	1 058	724	908	1 298	1 840	1 167	691	1 140	1 277	1 456
1. COPD*	4 139	2 278	1 862	154	74	302	684	1 064	201	92	304	568	697
2. Asthma	1 691	928	764	186	244	300	105	93	123	170	278	107	86
I. Digestive diseases	10 265	6 354	3 911	555	316	2 399	2 182	900	603	279	1 455	1 057	517
1. Peptic ulcer	1 404	856	548	9	14	365	297	172	17	27	241	165	98
2. Cirrhosis of the liver	4 956	3 329	1 627	122	69	1 242	1 339	558	161	140	563	524	239
3. Appendicitis	685	387	298	19	119	229	14	5	18	102	163	12	4
J. Genito-urinary diseases	3 785	2 059	1 726	204	482	277	627	468	106	737	386	238	259
1. Nephritis and nephrosis	3 109	1 445	1 664	170	467	258	264	287	98	733	365	222	245
2. Benign prostatic hypertrophy	524	524	-	-	-	-	352	171	-	-	-	-	-
L. Musculo-skeletal diseases	2 171	867	1 304	5	15	318	364	164	4	10	439	548	304
1. Rheumatoid arthritis	194	58	136	2	2	31	10	13	-	2	58	54	21
2. Osteoarthritis	1 926	778	1 147	-	-	280	350	148	-	-	375	492	280

Annex Table 10c, continued. DALYs [0,0] by age, sex and cause (thousands): India, 1990

Cause	Total	Male	Female	Males 0-4	5-14	15-44	45-59	60+	Females 0-4	5-14	15-44	45-59	60+
M. Congenital anomalies	13 014	6 427	6 587	5 727	378	272	35	14	5 762	464	287	53	21
1. Abdominal wall defect	102	55	47	55	-	-	-	-	47	-	-	-	-
2. Anencephaly	3 721	1 464	2 257	1 464	-	-	-	-	2 257	-	-	-	-
3. Anorectal atresia	52	28	24	28	-	-	-	-	24	-	-	-	-
4. Cleft lip	90	56	35	56	-	-	-	-	35	-	-	-	-
5. Cleft palate	72	37	35	37	-	-	-	-	35	-	-	-	-
6. Oesophageal atresia	70	38	32	38	-	-	-	-	32	-	-	-	-
7. Renal agenesis	196	99	97	99	-	-	-	-	97	-	-	-	-
8. Down syndrome	1 117	634	483	396	106	131	1	-	265	104	113	1	-
9. Congenital heart anomalies	4 203	2 218	1 985	1 897	180	98	31	13	1 595	223	106	43	17
10. Spina bifida	1 676	897	779	861	34	3	-	-	706	44	24	4	1
N. Oral conditions	1 284	641	643	95	66	119	156	206	90	66	123	158	207
1. Dental caries	697	358	338	93	64	94	52	56	88	59	86	50	54
2. Periodontal disease	56	29	27	-	-	21	5	3	-	-	19	5	3
3. Edentulism	497	245	251	-	-	-	99	147	-	-	-	102	149
III. Injuries	73 163	40 516	32 647	9 793	14 670	12 690	2 615	747	8 330	11 123	10 462	1 965	767
A. Unintentional injuries	65 052	36 201	28 851	9 280	14 340	9 895	2 060	626	7 677	10 805	8 110	1 582	677
1. Road traffic accidents	10 689	7 571	3 118	1 462	1 799	3 587	562	161	432	1 336	864	347	140
2. Poisonings	1 868	938	931	409	193	280	44	12	289	149	384	100	9
3. Falls	16 109	9 822	6 288	1 868	6 652	969	237	95	2 184	2 971	758	290	84
4. Fires	10 064	2 897	7 166	954	769	953	184	37	841	2 447	3 547	226	106
5. Drownings	5 367	2 847	2 521	859	1 142	721	90	35	724	1 131	513	103	48
6. Other unintentional	20 955	12 127	8 828	3 728	3 784	3 386	944	285	3 206	2 770	2 044	518	290
B. Intentional injuries	8 110	4 315	3 795	513	331	2 795	555	121	653	318	2 352	382	90
1. Self-inflicted injuries	4 963	2 446	2 518	-	198	1 834	357	57	-	200	2 111	186	20
2. Violence	2 951	1 673	1 278	513	133	764	198	64	653	118	241	197	69
3. War	196	196	-	513	-	196	-	-	-	-	-	-	-

Notes:

A dash (-) symbol indicates fewer than 500 DALYs.

*IA6 is Bacterial meningitis and meningococcaemia; ID is Conditions arising during the perinatal period;
IIE6 is Dementia and other degenerative and hereditary CNS disorders; IIH1 is Chronic obstructive pulmonary disease.

Annex Table 10d. DALYs [0,0] by age, sex and cause (thousands): China, 1990

Cause	Total	Male	Female	Males 0-4	5-14	15-44	45-59	60+	Females 0-4	5-14	15-44	45-59	60+
Population (millions)	1 134	585	548	60	97	306	73	49	58	90	284	64	52
All causes	348 507	179 410	169 097	51 047	9 839	51 116	28 048	39 360	57 450	7 772	45 908	21 527	36 440
I. Communicable, maternal, perinatal and nutritional conditions	97 683	45 438	52 246	32 127	2 899	4 971	2 576	2 864	37 636	2 935	7 399	1 753	2 522
A. Infectious and parasitic diseases	28 466	14 901	13 566	6 160	1 765	3 113	2 059	1 804	6 720	1 747	2 463	1 203	1 433
1. Tuberculosis	7 331	4 220	3 110	222	44	1 317	1 378	1 259	256	147	1 193	761	753
2. STDs excluding HIV	87	22	65	4	-	14	2	2	3	1	58	1	2
a. Syphilis	13	8	5	2	-	2	1	2	2	1	1	1	2
b. Chlamydia	50	5	45	1	-	4	-	-	-	-	44	-	-
c. Gonorrhoea	23	9	15	1	-	7	-	-	1	-	13	-	-
3. HIV	3	2	-	-	-	2	-	-	-	-	-	-	-
4. Diarrhoeal diseases	6 594	3 028	3 565	2 042	192	456	121	217	2 702	174	382	103	205
5. Childhood-cluster diseases	5 110	2 651	2 459	2 371	182	84	10	4	2 245	159	48	6	2
a. Pertussis	1 745	885	860	805	80	-	-	-	783	78	-	-	-
b. Poliomyelitis	767	433	334	412	3	17	1	-	318	2	13	1	-
c. Diphtheria	17	8	8	8	1	-	-	-	7	1	-	-	-
d. Measles	1 208	608	601	527	63	16	2	1	522	61	15	2	1
e. Tetanus	1 373	717	656	620	36	51	7	3	615	17	20	3	1
6. Bacterial meningitis*	2 617	1 312	1 304	794	38	315	95	70	791	37	302	94	81
7. Hepatitis B and hepatitis C	1 197	794	403	148	22	359	202	64	125	21	127	44	86
8. Malaria	66	34	32	10	9	12	2	1	10	8	11	2	1
9. Tropical-cluster diseases	367	299	68	11	38	225	17	8	3	7	47	6	5
a. Trypanosomiasis	-	-	-	-	-	-	-	-	-	-	-	-	-
b. Chagas disease	-	-	-	-	-	-	-	-	-	-	-	-	-
c. Schistosomiasis	39	25	14	-	1	11	8	6	-	1	4	5	4
d. Leishmaniasis	2	1	1	-	1	1	-	-	-	-	1	-	-
e. Lymphatic filariasis	325	272	53	11	36	214	9	2	3	6	42	1	2
f. Onchocerciasis	-	-	-	-	-	-	-	-	-	-	-	-	-
10. Leprosy	11	5	5	-	-	-	-	-	-	-	-	-	-
11. Dengue	58	27	31	7	19	1	-	-	2	22	3	1	-
12. Japanese encephalitis	897	450	447	270	147	29	3	1	279	137	27	3	1
13. Trachoma	495	135	360	-	-	25	43	67	-	-	65	104	190
14. Intestinal nematode infections	2 098	1 066	1 032	18	1 001	35	8	5	18	969	32	7	5
a. Ascariasis	1 083	549	534	17	525	6	1	-	18	510	5	1	-
b. Trichuriasis	892	454	438	-	453	-	-	-	-	437	-	-	-
c. Ancylostomiasis and necatoriasis	123	63	60	-	23	29	7	5	-	22	27	6	5

Annex Table 10d, continued. DALYs [0,01] by age, sex and cause (thousands): China, 1990

Cause	Total	Male	Female	Males					Females				
				0–4	5–14	15–44	45–59	60+	0–4	5–14	15–44	45–59	60+
B. Respiratory infections	**28 428**	**12 961**	**15 467**	**11 368**	**441**	**289**	**154**	**710**	**13 931**	**446**	**302**	**93**	**694**
1. Lower respiratory infections	27 638	12 586	15 052	11 117	339	277	151	701	13 636	349	291	90	686
2. Upper respiratory infections	292	134	158	107	6	10	3	8	133	6	10	2	8
3. Otitis media	497	241	256	144	96	1	–	–	163	91	2	–	–
C. Maternal conditions	**3 504**		**3 504**								**3 437**	**67**	
1. Maternal haemorrhage	698		698								677	21	
2. Maternal sepsis	442		442								440	2	
3. Hypertensive disorders of pregnancy	155		155								150	5	
4. Obstructed labour	868		868								867	1	
5. Abortion	137		137								133	4	
D. Perinatal conditions*	**24 358**	**11 574**	**12 784**	**11 574**					**12 784**				
E. Nutritional deficiencies	**12 928**	**6 002**	**6 926**	**3 026**	**694**	**1 569**	**363**	**351**	**4 201**	**743**	**1 197**	**390**	**395**
1. Protein-energy malnutrition	4 479	1 786	2 693	1 709	5	18	9	44	2 623	6	21	5	38
2. Iodine deficiency	999	508	492	441	41	25	–	–	428	39	24	1	–
3. Vitamin A deficiency	749	379	370	269	97	14	–	–	265	92	13	–	–
4. Iron-deficiency anaemia	6 700	3 329	3 372	606	550	1 512	353	307	885	606	1 139	384	356
II. Noncommunicable diseases	**184 812**	**96 699**	**88 113**	**9 444**	**2 734**	**27 077**	**22 572**	**34 873**	**10 154**	**1 973**	**25 748**	**17 813**	**32 425**
A. Malignant neoplasms	**33 970**	**20 751**	**13 219**	**420**	**712**	**5 421**	**6 945**	**7 253**	**557**	**366**	**3 684**	**4 054**	**4 558**
1. Mouth and oropharynx cancers	1 030	691	339	17	15	302	192	164	–	1	144	109	86
2. Oesophagus cancer	3 433	2 332	1 100	–	–	309	868	1 155	–	–	78	357	665
3. Stomach cancer	6 339	4 007	2 332	–	15	467	1 562	1 963	–	15	561	697	1 059
4. Colon and rectum cancers	1 900	1 035	865	–	15	328	307	385	–	18	213	285	349
5. Liver cancer	7 358	5 441	1 917	17	45	2 044	2 120	1 215	18	44	528	701	626
6. Pancreas cancer	579	360	219	–	–	71	113	176	–	–	21	58	139
7. Trachea, bronchus, lung cancers	4 008	2 737	1 270	16	28	257	975	1 461	–	1	137	485	649
8. Melanoma and other skin cancers	26	16	11	–	1	5	4	5	–	–	3	3	4
9. Breast cancer	731	–	731						–	–	308	261	162
10. Cervix uteri cancer	522	–	522						–	–	143	207	172
11. Corpus uteri cancer	169	–	169						–	–	37	97	35
12. Ovary cancer	329	–	329						–	–	150	97	57
13. Prostate cancer	72	72	–	–	–	5	8	59					
14. Bladder cancer	325	256	69	–	–	32	58	165	–	–	6	13	49
15. Lymphomas and multiple myeloma	640	438	202	–	59	174	97	107	–	–	69	86	47
16. Leukaemia	3 020	1 564	1 456	235	357	724	169	78	258	189	746	165	98
C. Diabetes mellitus	**1 873**	**872**	**1 001**	**20**	**27**	**241**	**273**	**311**	**19**	**25**	**218**	**306**	**432**
D. Endocrine disorders	**857**	**231**	**626**	**31**	**20**	**80**	**53**	**47**	**221**	**44**	**256**	**43**	**62**

Annex Table 10d, continued. DALYs [0,0] by age, sex and cause (thousands): China, 1990

Cause	Total	Male	Female	Males 0-4	5-14	15-44	45-59	60+	Females 0-4	5-14	15-44	45-59	60+
E. Neuro-psychiatric conditions	**27 299**	**12 883**	**14 416**	**393**	**413**	**9 564**	**1 263**	**1 251**	**331**	**357**	**10 466**	**1 548**	**1 713**
1. Unipolar major depression	9 555	3 496	6 059	-	-	2 777	530	189	-	-	4 854	851	354
2. Bipolar disorder	2 683	1 386	1 297	-	-	1 244	96	46	-	-	1 154	86	56
3. Schizophrenia	4 000	2 168	1 832	39	89	2 119	20	30	35	85	1 780	29	23
4. Epilepsy	1 098	585	513	-	-	374	53	29	-	-	325	40	27
5. Alcohol use	1 190	1 104	86	-	-	976	104	24	-	-	76	7	3
6. Dementia*	2 795	1 283	1 512	96	36	96	261	794	94	26	90	262	1 040
7. Parkinson disease	176	86	90	-	-	-	30	56	-	-	-	30	60
8. Multiple sclerosis	481	209	272	-	11	172	25	12	-	-	219	36	17
9. Drug use	146	131	15	-	25	114	5	1	-	1	13	1	-
10. Post-traumatic stress disorder	350	136	214	16	-	83	10	3	26	40	130	14	4
11. Obsessive-compulsive disorders	1 757	777	980	-	89	609	46	32	-	111	751	72	45
12. Panic disorder	831	290	541	-	32	208	49	-	-	31	423	69	18
F. Sense organ diseases	**2 881**	**1 145**	**1 736**	**86**	**-**	**91**	**379**	**589**	**63**	**23**	**202**	**690**	**758**
1. Glaucoma	1 188	387	801	17	-	50	182	139	21	-	87	485	207
2. Cataracts	1 368	654	714	38	-	29	165	422	5	-	38	162	509
G. Cardiovascular diseases	**43 710**	**22 578**	**21 131**	**787**	**287**	**4 137**	**5 698**	**11 670**	**595**	**166**	**3 981**	**4 710**	**11 679**
1. Rheumatic heart disease	4 285	1 775	2 511	-	48	891	375	461	63	53	1 047	640	709
2. Ischaemic heart disease	11 644	6 073	5 572	-	-	993	1 577	3 503	-	-	748	1 203	3 621
3. Cerebrovascular disease	20 721	10 976	9 745	184	117	1 524	2 937	6 215	147	46	1 274	2 364	5 914
4. Inflammatory heart diseases	2 140	1 084	1 057	137	49	481	220	197	123	35	482	204	213
H. Respiratory diseases	**36 160**	**18 952**	**17 208**	**1 408**	**375**	**3 138**	**3 874**	**10 158**	**1 554**	**237**	**2 462**	**3 020**	**9 935**
1. COPD*	30 481	15 777	14 704	335	14	2 213	3 568	9 648	791	9	1 700	2 780	9 425
2. Asthma	2 959	1 652	1 307	283	319	656	210	184	179	192	581	185	172
I. Digestive diseases	**16 704**	**9 175**	**7 529**	**2 330**	**274**	**2 424**	**2 273**	**1 874**	**2 601**	**219**	**1 622**	**1 527**	**1 560**
1. Peptic ulcer	733	432	300	24	9	137	115	148	27	7	76	65	126
2. Cirrhosis of the liver	5 387	3 622	1 765	157	44	1 351	1 207	862	52	46	452	617	598
3. Appendicitis	636	370	266	12	104	233	15	6	12	80	158	11	5
J. Genito-urinary diseases	**4 338**	**2 644**	**1 694**	**158**	**129**	**928**	**887**	**543**	**165**	**88**	**725**	**326**	**389**
1. Nephritis and nephrosis	3 024	1 681	1 344	112	129	869	264	306	165	88	629	202	259
2. Benign prostatic hypertrophy	686	686	-	16	-	14	537	119	-	-	-	-	-
L. Musculo-skeletal diseases	**5 417**	**1 847**	**3 570**	**-**	**41**	**400**	**596**	**810**	**36**	**27**	**1 252**	**1 300**	**955**
1. Rheumatoid arthritis	737	236	501	-	1	67	108	59	1	5	140	197	158
2. Osteoarthritis	3 563	1 203	2 360	-	-	247	428	527	-	-	791	971	598

Annex Table 10d, continued. DALYs [0,0] by age, sex and cause (thousands): China, 1990

Cause	Total	Male	Female	Males					Females				
				0-4	5-14	15-44	45-59	60+	0-4	5-14	15-44	45-59	60+
M. Congenital anomalies	**8 023**	**3 843**	**4 180**	**3 172**	**323**	**339**	**9**	**-**	**3 386**	**332**	**451**	**11**	**-**
1. Abdominal wall defect	55	31	24	31	-	-	-	-	24	-	-	-	-
2. Anencephaly	3 165	1 200	1 965	1 200	-	-	-	-	1 965	-	-	-	-
3. Anorectal atresia	12	7	5	7	-	-	-	-	5	-	-	-	-
4. Cleft lip	58	35	23	35	-	-	-	-	23	-	-	-	-
5. Cleft palate	46	23	23	23	-	-	-	-	23	-	-	-	-
6. Oesophageal atresia	10	6	4	6	-	-	-	-	4	-	-	-	-
7. Renal agenesis	42	21	21	21	-	-	-	-	21	-	-	-	-
8. Down syndrome	856	391	465	219	68	100	4	-	225	83	150	6	-
9. Congenital heart anomalies	2 143	1 207	936	893	143	168	3	-	558	123	250	4	-
10. Spina bifida	965	534	431	467	63	3	-	-	351	76	5	-	-
N. Oral conditions	**1 728**	**846**	**882**	**425**	**32**	**47**	**140**	**201**	**409**	**33**	**72**	**136**	**231**
1. Dental caries	1 018	520	498	423	30	29	23	15	407	28	27	20	16
2. Periodontal disease	25	13	12	-	-	11	1	1	-	-	10	1	1
3. Edentulism	629	301	328	-	-	-	116	185	-	-	-	114	214
III. Injuries	***66 012***	***37 273***	***28 739***	***9 475***	***4 206***	***19 067***	***2 900***	***1 624***	***9 660***	***2 863***	***12 760***	***1 962***	***1 493***
A. Unintentional injuries	**48 500**	**29 775**	**18 725**	**9 040**	**3 955**	**13 722**	**2 055**	**1 004**	**8 831**	**2 622**	**5 355**	**1 048**	**869**
1. Road traffic accidents	7 351	5 089	2 262	350	587	3 390	544	218	263	571	1 043	280	105
2. Poisonings	2 965	1 677	1 287	553	117	665	244	98	175	167	791	70	84
3. Falls	7 181	3 925	3 256	1 153	501	1 836	250	185	1 602	358	749	232	316
4. Fires	1 305	728	578	274	124	250	35	45	197	187	100	37	56
5. Drownings	9 165	5 578	3 587	2 417	1 537	1 423	121	81	2 102	773	568	64	80
6. Other unintentional	20 533	12 777	7 756	4 293	1 090	6 157	860	377	4 492	566	2 104	365	228
B. Intentional injuries	**17 511**	**7 498**	**10 013**	**436**	**251**	**5 346**	**846**	**620**	**829**	**241**	**7 405**	**914**	**624**
1. Self-inflicted injuries	14 306	5 672	8 634	-	168	4 148	768	587	-	126	7 059	861	589
2. Violence	3 163	1 784	1 379	436	83	1 155	78	33	829	115	347	53	35
3. War	43	43	-	43	-	43	-	-	-	-	-	-	-

Notes:
A dash (-) symbol indicates fewer than 500 DALYs.
*IA6 is Bacterial meningitis and meningococcaemia; ID is Conditions arising during the perinatal period;
IIE6 is Dementia and other degenerative and hereditary CNS disorders; IIH1 is Chronic obstructive pulmonary disease.

Annex Table 10e. DALYs [0,0] by age, sex and cause (thousands): Other Asia and Islands, 1990

Cause	Total	Male	Female	Males					Females				
				0-4	5-14	15-44	45-59	60+	0-4	5-14	15-44	45-59	60+
Population (millions)	*683*	*343*	*340*	*44*	*84*	*161*	*34*	*20*	*42*	*80*	*160*	*35*	*23*
All causes	313 832	168 632	145 200	80 600	20 756	36 440	15 492	15 344	67 014	15 576	33 369	13 075	16 166
I. Communicable, maternal, perinatal and nutritional conditions	159 398	82 355	77 043	64 610	7 291	5 833	2 261	2 360	52 984	6 545	12 590	2 542	2 381
A. Infectious and parasitic diseases	78 593	41 560	37 033	29 006	4 618	4 618	1 934	1 384	23 700	4 148	5 672	2 043	1 470
1. Tuberculosis	9 342	4 600	4 742	91	162	1 904	1 390	1 053	34	168	1 941	1 473	1 126
2. STDs excluding HIV	4 921	2 065	2 856	1 585	7	419	21	33	1 212	33	1 534	34	43
a. Syphilis	2 676	1 510	1 166	1 380	1	78	19	33	1 001	1	96	26	42
b. Chlamydia	1 288	167	1 121	48	3	115	1	-	50	23	1 042	6	1
c. Gonorrhoea	957	388	569	157	4	225	1	-	161	9	396	3	-
3. HIV	104	66	38	7	1	54	3	1	7	1	30	-	-
4. Diarrhoeal diseases	31 429	17 691	13 738	16 430	937	168	71	84	12 567	716	276	98	81
5. Childhood-cluster diseases	18 267	9 448	8 818	8 151	947	288	44	18	7 483	949	317	52	19
a. Pertussis	2 974	1 545	1 429	1 420	125	-	-	-	1 314	115	-	-	-
b. Poliomyelitis	836	474	363	451	5	17	1	-	345	3	13	1	-
c. Diphtheria	187	98	89	88	9	1	-	-	81	8	1	-	-
d. Measles	9 005	4 681	4 324	4 126	547	7	1	-	3 827	490	6	-	-
e. Tetanus	5 263	2 650	2 613	2 066	261	263	42	17	1 916	334	296	50	19
6. Bacterial meningitis*	1 740	879	861	629	33	134	52	31	597	32	143	59	30
7. Hepatitis B and hepatitis C	741	417	324	123	58	118	72	46	94	51	103	37	39
8. Malaria	4 616	2 398	2 218	487	849	897	126	40	454	756	825	143	40
9. Tropical-cluster diseases	888	608	280	22	144	376	58	8	16	46	161	50	6
a. Trypanosomiasis													
b. Chagas disease													
c. Schistosomiasis	18	10	7	-	1	4	3	2	-	1	2	2	-
d. Leishmaniasis	120	74	46	4	23	44	3	1	2	14	28	2	2
e. Lymphatic filariasis	750	523	226	18	120	328	53	5	14	32	131	46	4
f. Onchocerciasis													
10. Leprosy	133	63	70	2	25	26	8	3	17	21	26	6	1
11. Dengue	504	236	268	59	171	4	1	-	69	193	5	2	-
12. Japanese encephalitis	326	170	157	102	55	10	1	-	95	50	10	1	-
13. Trachoma	64	17	47	-	-	3	5	8	-	-	9	15	23
14. Intestinal nematode infections	2 086	1 056	1 030	11	919	94	20	12	11	893	92	21	14
a. Ascariasis	800	406	394	10	394	2	-	-	10	382	2	-	-
b. Trichuriasis	930	472	458	-	472	-	-	-	-	457	-	-	-
c. Ancylostomiasis and necatoriasis	356	177	179	-	54	92	20	12	-	54	90	21	13

Annex Table 10e, continued. DALYs [0,0] by age, sex and cause (thousands): Other Asia and Islands, 1990

Cause	Total	Male	Female	Males 0-4	5-14	15-44	45-59	60+	Females 0-4	5-14	15-44	45-59	60+
B. Respiratory infections	**34 569**	**19 200**	**15 369**	**15 587**	**2 068**	**536**	**173**	**836**	**12 077**	**1 845**	**493**	**197**	**757**
1. Lower respiratory infections	33 724	18 741	14 982	15 271	1 950	522	171	827	11 826	1 734	480	194	748
2. Upper respiratory infections	358	199	160	153	23	11	3	9	118	20	10	3	8
3. Otitis media	487	260	227	162	95	3	–	–	133	91	2	–	–
C. Maternal conditions	**5 286**	**–**	**5 286**								**5 219**	**68**	
1. Maternal haemorrhage	688	–	688								672	15	
2. Maternal sepsis	830	–	830								820	10	
3. Hypertensive disorders of pregnancy	337	–	337								330	8	
4. Obstructed labour	1 329	–	1 329								1 324	5	
5. Abortion	826	–	826								817	9	
D. Perinatal conditions*	**28 738**	**15 692**	**13 046**	**15 692**					**13 046**				
E. Nutritional deficiencies	**12 211**	**5 903**	**6 308**	**4 326**	**605**	**679**	**153**	**140**	**4 160**	**553**	**1 207**	**234**	**154**
1. Protein-energy malnutrition	6 233	3 175	3 058	3 117	26	10	10	13	3 003	20	16	8	10
2. Iodine deficiency	346	175	172	150	19	5	–	–	148	18	6	–	–
3. Vitamin A deficiency	1 375	719	656	472	232	15	–	–	438	205	12	–	–
4. Iron-deficiency anaemia	4 257	1 834	2 423	587	328	648	144	127	571	310	1 173	226	144
II. Noncommunicable diseases	**109 698**	**56 954**	**52 744**	**9 297**	**7 178**	**16 347**	**11 586**	**12 546**	**8 137**	**5 808**	**15 394**	**9 911**	**13 493**
A. Malignant neoplasms	**16 988**	**8 916**	**8 073**	**581**	**1 244**	**1 775**	**2 549**	**2 767**	**599**	**849**	**2 135**	**2 183**	**2 307**
1. Mouth and oropharynx cancers	1 483	865	618	16	35	210	185	419	20	29	160	101	308
2. Oesophagus cancer	462	294	168	–	–	33	134	127	–	–	25	60	83
3. Stomach cancer	1 252	784	469	2	3	149	342	288	1	1	102	167	197
4. Colon and rectum cancers	860	425	435	6	12	109	88	210	7	9	98	92	229
5. Liver cancer	1 629	1 198	431	22	45	303	559	270	17	24	85	147	159
6. Pancreas cancer	197	118	79	–	–	24	46	48	2	3	8	28	39
7. Trachea, bronchus, lung cancers	1 694	1 240	454	7	15	146	534	538	7	9	58	156	225
8. Melanoma and other skin cancers	56	24	32	1	2	7	8	6	–	–	9	10	14
9. Breast cancer	831	–	831						5	7	307	342	170
10. Cervix uteri cancer	951	–	951						1	1	295	456	197
11. Corpus uteri cancer	98	–	98								16	40	35
12. Ovary cancer	374	–	374						23	32	172	90	57
13. Prostate cancer	199	199	–			4	34	153					
14. Bladder cancer	203	143	60			14	48	81			7	13	38
15. Lymphomas and multiple myeloma	796	500	296	74	155	127	56	88	3	4	77	36	94
16. Leukaemia	1 612	871	741	203	422	166	31	49	218	299	136	32	56
C. Diabetes mellitus	**2 120**	**957**	**1 162**	**23**	**52**	**264**	**326**	**292**	**24**	**51**	**263**	**378**	**447**
D. Endocrine disorders	**717**	**350**	**367**	**179**	**75**	**45**	**27**	**24**	**142**	**41**	**83**	**49**	**52**

Annex Table 10e, continued. DALYs [0,0] by age, sex and cause (thousands): Other Asia and Islands, 1990

Cause	Total	Male	Female	Males					Females				
				0-4	5-14	15-44	45-59	60+	0-4	5-14	15-44	45-59	60+
E. Neuro-psychiatric conditions	**18 040**	**9 006**	**9 033**	**348**	**600**	**6 528**	**859**	**671**	**351**	**559**	**6 254**	**952**	**918**
1. Unipolar major depression	4 893	1 703	3 191			1 388	239	76			2 596	443	151
2. Bipolar disorder	1 370	685	685			620	45	20			613	45	26
3. Schizophrenia	3 203	1 640	1 563			1 601	23	16			1 527	11	26
4. Epilepsy	966	508	458	37	158	235	56	22	40	163	204	32	19
5. Alcohol use	1 432	1 322	110			1 166	125	32			96	9	4
6. Dementia*	1 537	657	880	58	26	51	160	364	80	30	51	181	539
7. Parkinson disease	170	92	78				33	58				29	49
8. Multiple sclerosis	237	99	137			84	11	4			113	18	7
9. Drug use	708	637	71	1	57	549	24	6		6	61	3	1
10. Post-traumatic stress disorder	219	83	137	11	22	43	5	1	19	36	73	8	2
11. Obsessive-compulsive disorders	1 012	432	580		77	320	22	13		98	422	39	20
12. Panic disorder	470	160	310		27	109	23			27	237	38	8
F. Sense organ diseases	**2 115**	**870**	**1 244**	**11**	**8**	**54**	**359**	**439**	**13**		**84**	**582**	**566**
1. Glaucoma	710	207	502			15	131	62			47	350	104
2. Cataracts	1 379	644	736	3		36	227	377	8		36	231	460
G. Cardiovascular diseases	**34 199**	**17 508**	**16 691**	**2 527**	**3 074**	**3 971**	**3 011**	**4 926**	**2 330**	**2 638**	**3 274**	**2 480**	**5 970**
1. Rheumatic heart disease	268	110	157		16	38	19	38		24	54	28	51
2. Ischaemic heart disease	7 615	3 896	3 719			717	1 071	2 108			501	793	2 425
3. Cerebrovascular disease	8 487	4 241	4 247	319	582	896	880	1 565	294	450	663	818	2 023
4. Inflammatory heart diseases	4 104	2 130	1 974	489	688	633	193	127	549	619	496	158	153
H. Respiratory diseases	**7 179**	**3 995**	**3 185**	**1 314**	**582**	**644**	**514**	**941**	**1 065**	**410**	**635**	**321**	**753**
1. COPD*	2 140	1 257	884	185	49	193	263	566	164	42	139	132	406
2. Asthma	1 656	919	738	176	262	324	86	70	112	172	294	86	74
I. Digestive diseases	**13 530**	**7 951**	**5 579**	**1 267**	**775**	**1 874**	**2 453**	**1 582**	**1 023**	**591**	**1 132**	**1 488**	**1 345**
1. Peptic ulcer	558	343	215	15	22	94	102	110	11	17	50	49	89
2. Cirrhosis of the liver	3 989	2 856	1 134	97	85	914	1 199	560	67	80	257	407	323
3. Appendicitis	567	322	245	11	153	146	9	3	11	124	100	7	3
J. Genito-urinary diseases	**3 331**	**1 754**	**1 577**	**137**	**358**	**374**	**535**	**350**	**100**	**261**	**440**	**325**	**451**
1. Nephritis and nephrosis	2 442	1 189	1 253	107	313	325	199	245	100	230	343	236	344
2. Benign prostatic hypertrophy	308	308	-				274	34					
L. Musculo-skeletal diseases	**3 196**	**1 346**	**1 851**	**30**	**40**	**334**	**653**	**289**	**29**	**47**	**572**	**835**	**367**
1. Rheumatoid arthritis	247	73	173			5	20	49			41	33	98
2. Osteoarthritis	2 483	1 104	1 379			296	603	204			428	750	201

Annex Table 10e, continued. DALYs [0,0] by age, sex and cause (thousands): Other Asia and Islands, 1990

Cause	Total	Male	Female	Males					Females				
				0-4	5-14	15-44	45-59	60+	0-4	5-14	15-44	45-59	60+
M. Congenital anomalies	**5 673**	**3 042**	**2 631**	**2 673**	**213**	**129**	**19**	**7**	**2 291**	**205**	**103**	**23**	**9**
1. Abdominal wall defect	57	34	23	34	-	-	-	-	23	-	-	-	-
2. Anencephaly	1 564	604	960	604	-	-	-	-	960	-	-	-	-
3. Anorectal atresia	19	11	7	11	-	-	-	-	7	-	-	-	-
4. Cleft lip	60	40	20	40	-	-	-	-	20	-	-	-	-
5. Cleft palate	47	27	20	27	-	-	-	-	20	-	-	-	-
6. Oesophageal atresia	39	23	15	23	-	-	-	-	15	-	-	-	-
7. Renal agenesis	138	69	69	69	-	-	-	-	69	-	-	-	-
8. Down syndrome	452	286	166	202	39	44	-	-	107	31	28	-	-
9. Congenital heart anomalies	2 119	1 269	850	1 081	101	64	17	7	680	91	51	19	8
10. Spina bifida	449	242	206	211	30	1	-	-	154	42	8	1	1
N. Oral conditions	**1 701**	**807**	**894**	**69**	**41**	**277**	**207**	**213**	**67**	**43**	**300**	**228**	**257**
1. Dental caries	536	268	268	68	39	75	53	32	66	38	75	55	35
2. Periodontal disease	26	13	13	-	-	9	2	1	-	-	9	2	2
3. Edentulism	1 112	520	592	-	-	189	151	180	-	-	201	171	220
III. Injuries	***44 737***	***29 323***	***15 413***	***6 693***	***6 287***	***14 261***	***1 645***	***438***	***5 893***	***3 223***	***5 384***	***622***	***291***
A. Unintentional injuries	**37 627**	**24 845**	**12 783**	**6 458**	**5 915**	**10 873**	**1 272**	**326**	**5 636**	**2 982**	**3 439**	**492**	**234**
1. Road traffic accidents	8 514	5 810	2 704	1 107	1 255	3 010	335	103	1 036	655	795	144	73
2. Poisonings	1 942	995	948	198	186	502	81	28	183	196	498	44	26
3. Falls	6 467	4 135	2 331	1 572	947	1 389	184	43	1 255	456	509	82	30
4. Fires	956	471	485	163	150	137	15	6	228	172	73	7	5
5. Drownings	5 643	3 824	1 819	1 522	1 436	775	65	25	971	570	240	24	15
6. Other unintentional	14 105	9 610	4 495	1 896	1 941	5 060	592	121	1 963	933	1 324	190	85
B. Intentional injuries	**7 109**	**4 479**	**2 631**	**235**	**372**	**3 387**	**373**	**112**	**258**	**241**	**1 946**	**130**	**57**
1. Self-inflicted injuries	3 338	1 813	1 525	-	134	1 434	173	72	-	83	1 319	83	41
2. Violence	2 695	2 065	631	102	167	1 577	184	35	120	104	361	35	10
3. War	1 076	601	475	133	71	376	16	5	137	53	266	12	6

Notes:
A dash (-) symbol indicates fewer than 500 DALYs.
*IA6 is Bacterial meningitis and meningococcaemia; ID is Conditions arising during the perinatal period;
IIE6 is Dementia and other degenerative and hereditary CNS disorders; IIH1 is Chronic obstructive pulmonary disease.

Annex Table 10f. DALYs [0,0] by age, sex and cause (thousands): Sub-Saharan Africa, 1990

Cause	Total	Male	Female	Males					Females				
				0-4	5-14	15-44	45-59	60+	0-4	5-14	15-44	45-59	60+
Population (millions)	510	252	258	47	70	104	20	11	47	70	106	22	13
All causes	566 019	295 860	270 160	184 330	33 194	55 606	13 059	9 670	163 928	30 524	51 109	12 389	12 209
I. Communicable, maternal, perinatal and nutritional conditions	407 397	203 612	203 785	168 031	16 161	14 569	2 884	1 967	149 213	16 667	32 406	2 984	2 516
A. Infectious and parasitic diseases	262 114	135 186	126 928	105 853	12 054	13 564	2 646	1 068	92 937	12 265	17 775	2 663	1 287
1. Tuberculosis	18 438	8 441	9 997	1 465	799	4 491	1 259	427	1 638	1 176	5 438	1 282	463
2. STDs excluding HIV	8 742	3 636	5 106	3 020	11	516	33	56	2 978	52	1 934	56	86
a. Syphilis	5 801	2 889	2 912	2 678	2	124	31	55	2 609	2	172	44	85
b. Chlamydia	1 444	173	1 271	65	2	104			70	33	1 160	7	1
c. Gonorrhoea	1 497	573	923	276	7	289	2		298	18	603	5	
3. HIV	14 798	6 810	7 988	2 554	312	3 636	254	54	2 484	328	4 937	202	37
4. Diarrhoeal diseases	73 486	39 325	34 161	35 988	2 544	500	120	173	29 981	2 725	1 056	168	231
5. Childhood-cluster diseases	69 184	35 616	33 568	31 350	3 912	277	54	23	29 174	3 976	342	53	23
a. Pertussis	12 511	6 475	6 036	5 936	539				5 502	534	9	1	
b. Poliomyelitis	1 119	626	493	611	4	10	1		480	3	1	1	
c. Diphtheria	146	75	70	67	7	4	1		62	7	5		
d. Measles	45 604	23 461	22 143	20 398	3 058	4			19 074	3 063			
e. Tetanus	9 804	4 978	4 826	4 337	303	262	52	23	4 055	369	327	51	23
6. Bacterial meningitis*	2 064	1 016	1 048	841	27	99	32	16	824	28	133	40	23
7. Hepatitis B and hepatitis C	604	317	287	91	49	83	57	36	71	48	100	30	38
8. Malaria	59 507	31 624	27 883	27 805	2 102	1 440	216	61	23 415	2 173	1 947	261	86
9. Tropical-cluster diseases	7 393	4 429	2 964	184	1 573	2 081	478	113	212	996	1 320	357	78
a. Trypanosomiasis	2 595	1 226	1 369	40	474	535	154	23	81	502	651	115	18
b. Chagas disease													
c. Schistosomiasis	1 144	676	468	59	254	275	61	28	40	172	200	39	17
d. Leishmaniasis	752	478	274	26	274	169	8	1	12	142	113	6	
e. Lymphatic filariasis	2 042	1 557	485	47	498	902	104	6	68	119	202	87	9
f. Onchocerciasis	859	492	367	13	73	199	152	55	10	60	153	110	34
10. Leprosy	67	33	34	1	13	16	3		1	11	17	4	1
11. Dengue	42	19	23	4	14				5	18			
12. Japanese encephalitis													
13. Trachoma	458	116	342			25	40	52			69	115	158
14. Intestinal nematode infections	551	268	283	2	167	75	15	8	2	174	80	17	10
a. Ascariasis	146	71	75	2	69				2	72			
b. Trichuriasis	128	63	65		63					65			
c. Ancylostomiasis and necatoriasis	276	133	143		35	75	15	8		37	80	17	10

Annex Table 10f, continued. DALYs [0,0] by age, sex and cause (thousands): Sub-Saharan Africa, 1990

Cause	Total	Male	Female	Males					Females				
				0-4	5-14	15-44	45-59	60+	0-4	5-14	15-44	45-59	60+
B. Respiratory infections	**70 117**	**37 689**	**32 427**	**32 822**	**3 259**	**642**	**156**	**810**	**27 440**	**2 801**	**878**	**191**	**1 119**
1. Lower respiratory infections	68 663	36 914	31 749	32 195	3 135	629	154	802	26 909	2 684	861	188	1 107
2. Upper respiratory infections	709	381	328	326	35	3	2	9	272	30	12	3	12
3. Otitis media	745	395	350	302	90	3	–	–	259	86	5	–	–
C. Maternal conditions	**13 883**	**–**	**13 883**							**732**	**13 138**	**13**	**–**
1. Maternal haemorrhage	2 449		2 449							172	2 274	3	
2. Maternal sepsis	2 376		2 376							114	2 260	2	
3. Hypertensive disorders of pregnancy	1 219		1 219							86	1 132	1	
4. Obstructed labour	2 367		2 367							57	2 308	1	
5. Abortion	2 103		2 103							97	2 005	2	
D. Perinatal conditions*	**44 283**	**22 358**	**21 925**	**22 358**					**21 925**				
E. Nutritional deficiencies	**17 002**	**8 379**	**8 623**	**6 998**	**848**	**363**	**81**	**89**	**6 911**	**869**	**615**	**118**	**110**
1. Protein-energy malnutrition	11 233	5 614	5 619	5 456	72	39	17	29	5 394	80	94	17	34
2. Iodine deficiency	241	116	126	101	12	3	–	–	106	13	6	1	–
3. Vitamin A deficiency	2 597	1 307	1 290	895	396	16	–	–	861	407	21	–	–
4. Iron-deficiency anaemia	2 931	1 343	1 588	546	368	306	64	59	550	368	494	100	76
II. Noncommunicable diseases	*80 452*	*39 765*	*40 687*	*6 654*	*5 286*	*12 296*	*8 327*	*7 202*	*6 854*	*6 140*	*9 619*	*8 718*	*9 356*
A. Malignant neoplasms	**11 742**	**6 191**	**5 550**	**298**	**754**	**1 592**	**1 884**	**1 664**	**368**	**836**	**1 051**	**1 805**	**1 490**
1. Mouth and oropharynx cancers	518	290	227	2	7	74	68	140	11	31	40	38	107
2. Oesophagus cancer	526	386	141	–	–	75	202	109	–	–	20	57	64
3. Stomach cancer	734	416	318	1	3	82	195	136	–	–	48	162	108
4. Colon and rectum cancers	318	166	152	1	3	49	40	73	–	2	28	34	87
5. Liver cancer	1 582	1 179	403	7	20	535	450	168	9	22	106	150	117
6. Pancreas cancer	161	89	71	–	–	21	44	25	–	–	13	36	23
7. Trachea, bronchus, lung cancers	425	316	109	–	1	52	157	107	–	2	14	53	41
8. Melanoma and other skin cancers	181	73	107	–	1	13	36	23	–	3	10	43	52
9. Breast cancer	453	–	453								111	209	128
10. Cervix uteri cancer	835		835								170	402	260
11. Corpus uteri cancer	78		78							2	8	33	35
12. Ovary cancer	224		224						10	25	54	84	51
13. Prostate cancer	511	511	–			10	128	373					
14. Bladder cancer	291	183	108			30	72	80			21	42	45
15. Lymphomas and multiple myeloma	1 152	669	483	105	303	123	64	74	93	241	57	40	52
16. Leukaemia	380	155	225	19	55	44	13	25	41	106	29	25	25
C. Diabetes mellitus	**895**	**404**	**491**	**31**	**99**	**75**	**104**	**95**	**37**	**102**	**58**	**131**	**162**
D. Endocrine disorders	**1 565**	**727**	**838**	**278**	**70**	**179**	**136**	**64**	**177**	**139**	**171**	**174**	**177**

Annex Table 10f, continued. DALYs [0,0] by age, sex and cause (thousands): Sub-Saharan Africa, 1990

Cause	Total	Males						Females					
		Male	0-4	5-14	15-44	45-59	60+	Female	0-4	5-14	15-44	45-59	60+
E. Neuro-psychiatric conditions	10 391	5 048	286	444	3 581	471	267	5 343	340	452	3 531	552	467
1. Unipolar major depression	3 301	1 121			931	148	42	2 181			1 798	292	91
2. Bipolar disorder	939	461			422	28	11	478			431	30	16
3. Schizophrenia	591	303			293	6	3	288			279	4	6
4. Epilepsy	626	343	50	107	145	29	12	283	57	101	97	16	12
5. Alcohol use	1 308	1 049			931	96	22	259			219	28	12
6. Dementia*	610	198	24	11	21	41	102	412	66	27	29	49	241
7. Parkinson disease	85	44				16	28	40				15	25
8. Multiple sclerosis	144	61			51	7	3	83			65	13	5
9. Drug use	285	258		23	222	10	3	27		3	23	1	
10. Post-traumatic stress disorder	169	62	12	18	28	3	1	106	21	31	49	5	1
11. Obsessive-compulsive disorders	694	291		65	206	13	7	403		86	281	25	11
12. Panic disorder	320	108		23	71	14		212		24	160	24	4
F. Sense organ diseases	2 467	1 116	11	1	58	489	557	1 351	11	1	60	579	700
1. Glaucoma	551	217			1	92	124	334			2	152	180
2. Cataracts	1 907	894	11	1	52	397	433	1 014	11	1	55	427	520
G. Cardiovascular diseases	21 878	9 615	941	1 377	2 816	2 166	2 315	12 263	1 114	2 003	2 043	2 904	4 198
1. Rheumatic heart disease	1 164	520	2	230	263	19	5	644	4	357	236	35	11
2. Ischaemic heart disease	4 491	1 944			526	659	759	2 547	335		264	754	1 193
3. Cerebrovascular disease	8 768	3 759	151	439	1 140	922	1 107	5 009	176	444	724	1 420	2 245
4. Inflammatory heart diseases	2 637	1 117	249	226	312	179	150	1 521	415	406	266	175	260
H. Respiratory diseases	11 006	6 027	1 504	679	1 460	1 230	1 153	4 980	1 497	632	943	991	917
1. COPD*	3 038	1 811	191	67	409	510	633	1 227	212	74	175	339	426
2. Asthma	1 596	844	211	242	272	68	50	752	167	191	267	75	53
I. Digestive diseases	8 286	4 595	609	753	1 556	1 059	619	3 691	612	969	826	650	634
1. Peptic ulcer	444	285			168	79	36	159		2	55	57	44
2. Cirrhosis of the liver	1 100	763		63	316	248	136	337		33	104	112	87
3. Appendicitis	823	487	14	260	198	11	3	336	17	222	83	10	3
J. Genito-urinary diseases	4 515	2 525	516	692	514	525	277	1 990	407	579	362	363	279
1. Nephritis and nephrosis	3 479	1 869	458	592	435	184	201	1 610	397	510	260	244	199
2. Benign prostatic hypertrophy	276	276				262	14	-					
L. Musculo-skeletal diseases	1 507	492			228	170	94	1 015		2	360	462	191
1. Rheumatoid arthritis	85	24			12	8	5	61		2	30	20	9
2. Osteoarthritis	1 390	455			210	159	86	935			320	436	179

Annex Table 10f, continued. DALYs [0,0] by age, sex and cause (thousands): Sub-Saharan Africa, 1990

Cause	Total	Male	Female	Males					Females				
				0-4	5-14	15-44	45-59	60+	0-4	5-14	15-44	45-59	60+
M. Congenital anomalies	4 062	1 923	2 139	1 571	202	124	19	8	1 797	233	69	29	12
1. Abdominal wall defect	33	16	16	16	–	–	–	–	16	–	–	–	–
2. Anencephaly	969	360	609	360	–	–	–	–	609	–	–	–	–
3. Anorectal atresia	17	8	8	8	–	–	–	–	8	–	–	–	–
4. Cleft lip	29	16	13	16	–	–	–	–	13	–	–	–	–
5. Cleft palate	24	11	13	11	–	–	–	–	13	–	–	–	–
6. Oesophageal atresia	23	11	11	11	–	–	–	–	11	–	–	–	–
7. Renal agenesis	165	82	83	82	–	–	–	–	83	–	–	–	–
8. Down syndrome	423	233	190	118	55	60	–	–	98	56	36	–	–
9. Congenital heart anomalies	1 469	724	744	564	94	45	16	7	565	115	33	23	8
10. Spina bifida	373	182	192	168	12	1	–	–	169	15	5	2	1
N. Oral conditions	532	253	280	106	47	33	11	57	105	53	38	12	72
1. Dental caries	371	185	186	104	44	23	10	5	103	44	23	10	6
2. Periodontal disease	19	10	10	–	–	8	1	–	–	–	9	1	–
3. Edentulism	118	52	66	–	–	–	–	52	–	–	–	–	66
III. Injuries	*78 170*	*52 483*	*25 687*	*9 645*	*11 747*	*28 742*	*1 848*	*501*	*7 861*	*7 717*	*9 084*	*687*	*338*
A. Unintentional injuries	47 005	31 524	15 481	6 954	9 772	13 373	1 109	316	5 262	6 516	3 142	363	198
1. Road traffic accidents	10 095	7 180	2 915	809	2 617	3 319	338	97	577	1 262	936	110	30
2. Poisonings	2 700	1 573	1 128	1 126	286	124	25	11	853	146	117	7	5
3. Falls	3 106	1 807	1 299	373	864	468	68	35	424	555	220	40	60
4. Fires	6 398	3 121	3 277	1 328	1 044	656	65	28	1 179	1 482	527	52	37
5. Drownings	6 209	4 440	1 769	1 248	2 365	760	50	17	654	957	139	13	6
6. Other unintentional	18 496	13 403	5 093	2 070	2 595	8 046	562	130	1 577	2 114	1 201	141	59
B. Intentional injuries	31 165	20 958	10 206	2 690	1 976	15 368	739	184	2 599	1 201	5 942	324	140
1. Self-inflicted injuries	817	656	161	–	98	507	39	12	–	–	145	14	2
2. Violence	11 336	9 661	1 675	348	607	8 222	404	79	181	256	1 116	93	30
3. War	19 012	10 642	8 370	2 342	1 270	6 640	296	93	2 418	946	4 682	217	107

Notes:
A dash (–) symbol indicates fewer than 500 DALYs.
*IA6 is Bacterial meningitis and meningococcaemia; ID is Conditions arising during the perinatal period;
IIH1 is Chronic obstructive pulmonary disease.
IIE6 is Dementia and other degenerative and hereditary CNS disorders.

Annex Table 10g. DALYs [0,0] by age, sex and cause (thousands): Latin America and the Caribbean, 1990

Cause	Total	Male	Female	Males					Females				
				0-4	5-14	15-44	45-59	60+	0-4	5-14	15-44	45-59	60+
Population (millions)	*444*	*222*	*223*	*29*	*52*	*104*	*22*	*14*	*28*	*51*	*104*	*23*	*17*
All causes	*164 957*	*90 158*	*74 798*	*36 710*	*8 549*	*26 533*	*9 459*	*8 908*	*29 333*	*6 409*	*21 351*	*8 299*	*9 407*
I. Communicable, maternal, perinatal and nutritional conditions	*70 707*	*37 025*	*33 682*	*29 569*	*2 147*	*3 645*	*891*	*773*	*23 135*	*2 409*	*6 574*	*785*	*779*
A. Infectious and parasitic diseases	33 863	18 083	15 780	12 299	1 493	3 178	674	438	9 922	1 640	3 270	553	395
1. Tuberculosis	3 116	1 639	1 477	121	112	918	284	204	100	173	877	191	136
2. STDs excluding HIV	1 469	544	925	443	1	90	4	6	384	10	516	7	9
a. Syphilis	835	443	392	418	-	16	4	6	358	-	21	5	8
b. Chlamydia	424	35	389	6	-	28	-	-	7	7	373	1	-
c. Gonorrhoea	210	66	145	18	1	46	-	-	19	2	123	-	-
3. HIV	1 658	1 283	375	86	6	1 093	79	19	82	8	268	13	4
4. Diarrhoeal diseases	12 072	6 794	5 278	6 306	264	121	47	55	4 632	300	219	57	69
5. Childhood-cluster diseases	7 823	4 062	3 760	3 773	264	18	5	3	3 440	280	31	6	3
a. Pertussis	1 633	842	791	783	59				728	63			
b. Poliomyelitis	444	251	193	245	1	4	-	-	188	1	3	-	-
c. Diphtheria	35	17	18	11	5	1			9	8	1		
d. Measles	4 125	2 125	2 000	1 948	173	4			1 792	197	10		
e. Tetanus	1 586	828	758	785	26	10	5	3	722	11	16	5	3
6. Bacterial meningitis*	1 033	507	526	355	20	84	28	20	338	21	107	32	26
7. Hepatitis B and hepatitis C	239	103	136	45	28	20	6	4	34	31	56	10	4
8. Malaria	819	389	429	91	101	167	22	7	85	115	195	26	10
9. Tropical-cluster diseases	1 124	524	600	21	32	320	105	47	15	21	397	117	50
a. Trypanosomiasis													
b. Chagas disease	965	430	535	3	5	281	97	44	3	2	372	110	47
c. Schistosomiasis	74	37	36	2	8	20	5	2	2	9	18	5	2
d. Leishmaniasis	70	46	24	16	15	13	1		10	10	5	1	
e. Lymphatic filariasis	12	10	3			5	1				1		
f. Onchocerciasis	3	2	1			1					1		
10. Leprosy	85	42	43	2	15	18	5	3	1	15	20	5	2
11. Dengue	2	1	1							1			
12. Japanese encephalitis													
13. Trachoma													
14. Intestinal nematode infections	917	448	469	6	399	33	7	4	6	417	33	7	5
a. Ascariasis	373	182	192	5	175	1			5	185	1		
b. Trichuriasis	413	203	211		202	1				210	1		
c. Ancylostomiasis and necatoriasis	131	64	67		21	32	7	4		22	32	7	5

Annex Table 10g, continued. DALYs [0,0] by age, sex and cause (thousands): Latin America and the Caribbean, 1990

Cause	Total	Male	Female	Males					Females				
				0–4	5–14	15–44	45–59	60+	0–4	5–14	15–44	45–59	60+
B. Respiratory infections	**11 080**	**6 047**	**5 033**	**5 051**	**347**	**273**	**145**	**230**	**3 816**	**402**	**436**	**128**	**251**
1. Lower respiratory infections	10 794	5 901	4 893	4 972	292	266	143	228	3 749	345	425	126	247
2. Upper respiratory infections	115	62	52	48	4	6	2	3	35	5	7	2	3
3. Otitis media	172	84	88	31	51	1	–	–	32	52	4	–	–
C. Maternal conditions	**2 247**	**–**	**2 247**	**–**	**–**	**–**	**–**	**–**	**–**	**11**	**2 232**	**4**	**–**
1. Maternal haemorrhage	282	–	282	–	–	–	–	–	–	2	279	1	–
2. Maternal sepsis	294	–	294	–	–	–	–	–	–	2	293	–	–
3. Hypertensive disorders of pregnancy	177	–	177	–	–	–	–	–	–	1	174	1	–
4. Obstructed labour	640	–	640	–	–	–	–	–	–	2	639	–	–
5. Abortion	490	–	490	–	–	–	–	–	–	–	487	1	–
D. Perinatal conditions*	**17 107**	**9 781**	**7 326**	**9 779**	**2**	**–**	**–**	**–**	**7 325**	**1**	**–**	**–**	**–**
E. Nutritional deficiencies	**6 410**	**3 115**	**3 295**	**2 440**	**306**	**194**	**71**	**104**	**2 072**	**356**	**635**	**100**	**133**
1. Protein-energy malnutrition	3 747	2 001	1 746	1 794	72	48	31	55	1 462	100	85	30	69
2. Iodine deficiency	184	90	94	80	7	3	–	–	79	9	5	–	–
3. Vitamin A deficiency	406	204	201	152	47	5	–	–	142	54	6	–	–
4. Iron-deficiency anaemia	2 035	803	1 232	402	179	136	38	48	373	191	536	69	63
II. Noncommunicable diseases	***66 392***	***33 014***	***33 378***	***4 632***	***2 484***	***10 970***	***7 243***	***7 684***	***4 280***	***2 169***	***11 426***	***7 126***	***8 379***
A. Malignant neoplasms	**8 353**	**3 706**	**4 647**	**180**	**469**	**682**	**1 026**	**1 349**	**169**	**353**	**1 357**	**1 443**	**1 325**
1. Mouth and oropharynx cancers	282	203	79	1	3	46	92	60	1	3	15	26	34
2. Oesophagus cancer	188	132	56	–	–	14	62	55	–	–	5	18	33
3. Stomach cancer	708	420	287	–	–	69	152	198	–	–	51	88	149
4. Colon and rectum cancers	454	204	251	–	1	47	68	88	–	1	42	75	133
5. Liver cancer	110	55	55	1	3	12	18	20	1	3	8	17	28
6. Pancreas cancer	144	72	72	–	–	11	28	33	–	–	7	23	41
7. Trachea, bronchus, lung cancers	641	460	181	1	2	63	189	206	–	1	29	63	87
8. Melanoma and other skin cancers	80	36	43	–	1	15	12	8	1	2	16	14	12
9. Breast cancer	806	–	806	–	–	–	–	–	–	–	267	333	207
10. Cervix uteri cancer	705	–	705	–	–	–	–	–	–	–	286	277	142
11. Corpus uteri cancer	150	–	150	–	–	–	–	–	–	–	27	70	53
12. Ovary cancer	170	–	170	–	–	–	–	–	–	10	67	48	41
13. Prostate cancer	278	278	–	–	–	6	37	234	–	–	–	–	–
14. Bladder cancer	147	108	39	–	2	11	33	63	–	1	4	10	24
15. Lymphomas and multiple myeloma	528	304	224	33	80	100	51	40	21	51	58	41	53
16. Leukaemia	597	327	271	57	140	86	22	20	47	113	62	23	25
C. Diabetes mellitus	**2 482**	**1 032**	**1 450**	**28**	**52**	**243**	**335**	**373**	**27**	**45**	**297**	**478**	**604**
D. Endocrine disorders	**2 076**	**1 005**	**1 071**	**518**	**109**	**200**	**91**	**87**	**426**	**90**	**276**	**146**	**132**

Annex Table 10g, continued. DALYs [0,0] by age, sex and cause (thousands): Latin America and the Caribbean, 1990

Cause	Total	Male	Female	Males					Females				
				0-4	5-14	15-44	45-59	60+	0-4	5-14	15-44	45-59	60+
E. Neuro-psychiatric conditions	**14 452**	**7 874**	**6 578**	**401**	**598**	**5 568**	**763**	**545**	**370**	**539**	**4 417**	**617**	**635**
1. Unipolar major depression	3 063	1 057	2 007	-	-	860	148	49	-	-	1 621	282	103
2. Bipolar disorder	846	421	425	-	-	381	27	13	-	-	381	28	16
3. Schizophrenia	1 887	957	929	-	-	929	17	11	-	-	910	7	13
4. Epilepsy	735	384	351	32	119	180	37	15	30	107	180	20	14
5. Alcohol use	2 936	2 687	249	-	-	2 238	327	122	-	-	219	21	9
6. Dementia*	1 205	513	691	75	42	33	94	271	78	32	40	125	417
7. Parkinson disease	63	34	30	-	-	-	12	21	-	-	-	11	18
8. Multiple sclerosis	164	68	97	-	-	57	8	3	-	-	79	13	5
9. Drug use	847	549	298	-	49	472	21	6	-	27	257	11	3
10. Post-traumatic stress disorder	142	53	89	8	14	28	3	1	12	23	48	11	1
11. Obsessive-compulsive disorders	632	268	364	-	46	199	14	9	-	60	265	25	14
12. Panic disorder	284	96	189	-	16	66	14	-	-	16	144	23	6
F. Sense organ diseases	**810**	**368**	**442**	**36**	**6**	**17**	**72**	**238**	**26**	**9**	**19**	**94**	**294**
1. Glaucoma	125	44	81	-	-	1	20	23	-	-	3	43	35
2. Cataracts	603	280	323	6	-	9	50	214	6	1	9	49	258
G. Cardiovascular diseases	**14 796**	**7 451**	**7 345**	**318**	**227**	**1 518**	**2 165**	**3 223**	**282**	**206**	**1 681**	**1 784**	**3 392**
1. Rheumatic heart disease	322	101	221	3	26	44	18	10	3	38	112	45	23
2. Ischaemic heart disease	5 686	3 019	2 666	-	-	493	1 013	1 513	-	-	423	719	1 524
3. Cerebrovascular disease	4 671	2 267	2 404	26	42	490	688	1 021	22	39	574	643	1 126
4. Inflammatory heart diseases	842	411	431	61	48	155	83	65	65	45	175	75	71
H. Respiratory diseases	**5 815**	**2 986**	**2 829**	**999**	**261**	**565**	**477**	**684**	**898**	**221**	**737**	**417**	**556**
1. COPD*	1 744	965	779	138	16	170	228	414	137	14	166	165	297
2. Asthma	1 071	547	524	107	141	198	54	47	87	118	186	69	65
I. Digestive diseases	**5 866**	**3 348**	**2 518**	**417**	**178**	**1 097**	**1 045**	**611**	**322**	**135**	**812**	**656**	**593**
1. Peptic ulcer	254	153	101	3	5	52	45	48	4	3	29	26	40
2. Cirrhosis of the liver	1 936	1 386	550	27	18	568	546	227	21	17	189	196	127
3. Appendicitis	97	56	42	2	24	26	2	2	2	17	20	2	1
J. Genito-urinary diseases	**2 028**	**1 014**	**1 014**	**145**	**104**	**164**	**381**	**219**	**126**	**118**	**384**	**183**	**204**
1. Nephritis and nephrosis	1 123	514	609	93	86	123	91	121	84	94	202	104	125
2. Benign prostatic hypertrophy	281	281	-	-	-	-	250	30	-	-	-	-	-
L. Musculo-skeletal diseases	**4 504**	**1 740**	**2 764**	**13**	**36**	**657**	**788**	**246**	**8**	**46**	**1 053**	**1 161**	**495**
1. Rheumatoid arthritis	540	116	424	-	1	55	39	22	-	5	245	111	62
2. Osteoarthritis	3 426	1 497	1 928	-	1	567	727	203	-	-	566	977	384

Annex Table 10g, continued. DALYs [0,0] by age, sex and cause (thousands): Latin America and the Caribbean, 1990

Cause	Total	Male	Female	Males					Females				
				0-4	5-14	15-44	45-59	60+	0-4	5-14	15-44	45-59	60+
M. Congenital anomalies	**3 310**	**1 620**	**1 691**	**1 425**	**136**	**49**	**6**	**4**	**1 473**	**120**	**82**	**11**	**5**
1. Abdominal wall defect	40	20	21	20	–	–	–	–	21	–	–	–	–
2. Anencephaly	693	267	426	267	–	–	–	–	426	–	–	–	–
3. Anorectal atresia	12	6	6	6	–	–	–	–	6	–	–	–	–
4. Cleft lip	50	28	22	28	–	–	–	–	22	–	–	–	–
5. Cleft palate	41	19	22	19	–	–	–	–	22	–	–	–	–
6. Oesophageal atresia	27	13	14	13	–	–	–	–	14	–	–	–	–
7. Renal agenesis	75	37	37	37	–	–	–	–	37	–	–	–	–
8. Down syndrome	294	156	139	114	26	13	3	–	94	22	17	5	–
9. Congenital heart anomalies	1 115	588	527	497	62	24	2	3	423	51	45	4	4
10. Spina bifida	494	241	253	215	22	5	–	–	221	23	8	–	–
N. Oral conditions	**1 000**	**495**	**506**	**82**	**213**	**118**	**27**	**55**	**79**	**208**	**118**	**30**	**70**
1. Dental caries	827	417	410	81	211	114	7	4	78	206	114	7	5
2. Periodontal disease	18	9	10	–	–	2	4	2	–	–	2	4	3
3. Edentulism	143	63	79	–	–	–	16	48	–	–	–	18	61
III. Injuries	***27 858***	***20 120***	***7 738***	***2 509***	***3 917***	***11 918***	***1 325***	***451***	***1 919***	***1 831***	***3 351***	***388***	***249***
A. Unintentional injuries	**20 114**	**14 070**	**6 044**	**2 254**	**3 557**	**6 952**	**950**	**357**	**1 682**	**1 639**	**2 195**	**309**	**220**
1. Road traffic accidents	6 852	4 875	1 977	299	1 229	2 862	369	115	231	643	929	121	53
2. Poisonings	300	172	128	70	30	59	9	4	52	26	43	4	3
3. Falls	2 622	1 889	732	390	739	605	89	66	198	247	174	45	68
4. Fires	598	320	278	108	110	84	12	7	101	113	51	8	5
5. Drownings	1 685	1 275	410	234	405	580	45	12	153	147	100	7	3
6. Other unintentional	8 058	5 538	2 521	1 152	1 043	2 762	426	154	947	464	898	124	88
B. Intentional injuries	**7 744**	**6 050**	**1 694**	**255**	**361**	**4 966**	**375**	**94**	**237**	**192**	**1 157**	**79**	**30**
1. Self-inflicted injuries	1 037	666	371	–	31	521	79	34	–	26	304	30	12
2. Violence	5 447	4 680	767	100	247	4 004	276	54	76	103	542	34	11
3. War	1 259	704	555	155	82	441	19	6	161	63	310	14	7

Notes:
A dash (–) symbol indicates fewer than 500 DALYs.
*IA6 is Bacterial meningitis and meningococcaemia; ID is Conditions arising during the perinatal period;
IIE6 is Dementia and other degenerative and hereditary CNS disorders; IIH1 is Chronic obstructive pulmonary disease.

Annex Table 10h. DALYs [0,0] by age, sex and cause (thousands): Middle Eastern Crescent, 1990

Cause	Total	Male	Female	Males					Females				
				0-4	5-14	15-44	45-59	60+	0-4	5-14	15-44	45-59	60+
Population (millions)	503	256	247	41	65	114	22	14	40	62	107	22	15
All causes	283 005	144 423	138 582	85 118	14 052	25 535	9 797	9 922	83 262	12 366	24 624	7 936	10 394
I. Communicable, maternal, perinatal and nutritional conditions	156 478	76 197	80 282	67 931	3 827	2 571	833	1 035	66 669	3 947	7 800	838	1 028
A. Infectious and parasitic diseases	67 372	34 392	32 979	29 159	1 977	2 148	714	394	28 333	1 872	1 817	548	409
1. Tuberculosis	4 546	2 805	1 741	413	199	1 469	490	234	265	130	875	298	173
2. STDs excluding HIV	1 311	575	736	521	1	44	3	5	514	5	206	5	6
a. Syphilis	1 057	529	527	509		12	3	5	502		15	4	6
b. Chlamydia	178	20	158	4		15			4	4	150	1	
c. Gonorrhoea	76	26	51	8		17			9	1	41		
3. HIV	54	43	11	4		35	4		4		6		
4. Diarrhoeal diseases	34 596	17 447	17 149	16 751	567	85	23	22	16 363	600	138	27	21
5. Childhood-cluster diseases	19 844	10 015	9 829	9 207	753	39	11	5	8 987	721	96	21	4
a. Pertussis	4 593	2 314	2 279	2 138	176				2 099	180			
b. Poliomyelitis	991	559	432	546	3	9			423	2	7		
c. Diphtheria	96	49	48	44	4				43				
d. Measles	7 658	3 834	3 824	3 406	426	2			3 376	441	6		
e. Tetanus	6 506	3 259	3 246	3 074	144	27	10	4	3 046	94	82	20	4
6. Bacterial meningitis*	1 459	728	730	552	27	97	32	20	551	27	94	36	22
7. Hepatitis B and hepatitis C	505	273	232	86	38	70	49	30	70	39	69	26	28
8. Malaria	587	292	295	87	105	82	13	5	85	105	84	15	6
9. Tropical-cluster diseases	372	229	142	48	87	70	17	7	32	51	46	9	4
a. Trypanosomiasis													
b. Chagas disease													
c. Schistosomiasis	163	104	59	4	29	49	15	7	2	10	35	8	3
d. Leishmaniasis	191	112	78	43	57	11	1		30	40	8	1	
e. Lymphatic filariasis	18	13	5		1	10	2			1	3	1	
f. Onchocerciasis													
10. Leprosy	18	10	8	2	3	4	1				4	1	1
11. Dengue													
12. Japanese encephalitis													
13. Trachoma	343	91	252			20	29	42			50	80	121
14. Intestinal nematode infections	240	120	120	3	86	24	5	3	3	86	23	5	3
a. Ascariasis	149	75	75	2	72				2	72			
b. Trichuriasis	2	1	1		1					1			
c. Ancylostomiasis and necatoriasis	89	45	44		13	24	5	3		13	23	5	3

Annex Table 10h, continued. DALYs [0.0] by age, sex and cause (thousands): Middle Eastern Crescent, 1990

Cause	Total	Male	Female	Males 0-4	Males 5-14	Males 15-44	Males 45-59	Males 60+	Females 0-4	Females 5-14	Females 15-44	Females 45-59	Females 60+
B. Respiratory infections	**36 894**	**18 440**	**18 453**	**16 226**	**1 351**	**203**	**73**	**588**	**15 896**	**1 550**	**325**	**122**	**560**
1. Lower respiratory infections	36 048	18 016	18 032	15 902	1 264	197	72	582	15 579	1 462	317	120	554
2. Upper respiratory infections	371	185	186	158	14	5	1	6	155	16	7	2	6
3. Otitis media	474	239	235	165	73	1	-	-	162	72	2	-	-
C. Maternal conditions	**5 009**	**-**	**5 009**							**4**	**4 909**	**95**	
1. Maternal haemorrhage	651	-	651							1	628	22	
2. Maternal sepsis	870	-	870							1	854	15	
3. Hypertensive disorders of pregnancy	423	-	423							1	407	15	
4. Obstructed labour	1 496	-	1 496								1 488	7	
5. Abortion	400	-	400								392	7	
D. Perinatal conditions*	**34 463**	**17 293**	**17 169**	**17 293**					**17 169**				
E. Nutritional deficiencies	**12 741**	**6 071**	**6 671**	**5 253**	**499**	**219**	**46**	**53**	**5 271**	**521**	**749**	**72**	**59**
1. Protein-energy malnutrition	7 848	3 923	3 925	3 880	14	11	5	14	3 871	14	22	5	13
2. Iodine deficiency	492	242	250	214	22	6	-	-	213	24	11	1	1
3. Vitamin A deficiency	1 621	777	844	557	211	10	-	-	592	240	12	-	-
4. Iron-deficiency anaemia	2 780	1 128	1 652	602	253	193	41	39	595	242	704	66	45
II. Noncommunicable diseases	**91 415**	**46 123**	**45 292**	**11 979**	**5 691**	**11 788**	**8 041**	**8 624**	**11 663**	**5 918**	**11 870**	**6 685**	**9 155**
A. Malignant neoplasms	**6 711**	**3 475**	**3 236**	**221**	**566**	**829**	**1 016**	**844**	**195**	**547**	**934**	**829**	**731**
1. Mouth and oropharynx cancers	407	250	157	3	9	90	60	88	3	11	51	33	59
2. Oesophagus cancer	231	130	102	-	1	27	63	39	1	3	22	40	36
3. Stomach cancer	499	295	204	1	4	73	131	85	1	2	49	71	82
4. Colon and rectum cancers	300	146	154	1	3	51	35	56	2	6	40	29	77
5. Liver cancer	214	128	85	2	8	31	55	33	2	7	18	30	28
6. Pancreas cancer	109	65	44	-	-	17	30	18	-	-	7	18	18
7. Trachea, bronchus, lung cancers	682	537	144	3	10	95	269	161	3	9	26	52	54
8. Melanoma and other skin cancers	34	20	14	-	1	7	9	3	-	-	7	5	3
9. Breast cancer	401	-	401						1	4	166	156	74
10. Cervix uteri cancer	243	-	243							1	85	107	49
11. Corpus uteri cancer	52	-	52							1	10	22	19
12. Ovary cancer	134	-	134							12	61	39	19
13. Prostate cancer	78	78	-			5	20	51					
14. Bladder cancer	223	174	49	1	3	38	68	64	1	2	11	18	18
15. Lymphomas and multiple myeloma	380	243	137	25	82	84	26	27	16	53	36	12	20
16. Leukaemia	657	324	333	47	149	88	19	23	54	174	62	15	28
C. Diabetes mellitus	**2 423**	**1 136**	**1 287**	**74**	**136**	**302**	**343**	**281**	**71**	**139**	**289**	**383**	**406**
D. Endocrine disorders	**1 532**	**715**	**817**	**373**	**125**	**117**	**65**	**35**	**358**	**232**	**141**	**51**	**36**

Annex Table 10h, continued. DALYs [0,0] by age, sex and cause (thousands): Middle Eastern Crescent, 1990

Cause	Total	Male	Female	Males 0-4	5-14	15-44	45-59	60+	Females 0-4	5-14	15-44	45-59	60+
E. Neuro-psychiatric conditions	13 038	6 422	6 617	878	808	4 014	424	298	714	764	4 255	506	377
1. Unipolar major depression	3 322	1 191	2 131	-	-	985	156	51	-	-	1 747	281	102
2. Bipolar disorder	943	483	460	-	-	440	29	13	-	1	414	29	16
3. Schizophrenia	2 057	1 069	987	-	-	1 046	13	10	-	-	957	18	16
4. Epilepsy	738	379	360	70	131	144	23	11	56	147	130	19	8
5. Alcohol use	196	176	20	-	-	156	16	5	-	-	17	2	1
6. Dementia*	534	245	289	52	15	29	38	111	67	18	30	29	146
7. Parkinson disease	110	59	51	-	-	-	20	38	-	-	-	18	32
8. Multiple sclerosis	165	71	94	-	-	61	7	3	-	-	78	12	5
9. Drug use	711	640	71	1	57	552	24	6	-	6	61	3	1
10. Post-traumatic stress disorder	163	62	100	11	17	31	3	1	18	28	49	5	1
11. Obsessive-compulsive disorders	701	307	394	-	60	224	14	9	-	75	281	25	13
12. Panic disorder	308	108	200	-	20	74	14	-	-	20	152	23	5
F. Sense organ diseases	1 153	522	631	5	-	26	195	295	6	1	28	230	366
1. Glaucoma	146	55	91	-	-	1	33	21	-	-	2	60	29
2. Cataracts	992	461	531	4	-	22	161	274	4	-	23	168	336
G. Cardiovascular diseases	32 250	16 358	15 892	2 791	2 332	3 134	3 255	4 845	2 478	2 495	3 010	2 482	5 427
1. Rheumatic heart disease	1 368	576	792	2	204	336	27	7	4	290	441	44	13
2. Ischaemic heart disease	10 236	5 466	4 770	-	-	1 000	1 759	2 707	-	-	750	1 118	2 902
3. Cerebrovascular disease	4 669	2 271	2 397	150	370	450	502	799	121	345	344	501	1 085
4. Inflammatory heart diseases	3 499	1 732	1 766	533	446	455	172	127	585	445	448	150	139
H. Respiratory diseases	9 935	4 949	4 986	2 289	563	716	558	823	2 386	642	781	515	662
1. COPD*	2 479	1 231	1 248	341	49	167	183	490	412	91	193	217	335
2. Asthma	1 016	657	358	163	196	208	51	40	64	83	129	42	40
I. Digestive diseases	10 132	5 252	4 880	2 233	503	1 030	947	539	2 567	409	765	660	479
1. Peptic ulcer	205	141	64	1	8	59	45	28	2	3	25	19	15
2. Cirrhosis of the liver	1 450	779	670	30	71	235	275	168	23	143	156	194	154
3. Appendicitis	273	155	118	7	72	70	4	2	6	60	46	3	2
J. Genito-urinary diseases	4 726	2 623	2 103	252	284	820	823	445	206	301	787	472	338
1. Nephritis and nephrosis	1 460	698	762	122	151	211	106	108	105	217	257	98	85
2. Benign prostatic hypertrophy	277	277	-	1	1	2	243	31	-	-	-	-	-
L. Musculo-skeletal diseases	1 278	529	749	20	18	251	166	73	17	12	288	268	164
1. Rheumatoid arthritis	146	81	65	-	-	75	4	2	-	2	28	23	12
2. Osteoarthritis	953	369	583	-	-	151	154	65	-	-	211	230	142

Annex Table 10h, continued. DALYs [0,0] by age, sex and cause (thousands): Middle Eastern Crescent, 1990

Cause	Total	Male	Female	Males 0-4	Males 5-14	Males 15-44	Males 45-59	Males 60+	Females 0-4	Females 5-14	Females 15-44	Females 45-59	Females 60+
M. Congenital anomalies	5 753	2 938	2 815	2 593	191	129	18	7	2 431	226	122	26	10
1. Abdominal wall defect	71	46	25	46	-	-	-	-	25	-	-	-	-
2. Anencephaly	1 573	606	966	606	-	-	-	-	966	-	-	-	-
3. Anorectal atresia	23	14	8	14	-	-	-	-	8	-	-	-	-
4. Cleft lip	53	31	22	31	-	-	-	-	22	-	-	-	-
5. Cleft palate	43	20	22	20	-	-	-	-	22	-	-	-	-
6. Oesophageal atresia	48	31	17	31	-	-	-	-	17	-	-	-	-
7. Renal agenesis	139	70	70	70	-	-	-	-	70	-	-	-	-
8. Down syndrome	563	307	256	206	47	54	-	-	148	60	48	-	-
9. Congenital heart anomalies	2 137	1 205	931	1 035	95	55	15	6	746	107	48	22	9
10. Spina bifida	356	198	158	186	11	1	-	-	134	14	8	2	-
N. Oral conditions	1 879	924	956	194	93	335	192	109	187	91	339	208	131
1. Dental caries	829	420	409	193	92	71	35	30	186	87	67	35	34
2. Periodontal disease	14	7	7	-	-	7	-	-	-	-	6	-	-
3. Edentulism	1 016	491	525	-	-	255	157	79	-	-	256	173	97
III. Injuries	35 112	22 104	13 008	5 208	4 533	11 176	923	262	4 930	2 501	4 954	413	211
A. Unintentional injuries	18 113	12 204	5 908	3 235	3 011	5 259	553	147	2 851	1 447	1 314	195	101
1. Road traffic accidents	4 398	3 375	1 023	238	776	2 120	194	46	214	380	347	57	26
2. Poisonings	696	421	275	148	41	183	41	9	140	34	78	16	7
3. Falls	2 716	1 723	994	621	645	398	45	13	546	281	129	25	12
4. Fires	1 324	601	723	229	201	150	16	5	241	219	241	14	8
5. Drownings	1 827	1 246	581	450	391	378	22	6	396	114	64	5	2
6. Other unintentional	7 151	4 838	2 312	1 549	957	2 029	236	67	1 316	419	456	77	45
B. Intentional injuries	16 999	9 899	7 100	1 974	1 523	5 917	370	116	2 079	1 054	3 639	218	110
1. Self-inflicted injuries	2 390	1 605	784	-	574	866	124	41	-	273	424	53	34
2. Violence	2 366	1 450	915	464	146	766	58	17	521	159	200	27	9
3. War	12 244	6 844	5 400	1 510	803	4 286	188	58	1 558	622	3 015	139	67

Notes:
A dash (-) symbol indicates fewer than 500 DALYs.
*IA6 is Bacterial meningitis and meningococcaemia; ID is Conditions arising during the perinatal period;
*IIH1 is Chronic obstructive pulmonary disease.
IIE6 is Dementia and other degenerative and hereditary CNS disorders;

Annex Table 10i. DALYs [0,0] by age, sex and cause (thousands): World, 1990

Cause	Total	Male	Female	Males					Females				
				0-4	5-14	15-44	45-59	60+	0-4	5-14	15-44	45-59	60+
Population (millions)	*5 267*	*2 654*	*2 614*	*321*	*551*	*1 250*	*312*	*219*	*309*	*526*	*1 199*	*311*	*269*
All causes	2 480 237	1 289 843	1 190 393	593 673	120 390	285 191	132 807	157 784	560 802	105 013	254 076	106 159	164 344
I. Communicable, maternal, perinatal and nutritional conditions	1 252 540	618 058	634 482	492 204	44 053	49 005	16 470	16 325	465 847	46 922	92 105	14 096	15 512
A. Infectious and parasitic diseases	648 476	335 150	313 327	240 782	29 928	41 459	13 994	8 987	222 315	30 399	42 066	10 877	7 670
1. Tuberculosis	68 366	37 927	30 439	3 515	2 005	17 327	9 366	5 715	3 223	2 346	14 448	6 659	3 763
2. STDs excluding HIV	24 258	9 644	14 613	7 640	31	1 719	98	155	7 310	153	6 776	155	219
a. Syphilis	14 570	7 373	7 197	6 765	4	363	88	152	6 414	5	451	117	211
b. Chlamydia	5 573	659	4 914	196	10	449	3	1	200	106	4 580	25	4
c. Gonorrhoea	4 099	1 605	2 494	679	17	902	6	2	696	44	1 741	11	1
3. HIV	18 854	10 030	8 823	2 727	329	6 271	601	102	2 645	347	5 538	247	47
4. Diarrhoeal diseases	227 037	117 054	109 982	106 784	6 191	2 357	678	1 044	97 995	6 934	3 139	767	1 148
5. Childhood-cluster diseases	162 091	82 606	79 486	72 986	7 909	1 387	226	98	69 315	8 280	1 540	250	101
a. Pertussis	30 483	15 562	14 921	14 294	1 268				13 652	1 269			
b. Poliomyelitis	6 847	3 878	2 969	3 769	22	80	6	1	2 883	17	63	5	1
c. Diphtheria	834	423	412	376	42	5			361	44	6		
d. Measles	84 058	42 851	41 207	37 546	5 252	45	6	2	35 846	5 298	54	7	2
e. Tetanus	39 869	19 891	19 978	17 001	1 326	1 257	214	94	16 572	1 652	1 418	238	98
6. Bacterial meningitis*	12 954	6 512	6 442	4 697	223	1 034	335	222	4 573	225	1 038	352	255
7. Hepatitis B and hepatitis C	4 153	2 378	1 775	619	252	803	468	236	500	247	590	190	248
8. Malaria	67 578	35 746	31 832	28 818	3 458	2 905	431	134	24 353	3 495	3 331	492	161
9. Tropical-cluster diseases	15 129	9 462	5 667	515	3 163	4 796	789	199	413	1 780	2 613	701	160
a. Trypanosomiasis	2 595	1 226	1 369	40	474	535	154	23	81	502	651	115	18
b. Chagas disease	965	430	535	3	5	281	97	44	3	2	372	110	47
c. Schistosomiasis	1 438	853	585	65	293	359	92	44	44	193	260	59	28
d. Leishmaniasis	3 438	2 076	1 362	219	962	848	36	11	146	640	541	26	9
e. Lymphatic filariasis	5 832	4 383	1 449	175	1 355	2 573	259	21	129	382	635	279	23
f. Onchocerciasis	862	493	369	13	74	200	152	55	11	60	153	111	34
10. Leprosy	604	300	304	11	110	138	31	11	26	104	138	28	8
11. Dengue	1 485	673	811	165	492	12	4		197	595	14	5	
12. Japanese encephalitis	1 383	698	685	419	227	45	5	2	422	215	42	4	2
13. Trachoma	1 396	368	1 027			75	120	174			199	324	505
14. Intestinal nematode infections	6 851	3 446	3 405	43	2 891	379	83	50	44	2 850	370	85	55
a. Ascariasis	2 880	1 448	1 431	42	1 395	10	1		42	1 377	10	1	
b. Trichuriasis	2 546	1 284	1 261	1	1 282	1		1	2	1 259	2	1	
c. Ancylostomiasis and necatoriasis	1 423	713	710		214	368	82	49		214	358	83	55

Annex Table 10i, continued. DALYs[0,0] by age, sex and cause (thousands): World, 1990

Cause	Total	Male	Female	Males 0-4	5-14	15-44	45-59	60+	Females 0-4	5-14	15-44	45-59	60+
B. Respiratory infections	**264 651**	**133 696**	**130 955**	**112 562**	**10 013**	**3 471**	**1 492**	**6 159**	**107 912**	**11 468**	**3 711**	**1 420**	**6 443**
1. Lower respiratory infections	257 343	130 423	126 920	110 151	9 327	3 382	1 468	6 094	104 763	10 773	3 617	1 395	6 371
2. Upper respiratory infections	2 739	1 391	1 348	1 116	113	73	23	65	1 053	127	74	24	74
3. Otitis media	3 791	1 883	1 908	1 294	572	15	–	1	1 318	568	20	1	1
C. Maternal conditions	**41 220**	**–**	**41 220**	–	–	–	–	–	–	**747**	**40 111**	**362**	**–**
1. Maternal haemorrhage	6 323	–	6 323	–	–	–	–	–	–	175	6 059	89	–
2. Maternal sepsis	6 509	–	6 509	–	–	–	–	–	–	116	6 345	47	–
3. Hypertensive disorders of pregnancy	3 093	–	3 093	–	–	–	–	–	–	88	2 963	42	–
4. Obstructed labour	9 539	–	9 539	–	–	–	–	–	–	59	9 457	23	–
5. Abortion	5 912	–	5 912	–	–	–	–	–	–	99	5 774	40	–
D. Perinatal conditions*	**215 638**	**109 973**	**105 665**	**109 968**	**4**	**2**	–	–	**105 661**	**2**	**1**	–	–
E. Nutritional deficiencies	**82 554**	**39 238**	**43 316**	**28 893**	**4 109**	**4 073**	**985**	**1 179**	**29 958**	**4 305**	**6 216**	**1 437**	**1 399**
1. Protein-energy malnutrition	44 544	21 671	22 873	20 883	261	209	98	219	21 818	427	290	85	253
2. Iodine deficiency	3 095	1 549	1 546	1 353	139	55	1	–	1 332	143	65	4	2
3. Vitamin A deficiency	8 374	4 196	4 177	2 888	1 231	77	–	–	2 841	1 256	81	–	–
4. Iron-deficiency anaemia	26 363	11 744	14 618	3 727	2 468	3 721	877	951	3 926	2 470	5 755	1 340	1 127
II. Noncommunicable diseases	***862 432***	***440 677***	***421 755***	***56 292***	***29 014***	***118 835***	***100 865***	***135 672***	***54 950***	***27 856***	***110 631***	***84 418***	***143 899***
A. Malignant neoplasms	**133 683**	**72 859**	**60 825**	**2 215**	**4 438**	**14 726**	**23 568**	**27 912**	**2 202**	**3 382**	**14 325**	**19 077**	**21 838**
1. Mouth and oropharynx cancers	6 793	4 269	2 524	46	79	1 087	1 515	1 543	41	84	661	801	936
2. Oesophagus cancer	6 847	4 515	2 331	1	1	605	1 891	2 017	–	–	277	852	1 198
3. Stomach cancer	14 586	9 006	5 580	5	27	1 248	3 576	4 150	2	19	1 144	1 796	2 619
4. Colon and rectum cancers	8 774	4 459	4 315	9	35	878	1 286	2 251	11	37	664	1 195	2 409
5. Liver cancer	12 172	8 871	3 301	58	127	3 032	3 559	2 094	52	104	794	1 166	1 184
6. Pancreas cancer	3 084	1 761	1 323	–	–	257	650	852	4	5	123	393	798
7. Trachea, bronchus, lung cancers	17 035	12 619	4 416	32	59	1 187	5 072	6 269	11	22	474	1 561	2 348
8. Melanoma and other skin cancers	1 049	540	509	3	6	171	189	171	2	4	145	161	197
9. Breast cancer	7 982	–	7 982	–	–	–	–	–	8	14	2 323	3 222	2 414
10. Cervix uteri cancer	5 415	–	5 415	–	–	–	–	–	2	4	1 613	2 472	1 324
11. Corpus uteri cancer	1 246	–	1 246	–	–	–	–	–	4	7	181	514	540
12. Ovary cancer	2 688	–	2 688	–	–	–	–	–	54	98	830	900	805
13. Prostate cancer	2 624	2 624	–	–	–	45	395	2 174	–	–	–	–	–
14. Bladder cancer	2 309	1 737	572	6	9	157	472	1 093	3	6	64	144	355
15. Lymphomas and multiple myeloma	5 892	3 580	2 312	307	793	1 058	654	768	189	430	536	450	708
16. Leukaemia	8 720	4 624	4 096	721	1 368	1 547	480	508	720	1 040	1 369	456	512
C. Diabetes mellitus	**18 796**	**8 445**	**10 351**	**350**	**676**	**1 970**	**2 582**	**2 867**	**353**	**678**	**1 944**	**3 001**	**4 375**
D. Endocrine disorders	**9 230**	**4 070**	**5 159**	**1 616**	**493**	**933**	**513**	**515**	**1 544**	**617**	**1 324**	**824**	**850**

Annex Table 10i, continued. DALYs[0,0] by age, sex and cause (thousands): World, 1990

Cause	Total	Male	Female	Males 0-4	5-14	15-44	45-59	60+	Females 0-4	5-14	15-44	45-59	60+
E. Neuro-psychiatric conditions	**140 698**	**69 095**	**71 604**	**3 496**	**4 075**	**46 599**	**7 418**	**7 507**	**3 419**	**3 810**	**45 110**	**7 876**	**11 390**
1. Unipolar major depression	37 617	13 323	24 295	-	-	10 496	2 078	750	-	-	18 964	3 730	1 601
2. Bipolar disorder	10 372	5 247	5 125	-	2	4 665	383	197	1	2	4 466	377	279
3. Schizophrenia	19 020	9 867	9 154	-	-	9 600	131	136	1	-	8 892	92	170
4. Epilepsy	6 463	3 438	3 025	349	854	1 699	354	182	345	882	1 392	228	179
5. Alcohol use	12 904	11 343	1 561	-	-	9 346	1 498	498	-	-	1 253	199	110
6. Dementia*	16 300	6 605	9 695	495	202	397	1 267	4 245	596	200	392	1 416	7 090
7. Parkinson disease	1 982	917	1 065	-	1	2	286	628	1	-	2	313	749
8. Multiple sclerosis	2 048	865	1 183	-	-	697	112	55	-	-	921	172	90
9. Drug use	4 328	3 479	848	3	309	3 003	131	33	1	77	729	33	9
10. Post-traumatic stress disorder	1 629	620	1 009	84	145	337	42	12	138	234	548	67	22
11. Obsessive-compulsive disorders	7 627	3 289	4 337	-	502	2 452	195	141	-	637	3 126	343	231
12. Panic disorder	3 502	1 178	2 324	-	146	827	204	2	-	175	1 736	322	91
F. Sense organ diseases	**13 405**	**5 943**	**7 462**	**160**	**16**	**366**	**2 306**	**3 094**	**128**	**34**	**490**	**2 935**	**3 876**
1. Glaucoma	3 667	1 413	2 253	17	-	108	780	508	21	-	159	1 351	722
2. Cataracts	9 271	4 343	4 928	71	2	225	1 490	2 556	43	3	239	1 536	3 107
G. Cardiovascular diseases	**257 439**	**130 817**	**126 622**	**8 875**	**8 088**	**22 965**	**32 054**	**58 835**	**8 446**	**8 705**	**18 761**	**23 455**	**67 255**
1. Rheumatic heart disease	11 065	4 540	6 524	12	611	2 274	919	725	79	893	2 810	1 514	1 229
2. Ischaemic heart disease	91 689	49 295	42 394	-	-	6 260	15 133	27 902	335	-	3 615	8 664	29 780
3. Cerebrovascular disease	74 334	35 935	38 399	1 123	1 684	5 823	8 952	18 352	1 061	1 483	4 785	8 103	22 966
4. Inflammatory heart diseases	18 364	9 127	9 237	1 745	1 643	2 966	1 515	1 258	2 109	1 847	2 505	1 240	1 536
H. Respiratory diseases	**93 908**	**49 977**	**43 931**	**8 824**	**3 368**	**8 563**	**9 801**	**19 421**	**8 744**	**2 953**	**7 589**	**7 608**	**17 037**
1. COPD*	49 975	27 147	22 827	1 357	274	3 739	6 399	15 379	1 924	325	2 823	4 610	13 145
2. Asthma	11 901	6 539	5 362	1 243	1 562	2 345	736	653	804	1 027	2 100	732	699
I. Digestive diseases	**76 660**	**43 243**	**33 417**	**7 647**	**2 843**	**12 202**	**12 316**	**8 235**	**7 897**	**2 641**	**7 657**	**7 574**	**7 648**
1. Peptic ulcer	4 341	2 689	1 652	54	60	993	845	737	63	59	518	438	575
2. Cirrhosis of the liver	22 969	15 516	7 453	441	353	5 308	6 065	3 349	329	463	1 982	2 569	2 109
3. Appendicitis	3 148	1 815	1 333	66	738	917	63	32	66	609	579	49	30
J. Genito-urinary diseases	**26 347**	**14 421**	**11 926**	**1 465**	**2 065**	**3 416**	**4 261**	**3 214**	**1 149**	**2 104**	**3 438**	**2 389**	**2 846**
1. Nephritis and nephrosis	16 054	8 143	7 911	1 101	1 747	2 405	1 270	1 621	979	1 885	2 172	1 231	1 643
2. Benign prostatic hypertrophy	2 791	2 790	-	17	-	16	2 082	674	-	-	-	-	-
L. Musculo-skeletal diseases	**28 953**	**10 462**	**18 491**	**75**	**160**	**3 634**	**4 233**	**2 360**	**100**	**165**	**6 035**	**7 580**	**4 612**
1. Rheumatoid arthritis	3 578	976	2 602	3	5	344	322	303	1	24	974	738	864
2. Osteoarthritis	21 822	8 381	13 441	-	1	2 993	3 712	1 675	-	-	3 980	6 310	3 151

Annex Table 10i, continued. DALYs[0,0] by age, sex and cause (thousands): World, 1990

Cause	Total	Male	Female	Males					Females				
				0-4	5-14	15-44	45-59	60+	0-4	5-14	15-44	45-59	60+
M. Congenital anomalies	**44 574**	**22 371**	**22 203**	**19 410**	**1 551**	**1 213**	**137**	**60**	**19 015**	**1 683**	**1 239**	**185**	**81**
1. Abdominal wall defect	415	221	194	221	-	-	-	-	194	-	-	-	-
2. Anencephaly	11 960	4 610	7 350	4 610	-	-	-	-	7 350	-	-	-	-
3. Anorectal atresia	145	80	65	80	-	-	-	-	65	-	-	-	-
4. Cleft lip	407	242	166	242	-	-	-	-	166	-	-	-	-
5. Cleft palate	327	161	166	161	-	-	-	-	166	-	-	-	-
6. Oesophageal atresia	245	136	109	136	-	-	-	-	109	-	-	-	-
7. Renal agenesis	940	472	469	472	-	-	-	-	469	-	-	-	-
8. Down syndrome	3 934	2 134	1 801	1 344	353	408	22	6	1 007	362	398	28	5
9. Congenital heart anomalies	15 014	8 218	6 796	6 797	722	556	98	44	5 257	752	598	131	58
10. Spina bifida	4 629	2 442	2 188	2 233	184	22	1	1	1 882	225	66	11	4
N. Oral conditions	**9 935**	**4 777**	**5 158**	**1 037**	**574**	**1 216**	**936**	**1 014**	**999**	**581**	**1 297**	**1 025**	**1 256**
1. Dental caries	4 914	2 476	2 439	1 027	562	493	214	180	990	549	476	214	209
2. Periodontal disease	200	100	100	-	-	74	16	10	-	-	71	16	12
3. Edentulism	4 635	2 153	2 481	-	-	627	704	822	-	-	661	789	1 031
III. Injuries	***365 265***	***231 109***	***134 157***	***45 177***	***47 323***	***117 350***	***15 471***	***5 787***	***40 004***	***30 236***	***51 340***	***7 645***	***4 932***
A. Unintentional injuries	**264 637**	**169 329**	**95 308**	**38 740**	**42 255**	**73 340**	**10 934**	**4 060**	**33 007**	**26 820**	**26 832**	**5 071**	**3 578**
1. Road traffic accidents	59 756	42 719	17 038	4 485	8 917	24 936	3 274	1 107	2 909	5 227	6 813	1 408	681
2. Poisonings	12 637	7 411	5 226	2 633	888	2 801	842	246	1 787	744	2 137	365	194
3. Falls	42 163	25 710	16 452	6 213	10 620	6 875	1 257	746	6 379	4 983	2 962	995	1 134
4. Fires	21 497	8 677	12 820	3 168	2 495	2 450	400	165	2 878	4 699	4 615	373	256
5. Drownings	31 535	20 555	10 980	6 899	7 517	5 383	531	224	5 082	3 768	1 706	244	181
6. Other unintentional	97 049	64 257	32 792	15 342	11 819	30 894	4 631	1 571	13 974	7 400	8 599	1 686	1 133
B. Intentional injuries	**100 628**	**61 780**	**38 848**	**6 437**	**5 068**	**44 010**	**4 537**	**1 727**	**6 997**	**3 416**	**24 507**	**2 574**	**1 354**
1. Self-inflicted injuries	33 571	17 895	15 676	-	1 265	12 843	2 564	1 223	-	723	12 367	1 635	950
2. Violence	31 118	23 681	7 437	2 037	1 438	18 454	1 421	332	2 452	902	3 345	533	205
3. War	35 938	20 203	15 735	4 400	2 365	12 714	552	173	4 545	1 791	8 794	407	198

Notes:

A dash (-) symbol indicates fewer than 500 DALYs.

*IA6 is Bacterial meningitis and meningococcaemia; ID is Conditions arising during the perinatal period;
IIH1 is Chronic obstructive pulmonary disease.
IIE6 is Dementia and other degenerative and hereditary CNS disorders;

Annex Table 11. Population by age, sex and region (thousands), 1990-2020, baseline projections

Established Market Economies

Age group	1990	2000	2010	2020
Males				
0-4	26 384	28 709	28 992	29 008
5-9	26 490	28 294	28 775	28 945
10-14	26 858	26 188	28 547	28 871
15-19	29 308	26 376	28 185	28 674
20-24	31 495	26 616	25 964	28 318
25-29	32 904	28 936	26 049	27 856
30-34	31 371	31 034	26 238	25 618
35-39	29 951	32 329	28 453	25 642
40-44	29 034	30 684	30 383	25 726
45-49	24 136	29 067	31 399	27 683
50-54	21 908	27 773	29 370	29 124
55-59	20 095	22 459	27 095	29 318
60-64	18 613	19 566	24 942	26 523
65-69	15 555	16 894	19 157	23 436
70-74	10 655	14 264	15 433	20 196
75+	15 725	21 482	28 532	36 446
All ages	390 482	410 669	427 513	441 383
Females				
0-4	25 065	27 368	27 630	27 640
5-9	25 167	27 008	27 449	27 598
10-14	25 513	24 921	27 247	27 539
15-19	27 883	25 114	26 958	27 404
20-24	30 160	25 430	24 846	27 172
25-29	31 980	27 763	25 012	26 857
30-34	30 754	30 001	25 304	24 732
35-39	29 585	31 759	27 582	24 860
40-44	28 837	30 458	29 731	25 089
45-49	24 252	29 177	31 359	27 264
50-54	22 397	28 233	29 898	29 248
55-59	21 150	23 455	28 349	30 581
60-64	20 807	21 257	27 002	28 771
65-69	19 721	19 476	21 883	26 729
70-74	14 831	18 167	18 937	24 460
75+	29 206	38 631	47 681	58 053
All ages	407 308	428 217	446 869	463 999
Total	797 790	838 886	874 382	905 382

Formerly Socialist Economies of Europe

Age group	1990	2000	2010	2020
Males				
0-4	13 759	12 747	12 604	12 277
5-9	13 744	12 544	12 584	12 359
10-14	13 605	13 536	12 572	12 466
15-19	12 702	13 640	12 457	12 504
20-24	12 055	13 422	13 362	12 416
25-29	11 512	12 418	13 346	12 196
30-34	13 826	11 686	13 026	12 980
35-39	13 895	11 091	11 977	12 887
40-44	12 288	13 229	11 192	12 492
45-49	8 591	13 009	10 362	11 168
50-54	8 848	10 971	11 694	9 790
55-59	9 534	7 266	10 821	8 464
60-64	7 850	7 052	8 583	8 977
65-69	6 356	7 119	5 330	7 812
70-74	2 833	5 351	4 762	5 765
75+	3 924	5 935	7 674	7 052
All ages	165 322	171 016	172 347	171 605
Females				
0-4	13 135	12 170	12 026	11 708
5-9	13 343	12 018	12 040	11 810
10-14	13 078	12 981	12 048	11 929
15-19	12 251	13 289	11 974	11 998
20-24	11 528	13 004	12 912	11 985
25-29	11 203	12 162	13 197	11 892
30-34	13 575	11 426	12 896	12 807
35-39	13 869	11 080	12 037	13 068
40-44	12 533	13 383	11 274	12 734
45-49	9 033	13 575	10 864	11 820
50-54	9 877	12 081	12 946	10 944
55-59	11 096	8 532	12 897	10 380
60-64	10 041	9 064	11 190	12 103
65-69	10 089	9 759	7 618	11 686
70-74	5 920	8 224	7 569	9 540
75+	10 344	14 118	17 005	17 041
All ages	180 915	186 865	190 493	193 444
Total	346 237	357 881	362 840	365 049

India

Age group	1990	2000	2010	2020
Males				
0-4	59 789	56 727	55 311	52 006
5-9	54 590	55 453	53 743	51 093
10-14	47 162	55 060	53 527	53 020
15-19	45 014	53 550	54 658	53 130
20-24	40 573	46 333	54 154	52 752
25-29	35 892	44 118	52 467	53 634
30-34	31 387	39 598	45 197	52 926
35-39	26 281	34 776	42 686	50 892
40-44	21 378	30 019	37 778	43 268
45-49	18 075	24 617	32 429	39 858
50-54	15 837	19 373	27 078	33 953
55-59	13 655	15 613	21 107	27 633
60-64	10 974	12 722	15 407	21 351
65-69	8 172	9 803	11 089	14 821
70-74	5 536	6 712	7 749	9 343
75+	5 086	7 666	9 831	11 769
All ages	439 401	512 141	574 211	621 448
Females				
0-4	56 679	53 842	52 562	49 543
5-9	51 318	52 360	50 870	48 625
10-14	43 945	51 769	50 590	50 327
15-19	41 427	50 176	51 558	50 297
20-24	37 156	43 035	50 931	49 899
25-29	32 705	40 474	49 243	50 705
30-34	28 350	36 244	42 173	50 022
35-39	23 678	31 855	39 593	48 271
40-44	19 926	27 501	35 325	41 193
45-49	17 359	22 699	30 735	38 311
50-54	15 419	18 665	25 967	33 528
55-59	13 227	15 704	20 722	28 302
60-64	10 577	13 220	16 260	22 956
65-69	7 928	10 422	12 746	17 262
70-74	5 437	7 159	9 266	11 779
75+	4 982	8 108	11 258	14 756
All ages	410 113	483 233	549 799	605 777
Total	849 514	995 374	1 124 010	1 227 225

Annex Table 11, continued.   Population by age, sex and region (thousands), 1990-2020, baseline projections

China

Age group	1990	2000	2010	2020
Males				
0-4	60 243	58 700	50 352	56 472
5-9	47 467	60 957	51 827	53 051
10-14	49 530	58 673	57 666	49 727
15-19	63 349	47 068	60 555	51 535
20-24	65 728	48 972	58 099	57 148
25-29	55 048	62 456	46 477	59 842
30-34	43 876	64 626	48 226	57 256
35-39	44 901	53 872	61 186	45 556
40-44	33 403	42 653	62 871	46 938
45-49	26 191	43 066	51 654	58 620
50-54	24 345	31 241	39 756	58 359
55-59	22 138	23 502	38 373	45 652
60-64	17 908	20 398	25 979	32 783
65-69	13 518	16 553	17 470	28 377
70-74	9 089	11 267	12 874	16 516
75+	8 465	12 104	15 871	18 814
All ages	585 199	656 106	699 235	736 646
Females				
0-4	57 946	55 805	47 916	53 756
5-9	44 152	57 794	49 274	50 480
10-14	46 249	56 322	54 804	47 326
15-19	59 405	43 864	57 507	49 059
20-24	61 412	45 823	55 893	54 413
25-29	50 757	58 700	43 431	56 969
30-34	40 380	60 614	45 333	55 338
35-39	41 906	50 015	57 993	42 956
40-44	30 218	39 651	59 701	44 719
45-49	23 083	40 801	48 911	56 852
50-54	21 391	28 944	38 222	57 802
55-59	19 929	21 569	38 467	46 441
60-64	16 619	19 193	26 362	35 221
65-69	13 521	16 690	18 541	33 731
70-74	9 973	12 199	14 615	20 697
75+	11 553	16 351	21 550	27 057
All ages	548 494	624 334	678 518	732 818
Total	1 133 693	1 280 441	1 377 753	1 469 464

Other Asia and Islands

Age group	1990	2000	2010	2020
Males				
0-4	43 763	44 070	43 306	43 720
5-9	43 939	42 363	42 192	42 135
10-14	40 093	40 808	41 907	41 718
15-19	37 037	43 103	41 756	41 712
20-24	33 033	39 469	40 238	41 388
25-29	29 141	36 315	42 309	41 048
30-34	25 268	32 228	38 550	39 370
35-39	20 686	28 268	35 243	41 137
40-44	15 660	24 288	30 980	37 137
45-49	13 168	19 581	26 763	33 418
50-54	11 647	14 477	22 499	28 707
55-59	9 323	11 743	17 515	23 952
60-64	7 768	9 811	12 279	19 144
65-69	5 338	7 172	9 168	13 804
70-74	3 603	5 205	6 721	8 557
75+	3 499	5 541	8 125	11 086
All ages	342 966	404 442	459 549	508 034
Females				
0-4	41 988	42 279	41 483	41 831
5-9	42 061	41 084	40 760	40 597
10-14	38 156	39 694	40 646	40 324
15-19	35 601	41 450	40 662	40 446
20-24	32 762	37 732	39 333	40 332
25-29	29 675	35 132	40 985	40 256
30-34	25 630	32 221	37 203	38 842
35-39	20 361	29 082	34 537	40 371
40-44	15 582	24 988	31 532	36 501
45-49	13 358	19 661	28 243	33 657
50-54	11 913	14 824	23 992	30 439
55-59	9 819	12 446	18 543	26 863
60-64	8 091	10 705	13 563	22 233
65-69	5 920	8 290	10 796	16 411
70-74	4 112	6 128	8 388	10 924
75+	4 539	7 401	11 357	16 294
All ages	339 568	403 117	462 024	516 320
Total	682 534	807 558	921 573	1 024 354

Sub-Saharan Africa

Age group	1990	2000	2010	2020
Males				
0-4	47 484	65 868	77 573	90 247
5-9	38 434	53 067	66 484	79 230
10-14	31 824	40 910	58 916	71 430
15-19	26 555	36 658	51 188	64 589
20-24	22 212	30 123	38 956	56 449
25-29	18 045	24 779	34 336	48 261
30-34	14 858	20 504	27 928	36 401
35-39	12 075	16 542	22 804	31 891
40-44	10 019	13 477	18 667	25 695
45-49	8 210	10 800	14 839	20 674
50-54	6 771	8 792	11 885	16 597
55-59	5 327	6 954	9 229	12 792
60-64	4 111	5 415	7 102	9 690
65-69	2 910	3 889	5 139	6 872
70-74	1 880	2 588	3 466	4 584
75+	1 607	2 511	3 652	5 008
All ages	252 322	342 877	452 164	580 412
Females				
0-4	47 030	63 629	74 761	86 758
5-9	38 146	52 143	65 055	77 145
10-14	31 672	41 292	57 926	69 905
15-19	26 619	36 610	50 683	63 732
20-24	22 465	30 339	39 914	56 478
25-29	18 342	25 288	35 071	49 047
30-34	15 383	21 172	28 876	38 450
35-39	12 721	17 168	23 951	33 680
40-44	10 727	14 274	19 922	27 606
45-49	8 825	11 674	15 957	22 613
50-54	7 377	9 707	13 057	18 427
55-59	5 915	7 791	10 428	14 406
60-64	4 655	6 226	8 332	11 372
65-69	3 468	4 623	6 263	8 565
70-74	2 346	3 162	4 376	5 993
75+	2 261	3 507	4 995	7 000
All ages	257 952	348 604	459 566	591 176
Total	510 274	691 481	911 730	1 171 588

Annex Table 11, continued.   Population by age, sex and region (thousands), 1990-2020, baseline projections

Latin America and the Caribbean

Age group	1990	2000	2010	2020
Males				
0-4	28 721	29 315	27 917	29 071
5-9	27 072	29 601	27 284	28 363
10-14	25 052	27 481	28 353	27 229
15-19	23 583	26 675	29 236	26 999
20-24	21 382	24 546	26 948	27 870
25-29	19 126	22 970	25 967	28 542
30-34	15 956	20 736	23 790	26 209
35-39	13 432	18 460	22 177	25 172
40-44	10 807	15 271	19 867	22 910
45-49	8 801	12 701	17 468	21 100
50-54	7 360	10 036	14 212	18 571
55-59	6 088	7 937	11 508	15 913
60-64	5 016	6 360	8 727	12 456
65-69	3 773	4 935	6 493	9 517
70-74	2 580	3 668	4 718	6 584
75+	2 862	4 766	6 874	9 557
All ages	221 611	265 455	301 539	336 063
Females				
0-4	27 676	28 094	26 712	27 780
5-9	26 295	28 602	26 275	27 235
10-14	24 449	26 740	27 388	26 216
15-19	23 100	26 042	28 391	26 117
20-24	21 040	24 173	26 495	27 176
25-29	19 078	22 759	25 737	28 108
30-34	16 105	20 686	23 835	26 183
35-39	13 687	18 699	22 400	25 379
40-44	11 075	15 708	20 263	23 422
45-49	9 091	13 219	18 152	21 831
50-54	7 723	10 534	15 024	19 465
55-59	6 541	8 472	12 403	17 123
60-64	5 526	6 992	9 634	13 858
65-69	4 327	5 665	7 454	11 064
70-74	3 109	4 418	5 705	8 014
75+	3 862	6 486	9 577	13 450
All ages	222 684	267 306	305 445	342 421
Total	444 295	532 761	606 983	678 484

Middle Eastern Crescent

Age group	1990	2000	2010	2020
Males				
0-4	41 161	49 821	55 273	61 521
5-9	35 057	45 221	49 941	56 988
10-14	30 288	38 191	47 035	52 910
15-19	26 617	34 413	44 573	49 354
20-24	23 464	29 757	37 611	46 391
25-29	20 120	26 029	33 732	43 759
30-34	17 880	22 863	29 067	36 799
35-39	14 789	19 549	25 345	32 888
40-44	11 025	17 236	22 092	28 122
45-49	8 339	14 027	18 585	24 110
50-54	7 437	10 213	15 990	20 467
55-59	6 561	7 455	12 554	16 582
60-64	5 205	6 293	8 663	13 519
65-69	3 749	5 102	5 824	9 780
70-74	2 278	3 499	4 257	5 845
75+	2 419	3 756	5 393	6 550
All ages	256 389	333 426	415 934	505 587
Females				
0-4	39 734	47 538	52 777	58 753
5-9	33 510	43 224	47 833	54 621
10-14	28 489	36 961	45 067	50 764
15-19	25 044	32 963	42 719	47 411
20-24	21 986	28 074	36 556	44 664
25-29	19 091	24 604	32 522	42 246
30-34	16 688	21 553	27 652	36 101
35-39	13 887	18 684	24 200	32 076
40-44	10 515	16 270	21 137	27 202
45-49	8 191	13 416	18 179	23 641
50-54	7 477	10 012	15 611	20 384
55-59	6 624	7 629	12 616	17 210
60-64	5 502	6 720	9 131	14 391
65-69	4 083	5 609	6 612	11 127
70-74	2 681	4 120	5 169	7 173
75+	3 184	4 954	7 362	9 515
All ages	246 686	322 330	405 144	497 279
Total	503 075	655 756	821 078	1 002 865

World

Age group	1990	2000	2010	2020
Males				
0-4	321 304	345 955	351 328	374 321
5-9	286 793	327 500	332 829	352 163
10-14	264 412	300 847	328 521	337 372
15-19	264 165	281 481	322 608	328 497
20-24	249 942	259 237	295 332	322 732
25-29	221 788	258 019	274 684	315 139
30-34	194 422	243 275	252 022	287 558
35-39	176 010	214 887	249 872	266 066
40-44	143 614	186 858	233 830	242 288
45-49	115 511	166 869	203 499	236 632
50-54	104 153	132 875	172 484	215 569
55-59	92 721	102 929	148 202	180 307
60-64	77 445	87 618	111 681	144 442
65-69	59 371	71 466	79 669	114 419
70-74	38 454	52 552	59 980	77 389
75+	43 587	63 761	85 951	106 281
All ages	2 653 692	3 096 132	3 502 491	3 901 177
Females				
0-4	309 253	330 724	335 868	357 769
5-9	273 992	314 233	319 556	338 111
10-14	251 551	290 681	315 716	324 329
15-19	251 330	269 507	310 451	316 464
20-24	238 509	247 610	286 880	312 120
25-29	212 831	246 897	265 198	306 080
30-34	186 865	233 918	243 273	282 475
35-39	169 694	208 340	242 294	260 662
40-44	139 413	182 232	228 884	238 466
45-49	113 192	164 223	202 400	235 991
50-54	103 574	133 001	174 717	220 237
55-59	94 301	105 598	154 425	191 306
60-64	81 818	93 376	121 475	160 904
65-69	69 057	80 534	91 913	136 573
70-74	48 409	63 577	74 024	98 580
75+	49 931	99 556	130 785	163 166
All ages	2 613 720	3 064 007	3 497 857	3 943 234
Total	5 267 412	6 160 139	7 000 348	7 844 411

Annex Table 12a. Deaths by age, sex and cause (thousands): Established Market Economies, 2000, baseline scenario

Cause	Total	Male	Female	Males							Females						
				0-4	5-14	15-29	30-44	45-59	60-69	70+	0-4	5-14	15-29	30-44	45-59	60-69	70+
Population (millions)	*839*	*411*	*428*	*29*	*54*	*82*	*94*	*79*	*36*	*36*	*27*	*52*	*78*	*92*	*81*	*41*	*57*
All causes	7 932	4 147	3 784	48	12	104	210	565	727	2 482	37	8	34	88	254	382	2 982
I. Communicable, maternal, perinatal and nutritional conditions	*532*	*300*	*232*	*24*	*1*	*15*	*52*	*29*	*18*	*160*	*17*	*1*	*4*	*8*	*6*	*10*	*186*
A. Infectious and parasitic diseases	173	125	48	2	–	15	51	25	8	25	2	–	3	7	4	4	28
1. Tuberculosis	14	10	4	–	–	–	–	–	–	6	–	–	–	–	–	–	3
2. STDs excluding HIV	1	–	–	–	–	–	–	–	–	–	–	–	–	–	–	–	–
a. Syphilis																	
b. Chlamydia																	
c. Gonorrhoea																	
3. HIV	105	91	14	1	–	14	49	22	3	1	1	–	3	7	2	1	1
4. Diarrhoeal diseases	3	1	2	–	–	–	–	–	–	1	–	–	–	–	–	–	1
5. Childhood-cluster diseases	1	–	–	–	–	–	–	–	–	–	–	–	–	–	–	–	–
a. Pertussis																	
b. Poliomyelitis																	
c. Diphtheria																	
d. Measles																	
e. Tetanus																	
6. Bacterial meningitis*	4	2	2	1	–	–	–	–	–	1	1	–	–	–	–	–	1
7. Hepatitis B and hepatitis C	3	2	1	–	–	–	–	–	–	1	–	–	–	–	–	–	1
8. Malaria																	
9. Tropical-cluster diseases																	
a. Trypanosomiasis																	
b. Chagas disease																	
c. Schistosomiasis																	
d. Leishmaniasis																	
10. Leprosy																	
11. Dengue																	
12. Japanese encephalitis																	
13. Trachoma																	
14. Intestinal nematode infections																	
a. Ascariasis																	
b. Trichuriasis																	
c. Ancylostomiasis, necatoriasis																	
15. Other infectious and parasitic	44	19	24	–	–	–	1	1	2	15	–	–	–	–	1	2	21

Annex Table 12a, continued. Deaths by age, sex and cause (thousands): Established Market Economies, 2000, baseline scenario

Cause	Total	Male	Female	Males							Females						
				0-4	5-14	15-29	30-44	45-59	60-69	70+	0-4	5-14	15-29	30-44	45-59	60-69	70+
B. Respiratory infections	302	146	156	1	-	-	1	4	10	128	1	-	-	1	2	5	147
1. Lower respiratory infections	299	145	154	1	-	-	1	4	10	127	1	-	-	1	2	5	145
2. Upper respiratory infections	3	1	2	-	-	-	-	-	-	1	-	-	-	-	-	-	2
3. Otitis media	-	-	-	-	-	-	-	-	-	-	-	-	-	-	-	-	-
C. Maternal conditions	-	-	-	-	-	-	-	-	-	-	-	-	-	-	-	-	-
1. Maternal haemorrhage	-	-	-	-	-	-	-	-	-	-	-	-	-	-	-	-	-
2. Maternal sepsis	-	-	-	-	-	-	-	-	-	-	-	-	-	-	-	-	-
3. Hypertensive disorders*	-	-	-	-	-	-	-	-	-	-	-	-	-	-	-	-	-
4. Obstructed labour	-	-	-	-	-	-	-	-	-	-	-	-	-	-	-	-	-
5. Abortion	-	-	-	-	-	-	-	-	-	-	-	-	-	-	-	-	-
6. Other maternal	-	-	-	-	-	-	-	-	-	-	-	-	-	-	-	-	-
D. Perinatal conditions*	34	20	14	20	-	-	-	-	-	-	14	-	-	-	-	-	-
E. Nutritional deficiencies	22	9	13	-	-	-	-	-	1	7	-	-	-	-	-	1	12
1. Protein-energy malnutrition	6	2	4	-	-	-	-	-	-	2	-	-	-	-	-	-	4
2. Iodine deficiency	-	-	-	-	-	-	-	-	-	-	-	-	-	-	-	-	-
3. Vitamin A deficiency	-	-	-	-	-	-	-	-	-	-	-	-	-	-	-	-	-
4. Iron-deficiency anaemia	14	6	8	-	-	-	-	-	1	5	-	-	-	-	-	1	7
II. Noncommunicable diseases	6 942	3 547	3 395	19	5	20	94	479	679	2 250	16	4	11	59	226	357	2 722
A. Malignant neoplasms	1 973	1 111	862	1	2	6	32	201	272	596	1	1	4	33	131	167	524
1. Mouth and oropharynx cancers	37	28	9	-	-	-	2	10	8	9	-	-	-	-	2	2	5
2. Oesophagus cancer	47	36	11	-	-	-	1	9	10	15	-	-	-	1	1	2	7
3. Stomach cancer	158	96	63	-	-	-	2	16	22	55	-	-	-	2	7	9	44
4. Colon and rectum cancers	234	119	116	-	-	-	3	18	27	71	-	-	-	2	12	18	83
5. Liver cancer	41	30	11	-	-	-	1	8	10	11	-	-	-	-	1	3	7
6. Pancreas cancer	95	49	46	-	-	-	1	9	13	26	-	-	-	1	5	8	32
7. Trachea, bronchus, lung cancers	439	315	125	-	-	-	8	68	93	145	-	-	-	3	22	33	67
8. Melanoma and other skin cancers	24	14	10	-	-	-	2	3	3	6	-	-	-	1	2	2	6
9. Breast cancer	142	-	142	-	-	-	-	-	-	-	-	-	-	11	35	29	67
10. Cervix uteri cancer	16	-	16	-	-	-	-	-	-	-	-	-	-	2	4	3	6
11. Corpus uteri cancer	26	-	26	-	-	-	-	-	-	-	-	-	-	1	3	5	16
12. Ovary cancer	43	-	43	-	-	-	-	-	-	-	-	-	-	2	9	10	22
13. Prostate cancer	109	109	-	-	-	-	-	3	15	91	-	-	-	-	-	-	-
14. Bladder cancer	54	39	15	-	-	-	-	3	7	28	-	-	-	-	1	2	12
15. Lymphomas, multiple myeloma	87	47	40	-	-	1	3	8	10	24	-	-	1	1	5	7	26
16. Leukaemia	62	35	28	1	1	2	2	5	7	18	1	1	1	2	3	4	17
17. Other cancers	356	195	161	-	1	3	8	39	47	96	-	-	2	5	19	28	106

Annex Table 12a, continued. Deaths by age, sex and cause (thousands): Established Market Economies, 2000, baseline scenario

Cause	Total	Male	Female	Males 0-4	5-14	15-29	30-44	45-59	60-69	70+	Females 0-4	5-14	15-29	30-44	45-59	60-69	70+
B. Other neoplasms	39	19	20	-	-	-	1	3	3	11	-	-	-	1	2	2	15
C. Diabetes mellitus	164	63	102	-	-	-	2	7	11	42	-	-	-	1	5	11	84
D. Endocrine disorders	51	22	29	1	-	1	1	2	4	13	1	-	-	1	2	3	22
E. Neuro-psychiatric conditions	230	104	126	1	1	4	8	12	12	65	1	1	1	3	6	8	107
2. Bipolar disorder	1	-	-														
3. Schizophrenia	15	6	9			1		1	1	4							8
4. Epilepsy	7	4	3			1		1		1					1		1
5. Alcohol use	15	12	3				2	5	2	2					1		1
6. Dementia*	111	40	70				1	2	4	32	1				4	4	64
7. Parkinson disease	35	18	18						1	16						1	17
8. Multiple sclerosis	5	2	3					1	1	1					1	1	1
9. Drug use	3	3	1			2							1				
13. Other neuro-psychiatric	38	19	19	1	1	2	2	2	2	9	1	1	1	1	1	1	14
F. Sense organ diseases	-	-	-														
1. Glaucoma	-	-	-														
2. Cataracts	-	-	-														
G. Cardiovascular diseases	3 489	1 688	1 801	2	1	5	33	188	290	1 170	1	-	2	12	50	118	1 617
1. Rheumatic heart disease	21	7	14					1	2	3					1	2	10
2. Ischaemic heart disease	1 838	940	898			1	17	118	177	627				4	25	65	804
3. Cerebrovascular disease	870	368	502			1	6	29	47	284			1	4	14	27	457
4. Inflammatory heart diseases	70	37	33	1	0	1	3	8	5	20	1	0	1	1	2	2	27
5. Other cardiovascular	690	337	353			2	7	32	60	235				2	8	22	319
H. Respiratory diseases	409	243	165	1	-	1	3	14	37	188	-	-	1	2	10	21	132
1. COPD*	292	183	109				1	9	28	146				1	6	15	87
2. Asthma	26	12	14				1	2	2	7				1	2	2	9
3. Other respiratory	91	48	42			1	1	4	7	35				1	2	4	35
I. Digestive diseases	361	199	162	-	-	1	12	45	40	100	-	-	1	5	16	19	121
1. Peptic ulcer	38	20	18					2	3	14					1	1	16
2. Cirrhosis of the liver	134	91	43				9	33	23	26				3	11	9	19
3. Appendicitis	2	1	1							1							
4. Other digestive	187	86	101		1		3	10	13	59				2	5	8	86
J. Genito-urinary diseases	142	66	76	-	-	-	1	4	7	53	-	-	-	1	3	5	67
1. Nephritis and nephrosis	92	44	49				1	3	5	34				1	2	4	42
2. Benign prostatic hypertrophy	4	4	-							4							
3. Other genito-urinary	45	18	28					1	2	15					1	2	25
K. Skin diseases	14	4	10							4							9

Annex Table 12a, continued. Deaths by age, sex and cause (thousands): Established Market Economies, 2000, baseline scenario

Cause	Total	Male	Female	Males							Females						
				0-4	5-14	15-29	30-44	45-59	60-69	70+	0-4	5-14	15-29	30-44	45-59	60-69	70+
L. Musculo-skeletal diseases	36	10	26	-	-	-	-	1	1	7	-	-	-	1	2	2	21
1. Rheumatoid arthritis	10	2	8	-	-	-	-	-	-	2	-	-	-	-	1	1	6
3. Other musculo-skeletal	26	7	18	-	-	-	-	1	1	5	-	-	-	1	1	1	15
M. Congenital anomalies	33	18	15	13	1	1	1	1	-	1	11	1	1	-	-	-	2
N. Oral conditions	-	-	-	-	-	-	-	-	-	-	-	-	-	-	-	-	-
III. Injuries	*458*	*301*	*157*	*5*	*6*	*69*	*64*	*56*	*29*	*71*	*4*	*3*	*18*	*21*	*22*	*15*	*74*
A. Unintentional injuries	304	189	115	5	5	45	34	31	18	52	3	3	12	11	12	10	64
1. Road traffic accidents	126	86	40	2	3	34	17	13	6	12	1	2	10	7	6	4	9
2. Poisonings	12	8	4	-	-	2	3	2	1	1	-	-	-	1	1	-	1
3. Falls	77	35	43	-	-	1	3	5	4	22	-	-	-	1	1	2	38
4. Fires	10	6	4	-	-	1	1	1	1	2	1	-	-	-	1	-	2
5. Drownings	12	9	3	1	1	2	2	2	-	2	-	-	-	-	-	-	1
6. Other unintentional	66	45	21	2	1	6	8	8	6	14	1	-	1	2	2	2	12
B. Intentional injuries	154	111	42	1	1	24	30	26	12	19	1	-	6	9	10	5	11
1. Self-inflicted injuries	123	89	35	-	-	15	22	22	11	18	-	-	4	7	9	5	10
2. Violence	31	23	8	1	-	9	8	4	1	1	1	-	2	2	1	-	1
3. War	-	-	-	-	-	-	-	-	-	-	-	-	-	-	-	-	-

Notes:

Causes responsible for no deaths have been omitted from this table.

A dash (-) symbol indicates fewer than 500 deaths.

*IA6 is Bacterial meningitis and meningococcaemia; IC3 is Hypertensive disorders of pregnancy; ID is Conditions arising during the perinatal period; IIE6 is Dementia and other degenerative and hereditary CNS disorders; IIH1 is Chronic obstructive pulmonary disease.

Annex Table 12b. Deaths by age, sex and cause (thousands): Formerly Socialist Economies of Europe, 2000, baseline scenario

Cause	Total	Male	Female	Males							Females						
				0-4	5-14	15-29	30-44	45-59	60-69	70+	0-4	5-14	15-29	30-44	45-59	60-69	70+
Population (millions)	*358*	*171*	*187*	*13*	*26*	*39*	*36*	*31*	*14*	*11*	*12*	*25*	*38*	*36*	*34*	*19*	*22*
All causes	*4 687*	*2 476*	*2 211*	*51*	*14*	*87*	*157*	*538*	*469*	*1 160*	*38*	*8*	*27*	*50*	*189*	*271*	*1 629*
I. Communicable, maternal, perinatal and nutritional conditions	*205*	*103*	*101*	*28*	*1*	*2*	*5*	*11*	*8*	*49*	*19*	*1*	*2*	*2*	*3*	*5*	*71*
A. Infectious and parasitic diseases	**47**	**28**	**19**	**5**	–	**1**	**4**	**7**	**4**	**8**	**4**	–	–	**1**	**1**	**2**	**10**
1. Tuberculosis	18	15	3	–	–	1	3	6	3	3	–	–	–	–	1	1	2
2. STDs excluding HIV	–	–	–	–	–	–	–	–	–	–	–	–	–	–	–	–	–
a. Syphilis	–	–	–	–	–	–	–	–	–	–	–	–	–	–	–	–	–
b. Chlamydia	–	–	–	–	–	–	–	–	–	–	–	–	–	–	–	–	–
c. Gonorrhoea	–	–	–	–	–	–	–	–	–	–	–	–	–	–	–	–	–
3. HIV	4	2	2	1	–	–	–	–	–	–	1	–	–	–	–	–	–
4. Diarrhoeal diseases	3	2	1	1	–	–	–	–	–	–	1	–	–	–	–	–	–
5. Childhood-cluster diseases	–	–	–	–	–	–	–	–	–	–	–	–	–	–	–	–	–
a. Pertussis	–	–	–	–	–	–	–	–	–	–	–	–	–	–	–	–	–
b. Poliomyelitis	–	–	–	–	–	–	–	–	–	–	–	–	–	–	–	–	–
c. Diphtheria	–	–	–	–	–	–	–	–	–	–	–	–	–	–	–	–	–
d. Measles	–	–	–	–	–	–	–	–	–	–	–	–	–	–	–	–	–
e. Tetanus	–	–	–	–	–	–	–	–	–	–	–	–	–	–	–	–	–
6. Bacterial meningitis*	5	3	2	1	–	–	–	–	–	1	1	–	–	–	–	–	1
7. Hepatitis B and hepatitis C	1	1	1	–	–	–	–	–	–	–	–	–	–	–	–	–	–
8. Malaria	–	–	–	–	–	–	–	–	–	–	–	–	–	–	–	–	–
9. Tropical-cluster diseases	–	–	–	–	–	–	–	–	–	–	–	–	–	–	–	–	–
a. Trypanosomiasis	–	–	–	–	–	–	–	–	–	–	–	–	–	–	–	–	–
b. Chagas disease	–	–	–	–	–	–	–	–	–	–	–	–	–	–	–	–	–
c. Schistosomiasis	–	–	–	–	–	–	–	–	–	–	–	–	–	–	–	–	–
d. Leishmaniasis	–	–	–	–	–	–	–	–	–	–	–	–	–	–	–	–	–
10. Leprosy	–	–	–	–	–	–	–	–	–	–	–	–	–	–	–	–	–
11. Dengue	–	–	–	–	–	–	–	–	–	–	–	–	–	–	–	–	–
12. Japanese encephalitis	–	–	–	–	–	–	–	–	–	–	–	–	–	–	–	–	–
13. Trachoma	–	–	–	–	–	–	–	–	–	–	–	–	–	–	–	–	–
14. Intestinal nematode infections	–	–	–	–	–	–	–	–	–	–	–	–	–	–	–	–	–
a. Ascariasis	–	–	–	–	–	–	–	–	–	–	–	–	–	–	–	–	–
b. Trichuriasis	–	–	–	–	–	–	–	–	–	–	–	–	–	–	–	–	–
c. Ancylostomiasis, necatoriasis	–	–	–	–	–	–	–	–	–	–	–	–	–	–	–	–	–
15. Other infectious and parasitic	15	6	9	1	–	–	–	–	1	3	1	–	–	–	–	1	7

Annex Table 12b, continued. Deaths by age, sex and cause (thousands): Formerly Socialist Economies of Europe, 2000, baseline scenario

Cause	Total	Male	Female	Males							Females						
				0-4	5-14	15-29	30-44	45-59	60-69	70+	0-4	5-14	15-29	30-44	45-59	60-69	70+
B. Respiratory infections	**121**	**56**	**65**	**7**	-	-	**1**	**4**	**4**	**39**	**5**	-	-	-	-	**1**	**2**	**55**
1. Lower respiratory infections	121	56	65	7	-	-	1	4	4	39	5	-	-	-	-	1	2	55
2. Upper respiratory infections	1	-	-	-	-	-	-	-	-	-	-	-	-	-	-	-	-
3. Otitis media	-	-	-	-	-	-	-	-	-	-	-	-	-	-	-	-	-
C. Maternal conditions	**1**		**1**			-	-	-	-	-	-		-	**1**	**1**	-	-	-
1. Maternal haemorrhage	-		-			-	-	-	-	-	-		-	-	1	-	-	-
2. Maternal sepsis	-		-			-	-	1	-	-	-		-	1	-	-	-	-
3. Hypertensive disorders*	-		-			-	-	-	-	-	-		-	-	-	-	-	-
4. Obstructed labour	-		-			-	-	-	-	-	-		-	-	-	-	-	-
5. Abortion	-		-			-	-	-	-	-	-		-	-	-	-	-	-
6. Other maternal	1		1			-	-	-	-	-	-		-	-	-	-	-	-
D. Perinatal conditions*	**25**	**15**	**10**	**15**	-	-	-	-	-	-	**10**	-	-	-	-	-	-	-
E. Nutritional deficiencies.	**10**	**3**	**6**		-	-	-	-	-	**2**		-	-	-	-	-	-	**5**
1. Protein-energy malnutrition	2	1	2		-	-	-	-	-	1		-	-	-	-	-	-	1
2. Iodine deficiency	-	-	-		-	-	-	-	-	-		-	-	-	-	-	-	-
3. Vitamin A deficiency	-	-	-		-	-	-	-	-	-		-	-	-	-	-	-	-
4. Iron-deficiency anaemia	5	2	3		-	-	-	-	-	1		-	-	-	-	-	-	3
II. Noncommunicable diseases	**4 062**	**2 064**	**1 999**	**15**	**4**	**16**	**72**	**443**	**435**	**1 078**	**12**	**3**	**9**	**32**	**165**	**254**	**1 523**
A. Malignant neoplasms	**814**	**505**	**309**	**1**	**2**	**5**	**21**	**164**	**140**	**172**	**1**	**1**	**4**	**16**	**67**	**74**	**145**
1. Mouth and oropharynx cancers	22	19	3	-	-	-	1	9	4	4	-	-	-	-	1	1	2
2. Oesophagus cancer	13	11	2	-	-	-	-	5	3	3	-	-	-	-	-	-	2
3. Stomach cancer	126	80	47	-	-	-	3	26	21	29	-	-	-	2	8	11	26
4. Colon and rectum cancers	85	44	41	-	-	-	-	10	11	21	-	-	-	1	7	9	23
5. Liver cancer	25	15	11	-	-	-	1	4	5	5	-	-	-	-	2	3	6
6. Pancreas cancer	36	21	14	-	-	-	1	7	6	7	-	-	-	-	2	4	8
7. Trachea, bronchus, lung cancers	198	167	31	-	-	-	6	62	54	45	-	-	-	1	7	9	14
8. Melanoma and other skin cancers	10	5	5	-	-	-	1	2	1	2	-	-	-	-	1	1	3
9. Breast cancer	42	-	42	-	-	-	-	-	-	-	-	-	-	4	14	10	13
10. Cervix uteri cancer	16	-	16	-	-	-	-	-	-	-	-	-	-	2	4	4	6
11. Corpus uteri cancer	14	-	14	-	-	-	-	-	-	-	-	-	-	-	3	4	6
12. Ovary cancer	16	-	16	-	-	-	-	-	-	-	-	-	-	1	5	4	5
13. Prostate cancer	22	22	-	-	-	-	-	2	4	16	-	-	-	-	-	-	-
14. Bladder cancer	21	17	4	-	-	-	-	3	5	8	-	-	-	-	-	-	3
15. Lymphomas, multiple myeloma	19	12	7	-	-	-	2	4	3	3	-	-	1	1	2	-	3
16. Leukaemia	22	13	9	-	1	1	1	3	3	4	-	-	1	1	2	2	3
17. Other cancers	125	79	46	1	1	2	5	26	20	25	1	1	1	2	9	10	22

Annex Table 12b, continued. Deaths by age, sex and cause (thousands): Formerly Socialist Economies of Europe, 2000, baseline scenario

Cause	Total	Male	Female	Males							Females						
				0-4	5-14	15-29	30-44	45-59	60-69	70+	0-4	5-14	15-29	30-44	45-59	60-69	70+
B. Other neoplasms	7	4	4	–	–	–	–	–	–	1	–	–	–	–	1	1	1
C. Diabetes mellitus	32	12	20	–	–	–	1	2	3	6	–	–	–	–	2	5	12
D. Endocrine disorders	4	2	2	–	–	–	1	–	–	–	–	–	–	–	–	–	1
E. Neuro-psychiatric conditions	76	35	41	1	1	2	3	6	5	16	1	1	1	2	3	4	30
2. Bipolar disorder	7	2	6	–	–	–	–	–	–	1	–	–	–	1	–	–	5
3. Schizophrenia	5	2	2	–	–	–	–	1	–	1	–	–	–	–	–	–	2
4. Epilepsy	6	4	2	–	–	1	1	1	–	1	–	–	–	–	–	–	1
5. Alcohol use	8	7	1	–	–	–	1	3	1	2	–	–	–	–	–	–	–
6. Dementia*	21	7	14	–	–	–	–	–	1	5	–	–	–	–	–	1	13
7. Parkinson disease	9	4	5	–	–	–	–	–	–	3	–	–	–	–	–	–	5
8. Multiple sclerosis	4	2	3	–	–	–	–	–	–	1	–	–	–	1	1	1	1
9. Drug use	–	–	–	–	–	–	–	–	–	–	–	–	–	–	–	–	–
13. Other neuro-psychiatric	16	9	7	1	1	1	1	1	1	3	1	1	1	–	–	1	4
F. Sense organ diseases	–	–	–	–	–	–	–	–	–	–	–	–	–	–	–	–	–
1. Glaucoma	–	–	–	–	–	–	–	–	–	–	–	–	–	–	–	–	–
2. Cataracts	–	–	–	–	–	–	–	–	–	–	–	–	–	–	–	–	–
G. Cardiovascular diseases	2 640	1 208	1 432	1	–	5	35	208	226	733	1	–	2	9	68	139	1 213
1. Rheumatic heart disease	26	12	14	–	–	–	2	6	2	1	–	–	–	1	6	4	3
2. Ischaemic heart disease	1 315	636	678	–	–	1	20	127	119	369	–	–	–	4	30	64	581
3. Cerebrovascular disease	809	329	480	–	–	1	6	46	64	212	–	–	–	3	25	51	400
4. Inflammatory heart diseases	48	25	23	–	–	1	2	6	3	12	–	–	–	1	2	2	18
5. Other cardiovascular	442	205	236	0	0	1	5	23	37	139	–	0	1	1	5	18	211
H. Respiratory diseases	269	169	100	–	–	1	2	27	35	104	–	–	–	1	7	13	78
1. COPD*	138	86	51	–	–	–	1	13	18	55	–	–	–	–	3	6	42
2. Asthma	12	5	7	–	–	–	–	1	1	3	–	–	–	–	1	1	4
3. Other respiratory	119	77	42	–	–	–	1	13	16	46	–	–	–	–	3	6	32
I. Digestive diseases	143	85	57	1	–	1	7	28	20	29	–	–	1	2	10	12	31
1. Peptic ulcer	18	12	5	–	–	–	1	4	3	5	–	–	–	–	1	1	3
2. Cirrhosis of the liver	60	39	21	–	–	–	3	15	10	10	–	–	–	1	6	5	8
3. Appendicitis	1	1	–	1	–	–	–	–	–	–	–	–	–	–	–	–	–
4. Other digestive	64	33	31	1	–	1	3	8	6	14	–	–	1	1	4	5	20
J. Genito-urinary diseases	49	29	19	–	–	1	2	5	5	17	–	–	1	1	4	4	9
1. Nephritis and nephrosis	20	11	9	–	–	1	1	3	2	4	–	–	–	1	2	2	4
2. Benign prostatic hypertrophy	8	8	–	–	–	–	–	1	1	7	–	–	–	–	–	–	–
3. Other genito-urinary	20	9	11	–	–	–	–	2	2	5	–	–	–	–	2	2	5
K. Skin diseases	2	1	1	–	–	–	–	–	–	–	–	–	–	–	–	–	–

Annex Table 12b, continued. Deaths by age, sex and cause (thousands): Formerly Socialist Economies of Europe, 2000, baseline scenario

Cause	Total	Male	Female	Males							Females						
				0-4	5-14	15-29	30-44	45-59	60-69	70+	0-4	5-14	15-29	30-44	45-59	60-69	70+
L. Musculo-skeletal diseases	5	2	3	-	-	-	-	-	-	1	-	-	-	-	1	1	1
1. Rheumatoid arthritis	1	-	1	-	-	-	-	-	-	-	-	-	-	-	-	1	1
3. Other musculo-skeletal	4	1	3	-	-	-	-	-	-	1	-	-	-	-	1	1	1
M. Congenital anomalies	22	13	10	11	1	1	-	-	-	-	8	1	-	-	-	-	-
N. Oral conditions	-	-	-	-	-	-	-	-	-	-	-	-	-	-	-	-	-
III. Injuries	*420*	*309*	*111*	*8*	*9*	*70*	*79*	*84*	*25*	*33*	*6*	*4*	*17*	*16*	*21*	*12*	*35*
A. Unintentional injuries	271	201	70	5	7	43	50	57	17	22	3	3	8	8	13	8	27
1. Road traffic accidents	99	76	23	1	3	24	19	17	6	6	1	1	4	3	5	3	6
2. Poisonings	48	36	11	1	-	3	11	16	4	2	1	-	1	2	4	2	2
3. Falls	35	19	16	-	-	2	3	4	2	7	-	-	-	-	1	2	13
4. Fires	9	6	3	-	-	1	1	2	1	1	-	1	1	-	-	-	1
5. Drownings	24	20	4	1	2	5	5	4	1	1	1	1	1	-	-	-	1
6. Other unintentional	57	44	13	2	1	8	11	13	4	4	1	-	1	2	3	2	4
B. Intentional injuries	149	107	42	3	2	26	29	27	9	11	3	1	9	7	8	5	8
1. Self-inflicted injuries	88	68	21	-	-	12	18	21	7	10	-	-	2	3	5	3	7
2. Violence	31	23	8	-	-	7	8	5	1	1	-	-	2	2	2	1	1
3. War	29	17	12	3	2	8	3	1	-	-	3	1	5	2	1	-	-

Notes:
Causes responsible for no deaths have been omitted from this table.
A dash (-) symbol indicates fewer than 500 deaths.
"IA6 is Bacterial meningitis and meningococcaemia; IC3 is Hypertensive disorders of pregnancy; ID is Conditions arising during the perinatal period; IIE6 is Dementia and other degenerative and hereditary CNS disorders; IIH1 is Chronic obstructive pulmonary disease.

Annex Table 12c. Deaths by age, sex and cause (thousands): India, 2000, baseline scenario

Cause	Total	Male	Female	Males							Females						
				0-4	5-14	15-29	30-44	45-59	60-69	70+	0-4	5-14	15-29	30-44	45-59	60-69	70+
Population (millions)	*995*	*512*	*483*	*57*	*111*	*144*	*104*	*60*	*23*	*14*	*54*	*104*	*134*	*96*	*57*	*24*	*15*
All causes	9 476	5 141	4 334	1 060	184	290	467	877	885	1 379	1 039	190	284	278	544	631	1 367
I. Communicable, maternal, perinatal and nutritional conditions	3 669	1 984	1 685	874	74	119	210	237	167	303	875	93	121	132	140	95	230
A. Infectious and parasitic diseases	2 341	1 350	991	435	54	112	199	224	125	200	430	59	89	100	125	62	127
1. Tuberculosis	948	630	319	14	10	62	114	190	96	144	10	8	44	48	104	38	67
2. STDs excluding HIV	42	19	24	13	–	–	–	1	1	4	13	–	2	2	1	1	5
a. Syphilis	39	19	20	13	–	–	–	1	1	4	13	–	1	1	–	–	5
b. Chlamydia	3	–	3	–	–	–	–	–	–	–	–	–	1	1	–	–	–
c. Gonorrhoea	1	1		–	–	–	–	–	–	–	–	–	–	–	–	–	–
3. HIV	267	156	111	27	5	36	63	17	6	3	28	5	31	38	7	2	1
4. Diarrhoeal diseases	553	272	281	211	11	4	6	5	10	25	215	15	4	4	5	10	28
5. Childhood-cluster diseases	292	150	143	125	12	3	4	2	1	2	118	14	3	3	2	1	2
a. Pertussis	46	23	22	22	2	–	–	–	–	–	21	2	–	–	–	–	–
b. Poliomyelitis	6	4	3	4	–	–	–	–	–	–	3	–	–	–	–	–	–
c. Diphtheria	3	1	1	1	–	–	–	–	–	–	1	–	–	–	–	–	–
d. Measles	117	60	57	53	7	–	–	–	–	–	50	7	3	3	–	–	–
e. Tetanus	121	61	59	45	4	3	4	2	1	2	43	5	3	3	2	1	2
6. Bacterial meningitis*	26	14	12	7	–	1	2	1	1	1	7	–	–	1	1	1	1
7. Hepatitis B and hepatitis C	11	6	5	1	–	–	1	1	1	2	1	–	1	–	1	–	2
8. Malaria	14	8	6	2	2	1	2	1	–	1	2	2	1	1	1	–	1
9. Tropical-cluster diseases	17	11	6	1	4	3	2	–	–	–	1	3	2	1	–	–	–
a. Trypanosomiasis				–	–	–	–	–	–	–	–	–	–	–	–	–	–
b. Chagas disease				–	–	–	–	–	–	–	–	–	–	–	–	–	–
c. Schistosomiasis				–	–	–	–	–	–	–	–	–	–	–	–	–	–
d. Leishmaniasis	17	11	6	1	4	3	2	–	–	–	1	3	2	1	–	–	–
10. Leprosy	1			–	–	–	–	–	–	–	–	–	–	–	–	–	–
11. Dengue	6	3	3	1	2	–	–	–	–	–	1	2	–	–	–	–	–
12. Japanese encephalitis	1			–	–	–	–	–	–	–	–	–	–	–	–	–	–
13. Trachoma	–			–	–	–	–	–	–	–	–	–	–	–	–	–	–
14. Intestinal nematode infections	2	1	1	–	–	–	–	–	–	–	–	–	–	–	–	–	–
a. Ascariasis	1	1		–	–	–	–	–	–	–	–	–	–	–	–	–	–
b. Trichuriasis				–	–	–	–	–	–	–	–	–	–	–	–	–	–
c. Ancylostomiasis, necatoriasis	1			–	–	–	–	–	–	–	–	–	–	–	–	–	–
15. Other infectious and parasitic	160	80	79	34	7	3	5	5	8	18	35	9	2	2	4	8	21

Annex Table 12c, continued. Deaths by age, sex and cause (thousands): India, 2000, baseline scenario

Cause	Total	Male	Female	Males							Females						
				0-4	5-14	15-29	30-44	45-59	60-69	70+	0-4	5-14	15-29	30-44	45-59	60-69	70+
B. Respiratory infections	806	402	405	221	17	5	9	11	41	97	226	30	5	5	11	31	96
1. Lower respiratory infections	791	394	397	216	17	5	9	11	41	96	220	30	5	5	11	31	95
2. Upper respiratory infections	8	4	4	2	–	–	–	–	–	1	2	–	–	–	–	–	1
3. Otitis media	7	3	4	3	–	–	–	–	–	–	3	–	–	–	–	–	1
C. Maternal conditions	53	–	53	–	–	–	–	–	–	–	–	–	25	25	2	–	–
1. Maternal haemorrhage	13	–	13	–	–	–	–	–	–	–	–	–	6	6	1	–	–
2. Maternal sepsis	8	–	8	–	–	–	–	–	–	–	–	–	4	4	–	–	–
3. Hypertensive disorders*	4	–	4	–	–	–	–	–	–	–	–	–	2	2	–	–	–
4. Obstructed labour	2	–	2	–	–	–	–	–	–	–	–	–	1	1	–	–	–
5. Abortion	4	–	4	–	–	–	–	–	–	–	–	–	2	2	–	–	–
6. Other maternal	8	–	8	–	–	–	–	–	–	–	–	–	4	4	–	–	–
D. Perinatal conditions*	394	198	196	198	–	–	–	–	–	–	196	–	–	–	–	–	–
E. Nutritional deficiencies	76	35	40	20	3	1	1	1	2	6	24	4	1	1	2	2	7
1. Protein-energy malnutrition	42	19	23	14	1	–	1	–	1	2	17	1	1	1	1	1	3
2. Iodine deficiency	3	2	2	1	–	–	–	–	–	1	1	–	–	–	–	–	1
3. Vitamin A deficiency	11	6	5	4	2	–	–	–	–	–	4	1	–	–	–	–	–
4. Iron-deficiency anaemia	19	9	10	2	1	1	1	1	–	3	1	1	1	1	1	1	4
II. Noncommunicable diseases	4 850	2 601	2 248	116	37	49	134	544	687	1 035	113	38	61	83	348	507	1 099
A. Malignant neoplasms	703	371	332	4	6	13	30	120	81	117	2	3	21	29	117	73	88
1. Mouth and oropharynx cancers	104	63	41	–	–	2	4	22	15	20	–	–	1	3	16	10	11
2. Oesophagus cancer	67	35	32	–	–	–	2	12	8	13	–	–	–	1	12	8	11
3. Stomach cancer	58	37	21	–	1	1	2	13	8	12	–	–	1	1	6	5	8
4. Colon and rectum cancers	27	14	13	–	–	1	1	4	3	5	–	–	1	1	7	3	1
5. Liver cancer	17	12	5	–	–	1	1	4	2	4	–	–	–	1	1	1	2
6. Pancreas cancer	10	6	4	–	–	–	1	1	2	2	–	–	–	–	1	1	2
7. Trachea, bronchus, lung cancers	92	74	18	–	–	–	6	30	22	16	–	1	1	2	4	5	5
8. Melanoma and other skin cancers	1	1	1	–	–	–	–	–	–	1	–	–	–	–	–	–	–
9. Breast cancer	44	–	44	–	–	–	–	–	–	–	–	–	5	5	17	8	9
10. Cervix uteri cancer	61	–	61	–	–	–	–	–	–	–	–	–	4	5	30	12	10
11. Corpus uteri cancer	4	–	4	–	–	–	–	–	–	–	–	–	–	–	1	1	2
12. Ovary cancer	15	–	15	–	–	–	–	–	–	–	–	1	1	2	4	4	3
13. Prostate cancer	16	16	–	–	–	–	–	1	3	12	–	–	–	–	–	–	–
14. Bladder cancer	9	7	2	–	–	–	–	1	2	4	–	–	–	–	–	–	2
15. Lymphomas, multiple myeloma	24	15	9	1	1	1	3	4	2	3	1	–	1	1	2	2	2
16. Leukaemia	19	11	8	1	2	1	2	2	1	2	1	1	1	1	2	1	1
17. Other cancers	134	79	55	2	3	4	9	23	14	24	2	3	5	6	13	11	15

Annex Table 12c, continued. Deaths by age, sex and cause (thousands): India, 2000, baseline scenario

Cause	Total	Male	Female	Males 0-4	5-14	15-29	30-44	45-59	60-69	70+	Females 0-4	5-14	15-29	30-44	45-59	60-69	70+
B. Other neoplasms	5	3	2	–	–	–	1	–	–	–	–	–	–	–	–	–	–
C. Diabetes mellitus	106	48	58	2	3	1	4	10	12	17	2	3	1	2	10	17	23
D. Endocrine disorders	2	1	1	–	–	–	1	–	–	–	–	–	–	–	–	–	–
E. Neuro-psychiatric conditions	108	60	48	6	4	4	8	9	11	18	8	3	4	3	3	9	19
2. Bipolar disorder	3	1	2	–	–	–	–	–	–	1	–	–	–	–	–	1	1
3. Schizophrenia	5	3	2	–	1	1	–	–	1	–	–	–	1	–	–	1	–
4. Epilepsy	12	7	5	–	1	1	2	2	1	–	–	1	1	1	1	1	–
5. Alcohol use	12	11	1	–	–	3	8	–	–	–	–	–	–	–	–	–	1
6. Dementia*	24	11	13	–	–	–	–	1	1	7	–	–	–	–	1	2	8
7. Parkinson disease	7	4	3	–	–	–	–	–	1	3	–	–	–	–	1	1	2
8. Multiple sclerosis	3	1	2	–	–	–	1	–	–	–	–	–	1	1	–	–	–
9. Drug use	–	–	–	–	–	–	–	–	–	–	–	–	2	1	1	–	–
13. Other neuro-psychiatric	48	26	22	5	3	2	3	3	5	5	6	2	2	1	1	4	5
F. Sense organ diseases	–	–	–	–	–	–	–	–	–	–	–	–	–	–	–	–	–
1. Glaucoma	–	–	–	–	–	–	–	–	–	–	–	–	–	–	–	–	–
2. Cataracts	–	–	–	–	–	–	–	–	–	–	–	–	–	–	–	–	–
G. Cardiovascular diseases	3 006	1 576	1 430	17	7	14	54	293	478	714	15	10	16	29	158	353	849
1. Rheumatic heart disease	80	36	43	–	1	4	8	14	6	3	–	1	5	9	16	8	5
2. Ischaemic heart disease	1 591	849	743	–	–	1	17	159	274	399	–	–	1	9	75	191	466
3. Cerebrovascular disease	598	307	291	3	2	3	6	45	95	156	3	1	2	4	23	76	182
4. Inflammatory heart diseases	99	52	47	3	2	3	6	15	10	14	3	2	3	4	10	7	18
5. Other cardiovascular	638	332	306	10	3	5	18	60	94	142	9	5	5	4	34	70	179
H. Respiratory diseases	379	215	164	7	6	2	7	34	60	99	6	5	5	5	27	34	81
1. COPD*	210	125	85	2	1	–	2	18	37	65	2	1	1	1	13	19	49
2. Asthma	28	15	13	–	1	1	1	3	3	6	–	1	1	1	3	3	6
3. Other respiratory	141	75	66	5	4	2	4	14	20	28	5	4	4	3	12	12	27
I. Digestive diseases	264	182	82	3	2	10	26	66	30	44	3	2	8	10	23	13	23
1. Peptic ulcer	46	30	16	–	–	1	3	9	6	10	1	1	1	2	4	3	6
2. Cirrhosis of the liver	161	117	44	1	1	6	15	46	20	29	–	1	3	5	14	7	13
3. Appendicitis	10	6	4	–	1	2	1	1	1	–	–	1	1	–	–	–	–
4. Other digestive	47	29	18	2	1	1	6	10	4	5	2	–	2	2	5	3	4
J. Genito-urinary diseases	101	58	43	7	5	2	3	10	14	23	1	7	3	3	7	8	14
1. Nephritis and nephrosis	88	46	42	7	4	2	3	9	9	16	1	7	3	3	7	8	14
2. Benign prostatic hypertrophy	11	11	–	–	–	–	–	1	4	7	–	–	–	–	–	–	–
3. Other genito-urinary	2	1	1	–	–	–	–	–	–	1	–	–	–	–	–	–	–
K. Skin diseases	2	1	1	–	–	–	–	–	–	–	–	–	–	–	–	–	–

Annex Table 12c, continued. Deaths by age, sex and cause (thousands): India, 2000, baseline scenario

Cause	Total	Male	Female	Males							Females						
				0-4	5-14	15-29	30-44	45-59	60-69	70+	0-4	5-14	15-29	30-44	45-59	60-69	70+
L. Musculo-skeletal diseases	2	1	1	-	-	-	-	-	-	1	-	-	-	-	1	-	-
1. Rheumatoid arthritis	2	1	1	-	-	-	-	-	-	1	-	-	-	-	1	-	-
3. Other musculo-skeletal	1	-	-	-	-	-	-	-	-	-	-	-	-	-	-	-	-
M. Congenital anomalies	171	85	86	74	4	3	2	1	1	-	74	5	3	2	1	1	-
N. Oral conditions	-	-	-	-	-	-	-	-	-	-	-	-	-	-	-	-	-
III. Injuries	*957*	*556*	*401*	*69*	*73*	*121*	*123*	*96*	*31*	*42*	*51*	*60*	*102*	*63*	*57*	*29*	*39*
A. Unintentional injuries	765	446	319	64	69	87	94	72	25	35	45	55	69	47	43	25	36
1. Road traffic accidents	271	193	78	16	26	51	45	32	10	14	5	19	11	11	16	8	9
2. Poisonings	31	16	14	5	2	2	4	2	1	-	3	1	4	3	2	-	-
3. Falls	51	33	18	3	6	3	5	6	3	5	4	3	1	2	2	2	5
4. Fires	130	40	90	9	3	8	10	7	2	2	7	9	35	20	8	4	7
5. Drownings	86	47	39	10	13	8	7	4	2	3	8	11	6	4	4	2	4
6. Other unintentional	197	118	79	21	19	15	24	21	8	10	18	12	11	8	10	8	11
B. Intentional injuries	192	110	82	5	5	34	29	24	5	7	7	5	33	16	14	4	3
1. Self-inflicted injuries	122	66	56	-	3	24	18	15	2	4	-	3	30	14	7	1	1
2. Violence	66	40	26	5	2	8	10	9	3	3	7	2	3	2	8	4	2
3. War	4	4	-	-	-	3	1	-	-	-	-	-	-	-	-	-	-

Notes:
Causes responsible for no deaths have been omitted from this table.
A dash (-) symbol indicates fewer than 500 deaths.
*IA6 is Bacterial meningitis and meningococcaemia; IC3 is Hypertensive disorders of pregnancy; ID is Conditions arising during the perinatal period; IIE6 is Dementia and other degenerative and hereditary CNS disorders; IIH1 is Chronic obstructive pulmonary disease.

Annex Table 12d. Deaths by age, sex and cause (thousands): China, 2000, baseline scenario

Cause	Total	Male	Female	Males 0-4	5-14	15-29	30-44	45-59	60-69	70+	Females 0-4	5-14	15-29	30-44	45-59	60-69	70+
Population (millions)	*1 280*	*656*	*624*	*59*	*120*	*158*	*161*	*98*	*37*	*23*	*55*	*114*	*148*	*150*	*91*	*36*	*29*
All causes	10 317	5 820	4 497	322	74	205	447	1 080	1 311	2 381	337	52	152	247	586	733	2 388
I. Communicable, maternal, perinatal and nutritional conditions	856	449	407	175	7	6	16	37	43	165	194	8	9	14	21	27	135
A. Infectious and parasitic diseases	347	203	144	31	4	4	15	34	34	81	32	4	3	9	17	20	59
1. Tuberculosis	187	119	68	1	–	2	8	24	26	57	1	1	2	5	13	14	32
2. STDs excluding HIV	–	–	–	–	–	–	–	–	–	–	–	–	–	–	–	–	–
a. Syphilis	–	–	–	–	–	–	–	–	–	–	–	–	–	–	–	–	–
b. Chlamydia	–	–	–	–	–	–	–	–	–	–	–	–	–	–	–	–	–
c. Gonorrhoea	–	–	–	–	–	–	–	–	–	–	–	–	–	–	–	–	–
3. HIV	4	–	–	1	–	–	1	–	–	–	1	–	–	–	–	–	–
4. Diarrhoeal diseases	60	29	31	11	1	–	1	1	3	12	13	1	–	–	1	1	15
5. Childhood-cluster diseases	26	14	12	12	1	–	–	–	–	–	11	1	–	–	–	–	–
a. Pertussis	8	4	4	4	–	–	–	–	–	–	4	–	–	–	–	–	–
b. Poliomyelitis	1	1	1	1	–	–	–	–	–	–	1	–	–	–	–	–	–
c. Diphtheria	–	–	–	–	–	–	–	–	–	–	–	–	–	–	–	–	–
d. Measles	7	4	3	3	–	–	–	–	–	–	3	–	–	–	–	–	–
e. Tetanus	9	5	4	4	–	–	–	–	–	–	4	–	–	–	–	–	–
6. Bacterial meningitis*	22	11	11	3	–	–	2	2	2	2	3	–	–	2	2	2	2
7. Hepatitis B and hepatitis C	20	13	7	1	–	1	2	4	1	4	1	–	–	–	1	–	3
8. Malaria	–	–	–	–	–	–	–	–	–	–	–	–	–	–	–	–	–
9. Tropical-cluster diseases	1	1	–	–	–	–	1	–	–	–	–	–	–	–	–	–	–
a. Trypanosomiasis	–	–	–	–	–	–	–	–	–	–	–	–	–	–	–	–	–
b. Chagas disease	–	–	–	–	–	–	–	–	–	–	–	–	–	–	–	–	–
c. Schistosomiasis	1	1	–	–	–	–	1	–	–	–	–	–	–	–	–	–	–
d. Leishmaniasis	–	–	–	–	–	–	–	–	–	–	–	–	–	–	–	–	–
10. Leprosy	–	–	–	–	–	–	–	–	–	–	–	–	–	–	–	–	–
11. Dengue	–	–	–	–	–	–	–	–	–	–	–	–	–	–	–	–	–
12. Japanese encephalitis	1	1	1	–	–	–	–	–	–	–	–	–	–	–	–	–	–
13. Trachoma	–	–	–	–	–	–	–	–	–	–	–	–	–	–	–	–	–
14. Intestinal nematode infections	3	2	2	–	1	–	–	–	–	–	–	1	–	–	–	–	–
a. Ascariasis	2	1	1	–	1	–	–	–	–	–	–	1	–	–	–	–	–
b. Trichuriasis	1	1	1	–	1	–	–	–	–	–	–	1	–	–	–	–	–
c. Ancylostomiasis, necatoriasis	–	–	–	–	–	–	–	–	–	–	–	–	–	–	–	–	–
15. Other infectious and parasitic	22	12	10	1	–	–	–	–	–	6	1	–	–	–	–	–	6

Annex Table 12d, continued. Deaths by age, sex and cause (thousands): China, 2000, baseline scenario

Cause	Total	Male	Female	Males							Females						
				0-4	5-14	15-29	30-44	45-59	60-69	70+	0-4	5-14	15-29	30-44	45-59	60-69	70+
B. Respiratory infections	**315**	**158**	**157**	**66**	**2**	**1**	**1**	**3**	**7**	**77**	**76**	**2**	**1**	**1**	**2**	**6**	**69**
1. Lower respiratory infections	311	156	154	65	2	1	1	3	7	77	74	2	1	1	2	6	69
2. Upper respiratory infections	3	2	2	1	–	–	–	–	–	1	1	–	–	1	–	–	1
3. Otitis media	1	1	1	1	–	–	–	–	–	–	1	–	–	–	–	–	–
C. Maternal conditions	**9**		**9**										**5**	**3**	**1**		
1. Maternal haemorrhage	4		4										2	1			
2. Maternal sepsis	–																
3. Hypertensive disorders*	1		1											1			
4. Obstructed labour	–																
5. Abortion	–																
6. Other maternal	1		1										1				
D. Perinatal conditions*	**140**	**69**	**71**	**69**								**71**						
E. Nutritional deficiencies	**45**	**18**	**27**	**8**	**1**	**1**	**1**		**1**	**6**	**15**	**2**		**1**	**1**	**2**	**7**
1. Protein-energy malnutrition	23	9	13	4					1	4	9				1	1	3
2. Iodine deficiency	4	2	2	2								2					
3. Vitamin A deficiency	4	2	2	2	1						1	1					
4. Iron-deficiency anaemia	14	5	9	1					1	2	2			1		1	2
II. Noncommunicable diseases	***8 249***	***4 665***	***3 584***	***80***	***26***	***69***	***269***	***921***	***1 194***	***2 106***	***84***	***17***	***47***	***159***	***489***	***660***	***2 129***
A. Malignant neoplasms	**2 115**	**1 371**	**744**	**5**	**13**	**25**	**138**	**415**	**404**	**371**	**8**	**6**	**16**	**74**	**191**	**191**	**259**
1. Mouth and oropharynx cancers	52	37	16			1	8	11	9	8			1	3	5	4	3
2. Oesophagus cancer	275	191	84				10	50	63	67				1	17	31	34
3. Stomach cancer	464	310	153			1	14	88	104	102			2	13	32	43	64
4. Colon and rectum cancers	120	68	52		1	2	7	17	18	24			1	5	13	14	19
5. Liver cancer	432	319	112		1	5	63	123	75	52		1	1	13	33	27	36
6. Pancreas cancer	47	29	18				1	7	9	11				1	3	6	8
7. Trachea, bronchus, lung cancers	325	235	90			2	10	73	86	64			1	3	24	26	37
8. Melanoma and other skin cancers	2	1	1														
9. Breast cancer	37		37										1	9	12	6	8
10. Cervix uteri cancer	29		29											3	10	8	9
11. Corpus uteri cancer	9		9											1	4	2	2
12. Ovary cancer	14		14										1	3	5	2	3
13. Prostate cancer	7	7	–						3	4							
14. Bladder cancer	27	22	6					3	8	10				1	1	2	3
15. Lymphomas, multiple myeloma	31	21	10		1	2	1	6	7	4			1	1	4	2	3
16. Leukaemia	84	44	40	3	6	7	9	10	4	5	4	3	6	9	8	4	6
17. Other cancers	162	87	74	2	3	5	14	27	17	20	4	1	3	10	20	15	21

Annex Table 12d, continued. Deaths by age, sex and cause (thousands): China, 2000, baseline scenario

Cause	Total	Male	Female	M 0-4	M 5-14	M 15-29	M 30-44	M 45-59	M 60-69	M 70+	F 0-4	F 5-14	F 15-29	F 30-44	F 45-59	F 60-69	F 70+
B. Other neoplasms	20	11	10	1	-	1	1	3	3	2	1	-	-	1	2	3	2
C. Diabetes mellitus	64	27	36	-	-	1	3	6	7	10	-	-	1	1	7	11	16
D. Endocrine disorders	14	5	9	2	-	-	1	1	1	2	2	1	1	1	1	1	4
E. Neuro-psychiatric conditions	97	49	48	2	2	8	10	6	5	16	2	1	4	6	5	6	23
2. Bipolar disorder	3	1	2	-	-	-	1	-	-	-	-	-	-	-	1	1	-
3. Schizophrenia	15	9	5	-	-	2	4	1	1	1	-	-	1	1	1	1	1
4. Epilepsy	10	6	4	-	-	2	1	1	1	1	-	-	1	1	1	1	-
5. Alcohol use	5	4	-	-	-	-	2	2	-	-	-	-	-	-	-	-	-
6. Dementia*	30	12	19	-	-	-	1	2	2	7	-	-	-	-	3	3	13
7. Parkinson disease	6	3	3	-	-	-	-	-	-	3	-	-	-	-	-	-	3
8. Multiple sclerosis	5	2	3	-	-	-	1	-	-	-	-	-	2	-	1	-	-
9. Drug use	-	-	-	-	-	-	-	-	-	-	-	-	-	-	-	-	-
13. Other neuro-psychiatric	22	12	11	2	-	4	1	3	-	2	2	-	2	1	2	1	3
F. Sense organ diseases	18	10	9	1	-	-	-	3	3	3	-	-	2	-	2	3	2
1. Glaucoma	7	4	3	1	-	-	-	1	1	1	-	-	-	-	1	1	1
2. Cataracts	6	4	2	-	-	-	-	1	1	1	-	-	-	-	1	-	1
G. Cardiovascular diseases	3 307	1 789	1 518	10	3	16	62	306	444	950	6	1	12	44	171	254	1 030
1. Rheumatic heart disease	192	87	105	-	-	5	9	20	16	35	1	-	4	11	23	17	49
2. Ischaemic heart disease	993	527	467	-	1	3	20	85	126	292	-	-	2	12	44	75	335
3. Cerebrovascular disease	1 650	914	737	2	1	4	24	154	244	484	2	-	2	14	85	137	496
4. Inflammatory heart diseases	77	42	36	2	-	2	5	11	6	15	1	-	2	4	7	4	18
5. Other cardiovascular	394	220	173	6	1	1	4	35	51	123	3	0	2	2	11	22	133
H. Respiratory diseases	1 911	1 002	909	8	1	4	14	103	250	622	9	1	1	12	68	147	671
1. COPD*	1 795	939	856	3	-	2	10	95	239	589	6	-	1	10	63	140	637
2. Asthma	43	24	19	-	1	1	2	5	5	10	-	-	1	2	4	4	9
3. Other respiratory	73	39	34	4	-	1	2	3	6	23	3	-	1	1	1	3	25
I. Digestive diseases	428	255	173	9	2	4	30	66	60	84	10	2	4	11	32	30	84
1. Peptic ulcer	38	21	16	-	-	-	1	3	5	12	-	-	-	-	2	2	12
2. Cirrhosis of the liver	200	133	67	1	1	2	22	43	36	29	-	1	1	5	18	17	25
3. Appendicitis	8	5	3	-	1	1	2	-	-	-	-	1	1	-	-	-	-
4. Other digestive	182	96	86	8	1	1	5	19	20	43	9	1	2	4	12	11	47
J. Genito-urinary diseases	124	72	52	2	1	5	9	12	13	30	2	1	3	7	9	11	20
1. Nephritis and nephrosis	97	55	42	1	1	5	8	10	10	18	2	1	2	6	7	9	15
2. Benign prostatic hypertrophy	7	7	-	-	-	-	-	-	2	6	-	-	-	-	-	-	-
3. Other genito-urinary	20	10	10	-	1	-	-	2	2	5	-	-	1	-	2	3	5
K. Skin diseases	12	8	5	1	-	-	-	1	1	5	1	-	-	-	-	1	2

Annex Table 12d, continued. Deaths by age, sex and cause (thousands): China, 2000, baseline scenario

Cause	Total	Male	Female	Males							Females						
				0-4	5-14	15-29	30-44	45-59	60-69	70+	0-4	5-14	15-29	30-44	45-59	60-69	70+
L. Musculo-skeletal diseases	**39**	**17**	**21**	-	-	-	-	1	4	11	-	-	1	2	2	2	14
1. Rheumatoid arthritis	2	1	1	-	-	-	-	-	-	1	-	-	-	-	-	-	1
3. Other musculo-skeletal	37	17	20	-	-	-	-	1	4	11	-	-	1	1	2	2	14
M. Congenital anomalies	**101**	**49**	**52**	41	4	3	1	-	-	-	43	4	4	1	-	-	-
N. Oral conditions	-	-	-	-	-	-	-	-	-	-	-	-	-	-	-	-	-
III. Injuries	***1 212***	***707***	***505***	*67*	*41*	*130*	*162*	*122*	*74*	*110*	*60*	*27*	*96*	*75*	*77*	*46*	*124*
A. Unintentional injuries	**759**	**486**	**273**	62	37	83	104	82	45	72	52	24	29	26	37	23	82
1. Road traffic accidents	267	196	71	4	11	38	58	41	22	22	3	11	13	12	17	7	22
2. Poisonings	67	40	27	4	1	4	8	11	4	8	1	2	5	5	3	3	9
3. Falls	84	36	49	2	1	4	4	5	6	14	3	1	1	1	5	6	8
4. Fires	28	15	13	2	1	1	2	1	1	7	1	1	1	1	1	1	33
5. Drownings	129	79	50	27	17	13	7	5	3	7	21	8	4	3	3	3	9
6. Other unintentional	184	121	63	23	6	23	26	19	10	14	22	3	5	5	9	4	16
B. Intentional injuries	**453**	**221**	**232**	5	4	48	58	40	29	38	8	4	68	49	39	22	42
1. Self-inflicted injuries	397	188	209	-	3	36	48	37	27	37	-	2	66	44	37	21	40
2. Violence	55	32	23	5	1	11	9	4	2	1	8	2	2	5	2	1	2
3. War	1	1	-	-	-	-	-	-	-	-	-	-	-	-	-	-	-

Notes:
Causes responsible for no deaths have been omitted from this table.
A dash (-) symbol indicates fewer than 500 deaths.
*IA6 is Bacterial meningitis and meningococcaemia; IC3 is Hypertensive disorders of pregnancy; ID is Conditions arising during the perinatal period;
IIE6 is Dementia and other degenerative and hereditary CNS disorders; IIH1 is Chronic obstructive pulmonary disease.

Annex Table 12e. Deaths by age, sex and cause (thousands): Other Asia and Islands, 2000, baseline scenario

Cause	Total	Male	Female	Males 0-4	5-14	15-29	30-44	45-59	60-69	70+	Females 0-4	5-14	15-29	30-44	45-59	60-69	70+
Population (millions)	*808*	*404*	*403*	*44*	*83*	*119*	*85*	*46*	*17*	*11*	*42*	*81*	*114*	*86*	*47*	*19*	*14*
All causes	5 862	3 280	2 582	641	156	223	326	503	503	928	494	110	140	197	298	355	988
I. Communicable, maternal, perinatal and nutritional conditions	1 635	880	756	499	43	38	55	54	61	130	378	37	44	61	50	43	142
A. Infectious and parasitic diseases	926	504	422	237	26	33	52	49	38	70	179	22	29	43	43	32	74
1. Tuberculosis	260	133	128	1	1	8	12	31	28	52	-	1	6	11	30	25	54
2. STDs excluding HIV	31	15	16	11	-	-	-	-	1	3	8	-	1	2	1	1	4
a. Syphilis	28	15	13	11	-	-	-	-	1	3	8	-	1	1	1	1	4
b. Chlamydia	2	-	2	-							-						
c. Gonorrhoea	1	-	1														
3. HIV	121	70	50	12	2	17	29	7	2	1	7	1	16	21	3	1	-
4. Diarrhoeal diseases	255	146	108	131	6	1	1	2	2	4	94	5	4	2	2	1	5
5. Childhood-cluster diseases	141	75	66	63	6	1	2	1	-	1	54	6	-	2	1	-	1
a. Pertussis	21	11	10	11	1						9	1					
b. Poliomyelitis	2	1	1	1							1						
c. Diphtheria	1	1	-	1							-						
d. Measles	70	37	33	34	4	-	-	-			29	3	2	1			
e. Tetanus	47	24	22	17	2	1	2	1	-	1	15	2	1	1	-	-	1
6. Bacterial meningitis*	16	9	8	4	-	-	-	2	1	1	3	-	-	1	1	1	1
7. Hepatitis B and hepatitis C	14	8	6	1	-	-	1	2	1	3	1	-	-	1	1	1	2
8. Malaria	44	24	20	4	6	5	4	3	1	1	3	5	4	3	3	1	1
9. Tropical-cluster diseases	2	1	1	-													
a. Trypanosomiasis																	
b. Chagas disease																	
c. Schistosomiasis	-	-	-														
d. Leishmaniasis	1	1	-														
10. Leprosy	1	-	-								1						
11. Dengue	4	2	2	-	1	-	-				1	1					
12. Japanese encephalitis	1	-	-														
13. Trachoma	-	-	-														
14. Intestinal nematode infections	4	2	2	2	2						1	1					
a. Ascariasis	2	1	1	1	1						1	1					
b. Trichuriasis	1	1	1	1	1												
c. Ancylostomiasis, necatoriasis	1	1	-	1							-						
15. Other infectious and parasitic	33	18	15	10	2	-	1	1	1	4	7	1	-	1	1	1	4

Annex Table 12e, continued. Deaths by age, sex and cause (thousands): Other Asia and Islands, 2000, baseline scenario

Cause	Total	Male	Female	Males 0-4	5-14	15-29	30-44	45-59	60-69	70+	Females 0-4	5-14	15-29	30-44	45-59	60-69	70+
B. Respiratory infections	413	227	187	122	15	4	4	4	22	57	88	13	3	2	5	11	65
1. Lower respiratory infections	407	223	184	120	14	4	3	4	22	56	87	13	3	2	5	11	65
2. Upper respiratory infections	4	2	2	1	–	–	–	–	–	1	1	–	–	–	–	–	1
3. Otitis media	2	1	1	1	–	–	–	–	–	–	1	–	–	–	–	–	–
C. Maternal conditions	28		28									–	–	11	15	1	–	–
1. Maternal haemorrhage	7		7									–	–	3	4	–	–	–
2. Maternal sepsis	4		4									–	–	2	2	–	–	–
3. Hypertensive disorders*	2		2									–	–	1	1	–	–	–
4. Obstructed labour	1		1									–	–	–	1	–	–	–
5. Abortion	2		2									–	–	1	1	–	–	–
6. Other maternal	4		4									–	–	2	2	–	–	–
D. Perinatal conditions*	216	122	94	122							94						
E. Nutritional deficiencies	52	27	25	18	2	1	1	1	1	3	16	2	–	1	1	1	3
1. Protein-energy malnutrition	27	14	12	13	–	1	1	1	1	1	11	–	–	1	1	1	1
2. Iodine deficiency	2	1	1	1	–	–	–	–	–	–	1	–	–	–	–	–	–
3. Vitamin A deficiency	10	5	5	4	2	–	–	–	–	–	3	1	–	–	–	–	–
4. Iron-deficiency anaemia	13	6	7	1	–	1	1	1	1	2	1	–	1	1	1	1	3
II. Noncommunicable diseases	3 577	1 951	1 625	91	65	49	161	388	420	777	75	49	43	100	227	300	832
A. Malignant neoplasms	892	514	378	7	17	10	45	132	138	165	8	11	13	41	89	95	123
1. Mouth and oropharynx cancers	96	60	36	–	–	1	5	9	20	24	–	–	–	3	4	12	16
2. Oesophagus cancer	32	22	10	–	–	–	1	7	6	8	–	–	–	–	2	3	4
3. Stomach cancer	81	53	28	–	–	1	4	17	14	17	–	–	1	2	7	8	11
4. Colon and rectum cancers	57	30	27	–	–	1	3	4	10	12	–	–	1	2	4	9	12
5. Liver cancer	94	70	24	1	1	2	8	28	14	17	–	1	–	2	6	7	9
6. Pancreas cancer	14	9	5	–	–	–	1	2	2	3	–	–	–	–	2	2	3
7. Trachea, bronchus, lung cancers	131	99	32	–	–	1	5	32	27	33	–	–	–	1	8	10	13
8. Melanoma and other skin cancers	3	1	2	–	–	–	–	–	–	–	–	–	–	–	1	–	1
9. Breast cancer	37	–	37								–	–	1	6	14	7	9
10. Cervix uteri cancer	45		45								–	–	2	6	18	8	11
11. Corpus uteri cancer	6		6								–	–	–	–	2	2	2
12. Ovary cancer	14		14								–	–	–	3	4	2	3
13. Prostate cancer	18	18	–	–	–	–	–	2	7	9							
14. Bladder cancer	16	11	4	–	–	–	–	2	4	5	–	–	–	–	–	2	2
15. Lymphomas, multiple myeloma	33	20	14	1	2	1	3	3	5	6	–	1	1	1	1	4	5
16. Leukaemia	37	20	17	2	6	1	4	2	3	3	3	4	1	3	1	2	3
17. Other cancers	179	102	77	3	7	3	12	24	25	28	3	5	3	11	17	17	21

Annex Table 12e, continued. Deaths by age, sex and cause (thousands): Other Asia and Islands, 2000, baseline scenario

Cause	Total	Male	Female	Males 0-4	5-14	15-29	30-44	45-59	60-69	70+	Females 0-4	5-14	15-29	30-44	45-59	60-69	70+
B. Other neoplasms	10	5	5	1	1	-	-	1	1	1	1	-	1	-	1	1	1
C. Diabetes mellitus	66	28	38	-	1	1	3	7	7	11	-	-	1	1	7	11	17
D. Endocrine disorders	9	4	5	1	1	-	-	-	-	1	1	-	-	-	1	1	2
E. Neuro-psychiatric conditions	75	42	33	2	2	4	7	8	6	13	2	2	2	2	4	5	16
2. Bipolar disorder	2	1	1	-	-	-	-	1	-	-	-	-	-	-	-	-	1
3. Schizophrenia	6	3	3	-	-	-	-	1	1	1	-	-	1	-	-	1	1
4. Epilepsy	9	5	3	-	1	1	2	1	1	1	-	-	1	1	-	-	-
5. Alcohol use	6	5	1	-	-	1	2	2	1	1	-	-	-	-	1	-	-
6. Dementia*	21	9	12	-	-	-	-	1	2	6	-	-	-	-	2	2	8
7. Parkinson disease	5	3	2	-	-	-	-	-	1	2	-	-	-	-	-	-	1
8. Multiple sclerosis	2	1	1	-	-	-	1	-	-	-	-	-	-	-	-	-	-
9. Drug use	2	2	-	-	-	1	1	-	-	-	-	-	-	-	-	-	-
13. Other neuro-psychiatric	23	13	10	2	2	2	2	2	1	2	2	2	1	1	1	1	3
F. Sense organ diseases	-	-	-	-	-	-	-	-	-	-	-	-	-	-	-	-	-
1. Glaucoma	-	-	-	-	-	-	-	-	-	-	-	-	-	-	-	-	-
2. Cataracts	-	-	-	-	-	-	-	-	-	-	-	-	-	-	-	-	-
G. Cardiovascular diseases	1 756	904	852	31	29	24	65	143	182	430	24	23	18	37	83	133	535
1. Rheumatic heart disease	13	6	7	-	-	-	-	1	1	3	-	-	-	1	1	1	4
2. Ischaemic heart disease	643	331	312	-	6	5	20	50	75	184	3	4	3	11	27	53	221
3. Cerebrovascular disease	523	259	264	4	6	5	14	41	60	128	5	5	3	8	26	47	172
4. Inflammatory heart diseases	87	48	39	6	-	-	8	9	4	10	-	-	-	5	5	3	12
5. Other cardiovascular	490	261	230	21	17	13	22	42	42	103	15	13	11	13	24	29	125
H. Respiratory diseases	208	121	87	8	4	2	4	12	22	69	5	3	2	3	7	13	54
1. COPD*	115	69	46	2	1	-	1	6	14	46	1	-	1	1	3	8	32
2. Asthma	25	13	12	-	1	1	2	2	2	5	-	-	1	1	2	2	5
3. Other respiratory	68	39	29	6	2	1	1	4	6	19	4	2	1	1	2	3	17
I. Digestive diseases	368	236	131	7	5	4	29	74	53	64	5	4	3	10	27	28	54
1. Peptic ulcer	30	18	12	-	1	-	1	4	4	9	-	1	1	1	1	2	7
2. Cirrhosis of the liver	157	115	42	1	1	2	18	46	27	21	-	-	1	4	12	11	12
3. Appendicitis	8	5	3	-	-	1	1	-	-	-	-	-	1	1	-	-	-
4. Other digestive	173	99	74	6	3	1	9	24	22	34	4	3	2	5	13	14	34
J. Genito-urinary diseases	108	51	57	1	3	2	5	9	9	22	1	2	2	4	9	12	27
1. Nephritis and nephrosis	94	44	50	1	3	2	4	8	8	18	1	2	2	3	8	10	23
2. Benign prostatic hypertrophy	1	1	-	-	-	-	-	-	-	1	-	-	-	-	-	-	-
3. Other genito-urinary	14	7	7	-	-	1	1	1	1	3	-	-	-	1	1	2	4
K. Skin diseases	3	1	1	-	-	-	-	-	-	-	-	-	-	-	-	-	1

Annex Table 12e, continued. Deaths by age, sex and cause (thousands): Other Asia and Islands, 2000, baseline scenario

Cause	Total	Male	Female	Males							Females						
				0-4	5-14	15-29	30-44	45-59	60-69	70+	0-4	5-14	15-29	30-44	45-59	60-69	70+
L. Musculo-skeletal diseases	**10**	**4**	**6**	–	–	–	–	1	1	1	–	–	–	–	1	1	3
1. Rheumatoid arthritis	1	–	1	–	–	–	–	–	–	1	–	–	–	–	1	1	1
3. Other musculo-skeletal	9	3	6	–	–	–	–	1	1	1	–	–	–	–	1	–	3
M. Congenital anomalies	**71**	**38**	**32**	32	2	1	1	1	–	–	27	2	1	1	1	–	–
N. Oral conditions	**–**	**–**	**–**	–	–	–	–	–	–	–	–	–	–	–	–	–	–
III. Injuries	***650***	***448***	***201***	*50*	*48*	*136*	*110*	*60*	*22*	*22*	*42*	*24*	*53*	*36*	*20*	*12*	*14*
A. Unintentional injuries	**482**	**334**	**148**	48	43	94	76	43	16	15	39	21	30	22	15	10	11
1. Road traffic accidents	183	130	53	13	15	41	32	17	7	6	12	8	11	9	6	4	4
2. Poisonings	39	21	18	2	2	6	5	4	2	1	2	2	6	3	2	1	1
3. Falls	38	27	10	4	2	6	7	5	2	2	3	1	1	1	1	1	2
4. Fires	10	6	4	2	1	1	1	1	–	–	2	1	1	–	–	–	–
5. Drownings	77	54	24	17	15	10	6	3	1	2	11	6	3	2	1	–	–
6. Other unintentional	135	97	38	11	9	29	25	14	5	4	11	4	7	6	4	3	3
B. Intentional injuries	**168**	**114**	**54**	3	5	42	34	17	6	7	3	3	23	14	5	3	3
1. Self-inflicted injuries	85	52	34	–	2	20	14	8	4	4	–	1	16	9	3	2	3
2. Violence	65	52	13	1	2	18	18	9	2	2	1	1	4	4	1	–	–
3. War	18	10	7	2	1	4	2	1	–	–	2	1	3	2	–	–	1

Notes:
Causes responsible for no deaths have been omitted from this table.
A dash (–) symbol indicates fewer than 500 deaths.
*IA6 is Bacterial meningitis and meningococcaemia; IC3 is Hypertensive disorders of pregnancy; ID is Conditions arising during the perinatal period; IIE6 is Dementia and other degenerative and hereditary CNS disorders; IIH1 is Chronic obstructive pulmonary disease.

Annex Table 12f. Deaths by age, sex and cause (thousands): Sub-Saharan Africa, 2000, baseline scenario

Cause	Total	Male	Female	Males 0-4	5-14	15-29	30-44	45-59	60-69	70+	Females 0-4	5-14	15-29	30-44	45-59	60-69	70+
Population (millions)	691	343	349	66	94	92	51	27	9	5	64	93	92	53	29	11	7
All causes	9 205	4 997	4 208	2 289	362	607	489	419	327	503	1 865	314	437	357	341	293	600
I. Communicable, maternal, perinatal and nutritional conditions	5 507	2 853	2 653	2 072	163	175	170	104	60	109	1 682	169	286	246	93	59	120
A. Infectious and parasitic diseases	3 784	1 986	1 798	1 344	124	169	166	99	43	42	1 086	129	227	187	87	39	43
1. Tuberculosis	522	251	271	25	14	67	48	57	25	14	27	21	78	54	53	23	14
2. STDs excluding HIV	82	40	43	33	-	-	-	1	1	4	29	-	3	2	1	1	5
a. Syphilis	77	40	38	33	-	-	-	1	1	4	29	-	1	1	1	1	5
b. Chlamydia	3	-	3	-	-	-	-	-	-	-	-	-	1	1	-	-	-
c. Gonorrhoea	2	-	2	-	-	-	-	-	-	-	-	-	1	-	-	-	-
3. HIV	658	310	348	88	12	79	98	23	6	3	83	12	121	110	17	4	2
4. Diarrhoeal diseases	892	496	397	447	25	3	3	3	4	12	339	25	5	5	4	4	14
5. Childhood-cluster diseases	803	431	372	386	39	1	2	1	1	1	328	38	2	2	1	1	1
a. Pertussis	140	76	64	71	5	-	-	-	-	-	60	4	-	-	-	-	-
b. Poliomyelitis	5	3	2	3	-	-	-	-	-	-	2	-	-	-	-	-	-
c. Diphtheria	2	1	1	1	-	-	-	-	-	-	1	-	-	-	-	-	-
d. Measles	536	287	248	256	31	1	2	1	-	-	219	29	2	2	1	-	1
e. Tetanus	121	64	56	55	3	1	1	1	1	1	47	4	2	1	1	1	1
6. Bacterial meningitis*	23	12	11	9	-	-	1	1	1	-	8	-	1	1	-	-	-
7. Hepatitis B and hepatitis C	12	7	5	1	-	-	1	1	2	2	1	-	1	1	1	1	2
8. Malaria	668	372	296	325	21	11	7	5	2	1	247	20	12	7	5	2	2
9. Tropical-cluster diseases	42	23	19	1	7	5	4	4	1	1	1	6	5	3	3	1	-
a. Trypanosomiasis	32	17	15	1	5	4	3	4	1	1	1	5	4	3	2	1	1
b. Chagas disease																	
c. Schistosomiasis	2	2	1	-	-	1	1	-	-	-	-	1	1	-	-	-	-
d. Leishmaniasis	7	2	5	2	2	1	1	-	-	-	-	1	1	-	-	-	-
10. Leprosy																	
11. Dengue																	
12. Japanese encephalitis																	
13. Trachoma																	
14. Intestinal nematode infections	1	1	1	1	-	-	-	-	-	-	1	-	-	-	-	-	-
a. Ascariasis																	
b. Trichuriasis																	
c. Ancylostomiasis, necatoriasis	1	1															
15. Other infectious and parasitic	80	44	36	30	5	2	2	2	1	3	23	5	2	2	2	1	2

Annex Table 12f, continued. Deaths by age, sex and cause (thousands): Sub-Saharan Africa, 2000, baseline scenario

Cause	Total	Male	Female	Males							Females						
				0-4	5-14	15-29	30-44	45-59	60-69	70+	0-4	5-14	15-29	30-44	45-59	60-69	70+
B. Respiratory infections	**978**	**534**	**444**	**406**	**34**	**5**	**4**	**4**	**17**	**64**	**309**	**28**	**6**	**4**	**4**	**19**	**74**
1. Lower respiratory infections	962	525	437	399	34	5	3	4	16	63	303	28	6	4	4	19	73
2. Upper respiratory infections	10	5	4	4	-	-	-	-	-	1	3	-	-	-	-	-	1
3. Otitis media	6	4	3	3	-	-	-	-	-	-	2	-	-	-	-	-	-
C. Maternal conditions	**111**		**111**								-	**7**	**51**	**54**	-	-	-
1. Maternal haemorrhage	27		27									2	12	13			
2. Maternal sepsis	18		18									1	8	9			
3. Hypertensive disorders*	9		9									1	4	4			
4. Obstructed labour	4		4										2	2			
5. Abortion	9		9									1	4	4			
6. Other maternal	15		15									1	7	7			
D. Perinatal conditions*	**496**	**262**	**234**	**262**								**234**						
E. Nutritional deficiencies	**137**	**71**	**66**	**60**	**5**	**1**	-	**1**	**1**	**3**	**53**	**5**	**2**	**1**	**1**	**1**	**3**
1. Protein-energy malnutrition	97	51	46	47	1	1	-	1	1	2	41	1	1	1	1	1	2
2. Iodine deficiency	1	1	1	1							1						
3. Vitamin A deficiency	29	15	14	11	4	-	-	-	-	-	10	4	1	-	-	-	-
4. Iron-deficiency anaemia	10	4	5	2	1	-	-	-	-	1	2	1	1	1	1	-	1
II. Noncommunicable diseases	**2 352**	**1 200**	**1 152**	**82**	**62**	**51**	**139**	**249**	**242**	**376**	**80**	**68**	**34**	**55**	**226**	**222**	**468**
A. Malignant neoplasms	**571**	**326**	**245**	**5**	**13**	**11**	**36**	**84**	**79**	**96**	**7**	**14**	**8**	**18**	**71**	**57**	**71**
1. Mouth and oropharynx cancers	31	19	12	-	-	-	2	3	6	8	-	-	-	1	1	1	1
2. Oesophagus cancer	31	23	8	-	-	1	2	9	5	7	-	-	-	-	3	2	2
3. Stomach cancer	42	25	17	-	-	1	2	9	6	8	-	-	-	1	2	2	3
4. Colon and rectum cancers	20	11	9	-	-	-	1	2	3	4	-	-	-	-	6	3	4
5. Liver cancer	75	55	19	-	-	4	12	20	8	10	2	4	1	2	6	3	5
6. Pancreas cancer	9	5	4	-	-	-	-	2	1	2	-	-	-	-	2	1	2
7. Trachea, bronchus, lung cancers	29	20	8	-	-	-	2	7	5	6	-	-	-	1	7	5	6
8. Melanoma and other skin cancers	11	4	6	-	-	-	-	2	1	1	-	-	-	-	2	1	1
9. Breast cancer	22	-	22	-	-	-	-	-	-	-	-	-	1	2	8	5	6
10. Cervix uteri cancer	42	-	42	-	-	-	-	-	-	-	-	-	1	3	16	10	13
11. Corpus uteri cancer	5		5								-	-	-	-	1	1	2
12. Ovary cancer	10		10								-	-	-	1	3	2	3
13. Prostate cancer	45	45	-	-	-	-	-	6	17	22							
14. Bladder cancer	18	12	6	-	-	-	1	3	4	5	-	-	-	-	2	2	2
15. Lymphomas, multiple myeloma	35	22	13	2	5	4	3	3	4	5	4	1	-	1	2	2	3
16. Leukaemia	12	6	6	1	2	-	1	1	1	2	1	2	-	-	1	1	1
17. Other cancers	134	76	58	3	6	3	11	19	16	18	4	7	2	5	15	12	13

Annex Table 12f, continued. Deaths by age, sex and cause (thousands): Sub-Saharan Africa, 2000, baseline scenario

Cause	Total	Male	Female	Males							Females						
				0-4	5-14	15-29	30-44	45-59	60-69	70+	0-4	5-14	15-29	30-44	45-59	60-69	70+
B. Other neoplasms	10	5	5	-	2	-	1	1	1	1	1	1	-	-	2	1	1
C. Diabetes mellitus	24	11	14	1	1	-	1	2	2	3	1	1	1	-	2	4	5
D. Endocrine disorders	25	11	14	3	1	1	2	2	1	2	2	1	1	1	2	2	5
E. Neuro-psychiatric conditions	44	26	18	2	3	3	5	4	3	6	3	3	1	1	2	3	6
2. Bipolar disorder	1	1	1	-	-	-	-	-	-	-	-	-	-	-	-	-	-
3. Schizophrenia	1	-	1	-	-	-	-	-	-	-	-	-	-	-	-	-	-
4. Epilepsy	6	4	2	-	1	1	1	1	1	-	-	-	-	-	1	-	-
5. Alcohol use	5	4	1	-	-	1	1	1	1	1	-	-	1	-	-	1	-
6. Dementia*	9	4	5	-	-	-	-	-	1	2	-	-	-	-	-	1	3
7. Parkinson disease	2	1	1	-	-	-	-	-	-	1	-	-	-	-	-	-	-
8. Multiple sclerosis	1	1	1	-	-	-	-	-	-	-	-	-	-	-	-	-	-
9. Drug use	1	1	-	-	-	-	-	-	-	-	-	-	-	-	-	-	-
13. Other neuro-psychiatric	17	10	7	2	2	2	2	1	1	1	2	2	1	-	1	-	1
F. Sense organ diseases	-	-	-	-	-	-	-	-	-	-	-	-	-	-	-	-	-
1. Glaucoma	-	-	-	-	-	-	-	-	-	-	-	-	-	-	-	-	-
2. Cataracts	-	-	-	-	-	-	-	-	-	-	-	-	-	-	-	-	-
G. Cardiovascular diseases	1 034	451	583	16	17	18	51	91	93	165	16	23	13	23	102	115	292
1. Rheumatic heart disease	19	10	10	-	3	3	2	1	1	-	-	4	2	1	1	1	-
2. Ischaemic heart disease	273	124	149	-	-	1	13	27	30	52	5	-	-	5	26	34	79
3. Cerebrovascular disease	496	201	294	3	6	7	21	39	44	81	3	6	4	10	50	60	163
4. Inflammatory heart diseases	76	35	41	4	3	1	5	7	6	9	6	4	2	2	6	7	14
5. Other cardiovascular	169	80	89	9	6	5	9	17	12	23	3	9	5	4	19	13	36
H. Respiratory diseases	298	173	125	11	6	5	17	29	35	69	9	6	3	5	24	21	58
1. COPD*	153	91	63	2	1	1	4	15	22	45	2	1	-	1	11	12	35
2. Asthma	19	10	8	-	1	1	2	2	2	5	2	-	2	1	2	2	3
3. Other respiratory	126	71	54	8	5	3	11	13	12	20	6	5	2	3	11	7	20
I. Digestive diseases	166	103	63	4	7	7	19	27	18	20	4	10	4	5	12	12	17
1. Peptic ulcer	15	9	6	-	-	1	2	3	1	2	-	-	1	1	2	1	3
2. Cirrhosis of the liver	39	27	11	-	1	1	5	9	6	5	-	-	1	1	3	3	3
3. Appendicitis	12	7	5	-	3	2	2	-	-	-	-	2	1	1	-	-	1
4. Other digestive	100	59	41	4	4	3	10	14	11	13	4	7	2	3	7	8	11
J. Genito-urinary diseases	101	56	45	8	8	4	7	8	8	13	6	7	2	3	9	7	11
1. Nephritis and nephrosis	87	48	39	7	7	3	6	7	7	11	6	6	2	2	8	6	9
2. Benign prostatic hypertrophy	1	1	-	-	-	-	-	-	-	1							
3. Other genito-urinary	13	7	6	1	1	1	1	1	1	1	-	1	1	-	1	1	2
K. Skin diseases	9	5	4	5	-	-	-	-	-	-	3	-	-	-	-	-	-

Annex Table 12f, continued. Deaths by age, sex and cause (thousands): Sub-Saharan Africa, 2000, baseline scenario

Cause	Total	Male	Female	Males							Females						
				0-4	5-14	15-29	30-44	45-59	60-69	70+	0-4	5-14	15-29	30-44	45-59	60-69	70+
L. Musculo-skeletal diseases																	
1. Rheumatoid arthritis	1	1	–					1									
3. Other musculo-skeletal	1	–	–														
M. Congenital anomalies	69	34	36	27	3	1	1	1	–	–	30	3	1	–	1	–	–
N. Oral conditions	–	–	–														
III. Injuries	*1 346*	*944*	*402*	*136*	*137*	*381*	*181*	*67*	*25*	*17*	*104*	*77*	*116*	*57*	*22*	*13*	*13*
A. Unintentional injuries	**681**	**476**	**205**	**92**	**103**	**140**	**78**	**37**	**14**	**12**	**64**	**58**	**38**	**19**	**11**	**6**	**10**
1. Road traffic accidents	211	153	58	13	38	49	30	14	6	3	9	19	16	7	4	1	1
2. Poisonings	48	29	20	19	4	2	1	1	1	1	14	2	2	1	–	1	–
3. Falls	23	14	9	1	2	4	2	2	1	2	1	1	1	1	–	–	4
4. Fires	85	44	41	18	6	9	4	3	1	2	16	9	7	3	2	1	2
5. Drownings	107	78	29	22	34	13	5	1	1	1	11	13	2	1	1	–	2
6. Other unintentional	207	158	49	19	18	63	36	14	4	4	13	14	9	5	3	2	2
B. Intentional injuries	**665**	**468**	**197**	**43**	**34**	**242**	**103**	**31**	**11**	**5**	**39**	**19**	**79**	**38**	**12**	**7**	**3**
1. Self-inflicted injuries	21	18	4	–	2	8	4	2	1	–	–	–	2	1	1	–	–
2. Violence	279	240	39	6	10	144	54	18	5	2	3	4	17	8	4	1	1
3. War	364	210	154	37	22	89	44	11	5	2	37	14	59	29	7	5	2

Notes:
Causes responsible for no deaths have been omitted from this table.
A dash (–) symbol indicates fewer than 500 deaths.
*IA6 is Bacterial meningitis and meningococcaemia; IC3 is Hypertensive disorders of pregnancy; ID is Conditions arising during the perinatal period; IIE6 is Dementia and other degenerative and hereditary CNS disorders; IIH1 is Chronic obstructive pulmonary disease.

Annex Table 12g. Deaths by age, sex and cause (thousands): Latin America and the Caribbean, 2000, baseline scenario

Cause	Total	Male	Female	Males							Females						
				0-4	5-14	15-29	30-44	45-59	60-69	70+	0-4	5-14	15-29	30-44	45-59	60-69	70+
Population (millions)	533	265	267	29	57	74	54	31	11	8	28	55	73	55	32	13	11
All causes	3 537	1 987	1 551	307	63	199	238	302	269	609	229	44	93	124	211	201	650
I. Communicable, maternal, perinatal and nutritional conditions	835	491	345	248	12	60	58	34	23	55	179	14	32	28	19	16	58
A. Infectious and parasitic diseases	472	296	176	108	8	58	55	28	17	22	81	9	21	20	14	10	20
1. Tuberculosis	59	35	24	1	1	6	4	8	7	7	1	1	5	4	5	4	5
2. STDs excluding HIV	9	5	5	4	–	–	–	–	1	1	3	–	–	–	–	1	1
a. Syphilis	9	5	4	4	–	–	–	–	1	1	3	–	–	–	–	1	1
b. Chlamydia	–	–	–	–							–						
c. Gonorrhoea	–	–	–	–							–						
3. HIV	147	118	29	5	–	48	45	13	4	2	5	–	11	9	2	–	1
4. Diarrhoeal diseases	112	64	48	54	1	–	1	–	1	5	37	1	1	1	1	1	5
5. Childhood-cluster diseases	63	34	30	31	2	–	–	–	–	–	27	2	–	–	–	–	–
a. Pertussis	12	6	6	6	–						5	2					
b. Poliomyelitis	1	1	–	1	–						–	–					
c. Diphtheria	–	–	–	–							–						
d. Measles	36	19	17	17	2						15	2					
e. Tetanus	14	8	7	7	–						6	–					
6. Bacterial meningitis*	11	5	5	2	–	–	1	1	1	1	2	–	1	1	1	1	1
7. Hepatitis B and hepatitis C	3	1	2	–							–			1			
8. Malaria	9	4	5	1	1	1	1	–	–	–	1	1	1	1	1	–	–
9. Tropical-cluster diseases	16	8	8	–	–	–	1	2	2	2	–	–	–	2	3	1	2
a. Trypanosomiasis	–	–	–														
b. Chagas disease	15	7	8	–	–	–	1	2	2	2	–	–	–	2	3	1	2
c. Schistosomiasis	–	–	–														
d. Leishmaniasis	–	–	–														
10. Leprosy	1	1	–	–							–						
11. Dengue	–	–	–														
12. Japanese encephalitis	–	–	–														
13. Trachoma	–	–	–														
14. Intestinal nematode infections	2	1	1	–	1	–	–	–	–	–	–	1	–	–	–	–	–
a. Ascariasis	1	1	–	–	1						–	1					
b. Trichuriasis	1	1	–	–	–						–	–					
c. Ancylostomiasis, necatoriasis	–	–	–														
15. Other infectious and parasitic	41	21	20	9	1	1	2	2	2	5	6	1	2	2	2	1	6

Annex Table 12g, continued. Deaths by age, sex and cause (thousands): Latin America and the Caribbean, 2000, baseline scenario

Cause	Total	Male	Female	Males							Females						
				0-4	5-14	15-29	30-44	45-59	60-69	70+	0-4	5-14	15-29	30-44	45-59	60-69	70+
B. Respiratory infections	151	81	70	42	3	1	2	4	5	24	29	3	2	3	3	4	26
1. Lower respiratory infections	149	80	69	41	3	1	2	4	5	24	28	3	2	3	3	4	26
2. Upper respiratory infections	2	1	1	-	-	-	-	-	-	-	-	-	-	-	-	-	-
3. Otitis media	-	-	-	-	-	-	-	-	-	-	-	-	-	-	-	-	-
C. Maternal conditions	11	-	11	-	-	-	-	-	-	-	-	-	7	4	-	-	-
1. Maternal haemorrhage	3	-	3	-	-	-	-	-	-	-	-	-	2	1	-	-	-
2. Maternal sepsis	1	-	1	-	-	-	-	-	-	-	-	-	1	-	-	-	-
3. Hypertensive disorders*	1	-	1	-	-	-	-	-	-	-	-	-	-	1	-	-	-
4. Obstructed labour	1	-	1	-	-	-	-	-	-	-	-	-	1	-	-	-	-
5. Abortion	1	-	1	-	-	-	-	-	-	-	-	-	1	-	-	-	-
6. Other maternal	3	-	3	-	-	-	-	-	-	-	-	-	2	1	-	-	-
D. Perinatal conditions*	140	83	57	83	-	-	-	-	-	-	57	-	-	-	-	-	-
E. Nutritional deficiencies	61	31	31	16	2	1	1	1	2	9	12	2	1	1	2	2	11
1. Protein-energy malnutrition	43	22	20	13	1	1	1	1	1	6	9	1	-	1	1	1	8
2. Iodine deficiency	1	-	-	-	-	-	-	-	-	-	-	-	-	-	-	-	-
3. Vitamin A deficiency	3	2	2	1	-	-	-	-	-	-	1	-	-	-	-	-	-
4. Iron-deficiency anaemia	14	6	8	1	1	-	-	1	1	2	1	1	1	1	1	-	3
II. Noncommunicable diseases	2 225	1 138	1 086	41	19	18	83	219	228	531	36	15	26	74	180	178	577
A. Malignant neoplasms	477	238	240	2	7	4	15	51	56	102	2	5	7	27	63	52	85
1. Mouth and oropharynx cancers	17	12	5	-	-	-	1	1	3	4	-	-	-	-	1	1	3
2. Oesophagus cancer	14	10	5	-	-	-	-	3	3	4	-	-	-	-	1	1	3
3. Stomach cancer	53	32	21	-	-	-	1	7	9	14	-	-	-	1	4	5	11
4. Colon and rectum cancers	32	15	17	-	-	-	1	3	3	7	-	-	-	1	3	4	9
5. Liver cancer	8	4	4	-	-	-	-	1	1	2	-	1	-	1	-	-	2
6. Pancreas cancer	11	6	6	-	-	-	-	1	2	2	-	-	-	-	1	2	3
7. Trachea, bronchus, lung cancers	53	37	15	-	-	-	2	11	10	14	-	-	-	1	5	6	3
8. Melanoma and other skin cancers	4	2	2	-	-	-	-	1	-	1	-	-	1	-	-	-	1
9. Breast cancer	40	-	40	-	-	-	-	-	-	-	-	-	1	5	14	8	12
10. Cervix uteri cancer	33	-	33	-	-	-	-	-	-	-	-	-	1	6	12	6	8
11. Corpus uteri cancer	9	-	9	-	-	-	-	-	-	-	-	-	-	1	3	2	3
12. Ovary cancer	8	-	8	-	-	-	-	-	-	-	-	-	-	1	2	2	3
13. Prostate cancer	29	29	-	-	-	-	-	2	9	18	-	-	-	-	-	-	-
14. Bladder cancer	12	9	3	-	-	-	-	2	2	5	-	-	-	-	-	1	2
15. Lymphomas, multiple myeloma	21	12	10	-	1	1	2	2	2	3	-	-	1	1	2	2	4
16. Leukaemia	16	9	7	1	2	1	1	1	1	2	1	2	1	1	-	1	1
17. Other cancers	116	63	53	1	3	1	4	13	12	28	1	2	2	8	13	10	16

Annex Table 12g, continued. Deaths by age, sex and cause (thousands): Latin America and the Caribbean, 2000, baseline scenario

Cause	Total	Male	Female	Males 0-4	5-14	15-29	30-44	45-59	60-69	70+	Females 0-4	5-14	15-29	30-44	45-59	60-69	70+
B. Other neoplasms	10	5	5	–	1	–	1	1	1	1	–	–	–	1	1	1	2
C. Diabetes mellitus	103	41	63	–	–	–	3	9	10	18	–	–	1	2	11	16	32
D. Endocrine disorders	30	14	16	4	1	1	2	–	1	5	3	1	1	1	2	1	7
E. Neuro-psychiatric conditions	53	32	21	3	3	2	7	7	3	7	3	2	3	3	2	2	6
2. Bipolar disorder	4	2	1	–	–	–	1	1	–	–	–	–	–	–	–	–	1
3. Schizophrenia	4	2	2	–	–	–	1	1	–	–	–	–	–	–	1	1	–
4. Epilepsy	6	3	3	1	–	1	1	–	–	–	1	–	1	1	–	–	–
5. Alcohol use	12	11	1	–	–	1	4	4	1	1	–	–	–	1	–	–	–
6. Dementia*	9	4	5	–	–	–	–	–	1	3	–	–	–	–	1	1	3
7. Parkinson disease	2	1	1	–	–	–	–	–	–	1	–	–	–	–	–	–	1
8. Multiple sclerosis	2	1	1	–	–	1	–	–	–	–	–	–	–	1	–	–	–
9. Drug use	2	1	1	2	2	1	1	1	–	–	2	2	1	–	–	–	–
13. Other neuro-psychiatric	14	7	6	–	–	1	1	1	–	1	2	2	1	–	1	–	–
F. Sense organ diseases	1	–	–	–	–	–	–	–	–	–	–	–	–	–	–	–	–
1. Glaucoma	–	–	–	–	–	–	–	–	–	–	–	–	–	–	–	–	–
2. Cataracts	–	–	–	–	–	–	–	–	–	–	–	–	–	–	–	–	–
G. Cardiovascular diseases	1 083	550	533	4	3	5	33	101	114	291	3	2	7	26	70	77	349
1. Rheumatic heart disease	9	3	6	–	–	1	1	–	–	1	–	–	1	1	2	1	1
2. Ischaemic heart disease	484	252	233	–	–	1	13	47	54	137	–	–	1	8	28	35	160
3. Cerebrovascular disease	342	170	172	1	–	1	10	32	35	90	–	1	2	10	25	26	110
4. Inflammatory heart diseases	31	16	15	–	1	1	2	2	4	6	1	–	1	2	3	1	7
5. Other cardiovascular	216	109	107	3	1	2	6	17	21	59	2	1	3	5	12	14	71
H. Respiratory diseases	176	94	82	6	1	1	4	10	16	55	4	1	2	4	12	13	47
1. COPD*	97	54	43	1	–	1	1	5	10	36	1	–	–	1	5	8	28
2. Asthma	19	8	10	–	–	1	1	1	1	4	–	–	1	1	2	2	5
3. Other respiratory	60	32	29	5	–	1	2	4	5	15	3	–	1	2	4	4	14
I. Digestive diseases	176	108	67	2	1	2	17	33	20	32	2	1	2	7	14	12	31
1. Peptic ulcer	15	9	6	–	–	–	1	2	1	5	–	–	–	–	1	1	4
2. Cirrhosis of the liver	78	57	21	–	–	1	12	23	11	10	–	–	1	3	7	4	6
3. Appendicitis	2	1	1	–	–	1	–	–	–	–	–	–	1	–	–	–	–
4. Other digestive	81	42	39	2	1	1	4	9	8	17	2	–	1	3	6	6	21
J. Genito-urinary diseases	61	31	30	1	1	1	2	4	5	17	1	1	2	3	5	4	14
1. Nephritis and nephrosis	44	22	22	1	1	1	2	4	4	10	1	1	1	2	4	3	10
2. Benign prostatic hypertrophy	2	2	–	–	–	–	–	–	1	2	–	–	–	–	–	–	–
3. Other genito-urinary	14	7	8	–	–	–	1	1	1	4	1	–	1	1	1	1	4
K. Skin diseases	4	1	2	–	–	–	–	–	–	1	–	–	–	–	–	1	1

Annex Table 12g, continued. Deaths by age, sex and cause (thousands): Latin America and the Caribbean, 2000, baseline scenario

Cause	Total	Male	Female	Males							Females						
				0-4	5-14	15-29	30-44	45-59	60-69	70+	0-4	5-14	15-29	30-44	45-59	60-69	70+
L. Musculo-skeletal diseases	10	3	7	–	–	–	–	–	–	2	–	–	1	1	1	1	3
1. Rheumatoid arthritis	2	1	1	–	–	–	–	–	–	–	–	–	1	1	1	1	1
3. Other musculo-skeletal	8	2	6	–	–	–	–	–	–	1	–	–	1	–	–	–	2
M. Congenital anomalies	41	20	20	17	2	1	–	–	–	–	17	1	1	–	–	–	–
N. Oral conditions	–	–	–	–	–	–	–	–	–	–	–	–	–	–	–	–	–
III. Injuries	*477*	*358*	*120*	*18*	*31*	*121*	*97*	*50*	*18*	*24*	*14*	*15*	*35*	*21*	*12*	*7*	*16*
A. Unintentional injuries	302	215	87	15	26	58	51	32	13	19	11	13	21	13	9	5	15
1. Road traffic accidents	143	104	39	3	13	32	27	16	6	6	3	7	12	8	5	2	3
2. Poisonings	5	3	2	1	–	–	1	–	–	–	–	–	1	–	–	–	–
3. Falls	24	15	9	1	1	2	3	2	1	5	–	–	–	–	1	1	6
4. Fires	8	4	3	1	1	1	1	1	–	1	1	–	1	1	–	–	–
5. Drownings	29	23	6	3	5	8	5	2	1	1	2	2	1	1	–	–	–
6. Other unintentional	92	65	27	7	6	15	16	11	4	7	5	3	6	4	3	2	5
B. Intentional injuries	176	143	33	3	5	63	45	18	5	4	3	2	14	8	3	1	1
1. Self-inflicted injuries	29	20	8	–	–	7	6	4	2	2	–	–	4	2	1	1	1
2. Violence	126	111	16	1	3	51	37	13	3	2	1	1	7	4	1	1	1
3. War	20	12	9	2	1	5	3	1	–	–	2	1	3	2	–	–	–

Notes:
Causes responsible for no deaths have been omitted from this table.
A dash (-) symbol indicates fewer than 500 deaths.
*IA6 is Bacterial meningitis and meningococcaemia; IC3 is Hypertensive disorders of pregnancy; ID is Conditions arising during the perinatal period; IIE6 is Dementia and other degenerative and hereditary CNS disorders; IIH1 is Chronic obstructive pulmonary disease.

Annex Table 12h. Deaths by age, sex and cause (thousands): Middle Eastern Crescent, 2000, baseline scenario

Cause	Total	Male	Female	Males							Females						
				0-4	5-14	15-29	30-44	45-59	60-69	70+	0-4	5-14	15-29	30-44	45-59	60-69	70+
Population (millions)	*656*	*333*	*322*	*50*	*83*	*90*	*60*	*32*	*11*	*7*	*47*	*80*	*86*	*57*	*31*	*12*	*9*
All causes	**5 101**	**2 777**	**2 324**	**895**	**149**	**187**	**204**	**346**	**329**	**666**	**813**	**126**	**129**	**122**	**204**	**228**	**702**
I. Communicable, maternal, perinatal and nutritional conditions	*1 692*	*878*	*813*	*708*	*34*	*17*	*18*	*22*	*30*	*48*	*646*	*33*	*24*	*24*	*17*	*20*	*48*
A. Infectious and parasitic diseases	**750**	**407**	**344**	**314**	**18**	**15**	**16**	**20**	**12**	**12**	**284**	**15**	**8**	**7**	**11**	**7**	**10**
1. Tuberculosis	84	54	30	5	2	10	9	14	8	7	3	1	5	4	7	5	5
2. STDs excluding HIV	12	6	6	6	–	–	–	–	–	–	5	–	–	–	–	–	–
a. Syphilis	12	6	6	6	–	–	–	–	–	–	5	–	–	–	–	–	–
b. Chlamydia	–	–	–	–	–	–	–	–	–	–	–	–	–	–	–	–	–
c. Gonorrhoea	–	–	–	–	–	–	–	–	–	–	–	–	–	–	–	–	–
3. HIV	12	10	2	1	–	3	4	2	–	–	1	–	–	1	–	–	–
4. Diarrhoeal diseases	368	192	176	184	5	–	–	–	–	1	167	5	1	–	–	–	1
5. Childhood-cluster diseases	202	105	97	97	7	–	–	–	–	–	89	6	1	–	–	–	–
a. Pertussis	45	24	22	22	2	–	–	–	–	–	20	1	1	–	–	–	–
b. Poliomyelitis	3	2	1	2	–	–	–	–	–	–	1	–	–	–	–	–	–
c. Diphtheria	1	1	–	–	1	–	–	–	–	–	–	–	–	–	–	–	–
d. Measles	82	43	39	38	4	1	–	–	–	–	35	4	–	–	–	–	–
e. Tetanus	71	37	34	35	1	1	–	–	–	–	32	1	1	–	–	–	–
6. Bacterial meningitis*	15	8	7	4	–	1	1	1	1	1	4	1	1	–	1	1	1
7. Hepatitis B and hepatitis C	11	6	5	1	–	1	1	1	1	2	1	–	1	1	1	1	1
8. Malaria	5	3	2	1	1	1	–	–	–	–	1	1	1	–	–	–	1
9. Tropical-cluster diseases	3	2	1	–	–	1	1	1	1	1	–	–	1	1	1	1	1
a. Trypanosomiasis	–	–	–	–	–	–	–	–	–	–	–	–	–	–	–	–	–
b. Chagas disease	–	–	–	–	–	–	–	–	–	–	–	–	–	–	–	–	–
c. Schistosomiasis	2	1	1	–	–	–	–	1	–	–	–	–	–	1	–	–	–
d. Leishmaniasis	1	1	1	–	–	1	1	–	–	–	–	–	1	–	–	–	–
10. Leprosy	–	–	–	–	–	–	–	–	–	–	–	–	–	–	–	–	–
11. Dengue	–	–	–	–	–	–	–	–	–	–	–	–	–	–	–	–	–
12. Japanese encephalitis	–	–	–	–	–	–	–	–	–	–	–	–	–	–	–	–	–
13. Trachoma	–	–	–	–	–	–	–	–	–	–	–	–	–	–	–	–	–
14. Intestinal nematode infections	1	1	–	–	–	1	–	1	1	1	–	–	–	–	1	–	1
a. Ascariasis	–	–	–	–	–	–	–	–	–	–	–	–	–	–	–	–	–
b. Trichuriasis	–	–	–	–	–	–	–	–	–	–	–	–	–	–	–	–	–
c. Ancylostomiasis, necatoriasis	–	–	–	–	–	–	–	–	–	–	–	–	–	–	–	–	–
15. Other infectious and parasitic	37	20	17	15	1	1	1	1	1	1	14	1	1	–	1	1	1

Annex Table 12h, continued. Deaths by age, sex and cause (thousands): Middle Eastern Crescent, 2000, baseline scenario

Cause	Total	Male	Female	Males							Females						
				0-4	5-14	15-29	30-44	45-59	60-69	70+	0-4	5-14	15-29	30-44	45-59	60-69	70+
B. Respiratory infections	**478**	**248**	**230**	**176**	**14**	**2**	**1**	**2**	**18**	**35**	**160**	**15**	**2**	**1**	**3**	**12**	**36**
1. Lower respiratory infections	470	244	226	173	14	2	1	2	18	35	157	15	2	1	3	12	36
2. Upper respiratory infections	5	2	2	2	-	-	-	-	-	-	2	-	-	-	-	-	-
3. Otitis media	3	2	1	1	-	-	-	-	-	-	1	-	-	-	-	-	-
C. Maternal conditions	**30**	-	**30**	-	-	-	-	-	-	-	-	-	**13**	**15**	**2**	-	-
1. Maternal haemorrhage	7	-	7	-	-	-	-	-	-	-	-	-	3	4	-	-	-
2. Maternal sepsis	5	-	5	-	-	-	-	-	-	-	-	-	2	2	1	-	-
3. Hypertensive disorders*	3	-	3	-	-	-	-	-	-	-	-	-	1	2	-	-	-
4. Obstructed labour	2	-	2	-	-	-	-	-	-	-	-	-	1	1	-	-	-
5. Abortion	2	-	2	-	-	-	-	-	-	-	-	-	1	1	-	-	-
6. Other maternal	2	-	2	-	-	-	-	-	-	-	-	-	1	1	-	-	-
D. Perinatal conditions*	**351**	**182**	**169**	**182**	-	-	-	-	-	-	-	**169**	-	-	-	-	-	-
E. Nutritional deficiencies	**82**	**42**	**41**	**36**	**3**	-	-	-	-	**2**	**33**	**3**	**1**	**1**	-	-	**2**
1. Protein-energy malnutrition	55	29	27	27	1	-	-	-	-	1	25	1	-	-	-	-	1
2. Iodine deficiency	3	2	1	1	-	-	-	-	-	-	1	-	-	-	-	-	-
3. Vitamin A deficiency	17	8	8	6	2	-	-	-	-	-	6	2	-	-	-	-	-
4. Iron-deficiency anaemia	8	3	4	2	-	-	-	-	-	1	1	-	1	1	-	-	1
II. Noncommunicable diseases	**2 830**	**1 521**	**1 309**	**132**	**64**	**47**	**99**	**286**	**286**	**607**	**115**	**65**	**47**	**65**	**173**	**200**	**644**
A. Malignant neoplasms	**320**	**187**	**133**	**3**	**10**	**7**	**17**	**56**	**45**	**49**	**3**	**8**	**7**	**16**	**34**	**30**	**35**
1. Mouth and oropharynx cancers	21	14	7	-	-	1	2	3	4	4	-	-	-	1	1	2	3
2. Oesophagus cancer	13	8	5	-	-	-	1	3	2	2	-	-	-	-	-	2	3
3. Stomach cancer	28	17	11	-	-	1	2	6	4	4	-	-	-	1	2	4	4
4. Colon and rectum cancers	17	9	8	-	-	-	1	2	3	3	-	-	-	-	2	3	3
5. Liver cancer	11	7	4	-	-	-	1	3	2	1	-	-	-	-	1	1	2
6. Pancreas cancer	6	4	2	-	-	-	1	1	1	1	-	-	-	-	-	1	1
7. Trachea, bronchus, lung cancers	64	50	14	-	-	1	3	19	12	14	-	-	-	1	4	4	5
8. Melanoma and other skin cancers	2	1	1	-	-	-	-	-	-	1	-	-	-	-	-	-	1
9. Breast cancer	16	-	16	-	-	-	-	-	-	-	-	-	1	3	6	3	3
10. Cervix uteri cancer	10	-	10	-	-	-	-	-	-	-	-	-	1	1	4	2	2
11. Corpus uteri cancer	3	-	3	-	-	-	-	-	-	-	-	-	-	-	1	1	1
12. Ovary cancer	5	-	5	-	-	-	-	-	-	-	-	-	-	1	2	1	1
13. Prostate cancer	6	6	-	-	-	-	-	1	2	3	-	-	-	-	-	-	-
14. Bladder cancer	13	11	2	-	-	-	2	3	3	3	-	-	-	-	-	1	1
15. Lymphomas, multiple myeloma	12	8	4	-	-	1	2	1	3	1	-	1	-	1	1	1	1
16. Leukaemia	17	9	8	1	3	2	1	1	1	-	2	4	1	-	-	1	-
17. Other cancers	76	44	31	2	5	2	4	11	9	10	2	4	2	5	7	6	6

Annex Table 12h, continued. Deaths by age, sex and cause (thousands): Middle Eastern Crescent, 2000, baseline scenario

				Males							Females						
Cause	Total	Male	Female	0-4	5-14	15-29	30-44	45-59	60-69	70+	0-4	5-14	15-29	30-44	45-59	60-69	70+
B. Other neoplasms	7	3	3	–	1	–	–	1	–	1	–	1	1	–	1	–	1
C. Diabetes mellitus	67	31	36	1	2	1	3	7	7	10	1	2	1	2	7	9	14
D. Endocrine disorders	18	9	9	3	1	1	1	1	1	1	3	2	1	2	1	1	1
E. Neuro-psychiatric conditions	66	35	30	8	6	4	3	4	3	7	6	6	3	2	3	2	8
2. Bipolar disorder	1	–	1	–	–	–	–	–	–	–	–	–	–	–	1	–	–
3. Schizophrenia	4	2	2	–	–	–	1	1	–	–	–	–	–	1	–	–	1
4. Epilepsy	9	5	4	1	1	1	1	1	–	–	–	1	1	–	1	–	–
5. Alcohol use	1	1	–	–	–	–	–	1	–	–	–	–	–	–	–	–	–
6. Dementia*	11	5	6	–	–	–	–	–	1	3	–	–	–	–	1	1	4
7. Parkinson disease	3	2	1	–	–	–	–	–	–	2	–	–	–	–	–	–	1
8. Multiple sclerosis	2	1	1	–	–	–	–	–	–	1	–	–	–	–	–	–	–
9. Drug use	2	2	–	–	–	2	–	–	–	–	–	–	–	–	–	–	–
13. Other neuro-psychiatric	33	18	15	7	5	2	1	1	–	1	5	5	2	1	1	–	1
F. Sense organ diseases	–	–	–	–	–	–	–	–	–	–	–	–	–	–	–	–	–
1. Glaucoma	–	–	–	–	–	–	–	–	–	–	–	–	–	–	–	–	–
2. Cataracts	–	–	–	–	–	–	–	–	–	–	–	–	–	–	–	–	–
G. Cardiovascular diseases	1 755	920	834	41	30	22	52	158	180	438	31	28	22	31	92	124	507
1. Rheumatic heart disease	25	12	13	–	3	4	3	1	1	–	–	3	4	3	2	1	1
2. Ischaemic heart disease	863	462	401	–	–	3	25	86	100	248	–	–	3	12	42	66	277
3. Cerebrovascular disease	291	139	152	2	5	3	6	24	29	70	2	4	2	4	18	24	99
4. Inflammatory heart diseases	85	46	39	8	6	4	5	8	4	11	7	5	4	4	5	3	11
5. Other cardiovascular	490	261	228	31	17	8	12	39	46	109	22	16	9	8	25	30	119
H. Respiratory diseases	241	133	108	17	5	2	5	20	24	61	15	7	3	4	13	16	50
1. COPD*	122	71	51	4	1	–	1	10	15	40	4	1	–	1	6	9	30
2. Asthma	15	8	7	–	–	–	1	1	1	3	–	–	–	1	1	1	3
3. Other respiratory	103	54	49	13	3	2	3	8	8	17	11	6	2	2	5	5	17
I. Digestive diseases	168	97	71	16	4	4	10	26	17	19	17	4	3	5	14	11	17
1. Peptic ulcer	7	5	2	–	–	1	1	1	1	2	–	–	–	–	–	–	1
2. Cirrhosis of the liver	54	32	23	–	1	1	4	11	7	7	–	1	1	2	6	5	7
3. Appendicitis	4	2	2	–	1	1	–	–	–	–	–	–	–	–	–	–	–
4. Other digestive	102	58	45	15	3	2	5	13	9	10	17	2	2	3	7	5	9
J. Genito-urinary diseases	98	58	40	3	3	4	7	13	9	20	2	3	4	4	8	6	12
1. Nephritis and nephrosis	42	23	18	2	2	2	3	4	3	8	1	2	2	2	3	3	5
2. Benign prostatic hypertrophy	2	2	–	–	–	–	–	–	1	1	–	–	–	–	–	–	–
3. Other genito-urinary	55	33	22	1	1	2	4	8	6	10	1	1	2	3	5	4	7
K. Skin diseases	2	1	1	–	–	–	–	–	–	–	–	–	–	–	–	–	–

Annex Table 12h, continued. Deaths by age, sex and cause (thousands): Middle Eastern Crescent, 2000, baseline scenario

Cause	Total	Male	Female	Males							Females						
				0-4	5-14	15-29	30-44	45-59	60-69	70+	0-4	5-14	15-29	30-44	45-59	60-69	70+
L. Musculo-skeletal diseases	2	1	1	-	-	-	-	-	-	-	-	-	-	-	-	-	-
1. Rheumatoid arthritis	-	-	1	-	-	-	-	-	-	-	-	-	-	-	-	-	-
3. Other musculo-skeletal	2	1	1	-	-	-	-	-	-	-	-	-	-	-	-	-	-
M. Congenital anomalies	86	45	41	38	2	2	1	1	-	-	35	3	1	1	1	-	-
N. Oral conditions	-	-	-	-	-	-	-	-	-	-	-	-	-	-	-	-	-
III. Injuries	*579*	*377*	*202*	*55*	*51*	*123*	*88*	*37*	*13*	*11*	*52*	*28*	*57*	*33*	*14*	*8*	*9*
A. Unintentional injuries	248	176	72	28	25	48	43	20	6	6	24	11	13	9	6	3	5
1. Road traffic accidents	91	71	20	3	10	24	21	8	2	2	3	5	4	4	2	1	1
2. Poisonings	16	10	5	2	1	2	3	2	1	-	2	-	1	1	1	-	1
3. Falls	14	10	4	2	1	2	2	1	1	1	2	1	1	-	1	-	1
4. Fires	18	8	10	3	1	2	1	1	-	-	3	1	3	1	1	-	1
5. Drownings	32	23	9	7	6	6	3	1	-	-	6	2	1	-	-	-	-
6. Other unintentional	77	54	23	12	7	13	12	6	2	2	10	3	3	3	2	1	2
B. Intentional injuries	331	202	129	28	26	75	45	16	6	5	28	16	44	24	8	5	4
1. Self-inflicted injuries	62	43	19	-	10	12	9	6	2	3	-	5	6	3	2	1	2
2. Violence	50	32	17	7	3	10	8	3	1	1	8	3	3	2	1	-	1
3. War	219	126	93	21	13	53	28	7	3	1	20	9	35	19	5	3	1

Notes:
Causes responsible for no deaths have been omitted from this table.
A dash (-) symbol indicates fewer than 500 deaths.
*IA6 is Bacterial meningitis and meningococcaemia; IC3 is Hypertensive disorders of pregnancy; ID is Conditions arising during the perinatal period; IIE6 is Dementia and other degenerative and hereditary CNS disorders; IIH1 is Chronic obstructive pulmonary disease.

Annex Table 12i. Deaths by age, sex and cause (thousands): World, 2000, baseline scenario

Cause	Total	Male	Female	Males 0-4	5-14	15-29	30-44	45-59	60-69	70+	Females 0-4	5-14	15-29	30-44	45-59	60-69	70+
Population (millions)	6 160	3 096	3 064	346	628	799	645	403	159	116	330	604	764	624	403	174	163
All causes	56 116	30 625	25 491	5 613	1 014	1 903	2 539	4 630	4 819	10 108	4 853	852	1 295	1 463	2 627	3 094	11 306
I. Communicable, maternal, perinatal and nutritional conditions	14 931	7 938	6 993	4 628	336	432	583	528	411	1 019	3 990	356	522	515	348	273	989
A. Infectious and parasitic diseases	8 841	4 900	3 942	2 477	234	408	557	485	280	460	2 099	239	382	375	302	175	371
1. Tuberculosis	2 092	1 245	847	47	28	156	198	331	194	291	42	33	140	126	213	111	182
2. STDs excluding HIV	178	85	93	66		1	1	2	3	12	58		6	7	3	3	16
a. Syphilis	166	85	81	66		1	1	2	3	12	58			1	2	3	15
b. Chlamydia	8	-	8										4	4			
c. Gonorrhoea	4	-	4										2	2			
3. HIV	1 318	759	559	137	19	197	289	84	22	11	127	19	184	187	31	8	4
4. Diarrhoeal diseases	2 246	1 202	1 044	1 040	49	8	11	12	21	59	868	53	11	12	13	18	70
5. Childhood-cluster diseases	1 529	810	719	714	68	6	9	5	3	5	627	67	6	7	5	2	5
a. Pertussis	272	145	127	136	9						119	8					
b. Poliomyelitis	19	11	8	11							8						
c. Diphtheria	7	4	3	3							3						
d. Measles	848	450	398	402	48						351	46					
e. Tetanus	383	200	183	162	11	6	9	5	3	5	146	12	6	7	5	2	5
6. Bacterial meningitis*	122	64	58	32	2	2	9	7	7	7	28	2	1	8	7	6	8
7. Hepatitis B and hepatitis C	76	44	32	5	2	3	6	10	6	13	4	2	2	3	4	5	11
8. Malaria	740	411	330	331	29	19	14	10	4	4	253	29	18	13	10	4	4
9. Tropical-cluster diseases	80	45	35	2	12	9	8	8	3	3	2	9	7	6	6	3	3
a. Trypanosomiasis	32	17	15		5	4	3	4	1	1	1	5	4	3	2	1	2
b. Chagas disease	15	7	8				1	2	2	2				2	3		
c. Schistosomiasis	6	4	2				1	1	1					1			
d. Leishmaniasis	28	17	10	2	7	5	3	1			1	4	2	1			
10. Leprosy	2	1	1														
11. Dengue	11	5	6	1	3						1						
12. Japanese encephalitis	3	1	1	1							1						
13. Trachoma	-	-	-														
14. Intestinal nematode infections	12	6	6		5							4					
a. Ascariasis	6	3	3		3							3					
b. Trichuriasis	4	2	2		2							2					
c. Ancylostomiasis, necatoriasis	3	2	2														
15. Other infectious and parasitic	432	221	211	100	16	8	12	15	17	54	87	18	6	7	10	15	68

Annex Table 12i, continued. Deaths by age, sex and cause (thousands): World, 2000, baseline scenario

Cause	Total	Male	Female	Males							Females						
				0-4	5-14	15-29	30-44	45-59	60-69	70+	0-4	5-14	15-29	30-44	45-59	60-69	70+
B. Respiratory infections	3 564	1 851	1 714	1 041	85	19	22	38	124	522	893	92	21	18	32	90	569
1. Lower respiratory infections	3 510	1 823	1 687	1 021	84	19	22	37	122	517	875	90	20	17	31	89	563
2. Upper respiratory infections	35	18	17	11	1	–	–	–	1	5	9	1	–	–	–	1	5
3. Otitis media	20	10	10	9	1	–	–	–	–	–	9	1	–	–	–	–	–
C. Maternal conditions	244	–	244								–	7	113	117	7	–	–
1. Maternal haemorrhage	60		60									2	28	28	2		
2. Maternal sepsis	37		37									1	17	18	1		
3. Hypertensive disorders*	21		21									1	9	10	1		
4. Obstructed labour	10		10										5	5			
5. Abortion	19		19										9	9	1		
6. Other maternal	33		33									1	15	16	1		
D. Perinatal conditions*	1 797	951	846	951								846						
E. Nutritional deficiencies	484	236	248	159	17	5	4	6	8	38	152	18	7	6	7	8	50
1. Protein-energy malnutrition	295	147	148	117	2	1	1	2	4	20	112	3	1	1	2	3	24
2. Iodine deficiency	14	7	7	6	1	–	–	–	–	–	5	1	–	–	–	–	–
3. Vitamin A deficiency	75	39	36	27	11	1	–	–	–	–	25	10	1	–	–	–	–
4. Iron-deficiency anaemia	97	41	56	8	3	3	3	3	4	17	9	4	4	5	5	5	24
II. Noncommunicable diseases	35 086	18 688	16 399	576	283	318	1 052	3 528	4 170	8 760	530	258	279	626	2 033	2 679	9 993
A. Malignant neoplasms	7 865	4 623	3 242	30	69	82	335	1 223	1 215	1 669	31	50	79	252	762	738	1 329
1. Mouth and oropharynx cancers	381	252	129	1	1	6	24	71	69	81	1	1	4	10	31	35	46
2. Oesophagus cancer	493	336	157	–	–	2	16	98	101	118	–	–	2	4	36	49	66
3. Stomach cancer	1 010	649	360	–	–	5	31	183	188	242	–	1	5	23	73	88	172
4. Colon and rectum cancers	592	309	283	–	1	5	18	60	79	147	–	–	3	13	45	64	158
5. Liver cancer	703	512	191	1	2	11	86	191	116	104	1	2	3	18	52	47	69
6. Pancreas cancer	228	129	99	–	–	–	5	32	35	55	–	–	–	2	15	24	58
7. Trachea, bronchus, lung cancers	1 331	997	333	–	1	5	41	303	310	337	–	–	2	12	76	94	149
8. Melanoma and other skin cancers	58	30	28	–	–	1	3	8	6	11	–	–	1	2	6	6	13
9. Breast cancer	380	–	380	–	–	–	–	–	–	–	–	–	10	44	120	76	129
10. Cervix uteri cancer	253		253								–	–	10	28	98	52	65
11. Corpus uteri cancer	76		76								–	–	1	3	19	18	35
12. Ovary cancer	125		125								–	1	5	14	34	28	42
13. Prostate cancer	253	253	–	–	–	–	1	17	61	173							
14. Bladder cancer	170	128	42	–	–	–	3	22	35	67	–	–	–	1	5	10	26
15. Lymphomas, multiple myeloma	263	155	108	1	2	8	17	31	33	48	3	7	4	8	18	22	47
16. Leukaemia	270	147	123	9	21	13	24	24	20	36	10	15	11	18	19	16	34
17. Other cancers	1 281	725	556	14	30	23	67	182	161	249	16	22	20	52	116	110	220

Annex Table 12i, continued. Deaths by age, sex and cause (thousands): World, 2000, baseline scenario

Cause	Total	Male	Female	Males							Females						
				0-4	5-14	15-29	30-44	45-59	60-69	70+	0-4	5-14	15-29	30-44	45-59	60-69	70+
B. Other neoplasms	109	55	53	3	5	3	5	10	9	19	3	4	3	4	8	9	23
C. Diabetes mellitus	627	261	366	5	7	4	18	50	60	116	5	7	5	10	51	85	204
D. Endocrine disorders	152	68	84	13	4	3	6	9	9	25	12	5	4	4	9	9	42
E. Neuro-psychiatric conditions	749	383	366	26	22	32	52	56	47	148	25	18	20	21	28	39	215
2. Bipolar disorder	18	5	13	–	–	1	1	1	1	1	–	–	1	2	1	1	10
3. Schizophrenia	56	29	27	–	–	2	6	5	4	12	–	–	7	5	3	4	17
4. Epilepsy	65	38	26	2	4	7	10	7	3	5	2	3	1	1	3	2	4
5. Alcohol use	57	49	9	–	–	1	14	19	8	6	–	–	–	1	3	2	2
6. Dementia*	237	93	145	3	1	2	2	7	13	65	4	1	1	2	6	14	117
7. Parkinson disease	70	37	33	–	–	–	–	1	5	31	–	–	–	–	1	3	29
8. Multiple sclerosis	25	11	15	–	–	–	3	4	2	2	–	–	1	2	5	3	4
9. Drug use	10	8	2	–	–	4	3	1	–	–	–	–	1	1	–	–	–
13. Other neuro-psychiatric	211	114	98	21	16	15	13	12	12	24	19	14	10	7	6	9	32
F. Sense organ diseases	20	11	10	1	–	–	–	3	3	3	–	–	–	1	2	3	3
1. Glaucoma	7	4	3	–	–	–	–	1	1	1	–	–	–	–	1	1	1
2. Cataracts	6	4	3	–	–	–	–	1	1	1	–	–	–	–	1	1	1
G. Cardiovascular diseases	18 069	9 087	8 982	120	90	107	385	1 488	2 007	4 891	96	87	92	210	792	1 312	6 392
1. Rheumatic heart disease	385	173	213	–	7	18	26	46	29	47	1	9	17	28	52	33	72
2. Ischaemic heart disease	8 000	4 120	3 881	–	–	11	145	699	956	2 309	–	–	7	66	296	583	2 923
3. Cerebrovascular disease	5 580	2 687	2 893	15	20	24	93	411	619	1 504	12	17	16	56	266	447	2 079
4. Inflammatory heart diseases	574	301	273	23	17	18	36	68	41	96	24	18	15	21	40	30	125
5. Other cardiovascular	3 529	1 807	1 722	81	45	36	84	264	362	935	54	44	37	39	137	219	1 192
H. Respiratory diseases	3 890	2 149	1 742	57	23	18	55	249	479	1 266	50	23	18	36	167	277	1 172
1. COPD*	2 923	1 618	1 305	15	4	4	20	171	383	1 022	16	4	2	14	110	217	940
2. Asthma	187	96	91	1	4	4	10	17	18	42	1	2	3	7	16	17	45
3. Other respiratory	780	434	346	41	16	10	25	62	78	202	33	17	12	14	41	43	186
I. Digestive diseases	2 072	1 266	807	42	22	34	150	365	258	393	42	23	26	54	148	136	377
1. Peptic ulcer	208	126	82	–	3	3	10	29	25	57	–	–	2	4	11	12	52
2. Cirrhosis of the liver	882	611	271	3	–	13	87	226	140	139	1	4	8	24	77	62	93
3. Appendicitis	46	27	18	1	7	7	7	3	2	1	2	6	4	4	2	1	1
4. Other digestive	937	502	436	38	12	11	45	108	92	196	39	12	12	22	58	61	231
J. Genito-urinary diseases	784	421	363	18	21	19	36	64	70	193	14	21	17	24	53	59	175
1. Nephritis and nephrosis	563	293	271	15	18	16	28	47	49	119	13	19	13	19	40	44	123
2. Benign prostatic hypertrophy	37	37	–	–	–	–	–	1	6	29	–	–	–	–	–	–	–
3. Other genito-urinary	183	92	92	3	3	3	8	16	15	44	1	2	4	5	13	14	52
K. Skin diseases	48	23	25	6	1	1	1	2	2	10	5	–	1	1	2	2	14

Annex Table 12i, continued. Deaths by age, sex and cause (thousands): World, 2000, baseline scenario

Cause	Total	Male	Female	Males							Females						
				0-4	5-14	15-29	30-44	45-59	60-69	70+	0-4	5-14	15-29	30-44	45-59	60-69	70+
L. Musculo-skeletal diseases	105	38	67	1	1	1	2	4	8	22	1	1	3	4	7	8	43
1. Rheumatoid arthritis	18	5	12	-	-	1	2	1	1	3	-	-	3	4	1	2	8
3. Other musculo-skeletal	87	33	54	1	-	1	1	3	7	19	1	1	3	4	6	6	35
M. Congenital anomalies	594	301	293	254	17	13	7	5	2	3	246	18	11	5	6	3	4
N. Oral conditions	2	1	1	-	-	-	-	-	-	-	-	-	-	-	-	-	-
III. Injuries	6 099	4 000	2 099	409	396	1 152	904	573	237	330	333	238	494	322	246	142	324
A. Unintentional injuries	3 812	2 524	1 288	319	314	598	531	374	155	234	241	188	219	156	146	89	249
1. Road traffic accidents	1 391	1 008	382	55	118	293	248	159	65	71	35	71	82	60	61	31	42
2. Poisonings	265	164	102	33	10	22	36	37	12	14	23	8	21	16	13	7	13
3. Falls	347	189	158	13	13	24	29	31	20	58	13	6	5	7	12	14	102
4. Fires	298	129	169	36	13	23	22	16	5	16	31	21	48	27	13	9	21
5. Drownings	497	332	165	87	92	64	40	24	10	16	59	42	19	11	10	6	17
6. Other unintentional	1 013	702	311	96	67	173	157	107	43	59	81	40	43	35	36	23	53
B. Intentional injuries	2 287	1 476	811	90	82	554	373	199	83	96	92	51	276	166	100	53	75
1. Self-inflicted injuries	929	543	386	-	22	134	139	115	55	78	-	12	130	82	65	34	63
2. Violence	702	553	150	26	22	258	152	64	18	13	29	13	40	30	21	9	9
3. War	656	380	275	64	39	161	82	20	10	4	63	26	106	54	13	10	4

Notes:
Causes responsible for no deaths have been omitted from this table.
A dash (-) symbol indicates fewer than 500 deaths.
*IA6 is Bacterial meningitis and meningococcaemia; IC3 is Hypertensive disorders of pregnancy; ID is Conditions arising during the perinatal period;
IIE6 is Dementia and other degenerative and hereditary CNS disorders; IIH1 is Chronic obstructive pulmonary disease.

Annex Table 13a. DALYs by age, sex and cause (thousands): Established Market Economies, 2000, baseline scenario

Cause	Total	Male	Female	Males					Females				
				0-4	5-14	15-44	45-59	60+	0-4	5-14	15-44	45-59	60+
Population (millions)	*839*	*411*	*428*	*29*	*54*	*176*	*79*	*72*	*27*	*52*	*171*	*81*	*98*
All causes	*100 545*	*56 831*	*43 714*	*2 640*	*1 258*	*21 281*	*13 384*	*18 269*	*2 146*	*942*	*14 266*	*9 037*	*17 323*
I. Communicable, maternal, perinatal and nutritional conditions	7 192	4 401	2 791	1 052	105	2 082	488	675	822	102	1 013	190	665
A. Infectious and parasitic diseases	3 755	2 717	1 038	152	33	1 975	402	155	124	35	662	84	133
1. Tuberculosis	91	66	25	–	–	13	19	34	–	–	4	6	15
2. STDs excluding HIV	296	19	277	1	–	17	1	1	–	2	270	2	2
a. Syphilis	5	3	2	1	–	1	–	1	–	–	1	–	–
b. Chlamydia	256	11	245	–	–	10	–	–	–	3	241	1	–
c. Gonorrhoea	33	6	27	–	–	6	–	–	–	–	26	–	–
3. HIV	2 690	2 302	388	43	7	1 875	345	33	31	7	305	38	7
4. Diarrhoeal diseases	157	80	76	33	6	23	8	9	30	6	19	8	13
5. Childhood-cluster diseases	26	14	11	11	1	1	–	1	8	1	–	–	1
a. Pertussis	15	8	7	8	1	–	–	–	7	–	–	–	–
b. Poliomyelitis	2	1	1	–	–	1	–	1	–	–	–	–	1
c. Diphtheria	–	–	–	–	–	–	–	–	–	–	–	–	–
d. Measles	8	5	3	3	1	–	–	–	1	1	–	–	–
e. Tetanus	1	–	1	–	–	–	–	–	–	–	–	–	–
6. Bacterial meningitis*	127	69	58	46	7	8	4	4	39	7	5	3	5
7. Hepatitis B and hepatitis C	36	23	13	1	–	9	7	6	1	–	4	3	5
8. Malaria	1	1	–	–	–	–	–	–	–	–	–	–	–
9. Tropical-cluster diseases	1	1	–	–	–	–	–	–	–	–	–	–	–
a. Trypanosomiasis	–	–	–	–	–	–	–	–	–	–	–	–	–
b. Chagas disease	–	–	–	–	–	–	–	–	–	–	–	–	–
c. Schistosomiasis	–	–	–	–	–	–	–	–	–	–	–	–	–
d. Leishmaniasis	1	–	–	–	–	–	–	–	–	–	–	–	–
e. Lymphatic filariasis	–	–	–	–	–	–	–	–	–	–	–	–	–
f. Onchocerciasis	–	–	–	–	–	–	–	–	–	–	–	–	–
10. Leprosy	1	–	–	–	–	–	–	–	–	–	–	–	–
11. Dengue	–	–	–	–	–	–	–	–	–	–	–	–	–
12. Japanese encephalitis	–	–	–	–	–	–	–	–	–	–	–	–	–
13. Trachoma	–	–	–	–	–	–	–	–	–	–	–	–	–
14. Intestinal nematode infections	–	–	–	–	–	–	–	–	–	–	–	–	–
a. Ascariasis	–	–	–	–	–	–	–	–	–	–	–	–	–
b. Trichuriasis	–	–	–	–	–	–	–	–	–	–	–	–	–
c. Ancylostomiasis and necatoriasis	–	–	–	–	–	–	–	–	–	–	–	–	–

Annex Table 13a, continued. DALYs by age, sex and cause (thousands): Established Market Economies, 2000, baseline scenario

Cause	Total	Male	Female	Males 0-4	Males 5-14	Males 15-44	Males 45-59	Males 60+	Females 0-4	Females 5-14	Females 15-44	Females 45-59	Females 60+
B. Respiratory infections	**1 240**	**660**	**580**	**55**	**33**	**56**	**66**	**449**	**39**	**31**	**34**	**38**	**437**
1. Lower respiratory infections	1 142	610	533	42	9	50	64	444	29	9	29	36	430
2. Upper respiratory infections	40	21	19	6	2	6	2	5	3	2	5	2	6
3. Otitis media	58	30	28	7	22	-	-	-	6	21	-	-	-
C. Maternal conditions	**156**	-	**156**	-	-	**156**	-	-	-	-	-	-	-
1. Maternal haemorrhage	10	-	10	-	-	10	-	-	-	-	-	-	-
2. Maternal sepsis	17	-	17	-	-	17	-	-	-	-	-	-	-
3. Hypertensive disorders of pregnancy	7	-	7	-	-	7	-	-	-	-	-	-	-
4. Obstructed labour	107	-	107	-	-	107	-	-	-	-	-	-	-
5. Abortion	6	-	6	-	-	6	-	-	-	-	-	-	-
D. Perinatal conditions*	**1 412**	**798**	**615**	**797**	**1**	-	-	-	**614**	-	-	-	-
E. Nutritional deficiencies	**630**	**226**	**403**	**49**	**37**	**50**	**19**	**70**	**45**	**35**	**161**	**67**	**95**
1. Protein-energy malnutrition	70	34	36	25	-	1	1	7	23	-	1	1	11
2. Iodine deficiency	-	-	-	-	-	-	-	-	-	-	-	-	-
3. Vitamin A deficiency	-	-	-	-	-	-	-	-	-	-	-	-	-
4. Iron-deficiency anaemia	553	189	364	24	37	48	17	62	22	35	159	66	82
II. Noncommunicable diseases	**82 250**	**44 625**	**37 626**	**1 307**	**735**	**13 812**	**11 757**	**17 012**	**1 127**	**606**	**11 461**	**8 286**	**16 147**
A. Malignant neoplasms	**15 965**	**9 234**	**6 731**	**34**	**82**	**1 074**	**3 209**	**4 836**	**29**	**60**	**1 082**	**2 225**	**3 335**
1. Mouth and oropharynx cancers	390	316	74	-	-	48	161	106	-	-	12	27	34
2. Oesophagus cancer	376	308	69	-	-	23	142	143	-	-	4	21	44
3. Stomach cancer	1 140	737	403	-	-	72	255	410	-	-	64	112	226
4. Colon and rectum cancers	1 737	951	786	-	-	79	308	564	-	-	67	217	502
5. Liver cancer	343	270	73	1	1	23	125	121	1	1	7	21	44
6. Pancreas cancer	635	370	265	-	-	31	137	202	-	-	17	76	172
7. Trachea, bronchus, lung cancers	3 530	2 560	970	-	-	199	1 053	1 308	-	-	78	359	533
8. Melanoma and other skin cancers	256	156	100	-	-	51	54	50	-	-	36	31	33
9. Breast cancer	1 436	-	1 436	-	-	-	-	-	-	-	317	594	525
10. Cervix uteri cancer	191	-	191	-	-	-	-	-	-	-	75	65	50
11. Corpus uteri cancer	187	-	187	-	-	-	-	-	-	-	24	70	94
12. Ovary cancer	377	-	377	-	-	-	-	-	-	-	59	155	163
13. Prostate cancer	651	651	-	-	-	-	72	575	-	-	-	-	-
14. Bladder cancer	408	331	78	-	-	4	63	259	-	-	4	13	60
15. Lymphomas and multiple myeloma	720	429	291	2	9	116	133	169	1	4	59	77	151
16. Leukaemia	597	349	248	11	33	111	78	116	10	22	73	55	88
C. Diabetes mellitus	**2 267**	**1 064**	**1 203**	**2**	**3**	**226**	**375**	**459**	**2**	**4**	**177**	**336**	**684**
D. Endocrine disorders	**1 102**	**478**	**624**	**84**	**51**	**144**	**71**	**128**	**80**	**39**	**165**	**161**	**180**

Annex Table 13a, continued. DALYs by age, sex and cause (thousands): Established Market Economies, 2000, baseline scenario

Cause	Total	Male	Female	Males 0-4	Males 5-14	Males 15-44	Males 45-59	Males 60+	Females 0-4	Females 5-14	Females 15-44	Females 45-59	Females 60+
E. Neuro-psychiatric conditions	24 682	12 793	11 889	122	305	9 066	1 757	1 544	104	257	7 315	1 745	2 467
1. Unipolar major depression	6 721	2 350	4 370	–	–	1 749	456	145	–	–	3 197	843	331
2. Bipolar disorder	1 673	843	830			736	76	31			713	77	40
3. Schizophrenia	2 151	1 123	1 028			1 095	10	18			1 000	3	25
4. Epilepsy	427	235	192	7	42	125	43	18	7	44	83	34	24
5. Alcohol use	4 611	3 894	717			3 216	549	129			582	98	37
6. Dementia*	3 286	1 295	1 991	39	16	46	278	916	37	14	36	293	1 610
7. Parkinson disease	523	238	285				77	161				85	200
8. Multiple sclerosis	222	95	127			75	14	6			97	20	9
9. Drug use	1 455	1 100	355	–	86	969	39	6	–	29	311	13	2
10. Post-traumatic stress disorder	268	101	167	4	16	68	11	2	6	26	112	17	5
11. Obsessive-compulsive disorders	1 437	612	825			480	49	29			618	88	51
12. Panic disorder	689	229	460			160	51	–			339	82	20
F. Sense organ diseases	123	57	66	–	–	4	24	28	–	–	2	26	38
1. Glaucoma	83	37	46			2	20	15			1	22	23
2. Cataracts	35	17	18			1	4	12			1	3	14
G. Cardiovascular diseases	19 112	11 377	7 735	58	24	1 293	3 286	6 717	45	17	605	1 015	6 052
1. Rheumatic heart disease	153	61	92			12	21	27			12	24	55
2. Ischaemic heart disease	9 401	5 994	3 407			457	1 925	3 613			117	416	2 874
3. Cerebrovascular disease	5 166	2 656	2 510	9	6	357	668	1 617	7	4	261	377	1 861
4. Inflammatory heart diseases	666	421	246	11	6	147	134	123	13	4	68	45	116
H. Respiratory diseases	5 082	2 905	2 177	85	125	570	631	1 494	52	88	515	518	1 004
1. COPD*	2 564	1 610	953	4	1	107	362	1 136	2	1	57	248	645
2. Asthma	1 201	617	585	36	106	298	104	72	20	77	288	115	85
I. Digestive diseases	4 681	2 736	1 945	44	16	631	1 135	909	32	14	411	606	882
1. Peptic ulcer	265	164	101	1	1	40	53	71	1	1	22	23	56
2. Cirrhosis of the liver	1 746	1 246	500			281	631	333			107	216	176
3. Appendicitis	33	20	13	–	3	9	3	4	–	2	6	2	4
J. Genito-urinary diseases	1 149	660	489	16	2	68	203	369	13	4	60	88	325
1. Nephritis and nephrosis	449	242	207	13	1	39	46	143	10	3	16	29	149
2. Benign prostatic hypertrophy	245	245	–			–	120	125					–
L. Musculo-skeletal diseases	4 484	1 525	2 958	2	3	395	829	296	1	10	791	1 304	852
1. Rheumatoid arthritis	1 005	244	762			55	105	83		4	315	189	253
2. Osteoarthritis	3 043	1 173	1 870	–	–	308	693	171	–	–	353	1 032	485

Annex Table 13a, continued. DALYs by age, sex and cause (thousands): Established Market Economies, 2000, baseline scenario

Cause	Total	Male	Female	Males					Females				
				0-4	5-14	15-44	45-59	60+	0-4	5-14	15-44	45-59	60+
M. Congenital anomalies	**1 745**	**931**	**814**	**829**	**26**	**55**	**12**	**8**	**737**	**23**	**33**	**11**	**9**
N. Oral conditions	**922**	**442**	**480**	**14**	**71**	**173**	**96**	**88**	**14**	**68**	**169**	**104**	**126**
1. Dental caries	415	207	208	14	71	84	19	20	13	68	81	19	27
2. Periodontal disease	34	17	17	-	-	15	1	1	-	-	15	1	1
3. Edentulism	466	215	251	-	-	73	75	66	-	-	72	82	96
III. Injuries	***11 102***	***7 806***	***3 297***	***280***	***418***	***5 386***	***1 139***	***582***	***198***	***234***	***1 792***	***561***	***512***
A. Unintentional injuries	**7 953**	**5 484**	**2 468**	**255**	**383**	**3 677**	**744**	**425**	**174**	**214**	**1 262**	**388**	**432**
1. Road traffic accidents	4 008	2 788	1 220	60	180	2 188	257	102	45	117	845	137	75
2. Poisonings	250	180	70	4	3	142	23	8	3	2	47	12	7
3. Falls	1 301	732	569	43	67	357	142	124	28	31	161	138	212
4. Fires	230	138	91	22	29	56	19	12	17	27	27	10	10
5. Drownings	235	186	50	27	27	97	22	12	14	7	16	6	6
6. Other unintentional	1 928	1 460	468	98	78	836	281	166	67	30	166	84	121
B. Intentional injuries	**3 150**	**2 321**	**828**	**25**	**35**	**1 710**	**395**	**156**	**24**	**21**	**530**	**174**	**80**
1. Self-inflicted injuries	2 189	1 593	596	-	14	1 102	335	143	-	4	366	153	73
2. Violence	958	726	232	25	21	607	60	13	24	16	164	21	7
3. War	2	2	-	-	-	1	-	-	-	-	-	-	-

Notes:
A dash (-) symbol indicates fewer than 500 DALYs.
*IA6 is Bacterial meningitis and meningococcaemia; ID is Conditions arising during the perinatal period;
IIE6 is Dementia and other degenerative and hereditary CNS disorders; IIH1 is Chronic obstructive pulmonary disease.

Annex Table 13b. DALYs by age, sex and cause (thousands): Formerly Socialist Economies of Europe, 2000, baseline scenario

Cause	Total	Male	Female	Males					Females				
				0-4	5-14	15-44	45-59	60+	0-4	5-14	15-44	45-59	60+
Population (millions)	*358*	*171*	*187*	*13*	*26*	*75*	*31*	*25*	*12*	*25*	*74*	*34*	*41*
All causes	**65 264**	**38 732**	**26 532**	**2 482**	**1 042**	**14 299**	**11 174**	**9 735**	**1 952**	**686**	**8 223**	**5 785**	**9 886**
I. Communicable, maternal, perinatal and nutritional conditions	***4 123***	***1 994***	***2 129***	***1 187***	***108***	***271***	***179***	***249***	***893***	***102***	***763***	***83***	***288***
A. Infectious and parasitic diseases	**1 264**	**622**	**642**	**228**	**31**	**190**	**110**	**64**	**190**	**31**	**333**	**31**	**57**
1. Tuberculosis	**253**	**218**	**35**	**2**	-	**96**	**86**	**34**	**1**	**1**	**13**	**10**	**11**
2. STDs excluding HIV	**296**	**42**	**254**	**4**	**1**	**35**	**1**	-	**4**	**3**	**244**	**1**	**1**
a. Syphilis	3	1	1	-	-	1	-	-	-	-	1	-	-
b. Chlamydia	229	16	213	2	-	14	-	-	2	3	207	1	-
c. Gonorrhoea	60	21	39	3	-	18	-	-	3	-	36	-	-
3. HIV	**129**	**70**	**59**	**41**	**6**	**21**	**2**	-	**41**	**6**	**11**	**1**	-
4. Diarrhoeal diseases	**160**	**84**	**75**	**63**	**4**	**11**	**4**	**3**	**55**	**3**	**9**	**4**	**4**
5. Childhood-cluster diseases	**25**	**12**	**12**	**9**	**1**	**1**	**1**	-	**9**	**2**	-	**1**	-
a. Pertussis	15	6	8	6	-	-	-	-	6	2	-	-	-
b. Poliomyelitis	-	-	-	-	-	-	-	-	-	-	-	-	-
c. Diphtheria	1	1	-	-	-	-	-	-	-	-	-	-	-
d. Measles	7	4	3	3	-	1	-	-	2	1	-	-	-
e. Tetanus	1	1	1	-	-	-	-	-	-	-	-	-	-
6. Bacterial meningitis*	**156**	**90**	**66**	**57**	**6**	**13**	**7**	**7**	**44**	**5**	**7**	**4**	**5**
7. Hepatitis B and hepatitis C	**25**	**14**	**11**	**5**	**1**	**4**	**2**	**2**	**4**	**1**	**4**	**1**	**1**
8. Malaria	-	-	-	-	-	-	-	-	-	-	-	-	-
9. Tropical-cluster diseases	-	-	-	-	-	-	-	-	-	-	-	-	-
a. Trypanosomiasis	-	-	-	-	-	-	-	-	-	-	-	-	-
b. Chagas disease	-	-	-	-	-	-	-	-	-	-	-	-	-
c. Schistosomiasis	-	-	-	-	-	-	-	-	-	-	-	-	-
d. Leishmaniasis	-	-	-	-	-	-	-	-	-	-	-	-	-
e. Lymphatic filariasis	-	-	-	-	-	-	-	-	-	-	-	-	-
f. Onchocerciasis	-	-	-	-	-	-	-	-	-	-	-	-	-
10. Leprosy	-	-	-	-	-	-	-	-	-	-	-	-	-
11. Dengue	-	-	-	-	-	-	-	-	-	-	-	-	-
12. Japanese encephalitis	-	-	-	-	-	-	-	-	-	-	-	-	-
13. Trachoma	-	-	-	-	-	-	-	-	-	-	-	-	-
14. Intestinal nematode infections	**1**	-	**1**	-	-	-	-	-	-	-	**1**	-	-
a. Ascariasis	-	-	-	-	-	-	-	-	-	-	-	-	-
b. Trichuriasis	-	-	-	-	-	-	-	-	-	-	-	-	-
c. Ancylostomiasis and necatoriasis	-	-	-	-	-	-	-	-	-	-	-	-	-

Annex Table 13b, continued. DALYs by age, sex and cause (thousands): Formerly Socialist Economies of Europe, 2000, baseline scenario

Cause	Total	Male	Female	Males 0-4	5-14	15-44	45-59	60+	Females 0-4	5-14	15-44	45-59	60+
B. Respiratory infections	**995**	**550**	**444**	**244**	**31**	**58**	**59**	**158**	**186**	**28**	**26**	**19**	**185**
1. Lower respiratory infections	945	524	421	236	19	55	58	157	179	17	24	18	184
2. Upper respiratory infections	17	9	8	3	1	2	1	1	3	1	2	1	2
3. Otitis media	32	17	15	5	11	-	-	-	4	11	-	1	-
C. Maternal conditions	**322**	**-**	**322**						**-**	**-**	**322**	**-**	**-**
1. Maternal haemorrhage	8		8								8		
2. Maternal sepsis	64		64								64		
3. Hypertensive disorders of pregnancy	6		6								6		
4. Obstructed labour	86		86								86		
5. Abortion	89		89								89		
D. Perinatal conditions*	**1 100**	**646**	**454**	**646**					**454**				
E. Nutritional deficiencies*	**443**	**176**	**267**	**69**	**46**	**24**	**10**	**27**	**64**	**43**	**82**	**33**	**45**
1. Protein-energy malnutrition	79	39	40	36	-	-	1	2	34	-	-	-	5
2. Iodine deficiency	-												
3. Vitamin A deficiency	-												
4. Iron-deficiency anaemia	314	115	198	24	42	20	7	22	22	40	72	29	35
II. Noncommunicable diseases	***49 427***	***27 746***	***21 681***	***871***	***416***	***7 990***	***9 360***	***9 109***	***733***	***337***	***6 070***	***5 221***	***9 320***
A. Malignant neoplasms	**8 473**	**5 460**	**3 013**	**39**	**73**	**753**	**2 619**	**1 977**	**32**	**45**	**571**	**1 140**	**1 225**
1. Mouth and oropharynx cancers	290	258	32	-	1	42	157	58	-	-	7	12	13
2. Oesophagus cancer	144	127	17	-	-	13	78	36	-	-	2	6	8
3. Stomach cancer	1 214	832	381	-	-	97	422	314	-	-	54	136	191
4. Colon and rectum cancers	775	428	347	-	-	49	178	200	-	-	38	121	188
5. Liver cancer	220	141	79	1	1	15	66	58	1	1	8	26	44
6. Pancreas cancer	324	215	109			25	108	81			10	39	60
7. Trachea, bronchus, lung cancers	2 059	1 785	274	1	1	158	970	655		1	31	108	134
8. Melanoma and other skin cancers	114	63	51			20	25	18			18	15	17
9. Breast cancer	508		508								118	243	147
10. Cervix uteri cancer	184		184								56	70	58
11. Corpus uteri cancer	135		135								20	61	54
12. Ovary cancer	189		189								40	90	59
13. Prostate cancer	146	146				4	33	109					
14. Bladder cancer	185	155	31			6	58	89			3	9	19
15. Lymphomas and multiple myeloma	271	176	95	5	14	64	59	34	3	5	35	26	26
16. Leukaemia	316	191	125	13	28	61	50	39	10	18	40	29	29
C. Diabetes mellitus	**614**	**268**	**346**	**1**	**1**	**67**	**100**	**99**	**1**	**2**	**56**	**105**	**182**
D. Endocrine disorders	**207**	**87**	**120**	**19**	**7**	**42**	**14**	**6**	**18**	**7**	**50**	**32**	**14**

Annex Table 13b, continued. DALYs by age, sex and cause (thousands): Formerly Socialist Economies of Europe, 2000, baseline scenario

Cause	Total	Male	Female	Males 0-4	5-14	15-44	45-59	60+	Females 0-4	5-14	15-44	45-59	60+
E. Neuro-psychiatric conditions	**10 729**	**5 474**	**5 255**	**106**	**204**	**3 958**	**723**	**482**	**92**	**163**	**3 337**	**758**	**906**
1. Unipolar major depression	3 179	1 086	2 093	-	-	825	200	60	-	-	1 538	393	162
2. Bipolar disorder	842	414	428	-	-	360	37	18	-	-	353	39	36
3. Schizophrenia	846	440	406	-	-	425	9	7	-	-	394	4	8
4. Epilepsy	320	201	120	8	46	106	29	12	7	33	48	19	12
5. Alcohol use	1 763	1 554	209	-	-	1 285	217	52	-	-	182	17	9
6. Dementia*	1 069	386	683	18	9	19	93	247	17	8	17	115	527
7. Parkinson disease	146	59	87	-	-	-	21	38	-	-	-	25	61
8. Multiple sclerosis	114	49	65	-	-	36	8	5	-	8	48	10	8
9. Drug use	528	422	105	-	32	373	15	3	-	13	93	4	1
10. Post-traumatic stress disorder	117	44	74	2	8	29	4	1	3	-	49	7	2
11. Obsessive-compulsive disorders	649	272	376	-	27	214	20	11	-	34	281	39	23
12. Panic disorder	313	103	211	-	9	72	21	-	-	9	156	37	9
F. Sense organ diseases	**74**	**32**	**42**	-	-	**1**	**8**	**22**	-	-	**2**	**15**	**25**
1. Glaucoma	34	12	22	-	-	-	4	7	-	-	1	12	10
2. Cataracts	40	20	19	-	-	1	4	15	-	-	1	3	15
G. Cardiovascular diseases	**16 632**	**9 664**	**6 968**	**25**	**12**	**1 250**	**3 541**	**4 835**	**20**	**9**	**432**	**1 241**	**5 266**
1. Rheumatic heart disease	385	194	191	-	2	68	97	27	-	1	41	102	46
2. Ischaemic heart disease	8 267	5 213	3 055	-	-	607	2 149	2 457	-	-	103	513	2 438
3. Cerebrovascular disease	5 050	2 507	2 543	4	3	267	808	1 425	2	2	186	502	1 850
4. Inflammatory heart diseases	498	314	183	5	3	116	112	78	6	2	44	45	86
H. Respiratory diseases	**4 062**	**2 567**	**1 495**	**33**	**47**	**435**	**1 069**	**983**	**20**	**32**	**296**	**414**	**734**
1. COPD*	1 575	1 101	474	-	1	130	514	456	-	-	59	103	311
2. Asthma	551	287	264	17	45	129	58	38	9	29	120	59	46
I. Digestive diseases	**2 795**	**1 649**	**1 146**	**53**	**10**	**531**	**694**	**360**	**38**	**9**	**281**	**425**	**393**
1. Peptic ulcer	215	158	57	-	-	44	71	43	1	1	15	19	22
2. Cirrhosis of the liver	812	562	250	2	1	115	300	144	1	1	41	116	91
3. Appendicitis	16	10	7	-	1	5	2	2	-	1	3	1	1
J. Genito-urinary diseases	**914**	**471**	**443**	**7**	**6**	**127**	**170**	**161**	**5**	**7**	**126**	**175**	**131**
1. Nephritis and nephrosis	244	142	103	3	4	60	45	31	3	5	34	31	30
2. Benign prostatic hypertrophy	134	134	-	-	-	-	60	73	-	-	-	-	-
L. Musculo-skeletal diseases	**2 864**	**1 056**	**1 808**	**2**	**4**	**625**	**294**	**132**	**1**	**7**	**702**	**742**	**356**
1. Rheumatoid arthritis	516	123	393	-	-	68	33	23	-	3	216	110	64
2. Osteoarthritis	2 124	872	1 252	-	-	523	246	104	-	-	408	573	270

Annex Table 13b, continued. DALYs by age, sex and cause (thousands): Formerly Socialist Economies of Europe, 2000, baseline scenario

Cause	Total	Male	Female	Males					Females				
				0-4	5-14	15-44	45-59	60+	0-4	5-14	15-44	45-59	60+
M. Congenital anomalies	1 133	611	522	558	20	27	4	1	481	19	17	4	1
N. Oral conditions	504	230	274	15	20	95	70	30	14	29	99	82	50
1. Dental caries	247	115	132	15	20	45	22	13	14	29	44	24	20
2. Periodontal disease	17	7	10	-	-	5	2	1	-	-	8	1	1
3. Edentulism	239	108	131	-	-	45	46	16	-	-	47	56	29
III. Injuries	*11 714*	*8 992*	*2 722*	*424*	*518*	*6 037*	*1 635*	*378*	*326*	*247*	*1 390*	*481*	*278*
A. Unintentional injuries	8 035	6 335	1 700	310	419	4 134	1 205	266	214	181	757	337	210
1. Road traffic accidents	2 859	2 306	553	37	146	1 720	327	76	22	78	311	94	48
2. Poisonings	913	712	200	38	13	389	234	38	28	10	81	60	21
3. Falls	1 096	744	352	49	69	440	131	55	36	27	136	73	80
4. Fires	183	129	55	16	14	63	27	8	14	10	16	8	8
5. Drownings	572	487	85	29	72	308	65	13	13	25	32	10	5
6. Other unintentional	2 412	1 957	455	141	104	1 214	421	76	102	30	182	92	48
B. Intentional injuries	3 678	2 657	1 021	113	99	1 903	430	111	112	65	633	144	68
1. Self-inflicted injuries	1 661	1 329	332	-	18	896	324	91	-	4	185	93	50
2. Violence	856	659	197	9	9	541	85	15	7	8	133	36	12
3. War	1 161	669	492	104	71	466	21	5	105	53	315	15	5

Notes:
A dash (-) symbol indicates fewer than 500 DALYs.
*IA6 is Bacterial meningitis and meningococcaemia; ID is Conditions arising during the perinatal period;
IIE6 is Dementia and other degenerative and hereditary CNS disorders; IIH1 is Chronic obstructive pulmonary disease.

Annex Table 13c. DALYs by age, sex and cause (thousands): India, 2000, baseline scenario

Cause	Total	Male	Female	Males 0-4	5-14	15-44	45-59	60+	Females 0-4	5-14	15-44	45-59	60+
Population (millions)	*995*	*512*	*483*	*57*	*111*	*248*	*60*	*37*	*54*	*104*	*229*	*57*	*39*
All causes	**250 158**	**130 612**	**119 546**	**43 137**	**13 621**	**38 089**	**19 424**	**16 341**	**42 773**	**11 743**	**36 251**	**13 844**	**14 935**
I. Communicable, maternal, perinatal and nutritional conditions	*110 495*	*55 563*	*54 932*	*32 654*	*3 950*	*12 217*	*3 945*	*2 797*	*32 959*	*4 435*	*12 965*	*2 591*	*1 982*
A. Infectious and parasitic diseases	**64 748**	**34 968**	**29 780**	**15 573**	**2 699**	**11 103**	**3 641**	**1 953**	**15 520**	**2 698**	**8 258**	**2 147**	**1 158**
1. Tuberculosis	**16 901**	**10 749**	**6 151**	**476**	**430**	**5 364**	**3 016**	**1 463**	**368**	**336**	**3 105**	**1 689**	**653**
2. STDs excluding HIV	**3 701**	**1 285**	**2 416**	**655**	**9**	**589**	**12**	**21**	**662**	**35**	**1 675**	**16**	**28**
a. Syphilis	1 147	557	590	438	1	88	9	20	459	1	92	11	27
b. Chlamydia	1 495	233	1 262	52	3	177	1	-	49	25	1 183	4	1
c. Gonorrhoea	1 059	495	564	164	5	324	2	-	154	9	400	1	-
3. HIV	**8 362**	**4 718**	**3 644**	**916**	**175**	**3 284**	**276**	**66**	**944**	**187**	**2 383**	**109**	**21**
4. Diarrhoeal diseases	**16 860**	**8 228**	**8 632**	**7 163**	**464**	**329**	**90**	**181**	**7 452**	**620**	**268**	**89**	**202**
5. Childhood-cluster diseases	**10 358**	**5 293**	**5 065**	**4 560**	**486**	**200**	**31**	**16**	**4 309**	**544**	**164**	**32**	**18**
a. Pertussis	1 721	878	843	801	77	-	-	-	768	75	4	-	-
b. Poliomyelitis	768	448	319	438	2	7	-	-	313	1	-	-	-
c. Diphtheria	86	44	42	39	4	1	-	-	37	4	-	-	-
d. Measles	4 001	2 025	1 975	1 765	257	3	-	-	1 714	258	2	-	-
e. Tetanus	3 783	1 898	1 885	1 518	146	189	30	16	1 475	205	157	31	18
6. Bacterial meningitis*	**847**	**443**	**405**	**319**	**13**	**74**	**22**	**14**	**302**	**12**	**52**	**22**	**16**
7. Hepatitis B and hepatitis C	**193**	**109**	**84**	**26**	**14**	**35**	**19**	**15**	**21**	**13**	**25**	**9**	**15**
8. Malaria	**607**	**324**	**282**	**85**	**98**	**113**	**19**	**9**	**74**	**104**	**80**	**17**	**8**
9. Tropical-cluster diseases	**1 580**	**1 112**	**468**	**66**	**389**	**608**	**42**	**7**	**36**	**185**	**181**	**58**	**8**
a. Trypanosomiasis	-	-	-	-	-	-	-	-	-	-	-	-	-
b. Chagas disease	-	-	-	-	-	-	-	-	-	-	-	-	-
c. Schistosomiasis	-	-	-	-	-	-	-	-	-	-	-	-	-
d. Leishmaniasis	669	417	252	33	170	202	8	4	22	117	104	5	3
e. Lymphatic filariasis	911	696	216	33	219	406	34	3	14	68	77	52	5
f. Onchocerciasis	-	-	-	-	-	-	-	-	-	-	-	-	-
10. Leprosy	**131**	**67**	**64**	**1**	**22**	**37**	**6**	**2**	**2**	**21**	**34**	**5**	**1**
11. Dengue	**222**	**102**	**120**	**24**	**75**	**2**	**1**	**-**	**27**	**90**	**2**	**1**	**-**
12. Japanese encephalitis	**46**	**23**	**22**	**14**	**7**	**2**	**-**	**-**	**13**	**7**	**1**	**-**	**-**
13. Trachoma	**17**	**5**	**13**	**-**	**-**	**1**	**2**	**2**	**-**	**-**	**2**	**4**	**7**
14. Intestinal nematode infections	**472**	**249**	**223**	**2**	**122**	**97**	**18**	**10**	**2**	**114**	**80**	**17**	**10**
a. Ascariasis	115	59	56	2	57	-	-	-	2	54	-	-	-
b. Trichuriasis	74	38	36	-	38	-	-	-	-	35	-	-	-
c. Ancylostomiasis and necatoriasis	283	152	132	-	27	97	18	10	-	25	79	17	10

Annex Table 13c, continued. DALYs by age, sex and cause (thousands): India, 2000, baseline scenario

Cause	Total	Male	Female	Males					Females				
				0-4	5-14	15-44	45-59	60+	0-4	5-14	15-44	45-59	60+
B. Respiratory infections	**19 917**	**9 624**	**10 293**	**7 609**	**730**	**418**	**171**	**697**	**7 914**	**1 215**	**323**	**174**	**667**
1. Lower respiratory infections	19 354	9 353	10 001	7 424	665	406	168	689	7 711	1 146	314	171	659
2. Upper respiratory infections	210	102	107	73	9	11	3	8	76	14	8	3	7
3. Otitis media	353	169	184	112	56	1	-	-	127	56	1	-	-
C. Maternal conditions	**3 370**	**-**	**3 370**	**-**	**-**	**-**	**-**	**-**	**-**	**-**	**3 336**	**34**	**-**
1. Maternal haemorrhage	386		386								378	8	
2. Maternal sepsis	571		571								566	5	
3. Hypertensive disorders of pregnancy	189		189								185	4	
4. Obstructed labour	683		683								681	3	
5. Abortion	728		728								723	5	
D. Perinatal conditions*	**15 231**	**7 601**	**7 630**	**7 601**	**-**	**-**	**-**	**-**	**7 630**	**-**	**-**	**-**	**-**
E. Nutritional deficiencies	**7 229**	**3 369**	**3 859**	**1 870**	**522**	**696**	**134**	**148**	**1 895**	**522**	**1 048**	**237**	**157**
1. Protein-energy malnutrition	2 939	1 429	1 510	1 364	19	23	6	17	1 422	51	11	5	20
2. Iodine deficiency	214	111	103	97	10	4	-	-	89	10	3	-	-
3. Vitamin A deficiency	404	206	198	136	65	5	-	-	130	64	4	-	-
4. Iron-deficiency anaemia	3 672	1 623	2 049	273	428	664	127	130	254	398	1 030	231	137
II. Noncommunicable diseases	**96 757**	**50 214**	**46 543**	**6 025**	**2 057**	**15 751**	**13 372**	**13 009**	**6 040**	**2 091**	**16 247**	**9 776**	**12 390**
A. Malignant neoplasms	**9 559**	**4 760**	**4 799**	**141**	**230**	**1 252**	**1 907**	**1 230**	**76**	**114**	**1 543**	**1 961**	**1 106**
1. Mouth and oropharynx cancers	1 394	797	597	3	5	185	371	234	2	5	161	278	151
2. Oesophagus cancer	754	371	383	-	-	67	182	122	-	-	82	175	126
3. Stomach cancer	711	444	268	-	1	104	214	125	-	1	77	112	78
4. Colon and rectum cancers	338	182	157	-	1	66	63	52	-	1	38	63	55
5. Liver cancer	191	133	59	1	3	33	61	35	1	1	15	23	19
6. Pancreas cancer	113	66	46	-	-	15	32	19	-	-	13	18	16
7. Trachea, bronchus, lung cancers	1 114	901	213	-	1	171	463	266	-	1	52	88	72
8. Melanoma and other skin cancers	20	10	10	-	-	3	5	2	-	-	4	4	2
9. Breast cancer	685	-	685						-	-	270	289	126
10. Cervix uteri cancer	927	-	927						-	-	271	496	161
11. Corpus uteri cancer	47		47						-	-	6	23	18
12. Ovary cancer	223		223						-	1	103	67	52
13. Prostate cancer	101	101	-	-	-	3	21	76					
14. Bladder cancer	87	67	19	-	-	9	26	31	-	-	3	7	9
15. Lymphomas and multiple myeloma	384	266	119	23	41	110	62	30	5	8	42	32	32
16. Leukaemia	448	263	184	43	74	100	32	15	24	41	79	28	13
C. Diabetes mellitus	**2 113**	**1 038**	**1 075**	**72**	**115**	**258**	**324**	**268**	**73**	**111**	**202**	**323**	**366**
D. Endocrine disorders	**99**	**54**	**46**	**25**	**5**	**14**	**8**	**2**	**19**	**2**	**10**	**8**	**7**

Annex Table 13c, continued. DALYs by age, sex and cause (thousands): India, 2000, baseline scenario

Cause	Total	Male	Female	Males					Females				
				0-4	5-14	15-44	45-59	60+	0-4	5-14	15-44	45-59	60+
E. Neuro-psychiatric conditions	23 949	10 969	12 981	449	429	8 366	1 050	676	566	505	9 856	1 209	844
1. Unipolar major depression	10 064	3 673	6 390	-	-	3 132	438	103	-	-	5 438	759	194
2. Bipolar disorder	2 867	1 485	1 381	-	-	1 382	78	25	-	-	1 279	73	29
3. Schizophrenia	2 041	1 097	944	-	-	1 081	9	7	-	-	929	4	11
4. Epilepsy	848	463	385	39	96	268	38	21	46	139	167	13	19
5. Alcohol use	1 113	1 018	95	-	-	929	76	14	-	-	88	5	2
6. Dementia*	1 192	570	621	53	22	51	140	305	64	22	47	138	350
7. Parkinson disease	167	81	86	-	-	-	32	48	-	-	-	37	50
8. Multiple sclerosis	253	113	140	-	-	100	10	4	-	-	122	12	5
9. Drug use	93	84	9	-	6	75	2	-	-	1	8	-	-
10. Post-traumatic stress disorder	376	146	230	8	33	96	8	1	12	53	150	12	2
11. Obsessive-compulsive disorders	2 007	890	1 117	-	115	719	39	16	-	145	883	66	23
12. Panic disorder	914	296	618	-	4	250	42	-	-	40	505	64	9
F. Sense organ diseases	3 805	1 946	1 859	6	1	163	966	811	4	-	123	778	953
1. Glaucoma	721	411	309	-	-	42	286	83	-	-	16	201	93
2. Cataracts	3 083	1 533	1 550	4	1	121	680	727	4	-	107	577	861
G. Cardiovascular diseases	28 500	15 938	12 563	567	271	2 350	5 223	7 527	520	383	1 637	2 908	7 114
1. Rheumatic heart disease	1 569	714	855	1	31	369	243	69	1	43	425	290	96
2. Ischaemic heart disease	13 223	7 670	5 554	-	-	498	2 838	4 334	-	-	297	1 361	3 895
3. Cerebrovascular disease	5 223	2 793	2 430	111	47	294	819	1 523	101	53	276	462	1 538
4. Inflammatory heart diseases	1 872	1 021	851	104	64	412	280	162	114	95	280	195	167
H. Respiratory diseases	9 142	4 851	4 291	486	458	1 038	1 421	1 448	444	350	1 124	1 220	1 153
1. COPD*	3 418	1 979	1 439	51	33	327	750	818	56	36	288	535	524
2. Asthma	1 626	915	711	90	209	424	121	71	50	128	365	105	64
I. Digestive diseases	5 762	3 773	1 989	197	101	1 411	1 533	532	209	89	763	622	305
1. Peptic ulcer	869	568	301	2	6	249	212	100	4	9	137	95	55
2. Cirrhosis of the liver	2 736	1 955	781	36	20	676	900	323	47	44	269	286	135
3. Appendicitis	275	159	116	5	35	107	9	3	5	32	71	6	2
J. Genito-urinary diseases	1 901	1 132	768	97	196	158	448	234	51	280	183	119	136
1. Nephritis and nephrosis	1 418	687	730	76	189	144	142	136	46	278	171	108	127
2. Benign prostatic hypertrophy	391	391	-	-	-	-	298	93	-	-	-	-	-
L. Musculo-skeletal diseases	1 781	710	1 071	3	7	294	297	110	2	6	410	432	220
1. Rheumatoid arthritis	221	65	156	1	1	46	10	7	-	3	87	49	16
2. Osteoarthritis	1 532	628	904	-	-	244	284	101	-	-	320	382	202

Annex Table 13c, continued. DALYs by age, sex and cause (thousands): India, 2000, baseline scenario

Cause	Total	Male	Female	Males					Females				
				0-4	5-14	15-44	45-59	60+	0-4	5-14	15-44	45-59	60+
M. Congenital anomalies	8 529	4 203	4 326	3 893	144	141	19	7	3 994	170	126	26	11
N. Oral conditions	1 277	640	637	40	78	218	152	152	38	75	213	149	163
1. Dental caries	795	408	387	39	77	177	66	49	37	72	164	63	51
2. Periodontal disease	89	46	43	-	-	37	6	3	-	-	35	6	3
3. Edentulism	368	180	188	-	-	-	80	101	-	-	-	79	109
III. Injuries	*42 905*	*24 835*	*18 070*	*4 457*	*7 614*	*10 122*	*2 107*	*536*	*3 774*	*5 217*	*7 039*	*1 478*	*563*
A. Unintentional injuries	37 622	21 937	15 685	4 247	7 418	8 084	1 726	462	3 507	5 033	5 406	1 232	507
1. Road traffic accidents	8 784	6 322	2 462	600	1 398	3 570	602	152	177	1 026	830	303	126
2. Poisonings	953	461	492	162	83	180	29	8	112	57	221	94	7
3. Falls	8 742	5 374	3 368	967	3 366	791	186	64	1 103	1 357	600	245	63
4. Fires	5 255	1 551	3 704	412	357	631	128	24	355	1 023	2 108	147	71
5. Drownings	2 444	1 348	1 097	343	473	449	61	22	283	421	294	65	33
6. Other unintentional	11 444	6 880	4 563	1 763	1 741	2 463	720	193	1 477	1 148	1 353	377	208
B. Intentional injuries	5 283	2 898	2 385	211	195	2 037	381	73	267	184	1 633	245	55
1. Self-inflicted injuries	3 426	1 718	1 708	-	115	1 324	244	34	-	114	1 462	119	13
2. Violence	1 713	1 035	677	211	80	569	137	39	267	70	171	127	43
3. War	145	145	-	-	-	145	-	-	-	-	-	-	-

Notes:
A dash (-) symbol indicates fewer than 500 DALYs.
*IA6 is Bacterial meningitis and meningococcaemia; ID is Conditions arising during the perinatal period;
IIE6 is Dementia and other degenerative and hereditary CNS disorders; IIH1 is Chronic obstructive pulmonary disease.

Annex Table 13d. DALYs by age, sex and cause (thousands): China, 2000, baseline scenario

Cause	Total	Male	Female	Males					Females				
				0-4	5-14	15-44	45-59	60+	0-4	5-14	15-44	45-59	60+
Population (millions)	*1 280*	*656*	*624*	*59*	*120*	*320*	*98*	*60*	*56*	*114*	*299*	*91*	*64*
All causes	**200 814**	**109 881**	**90 933**	**16 526**	**5 182**	**38 410**	**24 549**	**25 214**	**16 930**	**3 957**	**32 353**	**17 002**	**20 691**
I. Communicable, maternal, perinatal and nutritional conditions	*25 178*	*12 484*	*12 694*	*7 224*	*1 115*	*2 038*	*931*	*1 176*	*7 783*	*1 105*	*2 048*	*718*	*1 040*
A. Infectious and parasitic diseases	**7 720**	**4 205**	**3 514**	**1 371**	**590**	**919**	**650**	**675**	**1 376**	**575**	**614**	**404**	**545**
1. Tuberculosis	2 059	1 262	797	48	12	339	413	451	51	39	226	230	251
2. STDs excluding HIV	63	14	49	2		11		1	1	1	46		1
a. Syphilis	4	2	2					1					1
b. Chlamydia	41	4	36			4				1	35		
c. Gonorrhoea	19	8	11	1		7					10		1
3. HIV	131	72	59	25	4	38	4	1	30	5	24	1	
4. Diarrhoeal diseases	1 699	825	874	427	70	183	54	91	523	64	143	50	93
5. Childhood-cluster diseases	1 086	586	500	519	46	17	3	1	450	40	8	2	1
a. Pertussis	376	198	179	177	21				158	20			
b. Poliomyelitis	176	103	73	98	1	4			69	1	2		
c. Diphtheria	3	2	2	2					1				
d. Measles	248	130	118	111	15	3	1		100	15	2	1	
e. Tetanus	283	154	129	132	9	10	2	1	121	4	3	1	
6. Bacterial meningitis*	599	315	284	181	10	74	27	23	166	10	56	27	25
7. Hepatitis B and hepatitis C	285	195	90	31	5	77	58	24	25	5	20	13	28
8. Malaria	23	12	11	2	4	4	1	1	2	4	3	1	2
9. Tropical-cluster diseases	94	79	16	3	11	56	5	3	1	2	9	2	2
a. Trypanosomiasis													
b. Chagas disease													
c. Schistosomiasis	13	8	5			3	2	2			1	2	1
d. Leishmaniasis	1		1								1		
e. Lymphatic filariasis	81	70	11	3	10	53	3	1	1	2	8		
f. Onchocerciasis													
10. Leprosy	4	2	2		1	1				1	1		
11. Dengue	13	6	7	2	5				2	5			
12. Japanese encephalitis	222	116	106	68	39	7	1		64	36	5	1	
13. Trachoma	223	62	161			8	18	36			17	45	99
14. Intestinal nematode infections	765	393	372	6	360	20	4	3	5	343	16	4	3
a. Ascariasis	355	182	173	6	174	2			5	166	1		
b. Trichuriasis	347	178	169		177					169			
c. Ancylostomiasis and necatoriasis	62	33	29		8	18	4	3		8	15	4	3

Annex Table 13d, continued. DALYs by age, sex and cause (thousands): China, 2000, baseline scenario

Cause	Total	Male	Female	Males 0-4	Males 5-14	Males 15-44	Males 45-59	Males 60+	Females 0-4	Females 5-14	Females 15-44	Females 45-59	Females 60+
B. Respiratory infections	6 305	3 019	3 286	2 443	151	73	50	303	2 756	153	64	31	282
1. Lower respiratory infections	6 080	2 907	3 172	2 390	103	68	49	299	2 697	106	60	30	278
2. Upper respiratory infections	72	35	37	23	2	5	2	4	26	2	4	1	4
3. Otitis media	154	77	77	31	46				32	44			
C. Maternal conditions	750		750								728	22	
1. Maternal haemorrhage	115		115								109	6	
2. Maternal sepsis	134		134								133	1	
3. Hypertensive disorders of pregnancy	26		26								24	1	
4. Obstructed labour	163		163								163		
5. Abortion	22		22								21	1	
D. Perinatal conditions*	5 411	2 673	2 738	2 673					2 738				
E. Nutritional deficiencies	4 992	2 587	2 405	738	375	1 046	231	197	913	377	642	261	213
1. Protein-energy malnutrition	997	428	570	403	1	3	3	17	550	1	3	1	15
2. Iodine deficiency	233	122	111	108	10	4			97	9	4		
3. Vitamin A deficiency	159	83	76	58	23	2			53	22	2		
4. Iron-deficiency anaemia	3 602	1 954	1 649	169	340	1 036	228	180	213	344	633	259	198
II. Noncommunicable diseases	138 687	75 492	63 195	5 445	1 754	24 250	21 149	22 894	5 487	1 270	23 157	14 636	18 645
A. Malignant neoplasms	25 575	16 608	8 967	186	482	4 414	6 466	5 061	267	239	2 522	3 145	2 795
1. Mouth and oropharynx cancers	816	574	242	7	11	265	175	116			102	86	53
2. Oesophagus cancer	2 568	1 844	724			270	771	803			52	270	403
3. Stomach cancer	4 813	3 202	1 611		10	409	1 410	1 373		10	402	543	655
4. Colon and rectum cancers	1 427	816	610		10	252	281	274		12	155	225	219
5. Liver cancer	5 825	4 492	1 332	8	30	1 733	1 879	843	9	28	380	533	383
6. Pancreas cancer	419	275	144			52	100	123	1		14	45	85
7. Trachea, bronchus, lung cancers	3 363	2 489	874			320	1 129	1 015	1		94	391	388
8. Melanoma and other skin cancers	19	12	7			4	4				2	2	3
9. Breast cancer	546		546								243	203	100
10. Cervix uteri cancer	371		371								106	160	106
11. Corpus uteri cancer	125		125								26	78	21
12. Ovary cancer	225		225						5	9	101	74	35
13. Prostate cancer	53	53				4	7	42					
14. Bladder cancer	239	194	45			24	52	117			4	11	30
15. Lymphomas and multiple myeloma	436	299	136		40	98	86	75			41	66	29
16. Leukaemia	1 889	1 019	871	104	242	469	150	54	122	123	439	126	61
C. Diabetes mellitus	1 062	516	546	9	11	147	186	163	8	10	99	193	235
D. Endocrine disorders	507	144	363	21	11	51	37	25	141	23	132	30	36

Annex Table 13d, continued. DALYs by age, sex and cause (thousands): China, 2000, baseline scenario

Cause	Total	Male	Female	Males 0-4	Males 5-14	Males 15-44	Males 45-59	Males 60+	Females 0-4	Females 5-14	Females 15-44	Females 45-59	Females 60+
E. Neuro-psychiatric conditions	**31 275**	**14 271**	**17 003**	**249**	**395**	**11 294**	**1 504**	**830**	**202**	**396**	**13 273**	**1 982**	**1 150**
1. Unipolar major depression	14 179	5 151	9 027	-	-	4 226	751	175	-	-	7 435	1 269	324
2. Bipolar disorder	3 959	2 042	1 917	-	-	1 872	131	39	-	-	1 750	122	44
3. Schizophrenia	2 706	1 475	1 231	18	72	1 450	11	14	17	76	1 204	16	11
4. Epilepsy	715	383	333	-	-	229	46	17	-	-	192	31	17
5. Alcohol use	1 636	1 519	117	-	-	1 383	119	17	-	-	109	7	1
6. Dementia*	1 837	857	980	63	27	62	226	479	60	22	57	228	613
7. Parkinson disease	122	61	62	-	-	-	27	34	-	-	-	25	36
8. Multiple sclerosis	346	153	193	-	-	132	16	6	-	-	163	22	8
9. Drug use	198	178	20	-	16	155	7	1	-	2	17	1	-
10. Post-traumatic stress disorder	472	182	289	8	36	123	13	2	13	58	195	20	3
11. Obsessive-compulsive disorders	2 592	1 141	1 451	-	125	925	64	27	-	159	1 150	105	38
12. Panic disorder	1 255	435	819	-	44	322	70	-	-	44	658	103	15
F. Sense organ diseases	**2 554**	**1 044**	**1 510**	**44**	**-**	**86**	**437**	**476**	**34**	**15**	**169**	**723**	**569**
1. Glaucoma	1 034	314	719	7	-	32	178	97	9	-	73	490	146
2. Cataracts	1 294	657	637	17	-	44	233	363	2	-	41	196	397
G. Cardiovascular diseases	**27 362**	**15 919**	**11 442**	**337**	**111**	**2 658**	**5 243**	**7 570**	**199**	**60**	**1 988**	**3 045**	**6 150**
1. Rheumatic heart disease	2 384	1 108	1 275	-	18	444	345	300	21	19	455	410	371
2. Ischaemic heart disease	7 559	4 455	3 104	-	-	656	1 495	2 304	-	-	393	775	1 936
3. Cerebrovascular disease	13 388	7 942	5 446	78	47	1 123	2 674	4 021	51	18	751	1 539	3 088
4. Inflammatory heart diseases	1 271	723	548	59	19	300	215	130	41	12	238	137	118
H. Respiratory diseases	**26 966**	**14 962**	**12 004**	**655**	**338**	**3 210**	**4 110**	**6 649**	**516**	**181**	**2 590**	**2 914**	**5 803**
1. COPD*	22 482	12 363	10 119	113	7	2 159	3 765	6 319	212	3	1 730	2 667	5 506
2. Asthma	2 907	1 655	1 252	138	305	847	245	120	71	159	730	195	97
I. Digestive diseases	**8 416**	**4 903**	**3 513**	**769**	**93**	**1 290**	**1 653**	**1 098**	**824**	**80**	**780**	**994**	**834**
1. Peptic ulcer	428	270	157	5	3	91	88	83	6	3	43	43	64
2. Cirrhosis of the liver	2 986	2 090	896	39	13	723	829	485	13	15	203	368	298
3. Appendicitis	224	131	93	3	31	84	9	3	2	27	56	6	3
J. Genito-urinary diseases	**2 392**	**1 564**	**828**	**79**	**58**	**446**	**701**	**280**	**77**	**40**	**308**	**199**	**205**
1. Nephritis and nephrosis	1 429	814	615	52	58	407	152	144	77	40	257	111	130
2. Benign prostatic hypertrophy	578	578	-	7	-	8	489	74	-	-	-	-	-
L. Musculo-skeletal diseases	**4 126**	**1 392**	**2 734**	**-**	**22**	**309**	**544**	**517**	**23**	**18**	**893**	**1 175**	**625**
1. Rheumatoid arthritis	812	261	552	-	1	88	130	43	-	7	181	245	117
2. Osteoarthritis	2 674	905	1 768	-	-	177	373	356	-	-	542	836	390

Annex Table 13d, continued. DALYs by age, sex and cause (thousands): China, 2000, baseline scenario

Cause	Total	Male	Female	Males					Females				
				0-4	5-14	15-44	45-59	60+	0-4	5-14	15-44	45-59	60+
M. Congenital anomalies	6 204	3 033	3 171	2 771	132	124	5	-	2 883	135	147	6	-
N. Oral conditions	1 150	566	584	184	43	67	133	139	175	43	82	129	155
1. Dental caries	613	314	299	183	42	46	31	13	174	40	43	29	14
2. Periodontal disease	36	18	17	-	-	16	2	1	-	-	15	2	1
3. Edentulism	464	225	238	-	-	-	100	125	-	-	-	98	140
III. Injuries	36 949	21 905	15 044	3 857	2 313	12 122	2 470	1 144	3 661	1 582	7 148	1 648	1 006
A. Unintentional injuries	26 648	17 325	9 323	3 672	2 146	8 883	1 848	777	3 322	1 421	2 947	975	658
1. Road traffic accidents	7 550	5 424	2 126	148	636	3 570	779	291	107	604	972	334	109
2. Poisonings	1 332	794	538	199	52	329	156	58	58	67	309	50	54
3. Falls	3 886	2 193	1 693	529	266	1 091	192	115	654	163	424	217	234
4. Fires	589	336	253	107	57	121	23	28	71	76	41	27	38
5. Drownings	3 568	2 256	1 311	895	640	596	77	48	715	286	211	46	52
6. Other unintentional	9 723	6 322	3 401	1 794	495	3 175	620	238	1 716	226	989	300	170
B. Intentional injuries	10 301	4 580	5 721	185	167	3 239	622	367	338	161	4 201	673	349
1. Self-inflicted injuries	8 577	3 552	5 025	-	111	2 530	564	347	-	83	3 980	634	329
2. Violence	1 699	1 003	696	185	56	685	58	20	338	78	221	39	20
3. War	25	25	-	-	-	25	-	-	-	-	-	-	-

Notes:
A dash (-) symbol indicates fewer than 500 DALYs.
*IA6 is Bacterial meningitis and meningococcaemia; ID is Conditions arising during the perinatal period;
IIE6 is Dementia and other degenerative and hereditary CNS disorders; IIH1 is Chronic obstructive pulmonary disease.

Annex Table 13e. DALYs by age, sex and cause (thousands): Other Asia and Islands, 2000, baseline scenario

Cause	Total	Male	Female	Males 0-4	5-14	15-44	45-59	60+	Females 0-4	5-14	15-44	45-59	60+
Population (millions)	*808*	*404*	*403*	*44*	*83*	*204*	*46*	*28*	*42*	*81*	*201*	*47*	*33*
All causes	**163 992**	**90 325**	**73 667**	**26 533**	**8 577**	**32 819**	**12 177**	**10 219**	**21 402**	**6 122**	**26 818**	**9 040**	**10 284**
I. Communicable, maternal, perinatal and nutritional conditions	***53 909***	***27 706***	***26 203***	***18 772***	***2 362***	***4 394***	***1 058***	***1 121***	***14 755***	***2 094***	***7 128***	***1 074***	***1 152***
A. Infectious and parasitic diseases	**28 515**	**15 165**	**13 350**	**8 551**	**1 472**	**3 609**	**882**	**650**	**6 607**	**1 294**	**3 951**	**815**	**683**
1. Tuberculosis	**3 556**	**1 853**	**1 704**	**25**	**50**	**761**	**544**	**473**	**9**	**49**	**607**	**535**	**503**
2. STDs excluding HIV	**2 861**	**1 018**	**1 843**	**538**	**7**	**448**	**9**	**16**	**419**	**26**	**1 364**	**13**	**21**
a. Syphilis	818	460	358	378	1	59	7	15	261	1	67	9	20
b. Chlamydia	1 188	173	1 015	37	2	132	1	-	37	19	957	3	-
c. Gonorrhoea	855	385	470	123	4	257	1	-	121	7	340	1	-
3. HIV	**3 764**	**2 146**	**1 618**	**417**	**75**	**1 511**	**117**	**26**	**256**	**51**	**1 247**	**54**	**10**
4. Diarrhoeal diseases	**8 603**	**4 920**	**3 683**	**4 514**	**259**	**80**	**30**	**37**	**3 288**	**197**	**116**	**41**	**41**
5. Childhood-cluster diseases	**4 973**	**2 640**	**2 333**	**2 269**	**250**	**97**	**16**	**8**	**1 977**	**245**	**85**	**18**	**9**
a. Pertussis	817	434	383	399	35	-	-	-	352	31	-	-	-
b. Poliomyelitis	257	150	107	142	1	6	-	-	101	-	4	-	-
c. Diphtheria	50	27	23	24	2	-	-	-	21	2	-	-	-
d. Measles	2 408	1 280	1 128	1 134	143	2	-	-	1 001	125	2	-	-
e. Tetanus	1 440	748	692	569	68	88	15	8	502	85	79	17	9
6. Bacterial meningitis*	**531**	**278**	**253**	**188**	**10**	**48**	**19**	**13**	**169**	**9**	**42**	**21**	**13**
7. Hepatitis B and hepatitis C	**233**	**137**	**97**	**34**	**15**	**40**	**27**	**20**	**25**	**13**	**28**	**13**	**18**
8. Malaria	**1 365**	**742**	**623**	**137**	**234**	**307**	**48**	**17**	**121**	**205**	**228**	**51**	**18**
9. Tropical-cluster diseases	**338**	**238**	**99**	**8**	**46**	**155**	**26**	**4**	**5**	**14**	**55**	**21**	**3**
a. Trypanosomiasis	-	-	-	-	-	-	-	-	-	-	-	-	-
b. Chagas disease	-	-	-	-	-	-	-	-	-	-	-	-	-
c. Schistosomiasis	8	5	3	-	1	2	1	1	-	-	1	-	-
d. Leishmaniasis	41	26	15	1	7	17	1	1	1	4	9	1	-
e. Lymphatic filariasis	289	208	81	7	38	136	24	3	5	10	45	20	2
f. Onchocerciasis	-	-	-	-	-	-	-	-	-	-	-	-	-
10. Leprosy	**56**	**28**	**28**	**1**	**9**	**14**	**4**	**1**	**5**	**8**	**13**	**3**	**-**
11. Dengue	**132**	**63**	**69**	**16**	**45**	**1**	**-**	**-**	**18**	**49**	**1**	**1**	**-**
12. Japanese encephalitis	**104**	**55**	**48**	**34**	**17**	**4**	**-**	**-**	**30**	**15**	**3**	**-**	**-**
13. Trachoma	**37**	**10**	**27**	**-**	**-**	**2**	**3**	**5**	**-**	**-**	**4**	**8**	**15**
14. Intestinal nematode infections	**923**	**475**	**448**	**4**	**364**	**84**	**15**	**8**	**4**	**344**	**75**	**15**	**9**
a. Ascariasis	288	148	140	4	143	1	-	-	4	135	1	-	-
b. Trichuriasis	389	200	189	-	199	83	15	8	-	189	74	15	9
c. Ancylostomiasis and necatoriasis	246	127	119	-	21	-	-	-	-	21	-	-	-

Annex Table 13e, continued. DALYs by age, sex and cause (thousands): Other Asia and Islands, 2000, baseline scenario

Cause	Total	Male	Female	Males 0-4	5-14	15-44	45-59	60+	Females 0-4	5-14	15-44	45-59	60+
B. Respiratory infections	**9 939**	**5 596**	**4 343**	**4 324**	**613**	**204**	**69**	**386**	**3 193**	**544**	**163**	**74**	**368**
1. Lower respiratory infections	9 656	5 442	4 214	4 237	560	195	68	382	3 127	494	157	73	364
2. Upper respiratory infections	112	63	49	42	7	8	1	4	31	7	6	2	4
3. Otitis media	171	91	79	45	46	1	-	-	35	44	1	-	-
C. Maternal conditions	**2 090**	-	**2 090**	-	-	-	-	-	-	-	**2 066**	**24**	-
1. Maternal haemorrhage	202	-	202	-	-	-	-	-	-	-	197	5	-
2. Maternal sepsis	367	-	367	-	-	-	-	-	-	-	364	4	-
3. Hypertensive disorders of pregnancy	98	-	98	-	-	-	-	-	-	-	96	3	-
4. Obstructed labour	470	-	470	-	-	-	-	-	-	-	468	2	-
5. Abortion	401	-	401	-	-	-	-	-	-	-	398	3	-
D. Perinatal conditions*	**8 280**	**4 552**	**3 727**	**4 552**	-	-	-	-	**3 727**	-	-	-	-
E. Nutritional deficiencies	**5 085**	**2 393**	**2 692**	**1 345**	**277**	**581**	**106**	**85**	**1 228**	**256**	**947**	**160**	**101**
1. Protein-energy malnutrition	1 878	983	895	963	7	3	3	6	878	5	4	3	5
2. Iodine deficiency	107	55	52	48	5	2	-	-	45	5	2	-	-
3. Vitamin A deficiency	368	197	172	132	61	5	-	-	116	52	3	-	-
4. Iron-deficiency anaemia	2 732	1 159	1 574	202	204	571	102	79	188	194	938	157	96
II. Noncommunicable diseases	**82 879**	**44 112**	**38 767**	**4 845**	**3 251**	**17 418**	**9 810**	**8 788**	**4 128**	**2 506**	**15 737**	**7 475**	**8 920**
A. Malignant neoplasms	**11 698**	**6 436**	**5 261**	**244**	**646**	**1 522**	**2 080**	**1 945**	**269**	**420**	**1 569**	**1 486**	**1 517**
1. Mouth and oropharynx cancers	1 075	655	420	7	19	185	148	297	9	15	124	70	202
2. Oesophagus cancer	340	220	120	-	-	27	105	88	-	-	23	41	57
3. Stomach cancer	917	601	316	1	2	124	271	203	-	1	74	113	128
4. Colon and rectum cancers	614	321	294	2	6	92	71	149	3	5	72	63	151
5. Liver cancer	1 180	901	278	9	23	247	435	188	8	12	60	97	102
6. Pancreas cancer	141	89	52	-	-	20	35	34	1	-	6	19	25
7. Trachea, bronchus, lung cancers	1 376	1 044	331	-	-	164	494	375	3	4	42	123	158
8. Melanoma and other skin cancers	40	18	22	-	-	6	7	4	-	-	6	7	9
9. Breast cancer	572	-	572	-	-	225	230	111	-	-	225	230	111
10. Cervix uteri cancer	650	-	650	-	-	-	-	-	-	1	216	305	128
11. Corpus uteri cancer	65	-	65	-	-	-	-	-	-	-	5	28	32
12. Ovary cancer	249	-	249	-	-	-	-	-	-	2	55	123	69
13. Prostate cancer	143	143	-	-	-	7	28	108	-	-	-	-	-
14. Bladder cancer	147	107	39	-	-	12	38	58	-	-	5	9	25
15. Lymphomas and multiple myeloma	503	322	182	31	81	104	44	61	17	25	55	24	61
16. Leukaemia	898	498	401	85	218	136	24	34	98	148	97	21	36
C. Diabetes mellitus	**1 335**	**638**	**697**	**10**	**19**	**203**	**232**	**175**	**10**	**19**	**162**	**237**	**270**
D. Endocrine disorders	**432**	**208**	**224**	**108**	**34**	**32**	**19**	**15**	**87**	**18**	**53**	**33**	**34**

Annex Table 13e, continued. DALYs by age, sex and cause (thousands): Other Asia and Islands, 2000, baseline scenario

Cause	Total	Male	Female	Males					Females				
				0-4	5-14	15-44	45-59	60+	0-4	5-14	15-44	45-59	60+
E. Neuro-psychiatric conditions	**23 448**	**11 722**	**11 726**	**206**	**442**	**9 668**	**924**	**480**	**206**	**420**	**9 321**	**1 093**	**685**
1. Unipolar major depression	8 527	2 982	5 545	-	-	2 566	338	78	-	-	4 760	624	160
2. Bipolar disorder	2 407	1 211	1 197	-	-	1 133	60	18	-	-	1 114	60	23
3. Schizophrenia	2 841	1 482	1 359	15	109	1 460	13	9	17	119	1 339	6	14
4. Epilepsy	758	411	346	-	-	228	45	14	-	-	172	25	13
5. Alcohol use	2 413	2 232	181	-	-	2 085	124	23	-	-	171	7	3
6. Dementia*	1 101	482	619	40	18	43	140	242	48	19	40	151	361
7. Parkinson disease	128	69	59	-	-	-	29	39	-	-	-	24	34
8. Multiple sclerosis	208	90	118	-	-	80	7	2	-	-	104	10	4
9. Drug use	1 148	1 035	113	6	63	933	33	6	10	7	102	4	1
10. Post-traumatic stress disorder	311	117	194	-	25	79	6	1	-	41	131	10	2
11. Obsessive-compulsive disorders	1 678	720	958	-	87	590	30	12	-	112	773	54	19
12. Panic disorder	801	268	533	-	30	205	32	-	-	31	442	53	8
F. Sense organ diseases	**2 199**	**952**	**1 246**	**6**	**4**	**80**	**456**	**405**	**6**	-	**106**	**628**	**505**
1. Glaucoma	705	209	496	-	-	17	139	53	-	-	53	354	90
2. Cataracts	1 477	731	746	2	-	60	317	352	4	-	53	274	415
G. Cardiovascular diseases	**19 656**	**10 888**	**8 768**	**1 074**	**1 127**	**2 897**	**2 432**	**3 358**	**850**	**872**	**1 920**	**1 483**	**3 643**
1. Rheumatic heart disease	159	73	86	-	6	26	15	26	-	8	30	17	32
2. Ischaemic heart disease	5 225	2 923	2 302	135	226	585	883	1 455	110	162	332	474	1 496
3. Cerebrovascular disease	5 237	2 809	2 428	209	251	677	709	1 062	200	201	426	503	1 226
4. Inflammatory heart diseases	2 061	1 172	889	-	-	461	162	89	-	-	292	98	97
H. Respiratory diseases	**5 156**	**2 916**	**2 240**	**613**	**376**	**718**	**486**	**723**	**418**	**250**	**664**	**304**	**604**
1. COPD*	1 610	968	641	61	21	203	251	432	45	17	136	123	321
2. Asthma	1 524	844	680	94	215	401	84	51	50	137	354	83	55
I. Digestive diseases	**8 343**	**5 053**	**3 290**	**493**	**267**	**1 293**	**1 930**	**1 071**	**403**	**213**	**749**	**1 050**	**874**
1. Peptic ulcer	370	238	133	4	7	79	79	69	3	6	39	33	52
2. Cirrhosis of the liver	2 547	1 904	642	29	25	599	893	357	20	25	151	256	190
3. Appendicitis	231	134	97	3	46	77	6	2	3	40	48	4	2
J. Genito-urinary diseases	**1 863**	**1 044**	**819**	**65**	**143**	**235**	**402**	**200**	**44**	**104**	**228**	**182**	**260**
1. Nephritis and nephrosis	1 228	614	614	47	122	199	116	131	44	90	167	123	191
2. Benign prostatic hypertrophy	269	269	-	-	-	-	243	26	-	-	-	-	-
L. Musculo-skeletal diseases	**2 647**	**1 129**	**1 519**	**18**	**18**	**299**	**577**	**217**	**18**	**22**	**497**	**700**	**282**
1. Rheumatoid arthritis	255	69	186	-	-	5	23	41	-	2	63	37	84
2. Osteoarthritis	2 106	957	1 150	-	-	269	533	155	-	-	368	629	153

Annex Table 13e, continued. DALYs by age, sex and cause (thousands): Other Asia and Islands, 2000, baseline scenario

Cause	Total	Male	Female	Males					Females				
				0-4	5-14	15-44	45-59	60+	0-4	5-14	15-44	45-59	60+
M. Congenital anomalies	3 920	2 059	1 860	1 895	78	72	11	4	1 722	74	47	12	5
N. Oral conditions	1 638	790	848	31	44	336	208	170	30	45	345	221	207
1. Dental caries	646	322	324	30	43	145	72	31	29	42	143	74	36
2. Periodontal disease	43	21	22	-	-	17	3	1	-	-	17	3	1
3. Edentulism	929	443	486	-	-	172	133	139	-	-	173	143	170
III. Injuries	27 204	18 507	8 697	2 915	2 964	11 008	1 309	311	2 520	1 522	3 953	491	211
A. Unintentional injuries	22 254	15 311	6 943	2 812	2 763	8 466	1 034	236	2 408	1 392	2 569	400	174
1. Road traffic accidents	6 180	4 378	1 802	488	771	2 731	303	85	449	419	750	125	59
2. Poisonings	1 032	540	492	74	75	317	56	18	67	78	299	30	18
3. Falls	3 896	2 560	1 336	760	467	1 155	149	30	586	217	437	74	22
4. Fires	455	235	220	63	66	92	11	4	92	73	46	5	4
5. Drownings	2 423	1 673	751	582	551	478	45	17	364	215	145	16	10
6. Other unintentional	8 267	5 925	2 342	846	834	3 694	469	83	850	389	892	149	61
B. Intentional injuries	4 950	3 196	1 754	104	201	2 542	275	75	112	130	1 384	91	37
1. Self-inflicted injuries	2 370	1 305	1 065	-	71	1 060	127	48	-	44	936	58	27
2. Violence	1 887	1 488	399	45	92	1 192	136	23	52	57	259	24	7
3. War	693	402	291	59	38	289	13	3	59	29	190	9	4

Notes:
A dash (-) symbol indicates fewer than 500 DALYs.
*IA6 is Bacterial meningitis and meningococcaemia; ID is Conditions arising during the perinatal period;
IIE6 is Dementia and other degenerative and hereditary CNS disorders; IIH1 is Chronic obstructive pulmonary disease.

Annex Table 13f. DALYs by age, sex and cause (thousands): Sub-Saharan Africa, 2000, baseline scenario

Cause	Total	Male	Female	Males 0-4	Males 5-14	Males 15-44	Males 45-59	Males 60+	Females 0-4	Females 5-14	Females 15-44	Females 45-59	Females 60+
Population (millions)	*691*	*343*	*349*	*66*	*94*	*142*	*27*	*14*	*64*	*93*	*145*	*29*	*18*
All causes	**318 560**	**172 957**	**145 603**	**87 577**	**18 407**	**50 477**	**9 904**	**6 592**	**72 775**	**15 963**	**40 443**	**8 838**	**7 583**
I. Communicable, maternal, perinatal and nutritional conditions	***193 184***	***98 776***	***94 408***	***75 359***	***7 427***	***12 969***	***1 931***	***1 090***	***62 141***	***7 405***	***21 759***	***1 828***	***1 275***
A. Infectious and parasitic diseases	**131 327**	**68 483**	**62 845**	**48 067**	**5 583**	**12 363**	**1 815**	**655**	**39 353**	**5 523**	**15 571**	**1 677**	**720**
1. Tuberculosis	**13 807**	**6 485**	**7 322**	**872**	**602**	**3 797**	**922**	**292**	**931**	**870**	**4 333**	**891**	**298**
2. STDs excluding HIV	**5 376**	**2 119**	**3 257**	**1 486**	**13**	**581**	**14**	**26**	**1 382**	**48**	**1 767**	**22**	**37**
a. Syphilis	2 468	1 274	1 194	1 133	2	102	12	26	1 015	2	124	16	37
b. Chlamydia	1 407	197	1 210	65	3	128	1	–	68	31	1 107	4	–
c. Gonorrhoea	1 501	648	853	288	8	351	1	–	299	15	536	2	–
3. HIV	**20 548**	**9 458**	**11 089**	**3 001**	**460**	**5 551**	**373**	**73**	**2 855**	**478**	**7 430**	**279**	**47**
4. Diarrhoeal diseases	**30 021**	**16 715**	**13 306**	**15 360**	**1 007**	**220**	**49**	**80**	**11 767**	**1 028**	**349**	**62**	**100**
5. Childhood-cluster diseases	**28 270**	**15 141**	**13 130**	**13 505**	**1 497**	**107**	**20**	**10**	**11 544**	**1 452**	**106**	**18**	**10**
a. Pertussis	5 205	2 799	2 406	2 583	216	5	–	–	2 203	203	3	–	–
b. Poliomyelitis	566	329	237	322	2	–	–	–	232	1	–	–	–
c. Diphtheria	59	32	27	29	3	–	–	–	24	3	–	–	–
d. Measles	18 485	9 881	8 604	8 717	1 162	2	–	–	7 491	1 111	2	–	–
e. Tetanus	3 956	2 100	1 856	1 855	115	101	20	10	1 594	134	100	18	10
6. Bacterial meningitis*	**892**	**462**	**430**	**391**	**13**	**39**	**12**	**7**	**353**	**13**	**42**	**14**	**9**
7. Hepatitis B and hepatitis C	**232**	**129**	**103**	**39**	**19**	**33**	**22**	**16**	**28**	**17**	**31**	**11**	**16**
8. Malaria	**24 848**	**13 742**	**11 106**	**12 206**	**826**	**597**	**86**	**27**	**9 525**	**814**	**634**	**96**	**36**
9. Tropical-cluster diseases	**3 805**	**2 404**	**1 401**	**92**	**823**	**1 180**	**245**	**64**	**99**	**481**	**604**	**175**	**42**
a. Trypanosomiasis	978	495	482	18	187	220	61	10	33	188	212	42	7
b. Chagas disease	863	529	335	25	199	249	39	17	16	130	153	25	11
c. Schistosomiasis	320	213	108	12	119	79	3	–	5	59	41	2	–
d. Leishmaniasis	1 035	807	228	30	257	467	49	3	39	57	87	39	4
e. Lymphatic filariasis	609	360	249	7	61	165	92	34	6	48	110	65	20
f. Onchocerciasis	36	18	18	1	7	9	1	–	–	6	9	2	–
10. Leprosy	**36**	**18**	**18**				1			6		2	
11. Dengue	**16**	**7**	**9**	2	5				2	6			
12. Japanese encephalitis	**–**	**–**	**–**										
13. Trachoma	**273**	**73**	**200**			18	23	32			40	65	94
14. Intestinal nematode infections	**370**	**188**	**182**	**1**	**93**	**77**	**11**	**5**	**1**	**91**	**72**	**12**	**6**
a. Ascariasis	73	37	36	1	35	–	–	–	1	35	–	–	–
b. Trichuriasis	73	37	36	1	37	–	–	–	1	36	–	–	–
c. Ancylostomiasis and necatoriasis	224	114	110	–	21	77	11	5	–	20	71	12	6

Annex Table 13f, continued. DALYs by age, sex and cause (thousands): Sub-Saharan Africa, 2000, baseline scenario

Cause	Total	Male	Female	Males 0-4	5-14	15-44	45-59	60+	Females 0-4	5-14	15-44	45-59	60+
B. Respiratory infections	**29 077**	**16 192**	**12 885**	**14 105**	**1 361**	**279**	**64**	**383**	**10 853**	**1 139**	**327**	**72**	**494**
1. Lower respiratory infections	28 426	15 835	12 591	13 836	1 285	271	63	379	10 644	1 068	319	71	489
2. Upper respiratory infections	299	166	133	139	16	6	1	4	107	13	6	1	5
3. Otitis media	352	191	161	129	60	1	–	–	102	57	2	–	–
C. Maternal conditions	**5 691**		**5 691**							**271**	**5 415**	**5**	**–**
1. Maternal haemorrhage	824		824							62	761	1	
2. Maternal sepsis	1 079		1 079							41	1 037	1	
3. Hypertensive disorders of pregnancy	408		408							31	376		
4. Obstructed labour	992		992							21	971		
5. Abortion	1 000		1 000							35	964		
D. Perinatal conditions*	**18 700**	**9 827**	**8 873**	**9 827**					**8 873**				
E. Nutritional deficiencies	**8 389**	**4 275**	**4 114**	**3 361**	**482**	**327**	**53**	**51**	**3 062**	**473**	**445**	**74**	**61**
1. Protein-energy malnutrition	5 201	2 712	2 489	2 649	27	15	6	14	2 411	29	29	6	15
2. Iodine deficiency	117	58	59	52	5				50	6	3		
3. Vitamin A deficiency	1 040	543	497	387	150	6			343	148	7		
4. Iron-deficiency anaemia	2 031	962	1 069	274	300	305	46	38	258	290	406	68	46
II. Noncommunicable diseases	***67 024***	***34 187***	***32 837***	***5 976***	***3 197***	***13 327***	***6 537***	***5 151***	***5 708***	***3 481***	***11 069***	***6 498***	***6 080***
A. Malignant neoplasms	**8 114**	**4 489**	**3 625**	**182**	**509**	**1 318**	**1 327**	**1 153**	**231**	**529**	**781**	**1 173**	**912**
1. Mouth and oropharynx cancers	368	218	150	1	5	65	49	98	7	21	32	25	65
2. Oesophagus cancer	369	278	90			61	142	75			15	36	39
3. Stomach cancer	510	304	205	1	2	68	139	95		1	35	105	66
4. Colon and rectum cancers	221	123	98	1	2	41	29	51			21	22	54
5. Liver cancer	1 139	881	258	4	13	434	315	115	5	14	74	95	70
6. Pancreas cancer	111	65	46			17	31	17			9	23	14
7. Trachea, bronchus, lung cancers	341	233	108			53	106	73			29	46	33
8. Melanoma and other skin cancers	120	53	68			11	26	16			7	27	31
9. Breast cancer	297		297								81	135	78
10. Cervix uteri cancer	541		541								124	258	158
11. Corpus uteri cancer	50		50							1	6	22	21
12. Ovary cancer	146		146						6	16	39	54	31
13. Prostate cancer	359	359				8	91	259					
14. Bladder cancer	203	133	70			25	51	55			15	27	27
15. Lymphomas and multiple myeloma	773	467	307	64	206	100	45	51	58	152	40	25	31
16. Leukaemia	254	110	144	11	37	36	9	17	25	67	21	16	15
C. Diabetes mellitus	**522**	**248**	**274**	**18**	**48**	**58**	**69**	**55**	**21**	**48**	**40**	**77**	**87**
D. Endocrine disorders	**1 168**	**582**	**586**	**272**	**40**	**137**	**95**	**38**	**169**	**77**	**122**	**115**	**104**

Annex Table 13f, continued. DALYs by age, sex and cause (thousands): Sub-Saharan Africa, 2000, baseline scenario

Cause	Total	Male	Female	Males					Females				
				0-4	5-14	15-44	45-59	60+	0-4	5-14	15-44	45-59	60+
E. Neuro-psychiatric conditions	**15 788**	**7 627**	**8 160**	**255**	**415**	**6 253**	**512**	**193**	**295**	**435**	**6 440**	**648**	**343**
1. Unipolar major depression	6 193	2 113	4 080	-	-	1 865	205	43	-	-	3 580	406	94
2. Bipolar disorder	1 785	881	904	-	-	834	36	10	-	-	850	40	13
3. Schizophrenia	611	318	293	-	-	313	3	2	-	-	289	2	3
4. Epilepsy	526	288	239	30	92	138	21	8	35	89	97	12	7
5. Alcohol use	2 387	1 931	456	-	-	1 816	101	14	-	-	427	21	7
6. Dementia*	453	145	308	22	9	16	33	66	58	25	29	38	158
7. Parkinson disease	63	33	30	-	-	-	14	18	-	-	-	13	17
8. Multiple sclerosis	140	60	80	-	-	54	4	1	-	-	70	7	2
9. Drug use	504	455	49	-	34	406	13	2	-	4	44	1	-
10. Post-traumatic stress disorder	260	96	164	9	28	55	4	1	14	48	95	6	1
11. Obsessive-compulsive disorders	1 268	535	733	-	98	413	17	7	-	130	559	34	10
12. Panic disorder	594	198	396	-	35	144	19	-	-	36	323	33	4
F. Sense organ diseases	**2 460**	**1 159**	**1 301**	**9**	**1**	**92**	**558**	**499**	**9**	**1**	**85**	**616**	**591**
1. Glaucoma	523	207	315	-	-	2	98	108	-	-	3	158	154
2. Cataracts	1 930	947	983	9	1	85	460	392	9	1	79	458	437
G. Cardiovascular diseases	**13 390**	**6 477**	**6 913**	**558**	**671**	**2 136**	**1 526**	**1 586**	**551**	**876**	**1 249**	**1 768**	**2 468**
1. Rheumatic heart disease	627	309	318	1	111	179	13	4	2	155	133	21	6
2. Ischaemic heart disease	2 925	1 414	1 511	-	-	414	475	526	-	-	176	464	709
3. Cerebrovascular disease	5 487	2 560	2 927	89	224	854	640	753	164	209	446	868	1 315
4. Inflammatory heart diseases	1 594	771	823	149	109	276	132	106	206	173	177	112	156
H. Respiratory diseases	**9 037**	**4 956**	**4 081**	**1 004**	**546**	**1 487**	**1 006**	**913**	**821**	**498**	**1 005**	**964**	**793**
1. COPD*	2 390	1 437	952	83	38	428	400	488	75	41	178	308	350
2. Asthma	1 612	831	781	126	262	345	59	39	84	216	358	80	44
I. Digestive diseases	**5 418**	**3 103**	**2 314**	**422**	**335**	**1 075**	**848**	**423**	**408**	**463**	**580**	**462**	**401**
1. Peptic ulcer	310	200	111	-	-	118	59	22	-	-	47	38	25
2. Cirrhosis of the liver	685	491	194	-	28	199	177	86	-	16	61	68	49
3. Appendicitis	382	232	150	6	104	113	8	2	7	93	42	6	2
J. Genito-urinary diseases	**2 651**	**1 561**	**1 090**	**340**	**370**	**324**	**376**	**151**	**247**	**296**	**204**	**199**	**144**
1. Nephritis and nephrosis	1 907	1 062	844	282	313	263	101	103	238	258	131	121	97
2. Benign prostatic hypertrophy	230	230	-	-	-	-	220	10	-	-	-	-	-
L. Musculo-skeletal diseases	**1 404**	**470**	**933**	-	-	**247**	**152**	**72**	-	**3**	**383**	**403**	**144**
1. Rheumatoid arthritis	118	33	85	-	-	21	8	3	-	3	52	23	7
2. Osteoarthritis	1 264	428	836	-	-	221	141	66	-	-	323	377	135

Annex Table 13f, continued. DALYs by age, sex and cause (thousands): Sub-Saharan Africa, 2000, baseline scenario

Cause	Total	Male	Female	Males					Females				
				0-4	5-14	15-44	45-59	60+	0-4	5-14	15-44	45-59	60+
M. Congenital anomalies	5 224	2 542	2 682	2 358	97	73	10	4	2 520	108	34	14	6
N. Oral conditions	534	257	277	66	67	65	14	45	64	71	71	15	56
1. Dental caries	388	194	194	64	65	47	13	5	62	65	48	14	6
2. Periodontal disease	37	18	19	-	-	16	1	-	-	-	17	-	-
3. Edentulism	90	40	50	-	-	-	-	40	-	-	-	-	50
III. Injuries	58 352	39 994	18 358	6 242	7 783	24 181	1 436	352	4 926	5 077	7 615	511	228
A. Unintentional injuries	34 156	23 375	10 780	4 578	6 342	11 336	894	226	3 393	4 193	2 775	282	138
1. Road traffic accidents	7 782	5 518	2 264	496	1 880	2 825	253	65	337	959	866	82	20
2. Poisonings	1 598	937	661	663	158	90	19	7	488	78	87	5	3
3. Falls	2 509	1 450	1 059	307	649	410	58	26	336	398	243	38	45
4. Fires	4 255	2 111	2 143	862	683	498	49	20	741	931	410	36	24
5. Drownings	3 617	2 619	998	737	1 287	546	37	12	375	508	102	9	4
6. Other unintentional	14 394	10 740	3 654	1 514	1 685	6 967	477	97	1 115	1 319	1 066	112	42
B. Intentional injuries	24 196	16 619	7 578	1 664	1 441	12 846	542	125	1 533	885	4 840	230	90
1. Self-inflicted injuries	643	516	127	-	69	411	28	8	-	-	116	10	1
2. Violence	8 972	7 726	1 246	214	445	6 723	291	54	106	186	872	64	19
3. War	14 581	8 376	6 205	1 450	927	5 712	223	64	1 427	699	3 852	157	69

Notes:
A dash (-) symbol indicates fewer than 500 DALYs.
*IA6 is Bacterial meningitis and meningococcaemia; ID is Conditions arising during the perinatal period;
IIE6 is Dementia and other degenerative and hereditary CNS disorders; IIH1 is Chronic obstructive pulmonary disease.

Annex Table 13g. DALYs by age, sex and cause (thousands): Latin America and the Caribbean, 2000, baseline scenario

Cause	Total	Male	Female	Males 0-4	Males 5-14	Males 15-44	Males 45-59	Males 60+	Females 0-4	Females 5-14	Females 15-44	Females 45-59	Females 60+
Population (millions)	533	265	267	29	57	129	31	20	28	55	128	32	24
All causes	102 108	58 064	44 044	13 196	4 773	26 202	7 831	6 062	10 304	3 474	17 973	6 359	5 933
I. Communicable, maternal, perinatal and nutritional conditions	27 959	15 460	12 499	9 355	940	4 171	575	418	7 052	984	3 718	373	372
A. Infectious and parasitic diseases	15 397	9 173	6 224	3 899	639	3 920	471	245	2 993	658	2 131	260	183
1. Tuberculosis	1 155	652	503	37	41	357	124	93	28	59	279	79	58
2. STDs excluding HIV	922	255	668	145	1	103	2	3	120	10	530	3	4
a. Syphilis	265	143	122	125	–	13	2	3	101	–	15	2	4
b. Chlamydia	444	40	404	5	1	34	–	–	5	7	391	1	–
c. Gonorrhoea	213	72	142	14	1	56	–	–	14	2	125	–	–
3. HIV	4 262	3 367	895	181	17	2 920	202	47	168	19	672	28	8
4. Diarrhoeal diseases	3 735	2 145	1 590	1 898	124	72	24	28	1 311	129	89	27	34
5. Childhood-cluster diseases	2 345	1 255	1 090	1 154	90	7	2	1	987	90	9	2	1
a. Pertussis	498	264	234	243	21	–	–	–	212	21	–	–	–
b. Poliomyelitis	146	85	61	83	–	2	2	1	59	–	1	–	–
c. Diphtheria	11	5	5	3	2	1	–	–	2	2	–	–	–
d. Measles	1 220	647	573	587	58	1	–	–	508	62	3	–	–
e. Tetanus	470	253	217	237	9	4	2	1	205	4	5	2	1
6. Bacterial meningitis*	347	177	169	116	8	34	12	9	104	7	35	13	11
7. Hepatitis B and hepatitis C	77	35	43	14	9	7	3	2	10	10	17	4	2
8. Malaria	286	144	141	28	37	65	10	3	25	40	62	11	4
9. Tropical-cluster diseases	513	266	247	7	15	175	48	21	4	10	163	49	21
a. Trypanosomiasis	422	210	212	1	2	145	42	20	1	1	146	45	20
b. Chagas disease	51	27	24	1	6	16	3	1	1	6	13	3	1
c. Schistosomiasis	33	23	9	5	7	11	1	–	3	3	3	–	–
d. Leishmaniasis	5	4	1	–	1	2	1	–	–	–	1	–	–
e. Lymphatic filariasis	2	1	1	–	–	1	–	–	–	–	1	–	–
f. Onchocerciasis													
10. Leprosy	37	19	18	1	6	9	2	1	–	6	9	2	1
11. Dengue	1	1		–	–	–							
12. Japanese encephalitis	–	–	–										
13. Trachoma	–	–	–										
14. Intestinal nematode infections	452	229	223	2	186	32	6	3	2	182	29	6	4
a. Ascariasis	155	78	77	2	76	–	–	–	2	74	–	–	–
b. Trichuriasis	201	102	99	–	101	–	–	–	–	99	–	–	–
c. Ancylostomiasis and necatoriasis	96	49	47	–	9	31	6	3	–	9	28	6	3

Annex Table 13g, continued. DALYs by age, sex and cause (thousands): Latin America and the Caribbean, 2000, baseline scenario

Cause	Total	Male	Female	Males 0-4	5-14	15-44	45-59	60+	Females 0-4	5-14	15-44	45-59	60+
B. Respiratory infections	**3 477**	**1 881**	**1 596**	**1 433**	**147**	**118**	**66**	**117**	**1 102**	**160**	**159**	**55**	**121**
1. Lower respiratory infections	3 349	1 815	1 534	1 409	112	113	65	116	1 083	126	153	53	119
2. Upper respiratory infections	43	23	19	14	2	4	1	2	10	2	4	1	2
3. Otitis media	85	43	42	9	33	–	–	–	9	32	1	–	–
C. Maternal conditions	**976**		**976**							**4**	**970**	**2**	–
1. Maternal haemorrhage	92		92							1	91	–	–
2. Maternal sepsis	168		168							–	168	–	–
3. Hypertensive disorders of pregnancy	57		57							–	56	–	–
4. Obstructed labour	237		237							1	237	–	–
5. Abortion	255		255							–	254	–	–
D. Perinatal conditions*	**5 565**	**3 241**	**2 325**	**3 241**					**2 325**				
E. Nutritional deficiencies	**2 544**	**1 166**	**1 379**	**783**	**154**	**134**	**38**	**56**	**632**	**163**	**458**	**57**	**69**
1. Protein-energy malnutrition	1 183	647	536	563	24	18	13	28	434	32	26	12	33
2. Iodine deficiency	64	32	32	28	2	1	–	–	26	3	2	–	–
3. Vitamin A deficiency	123	64	59	46	16	–	–	–	41	17	2	–	–
4. Iron-deficiency anaemia	1 162	418	744	142	112	112	25	28	126	111	426	45	35
II. Noncommunicable diseases	***55 795***	***29 077***	***26 719***	***2 742***	***1 706***	***13 118***	***6 184***	***5 328***	***2 441***	***1 492***	***11 720***	***5 675***	***5 390***
A. Malignant neoplasms	**5 737**	**2 631**	**3 106**	**75**	**267**	**545**	**813**	**930**	**74**	**185**	**969**	**1 050**	**828**
1. Mouth and oropharynx cancers	205	152	53	1	2	38	71	41	–	1	11	18	21
2. Oesophagus cancer	132	95	37	–	–	11	47	38	–	–	4	13	21
3. Stomach cancer	497	307	190	–	–	53	117	137	–	–	36	62	92
4. Colon and rectum cancers	319	152	168	1	1	36	53	62	–	–	30	54	84
5. Liver cancer	74	39	35	1	2	9	14	13	1	1	5	11	17
6. Pancreas cancer	99	52	47	–	–	8	21	23	–	–	5	16	25
7. Trachea, bronchus, lung cancers	552	382	170	–	1	68	172	140	–	1	31	76	63
8. Melanoma and other skin cancers	56	27	29	–	1	12	9	6	–	1	11	10	7
9. Breast cancer	552		552							–	189	235	128
10. Cervix uteri cancer	483		483							–	202	194	87
11. Corpus uteri cancer	103		103							–	20	51	32
12. Ovary cancer	113		113							5	47	33	25
13. Prostate cancer	197	197				5	29	163					
14. Bladder cancer	104	79	25	–	1	8	25	44	–	–	3	7	15
15. Lymphomas and multiple myeloma	339	202	137	14	46	76	39	27	9	26	40	29	32
16. Leukaemia	354	200	154	24	80	65	17	14	21	59	43	16	15
C. Diabetes mellitus	**1 515**	**683**	**832**	**11**	**22**	**185**	**242**	**222**	**10**	**19**	**173**	**292**	**337**
D. Endocrine disorders	**1 329**	**656**	**673**	**310**	**69**	**158**	**65**	**53**	**250**	**57**	**189**	**96**	**81**

Annex Table 13g, continued. DALYs by age, sex and cause (thousands): Latin America and the Caribbean, 2000, baseline scenario

Cause	Total	Male	Female	Males 0-4	Males 5-14	Males 15-44	Males 45-59	Males 60+	Females 0-4	Females 5-14	Females 15-44	Females 45-59	Females 60+
E. Neuro-psychiatric conditions	**18 718**	**10 517**	**8 200**	**229**	**473**	**8 542**	**875**	**398**	**207**	**437**	**6 367**	**730**	**458**
1. Unipolar major depression	5 237	1 815	3 423	–	–	1 549	215	50	–	–	2 908	409	106
2. Bipolar disorder	1 457	728	729	–	–	679	38	12	–	–	676	39	14
3. Schizophrenia	1 559	810	749			793	10	6			739	4	7
4. Epilepsy	610	341	269	13	90	192	35	11	12	84	149	15	9
5. Alcohol use	4 709	4 321	389	–	–	3 839	381	100			364	18	6
6. Dementia*	809	343	466	42	24	27	77	174	42	19	29	107	270
7. Parkinson disease	46	25	21				11	14				9	12
8. Multiple sclerosis	138	59	79			52	5	2			69	8	3
9. Drug use	1 353	881	472	–	60	787	29	5	–	32	422	16	3
10. Post-traumatic stress disorder	202	76	127	4	17	50	4	1	6	28	84	7	1
11. Obsessive-compulsive disorders	1 041	443	597	–	57	358	19	8	–	74	475	36	13
12. Panic disorder	480	160	320		19	120	20	–		20	262	34	5
F. Sense organ diseases	**768**	**357**	**411**	**21**	**4**	**23**	**92**	**217**	**15**	**7**	**24**	**109**	**256**
1. Glaucoma	114	41	73			1	21	19			3	42	28
2. Cataracts	596	286	310	3		16	69	198	3	1	14	66	227
G. Cardiovascular diseases	**9 777**	**5 323**	**4 454**	**139**	**103**	**1 197**	**1 713**	**2 171**	**105**	**82**	**1 046**	**1 213**	**2 009**
1. Rheumatic heart disease	189	65	124	1	12	31	14	7		15	64	30	13
2. Ischaemic heart disease	3 876	2 213	1 663			380	809	1 024			267	489	906
3. Cerebrovascular disease	3 160	1 658	1 502	11	19	402	541	686	8	16	372	440	666
4. Inflammatory heart diseases	553	297	256	27	22	136	68	45	24	18	118	53	44
H. Respiratory diseases	**4 602**	**2 312**	**2 290**	**481**	**220**	**639**	**437**	**534**	**357**	**186**	**752**	**512**	**483**
1. COPD*	1 432	768	663	47	8	179	213	322	38	7	160	204	255
2. Asthma	1 099	555	544	53	136	276	55	36	36	114	243	94	56
I. Digestive diseases	**4 014**	**2 372**	**1 643**	**179**	**89**	**812**	**870**	**421**	**136**	**71**	**589**	**476**	**371**
1. Peptic ulcer	182	115	67	1	2	43	38	31	7	1	23	19	23
2. Cirrhosis of the liver	1 330	994	336	9	7	390	440	148	7	6	117	134	73
3. Appendicitis	49	29	20	1	9	16	2	1	1	7	11	1	1
J. Genito-urinary diseases	**1 247**	**668**	**579**	**73**	**58**	**107**	**302**	**128**	**64**	**67**	**225**	**108**	**114**
1. Nephritis and nephrosis	599	284	315	42	47	74	56	66	39	52	100	57	66
2. Benign prostatic hypertrophy	238	238	–				217	20				–	–
L. Musculo-skeletal diseases	**3 862**	**1 493**	**2 370**	**8**	**23**	**590**	**692**	**180**	**5**	**32**	**998**	**982**	**354**
1. Rheumatoid arthritis	722	151	571		–	86	47	17	–	6	383	132	49
2. Osteoarthritis	2 783	1 256	1 527	–	–	478	629	150	–	–	451	801	275

Annex Table 13g, continued. DALYs by age, sex and cause (thousands): Latin America and the Caribbean, 2000, baseline scenario

Cause	Total	Male	Female	Males					Females				
				0-4	5-14	15-44	45-59	60+	0-4	5-14	15-44	45-59	60+
M. Congenital anomalies	2 460	1 225	1 235	1 134	58	27	4	2	1 139	49	38	6	2
N. Oral conditions	1 177	587	590	37	259	220	29	42	36	252	219	31	52
1. Dental caries	1 036	522	513	37	258	214	10	4	35	250	213	10	5
2. Periodontal disease	24	12	13	-	-	4	5	2	-	-	4	6	3
3. Edentulism	107	49	59	-	-	-	13	35	-	-	-	15	44
III. Injuries	*18 354*	*13 527*	*4 827*	*1 099*	*2 127*	*8 913*	*1 073*	*316*	*812*	*998*	*2 535*	*311*	*172*
A. Unintentional injuries	12 968	9 235	3 734	986	1 910	5 296	788	254	710	886	1 730	254	153
1. Road traffic accidents	4 994	3 568	1 426	134	750	2 296	308	81	100	400	791	100	36
2. Poisonings	153	89	64	26	14	39	7	3	19	12	28	3	2
3. Falls	1 679	1 209	470	186	400	498	77	48	91	133	155	43	49
4. Fires	308	170	138	44	54	57	9	8	40	54	35	6	3
5. Drownings	874	680	194	90	181	368	33	8	58	65	64	5	2
6. Other unintentional	4 960	3 519	1 441	505	510	2 039	354	110	403	221	658	98	61
B. Intentional injuries	5 386	4 293	1 093	113	217	3 616	285	62	102	112	805	56	18
1. Self-inflicted injuries	731	476	255	-	18	376	60	22	-	15	212	21	7
2. Violence	3 853	3 354	500	45	149	2 915	210	36	33	60	375	25	7
3. War	801	462	339	69	49	325	15	4	69	37	219	11	4

Notes:
A dash (-) symbol indicates fewer than 500 DALYs.
*IA6 is Bacterial meningitis and meningococcaemia: ID is Conditions arising during the perinatal period;
IIE6 is Dementia and other degenerative and hereditary CNS disorders; IIH1 is Chronic obstructive pulmonary disease.

Annex Table 13h. DALYs by age, sex and cause (thousands): Middle Eastern Crescent, 2000, baseline scenario

Cause	Total	Male	Female	Males 0-4	5-14	15-44	45-59	60+	Females 0-4	5-14	15-44	45-59	60+
Population (millions)	656	333	322	50	83	150	32	19	48	80	142	31	21
All causes	155 411	83 089	72 322	36 853	8 165	22 914	8 328	6 829	33 740	6 517	19 619	5 959	6 486
I. Communicable, maternal, perinatal and nutritional conditions	61 296	30 594	30 702	26 436	1 738	1 508	431	482	24 300	1 671	3 864	391	476
A. Infectious and parasitic diseases	25 914	13 750	12 164	11 162	841	1 204	361	182	10 111	741	870	248	195
1. Tuberculosis	1 815	1 182	633	157	81	623	220	101	94	49	298	120	71
2. STDs excluding HIV	677	259	419	203	1	51	1	2	187	5	221	2	3
a. Syphilis	399	206	193	192	–	11	1	2	177	–	12	2	3
b. Chlamydia	196	23	173	3	–	19	–	–	3	4	166	–	–
c. Gonorrhoea	82	29	53	8	–	21	–	–	7	1	44	–	–
3. HIV	340	269	71	33	2	203	29	3	33	2	33	3	–
4. Diarrhoeal diseases	12 767	6 664	6 103	6 347	241	54	13	10	5 783	235	61	13	10
5. Childhood-cluster diseases	7 367	3 855	3 513	3 536	296	16	5	2	3 209	263	31	8	2
a. Pertussis	1 722	898	824	826	72	–	–	–	756	68	–	–	–
b. Poliomyelitis	415	242	173	236	1	4	–	–	169	–	3	–	–
c. Diphtheria	35	18	17	17	2	–	–	–	15	2	–	–	–
d. Measles	2 809	1 457	1 352	1 290	166	1	–	–	1 191	159	2	–	–
e. Tetanus	2 387	1 240	1 147	1 167	56	11	4	2	1 078	34	26	8	1
6. Bacterial meningitis*	577	301	276	227	12	40	14	8	211	11	31	14	9
7. Hepatitis B and hepatitis C	194	111	84	33	15	28	22	14	25	14	23	10	12
8. Malaria	271	143	129	34	54	45	7	3	31	51	37	7	3
9. Tropical-cluster diseases	202	128	74	19	48	48	10	3	12	27	28	5	2
a. Trypanosomiasis	–	–	–	–	–	–	–	–	–	–	–	–	–
b. Chagas disease	–	–	–	–	–	–	–	–	–	–	–	–	–
c. Schistosomiasis	103	66	37	2	18	35	8	3	1	8	21	5	2
d. Leishmaniasis	91	55	35	17	29	8	1	–	11	19	5	–	–
e. Lymphatic filariasis	9	6	2	–	–	5	–	–	–	–	1	–	–
f. Onchocerciasis	–	–	–	–	–	–	–	–	–	–	–	–	–
10. Leprosy	9	5	4	1	1	2	–	–	–	1	2	–	–
11. Dengue	–	–	–	–	–	–	–	–	–	–	–	–	–
12. Japanese encephalitis	–	–	–	–	–	–	–	–	–	–	–	–	–
13. Trachoma	204	57	147	–	–	13	19	25	–	–	28	49	71
14. Intestinal nematode infections	143	74	68	1	42	25	4	2	1	39	22	4	2
a. Ascariasis	70	36	34	1	35	–	–	–	1	33	–	–	–
b. Trichuriasis	1	1	–	–	–	–	–	–	–	–	–	–	–
c. Ancylostomiasis and necatoriasis	71	38	34	–	7	25	4	2	–	6	21	4	2

Annex Table 13h, continued. DALYs by age, sex and cause (thousands): Middle Eastern Crescent, 2000, baseline scenario

Cause	Total	Male	Female	Males 0-4	5-14	15-44	45-59	60+	Females 0-4	5-14	15-44	45-59	60+
B. Respiratory infections	**13 911**	**7 189**	**6 722**	**6 200**	**590**	**95**	**34**	**269**	**5 664**	**631**	**128**	**51**	**248**
1. Lower respiratory infections	13 544	6 999	6 545	6 077	532	90	34	266	5 551	576	122	50	245
2. Upper respiratory infections	146	75	71	60	7	4	1	3	55	7	5	1	3
3. Otitis media	221	114	106	63	51	-	-	-	58	48	1	-	-
C. Maternal conditions	**2 243**		**2 243**						**-**	**2**	**2 203**	**39**	**-**
1. Maternal haemorrhage	227		227								218	8	
2. Maternal sepsis	474		474								468	6	
3. Hypertensive disorders of pregnancy	146		146								140	6	
4. Obstructed labour	617		617								614	3	
5. Abortion	219		219								216	3	
D. Perinatal conditions*	**13 364**	**6 886**	**6 478**	**6 886**					**6 478**				
E. Nutritional deficiencies	**5 864**	**2 769**	**3 096**	**2 187**	**306**	**210**	**35**	**30**	**2 048**	**297**	**663**	**53**	**34**
1. Protein-energy malnutrition	3 153	1 633	1 521	1 615	5	4	2	6	1 501	5	7	2	6
2. Iodine deficiency	213	107	106	94	10	3	-	-	88	10	6	1	-
3. Vitamin A deficiency	601	299	302	214	82	4	-	-	212	86	4	-	-
4. Iron-deficiency anaemia	1 898	730	1 168	264	210	199	33	24	248	196	646	50	28
II. Noncommunicable diseases	***69 812***	***36 825***	***32 987***	***7 539***	***3 503***	***12 484***	***7 129***	***6 169***	***6 796***	***3 237***	***11 832***	***5 249***	***5 873***
A. Malignant neoplasms	**4 810**	**2 686**	**2 123**	**115**	**372**	**709**	**887**	**603**	**105**	**328**	**678**	**572**	**440**
1. Mouth and oropharynx cancers	292	190	103	1	6	76	48	58	2	7	38	22	33
2. Oesophagus cancer	161	96	65	-	1	21	49	25	1	2	17	26	20
3. Stomach cancer	350	221	129	1	3	59	104	55	-	1	34	47	46
4. Colon and rectum cancers	206	109	97	-	2	42	28	37	1	4	28	19	44
5. Liver cancer	147	94	53	1	5	24	42	21	1	4	12	19	16
6. Pancreas cancer	76	48	27	-	-	13	23	12	-	-	5	12	10
7. Trachea, bronchus, lung cancers	741	583	157	2	6	115	300	160	-	5	33	61	56
8. Melanoma and other skin cancers	25	15	10	-	-	6	7	2	-	-	5	3	2
9. Breast cancer	265	-	265						-	2	118	103	42
10. Cervix uteri cancer	159		159						-	1	60	70	28
11. Corpus uteri cancer	34		34						-	-	7	15	11
12. Ovary cancer	88		88						-	1	43	26	10
13. Prostate cancer	54	54		-	-	4	16	34					
14. Bladder cancer	160	129	31	1	2	31	54	42		-	8	12	11
15. Lymphomas and multiple myeloma	255	171	84	13	54	67	20	17	9	32	25	8	10
16. Leukaemia	423	220	203	24	97	69	15	15	29	105	43	10	16
C. Diabetes mellitus	**1 492**	**748**	**744**	**37**	**65**	**229**	**254**	**163**	**35**	**63**	**181**	**245**	**221**
D. Endocrine disorders	**1 034**	**510**	**524**	**270**	**77**	**93**	**48**	**21**	**254**	**123**	**91**	**35**	**21**

Annex Table 13h, continued. DALYs by age, sex and cause (thousands): Middle Eastern Crescent, 2000, baseline scenario

Cause	Total	Male	Female	Males 0-4	5-14	15-44	45-59	60+	Females 0-4	5-14	15-44	45-59	60+
E. Neuro-psychiatric conditions	16 494	7 994	8 500	625	657	5 993	503	215	496	577	6 515	628	283
1. Unipolar major depression	6 068	2 175	3 892	-	-	1 890	233	52	-	-	3 376	412	104
2. Bipolar disorder	1 732	887	845	-	-	834	41	12	-	-	791	40	14
3. Schizophrenia	1 857	979	877	35	93	966	8	5	28	110	862	9	6
4. Epilepsy	507	268	239	-	-	115	18	7	-	-	83	12	4
5. Alcohol use	341	307	34	-	-	287	17	3	-	-	32	1	1
6. Dementia*	387	185	201	45	14	25	32	70	51	15	25	21	90
7. Parkinson disease	82	45	38	-	-	-	19	26	-	-	-	16	21
8. Multiple sclerosis	149	66	83	-	-	59	5	2	-	-	74	7	2
9. Drug use	1 214	1 092	121	-	81	971	34	6	-	9	108	4	1
10. Post-traumatic stress disorder	247	95	153	7	25	58	4	1	11	41	93	7	1
11. Obsessive-compulsive disorders	1 246	545	701	-	86	430	20	8	-	110	542	35	12
12. Panic disorder	559	194	365	-	29	143	21	-	-	29	298	33	5
F. Sense organ diseases	1 232	596	636	3	-	42	272	279	4	1	39	273	320
1. Glaucoma	144	55	89	-	-	1	37	17	-	-	2	63	24
2. Cataracts	1 076	535	541	2	-	37	234	261	2	-	33	210	296
G. Cardiovascular diseases	20 004	11 096	8 909	1 456	1 161	2 404	2 724	3 350	1 099	1 085	1 813	1 644	3 267
1. Rheumatic heart disease	769	359	411	1	103	228	22	4	2	128	245	29	7
2. Ischaemic heart disease	7 090	4 140	2 950	-	-	790	1 475	1 875	-	-	457	738	1 755
3. Cerebrovascular disease	3 059	1 612	1 447	77	194	371	419	550	55	162	239	339	652
4. Inflammatory heart diseases	2 000	1 088	912	279	219	353	147	90	260	189	276	101	86
H. Respiratory diseases	7 203	3 831	3 371	1 237	474	803	571	747	1 046	441	739	556	588
1. COPD*	1 848	961	887	132	28	196	165	440	132	50	184	233	288
2. Asthma	1 055	690	365	103	218	277	58	34	30	89	165	47	33
I. Digestive diseases	6 252	3 419	2 833	1 202	250	771	829	367	1 341	193	505	497	297
1. Peptic ulcer	157	110	47	-	4	50	38	17	1	2	21	14	9
2. Cirrhosis of the liver	902	522	381	13	30	151	222	107	10	66	87	130	88
3. Appendicitis	134	78	56	2	30	41	3	1	2	26	25	2	1
J. Genito-urinary diseases	3 124	1 862	1 262	161	168	620	652	260	129	156	477	310	189
1. Nephritis and nephrosis	800	403	396	67	86	130	64	56	58	112	133	52	42
2. Benign prostatic hypertrophy	257	257	-	-	-	1	234	21	-	-	-	-	-
L. Musculo-skeletal diseases	1 162	518	644	15	11	286	153	54	12	8	267	237	120
1. Rheumatoid arthritis	222	132	89	-	-	126	4	1	-	2	48	28	10
2. Osteoarthritis	819	329	490	-	-	139	142	48	-	-	188	198	104

Annex Table 13h, continued. DALYs by age, sex and cause (thousands): Middle Eastern Crescent, 2000, baseline scenario

Cause	Total	Male	Female	Males					Females				
				0-4	5-14	15-44	45-59	60+	0-4	5-14	15-44	45-59	60+
M. Congenital anomalies	4 775	2 454	2 322	2 273	91	75	11	3	2 141	102	59	14	5
N. Oral conditions	1 826	912	913	104	131	393	195	89	99	127	383	199	105
1. Dental caries	896	455	441	103	130	143	50	29	99	125	135	49	33
2. Periodontal disease	26	13	13	-	-	13	1	-	-	-	12	1	-
3. Edentulism	887	440	448	-	-	235	145	60	-	-	227	149	71
III. Injuries	24 303	15 671	8 632	2 879	2 923	8 922	769	178	2 644	1 609	3 923	319	137
A. Unintentional injuries	12 327	8 503	3 823	1 839	1 870	4 217	475	101	1 590	895	1 113	158	68
1. Road traffic accidents	3 251	2 514	737	126	516	1 687	155	29	109	263	304	44	16
2. Poisonings	428	268	161	72	23	133	33	6	68	18	58	12	5
3. Falls	1 927	1 239	688	391	434	362	42	10	337	185	132	24	9
4. Fires	827	372	455	123	120	112	13	3	127	128	184	11	5
5. Drownings	1 032	724	308	226	210	265	17	4	196	59	47	4	2
6. Other unintentional	4 862	3 387	1 475	900	566	1 657	215	49	752	242	388	63	31
B. Intentional injuries	11 976	7 167	4 809	1 039	1 053	4 705	293	76	1 054	714	2 810	161	69
1. Self-inflicted injuries	1 750	1 186	565	-	393	669	96	27	-	182	323	38	21
2. Violence	1 533	994	539	239	100	598	45	11	259	106	150	19	6
3. War	8 693	4 988	3 705	800	560	3 437	152	38	795	427	2 337	104	42

Notes:
A dash (-) symbol indicates fewer than 500 DALYs.
*IA6 is Bacterial meningitis and meningococcaemia; ID is Conditions arising during the perinatal period;
IIE6 is Dementia and other degenerative and hereditary CNS disorders; IIH1 is Chronic obstructive pulmonary disease.

Annex Table 13i. DALYs by age, sex and cause (thousands): World, 2000, baseline scenario

Cause	Total	Male	Female	Males 0-4	5-14	15-44	45-59	60+	Females 0-4	5-14	15-44	45-59	60+
Population (millions)	*6 160*	*3 096*	*3 064*	*346*	*628*	*1 444*	*403*	*275*	*331*	*605*	*1 389*	*403*	*337*
All causes	*1 356 851*	*740 492*	*616 360*	*228 943*	*61 025*	*244 491*	*106 772*	*99 261*	*202 023*	*49 405*	*195 947*	*75 864*	*93 121*
I. Communicable, maternal, perinatal and nutritional conditions	*483 337*	*246 978*	*236 359*	*172 040*	*17 745*	*39 649*	*9 537*	*8 006*	*150 704*	*17 899*	*53 257*	*7 248*	*7 250*
A. Infectious and parasitic diseases	278 639	149 082	129 557	89 003	11 888	35 281	8 331	4 579	76 273	11 554	32 391	5 665	3 674
1. Tuberculosis	39 638	22 467	17 171	1 617	1 217	11 349	5 344	2 941	1 482	1 404	8 865	3 559	1 861
2. STDs excluding HIV	14 193	5 011	9 182	3 033	32	1 836	40	70	2 776	131	6 118	60	97
a. Syphilis	5 108	2 646	2 461	2 268	3	275	32	68	2 013	4	312	40	92
b. Chlamydia	5 255	697	4 558	164	10	519	2	1	163	93	4 286	14	2
c. Gonorrhoea	3 822	1 664	2 158	600	18	1 040	5	1	600	35	1 517	6	1
3. HIV	40 226	22 401	17 825	4 657	747	15 403	1 347	247	4 358	755	12 105	513	94
4. Diarrhoeal diseases	74 001	39 662	34 339	35 805	2 176	971	271	440	30 210	2 283	1 054	295	497
5. Childhood-cluster diseases	54 450	28 795	25 655	25 564	2 667	446	78	40	22 493	2 637	403	81	41
a. Pertussis	10 368	5 484	4 884	5 043	442				4 463	421			
b. Poliomyelitis	2 330	1 360	970	1 320	8	29	2	1	944	6	18	2	1
c. Diphtheria	245	128	117	114	13	2			103	13	2		
d. Measles	29 185	15 429	13 756	13 610	1 803	13	2	1	12 007	1 733	13	2	40
e. Tetanus	12 321	6 394	5 928	5 477	402	403	74	38	4 976	465	370	77	40
6. Bacterial meningitis*	4 075	2 134	1 941	1 524	78	331	117	84	1 387	74	270	117	93
7. Hepatitis B and hepatitis C	1 276	752	524	183	79	234	159	98	137	74	152	64	96
8. Malaria	27 401	15 109	12 292	12 492	1 253	1 132	172	59	9 778	1 216	1 045	183	69
9. Tropical-cluster diseases	6 533	4 227	2 306	194	1 331	2 223	376	103	158	720	1 040	309	78
a. Trypanosomiasis	978	495	482	18	187	220	61	10	33	188	212	42	7
b. Chagas disease	422	210	212	1	2	145	42	20	1	1	146	45	20
c. Schistosomiasis	1 038	635	403	27	224	306	54	24	17	145	189	36	16
d. Leishmaniasis	1 154	735	420	68	331	317	13	5	42	203	162	9	4
e. Lymphatic filariasis	2 330	1 791	539	73	527	1 069	112	10	59	137	220	112	12
f. Onchocerciasis	610	361	250	7	62	165	93	34	6	48	110	66	20
10. Leprosy	275	140	135	4	46	72	14	4	7	43	69	13	3
11. Dengue	384	179	205	43	130	4	1	-	49	151	3	2	-
12. Japanese encephalitis	371	194	177	116	63	13	2	1	107	58	9	1	1
13. Trachoma	754	206	548	-	-	41	65	99	-	-	91	172	285
14. Intestinal nematode infections	3 125	1 609	1 517	17	1 167	336	58	30	16	1 114	294	59	34
a. Ascariasis	1 057	541	516	16	520	4	1	-	16	497	3	1	-
b. Trichuriasis	1 084	555	530	-	554	-	-	-	-	529	-	-	-
c. Ancylostomiasis and necatoriasis	983	513	470	-	93	332	58	30	-	89	290	58	33

Annex Table 13i, continued. DALYs by age, sex and cause (thousands): World, 2000, baseline scenario

Cause	Total	Male	Female	Males					Females				
				0-4	5-14	15-44	45-59	60+	0-4	5-14	15-44	45-59	60+
B. Respiratory infections	**84 860**	**44 712**	**40 148**	**36 412**	**3 657**	**1 300**	**580**	**2 762**	**31 706**	**3 902**	**1 225**	**515**	**2 801**
1. Lower respiratory infections	82 495	43 485	39 010	35 650	3 287	1 249	567	2 732	31 021	3 541	1 178	503	2 768
2. Upper respiratory infections	938	494	444	360	46	46	12	31	310	47	41	12	33
3. Otitis media	1 426	732	694	401	325	5	–	–	374	313	6	–	–
C. Maternal conditions	**15 598**		**15 598**							**276**	**15 196**	**126**	
1. Maternal haemorrhage	1 863		1 863							63	1 771	29	
2. Maternal sepsis	2 874		2 874							42	2 817	16	
3. Hypertensive disorders of pregnancy	936		936							32	890	14	
4. Obstructed labour	3 356		3 356							21	3 327	8	
5. Abortion	2 719		2 719							36	2 670	13	
D. Perinatal conditions*	**69 064**	**36 225**	**32 839**	**36 224**	**1**				**32 838**				
E. Nutritional deficiencies	**35 176**	**16 960**	**18 217**	**10 401**	**2 200**	**3 067**	**626**	**665**	**9 887**	**2 167**	**4 445**	**942**	**775**
1. Protein-energy malnutrition	15 501	7 904	7 597	7 618	83	69	36	97	7 253	123	81	30	110
2. Iodine deficiency	947	484	462	425	42	16	1	–	396	43	21	2	–
3. Vitamin A deficiency	2 695	1 392	1 303	973	396	24	–	–	895	388	21	–	–
4. Iron-deficiency anaemia	15 964	7 150	8 814	1 372	1 673	2 955	586	564	1 332	1 608	4 310	906	658
II. Noncommunicable diseases	*642 632*	*342 278*	*300 354*	*34 751*	*16 620*	*118 150*	*85 297*	*87 459*	*32 459*	*15 019*	*107 295*	*62 817*	*82 764*
A. Malignant neoplasms	**89 930**	**52 305**	**37 626**	**1 016**	**2 660**	**11 586**	**19 308**	**17 735**	**1 082**	**1 919**	**9 714**	**12 752**	**12 157**
1. Mouth and oropharynx cancers	4 831	3 160	1 671	20	48	904	1 180	1 007	21	49	488	539	573
2. Oesophagus cancer	4 845	3 340	1 505	–	1	493	1 516	1 329	–	2	198	587	718
3. Stomach cancer	10 152	6 649	3 503	3	17	985	2 932	2 712	1	12	777	1 230	1 484
4. Colon and rectum cancers	5 638	3 081	2 557	4	21	658	1 009	1 388	5	22	449	785	1 296
5. Liver cancer	9 119	6 952	2 167	26	77	2 519	2 937	1 393	26	62	560	825	695
6. Pancreas cancer	1 916	1 180	737	–	–	181	487	511	–	2	78	248	407
7. Trachea, bronchus, lung cancers	13 076	9 979	3 097	14	36	1 248	4 689	3 992	2	12	389	1 253	1 438
8. Melanoma and other skin cancers	650	353	297	1	3	112	136	101	5	–	89	99	105
9. Breast cancer	4 861		4 861						–	8	1 560	2 033	1 257
10. Cervix uteri cancer	3 505		3 505						–	3	1 108	1 617	776
11. Corpus uteri cancer	746		746							4	121	347	272
12. Ovary cancer	1 610		1 610						27	56	558	558	411
13. Prostate cancer	1 704	1 704				35	298	1 366					
14. Bladder cancer	1 533	1 194	339	2	6	123	368	695	2	3	44	94	195
15. Lymphomas and multiple myeloma	3 682	2 331	1 351	152	492	735	488	465	101	252	338	286	373
16. Leukaemia	5 179	2 850	2 330	314	809	1 047	375	304	339	584	834	301	273
C. Diabetes mellitus	**10 921**	**5 204**	**5 717**	**160**	**285**	**1 373**	**1 783**	**1 604**	**161**	**275**	**1 091**	**1 808**	**2 382**
D. Endocrine disorders	**5 879**	**2 719**	**3 160**	**1 108**	**294**	**671**	**358**	**288**	**1 018**	**345**	**811**	**509**	**477**

Annex Table 13i, continued. DALYs by age, sex and cause (thousands): World, 2000, baseline scenario

Cause	Total	Male	Female	Males 0-4	5-14	15-44	45-59	60+	Females 0-4	5-14	15-44	45-59	60+
E. Neuro-psychiatric conditions	**165 082**	**81 367**	**83 715**	**2 242**	**3 319**	**63 141**	**7 847**	**4 818**	**2 167**	**3 190**	**62 426**	**8 795**	**7 137**
1. Unipolar major depression	60 166	21 345	38 821			17 802	2 836	707		1	32 231	5 115	1 475
2. Bipolar disorder	16 722	8 491	8 231			7 830	496	165			7 527	490	213
3. Schizophrenia	14 614	7 726	6 888			7 583	74	68			6 755	48	86
4. Epilepsy	4 712	2 590	2 122	166	639	1 402	274	108	170	694	991	162	106
5. Alcohol use	18 973	16 777	2 196			14 839	1 584	353			1 955	175	67
6. Dementia*	10 135	4 264	5 871	320	138	287	1 019	2 499	379	143	280	1 090	3 979
7. Parkinson disease	1 278	611	668			1	230	379			1	234	432
8. Multiple sclerosis	1 569	684	885			588	68	28			747	96	42
9. Drug use	6 493	5 247	1 246		379	4 669	171	29		92	1 105	42	7
10. Post-traumatic stress disorder	2 253	856	1 397	46	188	557	55	10	75	308	909	87	17
11. Obsessive-compulsive disorders	11 917	5 158	6 759		650	4 130	258	119		832	5 281	456	190
12. Panic disorder	5 605	1 883	3 722		188	1 416	277	1		227	2 981	438	77
F. Sense organ diseases	**13 215**	**6 144**	**7 072**	**90**	**11**	**491**	**2 814**	**2 737**	**72**	**25**	**549**	**3 168**	**3 257**
1. Glaucoma	3 357	1 287	2 070	7		98	783	399	9		152	1 341	567
2. Cataracts	9 531	4 726	4 805	37	2	365	2 001	2 320	24	3	330	1 787	2 661
G. Cardiovascular diseases	**154 433**	**86 681**	**67 752**	**4 214**	**3 481**	**16 185**	**25 689**	**37 112**	**3 391**	**3 385**	**10 690**	**14 318**	**35 968**
1. Rheumatic heart disease	6 235	2 882	3 352	6	284	1 358	771	465	28	370	1 405	924	626
2. Ischaemic heart disease	57 566	34 021	23 545			4 385	12 048	17 587	164		2 143	5 229	16 009
3. Cerebrovascular disease	45 770	24 538	21 233	514	766	4 344	7 278	11 636	423	626	2 956	5 030	12 197
4. Inflammatory heart diseases	10 515	5 807	4 708	843	692	2 201	1 249	822	864	695	1 493	786	870
H. Respiratory diseases	**71 250**	**39 300**	**31 950**	**4 595**	**2 584**	**8 900**	**9 731**	**13 491**	**3 674**	**2 027**	**7 685**	**7 402**	**11 162**
1. COPD*	37 317	21 188	16 129	491	135	3 729	6 421	10 411	560	155	2 792	4 422	8 200
2. Asthma	11 577	6 394	5 182	657	1 496	2 996	784	461	350	949	2 622	779	481
I. Digestive diseases	**45 681**	**27 009**	**18 672**	**3 359**	**1 161**	**7 815**	**9 493**	**5 181**	**3 391**	**1 132**	**4 658**	**5 133**	**4 358**
1. Peptic ulcer	2 797	1 824	973	14	23	714	637	436	16	21	346	285	305
2. Cirrhosis of the liver	13 743	9 764	3 979	129	125	3 134	4 392	1 984	98	174	1 036	1 572	1 099
3. Appendicitis	1 343	792	551	20	259	452	43	18	20	226	262	28	15
J. Genito-urinary diseases	**15 240**	**8 962**	**6 278**	**838**	**1 002**	**2 085**	**3 255**	**1 783**	**629**	**955**	**1 809**	**1 380**	**1 505**
1. Nephritis and nephrosis	8 073	4 248	3 825	583	820	1 314	720	811	514	838	1 009	632	832
2. Benign prostatic hypertrophy	2 340	2 340		7		10	1 880	442					
L. Musculo-skeletal diseases	**22 331**	**8 294**	**14 037**	**47**	**87**	**3 045**	**3 538**	**1 577**	**63**	**105**	**4 941**	**5 976**	**2 952**
1. Rheumatoid arthritis	3 870	1 077	2 793	1	2	494	361	219	1	30	1 347	815	601
2. Osteoarthritis	16 345	6 549	9 796			2 358	3 039	1 151			2 953	4 828	2 015

Annex Table 13i, continued. DALYs by age, sex and cause (thousands): World, 2000, baseline scenario

Cause	Total	Male	Female	Males					Females				
				0–4	5–14	15–44	45–59	60+	0–4	5–14	15–44	45–59	60+
M. Congenital anomalies	33 990	17 058	16 932	15 711	647	595	77	30	15 619	680	502	92	39
N. Oral conditions	9 027	4 424	4 603	492	713	1 567	897	755	470	710	1 581	929	913
1. Dental caries	5 036	2 536	2 499	485	706	901	282	163	463	691	871	282	192
2. Periodontal disease	306	154	153	–	–	123	21	9	–	–	122	21	10
3. Edentulism	3 550	1 700	1 851	–	–	526	592	582	–	–	519	623	709
III. Injuries	*230 883*	*151 236*	*79 647*	*22 153*	*26 660*	*86 691*	*11 937*	*3 795*	*18 859*	*16 487*	*35 395*	*5 799*	*3 106*
A. Unintentional injuries	161 963	107 505	54 457	18 698	23 252	54 093	8 713	2 749	15 318	14 215	18 559	4 025	2 340
1. Road traffic accidents	45 409	32 819	12 590	2 088	6 277	20 588	2 984	882	1 345	3 866	5 669	1 220	490
2. Poisonings	6 659	3 980	2 679	1 238	421	1 620	557	145	844	323	1 129	267	116
3. Falls	25 037	15 501	9 536	3 233	5 718	5 104	976	470	3 171	2 512	2 288	851	714
4. Fires	12 103	5 043	7 060	1 649	1 380	1 630	280	103	1 457	2 321	2 867	251	164
5. Drownings	14 766	9 972	4 794	2 930	3 443	3 106	358	136	2 020	1 587	911	161	115
6. Other unintentional	57 990	40 190	17 800	7 561	6 013	22 045	3 559	1 013	6 481	3 606	5 695	1 275	742
B. Intentional injuries	68 920	43 730	25 190	3 454	3 408	32 598	3 224	1 046	3 542	2 272	16 836	1 774	766
1. Self-inflicted injuries	21 348	11 676	9 672	–	810	8 367	1 778	721	–	446	7 579	1 126	520
2. Violence	21 471	16 986	4 485	972	952	13 830	1 021	210	1 087	580	2 344	353	121
3. War	26 101	15 068	11 033	2 482	1 646	10 401	425	115	2 455	1 246	6 913	295	125

Notes:
A dash (–) symbol indicates fewer than 500 DALYs.
*IA6 is Bacterial meningitis and meningococcaemia; ID is Conditions arising during the perinatal period;
IIE6 is Dementia and other degenerative and hereditary CNS disorders; IIH1 is Chronic obstructive pulmonary disease.

Annex Table 14a. Deaths by age, sex and cause (thousands): Established Market Economies, 2010, baseline scenario

Cause	Total	Male	Female	Males 0-4	5-14	15-29	30-44	45-59	60-69	70+	Females 0-4	5-14	15-29	30-44	45-59	60-69	70+
Population (millions)	*874*	*428*	*447*	*29*	*57*	*80*	*85*	*88*	*44*	*44*	*28*	*55*	*77*	*83*	*90*	*49*	*67*
All causes	*8 195*	*4 364*	*3 831*	*35*	*10*	*95*	*174*	*606*	*790*	*2 653*	*26*	*7*	*30*	*73*	*243*	*385*	*3 067*
I. Communicable, maternal, perinatal and nutritional conditions	*512*	*286*	*225*	*17*	-	*13*	*43*	*23*	*16*	*175*	*12*	-	*3*	*6*	*5*	*8*	*190*
A. Infectious and parasitic diseases	**155**	**110**	**45**	**2**	-	**12**	**42**	**20**	**6**	**27**	**1**	-	**3**	**6**	**3**	**3**	**28**
1. Tuberculosis	**14**	**9**	**4**	-	-	-	-	**1**	**1**	**7**	-	-	-	-	-	**1**	**3**
2. STDs excluding HIV	**1**	-	-	-	-	-	-	-	-	-	-	-	-	-	-	-	-
a. Syphilis	-	-	-	-	-	-	-	-	-	-	-	-	-	-	-	-	-
b. Chlamydia	-	-	-	-	-	-	-	-	-	-	-	-	-	-	-	-	-
c. Gonorrhoea	-	-	-	-	-	-	-	-	-	-	-	-	-	-	-	-	-
3. HIV	**88**	**76**	**12**	**1**	-	**12**	**41**	**18**	**3**	**1**	**1**	-	**3**	**6**	**2**	**1**	**1**
4. Diarrhoeal diseases	**3**	**1**	**2**	-	-	-	-	-	-	**1**	-	-	-	-	-	-	**1**
5. Childhood-cluster diseases	**1**	-	-	-	-	-	-	-	-	-	-	-	-	-	-	-	-
a. Pertussis	-	-	-	-	-	-	-	-	-	-	-	-	-	-	-	-	-
b. Poliomyelitis	-	-	-	-	-	-	-	-	-	-	-	-	-	-	-	-	-
c. Diphtheria	-	-	-	-	-	-	-	-	-	-	-	-	-	-	-	-	-
d. Measles	-	-	-	-	-	-	-	-	-	-	-	-	-	-	-	-	-
e. Tetanus	-	-	-	-	-	-	-	-	-	-	-	-	-	-	-	-	-
6. Bacterial meningitis*	**3**	**2**	**1**	-	-	-	-	-	-	**1**	-	-	-	-	-	-	**1**
7. Hepatitis B and hepatitis C	**3**	**2**	**1**	-	-	-	-	-	-	**1**	-	-	-	-	-	-	**1**
8. Malaria	-	-	-	-	-	-	-	-	-	-	-	-	-	-	-	-	-
9. Tropical-cluster diseases	-	-	-	-	-	-	-	-	-	-	-	-	-	-	-	-	-
a. Trypanosomiasis	-	-	-	-	-	-	-	-	-	-	-	-	-	-	-	-	-
b. Chagas disease	-	-	-	-	-	-	-	-	-	-	-	-	-	-	-	-	-
c. Schistosomiasis	-	-	-	-	-	-	-	-	-	-	-	-	-	-	-	-	-
d. Leishmaniasis	-	-	-	-	-	-	-	-	-	-	-	-	-	-	-	-	-
10. Leprosy	-	-	-	-	-	-	-	-	-	-	-	-	-	-	-	-	-
11. Dengue	-	-	-	-	-	-	-	-	-	-	-	-	-	-	-	-	-
12. Japanese encephalitis	-	-	-	-	-	-	-	-	-	-	-	-	-	-	-	-	-
13. Trachoma	-	-	-	-	-	-	-	-	-	-	-	-	-	-	-	-	-
14. Intestinal nematode infections	-	-	-	-	-	-	-	-	-	-	-	-	-	-	-	-	-
a. Ascariasis	-	-	-	-	-	-	-	-	-	-	-	-	-	-	-	-	-
b. Trichuriasis	-	-	-	-	-	-	-	-	-	-	-	-	-	-	-	-	-
c. Ancylostomiasis, necatoriasis	-	-	-	-	-	-	-	-	-	-	-	-	-	-	-	-	-
15. Other infectious and parasitic	**43**	**19**	**24**	-	-	-	-	**1**	**2**	**16**	-	-	-	-	-	**2**	**22**

Annex Table 14a, continued. Deaths by age, sex and cause (thousands): Established Market Economies, 2010, baseline scenario

Cause	Total	Male	Female	Males 0-4	5-14	15-29	30-44	45-59	60-69	70+	Females 0-4	5-14	15-29	30-44	45-59	60-69	70+
B. Respiratory infections	311	154	158	1	-	-	1	3	9	140	1	-	-	-	2	4	150
1. Lower respiratory infections	308	153	156	1	-	-	1	3	8	139	1	-	-	-	2	4	149
2. Upper respiratory infections	3	1	2	-	-	-	-	-	-	1	-	-	-	-	-	-	1
3. Otitis media	-	-	-	-	-	-	-	-	-	-	-	-	-	-	-	-	-
C. Maternal conditions	-	-	-	-	-	-	-	-	-	-	-	-	-	-	-	-	-
1. Maternal haemorrhage	-	-	-	-	-	-	-	-	-	-	-	-	-	-	-	-	-
2. Maternal sepsis	-	-	-	-	-	-	-	-	-	-	-	-	-	-	-	-	-
3. Hypertensive disorders*	-	-	-	-	-	-	-	-	-	-	-	-	-	-	-	-	-
4. Obstructed labour	-	-	-	-	-	-	-	-	-	-	-	-	-	-	-	-	-
5. Abortion	-	-	-	-	-	-	-	-	-	-	-	-	-	-	-	-	-
6. Other maternal	-	-	-	-	-	-	-	-	-	-	-	-	-	-	-	-	-
D. Perinatal conditions*	24	14	10	14	-	-	-	-	-	-	10	-	-	-	-	-	-
E. Nutritional deficiencies	22	9	13	-	-	-	-	-	1	8	-	-	-	-	-	1	12
1. Protein-energy malnutrition	7	2	4	-	-	-	-	-	-	2	-	-	-	-	-	-	4
2. Iodine deficiency	-	-	-	-	-	-	-	-	-	-	-	-	-	-	-	-	-
3. Vitamin A deficiency	-	-	-	-	-	-	-	-	-	-	-	-	-	-	-	-	-
4. Iron-deficiency anaemia	14	6	8	-	-	-	-	-	-	5	-	-	-	-	-	-	7
II. Noncommunicable diseases	7 232	3 785	3 447	14	5	17	79	527	744	2 399	11	4	9	47	214	359	2 804
A. Malignant neoplasms	2 103	1 202	901	1	2	5	29	227	300	638	1	1	4	28	132	182	554
1. Mouth and oropharynx cancers	39	30	9	-	-	-	1	10	8	10	-	-	-	-	2	2	5
2. Oesophagus cancer	51	39	12	-	-	-	1	10	11	17	-	-	-	-	1	2	8
3. Stomach cancer	169	105	64	-	-	-	2	17	24	61	-	-	-	2	6	10	46
4. Colon and rectum cancers	249	130	119	-	-	-	2	19	29	79	-	-	-	2	12	19	86
5. Liver cancer	44	32	11	-	-	-	1	9	11	12	-	-	-	-	1	3	7
6. Pancreas cancer	100	53	47	-	-	-	1	10	14	29	-	-	-	-	4	9	33
7. Trachea, bronchus, lung cancers	491	340	152	-	-	-	9	85	104	141	-	-	-	3	26	42	80
8. Melanoma and other skin cancers	25	15	10	-	-	-	1	4	3	7	-	-	-	1	2	2	6
9. Breast cancer	143	-	143	-	-	-	-	-	-	-	-	-	-	9	34	30	70
10. Cervix uteri cancer	16	-	16	-	-	-	-	-	-	-	-	-	-	2	4	3	7
11. Corpus uteri cancer	27	-	27	-	-	-	-	-	-	-	-	-	-	-	3	6	17
12. Ovary cancer	44	-	44	-	-	-	-	-	-	-	-	-	-	1	9	11	22
13. Prostate cancer	120	120	-	-	-	-	-	4	17	100	-	-	-	-	-	-	-
14. Bladder cancer	58	43	15	-	-	-	-	4	8	31	-	-	-	-	1	2	12
15. Lymphomas, multiple myeloma	91	50	41	-	1	1	2	9	11	26	1	1	-	1	5	8	27
16. Leukaemia	64	37	28	-	1	1	2	5	7	20	-	1	1	1	3	4	17
17. Other cancers	373	209	164	1	1	2	7	42	52	105	1	1	1	4	19	30	109

690

Annex Table 14a, continued. Deaths by age, sex and cause (thousands): Established Market Economies, 2010, baseline scenario

Cause	Total	Male	Female	Males 0-4	5-14	15-29	30-44	45-59	60-69	70+	Females 0-4	5-14	15-29	30-44	45-59	60-69	70+
B. Other neoplasms	41	19	22	-	-	-	1	1	3	12	-	-	-	-	1	2	17
C. Diabetes mellitus	177	65	112	-	-	-	1	7	11	46	-	-	-	1	4	10	97
D. Endocrine disorders	53	22	31	1	-	1	1	1	4	14	1	-	-	-	2	2	25
E. Neuro-psychiatric conditions	245	107	139	1	1	4	6	11	12	72	1	1	1	2	5	7	122
2. Bipolar disorder	1	-	1	-	-	-	-	-	-	-	-	-	-	-	-	-	1
3. Schizophrenia	17	6	10	-	-	1	-	1	1	5	-	-	1	-	1	-	10
4. Epilepsy	6	4	3	-	-	1	-	1	1	1	-	-	1	-	1	-	1
5. Alcohol use	14	11	3	-	-	-	2	5	2	2	-	-	-	1	1	-	-
6. Dementia*	122	43	79	-	-	-	-	2	4	36	-	-	-	-	1	3	74
7. Parkinson disease	39	19	20	-	-	-	-	-	1	18	-	-	-	-	1	1	19
8. Multiple sclerosis	5	2	3	-	-	-	1	1	-	1	-	-	-	1	1	1	1
9. Drug use	3	2	-	-	-	1	2	-	-	-	-	-	-	-	-	-	-
13. Other neuro-psychiatric	39	18	20	1	-	2	-	2	2	10	-	-	-	-	1	1	16
F. Sense organ diseases	-	-	-	-	-	-	-	-	-	-	-	-	-	-	-	-	-
1. Glaucoma	-	-	-	-	-	-	-	-	-	-	-	-	-	-	-	-	-
2. Cataracts	-	-	-	-	-	-	-	-	-	-	-	-	-	-	-	-	-
G. Cardiovascular diseases	3 533	1 782	1 751	1	1	4	27	208	321	1 220	1	-	2	9	38	102	1 599
1. Rheumatic heart disease	20	7	13	-	1	-	-	2	2	4	-	-	1	3	1	2	10
2. Ischaemic heart disease	1 872	996	876	-	-	1	13	131	196	655	-	-	-	3	19	57	797
3. Cerebrovascular disease	878	388	490	-	0	1	5	33	53	297	-	-	1	1	11	23	453
4. Inflammatory heart diseases	70	38	32	1	0	1	2	8	6	21	1	-	-	-	2	2	27
5. Other cardiovascular	693	353	340	1	-	2	6	35	66	243	1	-	1	2	6	18	313
H. Respiratory diseases	443	260	183	-	-	1	2	14	38	205	-	-	1	2	11	25	145
1. COPD*	318	197	121	-	-	-	-	8	28	159	-	-	-	1	6	18	96
2. Asthma	27	12	15	-	-	1	1	1	2	7	-	-	1	1	2	3	10
3. Other respiratory	98	51	47	-	-	1	1	4	7	38	-	-	-	-	2	4	39
I. Digestive diseases	402	230	172	-	-	1	10	51	46	122	-	-	1	4	18	19	130
1. Peptic ulcer	43	24	19	-	-	-	-	3	4	18	-	-	-	-	1	1	17
2. Cirrhosis of the liver	148	103	45	-	-	-	7	37	27	32	-	-	-	3	11	10	21
3. Appendicitis	2	1	1	-	-	-	-	-	-	-	-	-	-	-	-	-	-
4. Other digestive	209	102	108	-	-	1	3	12	15	72	-	-	1	1	5	8	93
J. Genito-urinary diseases	154	69	85	-	-	1	1	4	7	57	-	-	1	1	2	5	77
1. Nephritis and nephrosis	100	46	54	-	-	-	1	3	5	37	-	-	-	1	1	3	49
2. Benign prostatic hypertrophy	5	5	-	-	-	-	-	-	-	5	-	-	-	-	-	-	-
3. Other genito-urinary	50	19	31	-	-	1	-	1	2	16	-	-	1	-	1	1	29
K. Skin diseases	16	5	11	-	-	-	-	-	-	4	-	-	-	-	-	-	11

Annex Table 14a, continued. Deaths by age, sex and cause (thousands): Established Market Economies, 2010, baseline scenario

Cause	Total	Male	Female	Males							Females						
				0-4	5-14	15-29	30-44	45-59	60-69	70+	0-4	5-14	15-29	30-44	45-59	60-69	70+
L. Musculo-skeletal diseases	39	10	29	-	-	-	-	1	1	8	-	-	-	-	1	2	25
1. Rheumatoid arthritis	11	2	9	-	-	-	-	-	-	2	-	-	-	-	1	1	7
3. Other musculo-skeletal	28	8	20	-	-	-	-	1	1	6	-	-	-	-	1	1	17
M. Congenital anomalies	26	14	12	9	1	1	1	1	1	1	8	1	-	1	1	1	2
N. Oral conditions	-	-	-	-	-	-	-	-	-	-	-	-	-	-	-	-	-
III. Injuries	*452*	*293*	*158*	*4*	*5*	*65*	*52*	*56*	*31*	*79*	*3*	*3*	*18*	*20*	*24*	*18*	*73*
A. Unintentional injuries	288	175	113	4	4	42	25	28	17	55	2	3	12	11	13	11	60
1. Road traffic accidents	115	74	40	2	3	33	12	10	5	10	1	2	10	7	7	4	9
2. Poisonings	11	7	4	-	-	1	3	2	1	1	-	-	-	1	1	1	1
3. Falls	77	36	41	-	-	1	2	4	4	25	-	-	1	1	1	2	36
4. Fires	10	6	4	-	-	1	1	1	1	2	-	-	-	-	1	1	2
5. Drownings	11	8	3	1	1	1	1	1	1	2	1	1	-	-	-	-	1
6. Other unintentional	64	43	20	1	1	5	6	9	6	15	-	-	1	2	3	3	11
B. Intentional injuries	163	118	45	1	1	23	27	28	14	24	1	-	6	8	11	7	12
1. Self-inflicted injuries	132	95	38	-	-	15	20	24	13	23	-	-	4	6	10	6	11
2. Violence	31	23	8	1	1	8	7	4	1	1	1	-	2	2	1	1	1
3. War	-	-	-	-	-	-	-	-	-	-	-	-	-	-	-	-	-

Notes:
Causes responsible for no deaths have been omitted from this table.
A dash (-) symbol indicates fewer than 500 deaths.
*IA6 is Bacterial meningitis and meningococcaemia; IC3 is Hypertensive disorders of pregnancy; ID is Conditions arising during the perinatal period; IIE6 is Dementia and other degenerative and hereditary CNS disorders; IIH1 is Chronic obstructive pulmonary disease.

Annex Table 14b. Deaths by age, sex and cause (thousands): Formerly Socialist Economies of Europe, 2010, baseline scenario

Cause	Total	Male	Female	Males 0-4	5-14	15-29	30-44	45-59	60-69	70+	Females 0-4	5-14	15-29	30-44	45-59	60-69	70+
Population (millions)	*363*	*172*	*190*	*13*	*25*	*39*	*36*	*33*	*14*	*12*	*12*	*24*	*38*	*36*	*37*	*19*	*25*
All causes	**4 825**	**2 633**	**2 192**	**39**	**12**	**84**	**154**	**623**	**483**	**1 239**	**29**	**7**	**26**	**47**	**181**	**237**	**1 665**
I. Communicable, maternal, perinatal and nutritional conditions	*169*	*82*	*87*	*19*	*1*	*1*	*3*	*7*	*5*	*47*	*13*	*1*	*2*	*1*	*2*	*3*	*66*
A. Infectious and parasitic diseases	**37**	**21**	**16**	**4**	-	**1**	**2**	**4**	**2**	**7**	**3**	-	**1**	**1**	**1**	**1**	**9**
1. Tuberculosis	12	10	2	-	-	-	1	3	2	3	-	-	-	-	-	-	2
2. STDs excluding HIV	-	-	-	-	-	-	-	-	-	-	-	-	-	-	-	-	-
a. Syphilis	-	-	-	-	-	-	-	-	-	-	-	-	-	-	-	-	-
b. Chlamydia	-	-	-	-	-	-	-	-	-	-	-	-	-	-	-	-	-
c. Gonorrhoea	-	-	-	-	-	-	-	-	-	-	-	-	-	-	-	-	-
3. HIV	5	3	2	2	-	-	1	-	-	-	2	-	-	-	-	-	-
4. Diarrhoeal diseases	2	1	1	1	-	-	-	-	-	-	1	-	-	-	-	-	-
5. Childhood-cluster diseases	-	-	-	-	-	-	-	-	-	-	-	-	-	-	-	-	-
a. Pertussis	-	-	-	-	-	-	-	-	-	-	-	-	-	-	-	-	-
b. Poliomyelitis	-	-	-	-	-	-	-	-	-	-	-	-	-	-	-	-	-
c. Diphtheria	-	-	-	-	-	-	-	-	-	-	-	-	-	-	-	-	-
d. Measles	-	-	-	-	-	-	-	-	-	-	-	-	-	-	-	-	-
e. Tetanus	-	-	-	-	-	-	-	-	-	-	-	-	-	-	-	-	-
6. Bacterial meningitis*	4	2	1	1	-	-	-	-	-	1	-	-	-	-	-	-	1
7. Hepatitis B and hepatitis C	1	1	-	-	-	-	-	-	-	-	-	-	-	-	-	-	-
8. Malaria	-	-	-	-	-	-	-	-	-	-	-	-	-	-	-	-	-
9. Tropical-cluster diseases	-	-	-	-	-	-	-	-	-	-	-	-	-	-	-	-	-
a. Trypanosomiasis	-	-	-	-	-	-	-	-	-	-	-	-	-	-	-	-	-
b. Chagas disease	-	-	-	-	-	-	-	-	-	-	-	-	-	-	-	-	-
c. Schistosomiasis	-	-	-	-	-	-	-	-	-	-	-	-	-	-	-	-	-
d. Leishmaniasis	-	-	-	-	-	-	-	-	-	-	-	-	-	-	-	-	-
10. Leprosy	-	-	-	-	-	-	-	-	-	-	-	-	-	-	-	-	-
11. Dengue	-	-	-	-	-	-	-	-	-	-	-	-	-	-	-	-	-
12. Japanese encephalitis	-	-	-	-	-	-	-	-	-	-	-	-	-	-	-	-	-
13. Trachoma	-	-	-	-	-	-	-	-	-	-	-	-	-	-	-	-	-
14. Intestinal nematode infections	-	-	-	-	-	-	-	-	-	-	-	-	-	-	-	-	-
a. Ascariasis	-	-	-	-	-	-	-	-	-	-	-	-	-	-	-	-	-
b. Trichuriasis	-	-	-	-	-	-	-	-	-	-	-	-	-	-	-	-	-
c. Ancylostomiasis, necatoriasis	-	-	-	-	-	-	-	-	-	-	-	-	-	-	-	-	-
15. Other infectious and parasitic	13	5	8	1	-	-	-	-	-	3	-	-	-	-	-	-	7

Annex Table 14b, continued. Deaths by age, sex and cause (thousands): Formerly Socialist Economies of Europe, 2010, baseline scenario

Cause	Total	Male	Female	Males							Females						
				0-4	5-14	15-29	30-44	45-59	60-69	70+	0-4	5-14	15-29	30-44	45-59	60-69	70+
B. Respiratory infections	**106**	**48**	**58**	**5**	**-**	**-**	**1**	**2**	**3**	**37**	**5**	**-**	**-**	**1**	**1**	**2**	**52**
1. Lower respiratory infections	106	48	58	4	-	-	1	2	3	37	4	-	-	1	1	2	52
2. Upper respiratory infections	1	-	-	-	-	-	-	-	-	-	-	-	-	-	-	-	-
3. Otitis media	-	-	-	-	-	-	-	-	-	-	-	-	-	-	-	-	-
C. Maternal conditions	**1**		**1**														
1. Maternal haemorrhage	-		-														
2. Maternal sepsis	-		-														
3. Hypertensive disorders*	-		-														
4. Obstructed labour	-		-														
5. Abortion	-		-														
6. Other maternal	-		-														
D. Perinatal conditions*	**17**	**10**	**7**	**10**	**-**	**-**	**-**	**-**	**-**	**-**	**7**	**-**	**-**	**-**	**-**	**-**	**-**
E. Nutritional deficiencies	**8**	**3**	**6**	**-**	**-**	**-**	**-**	**-**	**-**	**2**	**-**	**-**	**-**	**-**	**-**	**-**	**5**
1. Protein-energy malnutrition	2	1	1	-	-	-	-	-	-	2	-	-	-	-	-	-	1
2. Iodine deficiency	-	-	-	-	-	-	-	-	-	-	-	-	-	-	-	-	-
3. Vitamin A deficiency	-	-	-	-	-	-	-	-	-	-	-	-	-	-	-	-	-
4. Iron-deficiency anaemia	4	1	3	-	-	-	-	-	-	1	-	-	-	-	-	-	2
II. Noncommunicable diseases	**4 228**	**2 241**	**1 987**	**13**	**4**	**13**	**73**	**530**	**453**	**1 155**	**10**	**2**	**8**	**30**	**156**	**221**	**1 560**
A. Malignant neoplasms	**907**	**589**	**318**	**1**	**2**	**5**	**24**	**208**	**152**	**198**	**1**	**1**	**3**	**16**	**69**	**72**	**156**
1. Mouth and oropharynx cancers	26	23	3	-	-	-	1	12	5	4	-	-	-	-	1	1	2
2. Oesophagus cancer	15	13	2	-	-	-	1	7	3	3	-	-	-	-	-	1	1
3. Stomach cancer	140	92	48	-	-	-	4	34	22	32	-	-	-	2	8	10	28
4. Colon and rectum cancers	92	51	42	-	-	-	3	14	12	23	-	-	-	1	7	9	25
5. Liver cancer	28	17	11	-	-	-	2	6	5	6	-	-	-	-	2	3	6
6. Pancreas cancer	40	25	15	-	-	-	1	9	6	8	-	-	-	-	2	4	9
7. Trachea, bronchus, lung cancers	236	199	37	-	-	-	7	75	61	57	-	-	-	1	9	10	17
8. Melanoma and other skin cancers	11	6	5	-	-	-	1	2	1	2	-	-	-	-	1	1	3
9. Breast cancer	42	-	42	-	-	-	-	-	-	-	-	-	-	4	14	9	14
10. Cervix uteri cancer	16		16								-	-	-	2	4	4	6
11. Corpus uteri cancer	14		14								-	-	-	1	3	4	7
12. Ovary cancer	16		16								-	-	-	1	5	4	5
13. Prostate cancer	24	24	-	-	-	-	-	2	4	17							
14. Bladder cancer	23	19	4	-	-	-	-	2	5	9	-	-	-	-	-	1	3
15. Lymphomas, multiple myeloma	21	13	7	-	-	1	-	4	3	3	-	-	-	-	2	2	3
16. Leukaemia	23	15	9	1	1	1	1	4	3	4	-	-	1	1	2	2	3
17. Other cancers	137	91	46	-	1	2	5	34	21	28	-	1	2	2	9	8	24

Annex Table 14b, continued. Deaths by age, sex and cause (thousands): Formerly Socialist Economies of Europe, 2010, baseline scenario

Cause	Total	Male	Female	Males 0-4	Males 5-14	Males 15-29	Males 30-44	Males 45-59	Males 60-69	Males 70+	Females 0-4	Females 5-14	Females 15-29	Females 30-44	Females 45-59	Females 60-69	Females 70+
B. Other neoplasms	7	3	3							1					1	1	1
C. Diabetes mellitus	30	11	19				1	2	3	5					2	4	13
D. Endocrine disorders	3	1	2				1										1
E. Neuro-psychiatric conditions	73	32	41	1	1	2	3	6	4	15	1	1	1	1	2	3	32
2. Bipolar disorder	7	2	6					1	1	1							5
3. Schizophrenia	5	3	2				1	1		1							2
4. Epilepsy	5	3	2	1	1	1	1	1	1	1					1	1	1
5. Alcohol use	7	6	1			1	1	2	1	1						1	
6. Dementia*	21	6	15							5						1	13
7. Parkinson disease	9	3	5							3							5
8. Multiple sclerosis	4	2	3							1					1	1	1
9. Drug use	-	-	-														
13. Other neuro-psychiatric	14	7	7	1	1		1	1		3	1			1	1		4
F. Sense organ diseases	-	-	-														
1. Glaucoma	-	-	-														
2. Cataracts	-	-	-														
G. Cardiovascular diseases	2 667	1 268	1 400	1		4	34	245	231	752	1			8	58	112	1 220
1. Rheumatic heart disease	25	13	12				2	7	3	1				1	5	3	3
2. Ischaemic heart disease	1 337	671	666			1	19	150	121	379				3	25	52	585
3. Cerebrovascular disease	812	344	468			1	6	54	66	217				2	22	41	403
4. Inflammatory heart diseases	49	26	22			1	2	8	3	12				1	2	1	18
5. Other cardiovascular	445	213	232	0		1	5	27	38	142	0	0	0	1	4	14	212
H. Respiratory diseases	326	210	117			1	3	33	40	134				1	9	14	92
1. COPD*	167	108	60				1	16	21	70					3	7	49
2. Asthma	14	7	8				1	1	1	4					1	1	5
3. Other respiratory	144	95	49				1	16	18	59				1	4	6	38
I. Digestive diseases	145	89	57			1	6	30	19	32				2	10	10	33
1. Peptic ulcer	18	13	5				1	4	3	5					1	1	4
2. Cirrhosis of the liver	61	41	20				3	16	10	11				1	6	5	8
3. Appendicitis	1	1	-														
4. Other digestive	65	34	31			1	2	9	6	16				1	4	5	21
J. Genito-urinary diseases	45	27	18			1	1	4	4	16				1	3	4	10
1. Nephritis and nephrosis	18	10	8			1	1	3	2	4					2	2	4
2. Benign prostatic hypertrophy	8	8	-						1	7							
3. Other genito-urinary	19	9	10					2	2	5					2	2	6
K. Skin diseases	2	1	1														1

Annex Table 14b, continued. Deaths by age, sex and cause (thousands): Formerly Socialist Economies of Europe, 2010, baseline scenario

Cause	Total	Male	Female	Males							Females						
				0-4	5-14	15-29	30-44	45-59	60-69	70+	0-4	5-14	15-29	30-44	45-59	60-69	70+
L. Musculo-skeletal diseases	**4**	**1**	**3**	-	-	-	-	-	-	-	-	-	-	-	1	1	1
1. Rheumatoid arthritis	1	-	1	-	-	-	-	-	-	-	-	-	-	-	-	1	-
3. Other musculo-skeletal	4	2	2	-	-	-	-	-	-	-	-	-	-	-	1	-	1
M. Congenital anomalies	**19**	**10**	**8**	9	-	-	-	-	-	-	7	-	-	-	-	-	-
N. Oral conditions	-	-	-	-	-	-	-	-	-	-	-	-	-	-	-	-	-
III. Injuries	**428**	**309**	**118**	7	8	69	78	86	24	36	6	4	18	16	24	12	39
A. Unintentional injuries	**276**	**200**	**76**	4	5	43	49	58	16	25	3	3	9	9	15	8	30
1. Road traffic accidents	111	83	28	1	3	27	20	19	6	8	1	1	6	4	6	3	7
2. Poisonings	46	34	11	1	-	3	10	15	3	2	-	-	1	2	4	2	2
3. Falls	36	19	17	1	-	1	3	4	2	8	-	-	-	-	1	1	14
4. Fires	8	5	3	-	-	1	1	2	-	1	-	-	-	-	-	-	1
5. Drownings	21	18	4	1	1	4	5	4	1	1	-	1	1	-	1	-	1
6. Other unintentional	53	41	13	2	1	7	10	13	3	4	1	1	1	2	3	2	4
B. Intentional injuries	**152**	**110**	**43**	3	2	26	29	29	9	12	3	1	9	7	9	5	9
1. Self-inflicted injuries	91	69	22	-	-	12	18	22	7	11	-	-	2	3	6	3	7
2. Violence	32	23	9	-	-	7	8	5	1	1	-	-	2	2	2	1	2
3. War	29	17	12	3	2	8	3	1	-	-	3	1	5	2	2	-	-

Notes:
Causes responsible for no deaths have been omitted from this table.
A dash (-) symbol indicates fewer than 500 deaths.
*IA6 is Bacterial meningitis and meningococcaemia; IC3 is Conditions arising during the perinatal period; ID is Hypertensive disorders of pregnancy; IIH1 is Chronic obstructive pulmonary disease.
IIE6 is Dementia and other degenerative and hereditary CNS disorders; IIH1 is Chronic obstructive pulmonary disease.

Annex Table 14c. Deaths by age, sex and cause (thousands): India, 2010, baseline scenario

Cause	Total	Male	Female	Males							Females						
				0-4	5-14	15-29	30-44	45-59	60-69	70+	0-4	5-14	15-29	30-44	45-59	60-69	70+
Population (millions)	*1 124*	*574*	*550*	*55*	*107*	*161*	*126*	*81*	*26*	*18*	*53*	*101*	*152*	*117*	*77*	*29*	*21*
All causes	*10 264*	*5 709*	*4 556*	*744*	*133*	*321*	*566*	*1 233*	*1 070*	*1 643*	*705*	*126*	*281*	*308*	*667*	*672*	*1 798*
I. Communicable, maternal, perinatal and nutritional conditions	*3 058*	*1 713*	*1 345*	*565*	*43*	*134*	*251*	*268*	*148*	*305*	*549*	*50*	*121*	*146*	*149*	*80*	*251*
A. Infectious and parasitic diseases	2 174	1 284	891	295	33	130	245	259	119	203	284	34	106	131	139	56	140
1. Tuberculosis	966	635	330	11	8	57	113	211	92	144	8	6	41	48	115	38	73
2. STDs excluding HIV	28	13	16	8					1	4	8			1	1	1	5
a. Syphilis	27	13	14	8					1	4	8			1	1	1	5
b. Chlamydia	1		1														
c. Gonorrhoea	1		1														
3. HIV	503	294	209	43	7	67	122	37	11	7	44	7	60	77	15	4	2
4. Diarrhoeal diseases	350	173	177	129	5	2	3	4	7	25	127	7	1	2	3	6	31
5. Childhood-cluster diseases	172	89	82	76	6	1	2	1	1	2	69	6	1	1	1	1	2
a. Pertussis	27	14	13	13	1						12	1					
b. Poliomyelitis	4	2	2	2							2						
c. Diphtheria		1	1	1							1						
d. Measles	68	35	33	32	3						30	3					
e. Tetanus	71	37	34	28	2	1	2	1	1	2	26	2	1	1	1	1	2
6. Bacterial meningitis*	16	8	8	4			1	1	1	1	4			1	1	1	2
7. Hepatitis B and hepatitis C	8	4	4					1	1	2					1	1	1
8. Malaria	8	4	3	1	1		1	1			1	1			1		
9. Tropical-cluster diseases	8	5	3	1	2	2						1	1				
a. Trypanosomiasis																	
b. Chagas disease																	
c. Schistosomiasis																	
d. Leishmaniasis	8	5	3	1	2	2						1	1				
10. Leprosy																	
11. Dengue	3	1	2		1							1					
12. Japanese encephalitis																	
13. Trachoma																	
14. Intestinal nematode infections	1	1	1		1							1					
a. Ascariasis																	
b. Trichuriasis																	
c. Ancylostomiasis, necatoriasis	1	1															
15. Other infectious and parasitic	110	54	56	21	3	1	3	3	5	18	20	4	1	1	3	5	22

Annex Table 14c, continued. Deaths by age, sex and cause (thousands): India, 2010, baseline scenario

Cause	Total	Male	Female	Males 0-4	5-14	15-29	30-44	45-59	60-69	70+	Females 0-4	5-14	15-29	30-44	45-59	60-69	70+
B. Respiratory infections	569	283	286	135	9	3	5	8	28	96	133	15	3	3	8	22	103
1. Lower respiratory infections	559	278	281	132	8	3	5	8	28	95	130	14	2	3	8	22	102
2. Upper respiratory infections	6	3	3	1	-	-	-	-	-	1	1	-	-	-	-	-	1
3. Otitis media	4	2	2	2	-	-	-	-	-	-	2	-	-	-	-	-	-
C. Maternal conditions	24	-	24	-	-	-	-	-	-	-	-	-	11	11	1	-	-
1. Maternal haemorrhage	6	-	6	-	-	-	-	-	-	-	-	-	3	3	-	-	-
2. Maternal sepsis	4	-	4	-	-	-	-	-	-	-	-	-	2	2	-	-	-
3. Hypertensive disorders*	2	-	2	-	-	-	-	-	-	-	-	-	1	1	-	-	-
4. Obstructed labour	1	-	1	-	-	-	-	-	-	-	-	-	1	1	-	-	-
5. Abortion	2	-	2	-	-	-	-	-	-	-	-	-	1	1	-	-	-
6. Other maternal	4	-	4	-	-	-	-	-	-	-	-	-	2	2	-	-	-
D. Perinatal conditions*	242	123	119	123	-	-	-	-	-	-	119	-	-	-	-	-	-
E. Nutritional deficiencies	49	23	26	12	1	1	1	1	1	6	14	2	1	-	1	1	7
1. Protein-energy malnutrition	27	12	15	8	-	-	-	1	1	2	10	1	-	-	1	-	3
2. Iodine deficiency	2	1	1	1	-	-	-	-	-	-	1	-	-	-	-	-	-
3. Vitamin A deficiency	6	3	3	2	1	-	-	-	-	-	2	1	-	-	-	-	-
4. Iron-deficiency anaemia	14	6	7	1	-	1	1	-	-	3	1	1	1	-	-	1	4
II. Noncommunicable diseases	6 065	3 322	2 743	114	26	43	157	820	880	1 281	109	25	52	88	434	553	1 482
A. Malignant neoplasms	964	533	431	4	6	15	43	199	111	155	2	3	22	36	157	90	121
1. Mouth and oropharynx cancers	138	85	53	-	-	2	5	33	18	26	-	-	3	3	21	12	14
2. Oesophagus cancer	88	47	42	-	-	1	2	18	9	16	-	-	-	2	14	10	15
3. Stomach cancer	77	50	27	-	-	1	2	20	9	16	-	-	-	2	8	10	7
4. Colon and rectum cancers	36	19	17	-	-	1	2	6	4	7	-	-	1	1	9	6	5
5. Liver cancer	23	16	7	-	-	1	1	6	3	6	-	-	-	-	2	2	3
6. Pancreas cancer	13	8	5	-	-	-	-	3	1	3	-	-	-	-	2	1	2
7. Trachea, bronchus, lung cancers	167	141	27	-	-	1	11	64	42	23	-	-	-	2	9	8	7
8. Melanoma and other skin cancers	2	1	1	-	-	-	-	-	-	1	-	-	-	-	-	-	1
9. Breast cancer	56	-	56	-	-	-	-	-	-	-	-	-	4	6	23	10	13
10. Cervix uteri cancer	79	-	79	-	-	-	-	-	-	-	-	-	4	6	40	14	14
11. Corpus uteri cancer	6	-	6	-	-	-	-	-	-	-	-	-	-	-	2	2	2
12. Ovary cancer	19	-	19	-	-	-	-	-	-	-	-	-	2	2	5	4	5
13. Prostate cancer	21	21	-	-	-	-	-	2	3	15	-	-	-	-	-	-	-
14. Bladder cancer	12	10	3	-	-	-	-	2	2	5	-	-	-	-	1	1	1
15. Lymphomas, multiple myeloma	30	19	11	-	-	-	3	6	4	6	-	-	1	1	3	2	4
16. Leukaemia	24	14	10	2	2	1	3	3	1	2	1	1	1	2	2	1	2
17. Other cancers	173	104	70	2	3	5	11	35	16	31	2	1	5	7	21	14	20

Annex Table 14c, continued. Deaths by age, sex and cause (thousands): India, 2010, baseline scenario

Cause	Total	Male	Female	Males							Females						
				0-4	5-14	15-29	30-44	45-59	60-69	70+	0-4	5-14	15-29	30-44	45-59	60-69	70+
B. Other neoplasms	4	3	2	-	-	-	1	-	-	-	-	-	-	-	-	-	-
C. Diabetes mellitus	108	47	61	-	-	1	3	10	11	17	2	2	1	2	10	17	28
D. Endocrine disorders	2	1	1	-	-	-	-	-	-	-	-	-	-	-	-	-	-
E. Neuro-psychiatric conditions	108	58	51	6	3	3	8	10	10	19	8	2	3	2	3	9	23
2. Bipolar disorder	3	1	2	-	-	-	-	-	-	1	-	-	-	-	1	1	-
3. Schizophrenia	5	3	3	-	-	-	2	-	-	1	-	-	-	-	1	-	2
4. Epilepsy	11	7	5	1	1	1	2	1	-	1	1	1	1	-	1	-	1
5. Alcohol use	5	5	-	-	-	1	2	2	-	-	-	-	-	-	-	-	-
6. Dementia*	26	11	15	-	-	-	-	-	4	7	-	-	-	-	3	2	10
7. Parkinson disease	7	5	3	-	-	-	-	1	1	3	-	-	-	-	-	1	2
8. Multiple sclerosis	3	1	2	-	-	-	-	1	-	-	-	-	-	-	1	1	-
9. Drug use	-	-	-	-	-	-	-	-	-	-	-	-	-	-	-	-	-
13. Other neuro-psychiatric	47	25	22	5	2	2	3	4	5	5	6	2	2	1	1	4	7
F. Sense organ diseases	-	-	-	-	-	-	-	-	-	-	-	-	-	-	-	-	-
1. Glaucoma	-	-	-	-	-	-	-	-	-	-	-	-	-	-	-	-	-
2. Cataracts	-	-	-	-	-	-	-	-	-	-	-	-	-	-	-	-	-
G. Cardiovascular diseases	3 797	2 041	1 756	17	4	11	65	450	617	877	13	6	11	29	187	370	1 139
1. Rheumatic heart disease	93	47	46	-	-	3	10	22	8	4	-	1	3	9	19	8	6
2. Ischaemic heart disease	2 034	1 108	926	-	-	1	20	244	354	489	-	-	1	9	89	202	625
3. Cerebrovascular disease	754	394	360	3	1	1	7	68	122	192	1	1	1	4	27	80	244
4. Inflammatory heart diseases	119	66	53	3	1	3	7	23	12	17	3	-	2	3	12	8	24
5. Other cardiovascular	797	426	371	10	2	4	21	92	121	175	8	3	4	4	40	73	240
H. Respiratory diseases	525	298	227	5	4	2	8	57	84	137	4	4	5	6	41	44	123
1. COPD*	298	176	122	1	1	-	2	29	52	90	1	1	1	1	19	25	74
2. Asthma	39	21	18	-	-	-	2	5	5	9	-	-	-	1	4	4	9
3. Other respiratory	189	102	87	4	3	2	5	23	28	38	3	3	4	4	18	15	41
I. Digestive diseases	286	201	85	2	1	7	23	82	33	52	2	1	6	8	26	13	29
1. Peptic ulcer	51	34	18	-	-	-	3	12	7	12	-	-	1	1	5	3	8
2. Cirrhosis of the liver	178	132	46	-	-	4	13	57	21	35	-	1	2	4	15	7	16
3. Appendicitis	8	5	3	-	1	1	2	-	-	-	-	-	1	1	-	-	-
4. Other digestive	49	31	18	1	-	1	6	13	4	6	1	-	1	2	5	3	5
J. Genito-urinary diseases	98	56	43	2	3	1	3	10	13	23	1	4	2	2	7	8	17
1. Nephritis and nephrosis	85	44	42	2	3	1	3	10	9	15	1	4	2	2	7	8	17
2. Benign prostatic hypertrophy	11	11	-	-	-	-	-	-	4	7	-	-	-	-	-	-	-
3. Other genito-urinary	2	1	1	-	-	-	-	-	-	-	-	-	-	-	-	-	-
K. Skin diseases	2	1	1	-	-	-	-	-	-	-	-	-	-	-	-	-	-

Annex Table 14c, continued. Deaths by age, sex and cause (thousands): India, 2010, baseline scenario

Cause	Total	Male	Female	Males							Females						
				0-4	5-14	15-29	30-44	45-59	60-69	70+	0-4	5-14	15-29	30-44	45-59	60-69	70+
L. Musculo-skeletal diseases																	
1. Rheumatoid arthritis	2	1	1	-	-	-	-	-	-	1	-	-	-	-	1	-	-
3. Other musculo-skeletal	1	1	-	-	-	-	-	-	-	-	-	-	-	-	-	-	-
M. Congenital anomalies	168	83	85	74	3	2	2	1	1	1	75	3	2	1	2	1	1
N. Oral conditions	-	-	-	-	-	-	-	-	-	-	-	-	-	-	-	-	-
III. Injuries	**1 142**	**674**	**468**	**65**	**64**	**144**	**157**	**145**	**41**	**57**	**47**	**51**	**109**	**75**	**83**	**39**	**65**
A. Unintentional injuries	**914**	**544**	**371**	**60**	**60**	**106**	**122**	**112**	**35**	**49**	**41**	**46**	**71**	**55**	**64**	**33**	**61**
1. Road traffic accidents	401	283	118	15	30	72	67	61	18	21	4	22	17	16	27	13	18
2. Poisonings	31	16	15	4	1	2	4	3	1	1	3	1	4	3	3	-	-
3. Falls	56	35	22	3	4	3	6	8	4	7	3	2	1	2	3	3	8
4. Fires	135	42	93	8	2	7	11	9	2	3	7	6	33	21	11	5	11
5. Drownings	83	44	39	9	9	7	8	5	2	3	8	7	5	4	6	2	7
6. Other unintentional	207	123	85	20	13	14	26	27	9	14	16	8	10	9	14	10	17
B. Intentional injuries	**228**	**130**	**97**	**5**	**5**	**38**	**35**	**32**	**6**	**8**	**7**	**4**	**38**	**20**	**19**	**5**	**4**
1. Self-inflicted injuries	146	80	66	-	3	27	22	21	3	4	-	3	34	17	9	1	2
2. Violence	78	47	31	5	2	9	12	12	3	4	7	1	4	2	10	4	2
3. War	4	4	-	-	-	3	1	-	-	-	-	-	-	-	-	-	-

Notes:
Causes responsible for no deaths have been omitted from this table.
A dash (-) symbol indicates fewer than 500 deaths.
*IA6 is Bacterial meningitis and meningococcaemia; IC3 is Hypertensive disorders of pregnancy; ID is Conditions arising during the perinatal period; IIE6 is Dementia and other degenerative and hereditary CNS disorders; IIH1 is Chronic obstructive pulmonary disease.

Annex Table 14d. Deaths by age, sex and cause (thousands): China, 2010, baseline scenario

Cause	Total	Male	Female	Males							Females						
				0-4	5-14	15-29	30-44	45-59	60-69	70+	0-4	5-14	15-29	30-44	45-59	60-69	70+
Population (millions)	*1 378*	*699*	*679*	*50*	*109*	*165*	*172*	*130*	*43*	*29*	*48*	*104*	*157*	*163*	*126*	*45*	*36*
All causes	**11 557**	**6 714**	**4 844**	**185**	**52**	**196**	**464**	**1 520**	**1 546**	**2 750**	**189**	**37**	**145**	**232**	**694**	**773**	**2 774**
I. Communicable, maternal, perinatal and nutritional conditions	**595**	**317**	**278**	**85**	**3**	**3**	**8**	**22**	**27**	**169**	**91**	**3**	**4**	**6**	**13**	**18**	**142**
A. Infectious and parasitic diseases	**259**	**151**	**108**	**15**	**2**	**2**	**7**	**20**	**21**	**84**	**15**	**2**	**1**	**4**	**11**	**13**	**62**
1. Tuberculosis	**148**	**94**	**55**	1	-	1	3	14	16	59	1	-	1	2	8	9	34
2. STDs excluding HIV	-	-	-	-	-	-	-	-	-	-	-	-	-	-	-	-	-
a. Syphilis	-	-	-	-	-	-	-	-	-	-	-	-	-	-	-	-	-
b. Chlamydia	-	-	-	-	-	-	-	-	-	-	-	-	-	-	-	-	-
c. Gonorrhoea	-	-	-	-	-	-	-	-	-	-	-	-	-	-	-	-	-
3. HIV	**6**	**3**	**3**	1	-	1	1	1	-	-	1	-	-	1	-	-	-
4. Diarrhoeal diseases	**44**	**21**	**23**	5	-	-	-	1	2	13	6	-	-	-	-	1	15
5. Childhood-cluster diseases	**12**	**7**	**5**	6	-	-	-	-	-	-	5	-	-	-	-	-	-
a. Pertussis	4	2	2	2	-	-	-	-	-	-	2	-	-	-	-	-	-
b. Poliomyelitis	1	1	-	-	-	-	-	-	-	-	-	-	-	-	-	-	-
c. Diphtheria	-	-	-	-	-	-	-	-	-	-	-	-	-	-	-	-	-
d. Measles	3	2	2	2	-	-	-	-	-	-	1	-	-	-	-	-	-
e. Tetanus	4	2	2	2	-	-	-	-	-	-	2	-	-	-	-	-	-
6. Bacterial meningitis*	**13**	**7**	**6**	2	-	-	1	1	1	2	2	-	-	1	1	1	2
7. Hepatitis B and hepatitis C	**14**	**9**	**6**	-	-	-	1	2	1	4	-	-	-	1	2	1	3
8. Malaria	-	-	-	-	-	-	-	-	-	-	-	-	-	-	-	-	-
9. Tropical-cluster diseases	**1**	**1**	-	-	-	-	-	-	-	-	-	-	-	-	-	-	-
a. Trypanosomiasis	-	-	-	-	-	-	-	-	-	-	-	-	-	-	-	-	-
b. Chagas disease	-	-	-	-	-	-	-	-	-	-	-	-	-	-	-	-	-
c. Schistosomiasis	1	1	-	-	-	-	-	-	-	-	-	-	-	-	-	-	-
d. Leishmaniasis	-	-	-	-	-	-	-	-	-	-	-	-	-	-	-	-	-
10. Leprosy	-	-	-	-	-	-	-	-	-	-	-	-	-	-	-	-	-
11. Dengue	-	-	-	-	-	-	-	-	-	-	-	-	-	-	-	-	-
12. Japanese encephalitis	**1**	**1**	-	-	-	-	-	-	-	-	-	-	-	-	-	-	-
13. Trachoma	-	-	-	-	-	-	-	-	-	-	-	-	-	-	-	-	-
14. Intestinal nematode infections	**1**	**1**	**1**	-	-	-	-	-	-	-	-	1	-	-	-	-	-
a. Ascariasis	1	1	1	-	-	-	-	-	-	-	-	1	-	-	-	-	-
b. Trichuriasis	-	-	-	-	-	-	-	-	-	-	-	-	-	-	-	-	-
c. Ancylostomiasis, necatoriasis	-	-	-	-	-	-	-	-	-	-	-	-	-	-	-	-	-
15. Other infectious and parasitic	**18**	**10**	**9**	1	-	-	-	1	1	6	1	-	-	-	1	1	6

Annex Table 14d, continued. Deaths by age, sex and cause (thousands): China, 2010, baseline scenario

Cause	Total		Males							Females						
	Male	Female	0-4	5-14	15-29	30-44	45-59	60-69	70+	0-4	5-14	15-29	30-44	45-59	60-69	70+
B. Respiratory infections	**120**	**115**	**32**	**1**	**-**	**-**	**2**	**5**	**80**	**35**	**1**	**-**	**-**	**2**	**4**	**73**
1. Lower respiratory infections	119	114	31	1	-	-	2	5	79	35	1	-	-	2	4	73
2. Upper respiratory infections	1	1	-	-	-	-	-	-	1	-	1	-	-	-	-	1
3. Otitis media	1	-	-	-	-	-	-	-	-	-	-	-	-	-	-	-
C. Maternal conditions		**4**										**2**	**1**	**1**		
1. Maternal haemorrhage		1										1	1			
2. Maternal sepsis		-														
3. Hypertensive disorders*		-														
4. Obstructed labour		-														
5. Abortion		-														
6. Other maternal		-														
D. Perinatal conditions*	**34**	**34**	**34**	**-**	**-**	**-**	**-**	**-**	**-**	**34**	**-**	**-**	**-**	**-**	**-**	**-**
E. Nutritional deficiencies	**12**	**16**	**4**	**-**	**-**	**-**	**1**	**1**	**6**	**7**	**1**	**-**	**-**	**1**	**1**	**4**
1. Protein-energy malnutrition	7	8	2	-	-	-	1	1	4	4	1	-	-	1	1	-
2. Iodine deficiency	1	1	1	-	-	-	-	-	-	1	-	-	-	-	-	-
3. Vitamin A deficiency	1	1	1	-	-	-	-	-	-	1	-	-	-	-	-	-
4. Iron-deficiency anaemia	3	6	-	-	-	-	-	-	2	1	-	-	-	-	1	3
II. Noncommunicable diseases	**5 629**	**3 977**	**54**	**19**	**57**	**288**	**1 340**	**1 432**	**2 439**	**57**	**11**	**36**	**144**	**570**	**695**	**2 464**
A. Malignant neoplasms	**1 826**	**918**	**4**	**11**	**24**	**167**	**645**	**512**	**462**	**6**	**5**	**15**	**76**	**254**	**233**	**328**
1. Mouth and oropharynx cancers	47	19	-	-	1	9	16	11	10	-	-	1	3	6	5	4
2. Oesophagus cancer	251	105	-	-	1	12	75	78	85	-	-	1	1	22	37	43
3. Stomach cancer	408	189	-	-	2	17	133	128	129	-	-	2	13	42	51	81
4. Colon and rectum cancers	88	64	-	-	1	8	26	23	30	-	-	1	5	17	16	24
5. Liver cancer	424	138	-	1	5	74	185	93	67	-	1	1	14	44	33	46
6. Pancreas cancer	38	22	-	-	-	2	10	11	14	-	-	-	-	4	7	11
7. Trachea, bronchus, lung cancers	343	120	-	-	2	16	131	120	73	-	-	-	3	35	34	47
8. Melanoma and other skin cancers	1	1	-	-	-	-	-	-	-	-	-	-	-	-	-	-
9. Breast cancer	-	44	-	-	-	-	-	-	-	-	-	-	9	16	8	12
10. Cervix uteri cancer	-	36	-	-	-	-	-	-	-	-	-	-	4	13	9	10
11. Corpus uteri cancer	-	11	-	-	-	-	-	-	-	-	-	-	1	6	2	3
12. Ovary cancer	-	17	-	-	-	-	-	-	-	-	-	1	3	6	3	4
13. Prostate cancer	9	-	-	-	-	-	1	4	4	-	-	-	-	-	-	-
14. Bladder cancer	28	7	-	-	-	-	5	10	12	-	-	-	1	1	2	2
15. Lymphomas, multiple myeloma	26	13	-	1	2	1	8	8	6	-	-	1	1	5	2	4
16. Leukaemia	51	43	2	5	7	11	15	5	6	3	3	6	9	10	5	7
17. Other cancers	111	89	1	3	5	16	41	20	26	3	1	2	10	26	18	27

Annex Table 14d, continued. Deaths by age, sex and cause (thousands): China, 2010, baseline scenario

Cause	Total	Male	Female	Males 0-4	5-14	15-29	30-44	45-59	60-69	70+	Females 0-4	5-14	15-29	30-44	45-59	60-69	70+
B. Other neoplasms	19	10	9	1	-	1	1	3	2	2	1	-	-	1	2	3	3
C. Diabetes mellitus	64	26	38	-	-	-	2	6	7	10	-	-	-	1	6	11	19
D. Endocrine disorders	13	5	9	1	-	-	-	1	1	2	1	-	-	1	1	1	5
E. Neuro-psychiatric conditions	93	44	49	2	1	6	9	6	4	17	1	-	3	4	5	6	28
2. Bipolar disorder	3	1	2	-	-	-	-	-	-	-	-	-	-	-	-	-	2
3. Schizophrenia	13	9	5	-	-	1	3	1	1	3	-	-	-	1	1	1	2
4. Epilepsy	9	5	4	-	-	1	1	1	1	1	-	-	1	1	1	-	1
5. Alcohol use	4	4	-	-	-	-	2	1	-	-	-	-	-	-	-	-	-
6. Dementia*	32	11	21	-	-	-	-	1	2	7	-	-	-	2	1	3	16
7. Parkinson disease	7	3	3	-	-	-	-	-	-	3	-	-	-	-	-	1	3
8. Multiple sclerosis	5	2	3	-	-	-	-	1	-	1	-	-	-	-	1	1	1
9. Drug use	-	-	-	-	-	-	-	-	-	-	-	-	1	-	1	-	-
13. Other neuro-psychiatric	20	10	10	1	-	3	2	1	1	2	1	-	-	2	1	1	4
F. Sense organ diseases	18	9	9	1	-	-	-	3	3	3	1	-	-	-	2	3	3
1. Glaucoma	6	3	3	-	-	-	-	1	1	1	-	-	-	-	1	1	1
2. Cataracts	6	3	2	-	-	-	-	1	1	1	-	-	-	-	1	1	1
G. Cardiovascular diseases	3 806	2 159	1 647	7	2	11	63	450	536	1 091	4	1	7	35	169	239	1 192
1. Rheumatic heart disease	210	104	106	-	-	4	9	30	20	40	-	-	2	9	22	15	57
2. Ischaemic heart disease	1 149	637	513	-	-	2	20	126	153	336	-	-	1	10	43	71	388
3. Cerebrovascular disease	1 909	1 106	803	2	1	3	24	226	294	556	1	-	1	12	86	129	574
4. Inflammatory heart diseases	85	49	36	1	-	2	5	16	8	18	-	-	1	3	7	3	20
5. Other cardiovascular	452	263	189	4	0	1	4	51	61	141	2	0	1	1	11	21	153
H. Respiratory diseases	2 161	1 158	1 003	4	1	4	14	136	291	708	4	-	1	11	85	157	744
1. COPD*	2 035	1 089	947	2	-	2	10	126	278	671	3	-	1	9	78	150	706
2. Asthma	49	27	21	-	-	1	2	7	6	11	-	-	-	2	5	4	10
3. Other respiratory	77	42	35	2	-	1	2	3	7	26	1	-	1	1	1	3	28
I. Digestive diseases	445	266	179	4	1	3	24	76	62	97	4	1	3	9	35	30	98
1. Peptic ulcer	41	23	18	-	-	1	1	4	5	13	-	-	1	-	2	2	13
2. Cirrhosis of the liver	210	139	71	-	-	1	18	50	36	34	-	-	1	4	20	16	29
3. Appendicitis	6	4	3	-	-	1	1	1	-	-	-	-	1	1	-	-	-
4. Other digestive	188	100	88	3	1	1	4	22	20	50	3	-	1	3	13	11	55
J. Genito-urinary diseases	118	67	51	1	1	4	7	12	11	30	1	1	2	4	9	11	24
1. Nephritis and nephrosis	91	50	41	1	1	4	7	10	9	19	1	1	2	4	7	8	18
2. Benign prostatic hypertrophy	7	7	-	-	-	-	-	-	-	6	-	-	-	-	-	-	-
3. Other genito-urinary	20	9	11	-	-	-	-	2	2	5	-	-	-	-	2	3	6
K. Skin diseases	12	7	5	-	-	-	-	1	1	5	-	-	-	-	-	1	3

Annex Table 14d, continued. Deaths by age, sex and cause (thousands): China, 2010, baseline scenario

Cause	Total	Male	Female	Males							Females						
				0-4	5-14	15-29	30-44	45-59	60-69	70+	0-4	5-14	15-29	30-44	45-59	60-69	70+
L. Musculo-skeletal diseases	**40**	**17**	**23**	-	-	-	-	1	4	11	-	-	-	1	2	2	17
1. Rheumatoid arthritis	2	1	1	-	-	-	-	-	-	1	-	-	-	-	-	-	1
3. Other musculo-skeletal	38	16	22	-	-	-	-	1	4	11	-	-	-	1	2	2	16
M. Congenital anomalies	**74**	**36**	**38**	30	2	3	1	-	-	-	32	2	2	1	-	-	-
N. Oral conditions	**-**	**-**	**-**	-	-	-	-	-	-	-	-	-	-	-	-	-	-
III. Injuries	**1 356**	**767**	**590**	46	31	136	169	157	86	142	41	23	106	82	111	60	167
A. Unintentional injuries	**834**	**514**	**320**	42	27	87	107	104	53	95	34	19	34	30	57	32	114
1. Road traffic accidents	361	255	106	3	12	52	66	59	29	34	2	12	22	16	28	11	15
2. Poisonings	68	39	29	3	1	3	7	12	4	10	1	1	4	5	4	4	10
3. Falls	99	37	62	1	-	1	4	6	6	17	2	-	-	1	6	7	45
4. Fires	31	15	16	1	-	1	2	1	1	8	1	-	-	1	2	2	10
5. Drownings	105	61	44	17	10	10	6	6	3	9	14	5	4	2	4	3	12
6. Other unintentional	169	107	62	15	4	18	22	21	10	18	14	2	4	5	12	4	22
B. Intentional injuries	**523**	**253**	**270**	4	4	50	62	54	34	47	7	4	71	53	54	28	53
1. Self-inflicted injuries	464	218	246	-	3	38	52	49	32	46	-	2	69	47	51	26	51
2. Violence	58	34	23	4	1	11	10	5	2	1	7	2	2	5	3	2	2
3. War	1	1	-	-	-	-	-	-	-	-	-	-	-	-	-	-	-

Notes:
Causes responsible for no deaths have been omitted from this table.
A dash (-) symbol indicates fewer than 500 deaths.
*IA6 is Bacterial meningitis and meningococcaemia; IC3 is Hypertensive disorders of pregnancy; ID is Conditions arising during the perinatal period; IIE6 is Dementia and other degenerative and hereditary CNS disorders; IIH1 is Chronic obstructive pulmonary disease.

Annex Table 14e. Deaths by age, sex and cause (thousands): Other Asia and Islands, 2010, baseline scenario

				Males							Females						
Cause	Total	Male	Female	0-4	5-14	15-29	30-44	45-59	60-69	70+	0-4	5-14	15-29	30-44	45-59	60-69	70+
Population (millions)	*922*	*460*	*462*	*43*	*84*	*124*	*105*	*67*	*21*	*15*	*41*	*81*	*121*	*103*	*71*	*24*	*20*
All causes	**6 655**	**3 760**	**2 895**	**463**	**119**	**222**	**397**	**724**	**604**	**1 231**	**349**	**79**	**134**	**210**	**379**	**389**	**1 354**
I. Communicable, maternal, perinatal and nutritional conditions	*1 358*	*732*	*626*	*338*	*26*	*40*	*73*	*54*	*51*	*151*	*248*	*21*	*42*	*61*	*47*	*35*	*171*
A. Infectious and parasitic diseases	829	453	376	165	16	37	71	50	32	82	121	13	35	52	41	26	89
1. Tuberculosis	236	118	118	–	1	4	7	25	21	60	–	1	2	5	25	20	65
2. STDs excluding HIV	23	12	12	7	–	–	–	–	–	3	5	–	1	1	1	–	3
a. Syphilis	22	12	10	7	–	–	–	–	–	3	5	–	–	1	1	–	3
b. Chlamydia	–	–	1	–	–	–	–	–	–	–	–	–	–	–	–	–	–
c. Gonorrhoea	1	1	–	–	–	–	–	–	–	–	–	–	–	–	–	–	–
3. HIV	227	133	95	19	–	29	57	17	5	3	12	2	29	41	8	2	1
4. Diarrhoeal diseases	168	97	71	85	3	1	–	1	2	4	60	2	–	1	1	2	6
5. Childhood-cluster diseases	90	49	42	41	3	1	1	1	–	1	35	3	1	1	1	1	2
a. Pertussis	13	7	6	7	3	–	–	–	–	–	6	3	–	–	–	–	–
b. Poliomyelitis	–	–	–	1	–	–	–	–	–	–	1	–	–	–	–	–	–
c. Diphtheria	1	1	–	–	–	–	–	–	–	–	–	–	–	–	–	–	–
d. Measles	44	24	20	22	2	1	–	–	–	1	19	2	–	1	–	1	2
e. Tetanus	31	16	14	11	1	1	1	1	1	1	9	1	1	1	1	–	1
6. Bacterial meningitis*	12	6	6	2	3	1	–	1	1	1	2	2	–	1	1	1	–
7. Hepatitis B and hepatitis C	12	7	5	1	–	1	1	1	1	3	–	–	1	1	1	1	2
8. Malaria	28	15	13	2	3	3	2	2	1	1	2	3	2	2	2	1	–
9. Tropical-cluster diseases	1	1	–	–	–	–	–	–	–	–	–	–	–	–	–	–	–
a. Trypanosomiasis	–	–	–	–	–	–	–	–	–	–	–	–	–	–	–	–	–
b. Chagas disease	–	–	–	–	–	–	–	–	–	–	–	–	–	–	–	–	–
c. Schistosomiasis	–	–	–	–	–	–	–	–	–	–	–	–	–	–	–	–	–
d. Leishmaniasis	1	1	–	1	–	–	–	–	–	–	–	–	–	1	–	–	–
10. Leprosy	–	–	–	–	–	–	–	–	–	–	–	–	–	–	–	–	–
11. Dengue	2	1	1	–	1	–	–	–	–	–	1	–	–	1	–	–	–
12. Japanese encephalitis	1	1	–	1	–	–	–	–	–	–	–	1	–	–	–	–	–
13. Trachoma	–	–	–	–	–	–	–	–	–	–	–	–	–	–	–	–	–
14. Intestinal nematode infections	2	1	1	–	1	–	–	–	–	–	–	1	–	1	–	–	–
a. Ascariasis	1	1	–	–	–	–	–	–	–	–	–	–	–	–	–	–	–
b. Trichuriasis	1	–	–	–	–	–	–	–	–	–	–	–	–	–	–	–	–
c. Ancylostomiasis, necatoriasis	1	–	–	–	–	–	–	–	–	–	–	–	–	–	–	–	–
15. Other infectious and parasitic	25	14	12	6	1	1	–	1	1	4	5	1	1	1	1	1	5

Annex Table 14e, continued. Deaths by age, sex and cause (thousands): Other Asia and Islands, 2010, baseline scenario

Cause	Total	Male	Female	Males 0-4	5-14	15-29	30-44	45-59	60-69	70+	Females 0-4	5-14	15-29	30-44	45-59	60-69	70+
B. Respiratory infections	**336**	**179**	**157**	**80**	**8**	**2**	**2**	**4**	**18**	**66**	**56**	**7**	**1**	**1**	**4**	**9**	**79**
1. Lower respiratory infections	332	177	155	78	8	2	2	4	18	65	55	7	1	1	4	9	78
2. Upper respiratory infections	3	2	2	–	–	2	2	–	–	1	1	–	1	1	–	–	1
3. Otitis media	1	1	1	1	–	–	–	–	–	1	1	–	–	–	–	–	1
C. Maternal conditions	**14**	**–**	**14**								**–**	**–**	**5**	**8**	**1**	**–**	**–**
1. Maternal haemorrhage	3	–	3								–	–	1	2	–	–	–
2. Maternal sepsis	2	–	2								–	–	1	1	–	–	–
3. Hypertensive disorders*	1	–	1								–	–	–	1	–	–	–
4. Obstructed labour	1	–	1								–	–	1	1	–	–	–
5. Abortion	1	–	1								–	–	1	–	–	–	–
6. Other maternal	2	–	2								–	–	1	1	–	–	–
D. Perinatal conditions*	**142**	**81**	**61**	**81**	–	–	–	–	–	–	**61**	–	–	–	–	–	–
E. Nutritional deficiencies	**36**	**19**	**18**	**12**	**1**	–	–	**1**	**1**	**3**	**10**	**1**	–	–	**1**	–	**4**
1. Protein-energy malnutrition	18	10	8	8	1	–	–	–	1	1	8	1	–	–	–	–	–
2. Iodine deficiency	1	1	–	–	–	–	–	–	–	–	–	–	–	–	–	–	–
3. Vitamin A deficiency	6	3	3	2	1	–	–	–	–	–	2	1	–	–	–	–	–
4. Iron-deficiency anaemia	11	5	6	1	1	1	–	1	1	2	1	1	1	–	1	–	3
II. Noncommunicable diseases	***4 559***	***2 521***	***2 038***	***81***	***52***	***42***	***190***	***582***	***525***	***1 049***	***64***	***36***	***35***	***105***	***300***	***337***	***1 161***
A. Malignant neoplasms	**1 211**	**715**	**496**	**7**	**16**	**10**	**62**	**210**	**177**	**234**	**8**	**10**	**12**	**47**	**128**	**117**	**174**
1. Mouth and oropharynx cancers	129	82	48	–	–	1	6	14	26	34	–	–	–	3	6	15	23
2. Oesophagus cancer	44	31	13	–	–	–	1	10	8	11	–	–	–	–	3	4	6
3. Stomach cancer	111	74	37	–	–	–	5	26	18	24	–	–	–	2	9	10	13
4. Colon and rectum cancers	77	41	36	–	–	1	3	7	13	17	–	–	–	2	9	10	17
5. Liver cancer	130	98	32	–	1	2	10	43	18	24	–	–	1	2	5	8	8
6. Pancreas cancer	19	12	7	–	–	–	1	4	3	4	–	–	–	–	2	2	3
7. Trachea, bronchus, lung cancers	197	149	48	–	–	1	9	56	35	48	–	–	1	1	13	14	15
8. Melanoma and other skin cancers	4	2	3	–	–	–	–	1	–	–	–	–	–	1	1	–	1
9. Breast cancer	49	–	49								–	–	2	7	19	8	13
10. Cervix uteri cancer	59	–	59								–	–	2	7	26	10	15
11. Corpus uteri cancer	7	–	7								–	–	–	–	2	2	3
12. Ovary cancer	18	–	18								–	–	–	4	5	3	4
13. Prostate cancer	25	25	–	–	–	–	–	3	10	13							
14. Bladder cancer	21	16	6	–	–	–	–	4	5	7	–	–	–	–	1	2	3
15. Lymphomas, multiple myeloma	43	26	17	1	2	1	4	4	6	8	2	2	1	2	1	5	4
16. Leukaemia	43	24	19	2	6	1	5	2	3	4	2	4	1	3	2	3	4
17. Other cancers	234	137	97	3	7	3	16	37	32	40	3	4	3	13	23	21	29

Annex Table 14e, continued. Deaths by age, sex and cause (thousands): Other Asia and Islands, 2010, baseline scenario

Cause	Total	Male	Female	Males 0-4	5-14	15-29	30-44	45-59	60-69	70+	Females 0-4	5-14	15-29	30-44	45-59	60-69	70+
B. Other neoplasms	10	5	5	1	1	-	1	1	1	1	-	-	-	-	1	1	2
C. Diabetes mellitus	76	31	44	-	-	1	3	8	7	12	-	-	1	1	8	12	23
D. Endocrine disorders	10	4	6	1	-	-	-	1	-	1	1	-	-	-	1	1	3
E. Neuro-psychiatric conditions	82	45	38	2	2	4	7	9	6	15	2	2	2	2	4	5	21
2. Bipolar disorder	2	1	2	-	-	-	1	-	-	-	-	-	-	-	-	1	1
3. Schizophrenia	7	4	4	-	-	-	2	1	1	-	-	-	-	-	1	1	2
4. Epilepsy	8	5	4	-	-	1	2	1	1	-	-	-	1	1	1	-	1
5. Alcohol use	6	6	3	-	-	1	1	3	2	-	-	-	-	-	-	1	2
6. Dementia*	26	10	15	-	-	-	-	1	1	7	-	-	-	-	1	2	11
7. Parkinson disease	6	3	2	-	-	-	-	-	1	3	-	-	-	-	-	1	2
8. Multiple sclerosis	3	1	1	-	-	-	1	1	-	-	-	-	-	2	-	-	-
9. Drug use	2	1	-	-	1	2	2	-	-	-	-	-	1	-	-	-	-
13. Other neuro-psychiatric	23	13	10	2	1	1	-	2	1	3	1	1	1	1	1	1	3
F. Sense organ diseases	-	-	-	-	-	-	-	-	-	-	-	-	-	-	-	-	-
1. Glaucoma	-	-	-	-	-	-	-	-	-	-	-	-	-	-	-	-	-
2. Cataracts	-	-	-	-	-	-	-	-	-	-	-	-	-	-	-	-	-
G. Cardiovascular diseases	2 226	1 163	1 063	29	22	20	77	218	231	566	20	15	13	36	101	139	738
1. Rheumatic heart disease	17	8	9	-	-	-	1	1	2	4	-	-	1	1	1	1	5
2. Ischaemic heart disease	845	440	405	-	-	-	24	77	95	243	-	-	-	11	32	56	306
3. Cerebrovascular disease	673	338	335	4	5	4	17	62	76	169	2	3	2	8	33	49	238
4. Inflammatory heart diseases	97	56	41	6	5	4	9	13	5	14	5	3	2	4	6	3	17
5. Other cardiovascular	595	323	273	20	12	11	26	65	53	136	13	9	8	12	29	30	172
H. Respiratory diseases	294	168	127	6	3	2	5	19	27	106	3	2	2	4	12	18	87
1. COPD*	170	100	70	1	-	-	1	10	17	70	1	-	-	1	5	10	52
2. Asthma	35	18	17	-	-	1	2	3	3	8	-	-	1	2	3	3	8
3. Other respiratory	90	50	40	4	2	1	1	6	7	28	2	1	1	1	3	4	27
I. Digestive diseases	452	295	157	4	3	3	29	104	64	86	3	3	3	10	35	31	73
1. Peptic ulcer	39	24	15	-	-	-	1	5	5	12	-	-	-	-	2	2	10
2. Cirrhosis of the liver	197	146	51	-	-	1	18	65	32	29	-	-	-	4	16	12	17
3. Appendicitis	7	4	3	-	1	1	1	1	-	-	-	1	1	-	-	-	-
4. Other digestive	210	121	89	4	2	1	9	34	27	45	3	2	1	5	17	16	46
J. Genito-urinary diseases	121	55	66	1	2	2	5	10	9	25	1	2	2	3	10	12	36
1. Nephritis and nephrosis	104	47	57	1	2	2	4	9	8	20	1	1	2	3	9	11	31
2. Benign prostatic hypertrophy	1	1	-	-	-	-	-	-	-	1	-	-	-	-	-	-	-
3. Other genito-urinary	16	7	9	-	-	-	-	1	1	4	-	1	-	-	1	2	5
K. Skin diseases	3	1	1	-	-	-	-	-	-	-	-	-	-	-	-	-	1

Annex Table 14e, continued. Deaths by age, sex and cause (thousands): Other Asia and Islands, 2010, baseline scenario

Cause	Total	Male	Female	Males							Females						
				0-4	5-14	15-29	30-44	45-59	60-69	70+	0-4	5-14	15-29	30-44	45-59	60-69	70+
L. Musculo-skeletal diseases	11	4	7	-	-	-	-	1	1	1	-	-	-	1	1	1	4
1. Rheumatoid arthritis	1	-	1	-	-	-	-	-	-	-	-	-	-	-	-	1	-
3. Other musculo-skeletal	10	4	6	-	-	-	-	1	1	1	-	-	-	1	1	1	4
M. Congenital anomalies	63	34	29	29	2	1	-	1	-	1	25	1	1	-	1	-	1
N. Oral conditions	-	-	-	-	-	-	-	-	-	-	-	-	-	-	-	-	-
III. Injuries	*738*	*507*	*231*	*44*	*41*	*140*	*134*	*88*	*28*	*31*	*37*	*22*	*57*	*44*	*32*	*17*	*22*
A. Unintentional injuries	539	371	168	42	36	95	92	63	21	22	34	19	33	27	24	13	17
1. Road traffic accidents	233	163	71	13	15	49	41	26	9	9	11	9	15	12	11	6	6
2. Poisonings	42	22	19	1	1	5	5	5	2	2	1	1	6	4	3	2	2
3. Falls	41	30	11	3	1	5	8	7	2	3	2	1	1	1	1	1	3
4. Fires	10	6	4	1	-	1	1	1	1	1	2	1	1	-	-	-	1
5. Drownings	71	49	22	14	11	9	6	4	2	2	9	4	3	2	2	1	1
6. Other unintentional	141	101	40	9	7	26	29	19	6	5	9	3	7	7	6	3	4
B. Intentional injuries	199	136	63	3	5	44	42	25	7	9	3	3	25	17	8	3	4
1. Self-inflicted injuries	102	62	40	-	2	21	17	12	5	6	-	1	17	10	5	2	3
2. Violence	77	62	15	1	2	19	22	12	2	3	1	1	5	5	2	1	-
3. War	20	11	8	1	1	5	3	1	-	-	1	1	3	2	1	-	-

Notes:
Causes responsible for no deaths have been omitted from this table.
A dash (-) indicates fewer than 500 deaths.
*IA6 is Bacterial meningitis and meningococcaemia; IC3 is Hypertensive disorders of pregnancy; ID is Conditions arising during the perinatal period;
IIE6 is Dementia and other degenerative and hereditary CNS disorders; IIH1 is Chronic obstructive pulmonary disease.

Annex Table 14f. Deaths by age, sex and cause (thousands): Sub-Saharan Africa, 2010, baseline scenario

Cause	Total	Male	Female	Males 0-4	5-14	15-29	30-44	45-59	60-69	70+	Females 0-4	5-14	15-29	30-44	45-59	60-69	70+
Population (millions)	*912*	*452*	*460*	*78*	*125*	*124*	*69*	*36*	*12*	*7*	*75*	*123*	*126*	*73*	*39*	*15*	*9*
All causes	*9 622*	*5 330*	*4 293*	*1 977*	*355*	*754*	*607*	*534*	*417*	*685*	*1 570*	*286*	*472*	*375*	*416*	*351*	*822*
I. Communicable, maternal, perinatal and nutritional conditions	*4 828*	*2 527*	*2 302*	*1 725*	*129*	*189*	*179*	*117*	*62*	*125*	*1 359*	*133*	*277*	*231*	*105*	*60*	*136*
A. Infectious and parasitic diseases	3 421	1 798	1 623	1 125	100	185	176	114	48	50	885	104	242	197	100	44	51
1. Tuberculosis	700	337	363	30	19	92	66	78	33	20	31	27	107	75	72	31	19
2. STDs excluding HIV	67	33	34	27	-	-	-	1	1	5	23	-	1	1	1	1	6
a. Syphilis	65	33	31	27	-	-	-	1	1	5	23	-	1	1	1	1	6
b. Chlamydia	2	-	2	-	-	-	-	-	-	-	-	-	-	-	-	-	-
c. Gonorrhoea	1	1	1	-	-	-	-	-	-	-	-	-	-	-	-	-	-
3. HIV	653	307	345	87	12	78	97	23	6	3	82	12	119	109	17	4	2
4. Diarrhoeal diseases	717	405	312	366	17	2	2	2	3	13	268	17	3	3	2	3	15
5. Childhood-cluster diseases	637	348	289	316	27	1	2	-	1	1	259	25	1	1	-	-	1
a. Pertussis	112	62	50	58	3	-	-	-	-	-	47	3	-	-	-	-	-
b. Poliomyelitis	4	2	2	2	-	-	-	-	-	-	1	-	-	-	-	-	-
c. Diphtheria	1	1	-	1	-	-	-	-	-	-	1	-	-	-	-	-	-
d. Measles	425	232	193	210	22	-	-	-	-	-	173	20	-	-	-	-	-
e. Tetanus	95	52	43	45	2	-	1	-	1	1	37	2	1	1	1	1	1
6. Bacterial meningitis*	18	9	9	7	-	-	1	1	-	-	6	-	-	1	-	1	2
7. Hepatitis B and hepatitis C	10	6	4	1	-	-	-	1	1	2	1	-	-	-	-	-	2
8. Malaria	526	299	227	266	15	7	5	4	2	2	195	14	6	4	4	2	2
9. Tropical-cluster diseases	28	16	12	1	5	3	2	3	1	1	1	4	2	2	2	1	1
a. Trypanosomiasis	21	12	10	-	3	3	2	3	1	1	1	3	2	1	2	1	1
b. Chagas disease	-	-	-	-	-	-	-	-	-	-	-	-	-	-	-	-	-
c. Schistosomiasis	2	1	1	-	-	-	-	-	-	-	-	-	1	-	-	-	-
d. Leishmaniasis	5	3	2	-	2	1	-	1	-	-	-	1	-	1	-	-	-
10. Leprosy	-	-	-	-	-	-	-	-	-	-	-	-	-	-	-	-	-
11. Dengue	-	-	-	-	-	-	-	-	-	-	-	-	-	-	-	-	-
12. Japanese encephalitis	-	-	-	-	-	-	-	-	-	-	-	-	-	-	-	-	-
13. Trachoma	-	-	-	-	-	-	-	-	-	-	-	-	-	-	-	-	-
14. Intestinal nematode infections	1	1	1	-	-	-	-	-	-	1	-	-	-	-	-	-	1
a. Ascariasis	-	-	-	-	-	-	-	-	-	-	-	-	-	-	-	-	-
b. Trichuriasis	-	-	-	-	-	-	-	-	-	-	-	-	-	-	-	-	-
c. Ancylostomiasis, necatoriasis	-	-	-	-	-	-	-	-	-	-	-	-	-	-	-	-	-
15. Other infectious and parasitic	63	35	28	25	3	1	1	1	1	3	18	3	1	1	1	1	2

Annex Table 14f, continued. Deaths by age, sex and cause (thousands): Sub-Saharan Africa, 2010, baseline scenario

Cause	Total	Male	Female	Males							Females						
				0-4	5-14	15-29	30-44	45-59	60-69	70+	0-4	5-14	15-29	30-44	45-59	60-69	70+
B. Respiratory infections	**824**	**452**	**371**	**333**	**26**	**4**	**3**	**3**	**14**	**71**	**244**	**21**	**4**	**2**	**3**	**15**	**81**
1. Lower respiratory infections	810	445	365	327	25	4	2	3	13	70	239	20	4	2	3	15	81
2. Upper respiratory infections	8	5	4	3	–	–	–	–	–	1	2	–	–	–	–	–	1
3. Otitis media	5	3	2	3	–	–	–	–	–	–	2	–	–	–	–	–	–
C. Maternal conditions	**66**	**–**	**66**								–	5	30	31	–	–	–
1. Maternal haemorrhage	16	–	16									1	7	7			
2. Maternal sepsis	11	–	11									1	5	5			
3. Hypertensive disorders*	5	–	5									1	2	2			
4. Obstructed labour	3	–	3										2	1			
5. Abortion	5	–	5										2	2			
6. Other maternal	9	–	9									1	4	4			
D. Perinatal conditions*	**407**	**218**	**189**	**218**							**189**						
E. Nutritional deficiencies	**110**	**58**	**52**	**49**	**4**	**1**	**–**	**–**	**1**	**4**	**42**	**4**	**1**	**–**	**–**	**1**	**4**
1. Protein-energy malnutrition	79	42	37	38	1	1	–	–	1	3	32	1	1	–	–	1	3
2. Iodine deficiency	1	1	1	–	–	–	–	–	–	–	–	–	–	–	–	–	–
3. Vitamin A deficiency	22	12	10	9	3	–	–	–	–	–	8	3	–	–	–	–	–
4. Iron-deficiency anaemia	8	4	4	1	–	–	–	–	–	1	1	–	–	–	–	–	1
II. Noncommunicable diseases	***3 038***	***1 566***	***1 472***	***94***	***62***	***56***	***179***	***322***	***320***	***534***	***90***	***64***	***34***	***65***	***281***	***273***	***666***
A. Malignant neoplasms	**773**	**449**	**323**	**7**	**17**	**15**	**52**	**112**	**108**	**138**	**9**	**16**	**10**	**24**	**91**	**75**	**97**
1. Mouth and oropharynx cancers	43	27	16	–	–	1	2	4	9	11	–	–	–	1	2	5	11
2. Oesophagus cancer	43	32	11	–	–	1	2	12	7	9	–	–	–	2	4	5	7
3. Stomach cancer	57	35	22	–	–	1	2	12	9	11	–	1	–	2	8	7	4
4. Colon and rectum cancers	27	15	12	–	–	–	3	2	5	6	–	–	–	1	2	5	7
5. Liver cancer	102	77	25	–	–	5	17	27	11	15	–	1	2	2	4	6	6
6. Pancreas cancer	12	7	5	–	–	–	1	3	2	2	–	–	–	–	3	2	–
7. Trachea, bronchus, lung cancers	41	28	13	–	–	–	3	9	7	8	–	–	–	1	3	4	2
8. Melanoma and other skin cancers	15	6	8	–	–	–	1	2	1	2	–	–	1	–	2	3	3
9. Breast cancer	28	–	28								–	–	1	1	10	6	8
10. Cervix uteri cancer	55		55								–	–	2	2	20	13	17
11. Corpus uteri cancer	6	–	6								–	–	–	–	2	2	2
12. Ovary cancer	13	–	13								–	–	1	1	4	3	3
13. Prostate cancer	63	63	–	–	–	–	–	8	24	31							
14. Bladder cancer	25	17	8	–	–	–	–	4	5	7	–	–	–	–	2	3	3
15. Lymphomas, multiple myeloma	47	30	17	2	7	1	4	4	5	7	2	5	1	1	2	3	3
16. Leukaemia	16	8	8	1	1	5	1	–	–	–	1	2	–	–	1	2	2
17. Other cancers	181	105	76	4	8	5	16	25	22	26	5	8	3	7	20	15	18

Annex Table 14f, continued. Deaths by age, sex and cause (thousands): Sub-Saharan Africa, 2010, baseline scenario

Cause	Total	Male	Female	Males							Females						
				0-4	5-14	15-29	30-44	45-59	60-69	70+	0-4	5-14	15-29	30-44	45-59	60-69	70+
B. Other neoplasms	11	6	5	–	2	1	1	1	1	1	1	1	–	–	1	1	1
C. Diabetes mellitus	26	11	15	1	1	–	1	2	2	4	1	1	–	1	2	4	6
D. Endocrine disorders	27	12	15	3	1	1	2	2	1	2	2	1	1	1	2	2	6
E. Neuro-psychiatric conditions	48	28	20	3	3	3	5	4	3	7	3	2	1	1	3	3	7
2. Bipolar disorder	1	1	1	–	–	–	1	–	–	–	–	–	–	1	–	–	–
3. Schizophrenia	2	1	1	–	–	–	1	–	–	–	–	–	–	1	–	–	–
4. Epilepsy	6	4	2	1	1	–	1	1	–	–	–	1	–	1	–	–	–
5. Alcohol use	5	4	1	–	–	1	1	1	1	–	–	–	–	1	–	–	–
6. Dementia*	11	5	6	–	–	–	–	1	1	3	–	–	–	–	1	2	3
7. Parkinson disease	3	2	1	–	–	–	–	–	1	1	–	–	–	–	–	–	1
8. Multiple sclerosis	2	1	1	–	–	–	–	–	–	1	–	–	–	–	1	–	–
9. Drug use	1	1	–	–	–	–	1	–	–	–	–	–	–	–	–	–	–
13. Other neuro-psychiatric	19	11	7	2	2	2	2	1	1	1	1	1	1	1	1	1	1
F. Sense organ diseases	–	–	–	–	–	–	–	–	–	–	–	–	–	–	–	–	–
1. Glaucoma	–	–	–	–	–	–	–	–	–	–	–	–	–	–	–	–	–
2. Cataracts	–	–	–	–	–	–	–	–	–	–	–	–	–	–	–	–	–
G. Cardiovascular diseases	1 332	595	737	19	16	19	67	119	126	229	16	19	12	26	121	133	410
1. Rheumatic heart disease	20	11	9	–	2	3	3	1	1	1	5	3	1	–	–	–	–
2. Ischaemic heart disease	360	168	192	–	–	1	18	35	41	73	–	–	1	12	31	39	111
3. Cerebrovascular disease	649	268	380	3	6	8	27	52	60	112	6	5	3	8	60	69	229
4. Inflammatory heart diseases	93	46	48	5	2	2	7	9	8	12	2	4	4	2	9	8	19
5. Other cardiovascular	211	103	108	11	6	5	11	22	16	32	3	7	4	5	22	15	51
H. Respiratory diseases	433	241	193	10	7	6	22	38	48	110	7	6	4	6	36	32	102
1. COPD*	232	131	101	2	1	1	6	19	30	73	2	1	1	1	17	18	61
2. Asthma	27	14	13	–	1	1	2	2	2	3	–	1	1	1	2	2	6
3. Other respiratory	174	95	79	7	5	4	15	16	16	32	5	5	3	4	17	11	35
I. Digestive diseases	187	119	69	4	5	7	20	34	23	27	3	8	3	5	13	14	22
1. Peptic ulcer	18	11	7	–	–	1	2	2	3	3	–	–	–	1	2	2	2
2. Cirrhosis of the liver	46	33	13	–	–	1	5	12	7	7	–	–	1	5	4	3	–
3. Appendicitis	11	7	4	–	2	2	2	1	–	–	–	2	1	–	–	–	–
4. Other digestive	112	68	44	3	3	3	10	18	13	17	3	5	2	3	8	10	14
J. Genito-urinary diseases	107	60	48	9	7	4	7	8	9	15	8	6	2	2	9	8	13
1. Nephritis and nephrosis	93	52	42	9	6	3	6	8	7	13	8	5	1	1	8	7	11
2. Benign prostatic hypertrophy	7	7	–	–	–	–	–	–	1	1	–	–	–	–	–	–	–
3. Other genito-urinary	13	7	6	1	1	1	1	1	1	1	–	1	–	1	2	1	2
K. Skin diseases	10	6	4	5	–	–	–	–	–	–	4	–	–	–	–	–	–

Annex Table 14f, continued. Deaths by age, sex and cause (thousands): Sub-Saharan Africa, 2010, baseline scenario

Cause	Total	Male	Female	Males							Females						
				0-4	5-14	15-29	30-44	45-59	60-69	70+	0-4	5-14	15-29	30-44	45-59	60-69	70+
L. Musculo-skeletal diseases	1	1	-	-	-	-	-	-	-	-	-	-	-	-	-	-	-
1. Rheumatoid arthritis	-	-	-	-	-	-	-	-	-	-	-	-	-	-	-	-	-
3. Other musculo-skeletal	1	-	-	-	-	-	-	-	-	-	-	-	-	-	-	-	-
M. Congenital anomalies	81	39	42	32	2	1	1	1	-	-	36	3	1	-	1	-	-
N. Oral conditions	-	-	-	-	-	-	-	-	-	-	-	-	-	-	-	-	-
III. Injuries	*1 756*	*1 237*	*519*	*158*	*164*	*510*	*249*	*95*	*34*	*26*	*121*	*89*	*160*	*80*	*31*	*17*	*20*
A. Unintentional injuries	867	608	259	107	118	181	108	53	20	20	75	65	53	27	16	8	16
1. Road traffic accidents	308	223	86	16	53	73	44	23	9	6	11	27	26	12	7	2	2
2. Poisonings	56	33	23	22	4	2	2	2	1	1	16	2	3	1	-	-	1
3. Falls	30	18	12	1	2	5	3	3	2	2	2	1	1	1	1	1	-
4. Fires	101	53	48	21	7	10	6	4	2	3	18	8	9	5	3	2	6
5. Drownings	119	88	32	25	35	15	7	3	1	2	13	13	3	1	1	-	4
6. Other unintentional	251	193	58	22	18	75	47	19	6	6	16	14	12	7	4	2	3
B. Intentional injuries	889	628	261	51	45	328	141	42	14	7	46	25	107	53	16	9	4
1. Self-inflicted injuries	29	24	5	-	2	11	6	2	1	1	-	-	3	1	1	-	-
2. Violence	378	325	53	7	14	196	74	25	6	3	3	6	24	11	5	2	2
3. War	482	279	203	44	29	121	61	14	7	3	43	19	81	41	10	7	3

Notes:
Causes responsible for no deaths have been omitted from this table.
A dash (-) symbol indicates fewer than 500 deaths.
*IA6 is Bacterial meningitis and meningococcaemia; IC3 is Hypertensive disorders of pregnancy; ID is Conditions arising during the perinatal period; IIE6 is Dementia and other degenerative and hereditary CNS disorders; IIH1 is Chronic obstructive pulmonary disease.

Annex Table 14g. Deaths by age, sex and cause (thousands): Latin America and the Caribbean, 2010, baseline scenario

Cause	Total	Male	Female	Males 0-4	5-14	15-29	30-44	45-59	60-69	70+	Females 0-4	5-14	15-29	30-44	45-59	60-69	70+
Population (millions)	*607*	*302*	*305*	*28*	*56*	*82*	*66*	*43*	*15*	*12*	*27*	*54*	*81*	*66*	*46*	*17*	*15*
All causes	**4 051**	**2 275**	**1 777**	**212**	**49**	**206**	**263**	**404**	**345**	**795**	**157**	**33**	**85**	**125**	**273**	**242**	**862**
I. Communicable, maternal, perinatal and nutritional conditions	*657*	*396*	*262*	*164*	*7*	*57*	*55*	*30*	*21*	*63*	*116*	*8*	*22*	*20*	*16*	*14*	*67*
A. Infectious and parasitic diseases	**384**	**250**	**134**	**72**	**5**	**55**	**53**	**25**	**15**	**26**	**53**	**5**	**17**	**15**	**11**	**9**	**23**
1. Tuberculosis	46	28	18	1	1	4	3	6	6	8	1	1	2	2	4	3	5
2. STDs excluding HIV	6	3	3	2	–	–	–	–	–	1	2	–	–	–	–	1	1
a. Syphilis	6	3	3	2	–	–	–	–	–	1	2	–	–	–	–	1	1
b. Chlamydia	–	–	–	–	–	–	–	–	–	–	–	–	–	–	–	–	–
c. Gonorrhoea	–	–	–	–	–	–	–	–	–	–	–	–	–	–	–	–	–
3. HIV	152	122	30	6	–	50	46	13	4	2	5	1	12	10	2	1	2
4. Diarrhoeal diseases	77	44	33	35	1	–	–	1	1	5	23	1	–	–	1	1	6
5. Childhood-cluster diseases	40	22	19	20	1	–	–	–	–	–	17	1	–	–	–	–	–
a. Pertussis	8	4	3	4	–	–	–	–	–	–	3	–	–	–	–	–	–
b. Poliomyelitis	1	1	–	–	–	–	–	–	–	–	–	–	–	–	–	–	–
c. Diphtheria	–	–	–	–	–	–	–	–	–	–	–	–	–	–	–	–	–
d. Measles	23	12	10	11	1	–	–	–	–	–	9	1	–	–	–	–	–
e. Tetanus	9	5	4	5	–	–	–	–	–	–	4	1	–	–	–	–	1
6. Bacterial meningitis*	8	4	4	1	–	–	1	1	1	1	1	–	–	1	1	1	1
7. Hepatitis B and hepatitis C	2	1	1	–	–	–	–	1	–	1	–	–	–	–	1	1	–
8. Malaria	6	3	3	–	–	1	–	–	1	2	–	–	1	–	2	1	2
9. Tropical-cluster diseases	13	7	7	–	–	–	1	2	1	2	–	–	–	1	2	1	2
a. Trypanosomiasis	–	–	–	–	–	–	1	–	1	–	–	–	–	1	–	1	–
b. Chagas disease	13	6	6	–	–	–	1	2	1	2	–	–	–	–	2	1	2
c. Schistosomiasis	–	–	–	–	–	–	–	–	–	–	–	–	–	–	–	–	–
d. Leishmaniasis	–	–	–	–	–	–	–	–	–	–	–	–	–	–	–	–	–
10. Leprosy	1	1	–	–	–	–	–	–	–	–	–	–	–	–	–	–	–
11. Dengue	–	–	–	–	–	–	–	–	–	–	–	–	–	–	–	–	–
12. Japanese encephalitis	–	–	–	–	–	–	–	–	–	–	–	–	–	–	–	–	–
13. Trachoma	–	–	–	–	–	–	–	–	–	–	–	–	–	–	–	–	–
14. Intestinal nematode infections	1	–	1	–	–	–	–	–	–	–	–	1	1	1	1	1	–
a. Ascariasis	–	–	–	–	–	–	–	–	–	–	–	–	–	–	–	–	–
b. Trichuriasis	–	–	–	–	–	–	–	–	–	–	–	–	–	–	–	–	–
c. Ancylostomiasis, necatoriasis	–	–	–	–	–	–	–	–	–	–	–	–	–	–	–	–	–
15. Other infectious and parasitic	32	17	15	5	1	1	1	2	1	5	4	1	1	1	1	1	7

Annex Table 14g, continued. Deaths by age, sex and cause (thousands): Latin America and the Caribbean, 2010, baseline scenario

Cause	Total	Male	Female	Males 0-4	5-14	15-29	30-44	45-59	60-69	70+	Females 0-4	5-14	15-29	30-44	45-59	60-69	70+
B. Respiratory infections	**126**	**66**	**59**	**27**	**2**	**1**	**2**	**4**	**4**	**28**	**18**	**2**	**1**	**2**	**3**	**3**	**31**
1. Lower respiratory infections	124	65	59	27	1	1	2	4	4	27	18	2	1	2	3	3	30
2. Upper respiratory infections	1	1	1	–	–	–	–	–	–	1	–	–	–	–	–	–	1
3. Otitis media	–	–	–	–	–	–	–	–	–	–	–	–	–	–	–	–	–
C. Maternal conditions	**6**	**–**	**6**										**4**	**2**			
1. Maternal haemorrhage	1		1											1			
2. Maternal sepsis	–		–														
3. Hypertensive disorders*	1		1										1				
4. Obstructed labour	–		–														
5. Abortion	–		–														
6. Other maternal	1		1										1				
D. Perinatal conditions*	**91**	**55**	**37**	**55**							**37**						
E. Nutritional deficiencies	**50**	**25**	**25**	**10**	**1**			**1**	**1**	**10**	**7**	**1**			**1**	**1**	**13**
1. Protein-energy malnutrition	35	18	17	8	1			1	1	7	6	1			1	1	9
2. Iodine deficiency	1	1	–														
3. Vitamin A deficiency	2	1	1	1							1						
4. Iron-deficiency anaemia	12	5	7	1						3	1						4
II. Noncommunicable diseases	**2 833**	**1 461**	**1 372**	**34**	**16**	**16**	**93**	**303**	**300**	**699**	**29**	**11**	**23**	**78**	**239**	**219**	**773**
A. Malignant neoplasms	**638**	**321**	**317**	**2**	**4**	**5**	**19**	**74**	**77**	**139**	**2**	**4**	**7**	**31**	**88**	**69**	**115**
1. Mouth and oropharynx cancers	23	16	6				1	6	4	5					1	2	3
2. Oesophagus cancer	20	13	6				1	4	4	5						1	5
3. Stomach cancer	71	43	28				2	10	12	19					5	7	16
4. Colon and rectum cancers	42	20	23				2	4	5	9				1	4	7	11
5. Liver cancer	10	5	5				1	1	1	2				1	1	1	1
6. Pancreas cancer	15	7	8					2	2	3					2	2	4
7. Trachea, bronchus, lung cancers	82	53	29				4	18	14	17			1		10	8	10
8. Melanoma and other skin cancers	5	3	3					1	1	1				1	1	1	
9. Breast cancer	52	–	52										1	6	19	11	15
10. Cervix uteri cancer	42		42										1	6	16	7	11
11. Corpus uteri cancer	12		12											1	4	3	5
12. Ovary cancer	10		10											2	3	2	3
13. Prostate cancer	40	40	–					2	12	25							
14. Bladder cancer	16	12	4				1	2	3	6						2	2
15. Lymphomas, multiple myeloma	27	15	12		1	1	3	3	2	4	1	1		1	2	3	5
16. Leukaemia	19	10	9	1	2	1	2	2	1	2	1	1		1	2	1	2
17. Other cancers	150	83	67	1	3	1	5	17	17	39	1	2	2	9	18	13	21

Annex Table 14g, continued. Deaths by age, sex and cause (thousands): Latin America and the Caribbean, 2010, baseline scenario

Cause	Total	Male	Female	Males							Females						
				0-4	5-14	15-29	30-44	45-59	60-69	70+	0-4	5-14	15-29	30-44	45-59	60-69	70+
B. Other neoplasms	11	5	6	-	-	-	1	1	1	2	-	-	-	-	1	1	2
C. Diabetes mellitus	119	46	73	-	-	-	3	10	11	21	-	-	1	2	12	17	41
D. Endocrine disorders	31	14	17	3	1	-	2	2	1	6	2	-	1	1	2	2	9
E. Neuro-psychiatric conditions	55	33	21	2	2	2	7	8	4	8	2	2	2	2	3	2	8
2. Bipolar disorder	1	-	1	-	-	-	-	-	-	1	-	-	-	-	-	-	1
3. Schizophrenia	5	3	2	-	-	-	-	1	-	-	-	-	-	-	-	-	-
4. Epilepsy	6	3	2	-	-	1	1	1	-	-	-	1	1	-	-	-	2
5. Alcohol use	13	12	1	-	-	-	4	5	2	1	1	-	-	-	-	1	-
6. Dementia*	10	5	6	1	-	-	-	1	1	2	-	-	-	-	-	1	4
7. Parkinson disease	3	2	1	-	-	-	-	-	-	1	-	-	-	-	-	-	1
8. Multiple sclerosis	2	1	1	-	-	-	1	-	-	-	-	-	-	1	-	-	-
9. Drug use	2	1	1	2	2	1	1	-	-	-	1	1	1	1	-	-	-
13. Other neuro-psychiatric	13	7	6	-	-	-	1	-	1	1	-	-	2	1	-	-	1
F. Sense organ diseases	1	-	-	-	-	-	-	-	-	-	-	-	-	-	-	-	-
1. Glaucoma	-	-	-	-	-	-	-	-	-	-	-	-	-	-	-	-	-
2. Cataracts	-	-	-	-	-	-	-	-	-	-	-	-	-	-	-	-	-
G. Cardiovascular diseases	1 387	719	668	4	2	4	37	142	153	376	2	1	5	26	87	87	458
1. Rheumatic heart disease	11	4	7	-	-	-	1	1	1	1	-	1	1	1	2	1	1
2. Ischaemic heart disease	627	331	295	-	-	1	15	66	73	176	-	-	1	8	35	40	211
3. Cerebrovascular disease	439	223	216	-	-	1	12	45	48	116	1	-	1	10	31	29	144
4. Inflammatory heart diseases	38	20	18	1	1	1	3	5	7	7	-	1	1	2	3	2	9
5. Other cardiovascular	273	141	132	3	1	1	7	25	29	75	2	1	2	5	15	16	93
H. Respiratory diseases	255	128	127	4	1	1	5	14	21	81	3	1	2	4	22	22	74
1. COPD*	145	76	69	1	-	-	1	7	13	54	1	-	-	1	10	12	44
2. Asthma	27	11	17	-	-	-	1	2	2	5	-	-	1	1	4	3	8
3. Other respiratory	82	41	42	3	1	1	2	5	6	22	2	1	1	2	8	6	22
I. Digestive diseases	218	137	81	1	1	2	17	47	26	44	1	1	2	7	17	14	40
1. Peptic ulcer	20	12	8	-	-	-	1	3	2	6	-	-	-	-	1	1	5
2. Cirrhosis of the liver	97	72	25	-	-	1	12	31	14	14	-	-	-	3	8	5	8
3. Appendicitis	2	1	1	-	-	-	-	-	-	-	-	-	1	-	-	-	-
4. Other digestive	100	52	48	1	-	1	4	13	10	23	1	1	1	3	8	7	27
J. Genito-urinary diseases	68	34	33	1	1	1	2	5	5	19	1	1	1	2	5	5	18
1. Nephritis and nephrosis	49	24	25	1	1	1	2	4	4	12	1	1	1	2	4	4	13
2. Benign prostatic hypertrophy	3	3	-	-	-	-	-	1	1	2	-	-	-	-	-	-	-
3. Other genito-urinary	16	7	9	-	-	-	-	1	1	5	-	-	-	1	1	1	5
K. Skin diseases	4	2	3	-	-	-	-	-	-	1	-	-	-	-	-	-	2

Annex Table 14g, continued. Deaths by age, sex and cause (thousands): Latin America and the Caribbean, 2010, baseline scenario

Cause	Total	Male	Female	Males							Females						
				0-4	5-14	15-29	30-44	45-59	60-69	70+	0-4	5-14	15-29	30-44	45-59	60-69	70+
L. Musculo-skeletal diseases	11	3	8	-	-	-	-	-	-	2	-	-	1	1	1	1	4
1. Rheumatoid arthritis	2	1	1	-	-	-	-	-	-	-	-	-	1	1	1	1	1
3. Other musculo-skeletal	9	3	6	-	-	-	-	-	-	1	-	-	1	1	1	1	3
M. Congenital anomalies	35	17	17	14	1	-	-	-	-	-	15	1	1	-	-	-	-
N. Oral conditions	-	-	-	-	-	-	-	-	-	-	-	-	-	-	-	-	-
III. Injuries	*561*	*418*	*144*	*15*	*27*	*133*	*115*	*70*	*24*	*33*	*12*	*14*	*41*	*27*	*18*	*9*	*23*
A. Unintentional injuries	354	249	105	12	22	64	61	45	17	28	9	11	26	17	14	8	21
1. Road traffic accidents	181	128	52	3	13	39	33	23	8	9	2	7	16	11	8	4	4
2. Poisonings	6	3	2	-	-	1	1	1	-	-	-	-	1	-	-	-	-
3. Falls	30	18	12	-	1	2	3	3	2	7	-	-	-	1	1	1	9
4. Fires	8	5	3	1	-	1	1	1	-	1	1	-	1	1	-	-	1
5. Drownings	29	23	6	2	4	7	5	3	1	1	1	1	2	-	-	-	-
6. Other unintentional	101	71	29	5	4	15	18	14	6	9	4	2	6	4	4	2	6
B. Intentional injuries	207	169	38	3	5	69	55	25	7	6	2	2	15	10	5	2	2
1. Self-inflicted injuries	35	25	10	-	-	7	7	5	2	3	-	-	4	3	2	1	1
2. Violence	149	131	18	1	3	57	45	19	4	3	1	1	8	5	2	1	1
3. War	23	13	10	2	1	5	3	1	-	-	2	1	4	2	1	-	-

Notes:
Causes responsible for no deaths have been omitted from this table.
A dash (-) symbol indicates fewer than 500 deaths.
*IA6 is Bacterial meningitis and meningococcaemia; IC3 is Hypertensive disorders of pregnancy; ID is Conditions arising during the perinatal period; IIE6 is Dementia and other degenerative and hereditary CNS disorders; IIH1 is Chronic obstructive pulmonary disease.

Annex Table 14h. Deaths by age, sex and cause (thousands): Middle Eastern Crescent, 2010, baseline scenario

Cause	Total	Male	Female	Males							Females						
				0-4	5-14	15-29	30-44	45-59	60-69	70+	0-4	5-14	15-29	30-44	45-59	60-69	70+
Population (millions)	*821*	*416*	*405*	*55*	*97*	*116*	*77*	*47*	*14*	*10*	*53*	*93*	*112*	*73*	*46*	*16*	*13*
All causes	**5 657**	**3 167**	**2 491**	**745**	**133**	**218**	**248**	**517**	**416**	**889**	**655**	**105**	**133**	**127**	**267**	**253**	**950**
I. Communicable, maternal, perinatal and nutritional conditions	*1 306*	*690*	*617*	*548*	*22*	*12*	*13*	*19*	*24*	*52*	*486*	*21*	*14*	*14*	*13*	*15*	*53*
A. Infectious and parasitic diseases	**571**	**314**	**256**	**242**	**11**	**11**	**12**	**17**	**9**	**12**	**213**	**9**	**5**	**4**	**9**	**6**	**11**
1. Tuberculosis	63	41	23	3	1	6	5	11	6	7	2	1	3	2	6	4	6
2. STDs excluding HIV	10	5	5	4	–	–	–	–	–	1	4	–	–	–	–	–	1
a. Syphilis	10	5	5	4	–	–	–	–	–	1	4	–	–	–	–	–	1
b. Chlamydia	–	–	–	–	–	–	–	–	–	–	–	–	–	–	–	–	–
c. Gonorrhoea	–	–	–	–	–	–	–	–	–	–	–	–	–	–	–	–	–
3. HIV	13	11	2	1	–	3	4	2	1	–	1	–	–	1	–	–	–
4. Diarrhoeal diseases	278	148	131	142	3	–	–	–	–	1	125	3	–	1	–	–	1
5. Childhood-cluster diseases	151	80	71	75	5	–	–	–	–	–	66	4	–	–	–	–	–
a. Pertussis	34	18	16	17	1	–	–	–	–	–	15	1	–	–	–	–	–
b. Poliomyelitis	2	1	1	1	–	–	–	–	–	–	1	–	–	–	–	–	–
c. Diphtheria	1	1	–	1	–	–	–	–	–	–	–	–	–	–	–	–	–
d. Measles	61	32	29	29	3	–	–	–	–	–	26	2	–	–	–	–	–
e. Tetanus	53	28	25	27	1	–	–	–	–	–	24	1	–	–	–	–	–
6. Bacterial meningitis*	12	6	5	3	–	–	–	1	1	1	3	–	–	–	1	–	1
7. Hepatitis B and hepatitis C	9	5	4	1	–	–	1	1	–	2	1	–	–	–	1	–	2
8. Malaria	3	2	2	–	–	–	–	–	–	–	–	–	–	–	–	–	–
9. Tropical-cluster diseases	2	1	1	–	–	–	–	–	–	–	–	–	–	–	–	–	–
a. Trypanosomiasis	–	–	–	–	–	–	–	–	–	–	–	–	–	–	–	–	–
b. Chagas disease	–	–	–	–	–	–	–	–	–	–	–	–	–	–	–	–	–
c. Schistosomiasis	1	1	–	–	–	–	–	–	–	–	–	–	–	–	–	–	–
d. Leishmaniasis	1	1	–	–	–	–	–	–	–	–	–	–	–	–	–	–	–
10. Leprosy	–	–	–	–	–	–	–	–	–	–	–	–	–	–	–	–	–
11. Dengue	–	–	–	–	–	–	–	–	–	–	–	–	–	–	–	–	–
12. Japanese encephalitis	–	–	–	–	–	–	–	–	–	–	–	–	–	–	–	–	–
13. Trachoma	–	–	–	–	–	–	–	–	–	–	–	–	–	–	–	–	–
14. Intestinal nematode infections	–	–	–	–	–	–	–	–	–	–	–	–	–	–	–	–	–
a. Ascariasis	–	–	–	–	–	–	–	–	–	–	–	–	–	–	–	–	–
b. Trichuriasis	–	–	–	–	–	–	–	–	–	–	–	–	–	–	–	–	–
c. Ancylostomiasis, necatoriasis	–	–	–	–	–	–	–	–	–	–	–	–	–	–	–	–	–
15. Other infectious and parasitic	28	15	13	12	1	–	–	–	–	1	10	1	–	–	–	–	1

Annex Table 14h, continued. Deaths by age, sex and cause (thousands): Middle Eastern Crescent, 2010, baseline scenario

Cause	Total	Male	Female	Males							Females						
				0-4	5-14	15-29	30-44	45-59	60-69	70+	0-4	5-14	15-29	30-44	45-59	60-69	70+
B. Respiratory infections	**384**	**200**	**184**	**136**	**9**	–	**1**	**2**	**14**	**38**	**119**	**10**	**1**	**1**	**3**	**10**	**40**
1. Lower respiratory infections	378	197	181	133	9	–	1	2	14	37	117	10	1	1	3	9	40
2. Upper respiratory infections	4	2	2	1	–	–	–	–	–	–	1	–	–	–	–	–	–
3. Otitis media	2	1	1	1	–	–	–	–	–	–	1	–	–	–	–	–	–
C. Maternal conditions	**18**	–	**18**	–	–	–	–	–	–	–	–	–	**7**	**8**	**2**	–	–
1. Maternal haemorrhage	4	–	4										2	2			
2. Maternal sepsis	3	–	3										2				
3. Hypertensive disorders*	2	–	2											1	1		
4. Obstructed labour	1	–	1										1	1			
5. Abortion	1	–	1										1				
6. Other maternal	1	–	1										1	1			
D. Perinatal conditions*	**272**	**143**	**129**	**143**	–	–	–	–	–	–	**129**	–	–	–	–	–	–
E. Nutritional deficiencies	**62**	**32**	**30**	**28**	**2**	–	–	–	–	**2**	**25**	**2**	**1**	–	–	–	**2**
1. Protein-energy malnutrition	42	22	20	21	–	–	–	–	–	1	19	–	1	–	–	–	1
2. Iodine deficiency	2	1	1	1	–	–	–	–	–	–	1	–	–	–	–	–	–
3. Vitamin A deficiency	12	6	6	5	1	–	–	–	–	–	4	1	–	–	–	–	–
4. Iron-deficiency anaemia	6	3	3	1	–	–	–	–	–	1	1	–	–	–	–	–	1
II. Noncommunicable diseases	***3 626***	***2 003***	***1 623***	***137***	***56***	***49***	***122***	***442***	***376***	***822***	***112***	***53***	***44***	***70***	***233***	***227***	***883***
A. Malignant neoplasms	**448**	**274**	**174**	**4**	**11**	**9**	**25**	**94**	**61**	**71**	**4**	**9**	**8**	**20**	**49**	**37**	**46**
1. Mouth and oropharynx cancers	28	19	10	–	–	1	2	4	5	6	–	–	–	1	2	3	3
2. Oesophagus cancer	18	11	7	–	–	–	1	5	2	3	–	–	–	–	2	2	3
3. Stomach cancer	38	23	14	–	–	1	1	10	5	6	–	–	–	1	2	2	2
4. Colon and rectum cancers	22	11	11	–	–	1	2	3	5	4	–	–	–	1	4	4	5
5. Liver cancer	16	10	6	–	–	–	1	4	3	2	–	–	–	1	2	3	5
6. Pancreas cancer	9	5	3	–	–	–	–	2	2	1	–	–	–	–	1	1	2
7. Trachea, bronchus, lung cancers	110	90	19	–	–	–	6	37	20	26	–	–	–	1	7	5	1
8. Melanoma and other skin cancers	2	1	1	–	–	1	–	–	–	–	–	–	–	–	–	–	1
9. Breast cancer	21	–	21	–	–	–	–	–	–	–	–	–	2	3	9	3	6
10. Cervix uteri cancer	14	–	14	–	–	–	–	–	–	–	–	–	1	2	6	2	3
11. Corpus uteri cancer	4	–	4	–	–	–	–	–	–	–	–	–	–	–	1	1	1
12. Ovary cancer	6	–	6	–	–	–	–	–	–	–	–	–	–	1	2	1	1
13. Prostate cancer	8	8	–	–	–	–	–	2	3	3	–	–	–	–	–	–	–
14. Bladder cancer	18	14	3	–	–	–	–	5	4	4	–	–	–	–	1	1	1
15. Lymphomas, multiple myeloma	16	11	5	–	–	–	–	2	2	2	–	–	–	1	1	1	1
16. Leukaemia	21	11	10	1	3	1	2	1	1	2	1	3	1	1	1	1	2
17. Other cancers	99	59	40	2	6	2	6	18	12	13	2	4	3	6	10	7	8

Annex Table 14h, continued. Deaths by age, sex and cause (thousands): Middle Eastern Crescent, 2010, baseline scenario

Cause	Total	Male	Female	Males							Females						
				0-4	5-14	15-29	30-44	45-59	60-69	70+	0-4	5-14	15-29	30-44	45-59	60-69	70+
B. Other neoplasms	7	4	3	-	-	-	-	1	-	1	-	-	-	-	1	-	1
C. Diabetes mellitus	72	33	39	1	1	1	3	9	7	11	1	1	1	1	8	10	17
D. Endocrine disorders	18	9	9	4	1	1	1	1	1	1	4	2	1	-	1	1	1
E. Neuro-psychiatric conditions	68	37	32	9	5	4	3	4	3	8	7	5	3	2	3	2	9
2. Bipolar disorder	1	-	1	-	-	-	-	-	-	-	-	-	-	-	-	-	1
3. Schizophrenia	4	2	2	-	-	-	1	-	-	1	-	-	-	-	1	-	1
4. Epilepsy	9	5	4	1	1	1	1	1	-	-	1	1	1	1	-	-	-
5. Alcohol use	1	1	-	-	-	-	1	-	-	-	-	-	-	-	-	-	-
6. Dementia*	13	6	7	-	-	-	-	1	1	4	-	-	-	-	1	1	5
7. Parkinson disease	4	2	2	-	-	-	-	-	-	2	-	-	-	-	-	-	2
8. Multiple sclerosis	2	1	1	-	-	-	1	-	-	-	-	-	-	1	-	-	-
9. Drug use	2	2	-	-	-	1	-	1	-	-	-	-	-	-	-	-	-
13. Other neuro-psychiatric	33	18	15	8	4	2	1	1	1	1	6	4	2	1	1	-	1
F. Sense organ diseases	-	-	-	-	-	-	-	-	-	-	-	-	-	-	-	-	-
1. Glaucoma	-	-	-	-	-	-	-	-	-	-	-	-	-	-	-	-	-
2. Cataracts	-	-	-	-	-	-	-	-	-	-	-	-	-	-	-	-	-
G. Cardiovascular diseases	2 271	1 224	1 047	47	25	22	66	247	238	579	30	21	19	33	121	135	689
1. Rheumatic heart disease	26	13	13	-	2	4	4	2	1	-	-	2	4	3	2	1	1
2. Ischaemic heart disease	1 150	630	520	-	-	3	31	134	133	328	-	-	1	13	55	72	377
3. Cerebrovascular disease	381	186	195	3	5	3	7	37	38	93	2	4	3	4	24	26	135
4. Inflammatory heart diseases	101	57	44	9	5	4	7	13	6	14	7	4	3	4	7	3	16
5. Other cardiovascular	614	338	276	35	14	8	15	61	61	144	22	12	8	8	33	32	161
H. Respiratory diseases	354	199	155	15	4	3	6	33	34	104	12	7	4	4	22	23	84
1. COPD*	192	112	80	3	1	-	2	17	21	68	3	1	-	1	10	13	51
2. Asthma	24	12	11	1	-	1	-	2	2	6	-	-	-	1	4	2	6
3. Other respiratory	139	74	65	11	3	2	4	14	11	29	9	5	3	3	8	8	28
I. Digestive diseases	187	112	75	12	3	4	10	38	21	25	13	3	3	5	18	12	21
1. Peptic ulcer	9	7	3	-	-	-	1	2	1	2	-	-	-	-	-	1	2
2. Cirrhosis of the liver	66	40	26	-	1	1	4	16	9	9	-	1	1	2	8	5	9
3. Appendicitis	4	2	2	-	1	1	-	-	-	-	-	1	1	-	-	-	-
4. Other digestive	108	63	45	12	1	2	5	19	10	13	13	1	2	3	9	6	11
J. Genito-urinary diseases	104	62	42	3	2	4	7	15	10	21	2	3	4	4	10	7	14
1. Nephritis and nephrosis	43	25	19	2	1	2	3	5	3	9	1	2	2	2	4	3	6
2. Benign prostatic hypertrophy	2	2	-	-	-	-	-	-	-	2	-	-	-	-	-	-	-
3. Other genito-urinary	59	35	23	1	1	2	4	10	6	11	1	1	2	2	6	4	8
K. Skin diseases	2	1	1	-	-	-	-	-	-	-	-	-	-	-	-	-	-

Annex Table 14h, continued. Deaths by age, sex and cause (thousands): Middle Eastern Crescent, 2010, baseline scenario

Cause	Total	Male	Female	Males							Females						
				0-4	5-14	15-29	30-44	45-59	60-69	70+	0-4	5-14	15-29	30-44	45-59	60-69	70+
L. Musculo-skeletal diseases	**2**	**1**	**1**	-	-	-	-	-	-	-	-	-	-	-	-	-	-
1. Rheumatoid arthritis	-	-	1	-	-	-	-	-	-	-	-	-	-	-	-	-	-
3. Other musculo-skeletal	2	1	1	-	-	-	-	-	-	-	-	-	-	-	-	-	-
M. Congenital anomalies	**92**	**48**	**44**	42	2	1	1	1	-	-	39	2	1	1	1	-	-
N. Oral conditions	-	-	-	-	-	-	-	-	-	-	-	-	-	-	-	-	-
III. Injuries	*725*	*474*	*251*	*60*	*55*	*157*	*113*	*56*	*16*	*16*	*57*	*31*	*75*	*44*	*21*	*11*	*14*
A. Unintentional injuries	**308**	**219**	**89**	29	25	60	55	32	8	9	26	12	18	13	9	4	8
1. Road traffic accidents	127	98	29	4	11	34	28	14	3	3	3	6	7	5	4	2	2
2. Poisonings	19	12	7	2	-	2	4	3	1	-	2	-	1	1	1	-	1
3. Falls	17	12	5	2	1	2	3	2	1	1	2	1	-	-	-	-	1
4. Fires	21	9	12	3	1	2	2	1	-	1	3	1	4	2	1	-	1
5. Drownings	35	25	10	7	5	6	4	2	-	-	6	1	1	1	-	-	-
6. Other unintentional	90	63	26	12	6	14	15	10	3	4	10	2	4	3	3	1	3
B. Intentional injuries	**417**	**254**	**162**	31	30	97	57	24	8	6	31	19	57	31	12	7	5
1. Self-inflicted injuries	80	55	25	-	12	16	12	9	3	3	-	6	7	4	3	2	3
2. Violence	62	41	21	8	3	13	10	4	1	1	8	3	3	3	2	-	1
3. War	275	159	117	23	15	68	36	11	4	2	23	10	46	24	7	4	2

Notes:
Causes responsible for no deaths have been omitted from this table.
A dash (-) symbol indicates fewer than 500 deaths.
[a]IA6 is Bacterial meningitis and meningococcaemia; IC3 is Hypertensive disorders of pregnancy; ID is Conditions arising during the perinatal period; IIE6 is Dementia and other degenerative and hereditary CNS disorders; IIH1 is Chronic obstructive pulmonary disease.

Annex Table 14i. Deaths by age, sex and cause (thousands): World, 2010, baseline scenario

Cause	Total	Male	Female	Males 0-4	5-14	15-29	30-44	45-59	60-69	70+	Females 0-4	5-14	15-29	30-44	45-59	60-69	70+
Population (millions)	7 000	3 502	3 498	351	661	893	736	524	191	146	336	635	863	714	532	213	205
All causes	60 828	33 950	26 878	4 401	864	2 096	2 873	6 161	5 671	11 886	3 682	680	1 307	1 498	3 120	3 300	13 292
I. Communicable, maternal, perinatal and nutritional conditions	12 483	6 743	5 740	3 461	231	448	624	540	354	1 086	2 874	238	484	484	349	234	1 077
A. Infectious and parasitic diseases	7 829	4 381	3 448	1 921	166	434	608	508	254	491	1 575	168	409	409	315	159	414
1. Tuberculosis	2 186	1 272	914	46	29	163	198	348	179	308	43	36	156	134	230	107	208
2. STDs excluding HIV	137	67	70	49	-	-	-	1	2	13	41	-	3	3	2	3	17
a. Syphilis	130	67	64	49	-	-	-	1	2	13	41	-	2	2	2	2	17
b. Chlamydia	4	-	4	-	-	-	-	-	-	-	-	-	2	1	-	-	-
c. Gonorrhoea	2	-	2	-	-	-	-	-	-	-	-	-	1	1	-	-	-
3. HIV	1 647	948	698	159	23	239	370	111	30	16	148	23	224	245	43	11	5
4. Diarrhoeal diseases	1 639	890	750	763	30	5	6	9	15	62	610	30	5	6	9	13	76
5. Childhood-cluster diseases	1 104	596	508	534	42	3	5	4	2	5	451	40	3	3	4	2	6
a. Pertussis	197	107	90	101	6	-	-	-	-	-	85	5	-	-	-	-	-
b. Poliomyelitis	13	8	5	7	-	-	-	-	-	-	5	-	-	-	-	-	-
c. Diphtheria	5	3	2	2	-	-	-	-	-	-	2	-	-	-	-	-	-
d. Measles	624	337	287	306	31	-	-	-	-	-	258	28	-	-	-	-	-
e. Tetanus	265	141	124	116	6	-	5	3	2	5	101	7	-	3	4	2	6
6. Bacterial meningitis*	85	45	41	22	-	1	5	5	5	7	19	-	1	3	5	5	8
7. Hepatitis B and hepatitis C	59	34	25	4	1	1	3	7	4	13	3	1	1	1	3	4	12
8. Malaria	571	323	248	270	19	11	8	7	3	4	199	18	9	7	7	3	5
9. Tropical-cluster diseases	54	31	23	2	7	5	5	6	3	4	1	6	3	3	4	2	3
a. Trypanosomiasis	21	12	10	-	3	3	2	3	1	1	-	3	2	1	2	1	2
b. Chagas disease	13	6	6	-	-	-	1	2	1	2	-	-	-	-	2	1	2
c. Schistosomiasis	4	3	2	-	-	-	-	1	1	1	-	-	-	1	2	-	1
d. Leishmaniasis	15	10	5	1	4	2	2	-	-	-	1	2	1	1	-	-	-
10. Leprosy	2	1	1	-	-	-	-	-	-	-	-	-	-	-	-	-	-
11. Dengue	6	3	3	1	2	-	-	-	-	-	1	2	-	-	-	-	-
12. Japanese encephalitis	1	1	1	-	-	-	-	-	-	-	-	-	-	-	-	-	-
13. Trachoma	-	-	-	-	-	-	-	-	-	-	-	-	-	-	-	-	-
14. Intestinal nematode infections	7	4	4	-	2	-	-	-	-	1	-	2	-	-	-	-	1
a. Ascariasis	3	1	1	-	1	-	-	-	-	-	-	1	-	-	-	-	-
b. Trichuriasis	2	1	1	-	1	-	-	-	-	-	-	1	-	-	-	-	-
c. Ancylostomiasis, necatoriasis	3	1	1	-	-	-	-	-	-	1	-	-	-	-	-	-	1
15. Other infectious and parasitic	333	169	164	71	9	4	6	10	12	56	59	9	3	3	7	11	72

Annex Table 14i, continued. Deaths by age, sex and cause (thousands): World, 2010, baseline scenario

Cause	Total	Male	Female	Males 0-4	5-14	15-29	30-44	45-59	60-69	70+	Females 0-4	5-14	15-29	30-44	45-59	60-69	70+
B. Respiratory infections	2 892	1 503	1 388	747	55	12	14	28	94	555	609	55	12	10	24	69	609
1. Lower respiratory infections	2 850	1 482	1 369	733	54	11	13	27	93	550	597	54	11	10	24	68	604
2. Upper respiratory infections	28	14	14	8	1	-	-	-	1	5	6	1	-	-	-	1	6
3. Otitis media	13	7	6	7	-	-	-	-	-	-	6	-	-	-	-	-	-
C. Maternal conditions	132	-	132	-	-	-	-	-	-	-	-	5	60	62	5	-	-
1. Maternal haemorrhage	32	-	32	-	-	-	-	-	-	-	-	1	15	15	1	-	-
2. Maternal sepsis	20	-	20	-	-	-	-	-	-	-	-	-	9	10	1	-	-
3. Hypertensive disorders*	11	-	11	-	-	-	-	-	-	-	-	-	5	5	1	-	-
4. Obstructed labour	6	-	6	-	-	-	-	-	-	-	-	-	3	3	-	-	-
5. Abortion	10	-	10	-	-	-	-	-	-	-	-	-	5	5	-	-	-
6. Other maternal	18	-	18	-	-	-	-	-	-	-	-	1	8	8	1	-	-
D. Perinatal conditions*	1 263	678	586	678	-	-	-	-	-	-	585	-	-	-	-	-	-
E. Nutritional deficiencies	366	181	186	115	10	3	2	4	6	40	105	10	3	3	5	6	54
1. Protein-energy malnutrition	226	114	111	86	1	1	1	2	3	21	78	2	1	1	2	2	26
2. Iodine deficiency	8	4	4	4	1	-	-	-	-	-	3	1	-	-	-	-	-
3. Vitamin A deficiency	50	27	24	20	6	-	-	-	-	-	18	6	-	-	-	-	-
4. Iron-deficiency anaemia	79	34	45	6	2	2	1	2	3	18	6	2	2	2	4	3	26
II. Noncommunicable diseases	41 188	22 529	18 659	541	238	294	1 181	4 867	5 031	10 378	483	206	240	626	2 426	2 884	11 793
A. Malignant neoplasms	9 786	5 909	3 877	29	71	87	422	1 767	1 497	2 036	33	50	81	277	970	876	1 591
1. Mouth and oropharynx cancers	491	328	163	1	1	6	29	100	85	107	1	-	5	12	40	43	61
2. Oesophagus cancer	634	437	197	-	-	3	20	141	124	150	-	-	2	5	47	59	84
3. Stomach cancer	1 260	830	429	-	-	3	36	261	227	299	-	1	5	24	92	103	206
4. Colon and rectum cancers	697	374	323	-	1	5	21	80	93	175	-	1	3	13	53	73	180
5. Liver cancer	913	678	235	1	2	12	105	281	144	134	1	2	3	19	67	56	87
6. Pancreas cancer	267	156	112	-	-	-	6	42	41	65	-	-	1	2	17	26	65
7. Trachea, bronchus, lung cancers	1 788	1 343	444	-	1	6	64	476	403	393	-	-	2	14	113	126	189
8. Melanoma and other skin cancers	67	35	32	-	-	1	3	11	7	13	-	-	1	2	7	7	15
9. Breast cancer	437	-	437	-	-	-	-	-	-	-	-	-	10	46	144	86	150
10. Cervix uteri cancer	318	-	318	-	-	-	-	-	-	-	-	-	10	32	128	63	84
11. Corpus uteri cancer	87	-	87	-	-	-	-	-	-	-	-	-	-	3	23	20	40
12. Ovary cancer	143	-	143	-	-	-	-	-	-	-	-	1	5	16	40	31	49
13. Prostate cancer	311	311	-	-	-	-	-	23	76	210	-	-	-	-	-	-	-
14. Bladder cancer	209	159	50	-	-	1	1	30	42	81	-	-	-	1	7	12	30
15. Lymphomas, multiple myeloma	313	189	124	1	1	4	4	42	39	59	-	1	4	9	21	25	55
16. Leukaemia	305	170	135	9	20	13	28	33	24	42	8	15	10	20	23	19	40
17. Other cancers	1 547	899	648	17	31	24	82	248	192	307	14	22	20	59	146	128	257

Annex Table 14i, continued. Deaths by age, sex and cause (thousands): World, 2010, baseline scenario

Cause	Total	Male	Female	M 0-4	M 5-14	M 15-29	M 30-44	M 45-59	M 60-69	M 70+	F 0-4	F 5-14	F 15-29	F 30-44	F 45-59	F 60-69	F 70+
B. Other neoplasms	**109**	**54**	**54**	**3**	**4**	**3**	**5**	**10**	**9**	**21**	**3**	**3**	**2**	**3**	**8**	**8**	**27**
C. Diabetes mellitus	**672**	**270**	**402**	**5**	**6**	**4**	**17**	**54**	**59**	**127**	**5**	**5**	**4**	**8**	**52**	**85**	**244**
D. Endocrine disorders	**158**	**69**	**89**	**13**	**3**	**3**	**6**	**9**	**9**	**27**	**11**	**4**	**3**	**3**	**9**	**9**	**49**
E. Neuro-psychiatric conditions	**773**	**383**	**390**	**26**	**17**	**28**	**48**	**58**	**45**	**161**	**25**	**14**	**16**	**17**	**28**	**38**	**252**
2. Bipolar disorder	20	6	14	–	–	–	1	1	1	3	–	–	1	2	1	1	12
3. Schizophrenia	58	29	29	–	–	2	5	5	4	13	–	–	1	4	3	4	20
4. Epilepsy	61	37	24	2	3	6	9	7	8	5	2	2	5	1	3	2	5
5. Alcohol use	57	48	8	–	–	1	13	19	8	7	–	–	1	1	3	2	2
6. Dementia*	261	97	163	3	–	–	1	8	12	71	3	–	–	1	6	14	137
7. Parkinson disease	77	39	38	–	–	–	–	1	4	34	–	–	–	–	1	3	34
8. Multiple sclerosis	25	11	14	–	–	–	1	2	2	2	–	–	–	2	5	3	4
9. Drug use	9	8	1	–	–	4	4	–	–	–	–	–	–	1	–	–	–
13. Other neuro-psychiatric	206	109	97	21	14	15	14	16	7	26	20	12	8	6	6	9	38
F. Sense organ diseases	**19**	**10**	**10**	**1**	–	–	–	**3**	**3**	**3**	**1**	–	–	–	**2**	**3**	**3**
1. Glaucoma	6	3	3	–	–	–	–	1	1	1	–	–	–	–	1	1	1
2. Cataracts	6	3	3	–	–	–	–	1	1	1	–	–	–	–	1	1	1
G. Cardiovascular diseases	**21 019**	**10 950**	**10 068**	**125**	**71**	**94**	**436**	**2 080**	**2 454**	**5 690**	**88**	**63**	**70**	**202**	**881**	**1 317**	**7 446**
1. Rheumatic heart disease	421	206	215	–	6	15	30	66	35	54	1	7	13	26	55	31	83
2. Ischaemic heart disease	9 374	4 980	4 393	–	–	10	162	964	1 166	2 680	5	–	6	63	329	590	3 400
3. Cerebrovascular disease	6 493	3 246	3 247	15	17	22	106	577	756	1 752	11	13	12	54	292	445	2 419
4. Inflammatory heart diseases	650	358	293	25	14	16	42	96	51	115	22	13	12	20	46	31	150
5. Other cardiovascular	4 080	2 160	1 920	85	35	32	97	377	445	1 089	49	31	28	39	160	219	1 394
H. Respiratory diseases	**4 793**	**2 660**	**2 133**	**46**	**21**	**19**	**65**	**342**	**583**	**1 585**	**33**	**20**	**18**	**38**	**236**	**334**	**1 452**
1. COPD*	3 557	1 988	1 569	11	3	4	23	232	460	1 255	10	4	2	15	150	254	1 134
2. Asthma	243	122	120	–	3	4	12	24	23	56	–	2	3	8	24	22	61
3. Other respiratory	993	550	443	34	14	10	31	87	100	274	23	15	13	16	63	58	257
I. Digestive diseases	**2 323**	**1 449**	**875**	**28**	**15**	**27**	**139**	**462**	**293**	**485**	**28**	**16**	**20**	**50**	**172**	**143**	**446**
1. Peptic ulcer	240	148	93	1	–	2	10	36	29	70	1	–	1	3	13	13	62
2. Cirrhosis of the liver	1 002	705	297	1	2	10	80	284	157	171	1	3	6	22	89	64	112
3. Appendicitis	39	24	16	1	4	6	7	3	2	1	1	4	3	4	2	1	1
4. Other digestive	1 042	572	470	26	8	9	43	139	106	242	25	9	9	21	68	65	271
J. Genito-urinary diseases	**816**	**430**	**386**	**19**	**16**	**13**	**34**	**69**	**68**	**207**	**15**	**16**	**13**	**19**	**55**	**59**	**209**
1. Nephritis and nephrosis	584	297	287	14	14	10	27	51	48	129	14	14	10	15	41	45	148
2. Benign prostatic hypertrophy	37	37	–	–	–	–	–	1	6	30	–	–	–	–	–	–	–
3. Other genito-urinary	195	96	99	5	2	3	7	17	15	48	1	2	3	4	14	14	61
K. Skin diseases	**51**	**24**	**27**	**7**	**1**	**1**	**1**	**2**	**2**	**3**	**5**	–	**1**	**1**	**2**	**2**	**17**

Annex Table 14i, continued. Deaths by age, sex and cause (thousands): World, 2010, baseline scenario

Cause	Total	Male	Female	Males 0-4	5-14	15-29	30-44	45-59	60-69	70+	Females 0-4	5-14	15-29	30-44	45-59	60-69	70+
L. Musculo-skeletal diseases	111	39	72	1	1	1	1	4	7	23	1	1	2	3	7	8	51
1. Rheumatoid arthritis	19	5	14	-	-	-	-	1	1	3	-	-	-	-	1	2	10
3. Other musculo-skeletal	91	33	58	-	1	1	1	3	6	20	1	1	2	3	5	6	41
M. Congenital anomalies	556	281	275	240	13	11	7	5	2	3	236	13	8	4	6	3	5
N. Oral conditions	2	1	1	-	-	-	-	-	-	-	-	-	-	-	-	-	-
III. Injuries	*7 157*	*4 678*	*2 479*	*399*	*395*	*1 354*	*1 068*	*754*	*286*	*422*	*324*	*236*	*583*	*388*	*345*	*182*	*421*
A. Unintentional injuries	4 380	2 880	1 500	300	298	678	619	495	187	303	224	177	255	189	212	117	326
1. Road traffic accidents	1 837	1 307	530	56	139	379	312	235	87	100	36	86	118	85	98	45	64
2. Poisonings	278	168	110	33	9	19	35	42	12	17	24	6	20	17	17	9	17
3. Falls	388	205	183	11	10	23	31	38	22	70	11	5	5	7	16	17	122
4. Fires	325	141	185	36	11	23	24	20	6	20	31	17	48	30	18	11	30
5. Drownings	475	316	159	77	75	60	43	29	11	20	51	33	18	12	14	8	23
6. Other unintentional	1 076	743	333	85	54	173	174	132	49	75	71	32	45	39	49	28	71
B. Intentional injuries	2 778	1 799	979	100	97	676	449	259	99	119	100	59	328	199	133	65	95
1. Self-inflicted injuries	1 080	628	452	-	24	146	152	145	65	96	-	12	142	92	86	41	78
2. Violence	864	686	178	27	26	321	188	86	22	18	28	15	48	36	28	11	11
3. War	834	484	350	73	48	209	108	28	13	5	72	32	139	71	19	13	5

Notes:
Causes responsible for no deaths have been omitted from this table.
A dash (-) symbol indicates fewer than 500 deaths.
*IA6 is Bacterial meningitis and meningococcaemia; IC3 is Hypertensive disorders of pregnancy; ID is Conditions arising during the perinatal period;
IIE6 is Dementia and other degenerative and hereditary CNS disorders; IIH1 is Chronic obstructive pulmonary disease.

Annex Table 15a. DALYs by age, sex and cause (thousands): Established Market Economies, 2010, baseline scenario

Cause	Total	Male	Female	Males					Females				
				0-4	5-14	15-44	45-59	60+	0-4	5-14	15-44	45-59	60+
Population (millions)	*874*	*428*	*447*	*29*	*57*	*165*	*88*	*88*	*28*	*55*	*159*	*90*	*116*
All causes	*98 553*	*56 234*	*42 320*	*1 892*	*1 116*	*18 971*	*14 320*	*19 934*	*1 540*	*875*	*12 590*	*9 063*	*18 252*
I. Communicable, maternal, perinatal and nutritional conditions	*5 722*	*3 597*	*2 125*	*731*	*74*	*1 708*	*392*	*692*	*566*	*72*	*682*	*144*	*661*
A. Infectious and parasitic diseases	3 053	2 258	795	110	23	1 645	331	149	88	24	491	64	128
1. Tuberculosis	73	52	20	–	–	7	13	33	–	–	2	4	15
2. STDs excluding HIV	214	15	199	–	–	13	–	1	–	2	194	2	2
a. Syphilis	3	2	1	–	–	1	–	1	–	–	1	1	–
b. Chlamydia	184	8	176	–	–	8	–	–	–	2	173	1	–
c. Gonorrhoea	24	5	19	–	–	4	–	–	–	–	19	–	–
3. HIV	2 280	1 951	329	36	6	1 590	292	28	26	6	259	32	6
4. Diarrhoeal diseases	105	54	51	23	4	12	6	10	20	4	8	6	13
5. Childhood-cluster diseases	18	10	8	7	1	–	–	1	6	1	–	–	1
a. Pertussis	10	5	5	5	–	–	–	–	5	–	–	–	–
b. Poliomyelitis	2	1	1	–	–	–	–	1	–	–	–	–	1
c. Diphtheria	–	–	–	–	–	–	–	–	–	–	–	–	–
d. Measles	5	3	2	2	1	–	–	–	1	1	–	–	–
e. Tetanus	1	–	–	–	–	–	–	–	–	–	–	–	–
6. Bacterial meningitis*	85	46	39	31	4	4	3	4	26	4	2	2	4
7. Hepatitis B and hepatitis C	25	16	9	1	–	4	5	6	–	–	2	2	4
8. Malaria	1	–	–	–	–	–	–	–	–	–	–	–	–
9. Tropical-cluster diseases	1	–	–	–	–	–	–	–	–	–	–	–	–
a. Trypanosomiasis	–	–	–	–	–	–	–	–	–	–	–	–	–
b. Chagas disease	–	–	–	–	–	–	–	–	–	–	–	–	–
c. Schistosomiasis	–	–	–	–	–	–	–	–	–	–	–	–	–
d. Leishmaniasis	1	–	–	–	–	–	–	–	–	–	–	–	–
e. Lymphatic filariasis	–	–	–	–	–	–	–	–	–	–	–	–	–
f. Onchocerciasis	–	–	–	–	–	–	–	–	–	–	–	–	–
10. Leprosy	1	–	–	–	–	–	–	–	–	–	–	–	–
11. Dengue	–	–	–	–	–	–	–	–	–	–	–	–	–
12. Japanese encephalitis	–	–	–	–	–	–	–	–	–	–	–	–	–
13. Trachoma	–	–	–	–	–	–	–	–	–	–	–	–	–
14. Intestinal nematode infections	–	–	–	–	–	–	–	–	–	–	–	–	–
a. Ascariasis	–	–	–	–	–	–	–	–	–	–	–	–	–
b. Trichuriasis	–	–	–	–	–	–	–	–	–	–	–	–	–
c. Ancylostomiasis and necatoriasis	–	–	–	–	–	–	–	–	–	–	–	–	–

Annex Table 15a, continued. DALYs by age, sex and cause (thousands): Established Market Economies, 2010, baseline scenario

Cause	Total			Males					Females				
	Total	Male	Female	0-4	5-14	15-44	45-59	60+	0-4	5-14	15-44	45-59	60+
B. Respiratory infections	**1 141**	**609**	**532**	**37**	**23**	**31**	**47**	**470**	**26**	**21**	**17**	**28**	**439**
1. Lower respiratory infections	1 072	573	498	29	6	28	45	465	20	6	15	26	432
2. Upper respiratory infections	30	15	14	4	1	3	2	5	2	1	3	2	6
3. Otitis media	39	20	19	5	15				4	15			
C. Maternal conditions	**79**		**79**								**79**		
1. Maternal haemorrhage	5		5								5		
2. Maternal sepsis	8		8								8		
3. Hypertensive disorders of pregnancy	3		3								3		
4. Obstructed labour	55		55								55		
5. Abortion	3		3								3		
D. Perinatal conditions*	**970**	**550**	**420**	**550**					**420**				
E. Nutritional deficiencies	**478**	**180**	**298**	**35**	**28**	**31**	**14**	**72**	**32**	**26**	**94**	**52**	**94**
1. Protein-energy malnutrition	53	25	28	17		1	1	7	16			1	11
2. Iodine deficiency													
3. Vitamin A deficiency													
4. Iron-deficiency anaemia	420	152	268	18	27	30	13	64	16	26	93	51	82
II. Noncommunicable diseases	*82 470*	*45 545*	*36 926*	*944*	*690*	*12 474*	*12 817*	*18 619*	*815*	*580*	*10 178*	*8 296*	*17 056*
A. Malignant neoplasms	**16 748**	**9 943**	**6 805**	**24**	**77**	**968**	**3 603**	**5 271**	**22**	**54**	**903**	**2 243**	**3 583**
1. Mouth and oropharynx cancers	402	329	72			41	171	117			10	27	35
2. Oesophagus cancer	396	327	69			19	151	157			4	20	45
3. Stomach cancer	1 181	784	397			61	272	451			53	109	236
4. Colon and rectum cancers	1 803	1 014	789			67	327	619			55	210	523
5. Liver cancer	358	285	73	1	1	19	133	132			5	21	46
6. Pancreas cancer	658	392	266			26	145	220			14	74	179
7. Trachea, bronchus, lung cancers	4 112	2 935	1 177			221	1 311	1 402			76	435	665
8. Melanoma and other skin cancers	250	156	94			44	58	55			29	30	34
9. Breast cancer	1 384		1 384								260	576	548
10. Cervix uteri cancer	177		177							1	61	63	52
11. Corpus uteri cancer	185		185								20	68	97
12. Ovary cancer	368		368								49	150	169
13. Prostate cancer	712	712				3	77	632					
14. Bladder cancer	438	360	79			7	67	286			3	13	63
15. Lymphomas and multiple myeloma	720	436	284	1		100	141	185	1	3	49	74	157
16. Leukaemia	579	345	234	8	31	96	83	127	8	20	62	53	91
C. Diabetes mellitus	**2 127**	**999**	**1 128**	**2**	**2**	**175**	**342**	**478**	**1**	**4**	**117**	**273**	**732**
D. Endocrine disorders	**947**	**417**	**531**	**60**	**43**	**116**	**65**	**133**	**57**	**33**	**113**	**134**	**194**

Annex Table 15a, continued. DALYs by age, sex and cause (thousands): Established Market Economies, 2010, baseline scenario

Cause	Total	Male	Female	Males					Females				
				0-4	5-14	15-44	45-59	60+	0-4	5-14	15-44	45-59	60+
E. Neuro-psychiatric conditions	**24 406**	**12 547**	**11 859**	**96**	**298**	**8 433**	**1 893**	**1 828**	**83**	**251**	**6 759**	**1 881**	**2 884**
1. Unipolar major depression	6 639	2 325	4 315			1 643	506	176			2 989	934	392
2. Bipolar disorder	1 612	813	799			691	84	38			667	85	47
3. Schizophrenia	2 021	1 056	965			1 027	9	19			934	3	28
4. Epilepsy	356	200	156	5	36	102	39	18	5	38	59	29	25
5. Alcohol use	4 441	3 755	686			3 009	594	152			540	103	42
6. Dementia*	3 780	1 491	2 290	35	16	40	302	1 098	34	14	31	319	1 892
7. Parkinson disease	600	273	327				85	188				93	234
8. Multiple sclerosis	204	88	115			69	13	6			88	18	9
9. Drug use	1 379	1 044	335	4	91	902	43	8	6	31	288	14	2
10. Post-traumatic stress disorder	263	100	164		17	64	12	3		28	104	19	6
11. Obsessive-compulsive disorders	1 405	597	808		56	451	54	36		72	578	97	61
12. Panic disorder	677	226	451		19	150	56	-		19	317	91	24
F. Sense organ diseases	**136**	**63**	**73**			**3**	**27**	**32**			**2**	**28**	**42**
1. Glaucoma	95	42	53			2	22	18			1	25	27
2. Cataracts	36	18	18			1	4	13			1	3	14
G. Cardiovascular diseases	**19 050**	**11 937**	**7 113**	**46**	**21**	**1 047**	**3 633**	**7 189**	**36**	**14**	**454**	**777**	**5 832**
1. Rheumatic heart disease	142	63	79			10	23	30			9	18	51
2. Ischaemic heart disease	9 553	6 375	3 179	8	5	369	2 128	3 878	6	3	88	314	2 777
3. Cerebrovascular disease	5 070	2 768	2 302	9	5	290	739	1 727	10	3	198	294	1 801
4. Inflammatory heart diseases	621	412	208			119	149	131			51	34	111
H. Respiratory diseases	**5 143**	**2 862**	**2 281**	**55**	**113**	**490**	**612**	**1 593**	**29**	**91**	**454**	**571**	**1 135**
1. COPD*	2 713	1 656	1 057	2	1	90	351	1 211	1	1	51	273	731
2. Asthma	1 123	555	568	23	96	258	101	76	11	80	254	127	96
I. Digestive diseases	**4 897**	**2 925**	**1 972**	**25**	**12**	**522**	**1 286**	**1 079**	**19**	**11**	**356**	**651**	**935**
1. Peptic ulcer	281	178	103			33	60	85			19	25	59
2. Cirrhosis of the liver	1 848	1 339	509	1		232	716	391			93	232	184
3. Appendicitis	31	19	12	-	2	7	4	5		1	5	2	4
J. Genito-urinary diseases	**1 166**	**684**	**482**	**12**	**2**	**53**	**209**	**408**	**9**	**4**	**40**	**73**	**356**
1. Nephritis and nephrosis	440	233	207	9	1	30	42	150	7	2	11	24	163
2. Benign prostatic hypertrophy	283	283	-				132	150					-
L. Musculo-skeletal diseases	**4 768**	**1 635**	**3 133**	**1**	**2**	**367**	**912**	**353**	**1**	**9**	**708**	**1 420**	**995**
1. Rheumatoid arthritis	1 070	268	803			52	116	100		4	294	208	297
2. Osteoarthritis	3 314	1 267	2 048			290	768	209			330	1 143	574

Annex Table 15a, continued. DALYs by age, sex and cause (thousands): Established Market Economies, 2010, baseline scenario

Cause	Total	Male	Female	Males					Females				
				0-4	5-14	15-44	45-59	60+	0-4	5-14	15-44	45-59	60+
M. Congenital anomalies	1 274	683	591	596	21	46	11	9	530	20	23	9	9
N. Oral conditions	972	465	507	14	75	162	107	107	14	71	158	115	149
1. Dental caries	426	212	213	14	75	79	21	24	13	71	76	21	32
2. Periodontal disease	33	17	17	-	-	14	2	1	-	-	14	2	1
3. Edentulism	506	233	273	-	-	69	83	81	-	-	68	91	114
III. Injuries	10 361	7 092	3 269	217	352	4 789	1 111	622	159	223	1 730	622	535
A. Unintentional injuries	7 228	4 788	2 439	192	315	3 175	673	433	135	202	1 234	430	440
1. Road traffic accidents	3 720	2 489	1 231	61	154	1 986	204	84	45	113	841	153	78
2. Poisonings	217	149	68	3	2	113	22	8	2	2	44	13	7
3. Falls	1 198	638	560	29	53	284	137	136	19	28	151	153	210
4. Fires	198	114	84	15	23	45	18	13	12	24	26	11	11
5. Drownings	197	152	45	18	22	78	21	13	10	7	15	7	7
6. Other unintentional	1 698	1 246	451	66	61	670	271	178	46	28	157	93	127
B. Intentional injuries	3 134	2 304	830	25	37	1 614	438	190	24	22	496	192	95
1. Self-inflicted injuries	2 198	1 596	602	-	15	1 037	371	174	-	4	341	169	86
2. Violence	934	706	227	25	22	576	67	16	24	17	154	23	9
3. War	2	2	-	-	-	1	-	1	-	-	-	-	-

Notes:

A dash (-) symbol indicates fewer than 500 DALYs.

*IA6 is Bacterial meningitis and meningococcaemia; ID is Conditions arising during the perinatal period;

IIE6 is Dementia and other degenerative and hereditary CNS disorders; IIH1 is Chronic obstructive pulmonary disease.

Annex Table 15b. DALYs by age, sex and cause (thousands): Formerly Socialist Economies of Europe, 2010, baseline scenario

Cause	Total	Male	Female	Males					Females				
				0-4	5-14	15-44	45-59	60+	0-4	5-14	15-44	45-59	60+
Population (millions)	*363*	*172*	*190*	*13*	*25*	*75*	*33*	*26*	*12*	*24*	*74*	*37*	*43*
All causes	*64 821*	*39 611*	*25 209*	*1 894*	*851*	*13 869*	*12 769*	*10 229*	*1 501*	*568*	*7 661*	*5 740*	*9 739*
I. Communicable, maternal, perinatal and nutritional conditions	*2 781*	*1 368*	*1 413*	*808*	*69*	*167*	*111*	*213*	*605*	*66*	*431*	*55*	*256*
A. Infectious and parasitic diseases	889	431	457	174	21	121	67	49	147	22	221	20	47
1. Tuberculosis	148	127	21	1	–	49	52	25	–	–	6	6	8
2. STDs excluding HIV	212	31	181	4	–	26	1	–	4	3	173	1	1
a. Syphilis	2	1	1	–	–	1	–	–	–	–	1	–	–
b. Chlamydia	164	12	152	1	–	10	–	–	1	2	147	1	–
c. Gonorrhoea	44	16	28	2	–	14	–	–	2	–	25	–	–
3. HIV	162	87	74	51	8	26	2	–	51	8	13	1	–
4. Diarrhoeal diseases	100	53	46	41	2	5	2	2	35	2	4	2	3
5. Childhood-cluster diseases	15	8	8	6	–	–	–	–	5	1	–	–	–
a. Pertussis	9	4	5	4	–	–	–	–	4	1	–	–	–
b. Poliomyelitis	–	–	–	–	–	–	–	–	–	–	–	–	–
c. Diphtheria	–	–	–	–	–	–	–	–	–	–	–	–	–
d. Measles	4	3	2	2	–	–	–	–	1	–	–	–	–
e. Tetanus	1	1	1	–	–	–	–	–	–	–	–	–	–
6. Bacterial meningitis*	97	56	41	37	3	6	4	5	28	3	3	3	4
7. Hepatitis B and hepatitis C	15	8	6	3	1	2	1	1	2	–	2	1	1
8. Malaria	–	–	–	–	–	–	–	–	–	–	–	–	–
9. Tropical-cluster diseases	–	–	–	–	–	–	–	–	–	–	–	–	–
a. Trypanosomiasis	–	–	–	–	–	–	–	–	–	–	–	–	–
b. Chagas disease	–	–	–	–	–	–	–	–	–	–	–	–	–
c. Schistosomiasis	–	–	–	–	–	–	–	–	–	–	–	–	–
d. Leishmaniasis	–	–	–	–	–	–	–	–	–	–	–	–	–
e. Lymphatic filariasis	–	–	–	–	–	–	–	–	–	–	–	–	–
f. Onchocerciasis	–	–	–	–	–	–	–	–	–	–	–	–	–
10. Leprosy	–	–	–	–	–	–	–	–	–	–	–	–	–
11. Dengue	–	–	–	–	–	–	–	–	–	–	–	–	–
12. Japanese encephalitis	–	–	–	–	–	–	–	–	–	–	–	–	–
13. Trachoma	1	–	1	–	–	–	–	–	–	–	1	–	–
14. Intestinal nematode infections	1	1	–	–	–	–	–	–	–	–	–	–	–
a. Ascariasis	–	–	–	–	–	–	–	–	–	–	–	–	–
b. Trichuriasis	–	–	–	–	–	–	–	–	–	–	–	–	–
c. Ancylostomiasis and necatoriasis	–	–	–	–	–	–	–	–	–	–	–	–	–

Annex Table 15b, continued. DALYs by age, sex and cause (thousands): Formerly Socialist Economies of Europe, 2010, baseline scenario

Cause	Total	Male	Female	Males 0-4	5-14	15-44	45-59	60+	Females 0-4	5-14	15-44	45-59	60+
B. Respiratory infections	715	387	328	159	18	32	37	140	119	16	13	12	168
1. Lower respiratory infections	684	371	313	153	11	31	37	139	114	10	12	12	166
2. Upper respiratory infections	11	6	6	2	-	1	1	1	2	-	1	1	2
3. Otitis media	19	10	9	3	7	-	-	-	3	6	1	-	-
C. Maternal conditions	151	-	151	-	-	-	-	-	-	-	151	-	-
1. Maternal haemorrhage	4	-	4	-	-	-	-	-	-	-	4	-	-
2. Maternal sepsis	30	-	30	-	-	-	-	-	-	-	30	-	-
3. Hypertensive disorders of pregnancy	3	-	3	-	-	-	-	-	-	-	3	-	-
4. Obstructed labour	40	-	40	-	-	-	-	-	-	-	40	-	-
5. Abortion	42	-	42	-	-	-	-	-	-	-	42	-	-
D. Perinatal conditions*	725	428	296	428	-	-	-	-	296	-	-	-	-
E. Nutritional deficiencies	302	121	181	47	30	14	7	24	43	28	46	23	41
1. Protein-energy malnutrition	53	26	27	23	-	-	-	2	22	-	-	-	4
2. Iodine deficiency	-	-	-	-	-	-	-	-	-	-	-	-	-
3. Vitamin A deficiency	-	-	-	-	-	-	-	-	-	-	-	-	-
4. Iron-deficiency anaemia	219	82	137	17	28	13	5	20	16	26	42	21	32
II. Noncommunicable diseases	***50 496***	***29 494***	***21 002***	***727***	***350***	***7 793***	***10 990***	***9 635***	***615***	***281***	***5 764***	***5 154***	***9 188***
A. Malignant neoplasms	9 455	6 427	3 027	33	68	825	3 318	2 183	29	40	556	1 170	1 232
1. Mouth and oropharynx cancers	346	314	31	-	1	47	205	62	-	-	7	12	13
2. Oesophagus cancer	171	155	17	-	-	14	101	39	-	-	2	6	8
3. Stomach cancer	1 370	992	378	-	-	106	549	337	-	-	52	136	190
4. Colon and rectum cancers	846	501	345	-	-	53	231	216	-	-	37	121	187
5. Liver cancer	245	167	78	1	1	17	86	63	1	-	7	26	44
6. Pancreas cancer	364	256	108	-	-	28	141	88	-	-	10	39	59
7. Trachea, bronchus, lung cancers	2 455	2 124	331	-	-	191	1 173	758	-	1	35	139	156
8. Melanoma and other skin cancers	124	74	50	-	-	22	32	20	-	1	17	15	18
9. Breast cancer	502	-	502	-	-	-	-	-	-	-	115	244	144
10. Cervix uteri cancer	181	-	181	-	-	-	-	-	-	-	54	70	57
11. Corpus uteri cancer	133	-	133	-	-	-	-	-	-	-	19	61	53
12. Ovary cancer	186	-	186	-	-	-	-	-	-	-	38	90	57
13. Prostate cancer	166	166	-	-	-	-	43	119	-	-	-	-	-
14. Bladder cancer	210	180	30	1	-	4	76	96	-	-	3	9	19
15. Lymphomas and multiple myeloma	289	197	92	4	13	66	77	36	3	4	33	26	26
16. Leukaemia	326	206	120	11	26	63	65	42	9	16	38	29	28
C. Diabetes mellitus	531	233	298	-	1	56	88	87	1	1	41	87	169
D. Endocrine disorders	168	73	96	16	5	35	12	5	15	5	36	27	13

Annex Table 15b, continued. DALYs by age, sex and cause (thousands): Formerly Socialist Economies of Europe, 2010, baseline scenario

Cause	Total	Male	Female	Males					Females				
				0-4	5-14	15-44	45-59	60+	0-4	5-14	15-44	45-59	60+
E. Neuro-psychiatric conditions	10 598	5 373	5 225	91	171	3 889	737	485	79	137	3 272	792	945
1. Unipolar major depression	3 227	1 097	2 130	–	–	824	210	63	–	–	1 537	422	171
2. Bipolar disorder	845	414	431	–	–	358	38	18	–	–	352	41	37
3. Schizophrenia	840	436	404	–	–	423	8	6	–	–	393	3	8
4. Epilepsy	261	166	95	6	35	89	25	11	6	25	36	16	11
5. Alcohol use	1 758	1 551	207	–	–	1 278	222	51	–	–	181	17	9
6. Dementia*	1 106	392	714	17	8	17	97	253	16	7	15	122	554
7. Parkinson disease	151	60	91	–	–	–	22	38	–	–	–	27	64
8. Multiple sclerosis	107	46	61	–	–	35	7	4	–	8	45	9	7
9. Drug use	527	421	105	–	31	372	15	3	–	12	93	4	1
10. Post-traumatic stress disorder	118	44	74	–	–	29	4	1	–	–	49	8	2
11. Obsessive-compulsive disorders	651	272	379	–	26	214	21	11	–	33	280	41	24
12. Panic disorder	317	103	213	–	9	72	22	–	–	9	156	39	10
F. Sense organ diseases	76	34	42	–	–	1	10	23	–	–	2	16	25
1. Glaucoma	35	12	23	–	–	–	5	7	–	–	1	12	10
2. Cataracts	41	22	19	–	–	1	5	16	–	–	1	3	15
G. Cardiovascular diseases	16 800	10 346	6 454	24	10	1 184	4 176	4 953	17	6	368	1 056	5 007
1. Rheumatic heart disease	367	207	161	–	1	63	115	28	–	1	35	86	38
2. Ischaemic heart disease	8 495	5 642	2 853	4	–	581	2 544	2 518	2	2	90	433	2 329
3. Cerebrovascular disease	5 007	2 661	2 346	5	2	252	943	1 460	5	1	161	432	1 750
4. Inflammatory heart diseases	490	326	163	–	–	107	132	80	–	–	37	38	82
H. Respiratory diseases	4 689	3 021	1 668	26	39	444	1 316	1 196	13	27	297	492	839
1. COPD*	1 863	1 323	540	–	–	134	632	556	–	–	60	123	357
2. Asthma	570	297	273	6	37	129	72	46	6	24	119	71	53
I. Digestive diseases	2 665	1 601	1 064	33	6	452	742	368	24	6	237	419	378
1. Peptic ulcer	211	157	53	–	–	38	76	43	–	–	13	19	21
2. Cirrhosis of the liver	802	566	236	–	–	99	321	145	–	–	35	114	85
3. Appendicitis	14	8	6	1	1	4	2	2	–	1	3	1	1
J. Genito-urinary diseases	794	426	368	4	5	106	160	150	4	5	91	147	121
1. Nephritis and nephrosis	205	121	84	2	3	50	39	28	2	4	25	26	27
2. Benign prostatic hypertrophy	135	135	–	–	–	–	63	72	–	–	–	–	–
L. Musculo-skeletal diseases	2 905	1 065	1 841	1	6	618	307	136	1	6	680	782	371
1. Rheumatoid arthritis	529	125	403	–	3	67	35	23	–	3	216	118	67
2. Osteoarthritis	2 196	888	1 308	–	–	522	258	107	–	–	408	616	285

Annex Table 15b, continued. DALYs by age, sex and cause (thousands): Formerly Socialist Economies of Europe, 2010, baseline scenario

Cause	Total	Male	Female	Males					Females				
				0-4	5-14	15-44	45-59	60+	0-4	5-14	15-44	45-59	60+
M. Congenital anomalies	**949**	**512**	**437**	**470**	**15**	**23**	**4**	**1**	**406**	**14**	**12**	**3**	**1**
N. Oral conditions	**515**	**234**	**282**	**15**	**20**	**95**	**73**	**31**	**14**	**28**	**99**	**88**	**53**
1. Dental caries	250	116	134	15	20	45	23	13	14	28	44	26	21
2. Periodontal disease	17	7	10	-	-	5	2	1	-	-	8	1	1
3. Edentulism	248	111	137	-	-	45	48	17	-	-	47	60	30
III. Injuries	*11 544*	*8 749*	*2 795*	*359*	*433*	*5 909*	*1 668*	*380*	*281*	*221*	*1 466*	*531*	*295*
A. Unintentional injuries	**7 842**	**6 076**	**1 766**	**247**	**337**	**4 010**	**1 216**	**267**	**171**	**159**	**835**	**376**	**225**
1. Road traffic accidents	3 176	2 489	688	36	141	1 871	358	82	22	80	414	115	56
2. Poisonings	845	653	192	29	9	350	229	36	22	8	76	65	21
3. Falls	1 001	661	339	38	50	391	127	55	28	21	128	78	85
4. Fires	162	113	49	13	10	56	27	8	11	8	15	8	8
5. Drownings	495	420	75	22	52	270	64	12	10	19	30	10	5
6. Other unintentional	2 163	1 740	423	109	75	1 072	411	74	79	23	172	99	49
B. Intentional injuries	**3 702**	**2 673**	**1 029**	**112**	**96**	**1 899**	**452**	**113**	**110**	**63**	**631**	**155**	**70**
1. Self-inflicted injuries	1 687	1 347	341	-	18	895	341	93	-	4	184	100	52
2. Violence	862	662	199	9	9	540	90	15	7	8	133	39	13
3. War	1 152	664	489	103	69	464	22	5	103	51	313	16	5

Notes:
A dash (-) symbol indicates fewer than 500 DALYs.
*IA6 is Bacterial meningitis and meningococcaemia; ID is Conditions arising during the perinatal period;
IIE6 is Dementia and other degenerative and hereditary CNS disorders; IIH1 is Chronic obstructive pulmonary disease.

Annex Table 15c. DALYs by age, sex and cause (thousands): India, 2010, baseline scenario

Cause	Total	Male	Female	Males 0-4	5-14	15-44	45-59	60+	Females 0-4	5-14	15-44	45-59	60+
Population (millions)	1 124	574	550	55	107	287	81	44	53	101	269	77	50
All causes	239 413	130 128	109 285	31 051	9 739	42 356	27 244	19 737	29 912	7 917	36 322	17 298	17 837
I. Communicable, maternal, perinatal and nutritional conditions	81 598	42 983	38 615	21 055	2 221	12 732	4 366	2 609	20 639	2 402	11 012	2 658	1 905
A. Infectious and parasitic diseases	54 288	30 234	24 055	10 517	1 577	12 088	4 150	1 902	10 221	1 535	8 803	2 342	1 154
1. Tuberculosis	16 728	10 621	6 107	380	342	5 130	3 339	1 430	294	268	2 987	1 876	682
2. STDs excluding HIV	2 514	900	1 614	440	7	427	8	18	430	24	1 123	11	26
a. Syphilis	719	354	365	268	1	61	6	18	271	1	61	7	26
b. Chlamydia	1 029	174	855	42	2	129	1	-	38	17	797	3	1
c. Gonorrhoea	766	372	394	130	4	237	1	-	121	6	266	1	-
3. HIV	14 328	8 020	6 308	1 445	267	5 596	583	128	1 520	285	4 222	237	44
4. Diarrhoeal diseases	9 953	4 945	5 008	4 369	210	160	58	148	4 388	273	109	58	180
5. Childhood-cluster diseases	6 010	3 132	2 879	2 782	220	98	20	13	2 537	239	67	20	15
a. Pertussis	1 009	523	485	488	35				452	33			
b. Poliomyelitis	459	272	187	267	2	4			184	1	2		
c. Diphtheria	50	26	24	24	2	1			22	2			
d. Measles	2 319	1 194	1 124	1 076	116	1			1 010	114	1		15
e. Tetanus	2 174	1 116	1 058	926	66	92	19	13	869	90	64	20	15
6. Bacterial meningitis*	494	262	232	195	6	37	14	11	178	5	22	14	13
7. Hepatitis B and hepatitis C	111	64	47	16	6	17	12	12	12	6	10	6	13
8. Malaria	311	171	140	52	44	55	12	7	43	46	33	11	7
9. Tropical-cluster diseases	780	555	225	40	179	302	28	5	21	83	77	38	7
a. Trypanosomiasis													
b. Chagas disease													
c. Schistosomiasis													
d. Leishmaniasis	317	203	114	20	77	98	5	3	13	52	43	4	2
e. Lymphatic filariasis	463	351	112	20	102	204	23	3	8	31	34	35	4
f. Onchocerciasis													
10. Leprosy	88	45	43	1	13	26	4	1	1	12	24	4	1
11. Dengue	107	50	57	14	34	1	-	-	16	40	1	-	-
12. Japanese encephalitis	25	13	12	8	3	1	-	-	8	3	-	-	-
13. Trachoma	13	3	10	-	-	-	1	2	-	-	1	3	6
14. Intestinal nematode infections	280	150	130	1	68	59	13	9	1	63	44	13	9
a. Ascariasis	63	33	30	1	32	-	-	-	1	29	-	-	-
b. Trichuriasis	41	21	20	-	21	-	-	-	-	20	-	-	-
c. Ancylostomiasis and necatoriasis	176	96	80	-	15	59	13	9	-	14	44	13	9

Annex Table 15c, continued. DALYs by age, sex and cause (thousands): India, 2010, baseline scenario

Cause	Total	Male	Female	Males 0-4	Males 5-14	Males 15-44	Males 45-59	Males 60+	Females 0-4	Females 5-14	Females 15-44	Females 45-59	Females 60+
B. Respiratory infections	**12 061**	**5 926**	**6 134**	**4 641**	**358**	**228**	**119**	**580**	**4 660**	**588**	**159**	**121**	**606**
1. Lower respiratory infections	11 735	5 767	5 968	4 528	326	222	117	574	4 541	554	154	119	600
2. Upper respiratory infections	126	63	64	44	4	6	2	6	45	7	4	2	7
3. Otitis media	199	96	102	68	27	1	–	–	75	27	1	–	–
C. Maternal conditions	**1 502**	**–**	**1 502**								**1 480**	**22**	**–**
1. Maternal haemorrhage	173		173								168	5	
2. Maternal sepsis	254		254								251	3	
3. Hypertensive disorders of pregnancy	84		84								82	2	
4. Obstructed labour	303		303								302	2	
5. Abortion	324		324								321	3	
D. Perinatal conditions*	**9 358**	**4 736**	**4 622**	**4 736**					**4 622**				
E. Nutritional deficiencies	**4 390**	**2 087**	**2 303**	**1 161**	**287**	**415**	**97**	**127**	**1 136**	**279**	**571**	**173**	**145**
1. Protein-energy malnutrition	1 756	870	886	832	8	11	4	14	838	22	5	3	18
2. Iodine deficiency	124	65	59	59	5	2	–	–	53	4	1	–	–
3. Vitamin A deficiency	221	115	106	83	29	2	–	–	77	28	1	–	–
4. Iron-deficiency anaemia	2 289	1 037	1 252	187	244	400	93	113	169	224	563	169	126
II. Noncommunicable diseases	**113 683**	**61 065**	**52 618**	**5 859**	**1 536**	**17 487**	**19 774**	**16 410**	**5 820**	**1 482**	**17 674**	**12 522**	**15 120**
A. Malignant neoplasms	**12 836**	**6 828**	**6 008**	**145**	**221**	**1 636**	**3 166**	**1 660**	**86**	**105**	**1 757**	**2 644**	**1 417**
1. Mouth and oropharynx cancers	1 829	1 078	751	3	5	227	559	285	3	4	184	370	190
2. Oesophagus cancer	992	506	486			82	275	148			93	232	161
3. Stomach cancer	940	603	336		1	127	323	152			88	150	99
4. Colon and rectum cancers	438	240	198			82	94	64			43	84	70
5. Liver cancer	253	179	74	2	2	41	92	43	1	1	17	31	24
6. Pancreas cancer	149	90	59			19	48	24			14	24	20
7. Trachea, bronchus, lung cancers	2 095	1 775	320		1	309	988	477		1	62	151	107
8. Melanoma and other skin cancers	26	13	13			4	7	2			4	6	3
9. Breast cancer	850	–	850								307	384	159
10. Cervix uteri cancer	1 170		1 170								307	660	203
11. Corpus uteri cancer	61		61								7	31	22
12. Ovary cancer	273		273								117	89	65
13. Prostate cancer	132	132				4	32	96					
14. Bladder cancer	114	90	25			12	39	39			4	9	11
15. Lymphomas and multiple myeloma	472	328	144	24	39	135	93	37	5	8	48	42	40
16. Leukaemia	512	304	208	44	71	123	48	18	27	38	90	37	17
C. Diabetes mellitus	**2 014**	**988**	**1 026**	**72**	**75**	**236**	**347**	**258**	**75**	**71**	**156**	**329**	**396**
D. Endocrine disorders	**94**	**51**	**44**	**25**	**3**	**12**	**9**	**2**	**19**	**1**	**8**	**9**	**7**

Annex Table 15c, continued. DALYs by age, sex and cause (thousands): India, 2010, baseline scenario

Cause	Total	Male	Female	Males 0-4	5-14	15-44	45-59	60+	Females 0-4	5-14	15-44	45-59	60+
E. Neuro-psychiatric conditions	**27 429**	**12 399**	**15 030**	**447**	**344**	**9 502**	**1 352**	**753**	**572**	**419**	**11 390**	**1 618**	**1 031**
1. Unipolar major depression	11 985	4 334	7 652	-	-	3 618	593	123	-	-	6 376	1 029	246
2. Bipolar disorder	3 363	1 730	1 634	-	-	1 596	104	29	-	-	1 499	98	36
3. Schizophrenia	2 366	1 262	1 103	-	-	1 245	10	7	-	-	1 087	4	12
4. Epilepsy	718	409	309	39	66	243	41	20	47	95	134	13	20
5. Alcohol use	1 283	1 172	111	-	-	1 063	95	15	-	-	103	6	2
6. Dementia*	1 420	666	754	52	20	54	185	356	64	20	49	183	439
7. Parkinson disease	207	96	111	-	-	-	43	53	-	-	-	50	61
8. Multiple sclerosis	286	128	159	-	-	113	11	3	-	-	139	14	6
9. Drug use	105	95	11	-	6	85	3	-	-	1	10	-	-
10. Post-traumatic stress disorder	422	163	259	7	32	111	11	2	12	52	176	17	3
11. Obsessive-compulsive disorders	2 311	1 015	1 295	-	112	831	53	20	-	141	1 036	89	29
12. Panic disorder	1 079	350	729	-	4	288	57	-	-	39	592	87	12
F. Sense organ diseases	**4 896**	**2 618**	**2 278**	**6**	-	**178**	**1 413**	**1 020**	**4**	-	**121**	**994**	**1 159**
1. Glaucoma	944	535	409	-	-	49	387	99	-	-	18	273	118
2. Cataracts	3 950	2 081	1 869	4	-	129	1 027	921	4	-	102	721	1 042
G. Cardiovascular diseases	**34 929**	**20 907**	**14 022**	**579**	**173**	**2 598**	**8 017**	**9 540**	**447**	**223**	**1 423**	**3 444**	**8 485**
1. Rheumatic heart disease	1 711	869	843	1	19	386	373	89	1	24	368	343	105
2. Ischaemic heart disease	17 011	10 455	6 555	-	-	590	4 370	5 495	-	-	284	1 609	4 662
3. Cerebrovascular disease	6 398	3 648	2 751	112	32	339	1 242	1 923	89	35	244	553	1 831
4. Inflammatory heart diseases	2 024	1 209	815	106	40	427	430	206	97	54	236	230	198
H. Respiratory diseases	**11 543**	**6 318**	**5 224**	**389**	**350**	**1 218**	**2 347**	**2 016**	**298**	**242**	**1 216**	**1 849**	**1 619**
1. COPD*	4 758	2 834	1 925	41	25	390	1 239	1 138	37	25	313	811	738
2. Asthma	1 794	1 024	770	72	159	494	200	99	34	88	400	160	89
I. Digestive diseases	**5 662**	**3 858**	**1 804**	**123**	**52**	**1 177**	**1 907**	**600**	**131**	**50**	**598**	**680**	**345**
1. Peptic ulcer	868	585	282	2	3	205	264	112	3	5	108	104	63
2. Cirrhosis of the liver	2 811	2 079	731	23	10	562	1 119	365	29	24	212	312	153
3. Appendicitis	203	119	84	3	18	83	11	3	3	18	54	6	2
J. Genito-urinary diseases	**1 805**	**1 161**	**644**	**97**	**128**	**141**	**563**	**231**	**52**	**181**	**140**	**123**	**149**
1. Nephritis and nephrosis	1 220	611	609	76	124	129	152	130	47	180	130	112	139
2. Benign prostatic hypertrophy	499	499	-	-	-	-	403	96	-	-	-	-	-
L. Musculo-skeletal diseases	**2 224**	**875**	**1 349**	**3**	**4**	**338**	**400**	**130**	**2**	**5**	**478**	**584**	**280**
1. Rheumatoid arthritis	264	75	189	1	1	52	14	8	-	3	101	65	21
2. Osteoarthritis	1 936	785	1 150	-	-	282	384	120	-	-	375	518	258

Annex Table 15c, continued. DALYs by age, sex and cause (thousands): India, 2010, baseline scenario

Cause	Total	Male	Female	Males					Females				
				0-4	5-14	15-44	45-59	60+	0-4	5-14	15-44	45-59	60+
M. Congenital anomalies	**8 424**	**4 127**	**4 297**	**3 885**	**94**	**121**	**20**	**6**	**4 054**	**110**	**96**	**27**	**11**
N. Oral conditions	**1 518**	**753**	**766**	**39**	**75**	**251**	**205**	**181**	**37**	**73**	**247**	**201**	**207**
1. Dental caries	914	465	449	38	74	205	89	58	36	70	192	85	65
2. Periodontal disease	106	55	52	-	-	43	8	3	-	-	40	8	3
3. Edentulism	474	228	246	-	-	-	108	120	-	-	-	108	138
III. Injuries	*44 131*	*26 079*	*18 052*	*4 137*	*5 982*	*12 137*	*3 104*	*718*	*3 453*	*4 033*	*7 636*	*2 118*	*812*
A. Unintentional injuries	**38 051**	**22 734**	**15 317**	**3 932**	**5 793**	**9 789**	**2 589**	**631**	**3 192**	**3 853**	**5 744**	**1 785**	**742**
1. Road traffic accidents	12 170	8 772	3 398	585	1 633	5 178	1 124	252	172	1 226	1 257	524	218
2. Poisonings	931	437	494	149	57	184	38	9	102	38	217	128	10
3. Falls	7 255	4 347	2 909	888	2 326	812	242	78	1 000	890	597	332	89
4. Fires	4 805	1 460	3 345	378	247	640	166	29	322	671	2 056	200	97
5. Drownings	2 153	1 197	956	315	327	449	79	27	257	276	288	88	46
6. Other unintentional	10 737	6 521	4 216	1 618	1 203	2 526	939	235	1 339	753	1 329	512	282
B. Intentional injuries	**6 080**	**3 345**	**2 734**	**206**	**190**	**2 347**	**515**	**87**	**261**	**179**	**1 892**	**333**	**69**
1. Self-inflicted injuries	3 988	2 005	1 982	-	112	1 522	331	41	-	111	1 693	162	16
2. Violence	1 928	1 175	752	206	78	661	185	47	261	68	199	172	53
3. War	165	165	-			165							-

Notes:
A dash (-) symbol indicates fewer than 500 DALYs.
*IA6 is Bacterial meningitis and meningococcaemia; ID is Conditions arising during the perinatal period;
IIE6 is Dementia and other degenerative and hereditary CNS disorders; IIH1 is Chronic obstructive pulmonary disease.

Annex Table 15d. DALYs by age, sex and cause (thousands): China, 2010, baseline scenario

Cause	Total	Male	Female	Males 0-4	5-14	15-44	45-59	60+	Females 0-4	5-14	15-44	45-59	60+
Population (millions)	*1 378*	*699*	*679*	*50*	*109*	*337*	*130*	*72*	*48*	*104*	*320*	*126*	*81*
All causes	**201 807**	**114 032**	**87 774**	**9 785**	**3 527**	**37 847**	**33 501**	**29 372**	**9 869**	**2 738**	**31 315**	**20 682**	**23 170**
I. Communicable, maternal, perinatal and nutritional conditions	**13 178**	**6 671**	**6 507**	**3 532**	**526**	**1 011**	**578**	**1 024**	**3 684**	**516**	**868**	**477**	**963**
A. Infectious and parasitic diseases	**4 211**	**2 300**	**1 911**	**666**	**272**	**422**	**387**	**554**	**645**	**263**	**265**	**255**	**483**
1. Tuberculosis	**1 237**	**768**	**469**	23	5	137	242	361	24	15	77	143	210
2. STDs excluding HIV	**41**	**10**	**31**	1	-	8	-	1	1	-	29	-	1
a. Syphilis	2	1	1	-	-	-	-	1	-	-	-	-	1
b. Chlamydia	26	3	23	-	-	3	-	-	-	-	23	-	-
c. Gonorrhoea	12	5	7	1	-	5	-	-	1	-	7	-	-
3. HIV	**163**	**89**	**74**	17	3	59	8	2	18	3	48	3	1
4. Diarrhoeal diseases	**855**	**417**	**438**	206	27	74	32	79	243	25	48	31	91
5. Childhood-cluster diseases	**506**	**277**	**229**	250	18	7	2	1	209	15	3	1	1
a. Pertussis	175	93	81	85	8				74	8			
b. Poliomyelitis	83	49	33	47	-				32				
c. Diphtheria	2	1	1	1					1				
d. Measles	114	61	54	53	6	-	1	-	47	6	1	-	1
e. Tetanus	133	73	59	63	3	4	1	1	56	2	1	1	-
6. Bacterial meningitis*	**290**	**154**	**136**	87	4	30	16	16	77	4	19	17	19
7. Hepatitis B and hepatitis C	**152**	**102**	**50**	15	2	31	34	20	11	2	7	8	22
8. Malaria	**10**	**5**	**5**	1	2	2	1	-	1	1	1	1	1
9. Tropical-cluster diseases	**42**	**35**	**7**	1	4	23	3	2	-	1	3	1	1
a. Trypanosomiasis	-	-	-										
b. Chagas disease	-	-	-										
c. Schistosomiasis	7	5	3	-	-	1	1	2	-	-	1	1	-
d. Leishmaniasis	-	-	-										
e. Lymphatic filariasis	34	30	4	1	4	22	2	1	1	-	3	-	-
f. Onchocerciasis	-	-	-										
10. Leprosy	**3**	**1**	**1**	-	-	1	1	-	-	-	1	-	-
11. Dengue	**5**	**3**	**3**	1	2	-	-	-	1	2	-	-	-
12. Japanese encephalitis	**98**	**52**	**46**	33	15	3	1	-	30	14	2	1	-
13. Trachoma	**176**	**47**	**129**	-	-	3	11	33	-	-	6	29	94
14. Intestinal nematode infections	**389**	**201**	**189**	3	181	11	3	3	3	172	8	3	3
a. Ascariasis	178	91	86	3	87	1	-	-	3	82	-	-	-
b. Trichuriasis	176	90	85	-	90	-	-	-	-	85	-	-	-
c. Ancylostomiasis and necatoriasis	36	19	17	-	4	10	3	2	-	4	7	3	3

Annex Table 15d, continued. DALYs by age, sex and cause (thousands): China, 2010, baseline scenario

Cause	Total	Male	Female	Males 0-4	5-14	15-44	45-59	60+	Females 0-4	5-14	15-44	45-59	60+
B. Respiratory infections	**3 264**	**1 592**	**1 672**	**1 175**	**64**	**33**	**32**	**288**	**1 281**	**65**	**26**	**21**	**278**
1. Lower respiratory infections	3 158	1 539	1 619	1 150	44	31	31	284	1 254	45	25	20	274
2. Upper respiratory infections	38	19	19	11	1	2	1	4	12	1	2	1	4
3. Otitis media	68	34	34	15	19	-	-	-	15	19	-	-	-
C. Maternal conditions	**280**		**280**						-	-	**267**	**14**	-
1. Maternal haemorrhage	44		44								40	4	
2. Maternal sepsis	49		49								49		
3. Hypertensive disorders of pregnancy	10		10								9	1	
4. Obstructed labour	60		60								60		
5. Abortion	8		8								8	1	
D. Perinatal conditions*	**2 637**	**1 320**	**1 317**	**1 320**					**1 317**				
E. Nutritional deficiencies	**2 786**	**1 459**	**1 327**	**371**	**190**	**557**	**159**	**182**	**440**	**188**	**310**	**187**	**203**
1. Protein-energy malnutrition	485	213	272	194	-	1	2	16	255	1	1	1	14
2. Iodine deficiency	108	58	50	52	4	2	-	-	45	4	1	-	-
3. Vitamin A deficiency	71	38	33	28	9	1	-	-	24	8	1	-	-
4. Iron-deficiency anaemia	2 122	1 151	971	98	177	553	157	166	115	175	307	186	188
II. Noncommunicable diseases	***152 447***	***86 331***	***66 116***	***3 661***	***1 279***	***24 616***	***29 798***	***26 978***	***3 717***	***923***	***22 776***	***17 825***	***20 875***
A. Malignant neoplasms	**32 717**	**22 114**	**10 603**	**134**	**411**	**5 135**	**10 044**	**6 391**	**209**	**196**	**2 551**	**4 192**	**3 456**
1. Mouth and oropharynx cancers	1 006	725	281	5	9	303	263	144	-	-	103	113	65
2. Oesophagus cancer	3 369	2 472	898			314	1 158	1 000			51	354	492
3. Stomach cancer	6 235	4 303	1 933			473	2 116	1 704			408	713	803
4. Colon and rectum cancers	1 782	1 052	730			281	421	341			158	295	268
5. Liver cancer	7 489	5 904	1 585	5	26	2 004	2 821	1 048	7	23	388	698	469
6. Pancreas cancer	538	361	177			57	151	153			14	58	104
7. Trachea, bronchus, lung cancers	5 091	3 903	1 188	5	16	492	2 031	1 359			99	579	510
8. Melanoma and other skin cancers	23	15	9			4	6	5			2	3	4
9. Breast cancer	640		640								250	266	123
10. Cervix uteri cancer	447		447								108	209	129
11. Corpus uteri cancer	154		154								26	103	26
12. Ovary cancer	254		254							7	101	98	43
13. Prostate cancer	67	67				4	11	52					
14. Bladder cancer	307	251	55			26	79	146			4	14	37
15. Lymphomas and multiple myeloma	520	358	163		35	100	130	93			40	87	36
16. Leukaemia	1 950	1 078	872	75	206	503	226	68	96	102	435	166	74
C. Diabetes mellitus	**980**	**474**	**506**	**6**	**7**	**120**	**188**	**152**	**6**	**6**	**67**	**184**	**242**
D. Endocrine disorders	**402**	**124**	**279**	**15**	**7**	**41**	**38**	**23**	**105**	**14**	**89**	**30**	**40**

Annex Table 15d, continued. DALYs by age, sex and cause (thousands): China, 2010, baseline scenario

Cause	Total	Male	Female	Males					Females				
				0-4	5-14	15-44	45-59	60+	0-4	5-14	15-44	45-59	60+
E. Neuro-psychiatric conditions	**33 709**	**15 132**	**18 577**	**189**	**318**	**11 704**	**1 954**	**967**	**157**	**329**	**13 995**	**2 677**	**1 420**
1. Unipolar major depression	15 781	5 666	10 115	-	-	4 461	996	209	-	-	7 963	1 745	407
2. Bipolar disorder	4 290	2 195	2 095	-	-	1 975	173	46	-	-	1 873	168	55
3. Schizophrenia	2 820	1 522	1 298	13	46	1 497	11	14	12	48	1 271	16	12
4. Epilepsy	555	308	247	-	-	186	47	16	-	-	138	31	17
5. Alcohol use	1 742	1 617	125	-	-	1 445	153	19	-	-	115	8	2
6. Dementia*	2 184	994	1 190	52	23	61	294	565	50	19	55	305	761
7. Parkinson disease	152	73	78	-	-	-	35	38	-	-	-	34	44
8. Multiple sclerosis	358	158	200	-	-	136	17	5	-	-	169	23	8
9. Drug use	207	186	21	-	14	162	9	1	-	2	18	1	-
10. Post-traumatic stress disorder	495	190	305	7	33	130	18	3	11	53	209	27	4
11. Obsessive-compulsive disorders	2 776	1 208	1 568	-	114	977	85	32	-	145	1 231	145	47
12. Panic disorder	1 377	472	905	-	40	339	92	-	-	40	704	141	19
F. Sense organ diseases	**3 069**	**1 272**	**1 798**	**34**	**-**	**86**	**596**	**556**	**27**	**12**	**167**	**943**	**649**
1. Glaucoma	1 319	382	937	5	-	32	233	112	7	-	79	670	181
2. Cataracts	1 516	814	702	12	-	44	331	426	2	-	35	227	439
G. Cardiovascular diseases	**30 677**	**19 458**	**11 219**	**239**	**63**	**2 484**	**7 723**	**8 948**	**130**	**31**	**1 486**	**3 010**	**6 561**
1. Rheumatic heart disease	2 404	1 265	1 139	-	10	389	511	355	13	9	331	400	386
2. Ischaemic heart disease	8 712	5 568	3 144	58	29	628	2 218	2 722	35	10	299	756	2 089
3. Cerebrovascular disease	15 279	9 835	5 444	42	10	1 077	3 915	4 757	26	6	583	1 542	3 274
4. Inflammatory heart diseases	1 253	788	465	-	-	265	318	154	-	-	172	134	126
H. Respiratory diseases	**29 545**	**16 781**	**12 764**	**355**	**228**	**3 086**	**5 459**	**7 654**	**239**	**120**	**2 421**	**3 636**	**6 349**
1. COPD*	25 496	14 422	11 074	61	4	2 081	5 001	7 274	98	2	1 623	3 327	6 023
2. Asthma	2 722	1 556	1 166	75	206	812	325	138	33	105	678	243	106
I. Digestive diseases	**7 454**	**4 459**	**2 996**	**337**	**45**	**991**	**1 913**	**1 172**	**372**	**40**	**596**	**1 099**	**889**
1. Peptic ulcer	417	265	153	2	1	70	102	90	3	1	32	47	69
2. Cirrhosis of the liver	2 946	2 060	886	17	6	566	960	511	6	7	158	406	308
3. Appendicitis	155	91	64	1	15	60	11	4	1	13	41	7	3
J. Genito-urinary diseases	**2 294**	**1 594**	**700**	**58**	**35**	**361**	**863**	**277**	**57**	**24**	**210**	**195**	**214**
1. Nephritis and nephrosis	1 192	692	501	38	35	329	154	135	57	24	175	109	136
2. Benign prostatic hypertrophy	744	744	-	5	-	7	648	84	-	-	-	-	-
L. Musculo-skeletal diseases	**4 891**	**1 624**	**3 267**	**-**	**13**	**314**	**709**	**588**	**17**	**13**	**889**	**1 578**	**770**
1. Rheumatoid arthritis	998	315	684	-	6	92	172	50	-	6	193	337	147
2. Osteoarthritis	3 328	1 107	2 221	-	-	187	494	426	-	-	580	1 150	491

Annex Table 15d, continued. DALYs by age, sex and cause (thousands): China, 2010, baseline scenario

Cause	Total		Males					Females				
	Male	Female	0-4	5-14	15-44	45-59	60+	0-4	5-14	15-44	45-59	60+
M. Congenital anomalies	**2 216**	**2 334**	**2 032**	**80**	**99**	**5**	**-**	**2 147**	**81**	**100**	**6**	**-**
N. Oral conditions	**610**	**648**	**158**	**39**	**70**	**176**	**167**	**150**	**39**	**86**	**178**	**195**
1. Dental caries	300	288	157	38	48	41	16	149	36	46	40	18
2. Periodontal disease	20	19	-	-	17	2	1	-	-	16	2	1
3. Edentulism	283	311	-	-	-	133	150	-	-	-	135	176
III. Injuries	***21 030***	***15 152***	***2 593***	***1 723***	***12 220***	***3 125***	***1 370***	***2 468***	***1 299***	***7 671***	***2 380***	***1 333***
A. Unintentional injuries	**16 040**	**8 870**	**2 434**	**1 570**	**8 804**	**2 299**	**932**	**2 178**	**1 153**	**3 191**	**1 454**	**894**
1. Road traffic accidents	6 783	3 010	127	656	4 484	1 117	399	92	661	1 512	573	172
2. Poisonings	670	479	130	32	272	173	63	38	40	262	69	70
3. Falls	1 735	1 495	347	161	888	213	127	425	98	364	298	309
4. Fires	262	215	70	35	99	25	33	46	45	35	38	51
5. Drownings	1 588	946	586	388	476	85	53	464	172	176	64	69
6. Other unintentional	5 002	2 727	1 174	299	2 585	686	257	1 113	136	841	413	223
B. Intentional injuries	**4 990**	**6 281**	**158**	**153**	**3 416**	**825**	**438**	**291**	**146**	**4 480**	**925**	**438**
1. Self-inflicted injuries	3 934	5 603	-	101	2 669	749	414	-	76	4 243	872	413
2. Violence	1 030	678	158	51	720	76	23	291	71	238	54	25
3. War	26	-	-	-	26	-	-	-	-	-	-	-

Note: the "Total" column also has overall total values: M. Congenital anomalies 4 550; N. Oral conditions 1 257; 1. Dental caries 588; 2. Periodontal disease 39; 3. Edentulism 594; III. Injuries 36 181; A. Unintentional injuries 24 910; 1. Road traffic accidents 9 792; 2. Poisonings 1 149; 3. Falls 3 230; 4. Fires 477; 5. Drownings 2 534; 6. Other unintentional 7 729; B. Intentional injuries 11 271; 1. Self-inflicted injuries 9 537; 2. Violence 1 708; 3. War 26.

Notes:
A dash (-) symbol indicates fewer than 500 DALYs.
*IA6 is Bacterial meningitis and meningococcaemia; ID is Conditions arising during the perinatal period;
IIE6 is Dementia and other degenerative and hereditary CNS disorders; IIH1 is Chronic obstructive pulmonary disease.

Annex Table 15e. DALYs by age, sex and cause (thousands): Other Asia and Islands, 2010, baseline scenario

Cause	Total	Male	Female	Males					Females				
				0–4	5–14	15–44	45–59	60+	0–4	5–14	15–44	45–59	60+
Population (millions)	*922*	*460*	*462*	*43*	*84*	*229*	*67*	*36*	*41*	*81*	*224*	*71*	*44*
All causes	*162 799*	*91 541*	*71 258*	*19 421*	*6 564*	*35 313*	*17 386*	*12 858*	*15 378*	*4 500*	*26 393*	*12 033*	*12 954*
I. Communicable, maternal, perinatal and nutritional conditions	*39 087*	*20 552*	*18 535*	*12 703*	*1 435*	*4 306*	*1 014*	*1 094*	*9 693*	*1 242*	*5 420*	*979*	*1 201*
A. Infectious and parasitic diseases	22 621	12 196	10 424	5 977	911	3 808	867	633	4 461	776	3 740	755	692
1. Tuberculosis	2 585	1 335	1 249	16	27	424	428	440	6	26	285	439	494
2. STDs excluding HIV	2 057	747	1 310	378	5	341	7	16	294	19	964	11	23
a. Syphilis	555	312	243	247	–	43	6	16	166	1	47	8	22
b. Chlamydia	858	134	724	30	2	101	–	–	30	14	678	3	–
c. Gonorrhoea	644	301	343	101	3	196	1	–	98	5	239	1	–
3. HIV	6 405	3 628	2 778	653	120	2 541	263	51	410	82	2 136	129	21
4. Diarrhoeal diseases	5 498	3 181	2 317	2 939	140	44	23	34	2 083	104	55	34	42
5. Childhood-cluster diseases	3 131	1 687	1 444	1 478	135	54	13	7	1 252	129	40	15	9
a. Pertussis	518	279	239	260	19	–	–	–	223	16	–	–	–
b. Poliomyelitis	164	97	67	93	1	3	–	–	64	1	2	–	–
c. Diphtheria	32	17	15	16	1	1	–	–	13	1	1	–	–
d. Measles	1 518	818	701	739	77	1	1	–	634	66	1	–	–
e. Tetanus	898	476	422	370	37	49	12	7	318	45	37	14	9
6. Bacterial meningitis*	343	182	161	122	5	29	15	11	107	5	20	17	12
7. Hepatitis B and hepatitis C	157	93	64	22	8	23	21	19	16	7	13	11	18
8. Malaria	782	434	348	89	126	166	38	15	77	108	105	42	17
9. Tropical-cluster diseases	201	142	59	5	25	87	21	4	3	8	27	18	3
a. Trypanosomiasis	–	–	–	–	–	–	–	–	–	–	–	–	–
b. Chagas disease	–	–	–	–	–	–	–	–	–	–	–	–	–
c. Schistosomiasis	6	3	2	–	–	1	1	1	–	–	1	1	–
d. Leishmaniasis	22	15	8	1	4	9	–	–	–	2	5	–	–
e. Lymphatic filariasis	173	123	49	4	21	76	19	3	3	5	22	16	3
f. Onchocerciasis	–	–	–	–	–	–	–	–	–	–	–	–	–
10. Leprosy	38	19	19	–	5	9	3	1	3	5	9	2	–
11. Dengue	75	36	39	11	24	1	–	–	11	26	1	1	–
12. Japanese encephalitis	63	34	29	22	9	2	–	–	19	8	1	–	–
13. Trachoma	33	8	25	–	–	1	2	4	–	–	2	7	16
14. Intestinal nematode infections	595	309	286	3	231	55	12	7	3	216	45	13	10
a. Ascariasis	181	94	87	3	90	–	–	–	3	84	–	–	–
b. Trichuriasis	246	127	119	–	127	–	–	–	–	119	–	–	–
c. Ancylostomiasis and necatoriasis	168	88	80	–	14	54	12	7	–	13	44	13	10

Annex Table 15e, continued. DALYs by age, sex and cause (thousands): Other Asia and Islands, 2010, baseline scenario

Cause	Total	Male	Female	Males					Females				
				0-4	5-14	15-44	45-59	60+	0-4	5-14	15-44	45-59	60+
B. Respiratory infections	6 613	3 726	2 887	2 816	354	120	58	378	2 022	309	88	65	402
1. Lower respiratory infections	6 435	3 628	2 807	2 759	323	115	57	373	1 981	281	85	64	398
2. Upper respiratory infections	74	42	33	27	4	4	1	4	19	4	3	1	5
3. Otitis media	103	56	47	29	26	1	-	-	22	25	-	-	-
C. Maternal conditions	1 051	-	1 051	-	-	-	-	-	-	-	1 031	20	-
1. Maternal haemorrhage	102	-	102	-	-	-	-	-	-	-	98	4	-
2. Maternal sepsis	184	-	184	-	-	-	-	-	-	-	181	3	-
3. Hypertensive disorders of pregnancy	50	-	50	-	-	-	-	-	-	-	48	2	-
4. Obstructed labour	235	-	235	-	-	-	-	-	-	-	234	1	-
5. Abortion	201	-	201	-	-	-	-	-	-	-	198	2	-
D. Perinatal conditions*	5 440	3 020	2 419	3 020	-	-	-	-	2 419	-	-	-	-
E. Nutritional deficiencies	3 363	1 609	1 754	889	171	377	89	83	791	156	561	139	107
1. Protein-energy malnutrition	1 209	641	568	627	4	2	3	5	556	3	2	2	5
2. Iodine deficiency	67	35	32	31	3	1	-	-	29	3	-	-	-
3. Vitamin A deficiency	223	121	103	86	33	2	-	-	74	28	1	-	-
4. Iron-deficiency anaemia	1 864	813	1 051	145	132	372	86	77	133	123	556	137	102
II. Noncommunicable diseases	95 548	51 826	43 721	4 196	2 635	19 165	14 476	11 354	3 491	1 931	16 558	10 286	11 456
A. Malignant neoplasms	15 164	8 662	6 502	223	627	1 944	3 293	2 576	267	386	1 733	2 140	1 975
1. Mouth and oropharynx cancers	1 391	873	519	6	18	230	227	392	9	14	137	99	260
2. Oesophagus cancer	467	311	156	-	-	34	161	117	-	-	25	58	73
3. Stomach cancer	1 248	840	408	1	2	154	415	268	-	1	82	160	166
4. Colon and rectum cancers	799	428	371	2	6	114	109	197	3	4	80	89	195
5. Liver cancer	1 604	1 251	353	8	22	306	666	248	8	11	66	137	131
6. Pancreas cancer	191	124	67	-	-	25	54	45	1	1	6	27	32
7. Trachea, bronchus, lung cancers	2 124	1 636	488	3	7	258	864	503	3	4	48	208	225
8. Melanoma and other skin cancers	52	24	28	-	1	8	10	5	-	-	7	10	11
9. Breast cancer	723	-	723	-	-	-	-	-	2	3	248	327	144
10. Cervix uteri cancer	836	-	836	-	-	-	-	-	-	1	238	432	165
11. Corpus uteri cancer	84	-	84	-	-	-	-	-	1	2	13	39	29
12. Ovary cancer	296	-	296	-	-	-	-	-	11	15	139	85	47
13. Prostate cancer	193	193	-	-	-	4	42	143	-	-	-	-	-
14. Bladder cancer	199	149	50	1	3	15	58	76	-	1	5	12	32
15. Lymphomas and multiple myeloma	599	386	212	29	79	130	67	81	17	23	61	34	78
16. Leukaemia	960	541	419	78	212	169	37	45	97	137	108	30	46
C. Diabetes mellitus	1 406	677	729	9	14	194	274	187	9	13	126	268	312
D. Endocrine disorders	399	188	210	96	25	29	22	16	79	13	41	38	41

Annex Table 15e, continued. DALYs by age, sex and cause (thousands): Other Asia and Islands, 2010, baseline scenario

Cause	Total	Male	Female	Males 0-4	5-14	15-44	45-59	60+	Females 0-4	5-14	15-44	45-59	60+
E. Neuro-psychiatric conditions	**26 604**	**13 229**	**13 375**	**188**	**392**	**10 749**	**1 297**	**603**	**189**	**369**	**10 302**	**1 606**	**909**
1. Unipolar major depression	9 961	3 481	6 480	-	-	2 886	493	102	-	-	5 321	942	218
2. Bipolar disorder	2 749	1 383	1 365	-	-	1 273	86	23	-	-	1 245	89	31
3. Schizophrenia	3 184	1 665	1 519	-	-	1 640	16	9	-	-	1 495	6	17
4. Epilepsy	664	378	287	14	83	212	53	15	16	89	138	29	15
5. Alcohol use	2 742	2 539	203	-	-	2 339	172	28	-	-	190	10	3
6. Dementia*	1 423	611	812	38	17	45	200	310	46	18	41	223	484
7. Parkinson disease	174	92	82	-	-	-	42	49	-	-	-	36	45
8. Multiple sclerosis	232	100	131	-	-	89	9	3	-	-	114	13	4
9. Drug use	1 285	1 159	126	-	64	1 041	47	7	-	7	113	5	1
10. Post-traumatic stress disorder	345	130	215	6	25	88	9	1	9	41	147	15	2
11. Obsessive-compulsive disorders	1 896	812	1 085	-	88	664	44	16	-	113	864	82	26
12. Panic disorder	924	309	615	-	31	230	47	-	-	31	494	79	11
F. Sense organ diseases	**2 962**	**1 299**	**1 663**	**6**	**4**	**88**	**678**	**524**	**6**	**-**	**110**	**897**	**650**
1. Glaucoma	1 005	291	714	-	-	20	202	69	-	-	59	533	122
2. Cataracts	1 941	997	944	1	-	65	475	455	3	-	51	363	527
G. Cardiovascular diseases	**22 349**	**12 970**	**9 379**	**1 028**	**838**	**3 063**	**3 703**	**4 339**	**722**	**582**	**1 688**	**1 814**	**4 573**
1. Rheumatic heart disease	179	87	91	-	4	26	23	33	-	5	26	21	39
2. Ischaemic heart disease	6 706	3 916	2 790	130	178	688	1 348	1 881	97	117	325	576	1 889
3. Cerebrovascular disease	6 230	3 476	2 754	200	184	721	1 075	1 372	169	132	388	622	1 530
4. Inflammatory heart diseases	2 004	1 212	792	-	-	467	246	115	-	-	250	119	122
H. Respiratory diseases	**5 908**	**3 325**	**2 582**	**465**	**313**	**808**	**726**	**1 012**	**269**	**205**	**700**	**494**	**914**
1. COPD*	2 153	1 279	873	46	17	233	375	607	29	14	145	199	486
2. Asthma	1 631	895	737	71	179	450	125	70	32	112	375	135	81
I. Digestive diseases	**9 296**	**5 785**	**3 511**	**309**	**164**	**1 244**	**2 727**	**1 342**	**256**	**137**	**668**	**1 378**	**1 071**
1. Peptic ulcer	429	281	149	3	4	75	111	88	2	4	34	43	66
2. Cirrhosis of the liver	3 053	2 324	729	18	16	585	1 262	442	13	16	139	335	225
3. Appendicitis	182	107	75	2	28	66	9	2	2	25	40	6	-
J. Genito-urinary diseases	**1 955**	**1 144**	**811**	**58**	**105**	**218**	**542**	**222**	**40**	**75**	**177**	**210**	**309**
1. Nephritis and nephrosis	1 195	593	602	42	90	184	136	141	40	65	130	142	226
2. Benign prostatic hypertrophy	387	387	-	-	-	-	354	34	-	-	-	-	-
L. Musculo-skeletal diseases	**3 456**	**1 474**	**1 983**	**16**	**13**	**331**	**835**	**279**	**16**	**16**	**532**	**1 043**	**375**
1. Rheumatoid arthritis	332	92	240	-	-	6	33	53	-	2	70	55	113
2. Osteoarthritis	2 849	1 282	1 567	-	-	302	777	202	-	-	411	948	208

Annex Table 15e, continued. DALYs by age, sex and cause (thousands): Other Asia and Islands, 2010, baseline scenario

Cause	Total	Male	Female	Males					Females				
				0-4	5-14	15-44	45-59	60+	0-4	5-14	15-44	45-59	60+
M. Congenital anomalies	**3 492**	**1 832**	**1 660**	**1 694**	**57**	**64**	**13**	**4**	**1 552**	**53**	**36**	**13**	**6**
N. Oral conditions	**2 052**	**980**	**1 073**	**31**	**45**	**378**	**304**	**223**	**29**	**45**	**384**	**333**	**281**
1. Dental caries	773	382	391	30	44	163	105	40	29	42	160	111	49
2. Periodontal disease	51	25	26	-	-	19	5	2	-	-	19	5	2
3. Edentulism	1 208	568	640	-	-	193	194	181	-	-	193	216	231
III. Injuries	***28 164***	***19 163***	***9 001***	***2 522***	***2 494***	***11 842***	***1 895***	***410***	***2 194***	***1 327***	***4 415***	***769***	***296***
A. Unintentional injuries	**22 573**	**15 524**	**7 049**	**2 421**	**2 291**	**9 006**	**1 494**	**313**	**2 084**	**1 195**	**2 891**	**632**	**247**
1. Road traffic accidents	7 464	5 230	2 234	479	801	3 347	481	122	440	459	1 029	216	90
2. Poisonings	1 015	529	486	62	56	311	78	23	57	59	302	46	24
3. Falls	3 643	2 394	1 249	635	349	1 165	207	38	491	165	450	112	30
4. Fires	405	213	192	53	49	91	15	5	77	55	47	8	5
5. Drownings	2 094	1 440	654	486	412	458	62	21	306	163	147	25	14
6. Other unintentional	7 951	5 719	2 233	706	624	3 634	650	104	713	295	916	225	83
B. Intentional injuries	**5 591**	**3 639**	**1 952**	**102**	**203**	**2 836**	**401**	**97**	**110**	**131**	**1 525**	**137**	**50**
1. Self-inflicted injuries	2 689	1 494	1 194	-	72	1 176	185	62	-	44	1 027	87	36
2. Violence	2 149	1 707	443	44	93	1 341	198	30	51	57	289	36	9
3. War	753	438	315	58	39	319	18	4	58	30	209	13	5

Notes:
A dash (-) symbol indicates fewer than 500 DALYs.
*IA6 is Bacterial meningitis and meningococcaemia; ID is Conditions arising during the perinatal period;
IIE6 is Dementia and other degenerative and hereditary CNS disorders; IIH1 is Chronic obstructive pulmonary disease.

Annex Table 15f. DALYs by age, sex and cause (thousands): Sub-Saharan Africa, 2010, baseline scenario

Cause	Total	Male	Female	Males					Females				
				0-4	5-14	15-44	45-59	60+	0-4	5-14	15-44	45-59	60+
Population (millions)	*912*	*452*	*460*	*78*	*125*	*194*	*36*	*19*	*75*	*123*	*198*	*39*	*24*
All causes	*320 228*	*178 546*	*141 682*	*76 767*	*18 189*	*62 375*	*12 563*	*8 652*	*62 308*	*14 844*	*43 772*	*10 942*	*9 816*
I. Communicable, maternal, perinatal and nutritional conditions	*163 608*	*84 923*	*78 685*	*62 745*	*5 853*	*13 081*	*2 077*	*1 168*	*50 218*	*5 808*	*19 344*	*1 950*	*1 365*
A. Infectious and parasitic diseases	114 858	60 068	54 789	40 241	4 462	12 643	1 988	735	32 052	4 450	15 641	1 837	810
1. Tuberculosis	18 429	8 648	9 780	1 027	803	5 180	1 249	389	1 094	1 145	5 933	1 205	405
2. STDs excluding HIV	4 333	1 772	2 560	1 250	11	476	10	25	1 131	39	1 338	16	37
a. Syphilis	1 991	1 046	945	929		82	9	25	803	2	92	11	36
b. Chlamydia	1 099	168	931	59	3	105	1	-	61	25	842	3	-
c. Gonorrhoea	1 243	558	685	261	6	289	-	-	267	12	403	2	-
3. HIV	20 095	9 248	10 848	2 973	455	5 382	366	71	2 829	472	7 228	273	46
4. Diarrhoeal diseases	23 868	13 549	10 319	12 584	710	143	35	77	9 293	693	191	44	98
5. Childhood-cluster diseases	22 391	12 215	10 176	11 065	1 056	70	14	10	9 117	980	58	13	9
a. Pertussis	4 145	2 268	1 877	2 116	152	-	-	-	1 740	137	-	-	-
b. Poliomyelitis	454	269	186	264	1	3	-	-	183	1	2	-	-
c. Diphtheria	47	26	21	23	2	-	-	-	19	-	-	-	-
d. Measles	14 629	7 963	6 666	7 142	819	1	-	-	5 916	749	1	-	-
e. Tetanus	3 116	1 690	1 426	1 519	81	66	14	10	1 259	90	55	13	9
6. Bacterial meningitis*	697	369	327	320	9	25	9	6	278	8	23	10	8
7. Hepatitis B and hepatitis C	170	97	73	32	13	21	16	15	22	12	17	7	15
8. Malaria	19 574	11 057	8 518	10 001	582	389	61	23	7 523	549	348	67	31
9. Tropical-cluster diseases	2 592	1 679	913	75	587	779	176	61	79	328	343	124	41
a. Trypanosomiasis	647	342	305	14	132	144	43	9	26	127	117	30	6
b. Chagas disease													
c. Schistosomiasis	590	372	218	20	143	165	28	16	12	89	89	18	10
d. Leishmaniasis	216	148	69	10	84	51	2	3	4	40	23	1	1
e. Lymphatic filariasis	711	558	154	25	185	310	36	-	31	39	51	28	4
f. Onchocerciasis	426	259	167	6	44	109	67	33	5	33	64	47	20
10. Leprosy	29	15	14	-	6	7	1	-	-	5	7	1	-
11. Dengue	11	5	6	1	4	-	-	-	2	4	-	-	-
12. Japanese encephalitis	-	-	-	-	-	-	-	-	-	-	-	-	-
13. Trachoma	222	60	163	-	-	12	17	31	-	-	24	46	93
14. Intestinal nematode infections	276	144	132	1	72	57	9	5	1	68	48	9	6
a. Ascariasis	55	28	27	1	27	-	-	-	1	26	-	-	-
b. Trichuriasis	56	29	27	-	29	-	-	-	-	27	-	-	-
c. Ancylostomiasis and necatoriasis	165	87	78	-	16	56	9	5	-	15	48	9	6

Annex Table 15f, continued. DALYs by age, sex and cause (thousands): Sub-Saharan Africa, 2010, baseline scenario

Cause	Total	Male	Female	Males 0-4	Males 5-14	Males 15-44	Males 45-59	Males 60+	Females 0-4	Females 5-14	Females 15-44	Females 45-59	Females 60+
B. Respiratory infections	23 380	13 215	10 165	11 556	1 028	199	49	382	8 571	834	212	54	494
1. Lower respiratory infections	22 864	12 927	9 937	11 336	971	194	48	378	8 406	782	207	53	489
2. Upper respiratory infections	239	135	104	114	12	4	1	4	84	10	4	1	5
3. Otitis media	276	153	124	106	46	1	-	-	81	42	1	-	-
C. Maternal conditions	3 386	-	3 386						-	183	3 201	2	-
1. Maternal haemorrhage	492	-	492						-	42	450	-	-
2. Maternal sepsis	641	-	641						-	28	613	-	-
3. Hypertensive disorders of pregnancy	244	-	244						-	21	222	-	-
4. Obstructed labour	588	-	588						-	14	574	-	-
5. Abortion	594	-	594						-	24	570	-	-
D. Perinatal conditions*	15 351	8 185	7 166	8 185	-	-	-	-	7 166	-	-	-	-
E. Nutritional deficiencies	6 633	3 455	3 178	2 763	362	239	41	51	2 429	342	290	56	60
1. Protein-energy malnutrition	4 176	2 218	1 958	2 170	19	10	5	13	1 904	20	16	4	15
2. Iodine deficiency	92	47	45	42	3	1	-	-	39	4	2	-	-
3. Vitamin A deficiency	800	427	374	317	106	4	-	-	271	100	4	-	-
4. Iron-deficiency anaemia	1 565	765	800	234	233	224	36	37	215	219	269	52	46
II. Noncommunicable diseases	82 704	42 606	40 098	6 757	3 293	17 102	8 465	6 989	6 343	3 370	13 974	8 284	8 126
A. Malignant neoplasms	10 827	6 119	4 709	227	659	1 862	1 775	1 596	311	636	1 025	1 522	1 215
1. Mouth and oropharynx cancers	495	300	195	2	6	91	66	135	10	25	42	32	87
2. Oesophagus cancer	499	381	118	-	-	86	191	104	-	-	20	46	52
3. Stomach cancer	684	416	267	1	2	95	186	131	1	-	46	134	87
4. Colon and rectum cancers	298	170	129	1	2	58	39	70	1	-	27	29	71
5. Liver cancer	1 548	1 213	335	5	17	609	423	160	7	17	97	122	92
6. Pancreas cancer	148	89	60	-	-	24	41	24	-	-	12	29	18
7. Trachea, bronchus, lung cancers	490	323	167	-	-	88	135	99	-	-	39	75	52
8. Melanoma and other skin cancers	160	72	88	-	-	15	34	22	-	-	10	35	42
9. Breast cancer	386	-	386						-	-	106	174	103
10. Cervix uteri cancer	704	-	704						-	-	162	331	208
11. Corpus uteri cancer	65	-	65						-	-	8	28	27
12. Ovary cancer	189	-	189						-	-	51	69	40
13. Prostate cancer	494	494	-	-	-	12	123	360					
14. Bladder cancer	273	182	91	-	-	35	69	77	-	-	20	35	36
15. Lymphomas and multiple myeloma	1 005	620	386	78	269	141	61	71	76	183	53	33	42
16. Leukaemia	331	148	183	14	47	50	13	24	34	82	27	20	20
C. Diabetes mellitus	540	261	279	22	44	61	74	59	26	43	36	77	97
D. Endocrine disorders	1 265	647	618	325	37	143	102	40	204	68	110	117	118

Annex Table 15f, continued. DALYs by age, sex and cause (thousands): Sub-Saharan Africa, 2010, baseline scenario

Cause	Total			Males					Females				
	Total	Male	Female	0-4	5-14	15-44	45-59	60+	0-4	5-14	15-44	45-59	60+
E. Neuro-psychiatric conditions	**20 993**	**10 093**	**10 900**	**304**	**476**	**8 405**	**665**	**243**	**354**	**498**	**8 743**	**852**	**453**
1. Unipolar major depression	8 462	2 880	5 582	-	-	2 544	277	58	-	-	4 904	549	129
2. Bipolar disorder	2 437	1 200	1 237	-	-	1 138	49	13	-	-	1 165	54	18
3. Schizophrenia	830	430	400	-	-	425	4	2	-	-	395	2	3
4. Epilepsy	538	301	237	36	89	145	22	8	42	83	92	12	8
5. Alcohol use	3 236	2 618	618	-	-	2 470	131	17	-	-	583	26	9
6. Dementia*	581	183	398	26	11	19	43	84	69	31	38	49	211
7. Parkinson disease	82	43	39	-	-	-	19	23	-	-	-	17	22
8. Multiple sclerosis	184	79	105	-	-	72	5	2	-	-	95	8	3
9. Drug use	680	613	67	-	45	548	17	3	-	5	60	2	-
10. Post-traumatic stress disorder	348	128	219	10	38	75	5	1	17	63	130	9	1
11. Obsessive-compulsive disorders	1 723	726	997	-	131	563	24	9	-	171	766	46	14
12. Panic disorder	809	269	540	-	46	197	26	-	-	48	442	45	6
F. Sense organ diseases	**3 206**	**1 530**	**1 676**	**10**	**1**	**113**	**729**	**677**	**10**	**1**	**95**	**783**	**788**
1. Glaucoma	708	280	429	-	-	2	133	145	-	-	4	214	211
2. Cataracts	2 489	1 245	1 244	10	1	105	596	532	10	1	87	569	577
G. Cardiovascular diseases	**15 975**	**8 100**	**7 875**	**688**	**620**	**2 621**	**2 006**	**2 164**	**580**	**724**	**1 283**	**2 108**	**3 181**
1. Rheumatic heart disease	613	326	287	2	100	202	18	5	2	124	128	25	8
2. Ischaemic heart disease	3 703	1 874	1 829	-	-	533	623	718	171	-	196	550	913
3. Cerebrovascular disease	6 752	3 252	3 500	109	219	1 053	843	1 028	97	188	477	1 040	1 700
4. Inflammatory heart diseases	1 795	940	855	184	98	342	173	144	215	139	171	132	197
H. Respiratory diseases	**11 252**	**6 065**	**5 187**	**950**	**588**	**1 910**	**1 287**	**1 329**	**656**	**506**	**1 234**	**1 480**	**1 311**
1. COPD*	3 275	1 901	1 374	79	40	557	512	713	60	42	219	474	580
2. Asthma	1 891	970	921	119	282	436	76	57	67	219	440	123	72
I. Digestive diseases	**5 558**	**3 303**	**2 256**	**350**	**254**	**1 083**	**1 081**	**536**	**337**	**370**	**545**	**519**	**485**
1. Peptic ulcer	343	223	120	-	-	119	75	29	-	-	46	43	31
2. Cirrhosis of the liver	764	558	206	-	21	201	226	109	-	13	58	77	59
3. Appendicitis	333	205	128	5	78	110	10	2	6	75	39	7	2
J. Genito-urinary diseases	**2 828**	**1 716**	**1 112**	**405**	**343**	**339**	**465**	**163**	**298**	**265**	**185**	**203**	**161**
1. Nephritis and nephrosis	1 988	1 120	868	337	290	274	108	111	287	230	118	123	109
2. Benign prostatic hypertrophy	311	311	-	-	-	-	298	13	-	-	-	-	-
L. Musculo-skeletal diseases	**1 901**	**636**	**1 265**	**-**	**-**	**335**	**205**	**96**	**-**	**4**	**521**	**544**	**197**
1. Rheumatoid arthritis	160	44	116	-	-	29	11	4	-	4	72	30	10
2. Osteoarthritis	1 720	582	1 138	-	-	302	191	89	-	4	443	510	185

Annex Table 15f, continued. DALYs by age, sex and cause (thousands): Sub-Saharan Africa, 2010, baseline scenario

Cause	Total	Male	Female	Males					Females				
				0-4	5-14	15-44	45-59	60+	0-4	5-14	15-44	45-59	60+
M. Congenital anomalies	6 185	2 993	3 192	2 812	90	76	11	4	3 044	97	31	14	6
N. Oral conditions	695	335	360	77	89	89	19	60	75	91	97	21	76
1. Dental caries	501	250	250	75	87	65	17	6	72	85	66	19	8
2. Periodontal disease	50	25	25	-	-	22	2	-	-	-	23	2	-
3. Edentulism	122	54	68	-	-	-	-	54	-	-	-	-	68
III. Injuries	73 916	51 016	22 900	7 265	9 044	32 192	2 021	495	5 747	5 666	10 454	707	325
A. Unintentional injuries	41 605	28 725	12 881	5 305	7 120	14 684	1 286	329	3 946	4 502	3 834	396	203
1. Road traffic accidents	11 214	7 904	3 310	584	2 604	4 213	400	103	396	1 366	1 389	127	31
2. Poisonings	1 839	1 075	764	766	160	112	26	10	567	76	110	6	5
3. Falls	2 839	1 631	1 209	355	657	502	81	36	390	386	315	51	67
4. Fires	4 767	2 395	2 372	997	691	612	68	28	861	903	524	49	35
5. Drownings	3 966	2 890	1 077	853	1 302	667	51	16	436	492	131	12	6
6. Other unintentional	16 979	12 830	4 149	1 751	1 705	8 578	661	135	1 295	1 279	1 364	151	60
B. Intentional injuries	32 311	22 292	10 019	1 960	1 923	17 508	734	167	1 801	1 164	6 621	311	122
1. Self-inflicted injuries	874	701	173	-	93	560	38	11	-	-	158	13	2
2. Violence	12 145	10 471	1 674	252	594	9 161	394	71	124	244	1 193	86	26
3. War	19 291	11 119	8 172	1 708	1 237	7 787	303	85	1 677	920	5 269	212	94

Notes:
A dash (-) symbol indicates fewer than 500 DALYs.
*IA6 is Bacterial meningitis and meningococcaemia; ID is Conditions arising during the perinatal period;
IIE6 is Dementia and other degenerative and hereditary CNS disorders; IIH1 is Chronic obstructive pulmonary disease.

Annex Table 15g. DALYs by age, sex and cause (thousands): Latin America and the Caribbean, 2010, baseline scenario

Cause	Total	Male	Female	Males					Females				
				0-4	5-14	15-44	45-59	60+	0-4	5-14	15-44	45-59	60+
Population (millions)	*607*	*302*	*305*	*28*	*56*	*148*	*43*	*27*	*27*	*54*	*147*	*46*	*32*
All causes	**104 152**	**59 979**	**44 173**	**9 334**	**3 759**	**28 442**	**10 548**	**7 896**	**7 227**	**2 677**	**18 079**	**8 525**	**7 665**
I. Communicable, maternal, perinatal and nutritional conditions	*19 664*	*11 398*	*8 266*	*6 166*	*559*	*3 743*	*506*	*424*	*4 560*	*574*	*2 440*	*309*	*384*
A. Infectious and parasitic diseases	11 493	7 209	4 283	2 594	378	3 578	419	240	1 959	383	1 548	214	180
1. Tuberculosis	747	441	306	24	23	209	98	87	18	32	140	63	54
2. STDs excluding HIV	670	184	485	97	1	81	2	3	79	7	392	3	4
a. Syphilis	176	96	80	81	-	10	1	3	64	-	11	2	4
b. Chlamydia	331	32	300	4	-	27	-	-	4	6	289	1	-
c. Gonorrhoea	163	57	105	12	1	44	-	-	12	2	92	-	-
3. HIV	4 333	3 421	912	187	17	2 963	206	48	174	20	682	29	8
4. Diarrhoeal diseases	2 383	1 386	997	1 227	68	42	19	29	827	69	45	21	35
5. Childhood-cluster diseases	1 481	803	679	746	50	4	2	1	622	48	5	2	1
a. Pertussis	314	169	145	157	12	-	-	-	134	11	-	-	-
b. Poliomyelitis	93	55	38	54	-	1	-	-	37	-	1	-	-
c. Diphtheria	6	3	3	2	1	-	-	-	-	1	-	-	-
d. Measles	768	413	355	380	32	1	2	1	320	34	1	-	-
e. Tetanus	300	163	137	153	5	2	2	1	129	2	2	2	1
6. Bacterial meningitis*	224	117	108	75	4	20	9	8	65	4	18	10	10
7. Hepatitis B and hepatitis C	47	22	25	9	5	4	2	2	6	5	9	3	2
8. Malaria	168	88	80	18	21	38	8	3	15	21	31	9	4
9. Tropical-cluster diseases	329	177	153	4	8	106	38	21	3	6	85	39	20
a. Trypanosomiasis	274	142	132	1	1	88	34	19	-	3	77	36	19
b. Chagas disease	31	17	14	1	3	10	3	1	-	3	7	2	1
c. Schistosomiasis	20	14	5	-	4	6	1	-	2	2	1	-	-
d. Leishmaniasis	3	3	1	3	1	1	-	-	-	-	-	-	-
e. Lymphatic filariasis	1	1	1	-	-	2	-	-	-	-	2	-	-
f. Onchocerciasis													
10. Leprosy	26	13	13	-	4	6	2	1	-	3	6	2	1
11. Dengue													
12. Japanese encephalitis													
13. Trachoma													
14. Intestinal nematode infections	295	152	144	2	120	22	5	3	2	115	18	5	4
a. Ascariasis	99	50	49	2	48	-	-	-	2	47	-	-	-
b. Trichuriasis	129	66	63	-	66	22	5	3	-	63	-	-	-
c. Ancylostomiasis and necatoriasis	68	36	32	-	6	22	5	3	-	6	18	5	4

Annex Table 15g, continued. DALYs by age, sex and cause (thousands): Latin America and the Caribbean, 2010, baseline scenario

Cause	Total	Male	Female	Males 0-4	Males 5-14	Males 15-44	Males 45-59	Males 60+	Females 0-4	Females 5-14	Females 15-44	Females 45-59	Females 60+
B. Respiratory infections	2 325	1 269	1 057	926	86	76	55	125	695	92	93	46	131
1. Lower respiratory infections	2 246	1 227	1 019	911	66	73	54	123	683	73	89	45	129
2. Upper respiratory infections	29	16	13	9	1	3	1	2	6	1	3	1	2
3. Otitis media	51	26	25	6	19	-	-	-	6	18	1	-	-
C. Maternal conditions	523	-	523	-	-	-	-	-	-	2	520	1	-
1. Maternal haemorrhage	49	-	49	-	-	-	-	-	-	-	49	-	-
2. Maternal sepsis	90	-	90	-	-	-	-	-	-	-	90	-	-
3. Hypertensive disorders of pregnancy	31	-	31	-	-	-	-	-	-	-	30	-	-
4. Obstructed labour	127	-	127	-	-	-	-	-	-	-	127	-	-
5. Abortion	137	-	137	-	-	-	-	-	-	-	136	-	-
D. Perinatal conditions*	3 631	2 132	1 500	2 132	-	-	-	-	1 500	-	-	-	-
E. Nutritional deficiencies	1 692	788	904	514	95	89	31	59	407	97	280	48	73
1. Protein-energy malnutrition	777	428	349	364	13	11	10	30	274	17	13	9	36
2. Iodine deficiency	40	20	20	18	-	1	-	-	17	2	1	-	-
3. Vitamin A deficiency	75	40	36	30	9	1	-	-	26	9	-	-	-
4. Iron-deficiency anaemia	791	296	495	100	71	76	20	29	88	69	264	38	37
II. Noncommunicable diseases	64 579	33 957	30 622	2 252	1 416	14 699	8 546	7 044	1 984	1 221	12 617	7 761	7 041
A. Malignant neoplasms	7 327	3 411	3 916	65	249	659	1 172	1 265	69	162	1 091	1 483	1 111
1. Mouth and oropharynx cancers	268	201	67	-	2	44	99	56	-	1	13	25	28
2. Oesophagus cancer	177	129	48	-	-	12	65	51	-	-	-	17	27
3. Stomach cancer	655	410	244	-	-	62	162	186	-	-	40	84	120
4. Colon and rectum cancers	416	200	215	-	-	42	73	84	-	-	33	73	109
5. Liver cancer	95	50	45	-	-	11	19	18	-	-	6	15	22
6. Pancreas cancer	130	69	61	-	-	9	29	31	-	-	6	22	33
7. Trachea, bronchus, lung cancers	897	579	318	-	-	106	282	190	-	-	36	163	119
8. Melanoma and other skin cancers	70	34	36	-	-	13	12	8	-	-	13	13	9
9. Breast cancer	697	-	697	-	-	-	-	-	-	-	212	318	166
10. Cervix uteri cancer	602	-	602	-	-	-	-	-	-	-	227	263	113
11. Corpus uteri cancer	133	-	133	-	-	-	-	-	-	-	22	69	41
12. Ovary cancer	137	-	137	-	-	-	-	-	2	5	53	45	32
13. Prostate cancer	268	268	-	-	-	6	41	222	-	-	-	-	-
14. Bladder cancer	138	106	33	-	-	10	35	59	-	-	4	10	19
15. Lymphomas and multiple myeloma	393	234	158	-	43	88	54	37	9	23	45	39	42
16. Leukaemia	376	214	162	21	74	76	23	19	19	53	48	22	20
C. Diabetes mellitus	1 607	734	873	10	16	178	279	250	9	13	141	313	397
D. Endocrine disorders	1 209	599	610	263	50	151	75	60	214	41	153	105	98

Annex Table 15g, continued. DALYs by age, sex and cause (thousands): Latin America and the Caribbean, 2010, baseline scenario

Cause	Total	Male	Female	Males					Females				
				0-4	5-14	15-44	45-59	60+	0-4	5-14	15-44	45-59	60+
E. Neuro-psychiatric conditions	21 406	12 042	9 363	198	391	9 735	1 193	526	180	361	7 192	1 010	621
1. Unipolar major depression	6 217	2 153	4 064	-	-	1 782	303	69	-	-	3 340	578	145
2. Bipolar disorder	1 699	849	850	-	-	781	53	16	-	-	776	55	19
3. Schizophrenia	1 789	929	860	-	-	911	12	7	-	-	847	4	8
4. Epilepsy	537	313	224	11	67	182	40	12	10	62	124	17	11
5. Alcohol use	5 496	5 050	446	-	-	4 397	521	132	-	-	414	24	8
6. Dementia*	1 030	428	602	38	20	29	107	234	38	16	30	149	369
7. Parkinson disease	63	33	29	-	-	-	15	18	-	-	-	13	16
8. Multiple sclerosis	156	67	89	-	-	59	6	2	-	-	77	9	3
9. Drug use	1 540	1 004	536	-	59	898	41	7	-	31	479	22	4
10. Post-traumatic stress disorder	226	84	141	4	17	57	6	1	6	27	96	10	2
11. Obsessive-compulsive disorders	1 192	507	685	-	56	412	27	11	-	72	545	50	18
12. Panic disorder	560	185	374	-	19	138	28	-	-	19	301	47	7
F. Sense organ diseases	986	462	524	19	4	24	127	287	13	6	24	148	332
1. Glaucoma	158	57	101	-	-	1	30	25	-	-	3	59	39
2. Cataracts	772	376	396	2	-	17	96	261	2	-	14	87	292
G. Cardiovascular diseases	11 953	6 805	5 148	129	77	1 312	2 425	2 863	87	54	992	1 515	2 499
1. Rheumatic heart disease	193	71	122	1	9	32	20	9	1	10	59	38	15
2. Ischaemic heart disease	4 923	2 921	2 002	10	15	425	1 145	1 352	7	11	261	609	1 131
3. Cerebrovascular disease	3 899	2 139	1 759	25	16	444	765	905	20	11	361	553	826
4. Inflammatory heart diseases	600	340	260	-	-	145	96	59	-	-	108	66	54
H. Respiratory diseases	5 543	2 603	2 940	355	180	726	587	755	224	152	817	969	778
1. COPD*	1 988	987	1 001	35	6	205	286	456	24	5	175	386	410
2. Asthma	1 241	590	652	39	111	315	74	50	23	93	267	178	91
I. Digestive diseases	4 466	2 726	1 740	111	55	793	1 212	556	85	46	548	600	462
1. Peptic ulcer	213	138	75	1	1	41	53	42	1	-	21	23	29
2. Cirrhosis of the liver	1 579	1 202	377	6	4	385	612	195	4	4	112	168	89
3. Appendicitis	41	24	17	-	6	15	2	1	-	4	10	2	1
J. Genito-urinary diseases	1 296	756	540	62	42	101	403	148	54	48	182	119	137
1. Nephritis and nephrosis	571	278	293	35	34	70	64	75	33	37	81	62	79
2. Benign prostatic hypertrophy	332	332	-	-	-	-	306	26	-	-	-	-	-
L. Musculo-skeletal diseases	4 876	1 907	2 969	6	16	673	970	241	4	24	1 089	1 372	480
1. Rheumatoid arthritis	887	188	699	-	-	98	66	23	-	6	439	186	67
2. Osteoarthritis	3 667	1 638	2 028	-	-	549	886	203	-	-	518	1 133	377

Annex Table 15g, continued. DALYs by age, sex and cause (thousands): Latin America and the Caribbean, 2010, baseline scenario

Cause	Total	Male	Female	Males					Females				
				0-4	5-14	15-44	45-59	60+	0-4	5-14	15-44	45-59	60+
M. Congenital anomalies	**2 084**	**1 036**	**1 047**	**963**	**42**	**25**	**4**	**2**	**973**	**35**	**31**	**6**	**3**
N. Oral conditions	**1 283**	**638**	**645**	**35**	**252**	**253**	**41**	**57**	**34**	**244**	**252**	**44**	**71**
1. Dental caries	1 093	552	542	35	251	246	14	6	33	242	245	14	7
2. Periodontal disease	32	15	17	-	-	5	7	3	-	-	5	8	4
3. Edentulism	148	67	81	-	-	-	19	48	-	-	-	21	60
III. Injuries	***19 908***	***14 625***	***5 284***	***916***	***1 783***	***10 000***	***1 497***	***428***	***683***	***882***	***3 022***	***456***	***241***
A. Unintentional injuries	**13 751**	**9 691**	**4 060**	**808**	**1 572**	**5 871**	**1 096**	**344**	**587**	**774**	**2 108**	**376**	**216**
1. Road traffic accidents	6 003	4 200	1 804	127	721	2 790	448	114	95	407	1 090	158	54
2. Poisonings	145	84	61	21	10	40	9	3	15	9	30	4	3
3. Falls	1 597	1 126	472	149	293	516	103	65	73	100	170	60	68
4. Fires	277	153	124	35	40	60	13	6	32	41	38	8	5
5. Drownings	804	630	174	72	133	370	45	10	47	49	68	7	3
6. Other unintentional	4 924	3 498	1 426	404	374	2 096	478	146	325	167	711	139	84
B. Intentional injuries	**6 158**	**4 934**	**1 224**	**108**	**211**	**4 130**	**401**	**84**	**97**	**108**	**914**	**80**	**25**
1. Self-inflicted injuries	858	563	295	-	18	431	84	30	-	14	240	30	10
2. Violence	4 420	3 860	560	42	145	3 329	295	48	31	59	426	35	10
3. War	880	510	370	66	48	370	21	5	65	36	248	15	6

Notes:
A dash (-) symbol indicates fewer than 500 DALYs.
*IA6 is Bacterial meningitis and meningococcaemia; ID is Conditions arising during the perinatal period;
IIE6 is Dementia and other degenerative and hereditary CNS disorders; IIH1 is Chronic obstructive pulmonary disease.

Annex Table 15h. DALYs by age, sex and cause (thousands): Middle Eastern Crescent, 2010, baseline scenario

Cause	Total	Male	Female	Males					Females				
				0-4	5-14	15-44	45-59	60+	0-4	5-14	15-44	45-59	60+
Population (millions)	*821*	*416*	*405*	*55*	*97*	*192*	*47*	*24*	*53*	*93*	*185*	*46*	*28*
All causes	**157 996**	**87 232**	**70 764**	**31 223**	**7 327**	**27 516**	**12 301**	**8 865**	**27 717**	**5 544**	**21 341**	**8 041**	**8 120**
I. Communicable, maternal, perinatal and nutritional conditions	*45 893*	*23 482*	*22 411*	*20 482*	*1 133*	*1 080*	*357*	*430*	*18 288*	*1 056*	*2 302*	*318*	*446*
A. Infectious and parasitic diseases	**19 388**	**10 460**	**8 927**	**8 613**	**529**	**864**	**298**	**156**	**7 567**	**449**	**536**	**199**	**177**
1. Tuberculosis	**1 238**	**824**	**414**	**121**	**51**	**392**	**176**	**84**	**70**	**30**	**158**	**95**	**61**
2. STDs excluding HIV	**522**	**203**	**319**	**158**	**1**	**41**	**1**	**2**	**141**	**4**	**169**	**2**	**3**
a. Syphilis	305	160	145	148	-	8	1	2	132	-	9	1	3
b. Chlamydia	151	19	133	3	-	16	-	-	3	3	126	-	-
c. Gonorrhoea	65	24	41	7	-	17	-	-	7	1	34	-	-
3. HIV	**372**	**294**	**78**	**36**	**2**	**222**	**31**	**3**	**36**	**2**	**36**	**3**	**-**
4. Diarrhoeal diseases	**9 607**	**5 093**	**4 514**	**4 890**	**150**	**34**	**10**	**9**	**4 321**	**141**	**32**	**10**	**10**
5. Childhood-cluster diseases	**5 503**	**2 924**	**2 579**	**2 724**	**185**	**10**	**4**	**2**	**2 398**	**157**	**16**	**6**	**1**
a. Pertussis	1 287	681	605	636	45	-	-	-	565	41	-	-	-
b. Poliomyelitis	314	185	129	182	1	3	-	-	127	1	1	-	-
c. Diphtheria	26	14	12	13	1	-	-	-	11	1	-	-	-
d. Measles	2 084	1 098	986	994	103	1	-	-	889	95	1	-	-
e. Tetanus	1 792	946	847	899	35	7	4	1	806	20	14	6	1
6. Bacterial meningitis*	**425**	**225**	**199**	**175**	**7**	**25**	**11**	**7**	**157**	**7**	**16**	**11**	**8**
7. Hepatitis B and hepatitis C	**139**	**81**	**58**	**25**	**9**	**18**	**17**	**12**	**19**	**8**	**12**	**8**	**11**
8. Malaria	**177**	**96**	**81**	**26**	**34**	**28**	**6**	**2**	**23**	**30**	**20**	**6**	**3**
9. Tropical-cluster diseases	**134**	**86**	**47**	**15**	**30**	**31**	**8**	**3**	**9**	**17**	**15**	**4**	**2**
a. Trypanosomiasis	-	-	-	-	-	-	-	-	-	-	-	-	-
b. Chagas disease	-	-	-	-	-	-	-	-	-	-	-	-	-
c. Schistosomiasis	67	44	23	1	12	22	7	3	1	5	12	4	3
d. Leishmaniasis	60	38	23	13	18	5	1	-	8	11	3	-	-
e. Lymphatic filariasis	6	4	2	-	-	3	-	-	-	-	1	-	-
f. Onchocerciasis	-	-	-	-	-	-	-	-	-	-	-	-	-
10. Leprosy	**7**	**4**	**3**	**1**	**1**	**2**	**-**	**-**	**-**	**1**	**2**	**-**	**-**
11. Dengue	**-**	**-**	**-**	**-**	**-**	**-**	**-**	**-**	**-**	**-**	**-**	**-**	**-**
12. Japanese encephalitis	**-**	**-**	**-**	**-**	**-**	**-**	**-**	**-**	**-**	**-**	**-**	**-**	**-**
13. Trachoma	**169**	**46**	**123**	**-**	**-**	**8**	**16**	**22**	**-**	**-**	**16**	**40**	**67**
14. Intestinal nematode infections	**102**	**54**	**48**	**1**	**30**	**18**	**3**	**2**	**1**	**27**	**14**	**3**	**2**
a. Ascariasis	49	26	23	1	24	-	-	-	1	22	-	-	-
b. Trichuriasis	1	-	-	-	-	-	-	-	-	-	-	-	-
c. Ancylostomiasis and necatoriasis	52	28	24	-	5	18	3	2	-	5	14	3	2

Annex Table 15h, continued. DALYs by age, sex and cause (thousands): Middle Eastern Crescent, 2010, baseline scenario

Cause	Total	Male	Female	Males 0-4	5-14	15-44	45-59	60+	Females 0-4	5-14	15-44	45-59	60+
B. Respiratory infections	**10 511**	**5 511**	**5 000**	**4 777**	**393**	**65**	**29**	**246**	**4 231**	**409**	**80**	**43**	**237**
1. Lower respiratory infections	10 244	5 371	4 873	4 682	354	62	29	243	4 147	373	76	43	234
2. Upper respiratory infections	109	57	52	46	5	3	1	3	41	5	3	1	3
3. Otitis media	157	83	75	49	34	-	-	-	43	31	-	-	-
C. Maternal conditions	**1 285**	**-**	**1 285**						**-**	**1**	**1 253**	**31**	**-**
1. Maternal haemorrhage	131		131								124	7	
2. Maternal sepsis	271		271								267	4	
3. Hypertensive disorders of pregnancy	84		84								80	4	
4. Obstructed labour	352		352								349	2	
5. Abortion	125		125								123	2	
D. Perinatal conditions*	**10 342**	**5 395**	**4 947**	**5 395**					**4 947**				
E. Nutritional deficiencies	**4 368**	**2 117**	**2 251**	**1 697**	**211**	**150**	**30**	**28**	**1 543**	**198**	**433**	**45**	**33**
1. Protein-energy malnutrition	2 393	1 258	1 135	1 244	3	3	2	6	1 121	3	4	1	6
2. Iodine deficiency	157	81	76	72	6	2	-	-	66	6	3	1	-
3. Vitamin A deficiency	430	218	212	165	51	2	-	-	158	51	2	-	-
4. Iron-deficiency anaemia	1 389	560	829	216	151	143	28	22	197	137	424	43	27
II. Noncommunicable diseases	***82 885***	***44 880***	***38 004***	***7 652***	***3 162***	***15 099***	***10 768***	***8 199***	***6 570***	***2 785***	***13 922***	***7 238***	***7 489***
A. Malignant neoplasms	**6 541**	**3 846**	**2 695**	**130**	**418**	**979**	**1 479**	**839**	**129**	**347**	**837**	**823**	**559**
1. Mouth and oropharynx cancers	386	256	130	2	7	100	73	73	2	7	47	31	42
2. Oesophagus cancer	220	135	85	-	1	28	75	32	1	2	21	36	26
3. Stomach cancer	479	310	169	1	3	78	159	71	-	1	42	66	59
4. Colon and rectum cancers	271	147	124	-	2	55	43	47	1	4	35	27	56
5. Liver cancer	199	131	68	1	6	32	65	27	2	5	15	27	20
6. Pancreas cancer	104	68	36	-	-	18	35	15	-	-	6	17	13
7. Trachea, bronchus, lung cancers	1 288	1 061	227	2	7	199	580	273	2	6	41	105	73
8. Melanoma and other skin cancers	34	22	13	-	-	8	11	3	-	-	6	4	2
9. Breast cancer	346	-	346						1	3	145	144	53
10. Cervix uteri cancer	208	-	208						-	1	74	98	35
11. Corpus uteri cancer	44	-	44						-	1	9	21	13
12. Ovary cancer	112	-	112						2	7	53	36	13
13. Prostate cancer	73	73	-	-	-	-	24	43					
14. Bladder cancer	220	180	41	-	1	41	83	53	-	1	9	16	13
15. Lymphomas and multiple myeloma	316	216	100	15	61	88	31	22	11	33	31	11	15
16. Leukaemia	504	269	235	27	110	91	22	19	35	112	54	14	20
C. Diabetes mellitus	**1 553**	**795**	**758**	**40**	**53**	**230**	**302**	**170**	**38**	**50**	**157**	**273**	**240**
D. Endocrine disorders	**1 049**	**529**	**521**	**293**	**63**	**93**	**57**	**22**	**280**	**98**	**80**	**40**	**23**

Annex Table 15h, continued. DALYs by age, sex and cause (thousands): Middle Eastern Crescent, 2010, baseline scenario

Cause	Total	Male	Female	Males					Females				
				0-4	5-14	15-44	45-59	60+	0-4	5-14	15-44	45-59	60+
E. Neuro-psychiatric conditions	**20 584**	**9 873**	**10 710**	**681**	**632**	**7 579**	**719**	**263**	**547**	**546**	**8 340**	**915**	**362**
1. Unipolar major depression	7 983	2 841	5 142	-	-	2 427	347	67	-	-	4 388	616	138
2. Bipolar disorder	2 251	1 146	1 105	-	-	1 070	61	15	-	-	1 027	59	18
3. Schizophrenia	2 388	1 253	1 135	-	-	1 238	10	6	-	-	1 117	11	7
4. Epilepsy	480	261	219	38	79	115	21	7	31	92	77	14	5
5. Alcohol use	438	394	44	-	-	366	24	4	-	-	41	2	1
6. Dementia*	471	226	245	49	15	29	45	87	56	16	29	29	115
7. Parkinson disease	110	59	51	-	-	-	28	31	-	-	-	23	27
8. Multiple sclerosis	188	83	105	-	-	75	6	2	-	-	94	8	2
9. Drug use	1 542	1 387	156	7	94	1 234	51	7	12	11	139	6	1
10. Post-traumatic stress disorder	310	118	192	-	29	74	6	1	-	47	121	10	1
11. Obsessive-compulsive disorders	1 596	693	902	-	100	552	30	11	-	128	705	53	16
12. Panic disorder	727	250	477	-	34	184	32	-	-	34	388	50	6
F. Sense organ diseases	**1 667**	**840**	**827**	**3**		**49**	**417**	**370**	**4**	**1**	**40**	**376**	**406**
1. Glaucoma	206	78	128	-	-	1	54	23	-	-	3	94	31
2. Cataracts	1 446	754	692	2	-	43	361	347	2	-	34	281	374
G. Cardiovascular diseases	**24 033**	**14 126**	**9 907**	**1 662**	**965**	**2 804**	**4 257**	**4 438**	**1 087**	**811**	**1 763**	**2 153**	**4 093**
1. Rheumatic heart disease	747	375	372	2	85	250	34	6	2	94	231	37	8
2. Ischaemic heart disease	9 397	5 761	3 636	-	-	968	2 308	2 484	-	-	466	964	2 207
3. Cerebrovascular disease	3 769	2 075	1 693	88	172	436	652	728	56	132	241	448	817
4. Inflammatory heart diseases	2 142	1 244	898	319	180	397	230	119	257	139	263	133	107
H. Respiratory diseases	**8 619**	**4 660**	**3 959**	**1 094**	**451**	**997**	**952**	**1 166**	**786**	**406**	**865**	**969**	**933**
1. COPD*	2 579	1 354	1 224	117	26	246	276	689	99	46	216	406	458
2. Asthma	1 227	794	433	91	207	345	97	54	23	82	194	82	52
I. Digestive diseases	**6 091**	**3 470**	**2 620**	**926**	**170**	**746**	**1 179**	**449**	**1 037**	**140**	**467**	**629**	**348**
1. Peptic ulcer	178	127	50	-	3	49	55	21	1	1	20	18	10
2. Cirrhosis of the liver	1 026	622	403	10	20	146	315	131	7	48	81	164	103
3. Appendicitis	113	67	46	2	20	39	5	1	2	19	22	3	1
J. Genito-urinary diseases	**3 291**	**2 049**	**1 242**	**175**	**137**	**619**	**843**	**275**	**142**	**125**	**415**	**353**	**207**
1. Nephritis and nephrosis	781	407	374	73	70	129	76	59	64	89	116	59	46
2. Benign prostatic hypertrophy	375	375	-	-	-	1	347	26	-	-	-	-	-
L. Musculo-skeletal diseases	**1 541**	**679**	**862**	**16**	**9**	**361**	**225**	**68**	**13**	**7**	**334**	**351**	**157**
1. Rheumatoid arthritis	292	170	121	-	-	162	6	2	-	3	63	42	13
2. Osteoarthritis	1 129	451	677	-	-	178	210	63	-	-	244	296	137

Annex Table 15h, continued. DALYs by age, sex and cause (thousands): Middle Eastern Crescent, 2010, baseline scenario

Cause	Total	Male	Female	Males 0-4	5-14	15-44	45-59	60+	Females 0-4	5-14	15-44	45-59	60+
M. Congenital anomalies	5 150	2 636	2 514	2 471	75	74	13	4	2 360	82	52	16	5
N. Oral conditions	2 367	1 178	1 190	116	152	504	291	115	110	147	497	297	138
1. Dental caries	1 108	561	547	115	151	183	74	37	110	145	176	73	44
2. Periodontal disease	34	17	17	-	-	16	1	-	-	-	15	1	-
3. Edentulism	1 207	595	612	-	-	302	216	77	-	-	295	222	94
III. Injuries	29 218	18 870	10 348	3 089	3 032	11 337	1 176	236	2 858	1 703	5 117	485	185
A. Unintentional injuries	14 278	9 916	4 362	1 936	1 807	5 295	740	138	1 688	875	1 460	244	95
1. Road traffic accidents	4 397	3 387	1 010	140	611	2 334	259	43	121	325	464	75	25
2. Poisonings	494	311	183	76	20	158	49	8	72	16	71	18	6
3. Falls	2 025	1 295	730	410	383	426	63	13	357	161	163	36	12
4. Fires	885	390	495	129	106	130	20	4	135	111	226	16	7
5. Drownings	1 087	762	325	237	186	307	26	6	208	52	57	6	2
6. Other unintentional	5 389	3 770	1 619	943	500	1 939	323	65	795	210	478	94	43
B. Intentional injuries	14 941	8 954	5 986	1 153	1 224	6 042	436	98	1 170	827	3 657	241	90
1. Self-inflicted injuries	2 211	1 494	717	-	457	859	143	35	-	210	421	57	28
2. Violence	1 872	1 232	640	266	116	768	67	14	287	122	194	28	8
3. War	10 858	6 229	4 629	888	651	4 415	226	49	883	495	3 042	156	54

Notes:
A dash (-) symbol indicates fewer than 500 DALYs.
*IA6 is Bacterial meningitis and meningococcaemia; ID is Conditions arising during the perinatal period;
IIE6 is Dementia and other degenerative and hereditary CNS disorders; IIH1 is Chronic obstructive pulmonary disease.

Annex Table 15i. DALYs by age, sex and cause (thousands): World, 2010, baseline scenario

Cause	Total	Male	Female	Males					Females				
				0-4	5-14	15-44	45-59	60+	0-4	5-14	15-44	45-59	60+
Population (millions)	*7 000*	*3 502*	*3 498*	*351*	*661*	*1 628*	*524*	*337*	*336*	*635*	*1 577*	*532*	*418*
All causes	*1 349 768*	*757 304*	*592 464*	*181 368*	*51 073*	*266 689*	*140 633*	*117 541*	*155 451*	*39 663*	*197 474*	*92 324*	*107 553*
I. Communicable, maternal, perinatal and nutritional conditions	*371 532*	*194 974*	*176 557*	*128 221*	*11 870*	*37 827*	*9 402*	*7 654*	*108 252*	*11 736*	*42 499*	*6 890*	*7 181*
A. Infectious and parasitic diseases	230 800	125 158	105 643	68 890	8 173	35 169	8 507	4 418	57 139	7 902	31 245	5 685	3 671
1. Tuberculosis	41 184	22 816	18 368	1 593	1 250	11 528	5 598	2 848	1 506	1 516	9 587	3 830	1 929
2. STDs excluding HIV	10 563	3 862	6 701	2 328	25	1 413	30	66	2 080	98	4 381	45	96
a. Syphilis	3 753	1 972	1 781	1 675	3	207	23	65	1 437	3	220	29	91
b. Chlamydia	3 843	549	3 294	139	8	399	2	1	137	70	3 074	11	2
c. Gonorrhoea	2 962	1 339	1 623	514	14	806	4	1	507	27	1 085	4	1
3. HIV	48 138	26 738	21 401	5 399	878	18 379	1 751	331	5 063	878	14 625	708	127
4. Diarrhoeal diseases	52 368	28 678	23 690	26 279	1 312	516	184	387	21 211	1 310	492	206	472
5. Childhood-cluster diseases	39 056	21 055	18 001	19 058	1 664	243	55	35	16 147	1 570	188	58	38
a. Pertussis	7 466	4 023	3 443	3 752	271				3 196	247			
b. Poliomyelitis	1 570	929	641	907	4	16	2	1	628	3	8	1	
c. Diphtheria	163	87	76	79	7	1			69	7			
d. Measles	21 442	11 552	9 890	10 388	1 155	7		1	8 817	1 064	6		
e. Tetanus	8 414	4 464	3 950	3 932	226	220	52	33	3 437	249	173	55	36
6. Bacterial meningitis*	2 655	1 412	1 243	1 042	43	177	81	68	917	40	124	83	78
7. Hepatitis B and hepatitis C	817	483	334	123	45	121	108	87	89	41	71	46	87
8. Malaria	21 023	11 851	9 172	10 187	809	679	126	51	7 683	755	537	135	62
9. Tropical-cluster diseases	4 078	2 673	1 405	141	834	1 328	274	96	115	441	550	224	74
a. Trypanosomiasis	647	342	305	14	132	144	43	9	26	127	117	30	6
b. Chagas disease	274	142	132	1		88	34	19			77	36	19
c. Schistosomiasis	702	442	260	22	158	200	40	22	13	98	108	26	15
d. Leishmaniasis	637	418	219	47	187	171	9	4	28	107	74	6	3
e. Lymphatic filariasis	1 390	1 069	321	51	313	616	81	9	43	76	110	80	11
f. Onchocerciasis	428	260	168	6	44	110	67	33	5	33	64	47	20
10. Leprosy	190	97	93	3	29	51	11	4	5	27	49	10	2
11. Dengue	199	94	105	27	64	2	1		30	72	1	1	
12. Japanese encephalitis	185	98	87	63	27	6	1	1	57	25	3	1	1
13. Trachoma	613	164	449			25	47	93			48	125	276
14. Intestinal nematode infections	1 938	1 009	929	12	702	221	46	28	11	661	177	47	33
a. Ascariasis	625	322	303	12	308	2			11	290	1		
b. Trichuriasis	648	333	314		333					314			
c. Ancylostomiasis and necatoriasis	665	354	311		61	219	45	28		57	175	46	33

Annex Table 15i, continued. DALYs by age, sex and cause (thousands): World, 2010, baseline scenario

Cause	Total	Male	Female	Males					Females				
				0-4	5-14	15-44	45-59	60+	0-4	5-14	15-44	45-59	60+
B. Respiratory infections	60 009	32 234	27 775	26 087	2 324	786	427	2 610	21 606	2 335	688	392	2 755
1. Lower respiratory infections	58 439	31 404	27 035	25 548	2 102	756	418	2 581	21 146	2 123	662	382	2 721
2. Upper respiratory infections	656	352	304	258	29	27	9	29	212	28	22	9	33
3. Otitis media	914	478	435	281	194	3	–	–	249	183	4	–	–
C. Maternal conditions	8 257	–	8 257							185	7 980	91	–
1. Maternal haemorrhage	999		999							43	936	21	
2. Maternal sepsis	1 528		1 528							28	1 488	12	
3. Hypertensive disorders of pregnancy	509		509							21	477	10	
4. Obstructed labour	1 761		1 761							14	1 741	6	
5. Abortion	1 433		1 433							24	1 400	9	
D. Perinatal conditions*	48 454	25 767	22 687	25 766					22 687				
E. Nutritional deficiencies	24 013	11 816	12 196	7 478	1 372	1 872	468	626	6 820	1 313	2 585	723	756
1. Protein-energy malnutrition	10 902	5 679	5 223	5 472	49	38	26	93	4 985	65	40	22	109
2. Iodine deficiency	587	305	282	275	22	8	1	–	248	22	10	2	–
3. Vitamin A deficiency	1 821	958	863	708	236	13	–	–	630	224	10	–	–
4. Iron-deficiency anaemia	10 659	4 855	5 804	1 015	1 063	1 810	439	529	950	999	2 519	696	639
II. Noncommunicable diseases	724 812	395 705	329 107	32 048	14 361	128 435	115 634	105 227	29 356	12 572	113 463	77 366	96 351
A. Malignant neoplasms	111 615	67 351	44 264	981	2 730	14 009	27 850	21 781	1 122	1 926	10 452	16 215	14 549
1. Mouth and oropharynx cancers	6 122	4 075	2 047	18	48	1 083	1 663	1 264	24	52	541	709	721
2. Oesophagus cancer	6 292	4 415	1 877		1	589	2 177	1 648		2	220	770	884
3. Stomach cancer	12 792	8 659	4 133	3	17	1 157	4 183	3 300	1	10	812	1 550	1 760
4. Colon and rectum cancers	6 653	3 753	2 900	4	20	752	1 337	1 639	6	20	467	928	1 479
5. Liver cancer	11 792	9 181	2 611	24	76	3 038	4 304	1 738	26	59	601	1 077	849
6. Pancreas cancer	2 283	1 449	834			205	645	599	2	2	82	290	458
7. Trachea, bronchus, lung cancers	18 553	14 337	4 216	11	34	1 865	7 366	5 061	6	11	436	1 856	1 906
8. Melanoma and other skin cancers	740	410	330	1	4	117	170	118	2	8	88	116	123
9. Breast cancer	5 528	–	5 528						4	8	1 642	2 434	1 439
10. Cervix uteri cancer	4 325	–	4 325								1 232	2 126	962
11. Corpus uteri cancer	859		859								124	418	310
12. Ovary cancer	1 814		1 814						28	56	601	661	468
13. Prostate cancer	2 106	2 106	–	1	4	41	393	1 667					
14. Bladder cancer	1 901	1 497	404	2	6	152	505	832	2	3	51	118	230
15. Lymphomas and multiple myeloma	4 313	2 775	1 538	164	548	847	653	562	121	277	360	345	434
16. Leukaemia	5 538	3 105	2 433	278	778	1 170	517	361	326	559	861	370	317
C. Diabetes mellitus	10 757	5 160	5 598	161	213	1 250	1 894	1 641	165	202	842	1 804	2 585
D. Endocrine disorders	5 534	2 627	2 907	1 093	233	620	380	302	973	273	630	498	534

Annex Table 15i, continued. DALYs by age, sex and cause (thousands): World, 2010, baseline scenario

Cause	Total	Male	Female	Males					Females				
				0-4	5-14	15-44	45-59	60+	0-4	5-14	15-44	45-59	60+
E. Neuro-psychiatric conditions	185 728	90 688	95 040	2 193	3 021	69 996	9 809	5 669	2 161	2 909	69 994	11 351	8 624
1. Unipolar major depression	70 255	24 776	45 479	-	-	20 184	3 724	868	-	-	36 818	6 815	1 846
2. Bipolar disorder	19 246	9 731	9 516	-	1	8 883	649	198	-	1	8 604	650	261
3. Schizophrenia	16 238	8 554	7 684	-	-	8 405	78	70	-	-	7 539	49	96
4. Epilepsy	4 110	2 335	1 775	163	501	1 274	288	108	170	532	2 168	160	113
5. Alcohol use	21 137	18 697	2 440	-	-	16 368	1 911	419	-	-	800	196	76
6. Dementia*	11 994	4 989	7 005	306	-	294	1 272	2 987	373	141	289	1 378	4 825
7. Parkinson disease	1 539	730	809	-	-	1	289	439	-	-	1	293	514
8. Multiple sclerosis	1 715	749	966	-	-	647	74	27	-	94	822	101	43
9. Drug use	7 265	5 908	1 357	-	404	5 242	226	36	-	323	1 199	54	9
10. Post-traumatic stress disorder	2 526	957	1 569	47	198	629	71	12	76	-	1 033	115	22
11. Obsessive-compulsive disorders	13 550	5 831	7 719	-	684	4 664	337	146	-	874	6 005	603	237
12. Panic disorder	6 470	2 164	4 305	-	201	1 600	362	2	-	238	3 393	580	95
F. Sense organ diseases	16 999	8 118	8 882	78	10	542	3 997	3 490	64	20	560	4 185	4 052
1. Glaucoma	4 471	1 677	2 794	5	-	107	1 065	499	7	-	168	1 880	739
2. Cataracts	12 190	6 307	5 884	33	2	405	2 895	2 971	23	2	324	2 253	3 280
G. Cardiovascular diseases	175 765	104 648	71 117	4 395	2 766	17 112	35 940	44 435	3 106	2 445	9 459	15 876	40 231
1. Rheumatic heart disease	6 357	3 263	3 093	6	229	1 358	1 116	554	20	269	1 186	968	650
2. Ischaemic heart disease	68 501	42 512	25 988	517	652	4 782	16 682	21 048	171	-	2 009	5 811	17 997
3. Cerebrovascular disease	52 405	29 855	22 549	888	534	4 611	10 175	13 900	388	498	2 653	5 483	13 527
4. Inflammatory heart diseases	10 928	6 472	4 456	-	-	2 269	1 773	1 007	799	486	1 288	886	996
H. Respiratory diseases	82 242	45 636	36 606	3 688	2 262	9 678	13 287	16 721	2 514	1 748	8 004	10 460	13 878
1. COPD*	44 825	25 757	19 068	381	122	3 936	8 673	12 645	348	135	2 803	6 000	9 782
2. Asthma	12 200	6 680	5 520	504	1 279	3 238	1 069	591	228	805	2 728	1 119	640
I. Digestive diseases	46 090	28 127	17 963	2 213	758	7 007	12 047	6 101	2 261	799	4 015	5 975	4 912
1. Peptic ulcer	2 940	1 954	986	8	13	629	794	510	9	13	293	323	348
2. Cirrhosis of the liver	14 829	10 751	4 078	75	79	2 778	5 531	2 288	61	114	889	1 810	1 205
3. Appendicitis	1 073	640	432	14	168	383	54	21	14	156	214	32	16
J. Genito-urinary diseases	15 429	9 530	5 899	873	797	1 939	4 048	1 874	657	726	1 438	1 422	1 656
1. Nephritis and nephrosis	7 592	4 054	3 538	614	646	1 196	771	828	537	631	787	657	926
2. Benign prostatic hypertrophy	3 066	3 066	-	6	-	8	2 551	502	-	-	-	-	-
L. Musculo-skeletal diseases	26 563	9 894	16 669	44	61	3 337	4 563	1 889	55	84	5 232	7 675	3 624
1. Rheumatoid arthritis	4 533	1 277	3 255	1	1	558	453	264	-	30	1 448	1 042	734
2. Osteoarthritis	20 139	8 000	12 139	-	-	2 611	3 969	1 420	-	-	3 309	6 314	2 515

Annex Table 15i, continued. DALYs by age, sex and cause (thousands): World, 2010, baseline scenario

Cause	Total	Male	Female	Males					Females				
				0–4	5–14	15–44	45–59	60+	0–4	5–14	15–44	45–59	60+
M. Congenital anomalies	32 108	16 035	16 073	14 924	474	526	82	30	15 065	491	381	95	42
N. Oral conditions	10 660	5 191	5 469	485	747	1 802	1 216	941	464	738	1 820	1 276	1 171
1. Dental caries	5 652	2 837	2 816	478	740	1 034	384	201	457	721	1 004	390	244
2. Periodontal disease	363	181	182	–	–	142	28	11	–	–	140	29	13
3. Edentulism	4 506	2 138	2 368	–	–	609	801	728	–	–	603	854	912
III. Injuries	253 424	166 625	86 800	21 098	24 841	100 428	15 597	4 660	17 844	15 355	41 512	8 068	4 021
A. Unintentional injuries	170 238	113 494	56 744	17 274	20 805	60 634	11 393	3 387	13 980	12 713	21 296	5 694	3 062
1. Road traffic accidents	57 937	41 254	16 683	2 139	7 322	26 202	4 391	1 200	1 384	4 637	7 996	1 941	725
2. Poisonings	6 635	3 908	2 728	1 236	347	1 541	624	161	874	248	1 112	349	145
3. Falls	22 788	13 825	8 963	2 850	4 272	4 984	1 173	547	2 784	1 849	2 340	1 121	869
4. Fires	11 978	5 102	6 876	1 689	1 200	1 733	353	126	1 496	1 858	2 965	338	219
5. Drownings	13 330	9 079	4 251	2 589	2 822	3 075	434	159	1 737	1 230	913	219	152
6. Other unintentional	57 569	40 326	17 244	6 771	4 842	23 099	4 419	1 194	5 707	2 891	5 970	1 725	952
B. Intentional injuries	83 187	53 131	30 055	3 824	4 036	39 793	4 204	1 274	3 864	2 642	20 216	2 374	960
1. Self-inflicted injuries	24 041	13 135	10 906	–	885	9 149	2 241	860	–	464	8 308	1 491	643
2. Violence	26 017	20 843	5 174	1 002	1 108	17 097	1 372	265	1 077	646	2 826	472	152
3. War	33 128	19 153	13 975	2 822	2 043	13 547	591	149	2 787	1 532	9 082	411	164

Notes:

A dash (–) symbol indicates fewer than 500 DALYs.

*IA6 is Bacterial meningitis and meningococcaemia; ID is Conditions arising during the perinatal period;
IIE6 is Dementia and other degenerative and hereditary CNS disorders; IIH1 is Chronic obstructive pulmonary disease.

Annex Table 16a. Deaths by age, sex and cause (thousands): Established Market Economies, 2020, baseline scenario

Cause	Total	Male	Female	Males 0-4	5-14	15-29	30-44	45-59	60-69	70+	Females 0-4	5-14	15-29	30-44	45-59	60-69	70+
Population (millions)	*905*	*441*	*464*	*29*	*58*	*85*	*77*	*86*	*50*	*57*	*28*	*55*	*81*	*75*	*87*	*55*	*83*
All causes	**8 651**	**4 632**	**4 018**	**25**	**9**	**95**	**151**	**584**	**805**	**2 964**	**19**	**6**	**29**	**63**	**207**	**370**	**3 325**
I. Communicable, maternal, perinatal and nutritional conditions	*533*	*299*	*234*	*12*	–	*12*	*41*	*21*	*13*	*200*	*8*	–	*3*	*6*	*4*	*7*	*206*
A. Infectious and parasitic diseases	**154**	**109**	**46**	**2**	–	**12**	**41**	**19**	**5**	**31**	**1**	–	**3**	**6**	**2**	**3**	**31**
1. Tuberculosis	14	10	4	–	–	–	–	–	1	8	–	–	–	–	–	–	4
2. STDs excluding HIV	1	–	–	–	–	–	–	–	–	–	–	–	–	–	–	–	–
a. Syphilis																	
b. Chlamydia																	
c. Gonorrhoea																	
3. HIV	86	74	12	1	–	12	40	18	2	1	1	–	3	6	2	1	–
4. Diarrhoeal diseases	3	1	2	–	–	–	–	–	–	1	–	–	–	–	–	–	2
5. Childhood-cluster diseases	1	1	–	1	–	–	–	–	–	–	1	–	–	–	–	–	–
a. Pertussis																	
b. Poliomyelitis																	
c. Diphtheria																	
d. Measles																	
e. Tetanus																	
6. Bacterial meningitis*	3	1	1	–	–	–	–	–	–	1	–	–	–	–	–	–	1
7. Hepatitis B and hepatitis C	2	1	1	–	–	–	–	–	–	1	–	–	–	–	–	–	1
8. Malaria	–	–	–	–	–	–	–	–	–	–	–	–	–	–	–	–	–
9. Tropical-cluster diseases																	
a. Trypanosomiasis																	
b. Chagas disease																	
c. Schistosomiasis																	
d. Leishmaniasis																	
10. Leprosy																	
11. Dengue																	
12. Japanese encephalitis																	
13. Trachoma																	
14. Intestinal nematode infections																	
a. Ascariasis																	
b. Trichuriasis																	
c. Ancylostomiasis, necatoriasis																	
15. Other infectious and parasitic	46	21	25	–	–	–	–	–	1	19	–	–	–	–	–	1	23

Annex Table 16a, continued. Deaths by age, sex and cause (thousands): Established Market Economies, 2020, baseline scenario

Cause	Total	Male	Female	Males 0-4	5-14	15-29	30-44	45-59	60-69	70+	Females 0-4	5-14	15-29	30-44	45-59	60-69	70+
B. Respiratory infections	339	171	168	1	–	–	–	2	7	161	–	–	–	–	1	4	163
1. Lower respiratory infections	336	170	166	1	–	–	–	2	7	160	–	–	–	–	1	4	161
2. Upper respiratory infections	3	1	2	–	–	–	–	–	–	1	–	–	–	–	–	–	2
3. Otitis media	–	–	–	–	–	–	–	–	–	–	–	–	–	–	–	–	–
C. Maternal conditions	–	–	–	–	–	–	–	–	–	–	–	–	–	–	–	–	–
1. Maternal haemorrhage	–	–	–	–	–	–	–	–	–	–	–	–	–	–	–	–	–
2. Maternal sepsis	–	–	–	–	–	–	–	–	–	–	–	–	–	–	–	–	–
3. Hypertensive disorders*	–	–	–	–	–	–	–	–	–	–	–	–	–	–	–	–	–
4. Obstructed labour	–	–	–	–	–	–	–	–	–	–	–	–	–	–	–	–	–
5. Abortion	–	–	–	–	–	–	–	–	–	–	–	–	–	–	–	–	–
6. Other maternal	–	–	–	–	–	–	–	–	–	–	–	–	–	–	–	–	–
D. Perinatal conditions*	16	10	7	9	–	–	–	–	–	–	7	–	–	–	–	–	–
E. Nutritional deficiencies	23	10	13	–	–	–	–	–	–	9	–	–	–	–	–	–	13
1. Protein-energy malnutrition	7	3	4	–	–	–	–	–	–	3	–	–	–	–	–	–	4
2. Iodine deficiency	–	–	–	–	–	–	–	–	–	–	–	–	–	–	–	–	–
3. Vitamin A deficiency	–	–	–	–	–	–	–	–	–	–	–	–	–	–	–	–	–
4. Iron-deficiency anaemia	15	7	9	–	–	–	–	–	–	6	–	–	–	–	–	–	8
II. Noncommunicable diseases	7 666	4 042	3 624	10	4	16	66	513	762	2 671	8	3	8	38	180	343	3 044
A. Malignant neoplasms	2 222	1 277	944	–	2	5	27	225	308	710	–	1	3	23	116	187	613
1. Mouth and oropharynx cancers	40	31	9	–	–	–	1	10	8	12	–	–	–	–	1	2	5
2. Oesophagus cancer	54	42	12	–	–	–	1	9	11	20	–	–	–	–	1	2	9
3. Stomach cancer	180	114	67	–	–	–	2	16	25	72	–	–	–	1	7	9	50
4. Colon and rectum cancers	266	142	124	–	–	–	2	18	30	92	–	–	–	1	10	19	94
5. Liver cancer	45	34	12	–	–	–	1	8	11	14	–	–	–	1	2	3	8
6. Pancreas cancer	105	57	48	–	–	–	–	9	14	33	–	–	–	–	4	8	36
7. Trachea, bronchus, lung cancers	527	345	182	–	–	2	9	93	109	133	–	–	–	3	28	50	101
8. Melanoma and other skin cancers	26	16	10	–	–	–	1	3	3	8	–	–	–	1	2	2	6
9. Breast cancer	141	–	141	–	–	–	–	–	–	–	–	–	–	7	28	30	76
10. Cervix uteri cancer	15	–	15	–	–	–	–	–	–	–	–	–	1	2	3	3	7
11. Corpus uteri cancer	27	–	27	–	–	–	–	–	–	–	–	–	–	1	4	5	18
12. Ovary cancer	44	–	44	–	–	–	–	–	–	–	–	–	–	2	8	11	24
13. Prostate cancer	137	137	–	–	–	–	–	3	17	116	–	–	–	–	–	–	–
14. Bladder cancer	64	48	16	–	–	–	–	3	8	37	–	–	–	–	1	2	13
15. Lymphomas, multiple myeloma	95	53	42	–	–	1	2	8	11	30	–	–	–	1	4	8	29
16. Leukaemia	67	39	28	–	1	1	2	5	7	23	–	1	1	1	3	4	19
17. Other cancers	389	221	168	–	1	2	6	39	53	120	–	–	1	3	16	29	118

Annex Table 16a, continued. Deaths by age, sex and cause (thousands): Established Market Economies, 2020, baseline scenario

Cause	Total	Male	Female	Males							Females						
				0-4	5-14	15-29	30-44	45-59	60-69	70+	0-4	5-14	15-29	30-44	45-59	60-69	70+
B. Other neoplasms	44	20	24	-	-	-	-	2	3	14	-	-	-	-	1	2	21
C. Diabetes mellitus	199	69	129	-	-	-	1	5	10	52	-	-	-	-	3	9	117
D. Endocrine disorders	58	23	35	-	-	1	1	1	4	16	-	-	-	-	1	2	30
E. Neuro-psychiatric conditions	274	113	161	1	1	4	4	9	11	83	1	-	1	1	3	6	148
2. Bipolar disorder	1	-	-	-	-	-	-	-	-	-	-	-	-	-	-	-	-
3. Schizophrenia	19	7	12	-	-	-	-	-	1	6	-	-	-	-	-	-	12
4. Epilepsy	6	4	2	-	-	1	1	1	-	1	-	-	-	-	-	-	2
5. Alcohol use	12	10	2	-	-	1	1	4	2	2	-	-	-	-	1	-	1
6. Dementia*	141	48	94	-	-	-	1	2	4	41	-	-	-	1	1	3	89
7. Parkinson disease	46	22	24	-	-	-	-	-	1	21	-	-	-	-	-	1	23
8. Multiple sclerosis	5	2	3	-	-	-	-	1	-	1	-	-	-	-	1	1	1
9. Drug use	2	2	-	-	-	2	-	-	-	-	-	-	-	-	-	-	-
13. Other neuro-psychiatric	41	19	23	-	-	2	1	2	2	11	-	-	-	1	1	1	20
F. Sense organ diseases	-	-	-	-	-	-	-	-	-	-	-	-	-	-	-	-	-
1. Glaucoma	-	-	-	-	-	-	-	-	-	-	-	-	-	-	-	-	-
2. Cataracts	-	-	-	-	-	-	-	-	-	-	-	-	-	-	-	-	-
G. Cardiovascular diseases	3 663	1 886	1 778	1	-	3	21	203	331	1 325	1	-	1	7	25	83	1 660
1. Rheumatic heart disease	20	7	12	-	-	-	-	1	2	4	-	-	-	-	-	2	10
2. Ischaemic heart disease	1 946	1 053	893	-	-	1	11	127	202	713	-	-	-	2	12	47	831
3. Cerebrovascular disease	914	415	499	-	-	1	4	32	54	323	-	-	1	2	7	19	470
4. Inflammatory heart diseases	70	39	31	-	-	1	2	8	6	22	-	-	-	1	1	1	28
5. Other cardiovascular	714	371	343	1	-	-	5	34	68	262	1	-	-	1	4	15	322
H. Respiratory diseases	495	285	210	-	-	1	2	12	36	234	-	-	1	1	10	28	169
1. COPD*	356	217	139	-	-	-	1	7	27	182	-	-	-	-	6	20	112
2. Asthma	30	13	17	-	-	1	1	1	2	8	-	-	-	-	2	3	12
3. Other respiratory	109	55	53	-	-	-	1	3	7	44	-	-	1	1	2	5	45
I. Digestive diseases	454	266	187	-	-	1	9	52	50	155	-	-	-	4	17	18	148
1. Peptic ulcer	50	29	21	-	-	-	-	3	4	22	-	-	-	-	1	1	19
2. Cirrhosis of the liver	160	113	46	-	-	1	6	37	29	40	-	-	-	3	11	9	23
3. Appendicitis	2	1	1	-	-	-	-	-	-	1	-	-	-	1	-	-	-
4. Other digestive	242	122	119	-	-	1	2	12	16	92	-	-	-	1	5	8	105
J. Genito-urinary diseases	175	76	99	-	-	-	1	3	6	65	-	-	-	-	2	4	93
1. Nephritis and nephrosis	113	50	63	-	-	-	1	2	5	42	-	-	-	-	1	3	59
2. Benign prostatic hypertrophy	5	5	-	-	-	-	-	-	-	5	-	-	-	-	-	-	-
3. Other genito-urinary	57	21	36	-	-	-	-	1	1	18	-	-	-	-	-	1	34
K. Skin diseases	18	5	13	-	-	-	-	-	-	4	-	-	-	-	-	-	13

Annex Table 16a, continued. Deaths by age, sex and cause (thousands): Established Market Economies, 2020, baseline scenario

Cause	Total	Male	Female	Males							Females						
				0-4	5-14	15-29	30-44	45-59	60-69	70+	0-4	5-14	15-29	30-44	45-59	60-69	70+
L. Musculo-skeletal diseases	44	11	33	-	-	-	-	1	1	9	-	-	-	-	2	1	30
1. Rheumatoid arthritis	13	3	10	-	-	-	-	-	1	2	-	-	-	-	1	1	9
3. Other musculo-skeletal	31	8	23	-	-	-	-	1	-	7	-	-	-	-	1	1	21
M. Congenital anomalies	20	11	9	6	-	1	-	1	1	1	5	-	1	-	1	-	2
N. Oral conditions	-	-	-	-	-	-	-	-	-	-	-	-	-	-	-	-	-
III. Injuries	*451*	*291*	*160*	*3*	*4*	*67*	*43*	*50*	*31*	*93*	*3*	*3*	*19*	*19*	*23*	*20*	*75*
A. Unintentional injuries	278	166	112	3	3	42	19	22	15	62	2	2	12	11	13	12	59
1. Road traffic accidents	106	65	40	3	3	34	9	7	4	9	2	2	10	8	7	4	9
2. Poisonings	11	7	4	2	-	1	2	1	1	1	1	-	1	1	1	1	1
3. Falls	80	39	41	-	-	1	2	4	4	29	-	-	1	1	1	3	36
4. Fires	10	6	4	-	-	1	1	1	1	2	-	-	-	1	1	1	2
5. Drownings	10	7	3	-	1	1	1	1	1	2	-	-	-	-	-	-	2
6. Other unintentional	62	42	20	1	1	4	5	8	6	18	1	-	1	1	3	3	11
B. Intentional injuries	173	125	48	1	1	24	24	28	16	31	1	-	6	8	11	7	15
1. Self-inflicted injuries	142	102	40	-	-	16	18	24	14	29	-	-	4	6	10	7	14
2. Violence	31	23	8	-	-	9	6	4	1	2	-	-	2	2	1	1	1
3. War	-	-	-	1	-	-	-	-	-	-	-	-	-	-	-	-	-

Notes:
Causes responsible for no deaths have been omitted from this table.
A dash (-) symbol indicates fewer than 500 deaths.
*IA6 is Bacterial meningitis and meningococcaemia; IC3 is Hypertensive disorders of pregnancy; ID is Conditions arising during the perinatal period; IIE6 is Dementia and other degenerative and hereditary CNS disorders; IIH1 is Chronic obstructive pulmonary disease.

Annex Table 16b. Deaths by age, sex and cause (thousands): Formerly Socialist Economies of Europe, 2020, baseline scenario

Cause	Total	Male	Female	Males 0-4	5-14	15-29	30-44	45-59	60-69	70+	Females 0-4	5-14	15-29	30-44	45-59	60-69	70+
Population (millions)	*365*	*172*	*193*	*12*	*25*	*37*	*38*	*29*	*17*	*13*	*12*	*24*	*36*	*39*	*33*	*24*	*27*
All causes	*4 854*	*2 713*	*2 141*	*29*	*10*	*77*	*157*	*613*	*605*	*1 222*	*22*	*6*	*25*	*48*	*145*	*259*	*1 637*
I. Communicable, maternal, perinatal and nutritional conditions	**140**	**65**	**75**	**12**	**-**	**1**	**2**	**4**	**4**	**42**	**9**	**-**	**-**	**1**	**1**	**3**	**62**
A. Infectious and parasitic diseases	**29**	**15**	**13**	**3**	**-**	**-**	**1**	**2**	**2**	**7**	**2**	**-**	**-**	**-**	**-**	**1**	**9**
1. Tuberculosis	**9**	**7**	**2**	**-**	**-**	**-**	**1**	**2**	**1**	**3**	**-**	**-**	**-**	**-**	**-**	**-**	**1**
2. STDs excluding HIV	-	-	-	-	-	-	-	-	-	-	-	-	-	-	-	-	-
a. Syphilis	-	-	-	-	-	-	-	-	-	-	-	-	-	-	-	-	-
b. Chlamydia	-	-	-	-	-	-	-	-	-	-	-	-	-	-	-	-	-
c. Gonorrhoea	-	-	-	-	-	-	-	-	-	-	-	-	-	-	-	-	-
3. HIV	**4**	**2**	**2**	**1**	**-**	**-**	**-**	**-**	**-**	**-**	**1**	**-**	**-**	**-**	**-**	**-**	**-**
4. Diarrhoeal diseases	**1**	**1**	**1**	**1**	**-**	**-**	**-**	**-**	**-**	**-**	**1**	**-**	**-**	**-**	**-**	**-**	**-**
5. Childhood-cluster diseases	-	-	-	-	-	-	-	-	-	-	-	-	-	-	-	-	-
a. Pertussis	-	-	-	-	-	-	-	-	-	-	-	-	-	-	-	-	-
b. Poliomyelitis	-	-	-	-	-	-	-	-	-	-	-	-	-	-	-	-	-
c. Diphtheria	-	-	-	-	-	-	-	-	-	-	-	-	-	-	-	-	-
d. Measles	-	-	-	-	-	-	-	-	-	-	-	-	-	-	-	-	-
e. Tetanus	-	-	-	-	-	-	-	-	-	-	-	-	-	-	-	-	-
6. Bacterial meningitis*	**3**	**2**	**1**	-	-	-	-	-	-	**1**	-	-	-	-	-	-	**1**
7. Hepatitis B and hepatitis C	**1**	**1**	**-**	-	-	-	-	-	-	-	-	-	-	-	-	-	-
8. Malaria	-	-	-	-	-	-	-	-	-	-	-	-	-	-	-	-	-
9. Tropical-cluster diseases	-	-	-	-	-	-	-	-	-	-	-	-	-	-	-	-	-
a. Trypanosomiasis	-	-	-	-	-	-	-	-	-	-	-	-	-	-	-	-	-
b. Chagas disease	-	-	-	-	-	-	-	-	-	-	-	-	-	-	-	-	-
c. Schistosomiasis	-	-	-	-	-	-	-	-	-	-	-	-	-	-	-	-	-
d. Leishmaniasis	-	-	-	-	-	-	-	-	-	-	-	-	-	-	-	-	-
10. Leprosy	-	-	-	-	-	-	-	-	-	-	-	-	-	-	-	-	-
11. Dengue	-	-	-	-	-	-	-	-	-	-	-	-	-	-	-	-	-
12. Japanese encephalitis	-	-	-	-	-	-	-	-	-	-	-	-	-	-	-	-	-
13. Trachoma	-	-	-	-	-	-	-	-	-	-	-	-	-	-	-	-	-
14. Intestinal nematode infections	-	-	-	-	-	-	-	-	-	-	-	-	-	-	-	-	-
a. Ascariasis	-	-	-	-	-	-	-	-	-	-	-	-	-	-	-	-	-
b. Trichuriasis	-	-	-	-	-	-	-	-	-	-	-	-	-	-	-	-	-
c. Ancylostomiasis, necatoriasis	-	-	-	-	-	-	-	-	-	-	-	-	-	-	-	-	-
15. Other infectious and parasitic	**11**	**4**	**7**	-	-	-	-	-	-	**3**	-	-	-	-	-	-	**6**

Annex Table 16b, continued. Deaths by age, sex and cause (thousands): Formerly Socialist Economies of Europe, 2020, baseline scenario

Cause	Total	Male	Female	Males 0-4	5-14	15-29	30-44	45-59	60-69	70+	Females 0-4	5-14	15-29	30-44	45-59	60-69	70+
B. Respiratory infections	93	41	53	3	-	-	-	-	2	34	2	-	-	-	-	1	49
1. Lower respiratory infections	93	40	52	3	-	-	-	-	2	33	2	-	-	-	-	1	48
2. Upper respiratory infections	-	-	-	-	-	-	-	-	-	-	-	-	-	-	-	-	-
3. Otitis media	-	-	-	-	-	-	-	-	-	-	-	-	-	-	-	-	-
C. Maternal conditions	-	-	-	-	-	-	-	-	-	-	-	-	-	-	-	-	-
1. Maternal haemorrhage	-	-	-	-	-	-	-	-	-	-	-	-	-	-	-	-	-
2. Maternal sepsis	-	-	-	-	-	-	-	-	-	-	-	-	-	-	-	-	-
3. Hypertensive disorders*	-	-	-	-	-	-	-	-	-	-	-	-	-	-	-	-	-
4. Obstructed labour	-	-	-	-	-	-	-	-	-	-	-	-	-	-	-	-	-
5. Abortion	-	-	-	-	-	-	-	-	-	-	-	-	-	-	-	-	-
6. Other maternal	-	-	-	-	-	-	-	-	-	-	-	-	-	-	-	-	-
D. Perinatal conditions*	11	7	4	7	-	-	-	-	-	-	4	-	-	-	-	-	-
E. Nutritional deficiencies	7	2	5	-	-	-	-	-	-	2	-	-	-	-	-	-	5
1. Protein-energy malnutrition	2	1	1	-	-	-	-	-	-	1	-	-	-	-	-	-	1
2. Iodine deficiency	-	-	-	-	-	-	-	-	-	-	-	-	-	-	-	-	-
3. Vitamin A deficiency	-	-	-	-	-	-	-	-	-	-	-	-	-	-	-	-	-
4. Iron-deficiency anaemia	4	1	2	-	-	-	-	-	-	1	-	-	-	-	-	-	2
II. Noncommunicable diseases	4 295	2 353	1 942	8	2	11	77	536	573	1 143	8	2	6	29	122	240	1 535
A. Malignant neoplasms	994	665	328	1	2	4	28	221	199	210	1	1	3	17	59	87	161
1. Mouth and oropharynx cancers	29	25	3	-	-	-	2	13	6	4	-	-	-	-	1	1	2
2. Oesophagus cancer	17	15	2	-	-	-	1	7	4	3	-	-	-	-	-	1	1
3. Stomach cancer	152	103	49	-	-	-	4	37	28	33	-	-	-	2	7	12	28
4. Colon and rectum cancers	99	56	43	-	-	-	2	15	15	24	-	-	-	1	6	10	26
5. Liver cancer	30	19	11	-	-	-	1	6	6	6	-	-	-	1	1	3	6
6. Pancreas cancer	43	28	15	-	-	-	-	10	8	8	-	-	-	-	2	4	9
7. Trachea, bronchus, lung cancers	277	233	44	-	-	-	8	76	83	65	-	-	-	1	9	15	19
8. Melanoma and other skin cancers	12	7	5	-	-	-	-	2	1	3	-	-	-	-	1	1	3
9. Breast cancer	41	-	41	-	-	-	-	-	-	-	-	-	-	4	12	11	15
10. Cervix uteri cancer	16	-	16	-	-	-	-	-	-	-	-	-	-	2	4	4	7
11. Corpus uteri cancer	14	-	14	-	-	-	-	-	-	-	-	-	-	1	3	4	7
12. Ovary cancer	16	-	16	-	-	-	-	-	-	-	-	-	-	1	5	5	5
13. Prostate cancer	26	26	-	-	-	-	-	3	6	18	-	-	-	-	-	-	-
14. Bladder cancer	26	21	4	-	-	-	-	5	6	10	-	-	-	-	-	-	3
15. Lymphomas, multiple myeloma	22	15	7	-	-	1	2	5	4	3	-	-	-	1	1	2	3
16. Leukaemia	25	16	9	-	1	-	1	5	4	4	-	1	-	1	1	2	3
17. Other cancers	148	101	47	-	1	2	6	37	27	29	-	1	1	2	7	11	24

Annex Table 16b, continued. Deaths by age, sex and cause (thousands): Formerly Socialist Economies of Europe, 2020, baseline scenario

				Males							Females						
Cause	Total	Male	Female	0-4	5-14	15-29	30-44	45-59	60-69	70+	0-4	5-14	15-29	30-44	45-59	60-69	70+
B. Other neoplasms	**6**	**3**	**3**					1	1	1					1	1	1
C. Diabetes mellitus	**29**	**10**	**19**				1	2	3	5					2	4	13
D. Endocrine disorders	**3**	**1**	**2**							1	1						1
E. Neuro-psychiatric conditions	**70**	**28**	**42**	1	1	1	3	4	4	14	1		1	1	2	3	34
2. Bipolar disorder	7	1	6							1							6
3. Schizophrenia	4	2	2			1				1							2
4. Epilepsy	5	3	2					1	1	1					1		1
5. Alcohol use	6	5	1				1	2	1	1							1
6. Dementia*	21	6	16					1	1	4					1	1	14
7. Parkinson disease	9	3	6							3						1	5
8. Multiple sclerosis	4	1	2							1							2
9. Drug use	-	-	-														
13. Other neuro-psychiatric	13	6	7	1		1		1	1	2	1				1	1	4
F. Sense organ diseases	**-**	**-**	**-**														
1. Glaucoma	-	-	-														
2. Cataracts	-	-	-														
G. Cardiovascular diseases	**2 608**	**1 274**	**1 334**	1		3	35	244	285	707			1	8	39	110	1 176
1. Rheumatic heart disease	24	13	10				2	7	3	1				1	3	3	3
2. Ischaemic heart disease	1 313	677	636			1	20	150	150	357				3	17	52	565
3. Cerebrovascular disease	791	346	446			1	6	53	81	205				2	15	40	388
4. Inflammatory heart diseases	47	26	21				2	8	4	11				1	1	1	17
5. Other cardiovascular	433	213	221	1		1	5	26	47	133			1	1	3	14	203
H. Respiratory diseases	**378**	**248**	**130**				3	33	54	158				1	8	18	102
1. COPD*	195	128	67				1	16	28	83					3	9	54
2. Asthma	16	8	9					1	2	4					1	2	6
3. Other respiratory	167	113	54				2	16	24	70				1	4	8	42
I. Digestive diseases	**146**	**90**	**56**			1	6	27	23	34				2	9	11	34
1. Peptic ulcer	18	13	5				1	4	3	5					1	1	4
2. Cirrhosis of the liver	61	41	20				3	15	12	12				1	5	5	9
3. Appendicitis	1	-	-														
4. Other digestive	66	35	31				2	8	7	16				1	3	5	21
J. Genito-urinary diseases	**41**	**24**	**18**			1	1	3	4	15				1	2	4	11
1. Nephritis and nephrosis	16	9	8				1	2	2	4				1	1	2	4
2. Benign prostatic hypertrophy	7	7	-						1	6							
3. Other genito-urinary	17	8	10					1	2	4				1	1	2	6
K. Skin diseases	**2**	**1**	**1**							1							1

Annex Table 16b, continued. Deaths by age, sex and cause (thousands): Formerly Socialist Economies of Europe, 2020, baseline scenario

Cause	Total	Male	Female	Males							Females						
				0-4	5-14	15-29	30-44	45-59	60-69	70+	0-4	5-14	15-29	30-44	45-59	60-69	70+
L. Musculo-skeletal diseases	4	1	3	-	-	-	-	-	-	-	-	-	-	-	1	1	1
1. Rheumatoid arthritis	1	-	1	-	-	-	-	-	-	-	-	-	-	-	-	-	1
3. Other musculo-skeletal	3	1	2	-	-	-	-	-	-	-	-	-	-	-	1	1	-
M. Congenital anomalies	15	8	6	7	-	-	-	-	-	-	6	-	-	-	-	-	-
N. Oral conditions	-	-	-	-	-	-	-	-	-	-	-	-	-	-	-	-	-
III. Injuries	*419*	*295*	*123*	*6*	*7*	*66*	*79*	*73*	*28*	*37*	*5*	*4*	*19*	*18*	*22*	*16*	*40*
A. Unintentional injuries	266	186	80	3	4	41	48	47	17	25	2	2	10	10	14	10	31
1. Road traffic accidents	116	83	33	1	2	28	21	16	6	8	1	1	8	5	6	4	8
2. Poisonings	41	30	11	-	-	2	9	12	4	2	1	-	1	2	3	2	2
3. Falls	35	18	17	-	-	1	3	4	2	8	-	-	1	1	1	-	14
4. Fires	8	5	3	-	-	1	1	1	1	1	-	-	1	-	1	-	1
5. Drownings	19	15	3	-	1	3	5	3	1	1	-	-	-	-	-	2	1
6. Other unintentional	48	36	12	1	1	6	10	11	4	4	1	1	-	2	2	2	4
B. Intentional injuries	153	109	44	3	2	25	31	26	10	12	3	1	8	8	8	6	10
1. Self-inflicted injuries	92	69	23	-	-	11	19	20	8	11	-	-	1	3	5	4	8
2. Violence	32	23	9	-	-	7	9	5	1	1	-	-	2	3	2	1	2
3. War	29	17	12	3	2	7	3	1	1	-	3	1	5	2	1	1	-

Notes:
Causes responsible for no deaths have been omitted from this table.
A dash (-) symbol indicates fewer than 500 deaths.
*IA6 is Bacterial meningitis and meningococcaemia; IC3 is Hypertensive disorders of pregnancy; ID is Conditions arising during the perinatal period; IIE6 is Dementia and other degenerative and hereditary CNS disorders; IIH1 is Chronic obstructive pulmonary disease.

Annex Table 16c. Deaths by age, sex and cause (thousands): India, 2020, baseline scenario

Cause	Total	Male	Female	Males							Females						
				0-4	5-14	15-29	30-44	45-59	60-69	70+	0-4	5-14	15-29	30-44	45-59	60-69	70+
Population (millions)	*1 227*	*621*	*606*	*52*	*104*	*160*	*147*	*101*	*36*	*21*	*50*	*99*	*151*	*139*	*100*	*40*	*27*
All causes	**11 430**	**6 515**	**4 915**	**506**	**102**	**282**	**591**	**1 616**	**1 509**	**1 909**	**469**	**92**	**231**	**305**	**776**	**808**	**2 235**
I. Communicable, maternal, perinatal and nutritional conditions	**2 461**	**1 402**	**1 059**	**348**	**25**	**96**	**218**	**263**	**151**	**301**	**332**	**28**	**84**	**123**	**149**	**78**	**265**
A. Infectious and parasitic diseases	**1 829**	**1 094**	**735**	**183**	**20**	**94**	**214**	**257**	**126**	**200**	**173**	**20**	**78**	**116**	**142**	**59**	**148**
1. Tuberculosis	**965**	**630**	**335**	9	6	46	108	217	103	142	6	5	33	47	122	43	78
2. STDs excluding HIV	21	9	12	5	-	-	-	-	-	4	5	-	-	1	-	1	5
a. Syphilis	20	9	11	5	-	-	-	-	-	4	5	-	-	1	-	1	5
b. Chlamydia																	
c. Gonorrhoea																	
3. HIV	**392**	**229**	**163**	28	5	45	100	33	11	6	30	5	42	67	13	4	2
4. Diarrhoeal diseases	**234**	**115**	**119**	78	2	1	2	2	5	25	75	3	1	1	2	5	32
5. Childhood-cluster diseases	**103**	**54**	**49**	46	3	1	1	1	1	2	41	3	3	1	1	1	3
a. Pertussis	16	8	8	8							7						
b. Poliomyelitis	2	1	1	1							1						
c. Diphtheria	1	1															
d. Measles	40	21	19	20	2						17	1	1				
e. Tetanus	44	23	21	17	1	1	1	1	1	2	15	1	1				3
6. Bacterial meningitis*	11	6	5	3	-	-	1	1	1	1	2	-	-	1	1	1	2
7. Hepatitis B and hepatitis C	7	3	3	-	-	-	1	1		2				1	1		2
8. Malaria	5	3	2	1	-	-	-	-	-	1	1	-	-	-	-	1	-
9. Tropical-cluster diseases	5	3	2	-	1	1						1					
a. Trypanosomiasis																	
b. Chagas disease																	
c. Schistosomiasis																	
d. Leishmaniasis	5	3	2	-	1	1						1					
10. Leprosy																	
11. Dengue	2	2	1	-	2	1						2	1				
12. Japanese encephalitis																	
13. Trachoma																	
14. Intestinal nematode infections	1	1			1							1					
a. Ascariasis	1	1															
b. Trichuriasis																	
c. Ancylostomiasis, necatoriasis	1	1															
15. Other infectious and parasitic	84	40	44	12	2	1	1	2	4	17	12	2	1	2	2	4	24

Annex Table 16c, continued. Deaths by age, sex and cause (thousands): India, 2020, baseline scenario

Cause	Total	Male	Female	Males							Females						
				0-4	5-14	15-29	30-44	45-59	60-69	70+	0-4	5-14	15-29	30-44	45-59	60-69	70+
B. Respiratory infections	**438**	**215**	**222**	**82**	**5**	**1**	**3**	**5**	**24**	**95**	**79**	**8**	**1**	**1**	**5**	**19**	**110**
1. Lower respiratory infections	431	212	219	80	4	1	3	5	24	94	77	8	1	1	5	18	108
2. Upper respiratory infections	4	2	2	1	–	–	–	–	–	1	1	–	–	–	–	–	1
3. Otitis media	2	1	1	1	–	–	–	–	–	–	1	–	–	–	–	–	–
C. Maternal conditions	**11**	**–**	**11**	–	–	–	–	–	–	–	–	–	5	5	1	–	–
1. Maternal haemorrhage	3	–	3	–	–	–	–	–	–	–	–	–	1	1	–	–	–
2. Maternal sepsis	2	–	2	–	–	–	–	–	–	–	–	–	1	1	–	–	–
3. Hypertensive disorders*	1	–	1	–	–	–	–	–	–	–	–	–	–	1	–	–	–
4. Obstructed labour	1	–	1	–	–	–	–	–	–	–	–	–	1	–	–	–	–
5. Abortion	2	–	2	–	–	–	–	–	–	–	–	–	1	1	–	–	–
6. Other maternal	3	–	3	–	–	–	–	–	–	–	–	–	1	1	–	–	–
D. Perinatal conditions*	**148**	**76**	**72**	**76**	–	–	–	–	–	–	**72**	–	–	–	–	–	–
E. Nutritional deficiencies	**35**	**16**	**19**	**8**	**1**	–	–	**1**	**1**	**6**	**8**	**1**	–	–	**1**	**1**	**8**
1. Protein-energy malnutrition	19	8	10	5	–	–	–	1	1	2	5	–	–	–	1	1	4
2. Iodine deficiency		1	–	–	–	–	–	–	–	–	–	–	–	–	–	–	–
3. Vitamin A deficiency	4	2	2	1	–	–	–	–	–	–	1	–	–	–	–	–	–
4. Iron-deficiency anaemia	11	5	6	1	–	–	–	–	–	3	1	–	–	–	–	–	4
II. Noncommunicable diseases	**7 627**	**4 322**	**3 305**	**102**	**20**	**35**	**183**	**1 157**	**1 296**	**1 530**	**97**	**17**	**41**	**92**	**512**	**672**	**1 874**
A. Malignant neoplasms	**1 301**	**756**	**545**	**4**	**5**	**14**	**58**	**304**	**173**	**197**	**3**	**2**	**20**	**42**	**199**	**124**	**156**
1. Mouth and oropharynx cancers	180	113	67	–	–	2	6	48	24	33	–	–	1	4	26	16	19
2. Oesophagus cancer	115	62	53	–	–	1	3	25	13	20	–	–	–	2	17	13	20
3. Stomach cancer	100	67	34	–	–	1	4	29	12	20	–	–	1	2	11	8	11
4. Colon and rectum cancers	46	25	21	–	–	1	3	8	5	8	–	–	1	1	6	5	8
5. Liver cancer	30	21	9	–	–	1	1	9	3	7	–	–	–	1	2	2	4
6. Pancreas cancer	17	11	7	–	–	–	1	4	2	3	–	–	–	–	–	2	3
7. Trachea, bronchus, lung cancers	280	240	40	–	–	1	18	109	79	33	–	–	–	2	15	13	10
8. Melanoma and other skin cancers	2	1	1	–	–	–	–	1	–	–	–	–	–	–	–	–	–
9. Breast cancer	69	–	69	–	–	–	–	–	–	–	–	–	4	7	29	14	16
10. Cervix uteri cancer	98	–	98	–	–	–	–	–	–	–	–	–	4	7	50	19	19
11. Corpus uteri cancer	7	–	7	–	–	–	–	–	–	–	–	–	–	–	2	2	3
12. Ovary cancer	24	–	24	–	–	–	–	–	–	–	–	–	1	3	7	6	7
13. Prostate cancer	27	27	–	–	–	–	–	3	5	19	–	–	–	–	–	–	–
14. Bladder cancer	16	13	3	–	–	–	–	3	3	6	–	–	–	–	1	–	–
15. Lymphomas, multiple myeloma	39	25	14	1	–	1	4	9	3	6	–	–	1	1	3	3	6
16. Leukaemia	28	17	11	1	2	1	4	4	2	3	1	1	1	2	3	1	2
17. Other cancers	222	136	86	2	2	5	15	51	22	39	1	1	4	9	26	19	26

Annex Table 16c, continued. Deaths by age, sex and cause (thousands): India, 2020, baseline scenario

Cause	Total	Male	Female	Males							Females						
				0-4	5-14	15-29	30-44	45-59	60-69	70+	0-4	5-14	15-29	30-44	45-59	60-69	70+
B. Other neoplasms	**4**	**3**	**2**	-	-	-	1	-	-	-	-	-	-	-	-	-	-
C. Diabetes mellitus	**114**	**47**	**67**	2	1	1	1	11	12	17	2	1	1	1	10	19	33
D. Endocrine disorders	**2**	**1**	**1**	-	-	-	-	-	-	-	-	-	-	-	-	-	-
E. Neuro-psychiatric conditions	**111**	**57**	**54**	7	1	2	8	10	11	19	7	1	2	2	3	10	28
2. Bipolar disorder	3	1	2	-	-	-	-	1	-	1	-	-	-	-	-	1	2
3. Schizophrenia	6	3	3	-	-	1	2	2	1	1	-	-	1	-	1	1	2
4. Epilepsy	11	7	4	1	1	1	2	2	1	1	1	-	1	1	1	-	1
5. Alcohol use	5	5	-	-	-	1	2	1	2	-	1	-	-	-	-	-	-
6. Dementia*	28	11	17	1	-	-	-	-	1	7	1	-	-	-	1	3	12
7. Parkinson disease	8	5	3	-	-	-	-	1	-	4	-	-	-	-	-	1	3
8. Multiple sclerosis	3	1	2	-	-	-	-	-	-	-	-	-	-	-	1	1	-
9. Drug use				6	-	-	-	-	-	5	6	1	-	-	1	4	-
13. Other neuro-psychiatric	46	24	22	4	1	1	3	4	5	5	-	1	1	1	1	-	8
F. Sense organ diseases	-	-	-	-	-	-	-	-	-	-	-	-	-	-	-	-	-
1. Glaucoma	-	-	-	-	-	-	-	-	-	-	-	-	-	-	-	-	-
2. Cataracts	-	-	-	-	-	-	-	-	-	-	-	-	-	-	-	-	-
G. Cardiovascular diseases	**4 774**	**2 669**	**2 105**	16	3	8	76	636	905	1 025	11	3	7	29	204	428	1 423
1. Rheumatic heart disease	110	61	49	-	-	2	11	31	12	4	-	-	2	9	21	9	8
2. Ischaemic heart disease	2 584	1 461	1 123	-	-	1	23	346	519	572	2	1	-	9	97	235	781
3. Cerebrovascular disease	945	511	434	3	1	1	8	96	178	224	2	-	1	4	30	92	305
4. Inflammatory heart diseases	144	84	59	3	1	2	8	33	18	20	-	1	1	3	13	9	30
5. Other cardiovascular	991	552	440	10	1	3	25	130	178	204	6	2	2	4	43	83	299
H. Respiratory diseases	**744**	**427**	**317**	4	3	2	10	85	137	185	3	3	4	7	59	65	176
1. COPD*	429	255	174	1	-	-	3	44	85	122	1	-	1	1	28	37	106
2. Asthma	55	30	25	-	-	-	2	7	7	12	-	-	-	1	6	5	12
3. Other respiratory	261	143	118	3	2	1	6	34	45	51	2	2	3	4	26	22	58
I. Digestive diseases	**323**	**231**	**92**	1	1	5	22	99	42	61	1	-	4	8	28	16	35
1. Peptic ulcer	59	40	20	-	-	1	3	14	9	14	-	-	2	1	5	3	9
2. Cirrhosis of the liver	204	153	51	-	-	3	12	69	28	41	-	-	1	4	17	8	20
3. Appendicitis	7	4	3	-	-	1	1	1	-	-	1	-	1	1	-	-	-
4. Other digestive	53	34	19	1	-	1	5	15	6	7	1	-	-	2	6	4	6
J. Genito-urinary diseases	**99**	**55**	**44**	2	2	1	3	10	14	22	1	3	1	2	7	9	20
1. Nephritis and nephrosis	86	43	43	2	2	1	3	10	10	15	1	3	1	2	7	9	20
2. Benign prostatic hypertrophy	11	11	-	-	-	-	-	-	4	7	-	-	-	-	-	-	-
3. Other genito-urinary	2	1	1	-	-	-	-	-	-	-	-	-	-	-	-	-	-
K. Skin diseases	**2**	**1**	**1**	-	-	-	-	-	-	-	-	-	-	-	-	-	-

Annex Table 16c, continued. Deaths by age, sex and cause (thousands): India, 2020, baseline scenario

Cause	Total	Male	Female	Males							Females						
				0-4	5-14	15-29	30-44	45-59	60-69	70+	0-4	5-14	15-29	30-44	45-59	60-69	70+
L. Musculo-skeletal diseases	**2**	**1**	**1**	–	–	–	–	–	–	–	–	–	–	–	–	–	–
1. Rheumatoid arthritis	2	1	1	–	–	–	–	–	–	1	–	–	–	–	1	–	–
3. Other musculo-skeletal	1	1	–	–	–	–	–	–	–	–	–	–	–	–	–	–	–
M. Congenital anomalies	**150**	**74**	**76**	66	2	2	2	1	–	1	68	2	1	1	2	1	1
N. Oral conditions	–	–	–	–	–	–	–	–	–	–	–	–	–	–	–	–	–
III. Injuries	**1 342**	**791**	**550**	56	58	151	190	196	62	79	40	46	106	89	114	58	96
A. Unintentional injuries	**1 085**	**644**	**441**	51	53	113	149	155	54	68	34	42	68	66	90	50	90
1. Road traffic accidents	546	377	168	14	32	85	89	93	30	33	4	25	21	24	42	22	30
2. Poisonings	31	16	15	3	1	2	5	3	1	1	2	1	3	3	4	1	1
3. Falls	64	38	26	5	1	2	6	10	5	9	–	1	1	2	5	2	14
4. Fires	141	43	98	5	1	6	11	11	5	4	9	4	29	23	14	8	11
5. Drownings	83	42	41	8	6	6	9	6	3	4	6	5	5	5	7	3	9
6. Other unintentional	222	127	94	16	9	11	29	32	12	17	13	6	9	9	18	14	25
B. Intentional injuries	**257**	**148**	**109**	5	5	38	41	41	8	10	6	4	38	23	25	7	6
1. Self-inflicted injuries	163	90	73	–	3	27	25	26	4	5	–	3	34	21	12	1	2
2. Violence	90	53	36	5	2	8	14	14	5	5	6	1	3	3	13	6	2
3. War	5	5	–	–	–	3	2	–	–	–	–	–	–	–	–	–	–

Notes:
Causes responsible for no deaths have been omitted from this table.
A dash (-) symbol indicates fewer than 500 deaths.
*IA6 is Bacterial meningitis and meningococcaemia; IC3 is Hypertensive disorders of pregnancy; ID is Conditions arising during the perinatal period; IIE6 is Dementia and other degenerative and hereditary CNS disorders; IIH1 is Chronic obstructive pulmonary disease.

Annex Table 16d. Deaths by age, sex and cause (thousands): China, 2020, baseline scenario

Cause	Total	Male	Female	Males 0-4	5-14	15-29	30-44	45-59	60-69	70+	Females 0-4	5-14	15-29	30-44	45-59	60-69	70+
Population (millions)	*1 469*	*737*	*733*	*56*	*103*	*169*	*150*	*163*	*61*	*35*	*54*	*98*	*160*	*143*	*161*	*69*	*48*
All causes	*13 938*	*8 204*	*5 734*	*150*	*41*	*190*	*399*	*2 046*	*2 199*	*3 179*	*152*	*30*	*145*	*187*	*791*	*1 038*	*3 391*
I. Communicable, maternal, perinatal and nutritional conditions	*540*	*285*	*255*	*62*	*1*	*2*	*4*	*15*	*24*	*177*	*64*	*2*	*2*	*3*	*9*	*17*	*158*
A. Infectious and parasitic diseases	239	136	103	11	1	1	3	14	19	87	10	1	1	2	8	12	69
1. Tuberculosis	141	87	54	-	-	-	1	10	14	61	-	-	-	1	6	9	38
2. STDs excluding HIV	-	-	-	-	-	-	-	-	-	-	-	-	-	-	-	-	-
a. Syphilis	-	-	-	-	-	-	-	-	-	-	-	-	-	-	-	-	-
b. Chlamydia	-	-	-	-	-	-	-	-	-	-	-	-	-	-	-	-	-
c. Gonorrhoea	-	-	-	-	-	-	-	-	-	-	-	-	-	-	-	-	-
3. HIV	5	3	2	-	-	-	1	1	-	-	-	-	1	1	-	-	-
4. Diarrhoeal diseases	42	19	23	4	-	-	-	-	2	13	4	-	1	1	-	1	17
5. Childhood-cluster diseases	9	5	4	4	-	-	-	-	-	-	3	-	-	-	-	-	-
a. Pertussis	3	1	1	1	-	-	-	-	-	-	1	-	-	-	-	-	-
b. Poliomyelitis	-	-	-	-	-	-	-	-	-	-	-	-	-	-	-	-	-
c. Diphtheria	-	-	-	-	-	-	-	-	-	-	-	-	-	-	-	-	-
d. Measles	2	1	1	1	-	-	-	-	-	-	1	-	-	-	-	-	-
e. Tetanus	3	2	1	1	-	-	-	-	-	-	1	-	-	-	-	-	-
6. Bacterial meningitis*	11	5	5	1	-	-	-	1	1	2	1	-	-	-	1	1	2
7. Hepatitis B and hepatitis C	13	7	5	-	-	-	-	1	1	4	-	-	-	-	-	1	4
8. Malaria	-	-	-	-	-	-	-	-	-	-	-	-	-	-	-	-	-
9. Tropical-cluster diseases	1	1	-	-	-	-	-	-	-	-	-	-	-	-	-	-	-
a. Trypanosomiasis	-	-	-	-	-	-	-	-	-	-	-	-	-	-	-	-	-
b. Chagas disease	-	-	-	-	-	-	-	-	-	-	-	-	-	-	-	-	-
c. Schistosomiasis	1	1	-	-	-	-	-	-	-	-	-	-	-	-	-	-	-
d. Leishmaniasis	-	-	-	-	-	-	-	-	-	-	-	-	-	-	-	-	-
10. Leprosy	-	-	-	-	-	-	-	-	-	-	-	-	-	-	-	-	-
11. Dengue	-	-	-	-	-	-	-	-	-	-	-	-	-	-	-	-	-
12. Japanese encephalitis	-	-	-	-	-	-	-	-	-	-	-	-	-	-	-	-	-
13. Trachoma	-	-	-	-	-	-	-	-	-	-	-	-	-	-	-	-	-
14. Intestinal nematode infections	1	1	-	-	-	-	-	-	-	-	-	-	-	-	-	-	-
a. Ascariasis	-	-	-	-	-	-	-	-	-	-	-	-	-	-	-	-	-
b. Trichuriasis	-	-	-	-	-	-	-	-	-	-	-	-	-	-	-	-	-
c. Ancylostomiasis, necatoriasis	-	-	-	-	-	-	-	-	-	-	-	-	-	-	-	-	-
15. Other infectious and parasitic	17	9	9	-	-	-	-	1	1	6	-	-	-	-	-	1	7

Annex Table 16d, continued. Deaths by age, sex and cause (thousands): China, 2020, baseline scenario

Age-group columns are grouped under **Males** (0-4, 5-14, 15-29, 30-44, 45-59, 60-69, 70+) and **Females** (0-4, 5-14, 15-29, 30-44, 45-59, 60-69, 70+). ("·" and "-" denote negligible or not-applicable values as printed.)

Cause	Total	Male	Female	M 0-4	M 5-14	M 15-29	M 30-44	M 45-59	M 60-69	M 70+	F 0-4	F 5-14	F 15-29	F 30-44	F 45-59	F 60-69	F 70+
B. Respiratory infections	**225**	**113**	**112**	**23**	-	-	-	**1**	**4**	**82**	**25**	**1**	-	-	**1**	**4**	**82**
1. Lower respiratory infections	222	112	110	22	-	-	-	1	4	83	24	-	-	-	1	4	81
2. Upper respiratory infections	2	2	1	-	-	-	-	-	-	1	-	-	-	-	-	-	1
3. Otitis media	-	-	1	-	-	-	-	-	-	-	-	-	-	-	-	-	-
C. Maternal conditions	**2**	-	**2**	-	-	-	-	-	-	-	-	-	**1**	**1**	-	-	-
1. Maternal haemorrhage	1	-	1	-	-	-	-	-	-	-	-	-	1	-	-	-	-
2. Maternal sepsis	-	-	-	-	-	-	-	-	-	-	-	-	-	-	-	-	-
3. Hypertensive disorders*	-	-	-	-	-	-	-	-	-	-	-	-	-	-	-	-	-
4. Obstructed labour	-	-	-	-	-	-	-	-	-	-	-	-	-	-	-	-	-
5. Abortion	-	-	-	-	-	-	-	-	-	-	-	-	-	-	-	-	-
6. Other maternal	1	-	1	-	-	-	-	-	-	-	-	-	-	1	-	-	-
D. Perinatal conditions*	**49**	**25**	**25**	**25**	-	-	-	-	-	-	**25**	-	-	-	-	-	-
E. Nutritional deficiencies	**25**	**11**	**14**	**5**	-	-	-	-	-	**6**	**5**	-	-	-	-	**1**	**8**
1. Protein-energy malnutrition	14	6	7	3	-	-	-	-	-	4	3	-	-	-	-	-	4
2. Iodine deficiency	1	-	1	-	-	-	-	-	-	-	1	-	-	-	-	-	-
3. Vitamin A deficiency	1	1	1	1	-	-	-	-	-	-	1	-	-	-	-	-	-
4. Iron-deficiency anaemia	9	3	6	-	-	-	-	-	-	2	-	-	-	-	-	1	4
II. Noncommunicable diseases	**11 890**	**7 111**	**4 779**	**48**	**15**	**50**	**257**	**1 847**	**2 062**	**2 832**	**50**	**8**	**29**	**110**	**635**	**928**	**3 019**
A. Malignant neoplasms	**3 583**	**2 444**	**1 139**	**4**	**9**	**23**	**163**	**933**	**761**	**551**	**6**	**4**	**14**	**63**	**306**	**337**	**410**
1. Mouth and oropharynx cancers	83	60	22	-	1	1	9	23	16	12	-	-	1	2	8	7	5
2. Oesophagus cancer	467	333	134	-	-	1	11	106	113	102	-	-	1	1	26	53	53
3. Stomach cancer	780	545	235	-	-	1	16	188	185	155	-	-	1	11	50	73	100
4. Colon and rectum cancers	193	115	78	-	-	2	8	36	33	36	-	-	1	4	20	23	30
5. Liver cancer	718	550	167	-	1	4	70	261	134	80	-	1	1	11	52	46	56
6. Pancreas cancer	77	50	28	-	-	-	2	14	17	17	-	-	-	3	4	10	13
7. Trachea, bronchus, lung cancers	677	507	170	-	-	2	19	208	195	83	-	-	-	3	48	55	63
8. Melanoma and other skin cancers	3	2	1	-	-	-	-	1	-	1	-	-	-	-	-	-	1
9. Breast cancer	52	-	52	-	-	-	-	-	-	-	-	-	1	7	19	11	14
10. Cervix uteri cancer	44	-	44	-	-	-	-	-	-	-	-	-	-	3	15	13	13
11. Corpus uteri cancer	13	-	13	-	-	-	-	-	-	-	-	-	-	1	3	4	5
12. Ovary cancer	20	-	20	-	-	-	-	-	-	-	-	-	1	2	7	4	5
13. Prostate cancer	12	12	-	-	-	-	-	1	5	5	-	-	-	-	-	-	-
14. Bladder cancer	45	37	9	-	-	-	1	7	14	15	-	-	-	1	1	3	4
15. Lymphomas, multiple myeloma	50	34	15	-	-	2	1	12	12	7	-	-	-	1	6	3	5
16. Leukaemia	105	59	46	2	5	6	10	21	8	7	3	2	5	8	12	7	9
17. Other cancers	245	141	105	1	2	4	15	57	30	31	3	2	2	9	31	25	33

Annex Table 16d, continued. Deaths by age, sex and cause (thousands): China, 2020, baseline scenario

Cause	Total	Male	Female	Males							Females						
				0-4	5-14	15-29	30-44	45-59	60-69	70+	0-4	5-14	15-29	30-44	45-59	60-69	70+
B. Other neoplasms	19	9	10	1	-	1	1	3	3	2	1	-	-	-	2	3	4
C. Diabetes mellitus	70	26	43	-	-	-	2	6	7	11	-	-	-	1	6	13	24
D. Endocrine disorders	14	5	9	1	-	-	-	1	1	2	1	-	-	-	1	1	6
E. Neuro-psychiatric conditions	96	42	54	2	1	5	6	6	5	18	1	-	2	3	5	7	35
2. Bipolar disorder	3	1	3	-	-	-	-	-	-	-	-	-	-	-	-	-	2
3. Schizophrenia	12	8	5	-	-	1	2	1	1	3	-	-	1	1	1	1	2
4. Epilepsy	8	4	4	-	-	1	1	1	-	1	-	-	1	1	1	-	1
5. Alcohol use	4	3	-	-	-	1	1	1	-	-	-	-	-	-	-	-	-
6. Dementia*	37	12	25	-	-	-	-	-	2	8	-	-	-	-	-	3	20
7. Parkinson disease	8	3	4	-	-	-	-	-	-	3	-	-	-	-	-	-	4
8. Multiple sclerosis	5	2	3	-	-	-	-	1	1	-	-	-	-	-	1	1	1
9. Drug use	-	-	-	-	-	-	-	-	-	-	-	-	-	-	-	-	-
13. Other neuro-psychiatric	19	9	10	1	-	3	1	1	1	2	1	-	1	1	1	1	5
F. Sense organ diseases	19	9	10	1	-	-	-	3	3	3	1	-	-	-	2	3	4
1. Glaucoma	7	3	4	-	-	-	-	1	1	1	-	-	-	-	1	1	2
2. Cataracts	6	3	3	-	-	-	-	1	1	1	-	-	-	-	1	1	1
G. Cardiovascular diseases	4 533	2 654	1 879	7	1	9	51	611	757	1 218	3	-	5	24	158	278	1 410
1. Rheumatic heart disease	238	125	113	-	1	3	8	41	28	45	-	-	2	6	21	18	67
2. Ischaemic heart disease	1 372	781	591	2	-	2	17	172	216	375	-	-	1	7	39	84	460
3. Cerebrovascular disease	2 288	1 368	920	1	1	2	20	305	416	622	1	-	-	8	81	149	680
4. Inflammatory heart diseases	97	59	38	-	-	1	4	22	11	11	1	-	-	2	6	4	24
5. Other cardiovascular	539	321	217	4	-	1	3	70	86	157	1	-	1	1	10	23	180
H. Respiratory diseases	2 795	1 490	1 305	3	1	3	11	179	429	864	3	-	1	9	106	232	953
1. COPD*	2 639	1 405	1 234	1	-	2	8	166	410	818	2	-	-	7	99	221	904
2. Asthma	61	34	27	-	-	1	2	9	9	14	-	-	1	1	6	6	13
3. Other respiratory	95	51	44	2	-	-	1	5	10	32	1	-	-	1	2	5	36
I. Digestive diseases	516	309	208	2	1	2	17	91	80	115	3	1	2	6	40	38	119
1. Peptic ulcer	49	28	22	-	-	-	1	5	6	16	-	-	-	-	2	3	16
2. Cirrhosis of the liver	243	161	83	-	-	1	13	60	47	40	-	-	-	3	23	21	35
3. Appendicitis	5	3	3	-	-	1	1	-	-	-	-	-	-	1	1	-	-
4. Other digestive	218	117	101	2	-	1	3	26	26	59	3	-	2	2	15	14	67
J. Genito-urinary diseases	122	66	56	1	-	4	5	12	12	31	1	-	-	3	8	13	30
1. Nephritis and nephrosis	93	49	44	1	-	3	5	10	10	19	1	-	-	2	7	10	22
2. Benign prostatic hypertrophy	7	7	-	-	-	-	-	-	-	7	-	-	-	-	-	-	-
3. Other genito-urinary	22	10	12	-	-	-	-	2	2	6	-	-	-	-	2	3	7
K. Skin diseases	12	7	5	-	-	-	-	1	1	5	-	-	-	-	-	1	3

Annex Table 16d, continued. Deaths by age, sex and cause (thousands): China, 2020, baseline scenario

Cause	Total	Male	Female	Males							Females						
				0-4	5-14	15-29	30-44	45-59	60-69	70+	0-4	5-14	15-29	30-44	45-59	60-69	70+
L. Musculo-skeletal diseases	**44**	**18**	**27**	-	-	-	-	1	4	12	-	-	-	1	2	3	21
1. Rheumatoid arthritis	2	1	1	-	-	-	-	-	-	1	-	-	-	-	-	-	1
3. Other musculo-skeletal	42	17	25	-	-	-	-	1	4	11	-	-	-	1	2	2	20
M. Congenital anomalies	**65**	**32**	**33**	28	1	-	-	-	-	-	29	1	2	-	-	-	-
N. Oral conditions	**-**	-	-	-	-	-	-	-	-	-	-	-	-	-	-	-	-
III. Injuries	***1 508***	***809***	***699***	*40*	*24*	*138*	*138*	*184*	*113*	*170*	*38*	*20*	*115*	*74*	*146*	*92*	*214*
A. Unintentional injuries	**911**	**524**	**387**	36	21	88	85	117	65	113	30	17	42	28	77	50	144
1. Road traffic accidents	409	270	139	4	10	59	54	67	36	40	3	11	30	17	40	18	20
2. Poisonings	74	40	34	2	-	3	5	13	5	11	1	1	4	4	6	5	13
3. Falls	119	40	79	1	-	2	3	6	6	20	1	1	4	1	8	11	53
4. Fires	35	16	19	1	-	1	1	2	1	10	1	-	-	-	3	3	12
5. Drownings	101	55	46	15	7	8	5	6	4	11	12	3	-	2	5	5	19
6. Other unintentional	173	103	70	13	2	15	17	23	13	21	12	1	3	4	15	7	27
B. Intentional injuries	**597**	**284**	**313**	4	4	51	54	67	48	57	8	3	73	46	69	43	70
1. Self-inflicted injuries	534	248	286	-	3	38	45	61	44	56	-	2	71	42	65	40	67
2. Violence	62	36	26	4	1	12	9	6	3	1	8	1	2	5	4	3	3
3. War	1	-	-	-	-	-	-	-	-	-	-	-	-	-	-	-	-

Notes:
Causes responsible for no deaths have been omitted from this table.
A dash (-) symbol indicates fewer than 500 deaths.
*IA6 is Bacterial meningitis and meningococcaemia; IC3 is Hypertensive disorders of pregnancy; ID is Conditions arising during the perinatal period; IIE6 is Dementia and other degenerative and hereditary CNS disorders; IIH1 is Chronic obstructive pulmonary disease.

Annex Table 16e. Deaths by age, sex and cause (thousands): Other Asia and Islands, 2020, baseline scenario

Cause	Total	Male	Female	Males							Females						
				0-4	5-14	15-29	30-44	45-59	60-69	70+	0-4	5-14	15-29	30-44	45-59	60-69	70+
Population (millions)	*1 024*	*508*	*516*	*44*	*84*	*124*	*118*	*86*	*33*	*20*	*42*	*81*	*121*	*116*	*91*	*39*	*27*
All causes	**7 736**	**4 418**	**3 318**	**341**	**93**	**199**	**408**	**931**	**888**	**1 557**	**254**	**60**	**114**	**199**	**419**	**532**	**1 740**
I. Communicable, maternal, perinatal and nutritional conditions	**1 105**	**587**	**518**	**229**	**15**	**26**	**54**	**42**	**51**	**169**	**165**	**12**	**27**	**43**	**36**	**36**	**198**
A. Infectious and parasitic diseases	**670**	**361**	**309**	**112**	**9**	**25**	**53**	**39**	**32**	**91**	**80**	**8**	**23**	**38**	**31**	**26**	**102**
1. Tuberculosis	**230**	**113**	**117**	-	-	2	4	18	21	67	-	-	1	3	18	20	75
2. STDs excluding HIV	**19**	**10**	**10**	5	-	-	-	-	-	4	3	-	-	-	-	-	5
a. Syphilis	19	10	9	5	-	-	-	-	-	4	3	-	-	-	-	-	5
b. Chlamydia	-	-	-	-	-	-	-	-	-	-	-	-	-	-	-	-	-
c. Gonorrhoea	-	-	-	-	-	-	-	-	-	-	-	-	-	-	-	-	-
3. HIV	**177**	**103**	**74**	13	2	20	45	15	5	3	8	1	21	33	7	2	1
4. Diarrhoeal diseases	**117**	**68**	**50**	58	2	-	-	1	2	5	39	1	-	-	1	1	7
5. Childhood-cluster diseases	**61**	**33**	**28**	28	2	-	1	1	-	1	23	2	1	1	1	1	2
a. Pertussis	9	5	4	5	-	-	-	-	-	-	4	-	-	-	-	-	-
b. Poliomyelitis	1	1	-	1	-	-	-	-	-	-	-	-	-	-	-	-	-
c. Diphtheria	1	-	-	-	-	-	-	-	-	-	-	-	-	-	-	-	-
d. Measles	29	16	13	15	1	-	-	-	-	-	12	1	-	-	-	-	-
e. Tetanus	21	11	10	7	1	-	1	1	-	1	6	-	-	-	-	-	2
6. Bacterial meningitis*	**9**	**5**	**5**	2	-	-	1	1	1	1	1	-	-	-	1	1	1
7. Hepatitis B and hepatitis C	**11**	**6**	**5**	-	-	-	-	1	1	3	-	-	-	-	1	-	3
8. Malaria	**19**	**10**	**9**	2	2	1	1	2	1	1	1	1	1	1	2	1	2
9. Tropical-cluster diseases	**1**	**1**	-	-	-	-	-	-	-	-	-	-	-	-	-	-	-
a. Trypanosomiasis	-	-	-	-	-	-	-	-	-	-	-	-	-	-	-	-	-
b. Chagas disease	-	-	-	-	-	-	-	-	-	-	-	-	-	-	-	-	-
c. Schistosomiasis	-	-	-	-	-	-	-	-	-	-	-	-	-	-	-	-	-
d. Leishmaniasis	-	-	1	-	-	-	-	-	-	-	-	-	-	-	-	-	-
10. Leprosy	-	-	-	-	-	-	-	-	-	-	-	-	-	-	-	-	-
11. Dengue	**1**	**1**	**1**	-	-	-	-	-	-	-	-	-	-	-	-	-	-
12. Japanese encephalitis	-	-	-	-	-	-	-	-	-	-	-	-	-	-	-	-	-
13. Trachoma	-	-	-	-	-	-	-	-	-	-	-	-	-	-	-	-	-
14. Intestinal nematode infections	**2**	**1**	**1**	-	-	-	-	-	-	-	-	-	-	-	-	-	-
a. Ascariasis	1	1	1	-	-	-	-	-	-	-	-	-	-	-	-	-	-
b. Trichuriasis	-	-	-	-	-	-	-	-	-	-	-	-	-	-	-	-	-
c. Ancylostomiasis, necatoriasis	1	-	-	-	-	-	-	-	-	-	-	-	-	-	-	-	-
15. Other infectious and parasitic	**21**	**11**	**10**	4	1	2	1	-	-	5	3	-	-	-	-	-	6

Annex Table 16e, continued. Deaths by age, sex and cause (thousands): Other Asia and Islands, 2020, baseline scenario

Cause	Total	Male	Female	Males							Females						
				0-4	5-14	15-29	30-44	45-59	60-69	70+	0-4	5-14	15-29	30-44	45-59	60-69	70+
B. Respiratory infections	302	156	146	54	5	1	1	3	18	74	37	4	1	1	3	9	91
1. Lower respiratory infections	298	154	144	53	5	1	1	3	18	73	36	4	1	1	3	9	90
2. Upper respiratory infections	3	2	1	1	–	–	–	–	–	1	–	–	–	–	–	–	1
3. Otitis media	1	–	–	–	–	–	–	–	–	–	–	–	–	–	–	–	–
C. Maternal conditions	7	–	7	–	–	–	–	–	–	–	–	–	3	4	–	–	–
1. Maternal haemorrhage	2	–	2	–	–	–	–	–	–	–	–	–	1	1	–	–	–
2. Maternal sepsis	1	–	1	–	–	–	–	–	–	–	–	–	–	1	–	–	–
3. Hypertensive disorders*	1	–	1	–	–	–	–	–	–	–	–	–	–	1	–	–	–
4. Obstructed labour	1	–	1	–	–	–	–	–	–	–	–	–	1	–	–	–	–
5. Abortion	1	–	1	–	–	–	–	–	–	–	–	–	1	–	–	–	–
6. Other maternal	2	–	2	–	–	–	–	–	–	–	–	–	1	1	–	–	–
D. Perinatal conditions*	97	56	41	56	–	–	–	–	–	–	41	–	–	–	–	–	–
E. Nutritional deficiencies	28	14	14	8	1	–	–	1	1	4	7	1	–	–	1	–	5
1. Protein-energy malnutrition	13	7	6	6	–	–	–	–	–	1	5	–	–	–	–	–	1
2. Iodine deficiency	–	–	–	–	–	–	–	–	–	–	–	–	–	–	–	–	–
3. Vitamin A deficiency	4	2	2	2	–	–	–	–	–	–	2	–	–	–	–	–	–
4. Iron-deficiency anaemia	10	5	6	–	1	–	–	1	–	3	–	1	–	–	1	–	4
II. Noncommunicable diseases	5 810	3 275	2 535	72	43	35	207	777	795	1 346	56	28	27	105	340	468	1 512
A. Malignant neoplasms	1 627	984	643	6	16	9	75	292	274	313	7	9	11	51	156	178	230
1. Mouth and oropharynx cancers	176	112	63	–	–	1	8	18	39	45	–	–	–	4	7	22	30
2. Oesophagus cancer	60	43	17	–	–	1	–	14	13	15	–	–	–	1	4	5	7
3. Stomach cancer	150	101	49	–	–	–	6	35	28	32	–	–	1	1	14	13	20
4. Colon and rectum cancers	104	56	48	–	–	1	6	9	19	22	–	–	–	2	11	15	22
5. Liver cancer	174	133	42	–	1	2	12	58	28	32	–	1	1	2	9	12	16
6. Pancreas cancer	26	16	9	–	–	–	1	5	5	6	–	–	–	–	2	3	4
7. Trachea, bronchus, lung cancers	291	219	71	–	–	1	13	84	56	66	–	–	–	8	13	24	26
8. Melanoma and other skin cancers	6	2	3	–	–	–	–	1	1	–	–	–	–	–	1	1	1
9. Breast cancer	62	–	62	–	–	–	–	–	–	–	–	–	–	5	23	18	17
10. Cervix uteri cancer	74	–	74	–	–	–	–	–	–	–	–	–	2	7	31	14	20
11. Corpus uteri cancer	10	–	10	–	–	–	–	–	–	–	–	–	–	–	3	3	4
12. Ovary cancer	22	–	22	–	–	–	–	–	–	–	–	–	–	2	5	9	6
13. Prostate cancer	35	35	–	–	–	–	–	3	15	17	–	–	–	–	–	–	–
14. Bladder cancer	29	22	8	–	–	–	–	5	8	9	–	–	–	–	1	4	3
15. Lymphomas, multiple myeloma	56	33	22	1	2	1	5	6	8	10	–	1	1	2	2	6	10
16. Leukaemia	51	29	22	2	3	1	6	3	5	6	3	3	1	3	2	4	6
17. Other cancers	303	182	121	2	7	2	19	50	49	53	3	4	3	14	28	31	38

Annex Table 16e, continued. Deaths by age, sex and cause (thousands): Other Asia and Islands, 2020, baseline scenario

Cause	Total	Male	Female	Males							Females						
				0-4	5-14	15-29	30-44	45-59	60-69	70+	0-4	5-14	15-29	30-44	45-59	60-69	70+
B. Other neoplasms	**10**	**5**	**5**	1	-	-	-	1	1	1	-	-	-	-	1	1	2
C. Diabetes mellitus	**89**	**35**	**54**	-	-	-	2	8	9	14	-	-	-	1	7	15	30
D. Endocrine disorders	**10**	**4**	**6**	1	-	-	-	1	1	1	1	-	-	1	1	1	3
E. Neuro-psychiatric conditions	**92**	**47**	**44**	2	1	3	7	9	7	17	2	1	1	2	4	7	28
2. Bipolar disorder	3	1	2	-	-	-	-	-	-	-	-	-	-	-	-	-	2
3. Schizophrenia	9	4	5	-	-	-	-	1	1	1	-	-	1	-	-	1	3
4. Epilepsy	8	5	3	-	-	1	2	1	1	1	-	-	-	1	-	1	1
5. Alcohol use	7	6	1	-	-	-	2	3	2	1	-	-	-	-	-	-	-
6. Dementia*	31	12	19	-	-	-	-	1	2	8	-	-	-	-	1	3	15
7. Parkinson disease	7	4	3	-	-	-	-	-	1	3	-	-	-	-	-	1	2
8. Multiple sclerosis	3	1	2	-	-	-	-	-	-	-	-	-	1	-	1	-	-
9. Drug use	1	1	-	-	-	-	1	-	-	-	-	-	1	1	-	-	-
13. Other neuro-psychiatric	23	12	10	1	1	1	2	2	1	3	1	1	-	1	1	1	4
F. Sense organ diseases	-	-	-	-	-	-	-	-	-	-	-	-	-	-	-	-	-
1. Glaucoma	-	-	-	-	-	-	-	-	-	-	-	-	-	-	-	-	-
2. Cataracts	-	-	-	-	-	-	-	-	-	-	-	-	-	-	-	-	-
G. Cardiovascular diseases	**2 782**	**1 490**	**1 292**	28	17	16	83	293	353	699	18	11	9	34	103	176	942
1. Rheumatic heart disease	20	10	10	-	-	-	1	2	2	5	-	-	-	1	1	1	7
2. Ischaemic heart disease	1 082	576	506	-	-	4	26	103	146	300	-	2	1	10	33	72	391
3. Cerebrovascular disease	852	439	413	4	4	4	18	83	117	210	3	2	2	7	34	62	304
4. Inflammatory heart diseases	108	65	44	5	4	3	10	18	8	17	4	6	6	4	6	4	22
5. Other cardiovascular	720	401	319	19	9	9	28	87	81	168	11	6	6	12	29	37	219
H. Respiratory diseases	**419**	**235**	**184**	5	2	2	6	24	41	155	2	2	2	4	16	30	128
1. COPD*	247	143	104	1	-	1	1	12	25	102	-	1	1	1	7	17	77
2. Asthma	49	24	24	-	-	1	3	4	4	11	1	-	1	2	5	5	12
3. Other respiratory	123	68	56	3	2	1	2	7	11	42	2	1	1	1	4	7	40
I. Digestive diseases	**571**	**378**	**193**	3	2	2	28	134	96	114	2	2	2	9	41	43	95
1. Peptic ulcer	50	31	19	-	-	-	1	7	8	16	-	-	-	-	2	3	13
2. Cirrhosis of the liver	250	188	63	-	-	1	17	83	48	38	-	-	1	4	19	17	22
3. Appendicitis	6	4	2	-	-	1	1	1	-	-	-	1	-	1	-	-	-
4. Other digestive	264	155	109	2	1	1	8	43	40	60	2	1	1	4	19	22	60
J. Genito-urinary diseases	**138**	**60**	**78**	1	2	1	4	11	12	29	1	1	1	2	10	16	46
1. Nephritis and nephrosis	119	51	67	1	2	1	4	10	10	23	1	1	1	2	9	14	40
2. Benign prostatic hypertrophy	1	1	-	-	-	-	-	-	1	-	-	-	-	-	-	-	-
3. Other genito-urinary	19	8	10	-	-	-	-	1	1	4	-	1	-	-	1	2	7
K. Skin diseases	**3**	**1**	**2**	-	-	-	-	-	-	1	-	-	-	-	-	-	1

Annex Table 16e, continued. Deaths by age, sex and cause (thousands): Other Asia and Islands, 2020, baseline scenario

Cause	Total	Male	Female	Males							Females						
				0-4	5-14	15-29	30-44	45-59	60-69	70+	0-4	5-14	15-29	30-44	45-59	60-69	70+
L. Musculo-skeletal diseases	12	4	8	-	-	-	-	1	1	2	-	-	-	-	1	1	5
1. Rheumatoid arthritis	1	-	1	-	-	-	-	-	-	-	-	-	-	-	-	1	-
3. Other musculo-skeletal	11	4	7	-	-	-	-	1	1	2	-	-	-	-	1	1	5
M. Congenital anomalies	56	30	26	25	1	1	1	1	-	-	22	1	1	-	1	1	1
N. Oral conditions	-	-	-	-	-	-	-	-	-	-	-	-	-	-	-	-	-
III. Injuries	*822*	*556*	*265*	*39*	*36*	*138*	*147*	*112*	*42*	*42*	*33*	*20*	*60*	*51*	*43*	*27*	*30*
A. Unintentional injuries	596	401	195	37	31	94	99	79	31	30	30	17	35	32	33	22	25
1. Road traffic accidents	283	192	92	13	15	54	47	35	14	13	11	9	19	16	16	11	10
2. Poisonings	45	24	21	2	1	4	6	6	3	2	1	1	6	4	4	3	3
3. Falls	45	32	13	1	1	4	9	9	3	4	2	-	1	2	3	2	4
4. Fires	11	6	4	2	-	1	1	1	-	1	1	-	1	1	1	-	1
5. Drownings	65	45	21	12	8	8	7	5	2	3	7	3	3	2	2	1	2
6. Other unintentional	146	103	43	7	5	22	30	23	8	7	7	3	7	8	8	5	6
B. Intentional injuries	226	155	71	3	5	44	48	32	11	12	3	3	25	19	10	5	6
1. Self-inflicted injuries	117	72	45	-	2	21	19	15	8	8	-	1	17	12	6	4	5
2. Violence	87	71	17	1	2	19	25	16	3	4	1	1	4	5	3	1	-
3. War	21	12	9	2	1	5	3	1	1	-	2	1	3	2	1	1	-

Notes:
Causes responsible for no deaths have been omitted from this table.
A dash (-) symbol indicates fewer than 500 deaths.
*IA6 is Bacterial meningitis and meningococcaemia; IC3 is Hypertensive disorders of pregnancy; ID is Conditions arising during the perinatal period; IIE6 is Dementia and other degenerative and hereditary CNS disorders; IIH1 is Chronic obstructive pulmonary disease.

Annex Table 16f. Deaths by age, sex and cause (thousands): Sub-Saharan Africa, 2020, baseline scenario

Cause	Total	Male	Female	Males							Females						
				0-4	5-14	15-29	30-44	45-59	60-69	70+	0-4	5-14	15-29	30-44	45-59	60-69	70+
Population (millions)	*1 172*	*580*	*591*	*90*	*151*	*169*	*94*	*50*	*17*	*10*	*87*	*147*	*169*	*100*	*55*	*20*	*13*
All causes	**10 353**	**5 837**	**4 516**	**1 641**	**335**	**935**	**741**	**709**	**558**	**917**	**1 274**	**252**	**500**	**388**	**534**	**435**	**1 133**
I. Communicable, maternal, perinatal and nutritional conditions	*4 014*	*2 111*	*1 903*	*1 350*	*92*	*181*	*160*	*126*	*64*	*138*	*1 034*	*96*	*245*	*197*	*115*	*62*	*154*
A. Infectious and parasitic diseases	**2 891**	**1 520**	**1 371**	**880**	**72**	**178**	**158**	**124**	**52**	**56**	**673**	**78**	**224**	**178**	**112**	**49**	**59**
1. Tuberculosis	848	408	441	31	21	113	81	98	40	25	33	30	130	93	91	39	24
2. STDs excluding HIV	55	28	27	21	–	–	–	–	–	5	17	–	1	–	–	–	–
a. Syphilis	53	28	26	21	–	–	–	–	–	5	17	–	1	–	–	–	–
b. Chlamydia	1	–	1	–	–	–	–	–	–	–	–	–	–	–	–	–	–
c. Gonorrhoea	1	1	–	–	–	–	–	–	–	–	–	–	–	–	–	–	–
3. HIV	465	219	246	62	9	56	69	17	5	2	59	9	85	78	12	3	1
4. Diarrhoeal diseases	553	317	237	285	11	1	1	1	2	14	202	10	2	2	2	3	17
5. Childhood-cluster diseases	481	267	214	246	17	1	1	1	–	2	195	15	2	1	1	–	1
a. Pertussis	85	47	37	45	2	–	–	–	–	–	36	2	–	–	–	–	–
b. Poliomyelitis	3	2	1	1	–	–	–	–	–	–	1	–	–	–	–	–	–
c. Diphtheria	1	1	–	–	–	–	–	–	–	–	–	–	–	–	–	–	–
d. Measles	320	177	142	164	14	–	–	–	–	–	130	12	–	–	–	–	–
e. Tetanus	73	40	32	35	1	1	1	1	–	2	28	1	1	1	–	–	1
6. Bacterial meningitis*	14	7	6	6	–	–	–	–	–	1	5	–	–	–	–	–	1
7. Hepatitis B and hepatitis C	9	5	4	1	–	–	–	–	2	2	–	–	–	–	–	1	2
8. Malaria	397	229	167	207	9	4	3	3	1	2	147	8	3	2	3	2	2
9. Tropical-cluster diseases	19	11	7	–	3	2	2	2	1	1	–	2	1	1	1	1	–
a. Trypanosomiasis	14	8	6	–	2	2	1	2	1	1	–	2	1	1	1	1	–
b. Chagas disease	–	–	–	–	–	–	–	–	–	–	–	–	–	–	–	–	–
c. Schistosomiasis	1	1	–	–	–	–	–	–	–	–	–	–	–	–	–	–	–
d. Leishmaniasis	3	2	1	–	1	1	–	–	–	–	–	–	1	–	–	–	–
10. Leprosy	–	–	–	–	–	–	–	–	–	–	–	–	–	–	–	–	–
11. Dengue	–	–	–	–	–	–	–	–	–	–	–	–	–	–	–	–	–
12. Japanese encephalitis	–	–	–	–	–	–	–	–	–	–	–	–	–	–	–	–	–
13. Trachoma	–	–	–	–	–	–	–	–	–	–	–	–	–	–	–	–	–
14. Intestinal nematode infections	1	–	1	–	–	–	–	–	–	–	–	–	–	–	–	–	–
a. Ascariasis	–	–	–	–	–	–	–	–	–	–	–	–	–	–	–	–	–
b. Trichuriasis	–	–	–	–	–	–	–	–	–	–	–	–	–	–	–	–	–
c. Ancylostomiasis, necatoriasis	–	–	–	–	–	–	–	–	–	–	–	–	–	–	–	–	–
15. Other infectious and parasitic	49	28	21	19	2	1	1	1	1	3	14	2	1	–	–	1	3

Annex Table 16f, continued. Deaths by age, sex and cause (thousands): Sub-Saharan Africa, 2020, baseline scenario

Cause	Total	Male	Female	Males							Females						
				0-4	5-14	15-29	30-44	45-59	60-69	70+	0-4	5-14	15-29	30-44	45-59	60-69	70+
B. Respiratory infections	**680**	**373**	**308**	**259**	**17**	**3**	**2**	**2**	**11**	**78**	**184**	**14**	**3**	**2**	**3**	**13**	**91**
1. Lower respiratory infections	670	367	303	255	17	3	2	2	11	77	180	13	3	2	3	13	90
2. Upper respiratory infections	7	4	3	3	-	-	-	-	-	1	2	-	-	-	-	-	1
3. Otitis media	4	2	2	2	-	-	-	-	-	-	1	-	-	-	-	-	-
C. Maternal conditions	**38**	**-**	**38**	**-**	**-**	**-**	**-**	**-**	**-**	**-**	**-**	**-**	**18**	**18**	**1**	**-**	**-**
1. Maternal haemorrhage	9	-	9	-	-	-	-	-	-	-	-	-	4	4	-	-	-
2. Maternal sepsis	6	-	6	-	-	-	-	-	-	-	-	-	3	3	-	-	-
3. Hypertensive disorders*	5	-	5	-	-	-	-	-	-	-	-	-	2	2	-	-	-
4. Obstructed labour	3	-	3	-	-	-	-	-	-	-	-	-	1	2	-	-	-
5. Abortion	5	-	5	-	-	-	-	-	-	-	-	-	2	2	-	-	-
6. Other maternal	10	-	10	-	-	-	-	-	-	-	-	-	5	5	-	-	-
D. Perinatal conditions*	**319**	**173**	**146**	**173**	**-**	**-**	**-**	**-**	**-**	**-**	**146**	**-**	**-**	**-**	**-**	**-**	**-**
E. Nutritional deficiencies	**85**	**46**	**40**	**38**	**2**	**-**	**-**	**-**	**1**	**4**	**31**	**2**	**-**	**-**	**1**	**1**	**4**
1. Protein-energy malnutrition	62	34	28	30	-	-	-	-	1	3	24	-	-	-	1	1	3
2. Iodine deficiency	1	-	1	-	-	-	-	-	-	-	-	-	-	-	-	-	-
3. Vitamin A deficiency	16	9	7	7	2	-	-	-	-	-	6	1	-	-	-	-	-
4. Iron-deficiency anaemia	6	3	3	1	-	-	-	-	-	1	1	1	-	-	-	-	1
II. Noncommunicable diseases	***4 032***	***2 087***	***1 944***	***111***	***59***	***62***	***233***	***440***	***443***	***739***	***103***	***56***	***36***	***80***	***373***	***348***	***948***
A. Malignant neoplasms	**1 068**	**629**	**440**	**8**	**21**	**20**	**76**	**157**	**152**	**195**	**12**	**18**	**12**	**33**	**126**	**103**	**136**
1. Mouth and oropharynx cancers	59	38	21	-	-	1	3	5	12	16	-	1	-	1	2	7	9
2. Oesophagus cancer	60	45	15	-	-	1	3	17	10	13	-	-	1	1	4	4	6
3. Stomach cancer	79	49	30	-	-	1	4	16	12	16	-	-	1	1	11	7	10
4. Colon and rectum cancers	38	21	17	-	-	1	2	3	6	8	-	-	-	1	2	6	8
5. Liver cancer	143	108	35	1	1	7	25	38	16	21	1	5	1	3	10	8	11
6. Pancreas cancer	17	10	7	-	-	-	1	4	2	3	-	-	-	1	1	2	3
7. Trachea, bronchus, lung cancers	58	38	20	-	-	1	5	11	10	11	-	-	-	2	8	6	5
8. Melanoma and other skin cancers	20	9	12	-	-	-	1	3	2	3	-	-	2	3	3	3	3
9. Breast cancer	39	-	39	-	-	-	-	-	-	-	-	-	1	3	14	8	12
10. Cervix uteri cancer	75	-	75	-	-	-	-	-	-	-	-	-	2	5	27	17	24
11. Corpus uteri cancer	8	-	8	-	-	-	-	-	-	-	-	-	-	-	2	2	3
12. Ovary cancer	17	-	17	-	-	-	-	-	-	-	-	1	1	2	6	3	5
13. Prostate cancer	89	89	-	-	-	-	-	11	33	44	-	-	-	-	-	-	-
14. Bladder cancer	35	24	11	-	-	-	1	6	7	9	-	-	-	1	3	3	4
15. Lymphomas, multiple myeloma	62	40	22	-	8	2	6	5	7	9	3	5	1	2	3	4	5
16. Leukaemia	22	11	11	1	2	1	2	1	2	3	2	2	-	1	1	2	2
17. Other cancers	247	146	101	5	10	6	22	35	32	37	7	9	4	10	27	21	25

Annex Table 16f, continued. Deaths by age, sex and cause (thousands): Sub-Saharan Africa, 2020, baseline scenario

Cause	Total	Male	Female	Males 0-4	5-14	15-29	30-44	45-59	60-69	70+	Females 0-4	5-14	15-29	30-44	45-59	60-69	70+
B. Other neoplasms	11	6	6	-	1	-	-	1	1	1	1	1	-	-	1	1	1
C. Diabetes mellitus	30	12	17	1	1	-	1	3	3	4	1	1	1	-	3	5	8
D. Endocrine disorders	31	14	17	4	1	1	2	3	1	2	2	1	1	1	2	2	8
E. Neuro-psychiatric conditions	54	31	23	3	2	3	6	5	3	8	4	2	1	1	3	3	9
2. Bipolar disorder	1	-	1	-	-	-	-	-	-	-	-	-	-	-	-	-	1
3. Schizophrenia	2	1	1	-	-	-	1	-	-	-	-	-	-	-	1	-	-
4. Epilepsy	7	4	2	-	-	1	1	1	1	-	-	-	1	-	1	-	-
5. Alcohol use	6	4	2	-	-	1	1	2	1	1	-	-	-	1	1	1	-
6. Dementia*	12	5	7	-	-	-	-	1	1	3	-	-	-	-	1	1	4
7. Parkinson disease	3	2	1	-	-	-	-	-	1	1	-	-	-	-	-	-	1
8. Multiple sclerosis	2	1	1	-	-	-	-	-	-	1	-	-	-	-	-	1	-
9. Drug use	1	1	-	-	-	2	-	-	-	-	-	-	-	-	-	-	-
13. Other neuro-psychiatric	20	12	8	3	2	2	2	1	1	1	3	2	-	-	1	1	2
F. Sense organ diseases	-	-	-	-	-	-	-	-	-	-	-	-	-	-	-	-	-
1. Glaucoma	-	-	-	-	-	-	-	-	-	-	-	-	-	-	-	-	-
2. Cataracts	-	-	-	-	-	-	-	-	-	-	-	-	-	-	-	-	-
G. Cardiovascular diseases	1 748	795	952	25	14	19	87	166	177	307	18	14	11	30	152	158	569
1. Rheumatic heart disease	21	12	9	-	2	3	4	1	1	-	-	2	1	2	2	2	1
2. Ischaemic heart disease	481	228	252	-	-	1	23	49	58	98	-	-	1	7	38	47	154
3. Cerebrovascular disease	859	360	499	4	5	8	36	72	84	150	5	5	3	14	76	82	317
4. Inflammatory heart diseases	118	60	58	6	2	2	9	13	11	17	3	3	2	2	8	10	27
5. Other cardiovascular	269	135	134	14	4	5	15	30	23	43	6	4	4	6	28	18	71
H. Respiratory diseases	642	339	304	10	7	7	31	51	66	168	6	6	5	8	59	49	171
1. COPD*	353	189	163	2	1	1	8	26	41	110	1	1	1	2	28	28	103
2. Asthma	40	20	20	-	-	1	3	3	3	8	-	-	1	2	4	4	10
3. Other respiratory	250	130	120	8	5	4	20	22	22	49	4	4	4	5	28	17	59
I. Digestive diseases	222	144	78	3	4	6	21	45	30	36	3	6	3	5	16	17	29
1. Peptic ulcer	23	14	9	-	-	1	2	5	2	4	-	-	1	1	2	1	4
2. Cirrhosis of the liver	57	41	15	-	-	1	5	16	10	9	-	-	1	1	5	4	4
3. Appendicitis	10	6	4	-	1	1	2	1	-	-	-	1	-	1	-	-	-
4. Other digestive	133	83	50	3	1	3	11	24	18	23	3	2	2	3	9	11	19
J. Genito-urinary diseases	118	65	53	11	6	4	8	10	10	16	9	5	2	2	10	9	16
1. Nephritis and nephrosis	103	56	46	10	6	4	7	8	8	14	9	4	2	2	8	8	14
2. Benign prostatic hypertrophy	1	1	-	-	-	-	-	-	-	1	-	-	-	-	-	-	-
3. Other genito-urinary	15	8	7	1	1	-	1	2	2	1	-	1	-	-	2	1	2
K. Skin diseases	12	7	5	6	1	-	-	-	-	-	4	-	-	-	-	-	-

Annex Table 16f, continued. Deaths by age, sex and cause (thousands): Sub-Saharan Africa, 2020, baseline scenario

Cause	Total	Male	Female	Males							Females						
				0-4	5-14	15-29	30-44	45-59	60-69	70+	0-4	5-14	15-29	30-44	45-59	60-69	70+
L. Musculo-skeletal diseases																	
1. Rheumatoid arthritis	1	1	–	–	–	–	–	–	–	1	–	–	–	–	–	–	–
3. Other musculo-skeletal	1	–	–	–	–	–	–	–	–	–	–	–	–	–	–	–	–
M. Congenital anomalies	**94**	**45**	**49**	**39**	**2**	**1**	**1**	**1**	–	–	**44**	**2**	**1**	–	**1**	**1**	**1**
N. Oral conditions	–	–	–	–	–	–	–	–	–	–	–	–	–	–	–	–	–
III. Injuries	***2 307***	***1 638***	***669***	***180***	***185***	***691***	***347***	***143***	***51***	***41***	***137***	***99***	***219***	***111***	***46***	***24***	***32***
A. Unintentional injuries	**1 128**	**801**	**328**	**120**	**131**	**245**	**156**	**85**	**32**	**31**	**84**	**70**	**75**	**39**	**24**	**11**	**26**
1. Road traffic accidents	479	349	130	18	72	118	71	42	16	11	12	37	42	19	12	4	4
2. Poisonings	64	38	26	25	4	2	2	2	1	1	18	2	3	1	1	–	1
3. Falls	39	23	16	2	2	6	4	4	3	3	2	1	1	1	1	–	9
4. Fires	119	62	56	24	6	12	8	5	2	5	20	7	11	6	4	2	6
5. Drownings	127	94	33	28	31	18	9	5	2	2	14	11	3	2	1	3	1
6. Other unintentional	301	235	66	24	16	88	62	27	8	9	17	12	14	9	6	3	5
B. Intentional injuries	**1 179**	**838**	**341**	**59**	**54**	**447**	**191**	**58**	**19**	**9**	**54**	**29**	**145**	**73**	**22**	**13**	**6**
1. Self-inflicted injuries	39	32	7	–	3	15	8	3	1	1	–	–	4	1	1	–	–
2. Violence	510	439	70	8	17	267	100	35	9	5	4	7	32	16	7	3	2
3. War	630	366	264	51	35	164	82	20	10	4	50	23	109	56	14	10	4

Notes:
Causes responsible for no deaths have been omitted from this table.
A dash (-) symbol indicates fewer than 500 deaths.
*IA6 is Bacterial meningitis and meningococcaemia; IC3 is Hypertensive disorders of pregnancy; ID is Conditions arising during the perinatal period;
IIE6 is Dementia and other degenerative and hereditary CNS disorders; IIH1 is Chronic obstructive pulmonary disease.

Annex Table 16g. Deaths by age, sex and cause (thousands): Latin America and the Caribbean, 2020, baseline scenario

Cause	Total	Male	Female	Males							Females						
				0-4	5-14	15-29	30-44	45-59	60-69	70+	0-4	5-14	15-29	30-44	45-59	60-69	70+
Population (millions)	678	336	342	29	56	83	74	56	22	16	28	53	81	75	58	25	21
All causes	4 735	2 642	2 093	155	41	189	260	492	470	1 036	114	26	77	121	320	313	1 123
I. Communicable, maternal, perinatal and nutritional conditions	519	308	211	112	4	39	38	22	18	74	78	4	13	12	11	12	79
A. Infectious and parasitic diseases	291	188	103	49	3	39	37	18	13	29	36	3	11	10	8	8	27
1. Tuberculosis	39	24	15	-	-	2	1	4	6	10	-	-	1	1	3	3	6
2. STDs excluding HIV	5	3	3	2	-	-	-	-	-	1	1	-	-	-	-	-	1
a. Syphilis	5	3	2	2	-	-	-	-	-	1	1	-	-	-	-	-	1
b. Chlamydia	-	-	-	-	-	-	-	-	-	-	-	-	-	-	-	-	-
c. Gonorrhoea	-	-	-	-	-	-	-	-	-	-	-	-	-	-	-	-	-
3. HIV	110	88	22	4	-	36	34	10	3	2	4	-	9	7	1	1	-
4. Diarrhoeal diseases	58	32	26	24	-	-	-	1	1	6	16	-	-	-	1	1	8
5. Childhood-cluster diseases	27	15	12	14	1	-	-	-	-	-	11	1	-	-	-	-	-
a. Pertussis	5	3	2	3	1	-	-	-	-	-	2	1	-	-	-	-	-
b. Poliomyelitis	-	-	-	-	-	-	-	-	-	-	-	-	-	-	-	-	-
c. Diphtheria	-	-	-	-	-	-	-	-	-	-	-	-	-	-	-	-	-
d. Measles	15	8	7	8	-	-	-	-	-	-	6	1	-	-	-	-	-
e. Tetanus	6	4	3	3	-	-	-	-	-	-	3	-	-	-	-	-	-
6. Bacterial meningitis*	6	3	3	1	-	-	-	-	1	1	1	-	-	-	-	1	1
7. Hepatitis B and hepatitis C	2	1	1	-	-	-	-	-	-	1	-	-	-	-	-	-	1
8. Malaria	4	2	2	-	-	-	-	1	1	-	-	-	-	-	1	1	-
9. Tropical-cluster diseases	12	6	6	-	-	-	1	1	1	3	-	-	-	-	1	1	2
a. Trypanosomiasis	-	-	-	-	-	-	-	-	-	-	-	-	-	-	-	-	-
b. Chagas disease	11	6	5	-	-	-	1	1	1	3	-	-	-	-	1	1	2
c. Schistosomiasis	-	-	-	-	-	-	-	-	-	-	-	-	-	-	-	-	-
d. Leishmaniasis	-	-	-	-	-	-	-	-	-	-	-	-	-	-	-	-	-
10. Leprosy	1	-	-	-	-	-	-	-	-	-	-	-	-	-	-	-	-
11. Dengue	-	-	-	-	-	-	-	-	-	-	-	-	-	-	-	-	-
12. Japanese encephalitis	-	-	-	-	-	-	-	-	-	-	-	-	-	-	-	-	-
13. Trachoma	-	-	-	-	-	-	-	-	-	-	-	-	-	-	-	-	-
14. Intestinal nematode infections	1	-	-	-	-	-	-	-	-	-	-	-	-	-	-	-	-
a. Ascariasis	-	-	-	-	-	-	-	-	-	-	-	-	-	-	-	-	-
b. Trichuriasis	-	-	-	-	-	-	-	-	-	-	-	-	-	-	-	-	-
c. Ancylostomiasis, necatoriasis	-	-	-	-	-	-	-	-	-	-	-	-	-	-	-	-	-
15. Other infectious and parasitic	28	14	14	4	-	1	1	1	1	6	3	-	-	1	1	1	8

Annex Table 16g, continued. Deaths by age, sex and cause (thousands): Latin America and the Caribbean, 2020, baseline scenario

Cause	Total	Male	Female	Males							Females						
				0-4	5-14	15-29	30-44	45-59	60-69	70+	0-4	5-14	15-29	30-44	45-59	60-69	70+
B. Respiratory infections	116	60	56	18	1	1	1	3	4	33	12	1	1	1	2	3	36
1. Lower respiratory infections	115	60	56	18	1	1	1	3	4	33	12	1	1	1	2	3	36
2. Upper respiratory infections	1	1	-	-	-	-	-	-	-	-	-	-	-	-	-	-	-
3. Otitis media	-	-	-	-	-	-	-	-	-	-	-	-	-	-	-	-	-
C. Maternal conditions	3		3	-	-	-	-	-	-	-	-	-	2	1	-	-	-
1. Maternal haemorrhage	1		1	-	-	-	-	-	-	-	-	-	-	1	-	-	-
2. Maternal sepsis	-		-	-	-	-	-	-	-	-	-	-	-	-	-	-	-
3. Hypertensive disorders*	-		-	-	-	-	-	-	-	-	-	-	-	-	-	-	-
4. Obstructed labour	-		-	-	-	-	-	-	-	-	-	-	-	-	-	-	-
5. Abortion	1		1	-	-	-	-	-	-	-	-	-	1	-	-	-	-
6. Other maternal	1		1	-	-	-	-	-	-	-	-	-	1	-	-	-	-
D. Perinatal conditions*	63	38	25	38	-	-	-	-	-	-	25	-	-	-	-	-	-
E. Nutritional deficiencies	45	22	24	7	1	-	-	1	1	12	5	1	-	-	1	1	15
1. Protein-energy malnutrition	32	16	16	6	-	-	-	1	1	8	4	1	-	-	1	1	11
2. Iodine deficiency	-	-	-	-	-	-	-	-	-	-	-	-	-	-	-	-	-
3. Vitamin A deficiency	1	1	1	1	-	-	-	-	-	-	1	-	-	-	-	-	-
4. Iron-deficiency anaemia	11	5	6	1	-	-	-	-	-	3	-	-	-	-	-	-	4
II. Noncommunicable diseases	*3 581*	*1 870*	*1 711*	*29*	*13*	*14*	*96*	*384*	*419*	*916*	*25*	*9*	*18*	*76*	*284*	*286*	*1 013*
A. Malignant neoplasms	841	429	412	2	6	4	22	96	110	189	2	4	6	34	113	99	155
1. Mouth and oropharynx cancers	30	22	8	-	-	-	1	7	5	7	-	-	-	-	2	2	4
2. Oesophagus cancer	26	18	8	-	-	-	-	5	5	7	-	-	-	-	1	2	5
3. Stomach cancer	94	58	36	-	-	-	2	13	17	26	-	-	1	1	6	9	20
4. Colon and rectum cancers	56	26	30	-	-	-	1	5	7	13	-	-	-	1	5	8	15
5. Liver cancer	13	7	7	-	-	-	-	2	2	3	-	-	-	-	1	2	3
6. Pancreas cancer	20	10	10	-	-	-	-	2	3	4	-	-	-	-	2	3	6
7. Trachea, bronchus, lung cancers	125	75	51	-	-	-	5	27	21	22	-	-	-	1	17	16	16
8. Melanoma and other skin cancers	7	3	4	-	-	-	-	1	1	1	-	-	-	-	1	1	1
9. Breast cancer	66		66	-	-	-	-	-	-	-	-	-	1	6	23	14	20
10. Cervix uteri cancer	52		52	-	-	-	-	-	-	-	-	-	1	7	19	10	14
11. Corpus uteri cancer	15		15	-	-	-	-	-	-	-	-	-	-	1	5	4	6
12. Ovary cancer	12		12	-	-	-	-	-	-	-	-	-	-	2	3	3	4
13. Prostate cancer	55	55	-	-	-	-	-	3	17	35	-	-	-	-	-	-	-
14. Bladder cancer	22	16	5	-	-	-	-	3	5	9	-	-	-	-	-	1	-
15. Lymphomas, multiple myeloma	33	18	15	-	1	1	3	4	3	6	-	1	-	1	3	4	6
16. Leukaemia	22	12	10	1	2	1	2	2	2	3	1	1	-	2	2	2	3
17. Other cancers	192	109	83	1	3	1	6	22	23	53	1	2	2	10	22	18	27

Annex Table 16g, continued. Deaths by age, sex and cause (thousands): Latin America and the Caribbean, 2020, baseline scenario

Cause	Total	Male	Female	Males							Females						
				0-4	5-14	15-29	30-44	45-59	60-69	70+	0-4	5-14	15-29	30-44	45-59	60-69	70+
B. Other neoplasms	11	5	6	-	-	-	-	1	1	2	-	-	-	-	1	1	3
C. Diabetes mellitus	141	52	89	-	-	-	2	10	13	26	-	-	1	1	11	20	55
D. Endocrine disorders	34	15	19	3	-	-	1	2	2	7	2	-	-	1	2	2	12
E. Neuro-psychiatric conditions	57	34	23	2	2	2	6	8	4	10	2	1	2	2	3	2	11
2. Bipolar disorder	1	-	1	-	-	-	-	-	-	-	-	-	-	-	-	-	1
3. Schizophrenia	6	3	3	-	-	-	1	1	-	1	-	-	-	-	-	1	2
4. Epilepsy	5	3	2	-	-	1	1	1	-	-	-	-	1	-	1	-	-
5. Alcohol use	14	12	1	-	-	-	3	5	2	2	-	-	-	-	1	-	-
6. Dementia*	12	5	7	-	-	-	-	1	1	3	-	-	-	-	1	1	5
7. Parkinson disease	4	2	2	-	-	-	-	-	-	2	-	-	-	-	-	-	2
8. Multiple sclerosis	2	1	1	-	-	-	-	1	-	-	-	-	-	-	1	-	-
9. Drug use	2	1	-	-	-	-	1	-	-	-	-	-	-	-	-	-	-
13. Other neuro-psychiatric	12	7	5	2	1	1	1	1	-	1	1	1	1	1	-	-	1
F. Sense organ diseases	1	-	-	-	-	-	-	-	-	-	-	-	-	-	-	-	-
1. Glaucoma	-	-	-	-	-	-	-	-	-	-	-	-	-	-	-	-	-
2. Cataracts	-	-	-	-	-	-	-	-	-	-	-	-	-	-	-	-	-
G. Cardiovascular diseases	1 739	928	811	3	1	3	39	184	217	480	2	1	4	24	93	102	584
1. Rheumatic heart disease	12	5	7	-	-	1	1	2	1	1	-	-	1	1	2	1	2
2. Ischaemic heart disease	793	431	362	-	-	-	15	86	104	225	-	-	-	8	37	47	270
3. Cerebrovascular disease	550	288	262	-	-	1	12	58	68	149	-	-	1	9	34	34	184
4. Inflammatory heart diseases	44	24	20	1	-	-	3	7	4	9	1	-	-	2	4	2	12
5. Other cardiovascular	339	180	159	2	1	1	8	32	41	96	1	1	1	4	16	18	118
H. Respiratory diseases	360	172	188	3	1	1	5	16	29	117	2	1	2	4	35	36	108
1. COPD*	209	105	104	-	-	1	1	8	18	77	-	-	1	1	16	21	65
2. Asthma	39	14	25	1	1	-	2	2	2	8	-	-	1	1	6	5	12
3. Other respiratory	112	53	59	3	1	1	2	6	9	32	1	1	-	3	12	10	31
I. Digestive diseases	272	174	98	1	-	1	16	59	36	60	1	-	1	6	20	17	53
1. Peptic ulcer	26	16	10	-	-	-	1	3	3	8	1	-	-	-	1	1	7
2. Cirrhosis of the liver	120	90	29	-	-	1	11	40	19	19	-	-	-	3	10	6	10
3. Appendicitis	2	1	1	-	-	-	-	-	-	-	-	-	-	-	-	-	-
4. Other digestive	125	67	58	1	-	1	4	16	14	32	1	-	1	3	9	9	35
J. Genito-urinary diseases	78	39	39	1	-	1	2	5	6	23	1	-	1	2	5	6	24
1. Nephritis and nephrosis	56	27	29	1	-	1	2	4	5	14	1	-	1	1	4	4	18
2. Benign prostatic hypertrophy	3	3	-	-	-	-	-	-	-	3	-	-	-	-	-	-	-
3. Other genito-urinary	19	8	10	-	-	-	-	1	1	6	-	-	-	1	1	1	7
K. Skin diseases	5	2	3	-	-	-	-	-	-	1	-	-	-	-	-	-	2

Annex Table 16g, continued. Deaths by age, sex and cause (thousands): Latin America and the Caribbean, 2020, baseline scenario

Cause	Total	Male	Female	Males							Females						
				0-4	5-14	15-29	30-44	45-59	60-69	70+	0-4	5-14	15-29	30-44	45-59	60-69	70+
L. Musculo-skeletal diseases	**13**	**4**	**9**	-	-	-	-	1	1	2	-	-	-	1	1	1	5
1. Rheumatoid arthritis	2	1	2	-	-	-	-	1	1	2	-	-	-	-	1	1	5
3. Other musculo-skeletal	10	3	7	-	-	-	-	-	-	1	-	-	-	1	1	1	4
M. Congenital anomalies	**30**	**15**	**15**	13	1	-	-	-	-	-	13	1	-	-	-	-	-
N. Oral conditions	-	-	-	-	-	-	-	-	-	-	-	-	-	-	-	-	-
III. Injuries	**636**	**464**	**171**	**14**	**24**	**135**	**126**	**87**	**33**	**46**	**11**	**13**	**45**	**33**	**24**	**14**	**31**
A. Unintentional injuries	**403**	**274**	**129**	11	19	65	64	54	23	38	8	11	30	22	19	11	29
1. Road traffic accidents	217	148	69	3	12	43	36	29	11	13	3	7	21	15	11	6	7
2. Poisonings	6	3	2	-	-	1	1	1	-	-	-	-	-	-	-	-	-
3. Falls	37	21	16	1	-	1	1	4	2	9	-	-	-	1	1	1	12
4. Fires	9	5	4	1	-	2	-	1	-	1	1	1	1	1	1	-	1
5. Drownings	27	22	6	2	3	6	5	4	1	1	1	1	1	-	1	1	1
6. Other unintentional	107	75	32	4	3	12	18	17	7	13	3	2	6	5	5	3	9
B. Intentional injuries	**233**	**190**	**42**	3	5	70	62	32	10	8	3	2	15	11	6	3	2
1. Self-inflicted injuries	42	30	12	-	-	7	8	7	4	4	-	-	4	3	2	1	1
2. Violence	166	146	20	1	3	58	50	24	6	4	1	1	8	6	3	1	1
3. War	25	14	10	2	1	5	4	1	1	-	2	1	4	3	1	1	-

Notes:
Causes responsible for no deaths have been omitted from this table.
A dash (-) symbol indicates fewer than 500 deaths.
*IA6 is Bacterial meningitis and meningococcaemia; IC3 is Hypertensive disorders of pregnancy; ID is Conditions arising during the perinatal period;
IIE6 is Dementia and other degenerative and hereditary CNS disorders; IIH1 is Chronic obstructive pulmonary disease.

Annex Table 16h. Deaths by age, sex and cause (thousands): Middle Eastern Crescent, 2020, baseline scenario

Cause	Total	Male	Female	Males							Females						
				0-4	5-14	15-29	30-44	45-59	60-69	70+	0-4	5-14	15-29	30-44	45-59	60-69	70+
Population (millions)	*1 003*	*506*	*497*	*62*	*110*	*140*	*98*	*61*	*23*	*12*	*59*	*105*	*134*	*95*	*61*	*26*	*17*
All causes	*6 639*	*3 826*	*2 813*	*617*	*122*	*246*	*309*	*698*	*680*	*1 153*	*525*	*91*	*138*	*145*	*317*	*361*	*1 239*
I. Communicable, maternal, perinatal and nutritional conditions	*992*	*530*	*462*	*408*	*13*	*8*	*9*	*13*	*23*	*55*	*352*	*12*	*8*	*8*	*9*	*15*	*58*
A. Infectious and parasitic diseases	422	235	187	180	7	7	8	12	9	13	153	5	2	2	6	5	12
1. Tuberculosis	49	31	18	3	1	4	3	7	6	8	1	-	1	1	4	4	6
2. STDs excluding HIV	7	4	4	3	-	-	-	-	-	-	3	-	-	-	-	-	-
a. Syphilis	7	4	4	3	-	-	-	-	-	-	3	-	-	-	-	-	-
b. Chlamydia	-	-	-	-	-	-	-	-	-	-	-	-	-	-	-	-	-
c. Gonorrhoea	-	-	-	-	-	-	-	-	-	-	-	-	-	-	-	-	-
3. HIV	11	9	2	1	-	3	3	2	-	-	1	-	-	-	-	-	-
4. Diarrhoeal diseases	203	109	94	105	2	-	-	-	-	1	90	2	-	-	-	-	1
5. Childhood-cluster diseases	109	59	51	55	3	-	-	-	-	-	48	2	-	-	-	-	-
a. Pertussis	24	13	11	13	-	-	-	-	-	-	11	-	-	-	-	-	-
b. Poliomyelitis	1	1	1	1	-	-	-	-	-	-	1	-	-	-	-	-	-
c. Diphtheria	-	-	-	-	-	-	-	-	-	-	-	-	-	-	-	-	-
d. Measles	44	23	20	22	2	-	-	-	-	-	19	1	-	-	-	-	-
e. Tetanus	39	21	18	20	1	-	-	-	-	-	17	1	-	-	-	-	-
6. Bacterial meningitis*	9	5	4	3	-	-	-	-	1	-	2	-	-	-	-	-	1
7. Hepatitis B and hepatitis C	8	4	3	1	-	-	-	1	1	1	-	-	-	-	-	-	2
8. Malaria	2	1	1	-	-	-	-	1	-	-	-	-	-	-	-	-	-
9. Tropical-cluster diseases	1	1	-	-	-	-	-	-	-	-	-	-	-	-	-	-	-
a. Trypanosomiasis	-	-	-	-	-	-	-	-	-	-	-	-	-	-	-	-	-
b. Chagas disease	-	-	-	-	-	-	-	-	-	-	-	-	-	-	-	-	-
c. Schistosomiasis	1	1	-	-	-	-	-	-	-	-	-	-	-	-	-	-	-
d. Leishmaniasis	1	1	-	-	-	-	-	-	-	-	-	-	-	-	-	-	-
10. Leprosy	-	-	-	-	-	-	-	-	-	-	-	-	-	-	-	-	-
11. Dengue	-	-	-	-	-	-	-	-	-	-	-	-	-	-	-	-	-
12. Japanese encephalitis	-	-	-	-	-	-	-	-	-	-	-	-	-	-	-	-	-
13. Trachoma	-	-	-	-	-	-	-	-	-	-	-	-	-	-	-	-	-
14. Intestinal nematode infections	-	-	-	-	-	-	-	-	-	-	-	-	-	-	-	-	-
a. Ascariasis	-	-	-	-	-	-	-	-	-	-	-	-	-	-	-	-	-
b. Trichuriasis	-	-	-	-	-	-	-	-	-	-	-	-	-	-	-	-	-
c. Ancylostomiasis, necatoriasis	-	-	-	-	-	-	-	-	-	-	-	-	-	-	-	-	-
15. Other infectious and parasitic	21	12	10	9	-	-	-	-	-	1	8	-	-	-	-	-	1

Annex Table 16h, continued. Deaths by age, sex and cause (thousands): Middle Eastern Crescent, 2020, baseline scenario

Cause	Total	Male	Female	Males							Females						
				0-4	5-14	15-29	30-44	45-59	60-69	70+	0-4	5-14	15-29	30-44	45-59	60-69	70+
B. Respiratory infections	**312**	**163**	**148**	**100**	**6**	**1**	**1**	**1**	**14**	**40**	**86**	**6**	**1**	**1**	**2**	**10**	**43**
1. Lower respiratory infections	307	161	146	99	6	1	1	1	14	39	84	6	1	1	2	9	43
2. Upper respiratory infections	3	2	1	1	·	1	·	·	·	·	1	·	·	·	·	·	·
3. Otitis media	2	1	1	1	·	·	·	·	·	·	1	·	·	·	·	·	·
C. Maternal conditions	**10**	**–**	**10**								·	·	**4**	**5**	**1**	·	·
1. Maternal haemorrhage	2	–	2								·	·	1	1	·	·	·
2. Maternal sepsis	2	–	2								·	·	1	1	·	·	·
3. Hypertensive disorders*	2	–	2								·	·	1	1	·	·	·
4. Obstructed labour	1	–	1								·	·	1	·	·	·	·
5. Abortion	1	–	1								·	·	1	·	·	·	·
6. Other maternal	3	–	3								·	·	·	1	1	·	·
D. Perinatal conditions*	**203**	**108**	**95**	108	·	·	·	·	·	·	95	·	·	·	·	·	·
E. Nutritional deficiencies	**46**	**24**	**22**	**20**	**1**	·	·	·	·	**2**	**18**	**1**	·	·	·	·	**2**
1. Protein-energy malnutrition	32	17	15	15	1	·	·	·	·	2	13	1	·	·	·	·	1
2. Iodine deficiency	2	2	1	·	·	·	·	·	·	1	·	·	·	·	·	·	·
3. Vitamin A deficiency	8	4	4	3	1	·	·	·	·	·	3	1	·	·	·	·	·
4. Iron-deficiency anaemia	5	2	2	1	·	·	·	·	·	1	1	·	·	·	·	·	1
II. Noncommunicable diseases	**4 750**	**2 709**	**2 042**	**144**	**49**	**47**	**154**	**608**	**630**	**1 076**	**112**	**44**	**40**	**79**	**278**	**328**	**1 161**
A. Malignant neoplasms	**640**	**407**	**232**	**4**	**12**	**11**	**36**	**138**	**107**	**99**	**5**	**9**	**9**	**25**	**64**	**59**	**61**
1. Mouth and oropharynx cancers	39	26	13	·	·	1	3	6	9	7	·	·	·	1	·	·	·
2. Oesophagus cancer	24	15	9	·	·	·	1	7	4	3	·	·	·	·	2	4	5
3. Stomach cancer	52	33	20	·	·	1	3	14	8	7	·	·	·	1	5	3	3
4. Colon and rectum cancers	31	16	15	·	·	1	2	4	5	5	·	·	·	·	2	6	7
5. Liver cancer	22	14	8	·	·	·	2	6	3	3	·	·	·	1	2	5	6
6. Pancreas cancer	12	7	5	·	·	·	1	3	2	2	·	·	·	·	·	2	2
7. Trachea, bronchus, lung cancers	180	153	27	·	·	1	11	60	39	42	·	·	·	2	10	9	7
8. Melanoma and other skin cancers	3	2	1	·	·	·	·	1	·	·	·	·	·	·	·	·	·
9. Breast cancer	28	–	28								·	·	2	4	11	5	6
10. Cervix uteri cancer	18	–	18								·	·	1	2	7	4	4
11. Corpus uteri cancer	5	–	5								·	·	·	·	1	1	·
12. Ovary cancer	8	–	8								·	·	·	·	·	·	·
13. Prostate cancer	12	12	–	·	·	·	·	2	5	4							
14. Bladder cancer	25	20	4	·	·	·	·	7	6	5	·	·	·	·	·	1	2
15. Lymphomas, multiple myeloma	21	14	7	·	·	·	·	3	3	2	·	·	·	1	1	·	1
16. Leukaemia	27	15	12	1	3	1	3	2	2	2	1	3	1	2	1	2	2
17. Other cancers	132	80	52	3	6	3	8	24	20	17	3	4	3	7	13	11	11

Annex Table 16h, continued. Deaths by age, sex and cause (thousands): Middle Eastern Crescent, 2020, baseline scenario

Cause	Total	Male	Female	Males							Females						
				0-4	5-14	15-29	30-44	45-59	60-69	70+	0-4	5-14	15-29	30-44	45-59	60-69	70+
B. Other neoplasms	**7**	**4**	**3**	·	·	·	·	1	1	1	·	·	·	·	1	·	1
C. Diabetes mellitus	**82**	**36**	**46**	1	1	1	3	9	9	12	1	1	1	1	8	13	21
D. Endocrine disorders	**19**	**10**	**9**	4	1	·	1	1	1	1	4	2	1	·	1	1	1
E. Neuro-psychiatric conditions	**72**	**38**	**34**	9	4	4	3	4	4	9	7	4	3	2	3	3	11
2. Bipolar disorder	1	·	1	·	·	·	·	·	·	·	·	·	·	·	1	·	·
3. Schizophrenia	5	2	3	·	·	·	1	1	·	·	·	·	1	·	1	1	·
4. Epilepsy	9	5	4	1	·	1	1	1	1	·	1	1	1	1	·	·	·
5. Alcohol use	1	1	·	·	·	·	1	·	·	·	·	·	·	·	·	·	·
6. Dementia*	15	6	8	·	·	·	·	·	1	4	·	·	·	·	1	1	6
7. Parkinson disease	4	3	2	·	·	·	·	·	1	2	·	·	·	·	·	1	1
8. Multiple sclerosis	2	1	1	·	·	·	·	·	·	·	·	·	·	1	·	·	·
9. Drug use	2	2	·	·	·	1	1	·	·	·	·	·	·	·	·	·	·
13. Other neuro-psychiatric	33	18	15	8	4	2	1	1	1	1	6	3	1	1	1	1	2
F. Sense organ diseases	·	·	·	·	·	·	·	·	·	·	·	·	·	·	·	·	·
1. Glaucoma	·	·	·	·	·	·	·	·	·	·	·	·	·	·	·	·	·
2. Cataracts	·	·	·	·	·	·	·	·	·	·	·	·	·	·	·	·	·
G. Cardiovascular diseases	**2 966**	**1 656**	**1 310**	54	21	20	83	343	402	733	30	16	15	36	137	184	892
1. Rheumatic heart disease	27	15	12	·	2	4	5	3	1	1	·	2	2	4	3	1	1
2. Ischaemic heart disease	1 537	870	667	·	·	3	40	187	225	415	·	·	2	15	62	100	488
3. Cerebrovascular disease	499	252	247	3	4	3	10	51	64	117	2	3	1	4	27	35	175
4. Inflammatory heart diseases	121	71	49	10	4	4	8	18	10	18	7	3	3	4	8	4	20
5. Other cardiovascular	783	448	334	41	11	7	19	85	103	183	22	8	6	9	37	44	208
H. Respiratory diseases	**532**	**303**	**229**	14	4	3	9	47	61	166	9	6	4	5	34	41	130
1. COPD*	300	177	122	3	1	·	2	24	38	109	2	1	1	1	16	23	78
2. Asthma	36	19	17	·	·	·	2	3	4	10	·	1	1	1	3	4	9
3. Other respiratory	196	107	89	10	3	2	5	20	19	47	7	5	3	4	15	14	43
I. Digestive diseases	**218**	**135**	**83**	9	2	3	10	47	32	31	10	2	2	5	20	17	27
1. Peptic ulcer	12	8	3	·	·	·	1	3	2	1	·	·	·	·	1	1	1
2. Cirrhosis of the liver	82	51	31	·	·	1	4	20	14	12	·	·	1	2	9	8	11
3. Appendicitis	4	2	1	·	·	1	·	·	·	·	·	1	·	·	·	·	·
4. Other digestive	121	73	47	9	1	1	5	24	16	17	10	1	3	3	10	8	14
J. Genito-urinary diseases	**113**	**67**	**46**	3	2	3	7	16	12	23	3	2	3	3	10	9	17
1. Nephritis and nephrosis	47	26	20	2	1	2	3	5	5	10	2	1	2	1	4	4	7
2. Benign prostatic hypertrophy	2	2	·	·	·	·	·	·	·	2	·	·	·	·	·	·	·
3. Other genito-urinary	64	38	26	1	1	2	5	10	7	12	1	1	1	2	6	5	10
K. Skin diseases	**2**	**1**	**1**	·	·	·	·	·	·	·	·	·	·	·	·	·	·

Annex Table 16h, continued. Deaths by age, sex and cause (thousands): Middle Eastern Crescent, 2020, baseline scenario

Cause	Total	Male	Female	Males							Females						
				0-4	5-14	15-29	30-44	45-59	60-69	70+	0-4	5-14	15-29	30-44	45-59	60-69	70+
L. Musculo-skeletal diseases	3	1	1	-	-	-	-	-	-	-	-	-	-	-	-	-	-
1. Rheumatoid arthritis	-	-	1	-	-	-	-	-	-	-	-	-	-	-	-	-	-
3. Other musculo-skeletal	2	1	1	-	-	-	-	-	-	-	-	-	-	-	-	-	-
M. Congenital anomalies	98	51	47	45	2	1	1	1	-	-	42	2	1	1	1	1	1
N. Oral conditions	-	-	-	-	-	-	-	-	-	-	-	-	-	-	-	-	-
III. Injuries	*896*	*587*	*309*	*64*	*60*	*191*	*147*	*76*	*27*	*22*	*61*	*34*	*90*	*58*	*29*	*18*	*20*
A. Unintentional injuries	386	276	110	30	25	74	74	45	15	14	26	12	22	17	13	7	12
1. Road traffic accidents	182	140	42	4	14	47	41	22	6	5	4	8	10	9	6	3	4
2. Poisonings	22	15	8	2	-	2	4	4	1	1	2	-	1	1	1	1	1
3. Falls	20	14	6	2	1	2	3	3	1	2	3	-	-	1	1	1	1
4. Fires	23	10	13	3	1	2	2	1	1	1	6	1	4	2	2	1	2
5. Drownings	37	26	10	7	4	6	5	2	1	1	6	1	1	1	1	-	1
6. Other unintentional	102	71	30	12	5	15	18	12	5	5	10	2	4	4	4	2	4
B. Intentional injuries	511	311	199	34	34	117	73	32	13	8	35	22	69	40	16	11	7
1. Self-inflicted injuries	100	68	31	-	14	19	15	12	4	4	-	6	9	5	4	3	4
2. Violence	75	50	25	9	3	16	13	6	2	1	9	4	4	4	2	1	1
3. War	336	193	143	26	17	82	46	14	7	2	25	12	56	32	9	7	2

Notes:
Causes responsible for no deaths have been omitted from this table.
A dash (-) symbol indicates fewer than 500 deaths.
*IA6 is Bacterial meningitis and meningococcaemia; IC3 is Hypertensive disorders of pregnancy; ID is Conditions arising during the perinatal period; IIE6 is Dementia and other degenerative and hereditary CNS disorders; IIH1 is Chronic obstructive pulmonary disease.

Annex Table 16i. Deaths by age, sex and cause (thousands): World, 2020, baseline scenario

Cause	Total	Male	Female	Males 0-4	5-14	15-29	30-44	45-59	60-69	70+	Females 0-4	5-14	15-29	30-44	45-59	60-69	70+
Population (millions)	*7 844*	*3 901*	*3 943*	*374*	*690*	*966*	*796*	*633*	*259*	*184*	*358*	*662*	*935*	*782*	*648*	*297*	*262*
All causes	*68 337*	*38 788*	*29 549*	*3 463*	*754*	*2 213*	*3 016*	*7 688*	*7 715*	*13 939*	*2 828*	*563*	*1 258*	*1 455*	*3 508*	*4 114*	*15 823*
I. Communicable, maternal, perinatal and nutritional conditions	*10 305*	*5 588*	*4 717*	*2 535*	*151*	*365*	*525*	*507*	*349*	*1 156*	*2 043*	*156*	*381*	*392*	*335*	*231*	*1 180*
A. Infectious and parasitic diseases	6 525	3 659	2 867	1 419	112	356	516	484	258	514	1 129	114	341	352	310	163	457
1. Tuberculosis	2 296	1 310	986	44	28	167	200	356	193	323	42	36	167	145	244	118	233
2. STDs excluding HIV	109	53	55	36	–	–	–	1	2	14	29	–	1	2	1	2	19
a. Syphilis	105	53	52	36	–	–	–	1	2	14	29	–	1	2	1	2	19
b. Chlamydia	2	–	2	–	–	–	–	–	–	–	–	–	1	–	–	–	–
c. Gonorrhoea	1	–	1	–	–	–	–	–	–	–	–	–	–	–	–	–	–
3. HIV	1 250	727	522	111	16	172	294	94	27	14	104	16	160	192	36	9	5
4. Diarrhoeal diseases	1 212	662	550	555	18	3	4	6	13	65	427	17	3	3	6	11	83
5. Childhood-cluster diseases	791	433	358	394	25	2	3	2	2	6	321	23	1	2	3	1	6
a. Pertussis	142	78	64	75	3	–	–	–	–	–	61	3	–	–	–	–	–
b. Poliomyelitis	9	5	4	5	–	–	–	–	–	–	3	–	–	–	–	–	–
c. Diphtheria	3	2	1	2	–	–	–	–	–	–	1	–	–	–	–	–	–
d. Measles	450	247	203	229	18	–	–	–	–	–	186	16	–	–	–	–	–
e. Tetanus	187	101	86	83	3	2	3	2	2	6	70	4	1	2	3	1	6
6. Bacterial meningitis*	65	34	32	15	–	–	3	3	4	7	13	–	–	2	3	4	9
7. Hepatitis B and hepatitis C	51	28	23	3	1	1	2	5	4	14	2	1	1	1	2	3	14
8. Malaria	427	246	181	210	12	7	5	5	3	4	149	11	5	3	5	3	5
9. Tropical-cluster diseases	38	22	16	1	4	3	3	4	2	4	1	3	2	2	3	2	4
a. Trypanosomiasis	14	8	6	1	2	2	1	–	–	1	1	2	1	1	–	–	1
b. Chagas disease	11	6	5	–	–	–	1	1	1	3	–	–	–	1	1	1	3
c. Schistosomiasis	3	2	1	–	–	1	–	1	–	1	–	–	–	–	–	–	1
d. Leishmaniasis	9	6	3	1	2	1	1	1	–	–	–	1	1	–	–	–	–
10. Leprosy	1	1	1	–	–	–	–	–	–	1	–	–	–	–	–	–	1
11. Dengue	3	2	2	1	1	–	–	–	–	–	1	1	–	–	–	–	–
12. Japanese encephalitis	1	1	–	–	1	–	–	–	–	–	–	1	–	–	–	–	–
13. Trachoma	–	–	–	–	–	–	–	–	–	–	–	–	–	–	–	–	–
14. Intestinal nematode infections	5	2	2	–	1	1	–	–	–	1	–	1	–	–	–	–	1
a. Ascariasis	2	1	2	–	1	–	–	–	–	–	–	1	–	–	–	–	–
b. Trichuriasis	1	1	1	–	1	–	–	–	–	–	–	1	–	–	–	–	–
c. Ancylostomiasis, necatoriasis	2	1	1	–	1	–	–	–	–	1	–	–	–	–	–	–	1
15. Other infectious and parasitic	277	138	139	50	5	2	4	7	10	60	40	5	1	2	5	9	78

Annex Table 16i, continued. Deaths by age, sex and cause (thousands): World, 2020, baseline scenario

Cause	Total	Male	Female	Males 0-4	5-14	15-29	30-44	45-59	60-69	70+	Females 0-4	5-14	15-29	30-44	45-59	60-69	70+
B. Respiratory infections	2 506	1 292	1 213	540	34	7	8	20	85	598	424	33	6	6	18	62	664
1. Lower respiratory infections	2 472	1 275	1 197	530	34	7	8	19	85	592	416	33	6	5	18	62	657
2. Upper respiratory infections	24	12	12	5	–	–	–	–	–	5	4	–	–	–	–	1	–
3. Otitis media	9	5	4	5	–	–	–	–	1	–	4	–	–	–	–	–	6
C. Maternal conditions	72	–	72	–	–	–	–	–	–	–	–	3	32	33	4	–	–
1. Maternal haemorrhage	17	–	17	–	–	–	–	–	–	–	–	1	8	8	1	–	–
2. Maternal sepsis	11	–	11	–	–	–	–	–	–	–	–	–	5	5	1	–	–
3. Hypertensive disorders*	9	–	9	–	–	–	–	–	–	–	–	–	4	4	–	–	–
4. Obstructed labour	6	–	6	–	–	–	–	–	–	–	–	–	2	3	–	–	–
5. Abortion	10	–	10	–	–	–	–	–	–	–	–	–	4	4	–	–	–
6. Other maternal	19	–	19	–	–	–	–	–	–	–	–	–	8	9	1	–	–
D. Perinatal conditions*	907	492	415	492	–	–	–	–	–	–	415	–	–	–	–	–	–
E. Nutritional deficiencies	295	145	150	84	6	1	1	3	5	44	74	6	1	1	4	5	59
1. Protein-energy malnutrition	181	91	89	63	1	1	1	1	3	23	55	1	1	1	1	2	29
2. Iodine deficiency	6	3	3	3	–	–	–	–	–	–	2	–	–	–	–	–	–
3. Vitamin A deficiency	34	18	16	15	4	1	–	–	–	–	12	3	1	–	–	–	–
4. Iron-deficiency anaemia	71	31	41	4	1	1	1	2	2	20	4	1	1	1	3	3	29
II. Noncommunicable diseases	49 652	27 769	21 883	526	205	272	1 272	6 262	6 978	12 254	458	168	204	609	2 725	3 614	14 105
A. Malignant neoplasms	12 275	7 592	4 683	29	72	91	486	2 366	2 084	2 465	36	49	79	287	1 137	1 173	1 921
1. Mouth and oropharynx cancers	635	428	207	1	1	6	33	131	120	136	1	1	4	13	49	60	79
2. Oesophagus cancer	823	573	250	–	–	3	21	191	173	184	–	–	2	5	57	82	104
3. Stomach cancer	1 588	1 069	519	–	–	6	40	347	315	362	–	–	5	23	106	139	246
4. Colon and rectum cancers	832	457	375	–	–	5	23	98	121	209	–	–	3	13	57	93	209
5. Liver cancer	1 174	885	289	1	2	14	111	388	204	166	1	–	3	18	80	78	107
6. Pancreas cancer	318	189	129	–	–	–	7	51	53	77	–	–	–	2	19	33	74
7. Trachea, bronchus, lung cancers	2 415	1 809	606	–	1	6	88	668	591	455	–	–	2	15	153	189	247
8. Melanoma and other skin cancers	79	42	37	–	–	1	4	13	9	16	–	–	1	2	8	8	18
9. Breast cancer	498	–	498	–	–	–	–	–	–	–	–	–	10	47	158	106	176
10. Cervix uteri cancer	394	–	394	–	–	–	–	–	–	–	–	–	10	35	156	86	108
11. Corpus uteri cancer	101	–	101	–	–	–	–	–	–	–	1	–	–	3	25	25	47
12. Ovary cancer	162	–	162	–	–	–	–	–	–	–	–	–	5	16	44	38	57
13. Prostate cancer	393	393	–	–	–	–	–	29	103	259	–	–	–	–	–	–	–
14. Bladder cancer	262	201	61	–	–	–	5	39	57	99	–	–	–	1	8	15	35
15. Lymphomas, multiple myeloma	377	232	145	1	16	9	25	53	52	73	4	8	4	10	24	32	64
16. Leukaemia	346	197	149	8	20	13	31	43	32	51	10	14	10	19	26	24	47
17. Other cancers	1 878	1 117	762	14	32	25	96	315	255	379	19	22	20	64	169	165	303

Annex Table 16i, continued. Deaths by age, sex and cause (thousands): World, 2020, baseline scenario

Cause	Total	Male	Female	M 0-4	M 5-14	M 15-29	M 30-44	M 45-59	M 60-69	M 70+	F 0-4	F 5-14	F 15-29	F 30-44	F 45-59	F 60-69	F 70+
B. Other neoplasms	113	55	58	3	3	2	4	10	10	23	3	2	2	2	7	9	33
C. Diabetes mellitus	753	289	464	5	4	3	15	54	66	142	5	4	3	6	49	98	300
D. Endocrine disorders	171	72	98	13	2	3	5	9	9	31	11	3	2	3	8	10	61
E. Neuro-psychiatric conditions	824	390	434	25	14	25	43	56	49	178	24	11	13	13	25	43	305
2. Bipolar disorder	22	6	16	-	-	-	1	1	1	3	-	-	-	1	-	1	14
3. Schizophrenia	63	29	34	-	-	2	4	5	4	15	-	-	1	3	3	4	25
4. Epilepsy	58	35	23	2	2	6	9	7	8	5	2	2	4	3	3	3	6
5. Alcohol use	55	47	8	-	-	1	12	18	8	8	-	-	1	1	1	2	3
6. Dementia*	298	105	193	2	1	1	2	7	13	79	3	1	1	1	6	15	166
7. Parkinson disease	88	44	45	-	-	-	-	1	5	38	-	-	-	-	4	-	41
8. Multiple sclerosis	25	10	15	-	-	-	2	1	2	2	-	-	1	1	4	4	5
9. Drug use	8	7	1	-	-	3	3	-	-	1	-	-	-	1	-	-	-
13. Other neuro-psychiatric	207	107	100	21	11	11	11	13	10	28	19	9	6	5	6	10	45
F. Sense organ diseases	21	10	11	1	-	-	-	3	3	3	1	-	-	-	2	3	4
1. Glaucoma	7	3	4	-	-	-	-	1	1	1	-	-	-	-	1	1	2
2. Cataracts	6	3	3	-	-	-	-	1	1	1	-	-	-	-	1	1	1
G. Cardiovascular diseases	24 813	13 352	11 461	135	57	82	475	2 680	3 428	6 495	83	46	53	192	911	1 519	8 657
1. Rheumatic heart disease	471	248	224	-	4	13	32	88	49	61	1	5	9	23	54	35	97
2. Ischaemic heart disease	11 107	6 077	5 030	-	-	8	175	1 221	1 618	3 056	5	-	4	60	336	684	3 940
3. Cerebrovascular disease	7 698	3 977	3 721	16	15	20	114	751	1 062	2 000	11	10	9	52	303	512	2 823
4. Inflammatory heart diseases	749	429	320	27	11	13	46	126	73	133	21	9	9	19	48	35	178
5. Other cardiovascular	4 788	2 621	2 168	91	27	27	108	495	627	1 245	45	22	21	38	170	253	1 618
H. Respiratory diseases	6 366	3 499	2 866	39	19	19	76	447	852	2 047	24	17	19	40	328	499	1 939
1. COPD*	4 726	2 620	2 107	10	3	4	24	303	671	1 604	7	3	3	14	203	377	1 500
2. Asthma	326	161	165	1	3	4	13	31	33	76	-	1	3	8	33	34	85
3. Other respiratory	1 313	718	595	29	13	11	38	113	147	367	17	13	13	18	92	88	354
I. Digestive diseases	2 722	1 726	996	20	10	21	128	554	389	605	20	11	15	46	189	176	539
1. Peptic ulcer	288	179	109	-	-	2	9	43	37	87	1	-	-	3	14	16	75
2. Cirrhosis of the liver	1 176	838	339	1	1	8	71	339	207	211	1	2	4	20	97	79	136
3. Appendicitis	36	22	14	-	3	5	6	4	2	2	-	3	2	3	2	-	1
4. Other digestive	1 222	687	535	18	5	7	41	169	142	305	18	7	7	19	76	81	327
J. Genito-urinary diseases	885	451	433	20	13	15	32	70	77	225	16	12	10	15	54	70	257
1. Nephritis and nephrosis	632	311	321	17	11	12	24	52	54	141	14	11	8	11	41	53	183
2. Benign prostatic hypertrophy	38	38	-	-	-	-	-	1	6	31							
3. Other genito-urinary	215	102	112	3	2	3	7	18	17	52	2	1	3	3	13	17	74
K. Skin diseases	57	25	31	8	-	-	1	2	2	11	6	-	1	-	2	2	21

Annex Table 16i, continued. Deaths by age, sex and cause (thousands): World, 2020, baseline scenario

Cause	Total	Male	Female	Males							Females						
				0-4	5-14	15-29	30-44	45-59	60-69	70+	0-4	5-14	15-29	30-44	45-59	60-69	70+
L. Musculo-skeletal diseases	123	40	82	1	1	1	1	4	8	25	1	1	1	2	6	9	63
1. Rheumatoid arthritis	21	6	15	-	-	-	1	-	1	4	-	-	-	-	1	2	12
3. Other musculo-skeletal	101	34	66	1	1	1	1	3	7	21	1	1	1	2	5	7	51
M. Congenital anomalies	529	266	263	229	10	9	6	6	2	4	229	10	6	3	6	3	6
N. Oral conditions	1	1	1	-	-	-	-	-	-	-	-	-	-	-	-	-	-
III. Injuries	*8 381*	*5 432*	*2 949*	*403*	*397*	*1 577*	*1 218*	*920*	*388*	*529*	*328*	*239*	*673*	*454*	*449*	*269*	*538*
A. Unintentional injuries	5 053	3 271	1 781	291	288	761	694	604	252	381	216	173	294	225	282	174	416
1. Road traffic accidents	2 338	1 623	715	59	160	469	369	310	124	133	38	101	161	113	140	71	91
2. Poisonings	293	172	121	34	7	17	35	43	16	20	24	5	20	17	20	13	22
3. Falls	439	225	214	10	8	21	32	42	27	85	10	4	5	8	20	24	144
4. Fires	354	152	202	37	9	23	27	23	8	25	32	13	46	33	23	15	40
5. Drownings	469	307	162	72	61	57	45	33	14	25	47	26	17	13	18	11	30
6. Other unintentional	1 160	792	368	79	43	174	188	153	63	94	65	25	45	42	61	40	90
B. Intentional injuries	3 328	2 161	1 167	112	110	816	524	315	136	148	111	66	379	228	166	94	122
1. Self-inflicted injuries	1 229	711	517	-	25	154	157	169	88	119	-	13	146	92	105	60	101
2. Violence	1 052	841	211	29	29	395	226	109	30	22	30	16	57	42	36	15	15
3. War	1 047	608	439	83	56	266	141	37	18	7	81	37	176	94	25	19	7

Notes:
Causes responsible for no deaths have been omitted from this table.
A dash (-) symbol indicates fewer than 500 deaths.
*IA6 is Bacterial meningitis and meningococcaemia; IC3 is Hypertensive disorders of pregnancy; ID is Conditions arising during the perinatal period;
IIE6 is Dementia and other degenerative and hereditary CNS disorders; IIH1 is Chronic obstructive pulmonary disease.

Annex Table 17a. DALYs by age, sex and cause (thousands): Established Market Economies, 2020, baseline scenario

Cause	Total	Male	Female	Males					Females				
				0-4	5-14	15-44	45-59	60+	0-4	5-14	15-44	45-59	60+
Population (millions)	*905*	*441*	*464*	*29*	*58*	*162*	*86*	*107*	*28*	*55*	*156*	*87*	*138*
All causes	*97 000*	*55 532*	*41 468*	*1 360*	*965*	*17 857*	*13 697*	*21 653*	*1 108*	*794*	*11 762*	*8 100*	*19 704*
I. Communicable, maternal, perinatal and nutritional conditions	*5 048*	*3 281*	*1 768*	*514*	*52*	*1 621*	*349*	*745*	*394*	*51*	*525*	*106*	*691*
A. Infectious and parasitic diseases	**2 824**	**2 146**	**678**	**85**	**17**	**1 582**	**309**	**153**	**67**	**18**	**413**	**51**	**129**
1. Tuberculosis	**62**	**45**	**18**	-	-	**3**	**8**	**33**	-	-	**1**	**2**	**14**
2. STDs excluding HIV	**159**	**11**	**148**	-	-	**10**	-	**1**	-	**1**	**143**	**1**	**2**
a. Syphilis	3	2	1	-	-	1	-	1	-	-	-	1	-
b. Chlamydia	136	6	130	-	-	6	-	-	-	2	127	-	-
c. Gonorrhoea	18	3	14	-	-	3	-	-	-	-	14	-	-
3. HIV	**2 223**	**1 903**	**320**	**35**	**6**	**1 549**	**285**	**27**	**25**	**6**	**252**	**31**	**6**
4. Diarrhoeal diseases	**75**	**38**	**37**	**15**	**3**	**7**	**3**	**10**	**13**	**2**	**4**	**4**	**13**
5. Childhood-cluster diseases	**12**	**7**	**5**	**5**	**1**	-	-	**1**	**4**	**1**	-	-	**1**
a. Pertussis	7	3	3	3	1	-	-	-	3	1	-	-	-
b. Poliomyelitis	1	1	-	-	-	-	-	-	-	-	-	-	-
c. Diphtheria	-	-	-	-	-	-	-	-	-	-	-	-	-
d. Measles	3	2	1	2	1	-	-	-	1	-	-	-	-
e. Tetanus	1	-	-	-	-	-	-	-	-	-	-	-	-
6. Bacterial meningitis*	**58**	**32**	**27**	**21**	**3**	**2**	**2**	**4**	**17**	**3**	**1**	**1**	**4**
7. Hepatitis B and hepatitis C	**18**	**11**	**7**	-	-	**2**	**3**	**5**	-	-	**1**	**1**	**4**
8. Malaria	-	-	-	-	-	-	-	-	-	-	-	-	-
9. Tropical-cluster diseases	-	-	-	-	-	-	-	-	-	-	-	-	-
a. Trypanosomiasis	-	-	-	-	-	-	-	-	-	-	-	-	-
b. Chagas disease	-	-	-	-	-	-	-	-	-	-	-	-	-
c. Schistosomiasis	-	-	-	-	-	-	-	-	-	-	-	-	-
d. Leishmaniasis	-	-	-	-	-	-	-	-	-	-	-	-	-
e. Lymphatic filariasis	-	-	-	-	-	-	-	-	-	-	-	-	-
f. Onchocerciasis	-	-	-	-	-	-	-	-	-	-	-	-	-
10. Leprosy	-	-	-	-	-	-	-	-	-	-	-	-	-
11. Dengue	-	-	-	-	-	-	-	-	-	-	-	-	-
12. Japanese encephalitis	-	-	-	-	-	-	-	-	-	-	-	-	-
13. Trachoma	-	-	-	-	-	-	-	-	-	-	-	-	-
14. Intestinal nematode infections	-	-	-	-	-	-	-	-	-	-	-	-	-
a. Ascariasis	-	-	-	-	-	-	-	-	-	-	-	-	-
b. Trichuriasis	-	-	-	-	-	-	-	-	-	-	-	-	-
c. Ancylostomiasis and necatoriasis	-	-	-	-	-	-	-	-	-	-	-	-	-

Annex Table 17a, continued. DALYs by age, sex and cause (thousands): Established Market Economies, 2020, baseline scenario

Cause	Total	Male	Female	Males					Females				
				0-4	5-14	15-44	45-59	60+	0-4	5-14	15-44	45-59	60+
B. Respiratory infections	**1 127**	**603**	**524**	**25**	**15**	**18**	**30**	**515**	**17**	**14**	**9**	**18**	**464**
1. Lower respiratory infections	1 077	578	499	19	4	16	29	509	13	4	8	17	457
2. Upper respiratory infections	24	12	12	3	1	2	1	5	2	1	2	1	7
3. Otitis media	26	14	13	3	10	-	-	-	3	10	-	-	-
C. Maternal conditions	**44**	**-**	**44**	-	-	-	-	-	-	-	**44**	-	-
1. Maternal haemorrhage	2	-	2	-	-	-	-	-	-	-	2	-	-
2. Maternal sepsis	4	-	4	-	-	-	-	-	-	-	4	-	-
3. Hypertensive disorders of pregnancy	2	-	2	-	-	-	-	-	-	-	2	-	-
4. Obstructed labour	31	-	31	-	-	-	-	-	-	-	31	-	-
5. Abortion	2	-	2	-	-	-	-	-	-	-	2	-	-
D. Perinatal conditions*	**667**	**380**	**288**	379	-	-	-	-	287	-	-	-	-
E. Nutritional deficiencies	**386**	**152**	**234**	**25**	**20**	**20**	**10**	**77**	**23**	**19**	**58**	**37**	**98**
1. Protein-energy malnutrition	43	20	23	11	-	-	1	8	10	-	-	-	12
2. Iodine deficiency	-	-	-	-	-	-	-	-	-	-	-	-	-
3. Vitamin A deficiency	-	-	-	-	-	-	-	-	-	-	-	-	-
4. Iron-deficiency anaemia	339	130	210	13	20	19	9	68	12	19	58	36	85
II. Noncommunicable diseases	***82 131***	***45 658***	***36 473***	***673***	***629***	***11 733***	***12 380***	***20 243***	***583***	***540***	***9 508***	***7 391***	***18 451***
A. Malignant neoplasms	**16 763**	**10 155**	**6 608**	**17**	**70**	**884**	**3 566**	**5 619**	**16**	**47**	**765**	**1 972**	**3 807**
1. Mouth and oropharynx cancers	386	319	67	-	-	35	160	124	-	-	8	22	36
2. Oesophagus cancer	392	325	66	-	-	16	141	169	-	-	3	17	46
3. Stomach cancer	1 176	796	380	-	-	51	253	491	-	-	44	91	245
4. Colon and rectum cancers	1 800	1 036	764	-	-	57	305	673	-	-	45	176	542
5. Liver cancer	349	280	69	-	1	16	124	139	-	1	5	17	47
6. Pancreas cancer	650	394	256	-	-	22	136	236	-	-	11	62	183
7. Trachea, bronchus, lung cancers	4 438	3 089	1 349	-	-	238	1 427	1 423	-	-	75	460	814
8. Melanoma and other skin cancers	235	150	85	-	-	37	54	58	-	-	25	25	35
9. Breast cancer	1 254	-	1 254	-	-	-	-	-	-	-	213	483	558
10. Cervix uteri cancer	157	-	157	-	-	-	-	-	-	-	51	53	53
11. Corpus uteri cancer	172	-	172	-	-	-	-	-	-	-	16	57	99
12. Ovary cancer	337	-	337	-	-	-	-	-	-	-	40	125	171
13. Prostate cancer	779	779	-	-	-	3	72	704	-	-	-	-	-
14. Bladder cancer	462	384	79	-	-	6	62	315	-	-	2	11	65
15. Lymphomas and multiple myeloma	695	427	268	1	8	88	131	199	1	3	42	62	160
16. Leukaemia	550	334	216	6	28	86	78	137	6	18	54	44	94
C. Diabetes mellitus	**2 015**	**921**	**1 094**	**1**	**2**	**139**	**277**	**502**	**1**	**3**	**81**	**194**	**814**
D. Endocrine disorders	**830**	**366**	**463**	**42**	**35**	**99**	**52**	**138**	**40**	**27**	**82**	**97**	**217**

Annex Table 17a, continued. DALYs by age, sex and cause (thousands): Established Market Economies, 2020, baseline scenario

Cause	Total	Male	Female	Males 0-4	5-14	15-44	45-59	60+	Females 0-4	5-14	15-44	45-59	60+
E. Neuro-psychiatric conditions	**24 604**	**12 527**	**12 078**	**75**	**281**	**8 195**	**1 811**	**2 163**	**67**	**237**	**6 560**	**1 790**	**3 422**
1. Unipolar major depression	6 620	2 318	4 303	-	-	1 609	496	214	-	-	2 927	907	469
2. Bipolar disorder	1 596	805	792	-	-	677	82	46	-	-	653	82	56
3. Schizophrenia	1 982	1 033	949	-	-	1 005	7	21	-	-	914	2	33
4. Epilepsy	299	170	128	4	30	87	32	19	4	32	45	21	27
5. Alcohol use	4 357	3 685	672	-	-	2 937	571	177	-	-	526	97	49
6. Dementia*	4 319	1 687	2 631	31	15	37	291	1 313	30	13	29	305	2 254
7. Parkinson disease	673	305	368	-	-	-	83	222	-	-	-	90	278
8. Multiple sclerosis	191	84	108	-	-	66	11	6	-	-	84	14	9
9. Drug use	1 348	1 021	327	-	92	878	42	9	-	31	280	14	3
10. Post-traumatic stress disorder	261	99	162	4	17	62	12	4	6	28	102	19	7
11. Obsessive-compulsive disorders	1 400	595	805	-	57	442	53	43	-	72	566	94	73
12. Panic disorder	669	222	447	-	19	147	55	1	-	19	310	89	29
F. Sense organ diseases	**145**	**67**	**78**	**-**	**-**	**3**	**26**	**37**	**-**	**-**	**2**	**27**	**48**
1. Glaucoma	103	46	57	-	-	2	22	22	-	-	1	24	32
2. Cataracts	37	19	18	-	-	1	4	14	-	-	-	2	15
G. Cardiovascular diseases	**18 810**	**12 087**	**6 723**	**37**	**18**	**860**	**3 539**	**7 633**	**29**	**10**	**350**	**518**	**5 816**
1. Rheumatic heart disease	129	62	67	-	-	8	22	31	-	-	7	12	47
2. Ischaemic heart disease	9 528	6 484	3 044	-	5	298	2 072	4 114	5	3	67	207	2 770
3. Cerebrovascular disease	4 988	2 819	2 169	6	4	239	720	1 849	8	2	154	200	1 808
4. Inflammatory heart diseases	574	393	181	7		99	145	138	8		39	22	109
H. Respiratory diseases	**5 186**	**2 810**	**2 376**	**35**	**98**	**437**	**523**	**1 717**	**16**	**93**	**413**	**552**	**1 303**
1. COPD*	2 836	1 686	1 149	2	1	77	300	1 307	1	1	46	264	838
2. Asthma	1 051	500	551	15	84	234	86	81	6	81	231	123	110
I. Digestive diseases	**5 004**	**3 033**	**1 970**	**14**	**9**	**441**	**1 297**	**1 272**	**12**	**8**	**319**	**618**	**1 013**
1. Peptic ulcer	296	190	106	-	-	28	60	102	-	-	17	24	65
2. Cirrhosis of the liver	1 855	1 361	493	-	-	195	721	445	-	-	83	220	189
3. Appendicitis	29	18	11	-	1	7	4	6	-	1	5	2	4
J. Genito-urinary diseases	**1 202**	**703**	**499**	**8**	**1**	**43**	**192**	**458**	**7**	**3**	**28**	**53**	**409**
1. Nephritis and nephrosis	444	227	217	7	1	24	34	161	5	2	8	17	186
2. Benign prostatic hypertrophy	310	310	-	-	-	-	130	180	-	-	-	-	-
L. Musculo-skeletal diseases	**4 886**	**1 666**	**3 220**	**1**	**2**	**355**	**889**	**419**	**1**	**8**	**671**	**1 362**	**1 178**
1. Rheumatoid arthritis	1 127	283	844	-	-	51	113	119	-	4	287	201	351
2. Osteoarthritis	3 410	1 289	2 121	-	-	284	753	253	-	-	324	1 111	686

Annex Table 17a, continued. DALYs by age, sex and cause (thousands): Established Market Economies, 2020, baseline scenario

Cause	Total	Male	Female	Males					Females				
				0-4	5-14	15-44	45-59	60+	0-4	5-14	15-44	45-59	60+
M. Congenital anomalies	**916**	**495**	**422**	**419**	**17**	**40**	**9**	**9**	**372**	**16**	**17**	**7**	**10**
N. Oral conditions	**1 012**	**482**	**530**	**14**	**75**	**159**	**105**	**129**	**14**	**72**	**154**	**112**	**178**
1. Dental caries	434	216	218	14	75	77	20	29	13	72	74	21	38
2. Periodontal disease	33	17	16	-	-	14	2	1	-	-	13	2	2
3. Edentulism	538	247	291	-	-	67	82	98	-	-	66	88	136
III. Injuries	***9 821***	***6 593***	***3 228***	***173***	***284***	***4 503***	***968***	***665***	***131***	***203***	***1 729***	***603***	***562***
A. Unintentional injuries	**6 676**	**4 280**	**2 396**	**147**	**246**	**2 907**	**539**	**440**	**106**	**181**	**1 243**	**416**	**450**
1. Road traffic accidents	3 528	2 303	1 225	61	124	1 915	138	65	45	103	852	146	78
2. Poisonings	192	124	68	2	2	94	19	8	1	2	44	13	8
3. Falls	1 107	560	547	19	40	234	117	150	13	25	149	148	212
4. Fires	172	94	78	10	17	37	16	14	8	21	26	11	11
5. Drownings	168	126	41	12	16	66	18	14	7	6	15	7	7
6. Other unintentional	1 510	1 072	438	44	47	562	231	188	32	24	157	91	134
B. Intentional injuries	**3 145**	**2 313**	**831**	**25**	**37**	**1 596**	**429**	**226**	**24**	**22**	**487**	**187**	**112**
1. Self-inflicted injuries	2 207	1 604	603	-	15	1 019	364	207	-	5	332	165	101
2. Violence	936	708	228	25	23	577	65	18	24	17	154	22	10
3. War	2	2	-	-	-	1	-	1	-	-	-	-	-

Notes:
A dash (-) symbol indicates fewer than 500 DALYs.
*IA6 is Bacterial meningitis and meningococcaemia; ID is Conditions arising during the perinatal period;
IIE6 is Dementia and other degenerative and hereditary CNS disorders; IIH1 is Chronic obstructive pulmonary disease.

Annex Table 17b. DALYs by age, sex and cause (thousands): Formerly Socialist Economies of Europe, 2020, baseline scenario

Cause	Total	Male	Female	Males 0-4	5-14	15-44	45-59	60+	Females 0-4	5-14	15-44	45-59	60+
Population (millions)	365	172	193	12	25	75	29	30	12	24	74	33	50
All causes	63 534	39 594	23 940	1 395	719	13 576	12 372	11 532	1 115	493	7 381	4 791	10 159
I. Communicable, maternal, perinatal and nutritional conditions	1 884	926	958	530	44	105	59	188	394	43	253	32	236
A. Infectious and parasitic diseases	609	288	320	120	14	78	35	41	102	15	150	11	42
1. Tuberculosis	88	74	14	1	-	26	27	21	-	-	2	3	8
2. STDs excluding HIV	153	24	130	3	-	20	-	-	3	2	123	1	1
a. Syphilis	1	1	1	-	-	1	-	-	-	-	-	-	-
b. Chlamydia	117	9	108	1	-	8	-	-	1	2	105	1	-
c. Gonorrhoea	33	12	20	2	-	10	-	-	2	-	18	-	-
3. HIV	132	72	61	42	7	21	2	-	42	7	11	1	-
4. Diarrhoeal diseases	62	33	29	26	1	3	1	2	22	1	2	1	3
5. Childhood-cluster diseases	10	5	5	4	-	-	-	-	3	1	-	-	-
a. Pertussis	6	3	3	3	-	-	-	-	3	1	-	-	-
b. Poliomyelitis	-	-	-	-	-	-	-	-	-	-	-	-	-
c. Diphtheria	-	-	-	-	-	-	-	-	1	-	-	-	-
d. Measles	3	2	1	1	-	-	-	-	-	-	-	-	-
e. Tetanus	1	-	-	-	-	-	-	-	-	-	-	-	-
6. Bacterial meningitis*	61	35	26	24	2	3	2	4	18	1	1	1	4
7. Hepatitis B and hepatitis C	9	5	4	2	-	1	1	1	2	-	1	-	1
8. Malaria	-	-	-	-	-	-	-	-	-	-	-	-	-
9. Tropical-cluster diseases	-	-	-	-	-	-	-	-	-	-	-	-	-
a. Trypanosomiasis	-	-	-	-	-	-	-	-	-	-	-	-	-
b. Chagas disease	-	-	-	-	-	-	-	-	-	-	-	-	-
c. Schistosomiasis	-	-	-	-	-	-	-	-	-	-	-	-	-
d. Leishmaniasis	-	-	-	-	-	-	-	-	-	-	-	-	-
e. Lymphatic filariasis	-	-	-	-	-	-	-	-	-	-	-	-	-
f. Onchocerciasis	-	-	-	-	-	-	-	-	-	-	-	-	-
10. Leprosy	-	-	-	-	-	-	-	-	-	-	-	-	-
11. Dengue	-	-	-	-	-	-	-	-	-	-	-	-	-
12. Japanese encephalitis	-	-	-	-	-	-	-	-	-	-	-	-	-
13. Trachoma	-	-	-	-	-	-	-	-	-	-	-	-	-
14. Intestinal nematode infections	-	-	-	-	-	-	-	-	-	-	-	-	-
a. Ascariasis	-	-	-	-	-	-	-	-	-	-	-	-	-
b. Trichuriasis	-	-	-	-	-	-	-	-	-	-	-	-	-
c. Ancylostomiasis and necatoriasis	-	-	-	-	-	-	-	-	-	-	-	-	-

Annex Table 17b, continued. DALYs by age, sex and cause (thousands): Formerly Socialist Economies of Europe, 2020, baseline scenario

Cause	Total	Male	Female	Males					Females				
				0-4	5-14	15-44	45-59	60+	0-4	5-14	15-44	45-59	60+
B. Respiratory infections	**527**	**275**	**252**	**101**	**11**	**18**	**20**	**125**	**74**	**9**	**7**	**7**	**155**
1. Lower respiratory infections	508	265	243	97	6	18	20	124	71	6	6	7	153
2. Upper respiratory infections	8	4	4	1	–	1	–	1	1	–	1	–	1
3. Otitis media	12	6	5	2	4	–	–	–	1	4	–	–	–
C. Maternal conditions	**70**	–	**70**	–	–	–	–	–	–	–	70	–	–
1. Maternal haemorrhage	2	–	2	–	–	–	–	–	–	–	2	–	–
2. Maternal sepsis	14	–	14	–	–	–	–	–	–	–	14	–	–
3. Hypertensive disorders of pregnancy	1	–	1	–	–	–	–	–	–	–	1	–	–
4. Obstructed labour	19	–	19	–	–	–	–	–	–	–	19	–	–
5. Abortion	20	–	20	–	–	–	–	–	–	–	20	–	–
D. Perinatal conditions*	**467**	**278**	**190**	278	–	–	–	–	190	–	–	–	–
E. Nutritional deficiencies	**211**	**85**	**125**	**31**	**20**	**8**	**4**	**22**	**28**	**18**	**24**	**14**	**38**
1. Protein-energy malnutrition	35	17	18	15	–	–	–	2	14	–	–	–	4
2. Iodine deficiency	–	–	–	–	–	–	–	–	–	–	–	–	–
3. Vitamin A deficiency	–	–	–	–	–	–	–	–	–	–	–	–	–
4. Iron-deficiency anaemia	156	60	96	13	19	8	3	18	12	17	24	13	30
II. Noncommunicable diseases	**50 618**	**30 463**	**20 156**	**569**	**304**	**7 745**	**10 914**	**10 931**	**484**	**245**	**5 577**	**4 267**	**9 583**
A. Malignant neoplasms	**10 251**	**7 236**	**3 015**	**26**	**63**	**929**	**3 535**	**2 683**	**25**	**35**	**553**	**998**	**1 403**
1. Mouth and oropharynx cancers	384	354	31	–	–	54	224	75	–	–	7	10	14
2. Oesophagus cancer	191	175	16	–	–	17	111	47	–	–	2	5	9
3. Stomach cancer	1 495	1 121	374	–	–	121	601	399	–	–	52	112	210
4. Colon and rectum cancers	910	567	343	–	–	60	253	254	–	–	37	100	206
5. Liver cancer	268	190	78	1	1	19	94	75	1	–	7	21	48
6. Pancreas cancer	398	291	107	–	–	32	154	105	–	–	10	32	66
7. Trachea, bronchus, lung cancers	2 815	2 418	397	–	1	236	1 186	995	–	–	42	146	209
8. Melanoma and other skin cancers	131	83	48	1	1	24	35	23	–	–	17	12	19
9. Breast cancer	479	–	479	–	–	–	–	–	–	–	116	202	161
10. Cervix uteri cancer	175	–	175	–	–	–	–	–	–	–	54	58	64
11. Corpus uteri cancer	129	–	129	–	–	–	–	–	–	–	19	50	59
12. Ovary cancer	177	–	177	–	–	–	–	–	–	–	38	74	64
13. Prostate cancer	186	186	–	–	–	4	47	135	–	–	–	–	–
14. Bladder cancer	235	204	31	1	1	7	83	113	–	–	2	7	21
15. Lymphomas and multiple myeloma	301	213	87	3	12	69	85	44	–	–	31	21	29
16. Leukaemia	330	217	113	9	24	64	71	50	8	14	36	24	31
C. Diabetes mellitus	**465**	**199**	**267**	–	**1**	**48**	**66**	**84**	**1**	**1**	**29**	**60**	**176**
D. Endocrine disorders	**133**	**59**	**74**	**13**	**4**	**29**	**9**	**5**	**12**	**4**	**26**	**19**	**13**

Annex Table 17b, continued. DALYs by age, sex and cause (thousands): Formerly Socialist Economies of Europe, 2020, baseline scenario

Cause	Total	Male	Female	Males 0-4	5-14	15-44	45-59	60+	Females 0-4	5-14	15-44	45-59	60+
E. Neuro-psychiatric conditions	10 433	5 237	5 196	73	150	3 846	641	528	65	121	3 232	698	1 080
1. Unipolar major depression	3 204	1 084	2 120			825	188	70			1 541	381	198
2. Bipolar disorder	842	411	431			358	34	19			352	37	42
3. Schizophrenia	838	434	404			422	6	6			394	2	8
4. Epilepsy	212	137	75	5	27	75	19	10	5	20	27	11	12
5. Alcohol use	1 731	1 526	205			1 277	194	55			181	14	10
6. Dementia*	1 187	405	782	15	7	16	86	280	14	6	14	110	638
7. Parkinson disease	157	60	97				19	41				24	72
8. Multiple sclerosis	101	43	58			34	5	4			43	7	8
9. Drug use	525	420	105		31	373	14	3		8	93	3	1
10. Post-traumatic stress disorder	117	43	73	2	7	29	4	1			49	7	3
11. Obsessive-compulsive disorders	651	272	379		25	214	19	13		32	281	37	28
12. Panic disorder	312	101	212		9	72	20			9	156	35	11
F. Sense organ diseases	79	36	42			1	9	26			2	14	27
1. Glaucoma	36	12	24				4	8			1	11	12
2. Cataracts	42	24	18			1	5	18			1	2	15
G. Cardiovascular diseases	16 576	10 667	5 909	21	8	1 156	4 155	5 327	14	4	325	720	4 845
1. Rheumatic heart disease	335	208	127		1	60	114	33		1	31	58	37
2. Ischaemic heart disease	8 469	5 832	2 637			575	2 539	2 717			81	293	2 263
3. Cerebrovascular disease	4 886	2 749	2 138	3	2	244	930	1 569	2	2	144	299	1 693
4. Inflammatory heart diseases	466	325	141	4	2	102	132	85	4	1	32	26	78
H. Respiratory diseases	5 133	3 342	1 792	19	33	457	1 322	1 511	8	24	302	474	984
1. COPD*	2 074	1 478	597			140	635	702			62	118	416
2. Asthma	577	300	277	10	31	129	72	59	4	21	120	68	63
I. Digestive diseases	2 499	1 514	984	19	4	405	673	413	14	4	214	352	400
1. Peptic ulcer	202	152	50	1		34	69	49			12	16	22
2. Cirrhosis of the liver	768	547	220			91	291	165		1	33	96	91
3. Appendicitis	13	8	5			3	2	2			2	1	1
J. Genito-urinary diseases	679	376	303	4	4	90	128	149	3	4	66	102	127
1. Nephritis and nephrosis	171	102	69	2	2	42	29	26	2	3	18	18	28
2. Benign prostatic hypertrophy	132	132	–				56	76					–
L. Musculo-skeletal diseases	2 838	1 042	1 796	1	2	614	272	152	1	5	666	696	429
1. Rheumatoid arthritis	527	125	403			67	31	26		3	216	106	77
2. Osteoarthritis	2 170	875	1 296			523	231	121			409	556	331

Annex Table 17b, continued. DALYs by age, sex and cause (thousands): Formerly Socialist Economies of Europe, 2020, baseline scenario

Cause	Total	Male	Female	Males					Females				
				0-4	5-14	15-44	45-59	60+	0-4	5-14	15-44	45-59	60+
M. Congenital anomalies	745	402	342	369	11	19	3	1	319	11	9	2	1
N. Oral conditions	511	230	281	14	19	95	66	35	14	28	99	79	61
1. Dental caries	249	114	134	14	19	45	21	15	14	28	44	24	25
2. Periodontal disease	17	7	10	-	-	5	1	1	-	-	8	1	1
3. Edentulism	244	108	136	-	-	45	43	19	-	-	47	54	35
III. Injuries	11 031	8 205	2 826	296	371	5 726	1 399	413	237	206	1 551	491	340
A. Unintentional injuries	7 381	5 571	1 810	187	277	3 831	994	283	130	144	928	352	257
1. Road traffic accidents	3 324	2 510	814	35	134	1 948	304	89	21	82	524	116	71
2. Poisonings	746	566	180	21	7	316	184	38	16	6	74	58	25
3. Falls	888	569	319	27	36	346	103	57	20	16	123	71	89
4. Fires	140	96	44	9	7	49	21	9	8	6	14	8	9
5. Drownings	418	352	66	16	38	234	51	13	7	15	28	9	6
6. Other unintentional	1 865	1 479	387	78	54	938	331	78	57	18	165	90	56
B. Intentional injuries	3 650	2 634	1 016	109	94	1 895	405	130	107	62	623	140	84
1. Self-inflicted injuries	1 673	1 331	341	-	18	902	305	107	-	4	185	90	62
2. Violence	854	655	199	9	9	540	80	17	7	8	134	35	15
3. War	1 123	647	476	100	68	453	20	6	101	51	304	14	6

Notes:
A dash (-) symbol indicates fewer than 500 DALYs.
*IA6 is Bacterial meningitis and meningococcaemia; ID is Conditions arising during the perinatal period;
IIE6 is Dementia and other degenerative and hereditary CNS disorders; IIH1 is Chronic obstructive pulmonary disease.

Annex Table 17c. DALYs by age, sex and cause (thousands): India, 2020, baseline scenario

Cause	Total	Male	Female	Males 0-4	5-14	15-44	45-59	60+	Females 0-4	5-14	15-44	45-59	60+
Population (millions)	1 227	621	606	52	104	307	101	57	50	99	290	100	67
All causes	236 741	133 164	103 577	21 738	7 386	42 117	35 798	26 124	20 551	5 886	34 220	20 753	22 167
I. Communicable, maternal, perinatal and nutritional conditions	57 756	31 308	26 448	13 016	1 296	10 114	4 260	2 623	12 491	1 363	8 053	2 593	1 948
A. Infectious and parasitic diseases	41 007	23 292	17 715	6 548	938	9 735	4 106	1 964	6 252	895	6 997	2 363	1 209
1. Tuberculosis	15 969	10 135	5 834	293	272	4 605	3 441	1 525	227	214	2 655	1 987	751
2. STDs excluding HIV	1 744	641	1 103	300	5	313	6	17	286	17	767	8	26
a. Syphilis	461	229	233	164	-	44	4	17	161	1	41	5	25
b. Chlamydia	720	130	590	33	2	95	1	-	30	12	545	2	1
c. Gonorrhoea	562	282	280	103	3	174	1	-	95	4	181	1	-
3. HIV	10 956	6 104	4 852	949	178	4 337	516	125	1 027	195	3 366	221	43
4. Diarrhoeal diseases	5 989	3 007	2 982	2 652	103	80	38	135	2 592	131	45	38	175
5. Childhood-cluster diseases	3 539	1 870	1 670	1 688	108	49	13	12	1 499	115	28	14	15
a. Pertussis	597	314	283	296	17	-	-	-	267	16	1	-	-
b. Poliomyelitis	275	165	110	162	-	2	-	-	109	-	-	-	-
c. Diphtheria	29	15	14	14	1	1	-	-	13	1	-	-	-
d. Measles	1 363	711	652	653	57	1	-	-	596	55	-	-	-
e. Tetanus	1 275	664	611	562	32	46	12	12	513	43	27	13	15
6. Bacterial meningitis*	296	158	138	118	3	19	9	9	105	3	10	9	11
7. Hepatitis B and hepatitis C	71	40	31	10	3	9	8	11	7	3	4	4	12
8. Malaria	171	95	75	32	22	28	8	6	26	22	14	7	7
9. Tropical-cluster diseases	408	290	118	25	89	153	18	5	13	40	33	26	6
a. Trypanosomiasis	-	-	-	-	-	-	-	-	-	-	-	-	-
b. Chagas disease	-	-	-	-	-	-	-	-	-	-	-	-	-
c. Schistosomiasis	-	-	-	-	-	-	-	-	-	-	-	-	-
d. Leishmaniasis	159	104	55	12	38	48	3	2	8	25	18	2	2
e. Lymphatic filariasis	249	186	63	12	51	105	15	2	5	15	15	24	4
f. Onchocerciasis	-	-	-	-	-	-	-	-	-	-	-	-	-
10. Leprosy	57	29	28	-	7	17	3	1	1	7	16	3	1
11. Dengue	56	26	29	9	17	1	-	-	9	19	-	-	-
12. Japanese encephalitis	14	7	7	5	2	-	-	-	5	2	-	-	-
13. Trachoma	11	3	8	-	-	-	1	2	-	-	-	2	6
14. Intestinal nematode infections	177	96	81	1	41	36	10	8	1	37	24	10	9
a. Ascariasis	37	20	18	1	19	-	-	-	1	17	-	-	-
b. Trichuriasis	24	13	12	-	13	-	-	-	-	12	-	-	-
c. Ancylostomiasis and necatoriasis	115	63	52	-	9	36	10	8	-	9	24	10	9

Annex Table 17c, continued. DALYs by age, sex and cause (thousands): India, 2020, baseline scenario

Cause	Total	Male	Female	Males					Females				
				0-4	5-14	15-44	45-59	60+	0-4	5-14	15-44	45-59	60+
B. Respiratory infections	7 576	3 754	3 821	2 817	190	126	82	540	2 753	308	78	87	597
1. Lower respiratory infections	7 382	3 658	3 723	2 748	173	123	81	534	2 682	290	76	85	590
2. Upper respiratory infections	79	40	40	27	2	3	1	6	26	3	2	1	6
3. Otitis media	115	56	59	41	14	-	-	-	44	14	-	-	-
C. Maternal conditions	677		677						-		663	15	-
1. Maternal haemorrhage	78		78								75	3	
2. Maternal sepsis	115		115								112	2	
3. Hypertensive disorders of pregnancy	38		38								37	2	
4. Obstructed labour	136		136								135	1	
5. Abortion	146		146								144	2	
D. Perinatal conditions*	5 734	2 932	2 802	2 932					2 802				
E. Nutritional deficiencies	2 763	1 330	1 432	719	169	253	71	119	684	161	316	129	142
1. Protein-energy malnutrition	1 058	530	527	505	4	6	3	13	495	11	2	2	18
2. Iodine deficiency	73	39	34	36	2	-	-	-	31	2	1	-	-
3. Vitamin A deficiency	125	66	59	50	14	1	-	-	45	13	1	-	-
4. Iron-deficiency anaemia	1 507	695	812	128	148	245	68	106	113	134	313	127	124
II. Noncommunicable diseases	133 700	74 890	58 810	5 203	1 216	18 592	27 409	22 471	5 149	1 133	18 227	15 280	19 020
A. Malignant neoplasms	16 882	9 608	7 274	134	209	2 023	4 835	2 408	87	95	1 857	3 338	1 899
1. Mouth and oropharynx cancers	2 363	1 450	913	2	4	264	805	375	3	4	193	461	252
2. Oesophagus cancer	1 286	687	600			96	396	195			98	289	212
3. Stomach cancer	1 222	813	409			148	465	199			93	186	131
4. Colon and rectum cancers	558	315	243			95	136	84			46	104	93
5. Liver cancer	329	239	90	1	2	47	132	56	1	1	18	38	32
6. Pancreas cancer	194	122	71			22	69	31			15	29	27
7. Trachea, bronchus, lung cancers	3 509	3 035	474			479	1 699	855			71	236	167
8. Melanoma and other skin cancers	33	17	15		1	4	10	2			4	7	4
9. Breast cancer	1 012		1 012								323	478	210
10. Cervix uteri cancer	1 413		1 413								324	821	269
11. Corpus uteri cancer	76		76								8	38	29
12. Ovary cancer	322		322								123	110	86
13. Prostate cancer	174	174					46	123					
14. Bladder cancer	151	121	30			13	57	50			4	11	15
15. Lymphomas and multiple myeloma	568	399	169	22	37	157	134	49	5	7	51	53	53
16. Leukaemia	568	344	224	40	68	143	69	24	27	34	95	46	22
C. Diabetes mellitus	1 968	955	1 012	65	52	212	353	274	68	49	116	321	458
D. Endocrine disorders	86	46	41	22	2	10	9	2	17	1	6	8	9

Annex Table 17c, continued. DALYs by age, sex and cause (thousands): India, 2020, baseline scenario

Cause	Total	Male	Female	Males					Females				
				0-4	5-14	15-44	45-59	60+	0-4	5-14	15-44	45-59	60+
E. Neuro-psychiatric conditions	**29 786**	**13 303**	**16 483**	**403**	**290**	**10 043**	**1 639**	**927**	**522**	**364**	**12 187**	**2 072**	**1 339**
1. Unipolar major depression	13 322	4 772	8 551	-	-	3 866	746	160	-	-	6 887	1 331	332
2. Bipolar disorder	3 666	1 873	1 793	-	-	1 705	131	37	-	-	1 619	126	47
3. Schizophrenia	2 538	1 346	1 191	-	-	1 329	10	8	-	-	1 173	4	14
4. Epilepsy	607	360	248	35	47	214	42	22	43	68	100	13	24
5. Alcohol use	1 379	1 259	120	-	-	1 130	112	17	-	-	110	7	2
6. Dementia*	1 742	802	940	49	19	54	229	452	59	19	48	232	581
7. Parkinson disease	262	118	144			-	54	65			-	64	80
8. Multiple sclerosis	304	135	169			119	12	4			148	15	7
9. Drug use	112	100	11		5	90	4	1		1	10	-	-
10. Post-traumatic stress disorder	449	172	277	7	31	118	14	2	11	50	190	22	4
11. Obsessive-compulsive disorders	2 500	1 089	1 411		109	888	66	26		138	1 119	115	40
12. Panic disorder	1 190	384	805		4	308	72	-		38	639	112	16
F. Sense organ diseases	**6 296**	**3 522**	**2 773**	**5**	**-**	**190**	**1 935**	**1 392**	**3**	**-**	**116**	**1 204**	**1 451**
1. Glaucoma	1 199	668	531			52	486	129			20	353	159
2. Cataracts	5 094	2 852	2 242	3		138	1 448	1 262	3		96	851	1 292
G. Cardiovascular diseases	**43 524**	**27 788**	**15 736**	**550**	**118**	**2 810**	**11 331**	**12 979**	**369**	**139**	**1 238**	**3 749**	**10 241**
1. Rheumatic heart disease	1 898	1 066	831	1	13	397	528	127	1	15	320	373	123
2. Ischaemic heart disease	22 021	14 356	7 665			674	6 195	7 488			271	1 747	5 647
3. Cerebrovascular disease	7 971	4 841	3 130	106	24	378	1 736	2 597	76	24	216	608	2 206
4. Inflammatory heart diseases	2 252	1 453	798	101	27	437	609	281	79	33	198	250	238
H. Respiratory diseases	**15 180**	**8 549**	**6 631**	**293**	**276**	**1 380**	**3 541**	**3 060**	**190**	**181**	**1 246**	**2 661**	**2 353**
1. COPD*	6 700	4 094	2 606	31	20	452	1 869	1 722	24	18	324	1 168	1 072
2. Asthma	2 052	1 185	867	54	126	555	301	149	21	66	421	230	129
I. Digestive diseases	**5 895**	**4 147**	**1 748**	**74**	**29**	**1 005**	**2 289**	**750**	**79**	**30**	**478**	**745**	**415**
1. Peptic ulcer	912	632	281	1	2	172	316	140	2	3	87	114	76
2. Cirrhosis of the liver	3 027	2 298	730	14	6	479	1 343	456	18	15	171	342	184
3. Appendicitis	160	95	64	2	10	66	13	4	2	11	42	7	3
J. Genito-urinary diseases	**1 790**	**1 222**	**568**	**87**	**88**	**123**	**669**	**255**	**47**	**124**	**102**	**122**	**173**
1. Nephritis and nephrosis	1 093	558	535	68	85	113	154	138	43	123	96	112	162
2. Benign prostatic hypertrophy	618	618	-			-	506	112					
L. Musculo-skeletal diseases	**2 685**	**1 035**	**1 650**	**3**	**3**	**360**	**503**	**167**	**2**	**4**	**515**	**752**	**376**
1. Rheumatoid arthritis	302	82	220	1	-	55	17	9	-	3	109	81	27
2. Osteoarthritis	2 362	940	1 422			301	483	156			405	670	347

Annex Table 17c, continued. DALYs by age, sex and cause (thousands): India, 2020, baseline scenario

Cause	Total	Male	Female	Males					Females				
				0-4	5-14	15-44	45-59	60+	0-4	5-14	15-44	45-59	60+
M. Congenital anomalies	7 550	3 678	3 872	3 487	65	99	20	7	3 689	75	69	26	13
N. Oral conditions	1 783	872	911	37	73	268	258	236	35	70	266	261	279
1. Dental caries	1 023	514	509	36	72	219	112	76	34	69	207	110	88
2. Periodontal disease	119	61	59	-	-	46	10	4	-	-	44	10	5
3. Edentulism	617	292	325	-	-	-	136	156	-	-	-	139	186
III. Injuries	*45 285*	*26 966*	*18 319*	*3 519*	*4 874*	*13 412*	*4 130*	*1 030*	*2 911*	*3 389*	*7 940*	*2 880*	*1 198*
A. Unintentional injuries	38 721	23 332	15 389	3 326	4 690	10 919	3 482	916	2 665	3 214	5 955	2 450	1 104
1. Road traffic accidents	15 314	10 884	4 430	550	1 753	6 437	1 722	423	162	1 374	1 705	819	369
2. Poisonings	897	402	495	123	40	180	46	12	84	26	206	165	14
3. Falls	6 155	3 566	2 589	736	1 643	795	291	101	829	623	582	430	125
4. Fires	4 399	1 342	3 058	314	174	616	200	38	267	470	1 927	258	136
5. Drownings	1 905	1 046	858	261	231	424	95	36	213	193	272	114	65
6. Other unintentional	10 051	6 093	3 958	1 342	850	2 467	1 128	306	1 110	527	1 263	662	395
B. Intentional injuries	6 564	3 633	2 931	193	184	2 493	649	114	246	175	1 985	431	94
1. Self-inflicted injuries	4 299	2 185	2 114	-	109	1 607	416	53	-	109	1 774	209	22
2. Violence	2 094	1 277	818	193	75	714	233	61	246	66	210	222	73
3. War	171	171	-	193	171	171	-	-	-	-	-	-	-

Notes:

A dash (-) symbol indicates fewer than 500 DALYs.

*IA6 is Bacterial meningitis and meningococcaemia; ID is Conditions arising during the perinatal period; IIE6 is Dementia and other degenerative and hereditary CNS disorders; IIH1 is Chronic obstructive pulmonary disease.

Annex Table 17d. DALYs by age, sex and cause (thousands): China, 2020, baseline scenario

Cause	Total	Male	Female	Males 0-4	5-14	15-44	45-59	60+	Females 0-4	5-14	15-44	45-59	60+
Population (millions)	1 469	737	733	56	103	318	163	96	54	98	303	161	117
All causes	220 667	127 595	93 072	8 063	2 684	33 901	44 178	38 769	8 120	2 181	28 313	24 417	30 040
I. Communicable, maternal, perinatal and nutritional conditions	9 536	4 830	4 706	2 555	303	543	408	1 021	2 605	294	425	353	1 029
A. Infectious and parasitic diseases	3 063	1 644	1 420	475	154	209	265	541	447	147	133	182	511
1. Tuberculosis	963	592	371	16	2	60	163	350	17	7	29	100	218
2. STDs excluding HIV	29	7	21	1	–	5	–	1	1	–	20	–	1
a. Syphilis	2	1	1					1					1
b. Chlamydia	18	2	16			2					15		
c. Gonorrhoea	9	4	5	1		3			1		4		
3. HIV	122	67	55	10	2	44	8	2	7	1	42	4	1
4. Diarrhoeal diseases	615	294	321	147	13	34	21	78	170	12	18	22	99
5. Childhood-cluster diseases	349	193	156	179	9	3	1	1	147	8	1	1	1
a. Pertussis	120	65	55	61	4				52	4			
b. Poliomyelitis	58	35	23	34		1			23				
c. Diphtheria	1	1		1									
d. Measles	78	42	36	38	3	1			33	3			
e. Tetanus	92	51	41	45	2	2	1		39	1		1	
6. Bacterial meningitis*	198	103	94	62	2	13	11	15	54	2	7	12	20
7. Hepatitis B and hepatitis C	108	68	40	11	1	14	23	19	8	1	3	6	23
8. Malaria	6	3	3	1	1	1			1	1	1		
9. Tropical-cluster diseases	23	18	4	1	2	11	2	2			1	1	1
a. Trypanosomiasis													
b. Chagas disease													
c. Schistosomiasis	5	3	2			1	1	1			1		1
d. Leishmaniasis				1		1							
e. Lymphatic filariasis	17	15	2			10	1	1			1	1	
f. Onchocerciasis													
10. Leprosy	2	1	1		1				1				
11. Dengue	3	1	2		1	1			1		1		
12. Japanese encephalitis	62	33	29	23	8	2			21	7	1		
13. Trachoma	167	42	125			2	7	33			3	21	102
14. Intestinal nematode infections	237	123	115	3	109	6	2	3	2	103	4	2	3
a. Ascariasis	107	55	52	3	52				2	49			
b. Trichuriasis	106	55	51		54					51			
c. Ancylostomiasis and necatoriasis	24	13	11		3	6	2	3		2	4	2	3

Annex Table 17d, continued. DALYs by age, sex and cause (thousands): China, 2020, baseline scenario

				Males					Females				
Cause	Total	Male	Female	0-4	5-14	15-44	45-59	60+	0-4	5-14	15-44	45-59	60+
B. Respiratory infections	**2 476**	**1 212**	**1 264**	**842**	**34**	**17**	**23**	**296**	**897**	**35**	**12**	**16**	**304**
1. Lower respiratory infections	2 406	1 177	1 229	824	23	16	22	292	878	24	11	15	300
2. Upper respiratory infections	28	14	14	8	1	1	1	4	8	1	1	1	4
3. Otitis media	42	21	21	11	10	1	-	-	10	10	1	-	-
C. Maternal conditions	**124**	**-**	**124**	**-**	**-**	**-**	**-**	**-**	**-**	**-**	**114**	**10**	**-**
1. Maternal haemorrhage	20	-	20	-	-	-	-	-	-	-	17	3	-
2. Maternal sepsis	21	-	21	-	-	-	-	-	-	-	21	-	-
3. Hypertensive disorders of pregnancy	4	-	4	-	-	-	-	-	-	-	4	-	-
4. Obstructed labour	26	-	26	-	-	-	-	-	-	-	26	-	-
5. Abortion	4	-	4	-	-	-	-	-	-	-	3	1	-
D. Perinatal conditions*	**1 912**	**965**	**947**	**965**	**-**	**-**	**-**	**-**	**947**	**-**	**-**	**-**	**-**
E. Nutritional deficiencies	**1 960**	**1 009**	**951**	**272**	**115**	**318**	**120**	**184**	**314**	**112**	**165**	**145**	**215**
1. Protein-energy malnutrition	352	157	195	139	-	1	1	16	179	-	-	1	15
2. Iodine deficiency	74	40	34	37	2	1	-	-	32	2	-	-	-
3. Vitamin A deficiency	46	25	21	20	4	1	-	-	17	4	-	-	-
4. Iron-deficiency anaemia	1 488	787	700	76	108	316	119	168	86	106	164	145	200
II. Noncommunicable diseases	*174 998*	*102 728*	*72 270*	*3 241*	*1 031*	*22 282*	*40 156*	*36 019*	*3 303*	*750*	*20 150*	*20 934*	*27 132*
A. Malignant neoplasms	**41 362**	**29 027**	**12 336**	**122**	**356**	**4 976**	**14 534**	**9 039**	**204**	**163**	**2 149**	**5 036**	**4 783**
1. Mouth and oropharynx cancers	1 181	873	308	5	8	288	372	200	-	-	86	133	89
2. Oesophagus cancer	4 444	3 313	1 131	-	-	298	1 636	1 378	-	-	44	415	672
3. Stomach cancer	8 069	5 797	2 273	-	7	450	2 990	2 349	-	8	341	836	1 089
4. Colon and rectum cancers	2 185	1 336	849	-	7	267	595	467	-	7	132	346	364
5. Liver cancer	9 183	7 378	1 805	5	22	1 903	3 985	1 463	7	19	322	820	637
6. Pancreas cancer	698	477	222	-	-	54	213	210	-	-	12	69	141
7. Trachea, bronchus, lung cancers	7 553	5 889	1 664	-	14	569	3 212	2 090	-	-	87	796	781
8. Melanoma and other skin cancers	28	18	10	-	-	4	8	6	-	-	2	4	4
9. Breast cancer	687	-	687	-	-	-	-	-	-	-	207	313	167
10. Cervix uteri cancer	512	-	512	-	-	-	-	-	-	-	90	246	177
11. Corpus uteri cancer	177	-	177	-	-	-	-	-	-	-	22	120	35
12. Ovary cancer	269	-	269	-	-	-	-	-	4	6	85	115	59
13. Prostate cancer	91	91	-	-	-	4	16	71	-	-	-	-	-
14. Bladder cancer	407	337	70	-	-	25	111	200	-	-	3	16	50
15. Lymphomas and multiple myeloma	624	439	184	-	31	95	183	130	-	-	34	102	48
16. Leukaemia	1 990	1 138	852	69	179	478	319	93	95	85	377	194	101
C. Diabetes mellitus	**966**	**451**	**515**	**6**	**5**	**87**	**188**	**166**	**6**	**4**	**43**	**171**	**291**
D. Endocrine disorders	**353**	**112**	**241**	**14**	**5**	**31**	**38**	**25**	**96**	**10**	**58**	**28**	**49**

Annex Table 17d, continued. DALYs by age, sex and cause (thousands): China, 2020, baseline scenario

Cause	Total	Male	Female	Males					Females				
				0-4	5-14	15-44	45-59	60+	0-4	5-14	15-44	45-59	60+
E. Neuro-psychiatric conditions	**34 062**	**15 060**	**19 002**	**182**	**276**	**10 922**	**2 414**	**1 266**	**154**	**293**	**13 157**	**3 392**	**2 005**
1. Unipolar major depression	16 114	5 736	10 379			4 208	1 248	280			7 554	2 238	586
2. Bipolar disorder	4 209	2 141	2 068			1 863	217	61			1 776	214	77
3. Schizophrenia	2 640	1 416	1 224	12	33	1 389	11	15	11	34	1 195	15	15
4. Epilepsy	447	255	191			146	47	18			96	29	21
5. Alcohol use	1 684	1 563	120			1 351	187	25			109	10	2
6. Dementia*	2 823	1 239	1 584	56	20	54	363	746	54	18	49	384	1 079
7. Parkinson disease	196	92	104				44	48				43	61
8. Multiple sclerosis	340	149	191			125	18	6			156	24	10
9. Drug use	198	177	20		13	152	11	2		2	17	1	
10. Post-traumatic stress disorder	488	187	302	8	31	123	22	3	12	50	199	35	6
11. Obsessive-compulsive disorders	2 735	1 178	1 558		107	921	106	43		136	1 168	185	68
12. Panic disorder	1 389	474	915		38	320	116	1		37	668	181	28
F. Sense organ diseases	**3 826**	**1 621**	**2 204**	**33**		**77**	**777**	**735**	**27**	**10**	**149**	**1 164**	**855**
1. Glaucoma	1 665	470	1 195	5		29	288	147	6		75	857	258
2. Cataracts	1 904	1 067	837	11		39	449	566	1		27	251	559
G. Cardiovascular diseases	**36 021**	**24 325**	**11 695**	**229**	**44**	**2 026**	**10 484**	**11 542**	**117**	**19**	**1 028**	**2 820**	**7 711**
1. Rheumatic heart disease	2 535	1 474	1 062		7	314	696	457	12	6	227	370	448
2. Ischaemic heart disease	10 412	7 036	3 375			513	3 026	3 497			205	699	2 472
3. Cerebrovascular disease	18 170	12 415	5 755	57	21	883	5 291	6 164	33	7	410	1 462	3 844
4. Inflammatory heart diseases	1 306	890	416	39	7	215	433	197	23	4	118	124	147
H. Respiratory diseases	**36 026**	**20 640**	**15 386**	**265**	**173**	**2 642**	**7 172**	**10 387**	**154**	**96**	**1 956**	**4 574**	**8 606**
1. COPD*	31 986	18 272	13 714	46	3	1 775	6 571	9 876	63	2	1 297	4 186	8 167
2. Asthma	2 643	1 527	1 116	56	156	698	427	190	21	84	558	305	147
I. Digestive diseases	**7 787**	**4 725**	**3 061**	**217**	**26**	**715**	**2 291**	**1 477**	**247**	**24**	**443**	**1 246**	**1 102**
1. Peptic ulcer	451	286	165	1		50	122	112	2	1	24	53	85
2. Cirrhosis of the liver	3 193	2 222	972	11	4	407	1 149	651	4	4	118	461	385
3. Appendicitis	121	71	50	1	9	44	13	5	1	8	30	7	3
J. Genito-urinary diseases	**2 336**	**1 690**	**646**	**53**	**24**	**273**	**1 026**	**314**	**52**	**16**	**133**	**185**	**260**
1. Nephritis and nephrosis	1 056	608	448	35	24	250	154	146	52	16	111	103	165
2. Benign prostatic hypertrophy	927	927	-	5		5	812	106					-
L. Musculo-skeletal diseases	**5 838**	**1 933**	**3 905**			**291**	**877**	**756**	**16**	**10**	**806**	**1 993**	**1 079**
1. Rheumatoid arthritis	1 200	368	831			87	215	66		6	183	432	211
2. Osteoarthritis	4 098	1 365	2 732			176	619	570			550	1 475	707

Annex Table 17d, continued. DALYs by age, sex and cause (thousands): China, 2020, baseline scenario

Cause	Total	Male	Female	Males					Females				
				0-4	5-14	15-44	45-59	60+	0-4	5-14	15-44	45-59	60+
M. Congenital anomalies	4 090	1 990	2 099	1 850	55	81	5	-	1 969	56	69	6	-
N. Oral conditions	1 517	723	794	177	37	66	221	223	168	36	81	228	281
1. Dental caries	650	329	321	176	36	45	51	21	167	34	43	51	26
2. Periodontal disease	39	20	19	-	-	16	3	1	-	-	15	3	1
3. Edentulism	794	367	427	-	-	-	166	200	-	-	-	173	254
III. Injuries	36 133	20 037	16 096	2 267	1 349	11 077	3 615	1 730	2 212	1 137	7 738	3 130	1 879
A. Unintentional injuries	24 304	14 849	9 455	2 089	1 206	7 834	2 580	1 139	1 886	999	3 384	1 943	1 243
1. Road traffic accidents	10 631	6 892	3 739	142	587	4 408	1 267	488	103	644	1 915	812	265
2. Poisonings	1 091	613	478	110	21	213	192	77	32	29	230	89	98
3. Falls	3 043	1 496	1 547	293	109	704	236	155	363	71	316	382	415
4. Fires	448	228	219	59	23	78	28	39	39	33	30	48	68
5. Drownings	2 154	1 300	854	494	263	383	95	65	397	124	157	82	94
6. Other unintentional	6 938	4 319	2 618	991	203	2 048	762	315	952	98	736	529	303
B. Intentional injuries	11 829	5 188	6 641	178	143	3 242	1 034	591	326	138	4 354	1 187	636
1. Self-inflicted injuries	10 037	4 115	5 922	-	95	2 524	939	558	-	71	4 134	1 118	599
2. Violence	1 766	1 047	719	178	48	693	96	33	326	67	221	69	37
3. War	26	26	-	-	-	26	-	-	-	-	-	-	-

Notes:
A dash (-) symbol indicates fewer than 500 DALYs.
*IA6 is Bacterial meningitis and meningococcaemia; ID is Conditions arising during the perinatal period;
IIE6 is Dementia and other degenerative and hereditary CNS disorders; IIH1 is Chronic obstructive pulmonary disease.

Annex Table 17e. DALYs by age, sex and cause (thousands): Other Asia and Islands, 2020, baseline scenario

Cause	Total	Male	Female	Males					Females				
				0-4	5-14	15-44	45-59	60+	0-4	5-14	15-44	45-59	60+
Population (millions)	*1 024*	*508*	*516*	*44*	*84*	*242*	*86*	*53*	*42*	*81*	*237*	*91*	*66*
All causes	*165 978*	*94 706*	*71 272*	*14 502*	*5 170*	*34 955*	*22 225*	*17 855*	*11 389*	*3 468*	*25 045*	*13 955*	*17 416*
I. Communicable, maternal, perinatal and nutritional conditions	*27 369*	*14 508*	*12 861*	*8 661*	*866*	*3 023*	*796*	*1 163*	*6 492*	*742*	*3 536*	*756*	*1 334*
A. Infectious and parasitic diseases	*16 108*	*8 673*	*7 435*	*4 071*	*546*	*2 709*	*680*	*667*	*2 988*	*462*	*2 645*	*580*	*760*
1. Tuberculosis	2 048	1 033	1 015	11	15	232	313	463	4	14	134	323	540
2. STDs excluding HIV	1 510	561	949	276	4	258	5	17	215	14	686	9	26
a. Syphilis	394	221	174	167	-	32	4	17	110	-	33	6	25
b. Chlamydia	625	104	521	25	1	77	-	-	24	10	483	2	1
c. Gonorrhoea	491	236	255	84	2	149	1	-	81	4	169	1	-
3. HIV	4 904	2 764	2 140	452	81	1 939	237	54	291	56	1 651	118	23
4. Diarrhoeal diseases	3 671	2 141	1 530	1 986	78	24	17	36	1 376	57	26	25	47
5. Childhood-cluster diseases	2 057	1 120	937	998	75	30	9	8	827	70	19	11	10
a. Pertussis	342	186	156	176	11	-	-	-	147	9	-	-	-
b. Poliomyelitis	109	65	44	63	-	2	-	-	42	-	1	-	-
c. Diphtheria	21	11	9	11	1	-	-	-	9	1	-	-	-
d. Measles	999	543	455	499	43	1	-	-	419	36	-	-	-
e. Tetanus	586	314	272	250	21	27	9	8	210	24	17	10	10
6. Bacterial meningitis*	233	124	109	82	3	16	11	11	71	3	10	12	13
7. Hepatitis B and hepatitis C	115	67	48	15	5	12	15	20	10	4	6	8	20
8. Malaria	469	262	207	60	70	89	28	15	51	59	49	31	18
9. Tropical-cluster diseases	122	85	37	3	14	48	16	4	2	4	13	13	4
a. Trypanosomiasis	-	-	-	-	-	-	-	-	-	-	-	-	-
b. Chagas disease	-	-	-	-	-	-	-	-	-	-	-	-	-
c. Schistosomiasis	4	2	2	-	-	1	1	-	-	-	1	1	-
d. Leishmaniasis	13	8	4	-	2	5	-	1	-	-	2	-	-
e. Lymphatic filariasis	105	74	31	-	12	42	14	3	-	3	11	12	3
f. Onchocerciasis	-	-	-	-	-	-	-	-	-	-	-	-	-
10. Leprosy	25	12	12	-	3	6	2	1	-	3	6	2	-
11. Dengue	44	21	22	7	14	-	-	-	8	14	-	1	-
12. Japanese encephalitis	40	22	18	15	5	1	-	-	13	4	1	-	-
13. Trachoma	31	7	24	-	-	1	2	5	-	-	1	5	18
14. Intestinal nematode infections	396	207	189	2	151	36	10	8	2	139	27	11	11
a. Ascariasis	117	61	56	2	58	-	-	-	2	54	-	-	-
b. Trichuriasis	161	83	77	-	83	-	-	-	-	77	-	-	-
c. Ancylostomiasis and necatoriasis	118	62	56	-	9	35	10	8	-	9	26	10	10

Annex Table 17e, continued. DALYs by age, sex and cause (thousands): Other Asia and Islands, 2020, baseline scenario

Cause	Total	Male	Female	Males					Females				
				0-4	5-14	15-44	45-59	60+	0-4	5-14	15-44	45-59	60+
B. Respiratory infections	**4 707**	**2 636**	**2 071**	**1 902**	**210**	**70**	**45**	**408**	**1 336**	**182**	**47**	**51**	**456**
1. Lower respiratory infections	4 590	2 571	2 019	1 864	192	67	44	404	1 308	165	45	50	451
2. Upper respiratory infections	52	29	23	18	3	3	1	5	13	2	2	1	5
3. Otitis media	65	36	29	20	16				15	15			
C. Maternal conditions	**526**		**526**								**512**	**15**	
1. Maternal haemorrhage	52		52								49	3	
2. Maternal sepsis	92		92								90	2	
3. Hypertensive disorders of pregnancy	25		25								24	2	
4. Obstructed labour	117		117								116	1	
5. Abortion	100		100								99	2	
D. Perinatal conditions*	**3 714**	**2 078**	**1 636**	**2 078**					**1 636**				
E. Nutritional deficiencies	**2 313**	**1 121**	**1 192**	**610**	**109**	**243**	**71**	**88**	**532**	**99**	**333**	**111**	**118**
1. Protein-energy malnutrition	812	435	377	424	2	1	2	6	367	1	1	2	6
2. Iodine deficiency	44	23	21	21	2				19	2			
3. Vitamin A deficiency	142	77	64	58	18	1			49	15			
4. Iron-deficiency anaemia	1 316	586	730	107	87	240	69	82	97	81	331	109	112
II. Noncommunicable diseases	*110 004*	*60 926*	*49 078*	*3 668*	*2 201*	*19 915*	*19 047*	*16 094*	*2 988*	*1 543*	*16 751*	*12 175*	*15 621*
A. Malignant neoplasms	**19 329**	**11 463**	**7 866**	**199**	**597**	**2 280**	**4 586**	**3 799**	**259**	**349**	**1 802**	**2 605**	**2 851**
1. Mouth and oropharynx cancers	1 818	1 166	652	5	17	262	307	574	9	12	142	118	370
2. Oesophagus cancer	626	427	199			38	218	171			26	69	104
3. Stomach cancer	1 646	1 134	513	1	2	176	562	393		1	85	191	236
4. Colon and rectum cancers	1 047	574	473	2	6	130	147	289	3	4	83	106	277
5. Liver cancer	2 080	1 644	436	7	21	350	902	364	8	10	69	164	187
6. Pancreas cancer	254	168	86			28	74	66			7	32	46
7. Trachea, bronchus, lung cancers	3 136	2 423	714	2	7	355	1 300	759	1	1	51	297	359
8. Melanoma and other skin cancers	66	31	35		1	9	14	8			7	12	16
9. Breast cancer	857		857							3	258	391	205
10. Cervix uteri cancer	999		999							1	247	516	235
11. Corpus uteri cancer	104		104								14	47	41
12. Ovary cancer	336		336							2	145	101	67
13. Prostate cancer	275	275				4	57	210					
14. Bladder cancer	273	207	66	1		17	79	112			6	14	45
15. Lymphomas and multiple myeloma	712	461	252	26	76	148	91	119	16	21	63	40	111
16. Leukaemia	1 015	582	434	70	202	193	50	66	94	125	112	36	66
C. Diabetes mellitus	**1 488**	**710**	**779**	**7**	**10**	**174**	**291**	**227**	**8**	**10**	**95**	**261**	**404**
D. Endocrine disorders	**371**	**171**	**199**	**85**	**19**	**25**	**24**	**19**	**69**	**10**	**30**	**37**	**53**

Annex Table 17e, continued. DALYs by age, sex and cause (thousands): Other Asia and Islands, 2020, baseline scenario

Cause	Total	Male	Female	Males					Females				
				0-4	5-14	15-44	45-59	60+	0-4	5-14	15-44	45-59	60+
E. Neuro-psychiatric conditions	**28 877**	**14 236**	**14 641**	**170**	**353**	**11 247**	**1 623**	**843**	**172**	**330**	**10 792**	**2 022**	**1 325**
1. Unipolar major depression	10 982	3 830	7 152	-	-	3 046	635	148	-	-	5 618	1 210	325
2. Bipolar disorder	2 961	1 488	1 474	-	-	1 344	111	33	-	-	1 314	114	45
3. Schizophrenia	3 362	1 756	1 606	-	-	1 728	17	11	-	-	1 578	6	22
4. Epilepsy	578	340	238	12	65	189	56	19	14	69	107	29	19
5. Alcohol use	2 930	2 714	216	-	-	2 462	213	39	-	-	200	12	4
6. Dementia*	1 889	794	1 095	38	17	45	254	440	45	17	41	282	710
7. Parkinson disease	234	122	112	-	-	-	54	67	-	-	-	47	66
8. Multiple sclerosis	244	106	138	-	-	93	10	3	-	-	119	14	6
9. Drug use	1 360	1 226	134	-	63	1 092	61	11	-	7	118	7	1
10. Post-traumatic stress disorder	367	138	229	6	25	93	12	2	10	41	155	20	3
11. Obsessive-compulsive disorders	2 036	868	1 168	-	88	701	56	24	-	113	912	105	39
12. Panic disorder	1 005	335	670	-	31	243	61	-	-	31	521	102	16
F. Sense organ diseases	**3 840**	**1 739**	**2 101**	**5**	**3**	**91**	**896**	**744**	**5**		**110**	**1 096**	**889**
1. Glaucoma	1 311	382	929	-	-	21	261	100	3	-	62	685	182
2. Cataracts	2 513	1 347	1 166	1	-	67	635	643	-	-	48	410	705
G. Cardiovascular diseases	**25 850**	**15 690**	**10 160**	**993**	**645**	**3 053**	**4 980**	**6 019**	**629**	**402**	**1 458**	**1 846**	**5 826**
1. Rheumatic heart disease	202	106	96	-	3	26	31	46	-	4	22	21	50
2. Ischaemic heart disease	8 455	5 152	3 303	127	144	731	1 816	2 606	88	87	303	582	2 418
3. Cerebrovascular disease	7 457	4 348	3 109	193	140	722	1 442	1 915	147	89	345	641	1 948
4. Inflammatory heart diseases	1 996	1 275	721	-	-	452	331	159	-	-	210	121	154
H. Respiratory diseases	**7 085**	**3 928**	**3 157**	**361**	**264**	**857**	**950**	**1 495**	**179**	**173**	**710**	**683**	**1 412**
1. COPD*	2 896	1 689	1 207	36	15	251	491	897	19	12	149	276	751
2. Asthma	1 763	948	814	55	151	476	163	103	22	95	383	187	128
I. Digestive diseases	**10 749**	**6 866**	**3 884**	**197**	**105**	**1 148**	**3 499**	**1 916**	**167**	**92**	**597**	**1 593**	**1 434**
1. Peptic ulcer	511	339	171	2	3	68	143	124	1	2	30	50	88
2. Cirrhosis of the liver	3 665	2 827	839	12	10	546	1 620	640	8	11	127	388	304
3. Appendicitis	151	90	61	1	18	56	12	3	1	17	33	7	3
J. Genito-urinary diseases	**2 083**	**1 250**	**834**	**51**	**78**	**192**	**656**	**273**	**35**	**56**	**133**	**209**	**401**
1. Nephritis and nephrosis	1 194	579	614	37	67	162	145	169	35	48	98	141	293
2. Benign prostatic hypertrophy	504	504	-	-	-	-	456	48	-	-	-	-	-
L. Musculo-skeletal diseases	**4 287**	**1 837**	**2 450**	**14**	**10**	**345**	**1 070**	**398**	**14**	**13**	**546**	**1 328**	**549**
1. Rheumatoid arthritis	439	125	314	-	-	6	42	77	-	2	74	70	168
2. Osteoarthritis	3 577	1 614	1 963	-	-	319	1 002	293	-	-	434	1 218	310

Annex Table 17e, continued. DALYs by age, sex and cause (thousands): Other Asia and Islands, 2020, baseline scenario

Cause	Total	Male	Female	Males					Females				
				0-4	5-14	15-44	45-59	60+	0-4	5-14	15-44	45-59	60+
M. Congenital anomalies	**3 062**	**1 604**	**1 457**	**1 488**	**43**	**54**	**14**	**5**	**1 370**	**40**	**27**	**13**	**7**
N. Oral conditions	**2 515**	**1 189**	**1 327**	**31**	**44**	**399**	**391**	**323**	**30**	**44**	**405**	**428**	**420**
1. Dental caries	896	440	456	30	44	173	136	58	29	42	169	143	72
2. Periodontal disease	58	28	29	-	-	20	6	2	-	-	20	6	3
3. Edentulism	1 542	716	826	-	-	204	250	263	-	-	204	278	344
III. Injuries	***28 605***	***19 272***	***9 333***	***2 172***	***2 103***	***12 017***	***2 382***	***598***	***1 909***	***1 183***	***4 757***	***1 024***	***461***
A. Unintentional injuries	**22 585**	**15 330**	**7 254**	**2 070**	**1 900**	**9 040**	**1 865**	**456**	**1 798**	**1 052**	**3 170**	**848**	**386**
1. Road traffic accidents	8 561	5 847	2 714	484	792	3 748	637	186	444	482	1 323	314	151
2. Poisonings	989	508	481	50	41	289	94	32	47	46	295	59	36
3. Falls	3 361	2 190	1 171	518	260	1 108	251	53	405	128	450	144	45
4. Fires	361	191	170	43	36	86	19	7	64	43	46	10	8
5. Drownings	1 803	1 228	575	397	307	419	76	30	252	126	144	32	21
6. Other unintentional	7 509	5 367	2 142	577	464	3 390	788	148	588	228	912	289	125
B. Intentional injuries	**6 020**	**3 941**	**2 079**	**103**	**202**	**2 977**	**518**	**142**	**110**	**131**	**1 587**	**176**	**75**
1. Self-inflicted injuries	2 905	1 630	1 275	-	72	1 229	238	91	-	44	1 065	112	54
2. Violence	2 326	1 853	473	45	92	1 416	256	44	52	57	305	47	14
3. War	789	459	331	58	39	331	24	7	59	29	217	17	8

Notes:
A dash (-) symbol indicates fewer than 500 DALYs.
*IIA6 is Bacterial meningitis and meningococcaemia; ID is Conditions arising during the perinatal period;
IIE6 is Dementia and other degenerative and hereditary CNS disorders; IIH1 is Chronic obstructive pulmonary disease.

Annex Table 17f. DALYs by age, sex and cause (thousands): Sub-Saharan Africa, 2020, baseline scenario

Cause	Total	Male	Female	Males					Females				
				0-4	5-14	15-44	45-59	60+	0-4	5-14	15-44	45-59	60+
Population (millions)	*1 172*	*580*	*591*	*90*	*151*	*263*	*50*	*26*	*87*	*147*	*269*	*55*	*33*
All causes	*329 566*	*188 386*	*141 179*	*65 206*	*17 253*	*77 603*	*16 703*	*11 620*	*51 956*	*13 271*	*48 498*	*14 413*	*13 042*
I. Communicable, maternal, perinatal and nutritional conditions	*131 037*	*68 737*	*62 301*	*49 158*	*4 146*	*12 019*	*2 180*	*1 233*	*38 234*	*4 199*	*16 322*	*2 083*	*1 463*
A. Infectious and parasitic diseases	94 062	49 310	44 752	31 488	3 211	11 707	2 110	794	24 403	3 310	14 153	1 993	892
1. Tuberculosis	22 065	10 370	11 696	1 081	873	6 366	1 574	476	1 148	1 238	7 275	1 532	502
2. STDs excluding HIV	**3 421**	**1 439**	**1 982**	**1 010**	**9**	**387**	**8**	**26**	**893**	**31**	**1 009**	**12**	**37**
a. Syphilis	1 546	824	722	726	1	65	6	25	607	-	69	9	37
b. Chlamydia	854	141	712	53	2	86	-	-	53	20	637	8	-
c. Gonorrhoea	1 022	474	548	232	5	236	1	-	233	10	303	1	-
3. HIV	**14 502**	**6 675**	**7 826**	**2 121**	**325**	**3 916**	**263**	**51**	**2 017**	**337**	**5 243**	**196**	**33**
4. Diarrhoeal diseases	**18 102**	**10 445**	**7 657**	**9 810**	**443**	**91**	**25**	**76**	**7 003**	**421**	**102**	**32**	**99**
5. Childhood-cluster diseases	**16 862**	**9 349**	**7 513**	**8 625**	**659**	**45**	**10**	**9**	**6 870**	**595**	**31**	**9**	**9**
a. Pertussis	3 139	1 745	1 394	1 649	95	2	-	-	1 311	83	1	-	-
b. Poliomyelitis	348	209	140	206	1	-	-	-	138	1	1	-	-
c. Diphtheria	35	20	16	18	1	2	-	-	15	-	-	-	-
d. Measles	10 993	6 080	4 913	5 567	512	1	-	-	4 458	455	-	-	-
e. Tetanus	2 347	1 296	1 051	1 184	51	42	10	9	949	55	29	9	9
6. Bacterial meningitis*	**524**	**283**	**241**	**250**	**6**	**16**	**6**	**5**	**210**	**5**	**12**	**7**	**7**
7. Hepatitis B and hepatitis C	**125**	**72**	**53**	**25**	**8**	**14**	**11**	**14**	**17**	**7**	**9**	**5**	**14**
8. Malaria	**14 738**	**8 473**	**6 265**	**7 796**	**363**	**249**	**45**	**20**	**5 669**	**333**	**186**	**49**	**28**
9. Tropical-cluster diseases	**1 706**	**1 124**	**582**	**59**	**371**	**505**	**129**	**60**	**59**	**201**	**190**	**91**	**40**
a. Trypanosomiasis	411	225	186	11	82	92	32	8	20	77	63	22	5
b. Chagas disease													
c. Schistosomiasis	388	250	138	16	91	107	21	16	9	55	50	13	11
d. Leishmaniasis	136	95	41	8	53	33	2	-	3	24	12	1	-
e. Lymphatic filariasis	470	368	102	19	117	202	26	3	24	24	29	21	4
f. Onchocerciasis	300	186	115	5	28	71	49	33	3	20	36	35	20
10. Leprosy	**22**	**11**	**11**		**4**	**6**	**1**	**-**	**1**	**4**	**6**	**1**	**-**
11. Dengue	**7**	**4**	**4**	**1**	**2**	**-**	**-**	**-**	**-**	**3**	**-**	**-**	**-**
12. Japanese encephalitis													
13. Trachoma	**193**	**51**	**142**	**-**	**-**	**8**	**12**	**31**	**-**	**-**	**13**	**34**	**94**
14. Intestinal nematode infections	**198**	**105**	**93**	**1**	**51**	**41**	**7**	**5**	**1**	**47**	**31**	**8**	**6**
a. Ascariasis	39	20	19	1	19	-	-	-	1	18	-	-	-
b. Trichuriasis	39	20	19	1	20	-	-	-	1	19	-	-	-
c. Ancylostomiasis and necatoriasis	121	65	56	-	12	41	7	5	-	11	31	8	6

Annex Table 17f, continued. DALYs by age, sex and cause (thousands): Sub-Saharan Africa, 2020, baseline scenario

Cause	Total	Male	Female	Males					Females				
				0-4	5-14	15-44	45-59	60+	0-4	5-14	15-44	45-59	60+
B. Respiratory infections	**17 958**	**10 263**	**7 695**	**9 008**	**689**	**140**	**38**	**388**	**6 459**	**550**	**134**	**43**	**509**
1. Lower respiratory infections	17 571	10 045	7 527	8 837	650	136	37	384	6 334	516	131	42	504
2. Upper respiratory infections	183	105	79	89	8	3	1	4	63	6	3	1	–
3. Otitis media	203	114	89	83	31	1	–	–	61	28	1	–	5
C. Maternal conditions	**1 961**		**1 961**								**1 847**	**2**	
1. Maternal haemorrhage	285		285							25	259	1	
2. Maternal sepsis	371		371							17	354		
3. Hypertensive disorders of pregnancy	141		141							13	128		
4. Obstructed labour	340		340							9	331		
5. Abortion	344		344							14	329		
D. Perinatal conditions*	**12 030**	**6 498**	**5 532**	**6 498**					**5 532**				
E. Nutritional deficiencies	**5 027**	**2 666**	**2 362**	**2 164**	**247**	**172**	**32**	**51**	**1 841**	**227**	**187**	**44**	**61**
1. Protein-energy malnutrition	3 200	1 727	1 473	1 692	12	6	3	14	1 435	12	8	3	15
2. Iodine deficiency	69	36	33	33	2	1	–	–	30	2	1	–	–
3. Vitamin A deficiency	582	316	266	247	66	3	–	–	204	60	2	–	–
4. Iron-deficiency anaemia	1 176	587	589	193	166	163	29	37	173	153	176	41	46
II. Noncommunicable diseases	**105 097**	**54 422**	**50 675**	**7 817**	**3 204**	**22 236**	**11 518**	**9 648**	**7 235**	**3 095**	**17 948**	**11 297**	**11 100**
A. Malignant neoplasms	**14 704**	**8 440**	**6 264**	**282**	**790**	**2 633**	**2 480**	**2 256**	**424**	**714**	**1 365**	**2 094**	**1 666**
1. Mouth and oropharynx cancers	680	422	259	2	7	129	92	192	13	28	55	44	118
2. Oesophagus cancer	696	536	160	–	–	121	268	147	–	–	27	63	71
3. Stomach cancer	948	586	363	1	3	134	262	186	1	–	61	183	119
4. Colon and rectum cancers	413	239	174	1	3	81	55	100	1	1	36	39	97
5. Liver cancer	2 152	1 703	450	6	20	855	594	227	10	19	129	166	126
6. Pancreas cancer	206	125	81	–	–	33	58	34	–	–	16	40	25
7. Trachea, bronchus, lung cancers	712	453	260	–	1	141	177	134	–	–	53	125	81
8. Melanoma and other skin cancers	221	102	119	–	1	21	48	31	–	–	13	48	57
9. Breast cancer	522	–	522						–	–	141	237	141
10. Cervix uteri cancer	954	–	954						–	–	216	451	284
11. Corpus uteri cancer	88	–	88						–	–	11	38	37
12. Ovary cancer	251	–	251						–	–	68	94	55
13. Prostate cancer	699	699	–	–	–	16	172	510					
14. Bladder cancer	380	256	124	–	1	49	97	109	–	–	27	48	49
15. Lymphomas and multiple myeloma	1 281	803	478	98	322	198	85	100	102	205	70	44	57
16. Leukaemia	425	196	229	18	57	70	18	34	46	92	37	27	27
C. Diabetes mellitus	**578**	**279**	**299**	**26**	**38**	**66**	**84**	**66**	**31**	**35**	**34**	**83**	**115**
D. Endocrine disorders	**1 405**	**730**	**674**	**387**	**32**	**152**	**115**	**45**	**246**	**57**	**102**	**128**	**142**

Annex Table 17f, continued. DALYs by age, sex and cause (thousands): Sub-Saharan Africa, 2020, baseline scenario

Cause	Total	Male	Female	Males 0-4	5-14	15-44	45-59	60+	Females 0-4	5-14	15-44	45-59	60+
E. Neuro-psychiatric conditions	**27 895**	**13 369**	**14 527**	**362**	**506**	**11 289**	**899**	**313**	**424**	**534**	**11 784**	**1 176**	**609**
1. Unipolar major depression	11 517	3 920	7 597	-	-	3 455	386	79	-	-	6 648	772	177
2. Bipolar disorder	3 309	1 630	1 679	-	-	1 544	68	18	-	-	1 579	76	24
3. Schizophrenia	1 121	580	541	-	-	574	4	2	-	-	535	2	4
4. Epilepsy	547	312	235	43	79	156	25	9	50	72	90	13	10
5. Alcohol use	4 378	3 545	833	-	-	3 346	177	22	-	-	788	34	12
6. Dementia*	752	233	519	30	12	23	57	110	81	36	50	66	286
7. Parkinson disease	109	56	53	-	-	-	27	29	-	-	-	24	29
8. Multiple sclerosis	244	104	140	-	-	96	6	2	-	-	128	9	3
9. Drug use	910	820	90	-	54	738	24	4	-	6	80	3	3
10. Post-traumatic stress disorder	451	167	285	12	45	102	7	1	19	75	177	12	2
11. Obsessive-compulsive disorders	2 294	967	1 327	-	157	765	33	12	-	204	1 039	64	20
12. Panic disorder	1 086	359	727	-	56	268	36	-	-	57	599	63	8
F. Sense organ diseases	**4 336**	**2 086**	**2 250**	**12**	**1**	**141**	**999**	**933**	**11**	**1**	**110**	**1 057**	**1 070**
1. Glaucoma	979	383	596	-	-	3	185	196	-	-	6	301	290
2. Cataracts	3 345	1 695	1 650	12	1	131	815	737	11	1	100	757	781
G. Cardiovascular diseases	**19 738**	**10 413**	**9 324**	**876**	**528**	**3 237**	**2 786**	**2 986**	**618**	**555**	**1 361**	**2 646**	**4 145**
1. Rheumatic heart disease	608	347	261	2	82	231	25	7	2	93	125	32	9
2. Ischaemic heart disease	4 824	2 542	2 282	-	-	686	865	991	182	-	224	687	1 189
3. Cerebrovascular disease	8 542	4 225	4 318	136	196	1 304	1 172	1 417	105	156	526	1 311	2 220
4. Inflammatory heart diseases	2 101	1 180	921	235	81	425	240	200	228	103	171	165	253
H. Respiratory diseases	**14 868**	**7 729**	**7 139**	**963**	**583**	**2 532**	**1 725**	**1 926**	**557**	**456**	**1 575**	**2 420**	**2 130**
1. COPD*	4 674	2 587	2 087	80	40	745	687	1 035	51	38	281	774	943
2. Asthma	2 289	1 154	1 135	121	280	569	102	82	57	198	563	202	116
I. Digestive diseases	**5 992**	**3 712**	**2 280**	**282**	**174**	**1 102**	**1 450**	**704**	**271**	**273**	**519**	**613**	**605**
1. Peptic ulcer	395	260	135	-	-	122	101	38	-	9	45	51	39
2. Cirrhosis of the liver	897	667	229	-	15	206	303	143	-	9	56	91	73
3. Appendicitis	287	181	106	4	54	107	13	3	5	55	36	8	3
J. Genito-urinary diseases	**3 088**	**1 924**	**1 164**	**483**	**292**	**361**	**604**	**183**	**360**	**220**	**171**	**222**	**192**
1. Nephritis and nephrosis	2 095	1 184	911	402	247	291	122	122	346	191	109	135	130
2. Benign prostatic hypertrophy	432	432	-	-	-	-	415	17	-	-	-	-	-
L. Musculo-skeletal diseases	**2 608**	**867**	**1 741**	-	-	**454**	**284**	**129**	-	**4**	**703**	**763**	**270**
1. Rheumatoid arthritis	217	60	157	-	-	39	15	6	-	4	97	42	13
2. Osteoarthritis	2 368	796	1 572	-	-	409	266	121	-	-	600	717	255

Annex Table 17f, continued. DALYs by age, sex and cause (thousands): Sub-Saharan Africa, 2020, baseline scenario

Cause	Total	Male	Female	Males 0-4	5-14	15-44	45-59	60+	Females 0-4	5-14	15-44	45-59	60+
M. Congenital anomalies	**7 325**	**3 526**	**3 799**	**3 354**	**77**	**79**	**12**	**5**	**3 667**	**80**	**28**	**16**	**8**
N. Oral conditions	**885**	**425**	**460**	**90**	**107**	**120**	**26**	**81**	**87**	**108**	**131**	**29**	**105**
1. Dental caries	625	312	313	87	105	88	24	9	84	102	90	26	11
2. Periodontal disease	68	33	34	-	-	31	3	-	-	-	31	3	-
3. Edentulism	166	72	94	-	-	-	-	72	-	-	-	-	94
III. Injuries	***93 431***	***65 227***	***28 204***	***8 232***	***9 903***	***43 348***	***3 005***	***739***	***6 486***	***5 978***	***14 229***	***1 033***	***478***
A. Unintentional injuries	**50 760**	**35 602**	**15 158**	**5 952**	**7 593**	**19 561**	**1 983**	**513**	**4 396**	**4 586**	**5 268**	**596**	**312**
1. Road traffic accidents	16 864	11 956	4 908	679	3 550	6 791	740	196	460	1 894	2 281	217	55
2. Poisonings	2 033	1 189	844	856	143	139	36	15	629	65	134	9	7
3. Falls	3 085	1 758	1 327	396	588	610	113	51	433	331	390	71	102
4. Fires	5 101	2 611	2 489	1 113	619	745	96	39	955	775	638	69	52
5. Drownings	4 111	3 021	1 091	952	1 166	808	72	23	483	422	160	17	8
6. Other unintentional	19 567	15 068	4 499	1 956	1 527	10 469	926	190	1 436	1 098	1 666	212	87
B. Intentional injuries	**42 672**	**29 625**	**13 046**	**2 280**	**2 311**	**23 787**	**1 022**	**225**	**2 090**	**1 392**	**8 960**	**437**	**167**
1. Self-inflicted injuries	1 174	939	235	-	111	761	53	14	-	-	214	18	2
2. Violence	16 306	14 098	2 207	293	713	12 448	548	97	144	292	1 614	121	36
3. War	25 192	14 588	10 604	1 987	1 486	10 579	421	114	1 946	1 100	7 132	298	129

Notes:
A dash (-) symbol indicates fewer than 500 DALYs.
*IA6 is Bacterial meningitis and meningococcaemia; ID is Conditions arising during the perinatal period;
IIE6 is Dementia and other degenerative and hereditary CNS disorders; IIH1 is Chronic obstructive pulmonary disease.

Annex Table 17g. DALYs by age, sex and cause (thousands): Latin America and the Caribbean, 2020, baseline scenario

Cause	Total	Male	Female	Males					Females				
				0-4	5-14	15-44	45-59	60+	0-4	5-14	15-44	45-59	60+
Population (millions)	*678*	*336*	*342*	*29*	*56*	*158*	*56*	*38*	*28*	*53*	*156*	*58*	*46*
All causes	**107 639**	**61 870**	**45 769**	**6 954**	**3 092**	**28 245**	**12 959**	**10 620**	**5 361**	**2 203**	**17 591**	**10 448**	**10 167**
I. Communicable, maternal, perinatal and nutritional conditions	***13 541***	***8 014***	***5 528***	***4 250***	***334***	***2 622***	***368***	***439***	***3 084***	***339***	***1 461***	***228***	***415***
A. Infectious and parasitic diseases	**7 949**	**5 063**	**2 886**	**1 780**	**225**	**2 522**	**303**	**234**	**1 319**	**225**	**1 000**	**155**	**187**
1. Tuberculosis	**489**	**297**	**192**	**16**	**12**	**111**	**70**	**88**	**12**	**17**	**63**	**45**	**55**
2. STDs excluding HIV	**482**	**136**	**346**	**69**	**1**	**62**	**1**	**3**	**56**	**6**	**279**	**2**	**5**
a. Syphilis	123	67	56	56		7		3	43		7	1	4
b. Chlamydia	239	24	214	3		21			3	4	206	1	
c. Gonorrhoea	121	44	76	10		34			10	1	65		
3. HIV	**3 170**	**2 504**	**667**	**135**	**13**	**2 170**	**151**	**35**	**125**	**14**	**500**	**21**	**6**
4. Diarrhoeal diseases	**1 607**	**943**	**664**	**837**	**38**	**23**	**13**	**32**	**551**	**38**	**20**	**15**	**39**
5. Childhood-cluster diseases	**987**	**541**	**446**	**509**	**28**	**2**	**1**	**1**	**415**	**26**	**2**	**1**	**1**
a. Pertussis	209	114	96	107	7				89	6			
b. Poliomyelitis	63	37	25	37					25				
c. Diphtheria	4	2	2	2	1	1			1	1			
d. Measles	510	277	233	259	18				214	18	1		
e. Tetanus	202	111	91	105	3	1		1	86	1	1		1
6. Bacterial meningitis*	**151**	**79**	**72**	**51**	**2**	**11**	**7**	**8**	**44**	**2**	**8**	**7**	**10**
7. Hepatitis B and hepatitis C	**30**	**15**	**15**	**6**	**3**	**2**	**2**	**2**	**4**	**3**	**4**	**2**	**2**
8. Malaria	**99**	**53**	**46**	**12**	**11**	**20**	**6**	**3**	**10**	**12**	**14**	**6**	**4**
9. Tropical-cluster diseases	**208**	**114**	**94**	**3**	**5**	**58**	**27**	**21**	**2**	**3**	**41**	**28**	**20**
a. Trypanosomiasis	175	93	82		1	49	24	19		2	37	26	19
b. Chagas disease	19	11	8		2	6	2	1			3	2	1
c. Schistosomiasis	12	9	3	2	2	4	1			1	1		
d. Leishmaniasis	2	2				1							
e. Lymphatic filariasis													
f. Onchocerciasis	1	1											
10. Leprosy	**17**	**9**	**8**		**2**	**4**	**1**	**1**		**2**	**4**	**1**	**1**
11. Dengue													
12. Japanese encephalitis													
13. Trachoma													
14. Intestinal nematode infections	**194**	**101**	**94**	**1**	**78**	**14**			**1**	**74**	**11**	**4**	**4**
a. Ascariasis	64	33	31		31					30			
b. Trichuriasis	83	43	40		43					40			
c. Ancylostomiasis and necatoriasis	47	25	22	1	4	14				4	10	4	4

Annex Table 17g, continued. DALYs by age, sex and cause (thousands): Latin America and the Caribbean, 2020, baseline scenario

Cause	Total	Male	Female	Males					Females				
				0-4	5-14	15-44	45-59	60+	0-4	5-14	15-44	45-59	60+
B. Respiratory infections	1 659	910	750	632	51	45	42	140	463	54	49	35	148
1. Lower respiratory infections	1 608	883	726	621	39	43	41	138	455	42	47	35	146
2. Upper respiratory infections	20	11	9	6	1	2	1	2	4	1	1	1	2
3. Otitis media	31	16	15	4	11	-	-	-	4	11	-	-	-
C. Maternal conditions	253	-	253	-	-	-	-	-	-	1	251	1	-
1. Maternal haemorrhage	24		24								24		
2. Maternal sepsis	44		44								43		
3. Hypertensive disorders of pregnancy	15		15								15		
4. Obstructed labour	61		61								61		
5. Abortion	66		66								66		
D. Perinatal conditions*	2 508	1 482	1 025	1 482					1 025				
E. Nutritional deficiencies	1 172	559	614	356	59	55	23	65	277	59	161	36	81
1. Protein-energy malnutrition	547	302	245	248	7	6	7	33	183	9	6	7	41
2. Iodine deficiency	26	13	13	12	1	1	-	-	11	1	1	-	-
3. Vitamin A deficiency	48	26	22	21	5	1	-	-	17	5	1	-	-
4. Iron-deficiency anaemia	545	215	330	74	46	48	16	32	64	44	154	29	40
II. Noncommunicable diseases	73 275	38 801	34 473	1 911	1 224	15 310	10 761	9 595	1 677	1 049	12 728	9 612	9 407
A. Malignant neoplasms	9 114	4 331	4 783	57	234	732	1 530	1 778	66	145	1 131	1 886	1 555
1. Mouth and oropharynx cancers	333	251	82	-	2	46	124	79	-	1	13	30	37
2. Oesophagus cancer	228	167	61	-	-	13	82	72	-	-	4	21	36
3. Stomach cancer	835	530	305	-	-	66	203	261	-	-	41	102	162
4. Colon and rectum cancers	525	255	270	-	-	45	92	118	-	-	35	89	146
5. Liver cancer	118	63	56	-	2	11	24	26	-	1	6	19	29
6. Pancreas cancer	167	90	77	-	-	10	37	43	-	-	6	27	44
7. Trachea, bronchus, lung cancers	1 370	831	539	-	1	145	413	272	-	-	39	279	220
8. Melanoma and other skin cancers	84	41	43	-	-	14	16	11	-	1	13	16	13
9. Breast cancer	831	-	831	-					-		220	387	224
10. Cervix uteri cancer	706	-	706	-					-		235	320	152
11. Corpus uteri cancer	163	-	163						-		23	84	56
12. Ovary cancer	160	-	160						2	4	55	55	44
13. Prostate cancer	367	367	-	-	-	6	51	310					
14. Bladder cancer	180	139	41	-	-	10	44	83	-	-	4	12	26
15. Lymphomas and multiple myeloma	445	265	180	11	41	94	67	52	8	21	47	47	57
16. Leukaemia	394	225	169	18	70	81	29	26	18	48	50	26	27
C. Diabetes mellitus	1 685	770	915	8	12	161	292	296	8	10	107	300	491
D. Endocrine disorders	1 108	550	558	229	37	135	78	71	187	30	115	102	124

Annex Table 17g, continued. DALYs by age, sex and cause (thousands): Latin America and the Caribbean, 2020, baseline scenario

Cause	Total	Male	Female	Males					Females				
				0-4	5-14	15-44	45-59	60+	0-4	5-14	15-44	45-59	60+
E. Neuro-psychiatric conditions	**23 212**	**13 036**	**10 175**	**176**	**337**	**10 300**	**1 494**	**730**	**161**	**312**	**7 550**	**1 272**	**880**
1. Unipolar major depression	6 886	2 386	4 500	-	-	1 899	390	97	-	-	3 551	741	208
2. Bipolar disorder	1 843	921	921	-	-	832	68	22	-	-	824	70	27
3. Schizophrenia	1 904	990	914	-	-	969	12	9	-	-	899	4	11
4. Epilepsy	462	280	182	9	52	162	42	14	9	47	96	16	13
5. Alcohol use	5 984	5 507	477	-	-	4 670	653	184	-	-	437	28	12
6. Dementia*	1 345	549	796	36	18	30	135	330	37	15	29	189	526
7. Parkinson disease	83	44	39	-	-	-	19	25	-	-	-	16	23
8. Multiple sclerosis	165	71	94	-	-	62	7	2	-	-	81	9	4
9. Drug use	1 641	1 071	570	-	59	951	52	9	-	31	505	28	5
10. Post-traumatic stress disorder	241	90	151	4	17	61	8	1	6	27	102	13	2
11. Obsessive-compulsive disorders	1 287	546	741	-	56	439	35	16	-	71	579	65	26
12. Panic disorder	612	203	410	-	19	147	37	-	-	19	320	61	10
F. Sense organ diseases	**1 263**	**599**	**663**	**19**	**4**	**25**	**162**	**391**	**13**	**6**	**24**	**182**	**440**
1. Glaucoma	211	76	135	-	-	1	38	36	-	-	4	76	55
2. Cataracts	995	494	501	2	-	17	121	354	2	-	13	103	383
G. Cardiovascular diseases	**14 193**	**8 502**	**5 691**	**121**	**58**	**1 322**	**3 135**	**3 866**	**76**	**37**	**868**	**1 613**	**3 098**
1. Rheumatic heart disease	192	77	115	1	7	31	26	12	1	7	50	40	18
2. Ischaemic heart disease	6 029	3 742	2 287	-	-	435	1 480	1 827	-	-	233	645	1 409
3. Cerebrovascular disease	4 640	2 685	1 956	10	12	450	988	1 224	6	8	324	595	1 022
4. Inflammatory heart diseases	634	381	253	23	12	143	124	79	17	8	92	70	66
H. Respiratory diseases	**6 779**	**2 908**	**3 871**	**266**	**150**	**749**	**683**	**1 061**	**144**	**130**	**819**	**1 205**	**1 205**
1. COPD*	2 676	1 217	1 459	26	5	213	333	641	15	5	178	627	635
2. Asthma	1 400	605	796	29	93	326	86	70	15	80	270	288	143
I. Digestive diseases	**4 991**	**3 132**	**1 859**	**70**	**35**	**733**	**1 532**	**763**	**55**	**30**	**493**	**690**	**591**
1. Peptic ulcer	248	163	85	-	1	38	67	57	-	1	19	27	37
2. Cirrhosis of the liver	1 823	1 408	415	3	3	360	774	268	3	3	104	194	112
3. Appendicitis	36	21	15	-	4	12	3	2	-	3	9	2	1
J. Genito-urinary diseases	**1 357**	**849**	**508**	**54**	**31**	**90**	**496**	**178**	**47**	**35**	**137**	**116**	**173**
1. Nephritis and nephrosis	551	273	277	31	25	63	67	88	29	27	61	61	99
2. Benign prostatic hypertrophy	428	428	-	-	-	-	393	34	-	-	-	-	-
L. Musculo-skeletal diseases	**5 873**	**2 313**	**3 560**	**6**	**12**	**712**	**1 244**	**338**	**4**	**19**	**1 115**	**1 742**	**680**
1. Rheumatoid arthritis	1 029	223	806	-	-	105	85	33	-	6	467	238	96
2. Osteoarthritis	4 557	2 014	2 543	-	-	585	1 140	289	-	-	551	1 452	540

Annex Table 17g, continued. DALYs by age, sex and cause (thousands): Latin America and the Caribbean, 2020, baseline scenario

Cause	Total	Male	Female	Males					Females				
				0-4	5-14	15-44	45-59	60+	0-4	5-14	15-44	45-59	60+
M. Congenital anomalies	**1 805**	**897**	**908**	**837**	**31**	**22**	**5**	**3**	**850**	**26**	**23**	**6**	**3**
N. Oral conditions	**1 396**	**692**	**704**	**37**	**252**	**269**	**52**	**82**	**35**	**243**	**268**	**56**	**102**
1. Dental caries	1 140	575	565	36	251	263	18	8	35	241	260	18	10
2. Periodontal disease	40	19	21	-	-	5	10	4	-	-	5	10	5
3. Edentulism	206	93	113	-	-	-	24	68	-	-	-	27	86
III. Injuries	**20 823**	**15 055**	**5 768**	**793**	**1 534**	**10 313**	**1 830**	**585**	**600**	**815**	**3 401**	**608**	**344**
A. Unintentional injuries	**14 196**	**9 733**	**4 463**	**681**	**1 323**	**5 950**	**1 315**	**465**	**499**	**707**	**2 444**	**505**	**308**
1. Road traffic accidents	6 927	4 652	2 275	133	697	3 112	554	157	98	423	1 444	226	83
2. Poisonings	134	76	58	17	8	37	11	5	13	7	29	5	4
3. Falls	1 500	1 023	477	120	216	479	121	87	59	78	170	77	94
4. Fires	248	136	112	28	29	56	15	8	26	32	37	11	7
5. Drownings	711	556	155	58	98	333	53	14	38	38	66	9	4
6. Other unintentional	4 676	3 290	1 387	325	275	1 933	561	195	265	129	698	178	117
B. Intentional injuries	**6 627**	**5 322**	**1 305**	**112**	**211**	**4 363**	**516**	**120**	**100**	**108**	**958**	**102**	**36**
1. Self-inflicted injuries	946	627	319	-	18	457	108	43	-	14	252	39	14
2. Violence	4 750	4 155	595	44	145	3 516	380	69	33	58	446	44	14
3. War	931	540	391	68	48	389	27	8	68	36	260	19	8

Notes:
A dash (-) symbol indicates fewer than 500 DALYs.
*IA6 is Bacterial meningitis and meningococcaemia; ID is Conditions arising during the perinatal period;
IIE6 is Dementia and other degenerative and hereditary CNS disorders; IIH1 is Chronic obstructive pulmonary disease.

824

Annex Table 17h. DALYs by age, sex and cause (thousands): Middle Eastern Crescent, 2020, baseline scenario

Cause	Total	Male	Female	Males 0-4	5-14	15-44	45-59	60+	Females 0-4	5-14	15-44	45-59	60+
Population (millions)	*1 003*	*506*	*497*	*62*	*110*	*237*	*61*	*36*	*59*	*105*	*230*	*61*	*42*
All causes	*167 710*	*95 296*	*72 414*	*26 380*	*6 725*	*32 645*	*16 321*	*13 226*	*22 739*	*4 886*	*23 806*	*9 825*	*11 157*
I. Communicable, maternal, perinatal and nutritional conditions	*33 320*	*17 391*	*15 929*	*15 270*	*708*	*721*	*255*	*437*	*13 275*	*648*	*1 312*	*229*	*465*
A. Infectious and parasitic diseases	**14 009**	**7 646**	**6 363**	**6 388**	**318**	**575**	**210**	**155**	**5 455**	**263**	**323**	**140**	**182**
1. Tuberculosis	830	556	274	90	30	232	121	83	51	17	78	66	62
2. STDs excluding HIV	391	155	236	118	1	33	1	2	103	3	126	1	3
a. Syphilis	225	120	106	110	-	7	1	2	95	-	6	1	3
b. Chlamydia	115	15	99	2	-	13	-	-	2	2	94	-	-
c. Gonorrhoea	51	20	31	6	-	14	-	-	6	1	25	-	-
3. HIV	307	243	64	30	1	184	26	2	30	2	30	3	-
4. Diarrhoeal diseases	6 976	3 750	3 226	3 624	89	20	7	9	3 112	81	16	7	10
5. Childhood-cluster diseases	3 970	2 139	1 831	2 019	110	6	3	1	1 727	91	8	5	1
a. Pertussis	928	498	430	472	27	-	-	-	407	23	-	-	-
b. Poliomyelitis	229	137	92	135	-	2	-	-	91	-	1	-	-
c. Diphtheria	19	10	9	10	1	-	-	-	8	1	-	-	-
d. Measles	1 495	799	696	737	61	-	-	-	641	55	1	-	-
e. Tetanus	1 299	695	604	666	21	4	2	1	580	12	7	4	1
6. Bacterial meningitis*	305	164	141	130	4	15	8	7	113	4	8	8	8
7. Hepatitis B and hepatitis C	100	59	41	19	6	11	12	12	13	5	6	6	11
8. Malaria	113	62	50	19	20	17	4	2	17	17	10	4	3
9. Tropical-cluster diseases	86	56	30	11	18	19	6	3	6	10	8	3	2
a. Trypanosomiasis	-	-	-	-	-	-	-	-	-	-	-	-	-
b. Chagas disease	-	-	-	-	-	-	-	-	-	-	-	-	-
c. Schistosomiasis	43	29	14	1	7	13	5	3	-	3	6	3	2
d. Leishmaniasis	39	25	15	10	11	3	1	-	6	7	1	-	-
e. Lymphatic filariasis	4	3	1	-	-	2	1	-	-	-	1	-	-
f. Onchocerciasis	-	-	-	-	-	-	-	-	-	-	-	-	-
10. Leprosy	5	3	2	-	1	1	-	-	-	1	1	-	-
11. Dengue	-	-	-	-	-	-	-	-	-	-	-	-	-
12. Japanese encephalitis	-	-	-	-	-	-	-	-	-	-	-	-	-
13. Trachoma	146	39	107	-	-	5	11	23	-	-	8	28	71
14. Intestinal nematode infections	71	38	33	1	20	13	3	2	1	18	9	3	2
a. Ascariasis	33	17	16	1	17	-	-	-	1	15	-	-	-
b. Trichuriasis	1	-	-	-	-	-	-	-	-	-	-	-	-
c. Ancylostomiasis and necatoriasis	37	20	17	-	3	13	3	2	-	3	9	3	2

Annex Table 17h, continued. DALYs by age, sex and cause (thousands): Middle Eastern Crescent, 2020, baseline scenario

Cause	Total	Male	Female	Males 0-4	Males 5-14	Males 15-44	Males 45-59	Males 60+	Females 0-4	Females 5-14	Females 15-44	Females 45-59	Females 60+
B. Respiratory infections	**7 739**	**4 108**	**3 631**	**3 541**	**250**	**42**	**22**	**253**	**3 047**	**255**	**46**	**32**	**249**
1. Lower respiratory infections	7 550	4 008	3 542	3 470	225	40	21	251	2 987	233	44	32	247
2. Upper respiratory infections	80	43	38	34	3	2	1	3	29	3	2	1	3
3. Otitis media	108	58	51	36	22	–	–	–	31	19	–	–	–
C. Maternal conditions	**693**	**–**	**693**	**–**	**–**	**–**	**–**	**–**	**–**	**1**	**671**	**21**	**–**
1. Maternal haemorrhage	71	–	71	–	–	–	–	–	–	–	66	5	–
2. Maternal sepsis	146	–	146	–	–	–	–	–	–	–	143	3	–
3. Hypertensive disorders of pregnancy	46	–	46	–	–	–	–	–	–	–	43	3	–
4. Obstructed labour	189	–	189	–	–	–	–	–	–	–	187	2	–
5. Abortion	67	–	67	–	–	–	–	–	–	–	66	2	–
D. Perinatal conditions*	**7 723**	**4 073**	**3 651**	**4 073**	**–**	**–**	**–**	**–**	**3 651**	**–**	**–**	**–**	**–**
E. Nutritional deficiencies	**3 156**	**1 565**	**1 592**	**1 269**	**140**	**104**	**23**	**29**	**1 122**	**129**	**272**	**35**	**34**
1. Protein-energy malnutrition	1 751	933	818	922	2	2	1	6	808	2	2	1	6
2. Iodine deficiency	112	58	53	54	4	1	–	–	47	4	2	1	–
3. Vitamin A deficiency	298	154	145	122	30	1	–	–	114	30	1	–	–
4. Iron-deficiency anaemia	995	420	576	171	105	100	21	23	153	94	268	33	28
II. Noncommunicable diseases	**99 961**	**55 588**	**44 374**	**7 869**	**2 875**	**17 946**	**14 486**	**12 411**	**6 453**	**2 427**	**16 157**	**8 938**	**10 399**
A. Malignant neoplasms	**8 932**	**5 488**	**3 444**	**144**	**464**	**1 330**	**2 170**	**1 380**	**156**	**364**	**1 024**	**1 058**	**841**
1. Mouth and oropharynx cancers	525	354	171	2	8	130	102	113	3	7	58	39	64
2. Oesophagus cancer	301	189	112	–	1	36	103	48	1	2	25	45	39
3. Stomach cancer	657	432	224	–	3	101	220	108	1	2	52	82	88
4. Colon and rectum cancers	372	206	167	1	2	71	60	72	2	4	42	34	84
5. Liver cancer	269	180	89	2	6	41	90	42	2	5	18	34	30
6. Pancreas cancer	143	95	49	–	–	23	49	23	–	–	7	21	20
7. Trachea, bronchus, lung cancers	2 092	1 764	328	2	8	317	926	511	2	6	52	157	111
8. Melanoma and other skin cancers	45	29	16	–	1	10	15	4	–	–	7	5	3
9. Breast cancer	442	–	442	–	–	–	–	–	1	3	177	182	80
10. Cervix uteri cancer	268	–	268	–	–	–	–	–	–	1	90	123	53
11. Corpus uteri cancer	58	–	58	–	–	–	–	–	–	–	11	26	20
12. Ovary cancer	140	–	140	–	–	–	–	–	–	8	65	45	20
13. Prostate cancer	107	107	–	–	–	8	33	66	–	–	–	–	–
14. Bladder cancer	306	252	54	1	–	56	114	81	–	–	11	13	22
15. Lymphomas and multiple myeloma	395	275	120	17	3	179	42	34	13	35	37	13	22
16. Leukaemia	604	330	274	30	68	172	31	29	43	118	66	17	30
C. Diabetes mellitus	**1 641**	**843**	**798**	**43**	**43**	**231**	**318**	**208**	**41**	**40**	**135**	**274**	**308**
D. Endocrine disorders	**1 063**	**543**	**520**	**315**	**51**	**91**	**61**	**27**	**304**	**78**	**67**	**41**	**29**

Annex Table 17h, continued. DALYs by age, sex and cause (thousands): Middle Eastern Crescent, 2020, baseline scenario

Cause	Total	Male	Female	Males					Females				
				0-4	5-14	15-44	45-59	60+	0-4	5-14	15-44	45-59	60+
E. Neuro-psychiatric conditions	**24 941**	**11 858**	**13 084**	**733**	**610**	**9 239**	**906**	**370**	**595**	**524**	**10 255**	**1 185**	**524**
1. Unipolar major depression	10 016	3 543	6 474	-	-	2 993	450	99	-	-	5 455	813	206
2. Bipolar disorder	2 801	1 420	1 381	-	-	1 319	79	22	-	-	1 276	78	26
3. Schizophrenia	2 948	1 542	1 406	-	-	1 525	10	7	-	-	1 386	11	9
4. Epilepsy	449	250	199	41	67	112	22	8	34	77	68	14	6
5. Alcohol use	541	486	55	-	-	451	30	6	-	-	51	2	1
6. Dementia*	599	284	315	55	16	34	57	123	62	17	34	35	166
7. Parkinson disease	150	79	70	-	-	-	36	43	-	-	-	30	39
8. Multiple sclerosis	228	100	128	-	-	91	7	2	-	-	116	9	3
9. Drug use	1 886	1 694	192	-	107	1 511	66	11	-	12	171	7	1
10. Post-traumatic stress disorder	375	142	233	8	33	92	8	1	13	54	150	13	2
11. Obsessive-compulsive disorders	1 966	850	1 116	-	114	681	40	16	-	145	876	70	25
12. Panic disorder	902	307	595	-	38	227	41	-	-	38	482	65	10
F. Sense organ diseases	**2 257**	**1 189**	**1 068**	**3**	-	**56**	**570**	**560**	**4**	**1**	**42**	**461**	**559**
1. Glaucoma	280	106	174	-	-	2	71	33	-	-	4	123	47
2. Cataracts	1 960	1 076	884	3	-	50	497	525	2	-	34	336	511
G. Cardiovascular diseases	**29 708**	**18 468**	**11 241**	**1 911**	**791**	**3 235**	**5 918**	**6 612**	**1 079**	**602**	**1 709**	**2 453**	**5 398**
1. Rheumatic heart disease	729	393	336	2	68	266	47	10	2	69	213	42	11
2. Ischaemic heart disease	12 588	8 094	4 494	-	-	1 180	3 215	3 698	-	-	481	1 095	2 918
3. Cerebrovascular disease	4 737	2 738	1 999	100	150	505	900	1 083	57	107	244	515	1 076
4. Inflammatory heart diseases	2 342	1 448	895	366	145	438	320	178	254	101	248	151	140
H. Respiratory diseases	**10 995**	**6 000**	**4 995**	**1 000**	**422**	**1 239**	**1 373**	**1 967**	**608**	**361**	**1 009**	**1 483**	**1 534**
1. COPD*	3 744	2 000	1 744	107	25	310	398	1 161	76	41	255	621	751
2. Asthma	1 471	938	532	83	194	430	140	91	18	73	229	126	87
I. Digestive diseases	**6 138**	**3 654**	**2 484**	**685**	**114**	**719**	**1 480**	**656**	**772**	**100**	**432**	**711**	**469**
1. Peptic ulcer	203	149	54	-	2	47	69	31	-	-	19	21	14
2. Cirrhosis of the liver	1 190	750	440	7	14	141	396	191	6	34	76	186	139
3. Appendicitis	97	58	39	1	14	35	6	2	1	13	20	3	1
J. Genito-urinary diseases	**3 454**	**2 219**	**1 235**	**188**	**111**	**612**	**973**	**335**	**154**	**99**	**355**	**361**	**266**
1. Nephritis and nephrosis	770	412	358	79	57	127	80	70	69	71	99	61	59
2. Benign prostatic hypertrophy	487	487	-	-	-	1	450	36	-	-	-	-	-
L. Musculo-skeletal diseases	**1 971**	**854**	**1 117**	**17**	**7**	**440**	**290**	**100**	**14**	**7**	**405**	**459**	**232**
1. Rheumatoid arthritis	368	211	157	-	3	200	8	3	-	3	78	56	20
2. Osteoarthritis	1 485	586	899	-	-	220	273	93	-	-	303	391	205

Annex Table 17h, continued. DALYs by age, sex and cause (thousands): Middle Eastern Crescent, 2020, baseline scenario

Cause	Total	Male	Female	Males					Females				
				0-4	5-14	15-44	45-59	60+	0-4	5-14	15-44	45-59	60+
M. Congenital anomalies	5 494	2 802	2 693	2 653	60	71	14	4	2 561	65	44	16	7
N. Oral conditions	2 974	1 470	1 504	129	173	622	377	170	123	167	617	391	206
1. Dental caries	1 343	676	667	128	172	226	96	55	122	165	219	96	65
2. Periodontal disease	42	21	21	-	-	20	1	-	-	-	19	1	-
3. Edentulism	1 568	767	802	-	-	373	280	114	-	-	367	294	141
III. Injuries	34 429	22 318	12 111	3 241	3 142	13 978	1 580	377	3 011	1 812	6 336	658	293
A. Unintentional injuries	16 431	11 523	4 908	1 958	1 754	6 571	1 014	226	1 709	873	1 832	340	154
1. Road traffic accidents	6 091	4 675	1 416	156	747	3 287	404	81	135	414	705	117	45
2. Poisonings	547	347	199	76	17	179	62	12	72	13	81	23	10
3. Falls	2 055	1 308	747	412	323	475	80	19	359	135	187	48	19
4. Fires	908	395	512	130	89	144	26	7	135	93	252	21	11
5. Drownings	1 098	771	327	238	156	335	33	9	209	43	64	7	3
6. Other unintentional	5 733	4 026	1 707	946	421	2 150	410	98	799	176	543	123	66
B. Intentional injuries	17 998	10 795	7 203	1 284	1 388	7 407	566	151	1 303	939	4 504	318	140
1. Self-inflicted injuries	2 687	1 813	875	-	518	1 057	185	53	-	239	518	76	43
2. Violence	2 230	1 481	749	296	132	945	88	21	320	139	241	37	12
3. War	13 080	7 501	5 579	988	738	5 405	294	77	983	561	3 745	205	85

Notes:
A dash (-) symbol indicates fewer than 500 DALYs.
*IA6 is Bacterial meningitis and meningococcaemia; ID is Conditions arising during the perinatal period;
IIE6 is Dementia and other degenerative and hereditary CNS disorders; IIH1 is Chronic obstructive pulmonary disease.

Annex Table 17i. DALYs by age, sex and cause (thousands): World, 2020, baseline scenario

Cause	Total	Male	Female	Males					Females				
				0-4	5-14	15-44	45-59	60+	0-4	5-14	15-44	45-59	60+
Population (millions)	*7 844*	*3 901*	*3 943*	*374*	*690*	*1 762*	*633*	*443*	*358*	*662*	*1 716*	*648*	*559*
All causes	*1 388 836*	*796 144*	*592 692*	*145 598*	*43 994*	*280 899*	*174 255*	*151 398*	*122 340*	*33 183*	*196 616*	*106 701*	*133 852*
I. Communicable, maternal, perinatal and nutritional conditions	*279 492*	*148 994*	*130 498*	*93 955*	*7 749*	*30 768*	*8 674*	*7 848*	*76 970*	*7 679*	*31 887*	*6 380*	*7 582*
A. Infectious and parasitic diseases	179 631	98 062	81 569	50 955	5 422	29 117	8 018	4 549	41 033	5 335	25 814	5 475	3 912
1. Tuberculosis	42 515	23 101	19 414	1 508	1 205	11 635	5 716	3 038	1 459	1 509	10 237	4 059	2 150
2. STDs excluding HIV	7 889	2 973	4 916	1 777	19	1 087	22	67	1 556	74	3 151	34	100
a. Syphilis	2 755	1 463	1 292	1 223	2	156	17	65	1 016	2	157	21	95
b. Chlamydia	2 824	433	2 391	118	6	307	2	1	114	53	2 213	9	2
c. Gonorrhoea	2 306	1 076	1 230	437	11	623	3	1	426	20	780	3	1
3. HIV	36 317	20 331	15 986	3 773	613	14 161	1 487	297	3 565	618	11 095	595	113
4. Diarrhoeal diseases	37 097	20 652	16 445	19 097	769	282	126	378	14 840	743	233	144	485
5. Childhood-cluster diseases	27 787	15 223	12 564	14 028	989	135	38	33	11 492	906	89	41	38
a. Pertussis	5 348	2 927	2 421	2 768	160				2 279	142			
b. Poliomyelitis	1 084	649	435	636	2	9	1	1	428	4	4	1	
c. Diphtheria	110	60	51	55	4				46	4			
d. Measles	15 443	8 456	6 987	7 756	695	3	1	1	6 361	622	3	1	1
e. Tetanus	5 802	3 132	2 671	2 813	128	122	36	32	2 378	136	82	39	36
6. Bacterial meningitis*	1 826	979	847	738	25	97	55	64	632	22	58	58	77
7. Hepatitis B and hepatitis C	576	337	238	87	26	65	74	85	62	23	34	33	88
8. Malaria	15 596	8 949	6 647	7 920	488	403	90	48	5 773	444	272	98	60
9. Tropical-cluster diseases	2 553	1 688	865	102	500	793	198	95	83	259	286	163	74
a. Trypanosomiasis	411	225	186	11	82	92	32	8	20	77	63	22	5
b. Chagas disease	175	93	82	1	1	49	24	19			37	26	19
c. Schistosomiasis	460	295	165	17	100	127	29	22	10	60	60	19	16
d. Leishmaniasis	360	241	118	32	106	93	6	3	18	58	34	4	3
e. Lymphatic filariasis	846	647	199	36	183	361	58	9	31	43	56	57	12
f. Onchocerciasis	301	186	115	5	28	71	49	33	3	20	36	35	20
10. Leprosy	128	65	63	2	18	34	8	4	3	17	33	8	2
11. Dengue	110	53	57	18	34	1	1		19	37	1	1	
12. Japanese encephalitis	116	62	54	44	14	3	1	1	38	13	1	1	1
13. Trachoma	549	142	406			15	33	94			26	90	290
14. Intestinal nematode infections	1 274	669	605	9	450	146	36	29	8	419	106	37	35
a. Ascariasis	397	206	191	9	195	1			8	182	1		
b. Trichuriasis	414	214	200		213					199			
c. Ancylostomiasis and necatoriasis	462	249	214		41	145	35	28		38	105	36	34

Annex Table 17i, continued. DALYs by age, sex and cause (thousands): World, 2020, baseline scenario

Cause	Total	Male	Female	Males					Females				
				0-4	5-14	15-44	45-59	60+	0-4	5-14	15-44	45-59	60+
B. Respiratory infections	**43 769**	**23 761**	**20 008**	**18 868**	**1 448**	**477**	**303**	**2 665**	**15 047**	**1 407**	**383**	**288**	**2 882**
1. Lower respiratory infections	42 692	23 184	19 508	18 481	1 313	459	296	2 635	14 730	1 280	369	282	2 848
2. Upper respiratory infections	475	257	218	187	18	16	6	30	147	17	12	7	34
3. Otitis media	602	320	282	200	118	2	-	-	170	110	2	-	-
C. Maternal conditions	**4 349**	**-**	**4 349**							**112**	**4 173**	**64**	**-**
1. Maternal haemorrhage	535		535							26	495	15	
2. Maternal sepsis	807		807							17	781	8	
3. Hypertensive disorders of pregnancy	273		273							13	253	7	
4. Obstructed labour	920		920							9	907	4	
5. Abortion	748		748							15	727	6	
D. Perinatal conditions*	**34 755**	**18 685**	**16 070**	**18 685**					**16 070**				
E. Nutritional deficiencies	**16 989**	**8 486**	**8 503**	**5 447**	**878**	**1 173**	**354**	**634**	**4 821**	**824**	**1 518**	**553**	**788**
1. Protein-energy malnutrition	7 798	4 121	3 677	3 956	28	21	18	97	3 490	35	20	16	117
2. Iodine deficiency	397	210	188	193	12	4	-	-	170	12	4	1	-
3. Vitamin A deficiency	1 242	663	578	518	138	7	-	-	446	128	5	-	-
4. Iron-deficiency anaemia	7 522	3 479	4 043	774	698	1 139	334	534	710	647	1 487	534	665
II. Noncommunicable diseases	**829 785**	**463 477**	**366 308**	**30 950**	**12 685**	**135 758**	**146 670**	**137 413**	**27 873**	**10 782**	**117 047**	**89 894**	**120 714**
A. Malignant neoplasms	**137 337**	**85 748**	**51 589**	**981**	**2 782**	**15 787**	**37 235**	**28 962**	**1 237**	**1 912**	**10 647**	**18 987**	**18 806**
1. Mouth and oropharynx cancers	7 670	5 188	2 482	17	47	1 207	2 186	1 732	28	53	563	857	980
2. Oesophagus cancer	8 164	5 819	2 345	-	1	635	2 955	2 228		2	229	925	1 189
3. Stomach cancer	16 049	11 209	4 840	3	16	1 246	5 557	4 387	1	9	769	1 783	2 278
4. Colon and rectum cancers	7 810	4 528	3 283	4	19	805	1 642	2 057	6	18	455	995	1 809
5. Liver cancer	14 749	11 677	3 072	23	75	3 243	5 945	2 390	28	55	574	1 279	1 136
6. Pancreas cancer	2 710	1 760	950			224	788	748	2	2	84	312	550
7. Trachea, bronchus, lung cancers	25 626	19 901	5 725	11	32	2 479	10 341	7 040	6	11	470	2 496	2 742
8. Melanoma and other skin cancers	844	472	372	1	4	124	200	143	1	2	88	129	151
9. Breast cancer	6 084	-	6 084							8	1 654	2 673	1 745
10. Cervix uteri cancer	5 184		5 184							3	1 307	2 587	1 285
11. Corpus uteri cancer	967		967							4	123	460	377
12. Ovary cancer	1 991		1 991						32	55	619	720	566
13. Prostate cancer	2 677	2 677	-			49	495	2 129					
14. Bladder cancer	2 394	1 900	495	2	6	181	647	1 064	2	3	59	140	291
15. Lymphomas and multiple myeloma	5 019	3 282	1 737	177	596	963	819	726	148	294	375	384	537
16. Leukaemia	5 878	3 367	2 511	260	749	1 233	665	459	337	534	827	416	398
C. Diabetes mellitus	**10 805**	**5 127**	**5 678**	**157**	**162**	**1 119**	**1 868**	**1 822**	**163**	**152**	**640**	**1 664**	**3 059**
D. Endocrine disorders	**5 347**	**2 577**	**2 770**	**1 106**	**183**	**571**	**386**	**332**	**971**	**216**	**486**	**461**	**636**

Annex Table 17i, continued. DALYs by age, sex and cause (thousands): World, 2020, baseline scenario

Cause	Total	Male	Female	Males					Females				
				0-4	5-14	15-44	45-59	60+	0-4	5-14	15-44	45-59	60+
E. Neuro-psychiatric conditions	**203 811**	**98 626**	**105 185**	**2 174**	**2 804**	**75 080**	**11 428**	**7 140**	**2 160**	**2 716**	**75 518**	**13 607**	**11 184**
1. Unipolar major depression	78 662	27 587	51 075	-	-	21 901	4 538	1 148	-	1	40 180	8 395	2 501
2. Bipolar disorder	21 227	10 689	10 538	-	-	9 642	789	258	-	-	9 394	798	344
3. Schizophrenia	17 332	9 097	8 236	-	-	8 941	77	78	-	-	8 073	47	116
4. Epilepsy	3 601	2 105	1 496	162	399	1 140	284	119	170	418	630	147	133
5. Alcohol use	22 983	20 285	2 698	-	-	17 623	2 136	525	-	-	2 403	204	91
6. Dementia*	14 656	5 993	8 663	309	124	294	1 472	3 795	383	140	295	1 604	6 241
7. Parkinson disease	1 865	876	988	-	-	1	335	540	-	1	339	648	
8. Multiple sclerosis	1 818	793	1 026	-	-	687	76	30	-	-	875	101	49
9. Drug use	7 979	6 530	1 449	-	424	5 785	272	49	-	97	1 276	64	12
10. Post-traumatic stress disorder	2 750	1 039	1 712	50	207	680	86	16	81	337	1 124	140	29
11. Obsessive-compulsive disorders	14 869	6 363	8 505	-	713	5 051	407	192	-	912	6 540	736	318
12. Panic disorder	7 165	2 385	4 780	-	213	1 732	438	2	-	248	3 695	709	128
F. Sense organ diseases	**22 041**	**10 861**	**11 180**	**78**	**9**	**585**	**5 373**	**4 817**	**64**	**18**	**554**	**5 205**	**5 340**
1. Glaucoma	5 785	2 143	3 642	5	-	110	1 355	672	6	-	171	2 430	1 035
2. Cataracts	15 890	8 573	7 317	33	2	444	3 974	4 121	23	2	319	2 712	4 261
G. Cardiovascular diseases	**204 420**	**127 941**	**76 479**	**4 738**	**2 211**	**17 698**	**46 328**	**56 965**	**2 930**	**1 768**	**8 337**	**16 364**	**47 080**
1. Rheumatic heart disease	6 628	3 733	2 895	7	182	1 334	1 489	722	18	193	994	947	743
2. Ischaemic heart disease	82 325	53 238	29 087	-	-	5 093	21 208	26 937	182	-	1 865	5 955	21 085
3. Cerebrovascular disease	61 392	36 819	24 573	545	553	4 726	13 178	17 818	371	392	2 363	5 631	15 816
4. Inflammatory heart diseases	11 671	7 346	4 325	969	418	2 311	2 332	1 316	761	342	1 108	928	1 185
H. Respiratory diseases	**101 252**	**55 907**	**45 345**	**3 202**	**1 998**	**10 293**	**17 289**	**23 124**	**1 856**	**1 513**	**8 031**	**14 419**	**19 526**
1. COPD*	57 587	33 023	24 563	327	109	3 963	11 283	17 341	250	116	2 592	8 034	13 572
2. Asthma	13 246	7 158	6 088	423	1 114	3 417	1 378	826	163	698	2 775	1 529	923
I. Digestive diseases	**49 054**	**30 784**	**18 270**	**1 557**	**498**	**6 268**	**14 511**	**7 950**	**1 616**	**561**	**3 496**	**6 568**	**6 029**
1. Peptic ulcer	3 219	2 171	1 048	5	8	559	946	652	6	8	253	355	426
2. Cirrhosis of the liver	16 418	12 080	4 339	48	51	2 425	6 597	2 958	39	77	767	1 977	1 478
3. Appendicitis	893	542	351	10	110	330	66	27	10	108	177	36	19
J. Genito-urinary diseases	**15 989**	**10 232**	**5 757**	**929**	**629**	**1 785**	**4 743**	**2 146**	**705**	**557**	**1 124**	**1 371**	**2 000**
1. Nephritis and nephrosis	7 374	3 943	3 430	660	507	1 071	785	921	581	482	599	648	1 122
2. Benign prostatic hypertrophy	3 838	3 838	-	5	-	6	3 218	609	-				
L. Musculo-skeletal diseases	**30 986**	**11 546**	**19 440**	**42**	**45**	**3 571**	**5 429**	**2 458**	**51**	**71**	**5 428**	**9 096**	**4 794**
1. Rheumatoid arthritis	5 210	1 477	3 732	1	1	610	527	339	-	31	1 511	1 226	964
2. Osteoarthritis	24 026	9 479	14 547	-	-	2 817	4 767	1 895	-	-	3 576	7 590	3 381

Annex Table 17i, continued. DALYs by age, sex and cause (thousands): World, 2020, baseline scenario

Cause	Total	Male	Female	Males					Females				
				0-4	5-14	15-44	45-59	60+	0-4	5-14	15-44	45-59	60+
M. Congenital anomalies	**30 986**	**15 394**	**15 592**	**14 456**	**358**	**465**	**82**	**33**	**14 797**	**368**	**285**	**93**	**49**
N. Oral conditions	**12 592**	**6 082**	**6 511**	**529**	**780**	**1 998**	**1 497**	**1 278**	**505**	**768**	**2 021**	**1 584**	**1 632**
1. Dental caries	6 360	3 178	3 182	522	773	1 135	477	271	498	752	1 106	490	335
2. Periodontal disease	416	207	210	-	-	156	35	15	-	-	156	36	18
3. Edentulism	5 675	2 661	3 014	-	-	689	981	991	-	-	684	1 054	1 276
III. Injuries	**279 559**	**183 673**	**95 886**	**20 693**	**23 560**	**114 373**	**18 910**	**6 137**	**17 497**	**14 722**	**47 682**	**10 427**	**5 556**
A. Unintentional injuries	**181 054**	**120 221**	**60 833**	**16 409**	**18 990**	**66 613**	**13 771**	**4 437**	**13 190**	**11 756**	**24 224**	**7 450**	**4 213**
1. Road traffic accidents	71 240	49 719	21 520	2 240	8 384	31 646	5 765	1 684	1 469	5 416	10 749	2 768	1 118
2. Poisonings	6 628	3 826	2 803	1 255	280	1 447	644	199	894	194	1 092	422	200
3. Falls	21 195	12 470	8 724	2 521	3 214	4 751	1 311	673	2 481	1 406	2 366	1 372	1 099
4. Fires	11 776	5 094	6 682	1 705	996	1 812	420	160	1 502	1 472	2 970	436	301
5. Drownings	12 367	8 399	3 967	2 429	2 275	3 002	492	202	1 606	968	907	277	209
6. Other unintentional	57 849	40 713	17 137	6 259	3 840	23 957	5 138	1 519	5 238	2 299	6 140	2 174	1 285
B. Intentional injuries	**98 505**	**63 452**	**35 052**	**4 284**	**4 570**	**47 760**	**5 139**	**1 699**	**4 308**	**2 966**	**23 458**	**2 977**	**1 344**
1. Self-inflicted injuries	25 928	14 245	11 683	-	955	9 556	2 607	1 126	-	485	8 474	1 827	897
2. Violence	31 262	25 274	5 988	1 082	1 237	20 849	1 745	361	1 152	704	3 325	597	210
3. War	41 315	23 934	17 381	3 202	2 378	17 355	787	212	3 156	1 777	11 658	553	237

Notes:
A dash (-) symbol indicates fewer than 500 DALYs.
*IA6 is Bacterial meningitis and meningococcaemia; ID is Conditions arising during the perinatal period;
IIE6 is Dementia and other degenerative and hereditary CNS disorders; IIH1 is Chronic obstructive pulmonary disease.

Annex Table 18a. Deaths by age, sex and cause (thousands): Established Market Economies, 2020, pessimistic scenario

Cause	Total	Male	Female	Males 0-4	5-14	15-29	30-44	45-59	60-69	70+	Females 0-4	5-14	15-29	30-44	45-59	60-69	70+
Population (millions)	*890*	*434*	*455*	*29*	*57*	*85*	*77*	*85*	*49*	*53*	*27*	*55*	*81*	*75*	*87*	*55*	*76*
All causes	**9 886**	**5 178**	**4 708**	**42**	**12**	**108**	**193**	**653**	**908**	**3 261**	**32**	**8**	**35**	**74**	**268**	**491**	**3 802**
I. Communicable, maternal, perinatal and nutritional conditions	*665*	*382*	*283*	*21*	*1*	*18*	*62*	*33*	*22*	*225*	*15*	*1*	*4*	*9*	*6*	*11*	*236*
A: Infectious and parasitic diseases	**214**	**155**	**59**	**3**	**-**	**18**	**61**	**29**	**9**	**35**	**2**	**-**	**4**	**9**	**4**	**5**	**35**
1. Tuberculosis	18	12	5	-	-	-	-	1	2	9	-	-	-	-	-	1	4
2. STDs excluding HIV	1	-	1	-	-	-	-	-	-	-	-	-	-	-	-	-	-
a. Syphilis																	
b. Chlamydia																	
c. Gonorrhoea																	
3. HIV	128	111	17	2	-	17	60	26	4	1	1	-	4	8	3	1	2
4. Diarrhoeal diseases	3	1	2	-	-	-	-	-	-	1	-	-	-	-	-	-	-
5. Childhood-cluster diseases	1	1	-	-	-	-	-	-	-	-	-	-	-	-	-	-	-
a. Pertussis																	
b. Poliomyelitis																	
c. Diphtheria																	
d. Measles																	
e. Tetanus																	
6. Bacterial meningitis*	4	2	2	1	-	-	-	-	-	1	1	-	-	-	-	-	1
7. Hepatitis B and hepatitis C	3	2	1	-	-	-	-	-	-	1	-	-	-	-	-	-	1
8. Malaria																	
9. Tropical-cluster diseases																	
a. Trypanosomiasis																	
b. Chagas disease																	
c. Schistosomiasis																	
d. Leishmaniasis																	
10. Leprosy																	
11. Dengue																	
12. Japanese encephalitis																	
13. Trachoma																	
14. Intestinal nematode infections																	
a. Ascariasis																	
b. Trichuriasis																	
c. Ancylostomiasis, necatoriasis																	
15. Other infectious and parasitic	55	25	30	-	-	-	-	1	2	21	-	-	-	-	1	2	27

Annex Table 18a, continued. Deaths by age, sex and cause (thousands): Established Market Economies, 2020, pessimistic scenario

Cause	Total	Male	Female	Males 0-4	5-14	15-29	30-44	45-59	60-69	70+	Females 0-4	5-14	15-29	30-44	45-59	60-69	70+
B. Respiratory infections	**395**	**199**	**196**	**1**	-	-	**1**	**4**	**12**	**181**	**1**	-	-	**1**	**4**	**6**	**186**
1. Lower respiratory infections	391	197	194	1	-	-	1	4	12	179	1	-	-	1	4	6	185
2. Upper respiratory infections	4	2	2	-	-	-	-	-	-	1	-	-	-	-	-	-	2
3. Otitis media	-	-	-	-	-	-	-	-	-	-	-	-	-	-	-	-	-
C. Maternal conditions	-	-	-	-	-	-	-	-	-	-	-	-	-	-	-	-	-
1. Maternal haemorrhage	-	-	-	-	-	-	-	-	-	-	-	-	-	-	-	-	-
2. Maternal sepsis	-	-	-	-	-	-	-	-	-	-	-	-	-	-	-	-	-
3. Hypertensive disorders*	-	-	-	-	-	-	-	-	-	-	-	-	-	-	-	-	-
4. Obstructed labour	-	-	-	-	-	-	-	-	-	-	-	-	-	-	-	-	-
5. Abortion	-	-	-	-	-	-	-	-	-	-	-	-	-	-	-	-	-
6. Other maternal	-	-	-	-	-	-	-	-	-	-	-	-	-	-	-	-	-
D. Perinatal conditions*	**29**	**17**	**12**	**17**	-	-	-	-	-	-	**12**	-	-	-	-	-	-
E. Nutritional deficiencies	**28**	**12**	**16**	-	-	-	-	-	**1**	**10**	-	-	-	-	-	**1**	**15**
1. Protein-energy malnutrition	8	3	5	-	-	-	-	-	-	3	-	-	-	-	-	-	5
2. Iodine deficiency	-	-	-	-	-	-	-	-	-	-	-	-	-	-	-	-	-
3. Vitamin A deficiency	-	-	-	-	-	-	-	-	-	-	-	-	-	-	-	-	-
4. Iron-deficiency anaemia	18	8	10	-	-	-	-	-	1	7	-	-	-	-	-	1	9
II. Noncommunicable diseases	**8 715**	**4 469**	**4 247**	**17**	**5**	**20**	**81**	**561**	**849**	**2 935**	**13**	**4**	**11**	**47**	**238**	**459**	**3 474**
A. Malignant neoplasms	**2 433**	**1 360**	**1 073**	**1**	**2**	**6**	**31**	**245**	**334**	**740**	**1**	**1**	**4**	**27**	**140**	**221**	**679**
1. Mouth and oropharynx cancers	45	35	10	-	-	-	-	11	10	13	-	-	-	-	2	2	6
2. Oesophagus cancer	60	46	14	-	-	-	1	11	13	21	-	-	-	-	1	3	10
3. Stomach cancer	202	125	77	-	-	-	2	18	28	76	-	-	-	2	7	12	57
4. Colon and rectum cancers	299	155	144	-	-	-	2	21	34	98	-	-	-	2	12	24	106
5. Liver cancer	52	38	14	-	-	-	1	9	12	15	-	-	-	-	1	3	9
6. Pancreas cancer	120	63	57	-	-	-	1	10	16	36	-	-	-	-	5	11	41
7. Trachea, bronchus, lung cancers	506	332	174	-	-	-	9	92	107	124	-	-	-	3	28	50	93
8. Melanoma and other skin cancers	30	18	12	-	-	-	1	4	4	8	-	-	-	1	2	2	7
9. Breast cancer	168	-	168	-	-	-	-	-	-	-	-	-	-	8	36	37	86
10. Cervix uteri cancer	19	-	19	-	-	-	-	-	-	-	-	-	-	2	4	4	8
11. Corpus uteri cancer	32	-	32	-	-	-	-	-	-	-	-	-	-	1	4	7	21
12. Ovary cancer	52	-	52	-	-	-	-	-	-	-	-	-	-	1	10	13	28
13. Prostate cancer	148	148	-	-	-	-	-	4	19	124	-	-	-	-	-	-	-
14. Bladder cancer	71	52	19	-	-	-	-	4	9	39	-	-	-	-	1	2	15
15. Lymphomas, multiple myeloma	108	59	50	-	-	1	3	10	13	32	-	-	1	1	5	10	33
16. Leukaemia	76	43	33	-	1	2	2	6	8	24	-	1	1	1	4	5	21
17. Other cancers	444	246	198	-	1	2	7	45	60	129	-	1	1	4	20	36	136

Annex Table 18a, continued. Deaths by age, sex and cause (thousands): Established Market Economies, 2020, pessimistic scenario

Cause	Total	Male	Female	Males							Females						
				0-4	5-14	15-29	30-44	45-59	60-69	70+	0-4	5-14	15-29	30-44	45-59	60-69	70+
B. Other neoplasms	50	24	26	-	-	-	1	3	4	16	-	-	-	-	2	3	20
C. Diabetes mellitus	216	82	134	-	-	-	1	7	14	59	-	-	-	1	4	14	115
D. Endocrine disorders	65	28	37	1	-	1	1	2	5	19	1	-	1	-	2	3	30
E. Neuro-psychiatric conditions	297	133	165	1	1	4	6	12	15	93	1	1	1	2	5	10	145
2. Bipolar disorder	1	-	-	-	-	-	-	-	-	-	-	-	-	-	-	-	-
3. Schizophrenia	20	8	12	-	-	-	-	1	1	6	-	-	-	-	-	1	11
4. Epilepsy	8	5	3	-	-	1	1	1	1	1	-	-	1	-	-	-	2
5. Alcohol use	16	13	3	-	-	-	2	5	3	3	-	-	-	-	1	1	1
6. Dementia*	149	55	94	-	-	-	-	3	5	46	-	-	-	-	2	5	87
7. Parkinson disease	49	25	24	-	-	-	-	-	2	23	-	-	-	-	-	1	23
8. Multiple sclerosis	6	2	4	-	-	1	1	-	-	-	-	-	-	1	1	1	1
9. Drug use	3	2	-	-	-	-	-	-	-	-	-	-	-	-	-	-	-
13. Other neuro-psychiatric	47	22	24	1	1	2	2	2	3	13	1	1	-	1	1	1	19
F. Sense organ diseases	-	-	-	-	-	-	-	-	-	-	-	-	-	-	-	-	-
1. Glaucoma	-	-	-	-	-	-	-	-	-	-	-	-	-	-	-	-	-
2. Cataracts	-	-	-	-	-	-	-	-	-	-	-	-	-	-	-	-	-
G. Cardiovascular diseases	4 385	2 171	2 213	2	1	4	27	218	368	1 551	1	-	2	10	49	141	2 009
1. Rheumatic heart disease	25	8	17	-	1	-	-	1	3	5	-	-	-	1	1	3	12
2. Ischaemic heart disease	2 315	1 209	1 107	-	-	1	14	137	224	833	-	-	-	3	24	79	1 000
3. Cerebrovascular disease	1 095	477	618	-	-	1	5	34	60	377	-	-	-	3	13	32	568
4. Inflammatory heart diseases	85	45	40	1	-	-	2	9	6	26	1	-	-	1	2	2	34
5. Other cardiovascular	864	432	432	1	-	2	6	37	75	311	-	-	2	2	8	26	395
H. Respiratory diseases	508	279	229	-	-	1	2	17	42	215	-	-	1	1	13	33	181
1. COPD*	363	211	152	1	-	-	1	11	32	167	-	-	-	-	8	24	120
2. Asthma	32	13	19	-	-	-	-	2	2	8	-	-	1	1	2	3	12
3. Other respiratory	113	55	58	-	-	1	1	5	8	40	-	-	1	-	3	5	49
I. Digestive diseases	473	267	206	-	-	1	10	51	54	151	-	-	1	3	18	24	159
1. Peptic ulcer	52	29	23	-	-	-	-	3	4	22	-	-	-	-	1	2	20
2. Cirrhosis of the liver	167	115	52	-	-	-	7	37	32	39	-	-	-	3	12	12	25
3. Appendicitis	2	1	1	-	-	-	-	-	-	1	-	-	1	-	-	-	-
4. Other digestive	252	122	130	-	-	1	3	12	17	89	-	-	-	1	5	10	113
J. Genito-urinary diseases	191	89	102	-	-	-	1	4	9	75	-	-	-	1	2	7	92
1. Nephritis and nephrosis	123	59	65	-	-	-	1	3	7	48	-	-	-	-	2	5	58
2. Benign prostatic hypertrophy	6	6	-	-	-	-	-	-	-	6	-	-	-	-	-	-	-
3. Other genito-urinary	61	24	37	-	-	-	1	1	2	21	-	-	-	1	-	2	34
K. Skin diseases	19	6	13	-	-	-	-	-	-	5	-	-	-	-	-	-	13

Annex Table 18a, continued. Deaths by age, sex and cause (thousands): Established Market Economies, 2020, pessimistic scenario

Cause	Total	Male	Female	Males							Females						
				0-4	5-14	15-29	30-44	45-59	60-69	70+	0-4	5-14	15-29	30-44	45-59	60-69	70+
L. Musculo-skeletal diseases	**47**	**13**	**34**	-	-	-	-	1	2	10	-	-	-	-	1	3	**29**
1. Rheumatoid arthritis	14	3	11	-	-	-	-	-	1	2	-	-	-	-	-	1	9
3. Other musculo-skeletal	34	10	24	-	-	-	-	1	1	8	-	-	-	-	1	2	20
M. Congenital anomalies	**30**	**16**	**14**	**11**	1	1	1	1	1	2	**9**	1	1	-	1	1	**2**
N. Oral conditions	**-**	-	-	-	-	-	-	-	-	-	-	-	-	-	-	-	-
III. Injuries	***505***	***327***	***178***	*5*	*6*	*70*	*50*	*58*	*37*	*101*	*3*	*3*	*19*	*17*	*23*	*20*	*92*
A. Unintentional injuries	**336**	**205**	**131**	**4**	**5**	**46**	**26**	**31**	**22**	**72**	**3**	**3**	**13**	**10**	**13**	**13**	**77**
1. Road traffic accidents	130	87	43	1	3	35	13	12	7	15	1	2	11	6	7	5	12
2. Poisonings	12	8	4	-	-	1	3	2	1	1	-	-	1	1	-	1	1
3. Falls	95	44	51	-	-	1	2	5	5	31	-	-	1	-	1	3	46
4. Fires	12	7	5	-	-	1	1	1	1	3	-	-	1	-	1	1	2
5. Drownings	13	9	4	1	1	2	1	2	1	2	1	-	1	-	-	-	2
6. Other unintentional	74	50	24	1	1	6	6	10	7	19	1	-	1	1	3	3	14
B. Intentional injuries	**169**	**122**	**47**	**1**	**1**	**24**	**24**	**27**	**16**	**29**	**1**	-	**6**	**8**	**11**	**7**	**14**
1. Self-inflicted injuries	138	99	39	-	-	16	18	24	14	27	-	-	4	6	10	7	13
2. Violence	31	23	8	1	-	9	6	4	1	1	1	-	2	2	1	-	1
3. War	-	-	-	-	-	-	-	-	-	-	-	-	-	-	-	-	-

Notes:
Causes responsible for no deaths have been omitted from this table.
A dash (-) symbol indicates fewer than 500 deaths.
*IA6 is Bacterial meningitis and meningococcaemia; IC3 is Hypertensive disorders of pregnancy; ID is Conditions arising during the perinatal period; IIE6 is Dementia and other degenerative and hereditary CNS disorders; IIH1 is Chronic obstructive pulmonary disease.

836

Annex Table 18b. Deaths by age, sex and cause (thousands): Formerly Socialist Economies of Europe, 2020, pessimistic scenario

Cause	Total	Male	Female	Males							Females						
				0-4	5-14	15-29	30-44	45-59	60-69	70+	0-4	5-14	15-29	30-44	45-59	60-69	70+
Population (millions)	*361*	*170*	*191*	*12*	*25*	*37*	*38*	*29*	*17*	*12*	*12*	*24*	*36*	*39*	*33*	*23*	*25*
All causes	**5 146**	**2 819**	**2 328**	**40**	**12**	**81**	**172**	**637**	**616**	**1 259**	**30**	**7**	**26**	**53**	**176**	**317**	**1 719**
I. Communicable, maternal, perinatal and nutritional conditions	*195*	*94*	*101*	*21*	*1*	*1*	*4*	*8*	*8*	*52*	*15*	*1*	*1*	*1*	*2*	*5*	*76*
A. Infectious and parasitic diseases	**44**	**25**	**19**	**5**	-	**1**	**3**	**5**	**4**	**8**	**4**	-	-	**1**	**1**	**2**	**11**
1. Tuberculosis	15	12	3	-	-	-	2	4	2	3	-	-	-	-	-	1	2
2. STDs excluding HIV	-	-	-	-	-	-	-	-	-	-	-	-	-	-	-	-	-
a. Syphilis	-	-	-	-	-	-	-	-	-	-	-	-	-	-	-	-	-
b. Chlamydia	-	-	-	-	-	-	-	-	-	-	-	-	-	-	-	-	-
c. Gonorrhoea	-	-	-	-	-	-	-	-	-	-	-	-	-	-	-	-	-
3. HIV	6	3	3	2	-	-	1	-	-	-	2	-	-	-	-	-	-
4. Diarrhoeal diseases	2	1	1	1	-	-	-	-	-	-	1	-	-	-	-	-	-
5. Childhood-cluster diseases	-	-	-	-	-	-	-	-	-	-	-	-	-	-	-	-	-
a. Pertussis	-	-	-	-	-	-	-	-	-	-	-	-	-	-	-	-	-
b. Poliomyelitis	-	-	-	-	-	-	-	-	-	-	-	-	-	-	-	-	-
c. Diphtheria	-	-	-	-	-	-	-	-	-	-	-	-	-	-	-	-	-
d. Measles	-	-	-	-	-	-	-	-	-	-	-	-	-	-	-	-	-
e. Tetanus	-	-	-	-	-	-	-	-	-	-	-	-	-	-	-	-	-
6. Bacterial meningitis*	4	3	2	1	-	-	-	-	-	1	1	-	-	-	-	-	1
7. Hepatitis B and hepatitis C	1	1	-	-	-	-	-	-	-	-	-	-	-	-	-	-	-
8. Malaria	-	-	-	-	-	-	-	-	-	-	-	-	-	-	-	-	-
9. Tropical-cluster diseases	-	-	-	-	-	-	-	-	-	-	-	-	-	-	-	-	-
a. Trypanosomiasis	-	-	-	-	-	-	-	-	-	-	-	-	-	-	-	-	-
b. Chagas disease	-	-	-	-	-	-	-	-	-	-	-	-	-	-	-	-	-
c. Schistosomiasis	-	-	-	-	-	-	-	-	-	-	-	-	-	-	-	-	-
d. Leishmaniasis	-	-	-	-	-	-	-	-	-	-	-	-	-	-	-	-	-
10. Leprosy	-	-	-	-	-	-	-	-	-	-	-	-	-	-	-	-	-
11. Dengue	-	-	-	-	-	-	-	-	-	-	-	-	-	-	-	-	-
12. Japanese encephalitis	-	-	-	-	-	-	-	-	-	-	-	-	-	-	-	-	-
13. Trachoma	-	-	-	-	-	-	-	-	-	-	-	-	-	-	-	-	-
14. Intestinal nematode infections	-	-	-	-	-	-	-	-	-	-	-	-	-	-	-	-	-
a. Ascariasis	-	-	-	-	-	-	-	-	-	-	-	-	-	-	-	-	-
b. Trichuriasis	-	-	-	-	-	-	-	-	-	-	-	-	-	-	-	-	-
c. Ancylostomiasis, necatoriasis	-	-	-	-	-	-	-	-	-	-	-	-	-	-	-	-	-
15. Other infectious and parasitic	15	5	10	1	-	-	-	-	1	4	-	-	-	-	-	1	8

Annex Table 18b, continued. Deaths by age, sex and cause (thousands): Formerly Socialist Economies of Europe, 2020, pessimistic scenario

Cause	Total	Male	Female	Males 0-4	5-14	15-29	30-44	45-59	60-69	70+	Females 0-4	5-14	15-29	30-44	45-59	60-69	70+
B. Respiratory infections	122	54	68	5	-	-	1	3	4	41	4	-	-	-	1	2	60
1. Lower respiratory infections	121	54	67	5	-	-	1	3	4	41	4	-	-	-	1	2	60
2. Upper respiratory infections	1	-	1	-	-	-	-	-	-	-	-	-	-	-	-	-	-
3. Otitis media	-	-	-	-	-	-	-	-	-	-	-	-	-	-	-	-	-
C. Maternal conditions	1		1								-	-	-	1	-	-	-
1. Maternal haemorrhage	1		1								-	-	-	1	-	-	-
2. Maternal sepsis	-		-								-	-	-	-	-	-	-
3. Hypertensive disorders*	-		-								-	-	-	-	-	-	-
4. Obstructed labour	-		-								-	-	-	-	-	-	-
5. Abortion	-		-								-	-	-	-	-	-	-
6. Other maternal	-		-								-	-	-	-	-	-	-
D. Perinatal conditions*	18	11	7	11	-	-	-	-	-	-	7	-	-	-	-	-	-
E. Nutritional deficiencies	10	3	7	-	-	-	-	-	-	3	-	-	-	-	-	-	6
1. Protein-energy malnutrition	2	1	2	-	-	-	-	-	-	2	-	-	-	-	-	-	2
2. Iodine deficiency	2	-	2	-	-	-	-	-	-	-	-	-	-	-	-	-	-
3. Vitamin A deficiency	-	-	-	-	-	-	-	-	-	-	-	-	-	-	-	-	-
4. Iron-deficiency anaemia	5	2	3	-	-	-	-	-	-	1	-	-	-	-	-	-	3
II. Noncommunicable diseases	*4 531*	*2 423*	*2 108*	*13*	*4*	*14*	*86*	*554*	*580*	*1 172*	*10*	*3*	*8*	*34*	*153*	*297*	*1 603*
A. Malignant neoplasms	1 016	666	350	1	2	4	30	226	199	206	1	1	3	18	67	94	167
1. Mouth and oropharynx cancers	30	26	4	-	-	-	2	14	6	4	-	-	-	-	1	1	2
2. Oesophagus cancer	17	15	2	-	-	-	1	7	4	3	-	-	-	-	-	1	1
3. Stomach cancer	156	104	52	-	-	-	4	39	28	33	-	-	-	2	8	13	29
4. Colon and rectum cancers	102	56	46	-	-	-	2	15	16	23	-	-	-	1	7	11	27
5. Liver cancer	31	19	12	-	-	-	1	6	6	6	-	-	-	-	2	3	7
6. Pancreas cancer	44	28	16	-	-	-	1	10	8	8	-	-	-	-	2	5	9
7. Trachea, bronchus, lung cancers	272	229	43	-	-	-	8	75	82	63	-	-	-	1	9	14	18
8. Melanoma and other skin cancers	13	7	6	-	-	-	1	2	1	2	-	-	-	-	1	1	3
9. Breast cancer	45	-	45								-	-	-	4	14	12	15
10. Cervix uteri cancer	18	-	18								-	-	-	2	4	5	7
11. Corpus uteri cancer	16		16								-	-	-	-	3	5	7
12. Ovary cancer	18		18								-	-	-	1	5	5	6
13. Prostate cancer	26	26	-	-	-	-	-	3	6	18							
14. Bladder cancer	26	21	5	-	-	-	-	5	6	10	-	-	-	-	-	-	3
15. Lymphomas, multiple myeloma	23	15	8	-	-	1	2	6	4	3	-	-	-	1	2	2	3
16. Leukaemia	26	16	10	-	1	1	1	5	4	4	-	-	1	1	2	2	4
17. Other cancers	153	103	50	-	1	2	6	38	27	28	-	1	1	2	8	13	25

Annex Table 18b, continued. Deaths by age, sex and cause (thousands): Formerly Socialist Economies of Europe, 2020, pessimistic scenario

Cause	Total	Male	Female	Males							Females						
				0-4	5-14	15-29	30-44	45-59	60-69	70+	0-4	5-14	15-29	30-44	45-59	60-69	70+
B. Other neoplasms	7	4	4							1						1	2
C. Diabetes mellitus	35	12	23					2	3	6					2	6	14
D. Endocrine disorders	4	2	2				1										1
E. Neuro-psychiatric conditions	81	35	47	1	1	2	3	6	5	16	1	1	1	1	2	5	36
2. Bipolar disorder	8	2	6							1							6
3. Schizophrenia	5	2	3							1							2
4. Epilepsy	6	3	2			1	1	1		1							1
5. Alcohol use	8	6	1				1		2	2							1
6. Dementia*	24	7	17						2	5							15
7. Parkinson disease	10	4	6						1	3						1	5
8. Multiple sclerosis	5	2	3							1							2
9. Drug use																	
13. Other neuro-psychiatric	16	8	8	1	1	1	1	1	1	3	1		1		1	1	4
F. Sense organ diseases																	
1. Glaucoma																	
2. Cataracts																	
G. Cardiovascular diseases	2 820	1 343	1 477	1		4	40	250	288	761			1	10	58	154	1 253
1. Rheumatic heart disease	28	14	14				2	7	3	1				1	5	4	3
2. Ischaemic heart disease	1 413	712	702			1	23	153	151	384				4	26	71	601
3. Cerebrovascular disease	859	364	495			1	7	54	82	220				3	22	56	414
4. Inflammatory heart diseases	51	28	24			1	3	8	4	12				1	2	2	18
5. Other cardiovascular	469	226	243			1	6	27	48	144			1	1	4	20	217
H. Respiratory diseases	339	229	111			1	3	38	55	131				1	8	18	83
1. COPD*	174	117	57				1	18	29	69					3	8	45
2. Asthma	15	7	8					2	2	4					1	2	5
3. Other respiratory	151	104	47				2	19	25	58				1	4	8	34
I. Digestive diseases	152	90	62	1		1	7	26	23	32				2	10	14	35
1. Peptic ulcer	19	13	6					4	3	5						1	4
2. Cirrhosis of the liver	63	41	22				3	15	12	11				1	5	6	9
3. Appendicitis	1																
4. Other digestive	69	35	34	1			3	8	7	16				1	4	6	22
J. Genito-urinary diseases	51	29	21				2	4	5	18				1	3	5	11
1. Nephritis and nephrosis	21	11	9				1	3	2	5				1	2	2	5
2. Benign prostatic hypertrophy	9	9							1	8							
3. Other genito-urinary	21	10	12					1	2	5					2	3	7
K. Skin diseases	2	1	1														1

Annex Table 18b, continued. Deaths by age, sex and cause (thousands): Formerly Socialist Economies of Europe, 2020, pessimistic scenario

Cause	Total	Male	Female	Males							Females						
				0-4	5-14	15-29	30-44	45-59	60-69	70+	0-4	5-14	15-29	30-44	45-59	60-69	70+
L. Musculo-skeletal diseases	5	1	3	-	-	-	-	-	-	-	-	-	-	-	-	1	1
1. Rheumatoid arthritis	1	-	1	-	-	-	-	-	-	-	-	-	-	-	-	1	1
3. Other musculo-skeletal	4	1	3	-	-	-	-	-	-	1	-	-	-	-	1	1	1
M. Congenital anomalies	19	10	8	9	-	1	-	-	-	-	7	-	-	-	-	-	-
N. Oral conditions	-	-	-	-	-	-	-	-	-	-	-	-	-	-	-	-	-
III. Injuries	*420*	*302*	*119*	*7*	*8*	*66*	*82*	*75*	*29*	*35*	*5*	*4*	*17*	*17*	*21*	*15*	*39*
A. Unintentional injuries	270	194	75	4	6	42	51	50	19	24	3	3	9	9	13	9	30
1. Road traffic accidents	109	81	28	1	3	26	21	16	7	8	3	1	6	4	5	4	7
2. Poisonings	44	33	11	1	-	3	10	13	4	2	-	-	1	2	4	2	2
3. Falls	36	18	17	-	-	1	3	4	2	8	-	-	-	-	1	1	14
4. Fires	8	5	3	-	-	1	1	2	1	1	-	1	-	-	1	-	1
5. Drownings	21	17	4	-	2	4	5	4	1	1	-	1	1	1	1	-	1
6. Other unintentional	52	39	13	2	1	7	11	11	4	4	-	1	1	2	3	2	4
B. Intentional injuries	151	108	43	3	2	25	31	25	10	12	1	1	8	8	8	6	9
1. Self-inflicted injuries	91	69	22	-	1	11	19	20	8	10	-	-	2	3	5	4	7
2. Violence	32	23	9	-	-	7	9	5	1	1	-	-	1	2	2	1	2
3. War	29	16	12	3	1	7	3	1	1	-	1	1	5	2	1	1	-

Notes:
Causes responsible for no deaths have been omitted from this table.
A dash (-) symbol indicates fewer than 500 deaths.
*IA6 is Bacterial meningitis and meningococcaemia; IC3 is Conditions arising during the perinatal period; ID is Conditions arising during the perinatal period; IC3 is Hypertensive disorders of pregnancy; ID is Conditions arising during the perinatal period;
IIE6 is Dementia and other degenerative and hereditary CNS disorders; IIH1 is Chronic obstructive pulmonary disease.

Annex Table 18c. Deaths by age, sex and cause (thousands): India, 2020, pessimistic scenario

Cause	Total	Male	Female	Males 0-4	5-14	15-29	30-44	45-59	60-69	70+	Females 0-4	5-14	15-29	30-44	45-59	60-69	70+
Population (millions)	*1 196*	*608*	*589*	*50*	*100*	*156*	*146*	*100*	*35*	*20*	*48*	*94*	*147*	*138*	*98*	*38*	*25*
All causes	**13 052**	**7 239**	**5 813**	**826**	**147**	**326**	**712**	**1 732**	**1 544**	**1 953**	**802**	**148**	**310**	**408**	**946**	**993**	**2 207**
I. Communicable, maternal, perinatal and nutritional conditions	*4 048*	*2 255*	*1 794*	*665*	*56*	*146*	*329*	*402*	*249*	*409*	*660*	*68*	*140*	*204*	*235*	*137*	*350*
A. Infectious and parasitic diseases	**2 878**	**1 700**	**1 178**	**341**	**42**	**140**	**319**	**386**	**195**	**278**	**335**	**44**	**116**	**173**	**216**	**94**	**200**
1. Tuberculosis	1 404	921	483	12	9	67	160	320	151	202	9	7	49	69	179	62	109
2. STDs excluding HIV	39	16	22	10	–	–	–	1	1	5	10	–	1	2	1	1	7
a. Syphilis	35	16	19	10	–	–	–	1	1	5	10	–	1	1	1	1	7
b. Chlamydia	2	–	2	–	–	–	–	–	–	–	–	–	1	1	–	–	–
c. Gonorrhoea	1	–	1	–	–	–	–	–	–	–	–	–	1	–	–	–	–
3. HIV	536	313	223	39	6	62	137	45	15	9	41	7	58	91	18	5	3
4. Diarrhoeal diseases	455	223	233	155	7	3	6	7	13	32	156	10	3	4	7	12	42
5. Childhood-cluster diseases	219	113	106	92	8	2	4	3	1	3	86	9	2	3	3	1	3
a. Pertussis	33	17	16	16	1	–	–	–	–	–	15	1	–	–	–	–	–
b. Poliomyelitis	5	3	2	3	–	–	–	–	–	–	2	–	–	–	–	–	–
c. Diphtheria	2	1	1	1	–	–	–	–	–	–	1	–	–	–	–	–	–
d. Measles	85	44	41	39	5	–	–	–	–	–	37	5	–	–	–	–	–
e. Tetanus	95	49	46	33	3	2	4	2	1	3	31	4	2	3	3	1	3
6. Bacterial meningitis*	24	12	11	5	–	–	2	2	1	1	5	–	–	1	2	2	2
7. Hepatitis B and hepatitis C	13	7	6	1	–	–	1	2	1	2	–	–	–	1	1	1	3
8. Malaria	12	7	6	1	1	1	2	1	–	1	1	1	1	1	1	–	1
9. Tropical-cluster diseases	14	9	5	1	3	2	2	1	–	–	1	2	1	1	–	–	–
a. Trypanosomiasis	–	–	–	–	–	–	–	–	–	–	–	–	–	–	–	–	–
b. Chagas disease	–	–	–	–	–	–	–	–	–	–	–	–	–	–	–	–	–
c. Schistosomiasis	–	–	–	–	–	–	–	–	–	–	–	–	–	–	–	–	–
d. Leishmaniasis	14	9	5	1	3	2	2	1	–	–	1	2	1	1	–	–	–
10. Leprosy	1	1	–	–	–	–	–	–	–	–	–	–	–	–	–	–	–
11. Dengue	4	2	2	1	1	–	–	–	–	–	–	2	–	–	–	–	–
12. Japanese encephalitis	–	–	–	–	–	–	–	–	–	–	–	–	–	–	–	–	–
13. Trachoma	–	–	–	–	–	–	–	–	–	–	–	–	–	–	–	–	–
14. Intestinal nematode infections	2	1	1	–	2	–	–	–	–	–	–	2	–	–	–	–	–
a. Ascariasis	–	–	–	–	–	–	–	–	–	–	–	–	–	–	–	–	–
b. Trichuriasis	1	1	1	–	–	–	–	–	–	–	–	–	–	–	–	–	–
c. Ancylostomiasis, necatoriasis	1	1	1	–	–	–	–	–	–	–	–	–	–	–	–	–	–
15. Other infectious and parasitic	155	76	79	25	5	2	5	6	10	23	25	6	2	1	5	10	30

Annex Table 18c, continued. Deaths by age, sex and cause (thousands): India, 2020, pessimistic scenario

Cause	Total	Male	Female	Males							Females						
				0-4	5-14	15-29	30-44	45-59	60-69	70+	0-4	5-14	15-29	30-44	45-59	60-69	70+
B. Respiratory infections	767	377	390	162	12	4	9	14	52	123	164	21	4	5	14	41	141
1. Lower respiratory infections	754	371	383	159	12	4	9	14	51	122	160	20	4	5	14	40	139
2. Upper respiratory infections	8	4	4	2	-	-	-	-	1	1	2	-	-	-	-	-	1
3. Otitis media	5	2	3	2	-	-	-	-	-	-	2	-	-	-	-	-	-
C. Maternal conditions	46	-	46	-	-	-	-	-	-	-	-	-	19	24	3	-	-
1. Maternal haemorrhage	11	-	11	-	-	-	-	-	-	-	-	-	5	6	1	-	-
2. Maternal sepsis	7	-	7	-	-	-	-	-	-	-	-	-	3	4	-	-	-
3. Hypertensive disorders*	5	-	5	-	-	-	-	-	-	-	-	-	2	3	-	-	-
4. Obstructed labour	4	-	4	-	-	-	-	-	-	-	-	-	2	2	-	-	-
5. Abortion	7	-	7	-	-	-	-	-	-	-	-	-	3	4	-	-	-
6. Other maternal	11	-	11	-	-	-	-	-	-	-	-	-	5	6	1	-	-
D. Perinatal conditions*	290	147	144	147	-	-	-	-	-	-	144	-	-	-	-	-	-
E. Nutritional deficiencies	67	31	36	15	2	1	1	2	2	7	17	3	1	1	2	2	10
1. Protein-energy malnutrition	36	16	20	10	2	1	1	1	1	3	12	1	-	-	1	1	5
2. Iodine deficiency	2	1	1	1	-	-	-	-	-	-	1	-	-	-	-	-	-
3. Vitamin A deficiency	8	4	4	3	1	-	-	-	-	-	3	1	-	-	-	-	-
4. Iron-deficiency anaemia	21	9	11	1	-	1	1	1	1	4	1	1	1	1	2	1	5
II. Noncommunicable diseases	7 780	4 273	3 507	102	29	49	208	1 164	1 245	1 477	98	29	59	112	611	808	1 790
A. Malignant neoplasms	1 247	710	538	4	5	14	57	295	160	174	2	3	22	41	206	121	142
1. Mouth and oropharynx cancers	170	104	66	-	-	2	6	46	21	28	-	-	2	4	27	16	17
2. Oesophagus cancer	109	57	52	-	-	1	3	25	11	18	-	-	1	2	18	13	18
3. Stomach cancer	95	61	33	-	-	1	4	28	11	17	-	-	1	2	12	8	10
4. Colon and rectum cancers	44	23	21	-	-	1	2	8	4	7	-	-	1	2	6	5	8
5. Liver cancer	28	19	8	-	-	-	1	8	3	6	-	-	1	1	2	2	4
6. Pancreas cancer	16	10	7	-	-	-	1	4	2	3	-	-	-	-	2	1	3
7. Trachea, bronchus, lung cancers	274	235	38	-	-	1	17	108	78	31	-	-	1	2	14	12	9
8. Melanoma and other skin cancers	2	1	1	-	-	-	-	1	-	-	-	-	-	-	-	-	-
9. Breast cancer	69	-	69	-	-	-	-	-	-	-	-	-	4	7	30	14	15
10. Cervix uteri cancer	99	-	99	-	-	-	-	-	-	-	-	-	4	7	52	19	17
11. Corpus uteri cancer	7	-	7	-	-	-	-	-	-	-	-	-	-	-	2	2	3
12. Ovary cancer	23	-	23	-	-	-	-	-	-	-	-	-	2	3	7	6	6
13. Prostate cancer	24	24	-	-	-	-	-	3	4	17	-	-	-	-	-	-	-
14. Bladder cancer	15	11	3	-	-	-	-	3	2	5	-	-	-	-	1	1	2
15. Lymphomas, multiple myeloma	37	23	14	1	1	1	4	8	3	5	-	-	1	1	3	3	5
16. Leukaemia	27	16	11	1	2	1	4	4	1	2	1	1	1	2	3	1	2
17. Other cancers	210	125	85	2	2	5	14	49	19	34	1	1	5	9	27	18	24

Annex Table 18c, continued. Deaths by age, sex and cause (thousands): India, 2020, pessimistic scenario

Cause	Total	Male	Female	Males 0-4	5-14	15-29	30-44	45-59	60-69	70+	Females 0-4	5-14	15-29	30-44	45-59	60-69	70+
B. Other neoplasms	6	4	2	-	-	-	1	1	-	1	-	-	-	-	-	-	-
C. Diabetes mellitus	145	63	83	2	2	1	4	15	16	22	2	2	1	2	15	25	35
D. Endocrine disorders	2	1	1	-	-	-	-	-	-	-	-	-	-	-	-	-	-
E. Neuro-psychiatric conditions	138	75	63	5	3	3	11	14	15	24	5	2	4	3	4	13	30
2. Bipolar disorder	4	1	3	-	-	1	-	-	-	-	-	-	-	-	-	1	2
3. Schizophrenia	7	3	4	-	-	1	-	1	1	1	-	-	1	1	1	1	2
4. Epilepsy	15	9	6	1	1	1	3	2	1	-	-	1	1	1	1	1	1
5. Alcohol use	7	7	1	-	-	-	3	2	1	1	-	-	-	-	-	1	-
6. Dementia*	34	15	19	-	-	-	-	2	3	9	-	-	-	-	1	3	13
7. Parkinson disease	10	6	4	-	-	-	-	1	1	4	-	-	-	-	-	1	3
8. Multiple sclerosis	5	2	3	-	-	1	-	1	1	-	-	-	1	1	1	1	-
9. Drug use	-	-	-	-	-	-	-	-	-	-	-	-	-	-	-	-	-
13. Other neuro-psychiatric	57	31	26	5	2	2	4	5	7	7	5	2	2	1	1	6	8
F. Sense organ diseases	-	-	-	-	-	-	-	-	-	-	-	-	-	-	-	-	-
1. Glaucoma	-	-	-	-	-	-	-	-	-	-	-	-	-	-	-	-	-
2. Cataracts	-	-	-	-	-	-	-	-	-	-	-	-	-	-	-	-	-
G. Cardiovascular diseases	4 852	2 580	2 272	15	5	13	84	616	843	1 003	13	7	14	39	274	550	1 375
1. Rheumatic heart disease	127	62	65	-	1	4	12	30	11	4	-	1	4	12	28	12	8
2. Ischaemic heart disease	2 602	1 405	1 197	-	-	1	26	335	483	560	-	-	4	12	131	299	754
3. Cerebrovascular disease	956	493	463	3	1	1	9	93	166	219	3	1	2	5	39	118	295
4. Inflammatory heart diseases	154	84	69	3	1	3	9	32	17	20	3	2	2	5	17	12	29
5. Other cardiovascular	1 014	536	478	9	3	5	27	126	166	200	7	4	5	6	58	109	290
H. Respiratory diseases	718	423	294	5	5	2	11	96	143	161	5	4	5	8	59	66	147
1. COPD*	407	249	158	1	1	-	3	49	88	106	1	1	1	2	28	38	89
2. Asthma	53	30	24	-	1	1	2	8	8	10	-	1	-	1	6	5	10
3. Other respiratory	258	145	113	4	3	2	6	39	46	45	4	3	4	5	26	23	49
I. Digestive diseases	380	263	117	2	2	9	32	110	46	62	3	2	7	12	37	19	36
1. Peptic ulcer	68	44	24	-	-	1	4	16	9	14	1	-	1	2	7	4	9
2. Cirrhosis of the liver	236	172	64	1	-	5	19	76	30	41	-	1	3	6	23	10	20
3. Appendicitis	10	6	4	-	1	2	2	1	1	-	-	1	1	1	-	-	-
4. Other digestive	65	41	25	2	1	1	8	17	6	7	2	1	2	3	8	5	6
J. Genito-urinary diseases	131	75	57	2	4	2	4	14	19	29	2	5	2	3	11	12	22
1. Nephritis and nephrosis	114	58	55	2	3	2	4	14	13	20	2	5	2	3	10	11	22
2. Benign prostatic hypertrophy	15	15	-	-	-	-	-	-	6	9	-	-	-	-	-	-	-
3. Other genito-urinary	3	2	1	-	-	-	-	-	-	-	-	-	-	-	1	-	-
K. Skin diseases	3	2	1	-	-	-	-	-	-	-	-	-	-	-	-	-	-

Annex Table 18c, continued. Deaths by age, sex and cause (thousands): India, 2020, pessimistic scenario

Cause	Total	Male	Female	Males							Females						
				0-4	5-14	15-29	30-44	45-59	60-69	70+	0-4	5-14	15-29	30-44	45-59	60-69	70+
L. Musculo-skeletal diseases	3	2	2	–	–	–	–	–	–	1	–	–	–	–	–	1	1
1. Rheumatoid arthritis	3	1	1	–	–	–	–	–	–	1	–	–	–	–	–	–	1
3. Other musculo-skeletal	1	–	–	–	–	–	–	–	–	–	–	–	–	–	–	–	–
M. Congenital anomalies	154	76	78	65	3	3	2	2	1	1	65	3	2	2	2	1	1
N. Oral conditions	–	–	–	–	–	–	–	–	–	–	–	–	–	–	–	–	–
III. Injuries	*1 224*	*712*	*512*	*60*	*62*	*132*	*175*	*166*	*50*	*67*	*44*	*51*	*111*	*91*	*100*	*48*	*67*
A. Unintentional injuries	972	566	406	55	58	95	134	126	41	57	38	46	74	68	76	41	62
1. Road traffic accidents	375	265	111	14	24	58	66	59	18	26	4	18	13	17	29	14	16
2. Poisonings	36	18	17	4	2	3	5	3	1	1	3	1	5	4	3	1	–
3. Falls	66	41	25	3	5	3	7	10	5	8	3	2	1	2	4	5	8
4. Fires	159	49	111	7	2	8	13	12	3	3	6	7	37	28	14	7	11
5. Drownings	95	50	45	9	10	8	10	7	2	4	7	9	6	6	7	3	7
6. Other unintentional	241	143	98	18	15	15	32	35	13	15	15	10	12	11	18	13	18
B. Intentional injuries	251	145	106	5	4	37	41	40	8	10	6	4	37	23	24	7	5
1. Self-inflicted injuries	160	89	71	–	3	26	25	26	4	5	–	3	33	20	11	1	5
2. Violence	87	52	35	5	2	8	14	14	5	5	6	1	3	3	13	6	3
3. War	5	5	–	–	–	3	2	–	–	–	–	–	–	–	–	–	–

Notes:
Causes responsible for no deaths have been omitted from this table.
A dash (-) symbol indicates fewer than 500 deaths.
*IA6 is Bacterial meningitis and meningococcaemia; IC3 is Hypertensive disorders of pregnancy; ID is Conditions arising during the perinatal period; IIE6 is Dementia and other degenerative and hereditary CNS disorders; IIH1 is Chronic obstructive pulmonary disease.

Annex Table 18d. Deaths by age, sex and cause (thousands): China, 2020, pessimistic scenario

Cause	Total	Male	Female	Males							Females						
				0-4	5-14	15-29	30-44	45-59	60-69	70+	0-4	5-14	15-29	30-44	45-59	60-69	70+
Population (millions)	*1 447*	*727*	*721*	*56*	*101*	*167*	*149*	*161*	*59*	*33*	*53*	*96*	*159*	*142*	*159*	*66*	*44*
All causes	*15 323*	*8 823*	*6 500*	*245*	*57*	*211*	*465*	*2 273*	*2 353*	*3 219*	*254*	*41*	*158*	*227*	*1 009*	*1 308*	*3 502*
I. Communicable, maternal, perinatal and nutritional conditions	*903*	*475*	*428*	*125*	*5*	*5*	*11*	*46*	*55*	*228*	*138*	*5*	*7*	*9*	*28*	*40*	*200*
A. Infectious and parasitic diseases	410	237	174	22	2	4	10	42	44	112	23	3	3	6	24	29	87
1. Tuberculosis	241	149	92	1	–	1	5	29	33	79	1	1	1	3	18	21	48
2. STDs excluding HIV	1	–	–														
a. Syphilis	1	–	–														
b. Chlamydia	–	–	–														
c. Gonorrhoea	–	–	–														
3. HIV	7	4	3	–	–	1	1	1	–	–	–	–	1	1	–	–	–
4. Diarrhoeal diseases	66	31	35	8	–	–	1	1	4	17	10	–	–	–	1	2	22
5. Childhood-cluster diseases	19	10	8	9	1	–	–	–	–	–	8	–	–	–	–	–	–
a. Pertussis	6	3	3	3	–	–	–	–	–	–	3	–	–	–	–	–	–
b. Poliomyelitis	1	1	–	1	–	–	–	–	–	–	–	–	–	–	–	–	–
c. Diphtheria																	
d. Measles	5	3	2	2	1	–	–	–	–	–	2	–	–	–	–	–	–
e. Tetanus	7	4	3	3	–	–	–	–	–	–	3	–	–	–	–	–	–
6. Bacterial meningitis*	22	11	11	2	–	–	1	2	2	2	2	–	–	1	2	3	3
7. Hepatitis B and hepatitis C	23	14	9	1	–	1	1	5	2	5	1	–	–	–	1	3	5
8. Malaria	–	–	–														
9. Tropical-cluster diseases	1	1	–	–	–	–	1	–	–	–	–	–	–	–	–	–	–
a. Trypanosomiasis																	
b. Chagas disease																	
c. Schistosomiasis	1	1	–	–	–	–	1	–	–	–	–	–	–	–	–	–	–
d. Leishmaniasis																	
10. Leprosy	–	–	–														
11. Dengue	–	–	–														
12. Japanese encephalitis	1	–	–														
13. Trachoma	–	–	–														
14. Intestinal nematode infections	2	1	1	–	1	–	–	–	–	–	–	1	–	–	–	–	–
a. Ascariasis	1	1	–	–	1	–	–	–	–	–	–	–	–	–	–	–	–
b. Trichuriasis	1	–	1	–	–	–	–	–	–	–	–	1	–	–	–	–	–
c. Ancylostomiasis, necatoriasis																	
15. Other infectious and parasitic	28	15	13	1	–	–	–	3	2	8	1	–	–	–	1	1	9

Annex Table 18d, continued. Deaths by age, sex and cause (thousands): China, 2020, pessimistic scenario

Cause	Total	Male	Female	Males							Females						
				0-4	5-14	15-29	30-44	45-59	60-69	70+	0-4	5-14	15-29	30-44	45-59	60-69	70+
B. Respiratory infections	341	171	170	47	1	1	1	4	10	107	54	1	1	1	2	9	103
1. Lower respiratory infections	337	169	168	47	1	1	1	4	10	106	53	1	1	1	2	8	102
2. Upper respiratory infections	3	2	2	–	–	–	–	–	–	1	1	–	–	–	–	–	1
3. Otitis media	1	–	–	–	–	–	–	–	–	–	–	–	–	–	–	–	–
C. Maternal conditions	7	–	7	–	–	–	–	–	–	–	–	–	4	2	1	–	–
1. Maternal haemorrhage	3	–	3	–	–	–	–	–	–	–	–	–	1	1	1	–	–
2. Maternal sepsis	–	–	–	–	–	–	–	–	–	–	–	–	–	–	–	–	–
3. Hypertensive disorders*	1	–	1	–	–	–	–	–	–	–	–	–	1	–	–	–	–
4. Obstructed labour	–	–	–	–	–	–	–	–	–	–	–	–	–	–	–	–	–
5. Abortion	1	–	1	–	–	–	–	–	–	–	–	–	1	–	–	–	–
6. Other maternal	3	–	3	–	–	–	–	–	–	–	–	–	1	1	1	–	–
D. Perinatal conditions*	101	50	51	50	–	–	–	–	–	–	51	–	–	–	–	–	–
E. Nutritional deficiencies	43	18	26	6	1	–	–	1	2	8	10	1	–	1	1	3	10
1. Protein-energy malnutrition	22	10	12	3	–	–	–	–	1	6	7	–	–	–	–	1	5
2. Iodine deficiency	3	1	1	1	–	–	–	–	–	–	1	–	–	–	–	–	–
3. Vitamin A deficiency	3	2	1	1	1	–	–	–	–	–	1	–	–	–	–	–	–
4. Iron-deficiency anaemia	15	5	10	1	–	–	–	1	1	2	2	1	–	1	1	2	5
II. Noncommunicable diseases	12 898	7 490	5 409	67	21	68	302	2 025	2 177	2 831	69	13	46	146	843	1 180	3 111
A. Malignant neoplasms	3 669	2 465	1 204	5	11	26	175	975	755	519	7	5	17	70	342	359	405
1. Mouth and oropharynx cancers	86	62	24	–	–	1	10	24	16	11	–	–	1	2	9	7	5
2. Oesophagus cancer	477	335	143	–	–	1	12	113	113	96	–	–	–	1	30	57	54
3. Stomach cancer	798	549	250	–	–	1	17	199	185	147	–	–	2	12	57	79	100
4. Colon and rectum cancers	199	116	84	–	–	2	7	38	33	34	–	–	1	5	23	25	30
5. Liver cancer	749	568	181	–	1	5	76	277	134	75	–	1	1	13	59	50	56
6. Pancreas cancer	79	50	29	–	–	–	2	15	16	16	–	–	–	–	5	11	13
7. Trachea, bronchus, lung cancers	657	494	162	–	–	2	19	205	189	78	–	–	–	3	48	53	58
8. Melanoma and other skin cancers	3	2	1	–	–	–	–	1	1	–	–	–	–	–	1	–	–
9. Breast cancer	56	–	56	–	–	–	–	–	–	–	–	–	1	8	21	12	14
10. Cervix uteri cancer	48	–	48	–	–	–	–	–	–	–	–	–	1	3	17	14	13
11. Corpus uteri cancer	15	–	15	–	–	–	–	–	–	–	–	–	–	1	8	3	3
12. Ovary cancer	22	–	22	–	–	–	–	–	–	–	–	–	1	3	8	4	5
13. Prostate cancer	11	11	–	–	–	–	–	1	5	5	–	–	–	–	–	–	–
14. Bladder cancer	46	36	9	–	–	–	1	7	14	14	–	–	–	–	1	4	4
15. Lymphomas, multiple myeloma	52	35	17	–	–	2	1	13	12	6	–	–	1	1	7	4	5
16. Leukaemia	113	62	51	3	5	7	11	22	8	7	3	3	6	9	14	8	9
17. Other cancers	258	145	113	1	3	5	17	61	30	29	1	1	3	10	35	28	34

Annex Table 18d, continued. Deaths by age, sex and cause (thousands): China, 2020, pessimistic scenario

Cause	Total	Male	Female	Males 0-4	5-14	15-29	30-44	45-59	60-69	70+	Females 0-4	5-14	15-29	30-44	45-59	60-69	70+
B. Other neoplasms	27	14	14	1	-	1	1	4	4	3	1	-	-	1	3	5	4
C. Diabetes mellitus	97	38	59	-	-	-	2	9	11	14	-	-	1	1	10	20	27
D. Endocrine disorders	19	7	12	-	-	-	-	1	1	3	1	-	1	1	1	1	7
E. Neuro-psychiatric conditions	128	58	69	2	1	8	9	9	7	22	2	1	4	5	8	11	39
2. Bipolar disorder	4	1	3	-	-	-	-	-	-	1	-	-	-	1	1	-	3
3. Schizophrenia	18	11	7	-	-	2	3	1	1	1	-	-	1	1	2	1	2
4. Epilepsy	11	6	5	-	-	2	1	1	1	1	-	-	1	1	1	1	1
5. Alcohol use	6	5	1	-	-	-	2	2	1	-	-	-	-	-	2	-	-
6. Dementia*	46	16	30	-	-	-	-	2	3	10	-	-	-	-	2	5	22
7. Parkinson disease	9	4	5	-	-	-	-	-	1	4	-	-	-	-	1	1	4
8. Multiple sclerosis	7	3	4	-	-	-	1	1	1	1	-	-	-	1	2	1	1
9. Drug use	-	-	-	-	-	-	-	-	-	-	-	-	-	-	-	-	-
13. Other neuro-psychiatric	26	12	13	1	1	4	2	1	1	3	1	-	2	2	1	2	5
F. Sense organ diseases	27	13	14	1	-	-	-	4	5	4	-	-	-	-	3	5	4
1. Glaucoma	10	5	5	-	-	-	-	1	2	1	-	-	-	-	1	2	2
2. Cataracts	9	5	4	-	-	-	-	2	2	1	-	-	-	-	1	2	1
G. Cardiovascular diseases	4 973	2 756	2 217	9	2	15	62	638	766	1 263	5	1	11	39	267	420	1 475
1. Rheumatic heart disease	281	133	148	-	-	5	9	43	28	47	1	-	4	10	36	27	70
2. Ischaemic heart disease	1 495	811	684	-	-	3	20	180	218	389	-	-	1	11	68	124	480
3. Cerebrovascular disease	2 500	1 413	1 087	2	1	4	24	318	420	644	1	-	2	13	134	226	710
4. Inflammatory heart diseases	112	64	49	2	-	2	5	24	11	20	1	-	2	4	11	6	25
5. Other cardiovascular	585	335	250	5	-	1	4	73	88	164	2	-	2	2	18	36	189
H. Respiratory diseases	2 997	1 598	1 399	7	1	4	16	252	503	815	7	-	2	12	136	282	960
1. COPD*	2 823	1 502	1 321	3	1	2	11	233	481	772	5	-	1	10	126	269	911
2. Asthma	71	40	31	-	-	1	3	13	11	13	-	-	1	1	8	7	13
3. Other respiratory	103	55	48	4	-	1	2	6	12	30	2	-	1	1	2	6	36
I. Digestive diseases	631	372	259	6	1	4	27	111	98	125	7	1	4	10	54	53	130
1. Peptic ulcer	58	32	26	-	-	-	1	6	8	17	-	-	-	-	3	4	18
2. Cirrhosis of the liver	301	196	105	1	1	2	20	72	58	43	-	-	1	5	31	29	39
3. Appendicitis	9	5	4	-	1	1	1	1	1	-	-	-	1	-	1	1	-
4. Other digestive	264	139	125	5	-	1	4	32	32	64	6	-	2	4	20	19	73
J. Genito-urinary diseases	171	94	77	1	1	5	8	18	19	41	2	1	3	5	14	20	33
1. Nephritis and nephrosis	132	71	61	1	1	5	7	16	15	25	2	1	2	5	11	15	25
2. Benign prostatic hypertrophy	10	10	-	-	-	-	1	-	1	9	-	-	-	-	-	-	-
3. Other genito-urinary	30	14	16	-	-	-	2	2	3	7	-	-	1	-	3	5	8
K. Skin diseases	17	10	7	-	-	-	-	1	1	6	-	-	1	-	1	1	4

Annex Table 18d, continued. Deaths by age, sex and cause (thousands): China, 2020, pessimistic scenario

Cause	Total	Male	Female	Males							Females						
				0-4	5-14	15-29	30-44	45-59	60-69	70+	0-4	5-14	15-29	30-44	45-59	60-69	70+
L. Musculo-skeletal diseases	**58**	**24**	**33**	-	-	-	-	2	6	15	-	-	1	1	3	4	24
1. Rheumatoid arthritis	3	1	2	-	-	-	-	-	-	1	-	-	-	1	-	-	1
3. Other musculo-skeletal	55	23	32	-	-	-	-	2	6	15	-	-	1	1	3	4	23
M. Congenital anomalies	**85**	**42**	**44**	35	3	3	1	1	-	-	36	3	3	1	1	-	-
N. Oral conditions	-	-	-	-	-	-	-	-	-	-	-	-	-	-	-	-	-
III. Injuries	**1 521**	**858**	**663**	52	32	139	152	202	121	161	47	23	105	72	138	87	191
A. Unintentional injuries	**939**	**580**	**359**	48	28	89	99	135	75	106	39	19	32	26	70	46	127
1. Road traffic accidents	380	272	108	4	10	47	59	75	41	38	3	10	17	13	33	16	16
2. Poisonings	81	47	35	3	1	4	7	16	6	11	1	1	5	4	6	6	11
3. Falls	118	44	73	2	1	4	4	8	8	19	2	-	1	1	8	11	50
4. Fires	36	17	19	2	-	-	2	2	1	9	1	-	1	-	3	2	11
5. Drownings	124	72	51	20	12	12	6	8	4	10	16	6	4	2	5	5	13
6. Other unintentional	201	127	73	18	4	21	22	28	15	20	17	2	5	5	15	7	24
B. Intentional injuries	**582**	**278**	**304**	4	4	50	53	66	46	54	8	3	72	46	68	41	65
1. Self-inflicted injuries	520	242	278	-	2	38	45	60	43	53	-	2	70	41	64	39	62
2. Violence	61	36	26	4	1	12	9	6	3	1	8	1	2	5	4	2	3
3. War	1	1	-	-	-	-	-	-	-	-	-	-	-	-	-	-	-

Notes:
Causes responsible for no deaths have been omitted from this table.
A dash (-) symbol indicates fewer than 500 deaths.
*IA6 is Bacterial meningitis and meningococcaemia; IC3 is Hypertensive disorders of pregnancy; ID is Conditions arising during the perinatal period; IIE6 is Dementia and other degenerative and hereditary CNS disorders; IIH1 is Chronic obstructive pulmonary disease.

Annex Table 18e. Deaths by age, sex and cause (thousands): Other Asia and Islands, 2020, pessimistic scenario

Cause	Total	Male	Female	Males 0-4	5-14	15-29	30-44	45-59	60-69	70+	Females 0-4	5-14	15-29	30-44	45-59	60-69	70+
Population (millions)	1 002	497	505	43	81	122	117	85	32	19	41	79	119	115	89	37	25
All causes	8 922	4 968	3 954	543	143	233	487	1 029	952	1 581	417	100	151	268	556	672	1 790
I. Communicable, maternal, perinatal and nutritional conditions	1 903	1 004	899	414	37	45	91	94	105	217	313	32	51	86	87	76	253
A. Infectious and parasitic diseases	1 160	622	539	201	23	41	87	86	66	118	151	19	39	68	75	56	131
1. Tuberculosis	409	203	206	1	1	6	14	49	46	87	5	1	5	11	49	44	96
2. STDs excluding HIV	34	16	18	9	–	–	–	1	1	5	6	–	1	2	1	1	7
a. Syphilis	31	16	15	9	–	–	–	1	1	5	6	–	1	1	1	1	7
b. Chlamydia	2	–	2	–	–	–	–	–	–	–	–	–	1	1	–	–	–
c. Gonorrhoea	1	–	1	–													
3. HIV	242	141	101	18	3	28	62	21	7	3	12	2	28	45	10	3	1
4. Diarrhoeal diseases	221	126	96	106	5	1	1	2	4	6	77	4	1	1	3	2	8
5. Childhood-cluster diseases	121	64	57	51	5	1	2	2	1	2	44	5	1	2	2	1	2
a. Pertussis	17	9	8	9	1						7	1					
b. Poliomyelitis	2	1	1	1	–						1	–					
c. Diphtheria	1	1	1	1	–	–					1	–					
d. Measles	57	31	27	27	3	–	–				24	3	–	2			
e. Tetanus	44	23	21	14	1	1	2	2	1	2	12	2	1	2	2	1	2
6. Bacterial meningitis*	19	10	9	3	–	–	2	2	2	1	3	–	1	1	2	1	2
7. Hepatitis B and hepatitis C	20	12	9	1	–	–	1	3	2	4	1	–	–	1	1	1	4
8. Malaria	47	25	22	3	5	5	5	5	2	2	2	4	3	4	5	2	3
9. Tropical-cluster diseases	2	1	1	–	–	–	–	–	–	–	–	–	–	–	–	–	–
a. Trypanosomiasis																	
b. Chagas disease																	
c. Schistosomiasis	1	1															
d. Leishmaniasis	1	1															
10. Leprosy	1	1	–				1										
11. Dengue	3	1	2	–	–	–	–				–	1					
12. Japanese encephalitis	1	1	–														
13. Trachoma	–	–	–														
14. Intestinal nematode infections	4	2	2	–	1	–	–	–	–	–	–	1	–	–	–	–	–
a. Ascariasis	1	1	1		1							1					
b. Trichuriasis	1	1	1		1							1					
c. Ancylostomiasis, necatoriasis	1	1	1		1							1					
15. Other infectious and parasitic	37	20	17	8	1	–	1	2	1	6	6	1	–	1	2	1	7

Annex Table 18e, continued. Deaths by age, sex and cause (thousands): Other Asia and Islands, 2020, pessimistic scenario

Cause	Total	Male	Female	Males 0-4	5-14	15-29	30-44	45-59	60-69	70+	Females 0-4	5-14	15-29	30-44	45-59	60-69	70+
B. Respiratory infections	486	257	230	99	12	3	3	7	37	95	72	11	2	3	8	19	116
1. Lower respiratory infections	480	253	227	98	12	3	3	7	37	94	70	11	2	3	7	19	115
2. Upper respiratory infections	5	3	2	1						1	1						1
3. Otitis media	2	1	1	1							1						
C. Maternal conditions	27		27										9	15	2		
1. Maternal haemorrhage	6		6										2	4	1		
2. Maternal sepsis	4		4										2	2			
3. Hypertensive disorders*	3		3										1	1	1		
4. Obstructed labour	2		2										1	1			
5. Abortion	4		4										1	2			
6. Other maternal	7		7										3	4	1		
D. Perinatal conditions*	177	100	77	100							77						
E. Nutritional deficiencies	51	26	25	15	2	1	1	1	1	5	13	2	1	1	2	1	6
1. Protein-energy malnutrition	24	13	11	10					1	1	9						1
2. Iodine deficiency	1	1	–	1													
3. Vitamin A deficiency	8	4	4	3	1						3	1					
4. Iron-deficiency anaemia	18	8	10	1		1	1	1	1	4	1		1		2	1	5
II. Noncommunicable diseases	*6 192*	*3 392*	*2 800*	*84*	*63*	*49*	*242*	*822*	*805*	*1 326*	*68*	*46*	*43*	*133*	*430*	*571*	*1 511*
A. Malignant neoplasms	1 628	960	668	6	16	10	78	296	264	290	7	10	13	54	171	186	227
1. Mouth and oropharynx cancers	174	108	65			1	8	19	38	42			1	4	7	23	29
2. Oesophagus cancer	60	42	18				1	14	12	14				1	4	6	7
3. Stomach cancer	150	99	51			1	6	36	27	30			1	3	12	16	20
4. Colon and rectum cancers	103	54	49				4	9	19	21			1	2	7	17	22
5. Liver cancer	175	131	44		1	2	12	60	27	30			1	2	11	13	16
6. Pancreas cancer	25	16	10				1	5	5	5					2	3	4
7. Trachea, bronchus, lung cancers	281	213	68			1	13	83	54	62				2	18	23	24
8. Melanoma and other skin cancers	6	2	3					1	1						1	1	1
9. Breast cancer	65		65										2	8	26	13	17
10. Cervix uteri cancer	79		79										2	8	34	16	20
11. Corpus uteri cancer	10		10												3	3	4
12. Ovary cancer	23		23											4	7	5	6
13. Prostate cancer	33	33	–					4	14	16							
14. Bladder cancer	29	21	8				1	5	7	8					1	3	4
15. Lymphomas, multiple myeloma	56	33	23	1	2	1	5	6	9	10		1		2	3	7	9
16. Leukaemia	52	29	23	2	6	1	7	3	5	5	3	4	1	4	2	4	5
17. Other cancers	306	179	128	3	7	3	19	51	47	48	3	5	3	15	31	33	38

Annex Table 18e, continued. Deaths by age, sex and cause (thousands): Other Asia and Islands, 2020, pessimistic scenario

Cause	Total	Male	Female	Males							Females						
				0-4	5-14	15-29	30-44	45-59	60-69	70+	0-4	5-14	15-29	30-44	45-59	60-69	70+
B. Other neoplasms	14	7	7	1	1	-	1	2	1	1	-	1	-	1	1	1	2
C. Diabetes mellitus	117	48	69	-	-	1	3	12	13	18	-	-	1	2	12	21	33
D. Endocrine disorders	13	6	8	1	1	-	-	1	1	1	1	-	1	-	1	1	4
E. Neuro-psychiatric conditions	119	64	55	2	2	4	10	14	10	22	2	2	2	3	6	9	30
2. Bipolar disorder	3	1	2	-	-	-	-	-	-	1	-	-	-	-	-	-	2
3. Schizophrenia	11	5	6	-	-	1	1	2	1	2	-	-	-	1	1	1	3
4. Epilepsy	12	8	4	-	1	1	2	2	1	1	-	-	1	1	1	1	1
5. Alcohol use	10	9	1	-	-	1	2	4	1	1	-	-	-	-	-	-	-
6. Dementia*	38	15	22	-	-	-	-	2	3	10	-	-	-	1	1	4	16
7. Parkinson disease	9	5	4	-	-	-	-	-	1	4	-	-	-	-	-	1	3
8. Multiple sclerosis	4	2	2	-	-	-	-	1	1	-	-	-	-	-	1	1	-
9. Drug use	2	2	-	-	-	1	1	-	-	-	-	-	-	-	-	-	-
13. Other neuro-psychiatric	31	17	14	2	2	2	3	3	2	4	2	2	1	1	2	2	5
F. Sense organ diseases	-	-	-	-	-	-	-	-	-	-	-	-	-	-	-	-	-
1. Glaucoma	-	-	-	-	-	-	-	-	-	-	-	-	-	-	-	-	-
2. Cataracts	-	-	-	-	-	-	-	-	-	-	-	-	-	-	-	-	-
G. Cardiovascular diseases	2 977	1 529	1 448	31	29	24	95	301	346	704	23	21	17	49	151	242	945
1. Rheumatic heart disease	22	10	12	-	-	-	1	2	2	5	-	-	-	1	2	2	7
2. Ischaemic heart disease	1 133	581	552	-	-	-	30	106	143	302	-	-	-	15	49	97	392
3. Cerebrovascular disease	904	446	458	4	6	5	20	85	114	211	3	4	3	10	48	85	305
4. Inflammatory heart diseases	127	71	55	6	6	5	11	18	8	17	5	5	3	6	9	9	22
5. Other cardiovascular	791	420	370	21	16	13	32	89	79	169	14	12	11	17	44	53	220
H. Respiratory diseases	394	225	169	8	3	2	7	30	43	132	5	2	2	5	17	31	108
1. COPD*	227	133	93	2	1	-	2	15	27	87	1	-	1	1	8	18	65
2. Asthma	48	24	24	-	1	1	3	5	5	10	1	-	-	2	5	6	10
3. Other respiratory	119	67	52	6	2	1	2	9	12	35	3	2	1	2	4	8	33
I. Digestive diseases	661	428	233	5	5	4	41	149	107	117	4	4	3	14	52	54	101
1. Peptic ulcer	56	34	22	-	-	-	2	8	8	16	-	-	-	1	3	4	14
2. Cirrhosis of the liver	290	213	77	1	1	2	25	92	54	39	-	1	1	6	24	22	24
3. Appendicitis	9	6	4	-	1	1	2	2	-	-	-	1	1	1	1	-	-
4. Other digestive	305	175	130	5	3	1	12	48	44	62	4	2	2	6	25	28	63
J. Genito-urinary diseases	182	82	100	1	3	2	6	16	17	37	1	2	2	5	15	22	52
1. Nephritis and nephrosis	157	70	87	1	3	2	6	14	15	30	1	2	2	4	14	20	45
2. Benign prostatic hypertrophy	1	1	-	-	-	-	-	-	-	1	-	-	-	-	-	-	-
3. Other genito-urinary	24	11	13	-	-	-	1	2	2	6	-	-	-	1	2	3	8
K. Skin diseases	4	2	2	-	-	-	-	-	-	-	-	-	-	-	-	-	1

Annex Table 18e, continued. Deaths by age, sex and cause (thousands): Other Asia and Islands, 2020, pessimistic scenario

Cause	Total	Male	Female	Males							Females						
				0-4	5-14	15-29	30-44	45-59	60-69	70+	0-4	5-14	15-29	30-44	45-59	60-69	70+
L. Musculo-skeletal diseases	**16**	**6**	**10**	–	–	–	–	1	2	2	–	–	–	1	1	2	6
1. Rheumatoid arthritis	1	–	1	–	–	–	–	–	–	–	–	–	–	–	–	–	1
3. Other musculo-skeletal	15	5	9	–	–	–	–	1	2	2	–	–	–	1	1	2	5
M. Congenital anomalies	**66**	**36**	**30**	28	2	1	1	1	1	1	24	2	1	1	1	1	1
N. Oral conditions	**–**	**–**	**–**	–	–	–	–	–	–	–	–	–	–	–	–	–	–
III. Injuries	***827***	***572***	***255***	*44*	*44*	*139*	*154*	*113*	*42*	*38*	*37*	*23*	*56*	*49*	*40*	*25*	*26*
A. Unintentional injuries	**606**	**420**	**186**	41	39	96	106	81	31	26	34	20	32	30	30	20	20
1. Road traffic accidents	246	173	73	12	14	44	46	33	13	11	11	8	12	12	13	9	7
2. Poisonings	50	27	23	1	2	6	7	9	3	2	1	2	7	4	4	2	2
3. Falls	50	36	14	3	2	6	10	9	3	3	2	1	1	1	3	2	3
4. Fires	12	7	5	1	–	1	2	1	–	1	2	1	–	1	1	–	1
5. Drownings	80	55	25	14	13	10	8	5	2	3	9	5	3	2	2	1	2
6. Other unintentional	168	121	47	9	8	29	35	25	8	6	9	4	8	8	8	5	5
B. Intentional injuries	**221**	**152**	**69**	3	5	44	47	32	11	11	3	3	24	19	10	5	5
1. Self-inflicted injuries	115	71	44	–	2	20	19	15	7	7	–	1	17	12	6	4	4
2. Violence	86	70	16	1	2	19	25	16	3	4	1	1	4	5	3	1	1
3. War	21	12	9	1	1	4	3	1	1	–	1	1	3	2	1	1	1

Notes:
Causes responsible for no deaths have been omitted from this table.
A dash (-) symbol indicates fewer than 500 deaths.
*IA6 is Bacterial meningitis and meningococcaemia; IC3 is Hypertensive disorders of pregnancy; ID is Conditions arising during the perinatal period; IIE6 is Dementia and other degenerative and hereditary CNS disorders; IIH1 is Chronic obstructive pulmonary disease.

Annex Table 18f. Deaths by age, sex and cause (thousands): Sub-Saharan Africa, 2020, pessimistic scenario

Cause	Total	Male	Female	Males 0-4	5-14	15-29	30-44	45-59	60-69	70+	Females 0-4	5-14	15-29	30-44	45-59	60-69	70+
Population (millions)	*1 120*	*555*	*565*	*85*	*140*	*163*	*93*	*49*	*16*	*9*	*82*	*137*	*163*	*98*	*54*	*19*	*12*
All causes	**12 759**	**6 998**	**5 761**	**2 564**	**450**	**993**	**801**	**733**	**556**	**901**	**2 053**	**376**	**630**	**515**	**608**	**492**	**1 087**
I. Communicable, maternal, perinatal and nutritional conditions	**6 536**	**3 391**	**3 145**	**2 288**	**185**	**247**	**226**	**172**	**94**	**179**	**1 821**	**189**	**373**	**318**	**155**	**91**	**197**
A. Infectious and parasitic diseases	**4 551**	**2 391**	**2 160**	**1 483**	**141**	**239**	**221**	**165**	**70**	**71**	**1 175**	**146**	**305**	**248**	**147**	**65**	**73**
1. Tuberculosis	**1 002**	**484**	**518**	**36**	**23**	**132**	**97**	**118**	**48**	**29**	**38**	**34**	**153**	**111**	**108**	**45**	**28**
2. STDs excluding HIV	**96**	**46**	**50**	**36**	-	-	-	**1**	**1**	**7**	**32**	-	**3**	**3**	**1**	**2**	**9**
a. Syphilis	91	46	44	36	-	-	-	1	1	7	32	-	2	1	1	2	9
b. Chlamydia	3	-	3	-	-	-	-	-	-	-	-	-	1	1	-	-	-
c. Gonorrhoea	2	-	2	-	-	-	-	-	-	-	-	-	-	1	-	-	-
3. HIV	**661**	**311**	**349**	**88**	**12**	**79**	**99**	**23**	**6**	**3**	**83**	**12**	**121**	**110**	**17**	**4**	**2**
4. Diarrhoeal diseases	**992**	**555**	**437**	**493**	**27**	**4**	**4**	**4**	**5**	**19**	**366**	**26**	**6**	**6**	**5**	**5**	**22**
5. Childhood-cluster diseases	**878**	**477**	**401**	**425**	**42**	**2**	**3**	**2**	**1**	**2**	**354**	**39**	**2**	**2**	**2**	**1**	**2**
a. Pertussis	153	84	69	78	5	-	-	-	-	-	65	5	-	-	-	-	-
b. Poliomyelitis	5	3	2	3	-	-	-	-	-	-	2	-	-	-	-	-	-
c. Diphtheria	2	1	1	1	-	-	-	-	-	-	1	-	-	-	-	-	-
d. Measles	583	316	267	283	33	-	-	-	-	-	236	31	-	-	-	-	-
e. Tetanus	134	73	62	60	3	2	3	2	1	2	50	4	2	1	1	1	2
6. Bacterial meningitis*	**26**	**14**	**13**	**10**	-	-	**1**	**1**	**1**	**1**	**8**	-	-	**1**	**1**	**1**	**1**
7. Hepatitis B and hepatitis C	**16**	**9**	**7**	**1**	**1**	-	**1**	**2**	**1**	**3**	**1**	-	**1**	**1**	**1**	**1**	**3**
8. Malaria	**737**	**414**	**323**	**358**	**22**	**13**	**9**	**7**	**3**	**2**	**266**	**21**	**13**	**9**	**7**	**3**	**3**
9. Tropical-cluster diseases	**49**	**28**	**21**	**1**	**8**	**6**	**5**	**6**	**2**	**1**	**1**	**6**	**5**	**4**	**4**	**1**	**1**
a. Trypanosomiasis	38	20	17	1	5	5	3	5	1	1	1	5	4	3	3	1	1
b. Chagas disease	-	-	-	-	-	-	-	-	-	-	-	-	-	-	-	-	-
c. Schistosomiasis	3	2	1	-	-	-	1	1	-	-	-	-	-	-	-	-	-
d. Leishmaniasis	8	6	3	-	3	1	1	1	-	-	-	1	1	-	-	-	-
10. Leprosy	-	-	-	-	-	-	-	-	-	-	-	-	-	-	-	-	-
11. Dengue	-	-	-	-	-	-	-	-	-	-	-	-	-	-	-	-	-
12. Japanese encephalitis	-	-	-	-	-	-	-	-	-	-	-	-	-	-	-	-	-
13. Trachoma	-	-	-	-	-	-	-	-	-	-	-	-	-	-	-	-	-
14. Intestinal nematode infections	**2**	**1**	**1**	-	-	-	-	-	-	-	-	-	-	-	-	-	-
a. Ascariasis	1	1	1	-	-	-	-	-	-	-	-	-	-	-	-	-	-
b. Trichuriasis	-	-	-	-	-	-	-	-	-	-	-	-	-	-	-	-	-
c. Ancylostomiasis, necatoriasis	1	1	-	-	-	-	-	-	-	-	-	-	-	-	-	-	-
15. Other infectious and parasitic	**92**	**51**	**41**	**33**	**5**	**2**	**2**	**2**	**2**	**4**	**25**	**5**	**2**	**2**	**2**	**1**	**4**

Annex Table 18f, continued. Deaths by age, sex and cause (thousands): Sub-Saharan Africa, 2020, pessimistic scenario

Cause	Total	Male	Female	Males 0-4	5-14	15-29	30-44	45-59	60-69	70+	Females 0-4	5-14	15-29	30-44	45-59	60-69	70+
B. Respiratory infections	1 155	629	526	448	38	7	5	6	23	102	333	31	8	5	6	26	118
1. Lower respiratory infections	1 136	618	518	440	38	7	5	6	22	101	327	30	8	5	6	25	117
2. Upper respiratory infections	12	6	5	4	-	-	-	-	-	1	3	-	-	-	-	-	1
3. Otitis media	7	4	3	4	-	-	-	-	-	-	3	-	-	-	-	-	-
C. Maternal conditions	130		130								-	7	59	64	-	-	-
1. Maternal haemorrhage	31		31								-	2	14	15	-	-	-
2. Maternal sepsis	21		21								-	1	9	10	-	-	-
3. Hypertensive disorders*	16		16								-	1	7	8	-	-	-
4. Obstructed labour	10		10								-	1	5	5	-	-	-
5. Abortion	18		18								-	1	8	9	-	-	-
6. Other maternal	34		34								-	2	16	17	-	-	-
D. Perinatal conditions*	546	291	255	291	-	-	-	-	-	-	255	-	-	-	-	-	-
E. Nutritional deficiencies	154	81	73	66	6	1	1	1	1	5	57	6	2	-	1	1	6
1. Protein-energy malnutrition	109	58	51	51	1	-	-	1	1	4	44	1	-	-	1	1	4
2. Iodine deficiency	2	1	1	1	-	-	-	-	-	-	1	-	-	-	-	-	-
3. Vitamin A deficiency	31	17	15	12	4	-	-	-	-	1	10	4	1	-	-	-	-
4. Iron-deficiency anaemia	12	5	7	2	1	1	1	-	-	-	2	1	1	1	-	-	2
II. Noncommunicable diseases	4 026	2 051	1 974	100	77	80	249	436	419	689	98	82	50	90	411	378	865
A. Malignant neoplasms	1 011	583	429	7	19	19	72	150	140	175	9	19	13	31	129	101	127
1. Mouth and oropharynx cancers	55	35	20	-	-	1	3	5	11	14	-	-	-	1	3	7	9
2. Oesophagus cancer	56	42	14	-	-	1	3	16	9	12	-	-	-	1	4	4	5
3. Stomach cancer	75	46	30	-	-	1	4	15	11	14	-	1	1	1	11	7	9
4. Colon and rectum cancers	36	19	16	-	-	1	2	3	6	8	-	1	1	1	2	5	7
5. Liver cancer	135	101	34	-	-	7	24	37	15	19	2	1	1	3	11	8	10
6. Pancreas cancer	16	10	7	-	-	-	1	4	2	3	-	-	-	-	2	2	3
7. Trachea, bronchus, lung cancers	56	37	20	-	-	1	5	11	10	11	-	-	-	1	8	6	4
8. Melanoma and other skin cancers	19	8	11	-	-	-	1	3	2	2	-	-	-	-	3	3	2
9. Breast cancer	38	-	38	-	-	-	-	-	-	-	-	-	1	3	15	8	11
10. Cervix uteri cancer	74		74								-	-	2	5	28	17	22
11. Corpus uteri cancer	8		8								-	-	-	1	2	2	3
12. Ovary cancer	17		17								-	-	1	2	6	3	4
13. Prostate cancer	81	81	-	-	-	-	-	10	31	40							
14. Bladder cancer	33	22	10	-	-	-	1	6	6	8	-	-	-	-	3	3	4
15. Lymphomas, multiple myeloma	58	37	21	1	8	2	5	5	6	8	-	5	1	1	3	3	5
16. Leukaemia	20	10	10	-	1	1	2	1	2	3	1	2	2	1	2	2	2
17. Other cancers	233	135	98	5	9	6	21	33	29	33	5	9	4	9	28	20	23

Annex Table 18f, continued. Deaths by age, sex and cause (thousands): Sub-Saharan Africa, 2020, pessimistic scenario

Cause	Total	Male	Female	Males							Females						
				0-4	5-14	15-29	30-44	45-59	60-69	70+	0-4	5-14	15-29	30-44	45-59	60-69	70+
B. Other neoplasms	15	8	7	–	2	1	1	1	1	2	1	2	1	–	1	1	1
C. Diabetes mellitus	37	16	21	1	2	–	1	3	4	5	1	1	–	–	4	6	8
D. Endocrine disorders	37	17	20	3	1	1	3	4	2	3	2	2	1	1	3	3	9
E. Neuro-psychiatric conditions	66	39	27	3	4	5	7	6	4	10	3	3	2	1	4	4	10
2. Bipolar disorder	2	1	1	–	–	–	–	–	–	–	–	–	–	–	–	–	1
3. Schizophrenia	2	1	1	–	–	1	–	–	–	–	–	–	–	–	–	–	–
4. Epilepsy	8	6	3	1	1	1	2	1	1	–	1	1	1	–	1	1	–
5. Alcohol use	8	6	2	–	–	1	1	2	1	1	–	–	–	–	1	–	–
6. Dementia*	15	7	8	–	–	–	–	1	1	4	–	–	–	–	1	1	5
7. Parkinson disease	4	2	1	–	–	–	–	–	–	2	–	–	–	–	–	–	1
8. Multiple sclerosis	2	1	1	–	–	–	–	1	1	–	–	–	1	–	1	–	–
9. Drug use	1	1	–	–	–	1	–	–	–	–	–	–	–	–	–	–	–
13. Other neuro-psychiatric	25	15	10	2	3	3	3	2	1	2	2	2	1	3	1	1	2
F. Sense organ diseases	–	–	–	–	–	–	–	–	–	–	–	–	–	–	–	–	–
1. Glaucoma	–	–	–	–	–	–	–	–	–	–	–	–	–	–	–	–	–
2. Cataracts	–	–	–	–	–	–	–	–	–	–	–	–	–	–	–	–	–
G. Cardiovascular diseases	1 798	786	1 012	20	21	27	93	160	163	302	18	25	18	37	183	190	540
1. Rheumatic heart disease	28	15	13	–	3	5	4	1	–	–	–	4	3	–	2	1	1
2. Ischaemic heart disease	486	222	263	–	–	2	25	47	53	96	6	–	–	8	47	56	146
3. Cerebrovascular disease	877	356	521	3	7	12	38	70	78	147	3	7	5	17	90	99	301
4. Inflammatory heart diseases	124	59	65	5	3	2	10	12	10	16	7	5	3	2	10	12	25
5. Other cardiovascular	284	134	149	11	7	7	16	29	21	42	3	10	7	7	34	22	67
H. Respiratory diseases	552	306	246	11	8	8	30	51	63	135	8	8	5	8	51	43	123
1. COPD*	294	166	128	3	1	1	8	26	39	89	2	1	1	2	24	25	74
2. Asthma	35	18	16	–	1	1	3	3	3	7	–	1	1	1	3	3	7
3. Other respiratory	223	121	102	8	6	5	20	22	21	39	6	6	4	5	24	15	42
I. Digestive diseases	259	163	96	5	8	10	29	46	30	35	4	11	5	7	20	20	29
1. Peptic ulcer	25	15	10	–	–	1	3	5	2	4	–	–	–	–	3	2	5
2. Cirrhosis of the liver	63	45	18	–	–	2	8	16	10	9	–	–	–	2	6	5	5
3. Appendicitis	16	10	6	1	3	3	3	–	–	–	–	3	2	1	–	–	–
4. Other digestive	155	93	62	4	4	4	15	25	18	22	4	8	3	4	11	13	19
J. Genito-urinary diseases	147	82	65	8	10	5	11	13	13	21	8	8	3	4	14	11	17
1. Nephritis and nephrosis	127	71	56	8	8	5	9	10	11	18	8	7	3	3	12	9	15
2. Benign prostatic hypertrophy	1	1	–	–	–	–	–	–	–	1	–	–	–	–	–	–	–
3. Other genito-urinary	19	10	9	–	1	–	2	2	2	2	–	1	–	1	2	2	3
K. Skin diseases	11	7	5	6	–	–	–	–	–	–	4	–	–	–	–	–	–

Annex Table 18f, continued. Deaths by age, sex and cause (thousands): Sub-Saharan Africa, 2020, pessimistic scenario

Cause	Total	Male	Female	Males							Females						
				0-4	5-14	15-29	30-44	45-59	60-69	70+	0-4	5-14	15-29	30-44	45-59	60-69	70+
L. Musculo-skeletal diseases	**1**	**1**	**1**	-	-	-	-	-	-	-	-	-	-	-	-	-	1
1. Rheumatoid arthritis	1	-	-	-	-	-	-	-	-	-	-	-	-	-	-	-	-
3. Other musculo-skeletal	1	-	-	-	-	-	-	-	-	-	-	-	-	-	-	-	-
M. Congenital anomalies	**90**	**44**	**46**	35	3	2	2	1	-	1	39	3	1	1	1	1	1
N. Oral conditions	**-**	**-**	**-**	-	-	-	-	-	-	-	-	-	-	-	-	-	-
III. Injuries	***2 197***	***1 556***	***641***	*176*	*189*	*666*	*326*	*124*	*43*	*32*	*135*	*105*	*206*	*107*	*41*	*22*	*25*
A. Unintentional injuries	**1 060**	**747**	**313**	120	138	237	137	67	24	23	84	77	67	36	20	10	19
1. Road traffic accidents	342	247	95	17	53	86	51	25	9	6	12	27	30	14	8	2	2
2. Poisonings	67	40	27	25	5	3	3	2	1	1	18	3	4	1	1	-	1
3. Falls	39	24	15	2	2	7	4	4	2	3	2	1	1	2	1	1	1
4. Fires	128	67	61	24	8	15	8	5	2	4	21	11	12	7	4	1	5
5. Drownings	151	111	40	28	45	21	9	5	2	2	14	17	4	2	1	-	1
6. Other unintentional	333	258	74	24	24	105	64	26	8	7	18	18	16	10	6	3	4
B. Intentional injuries	**1 136**	**809**	**328**	56	50	429	189	57	19	9	51	28	139	71	21	12	6
1. Self-inflicted injuries	38	31	7	-	3	15	8	3	1	1	-	-	4	1	1	-	-
2. Violence	493	425	68	7	15	256	99	34	9	5	4	6	31	15	7	3	2
3. War	606	353	253	48	32	158	81	20	9	4	47	21	104	54	13	10	4

Notes:
Causes responsible for no deaths have been omitted from this table.
A dash (-) symbol indicates fewer than 500 deaths.
*IA6 is Bacterial meningitis and meningococcaemia; IC3 is Hypertensive disorders of pregnancy; ID is Conditions arising during the perinatal period; IIE6 is Dementia and other degenerative and hereditary CNS disorders; IIH1 is Chronic obstructive pulmonary disease.

Annex Table 18g. Deaths by age, sex and cause (thousands): Latin America and the Caribbean, 2020, pessimistic scenario

Cause	Total	Male	Female	Males 0-4	5-14	15-29	30-44	45-59	60-69	70+	Females 0-4	5-14	15-29	30-44	45-59	60-69	70+
Population (millions)	*5 435*	*2 967*	*2 468*	*253*	*56*	*217*	*312*	*551*	*506*	*1 071*	*189*	*39*	*98*	*160*	*417*	*393*	*1 173*
All causes	**667**	**331**	**336**	**28**	**54**	**82**	**74**	**55**	**21**	**15**	**27**	**52**	**81**	**74**	**57**	**24**	**20**
I. Communicable, maternal, perinatal and nutritional conditions	*893*	*518*	*375*	*202*	*10*	*63*	*63*	*46*	*37*	*97*	*147*	*12*	*30*	*30*	*28*	*26*	*103*
A. Infectious and parasitic diseases	507	317	190	88	7	61	60	37	26	39	67	7	21	21	21	17	36
1. Tuberculosis	81	49	32	1	1	6	5	12	12	13	1	1	4	4	7	7	8
2. STDs excluding HIV	9	4	5	3	-	-	-	-	-	1	2	-	-	-	-	1	1
a. Syphilis	9	4	4	3	-	-	-	-	-	1	2	-	-	-	-	1	1
b. Chlamydia	-	-	-	-	-	-	-	-	-	-	-	-	-	-	-	-	-
c. Gonorrhoea	-	-	-	-	-	-	-	-	-	-	-	-	-	-	-	-	-
3. HIV	159	127	31	6	-	52	49	14	5	2	5	1	12	10	2	1	1
4. Diarrhoeal diseases	104	58	47	44	1	-	1	2	2	8	30	1	1	1	2	2	10
5. Childhood-cluster diseases	52	28	24	25	2	-	-	-	-	-	22	2	-	-	-	-	-
a. Pertussis	10	5	4	5	-	-	-	-	-	-	4	-	-	-	-	-	-
b. Poliomyelitis	1	1	-	1	-	-	-	-	-	-	-	-	-	-	-	-	-
c. Diphtheria	-	-	-	-	-	-	-	-	-	-	-	-	-	-	-	-	-
d. Measles	29	15	14	14	1	-	-	-	-	-	12	1	-	-	-	-	-
e. Tetanus	12	7	6	6	-	-	-	-	-	-	5	-	-	-	-	-	-
6. Bacterial meningitis*	13	6	7	2	-	1	1	1	1	1	2	-	-	1	1	1	1
7. Hepatitis B and hepatitis C	4	2	2	-	1	1	1	1	-	1	-	1	1	1	1	-	1
8. Malaria	10	5	5	1	1	1	1	1	-	-	-	-	1	1	1	-	1
9. Tropical-cluster diseases	24	12	12	-	-	-	1	4	3	3	-	1	-	2	4	3	3
a. Trypanosomiasis	-	-	-	-	-	-	-	-	-	-	-	-	-	-	-	-	-
b. Chagas disease	23	11	12	-	-	-	1	4	3	3	-	1	-	2	4	2	3
c. Schistosomiasis	1	-	-	-	-	-	-	-	-	-	-	-	-	-	-	-	-
d. Leishmaniasis	-	-	-	-	-	-	-	-	-	-	-	-	-	-	-	-	-
10. Leprosy	1	1	-	-	-	1	-	-	-	-	-	-	-	-	-	-	-
11. Dengue	-	-	-	-	-	-	-	-	-	-	-	-	-	-	-	-	-
12. Japanese encephalitis	-	-	-	-	-	-	-	-	-	-	-	-	-	-	-	-	-
13. Trachoma	-	-	-	-	-	-	-	-	-	-	-	-	-	-	-	-	-
14. Intestinal nematode infections	2	1	1	-	-	1	-	-	-	-	-	1	-	-	-	-	-
a. Ascariasis	1	1	1	-	-	1	-	-	-	-	-	1	-	-	-	-	-
b. Trichuriasis	-	-	-	-	-	-	-	-	-	-	-	-	-	-	-	-	-
c. Ancylostomiasis, necatoriasis	-	-	-	-	-	-	-	-	-	-	-	-	-	-	-	-	-
15. Other infectious and parasitic	50	25	25	7	1	1	2	3	3	8	5	1	1	2	3	2	10

Annex Table 18g, continued. Deaths by age, sex and cause (thousands): Latin America and the Caribbean, 2020, pessimistic scenario

Cause	Total	Male	Female	Males 0-4	5-14	15-29	30-44	45-59	60-69	70+	Females 0-4	5-14	15-29	30-44	45-59	60-69	70+
B. Respiratory infections	**186**	**97**	**89**	**34**	**2**	**1**	**3**	**7**	**8**	**43**	**23**	**2**	**2**	**3**	**5**	**6**	**47**
1. Lower respiratory infections	184	96	88	33	2	1	3	7	8	42	23	2	2	3	5	6	47
2. Upper respiratory infections	2	1	1	-	-	-	-	-	-	-	-	-	-	-	-	-	-
3. Otitis media	-	-	-	-	-	-	-	-	-	-	-	-	-	-	-	-	-
C. Maternal conditions	**11**		**11**								-	-	**6**	**4**	-	-	-
1. Maternal haemorrhage	3		3										1	1			
2. Maternal sepsis	1		1										1				
3. Hypertensive disorders*	2		2										1	1			
4. Obstructed labour	1		1										1				
5. Abortion	2		2										1	1			
6. Other maternal	2		2										1	1			
D. Perinatal conditions*	**114**	**68**	**47**	**68**	-	-	-	-	-	-	**47**	-	-	-	-	-	-
E. Nutritional deficiencies	**75**	**36**	**39**	**13**	**1**	**1**	**1**	**2**	**3**	**15**	**10**	**2**	**1**	**1**	**2**	**3**	**20**
1. Protein-energy malnutrition	51	26	26	10	1	1	1	1	2	11	7	1	-	1	1	1	14
2. Iodine deficiency	1																
3. Vitamin A deficiency	3	1	1	1	-	-	-	-	-	-	1	-	-	-	-	-	-
4. Iron-deficiency anaemia	19	8	11	1	1	1	-	1	1	4	1	1	1	1	1	1	6
II. Noncommunicable diseases	***3 907***	***1 973***	***1 934***	***36***	***18***	***19***	***117***	***416***	***435***	***931***	***31***	***14***	***28***	***100***	***366***	***354***	***1 042***
A. Malignant neoplasms	**862**	**424**	**438**	**2**	**7**	**5**	**23**	**99**	**108**	**181**	**2**	**4**	**7**	**36**	**125**	**105**	**158**
1. Mouth and oropharynx cancers	30	22	9	-	-	1	1	8	5	7	-	-	-	1	2	2	4
2. Oesophagus cancer	26	18	9	-	-	-	-	6	5	7	-	-	-	1	1	2	5
3. Stomach cancer	95	57	38	-	-	-	2	13	16	25	-	-	-	1	7	10	20
4. Colon and rectum cancers	57	26	31	-	-	-	1	6	6	12	-	-	-	1	6	9	16
5. Liver cancer	14	7	7	-	-	-	1	2	2	3	-	-	-	1	1	2	4
6. Pancreas cancer	21	10	11	-	-	-	-	2	3	4	-	-	-	-	2	3	6
7. Trachea, bronchus, lung cancers	122	73	49	-	-	-	5	26	20	21	-	-	-	1	17	16	15
8. Melanoma and other skin cancers	7	3	4	-	-	-	-	-	1	1	-	-	-	-	1	1	1
9. Breast cancer	71		71								-	-	2	7	26	15	21
10. Cervix uteri cancer	57		57								-	-	1	8	22	11	15
11. Corpus uteri cancer	16		16								-	-	-	-	5	4	6
12. Ovary cancer	13		13								-	-	-	2	4	3	4
13. Prostate cancer	54	54		-	-	-	-	3	17	33							
14. Bladder cancer	22	16	6	-	-	-	-	3	5	8	-	-	-	-	1	1	3
15. Lymphomas, multiple myeloma	35	18	16	-	-	-	3	5	3	5	-	1	-	2	3	4	6
16. Leukaemia	23	12	11	1	2	1	3	2	2	3	1	1	1	2	2	2	3
17. Other cancers	197	108	89	1	3	1	6	23	23	51	1	2	2	11	25	20	28

Annex Table 18g, continued. Deaths by age, sex and cause (thousands): Latin America and the Caribbean, 2020, pessimistic scenario

Cause	Total	Male	Female	Males 0-4	5-14	15-29	30-44	45-59	60-69	70+	Females 0-4	5-14	15-29	30-44	45-59	60-69	70+
B. Other neoplasms	16	7	9	-	-	-	1	1	1	2	-	-	-	1	2	2	3
C. Diabetes mellitus	186	71	115	-	1	1	4	15	18	33	-	1	1	3	18	29	63
D. Endocrine disorders	45	20	25	3	1	1	2	3	3	9	2	-	1	1	3	3	14
E. Neuro-psychiatric conditions	78	48	30	2	3	3	9	12	6	13	2	2	3	3	4	3	13
2. Bipolar disorder	2	1	1	-	-	-	-	1	-	-	-	-	-	-	1	-	-
3. Schizophrenia	8	4	4	-	-	1	1	1	1	-	-	-	-	1	1	1	1
4. Epilepsy	7	4	3	-	1	1	1	1	-	-	-	1	1	1	-	-	-
5. Alcohol use	20	18	2	-	-	1	5	7	3	2	-	-	-	-	1	1	-
6. Dementia*	15	7	8	-	-	-	-	-	1	6	-	-	-	-	1	1	6
7. Parkinson disease	4	2	2	-	-	-	-	-	-	2	-	-	-	-	-	-	2
8. Multiple sclerosis	3	1	2	-	-	-	1	-	-	-	-	-	-	1	-	1	-
9. Drug use	2	2	-	-	-	1	1	-	-	-	-	1	1	-	-	-	-
13. Other neuro-psychiatric	16	9	7	2	2	1	1	1	1	2	1	2	1	1	1	1	-
F. Sense organ diseases	1	-	-	-	-	-	-	-	-	-	-	-	-	-	-	-	-
1. Glaucoma	-	-	-	-	-	-	-	-	-	-	-	-	-	-	-	-	-
2. Cataracts	-	-	-	-	-	-	-	-	-	-	-	-	-	-	-	-	-
G. Cardiovascular diseases	1 893	960	933	4	2	5	45	192	216	496	3	2	7	35	139	143	603
1. Rheumatic heart disease	15	5	10	-	-	-	1	2	1	1	-	-	1	2	4	1	2
2. Ischaemic heart disease	856	444	412	-	-	1	18	90	103	232	-	-	1	11	56	65	278
3. Cerebrovascular disease	600	297	302	-	-	1	14	60	67	153	-	-	2	13	49	48	190
4. Inflammatory heart diseases	51	26	25	1	-	1	3	7	4	10	1	-	-	3	6	3	12
5. Other cardiovascular	371	188	184	3	1	2	9	33	41	99	2	1	3	6	24	26	122
H. Respiratory diseases	347	166	180	6	1	1	6	20	31	101	4	1	2	5	39	37	93
1. COPD*	196	99	97	1	-	-	2	10	19	66	1	1	2	1	18	21	56
2. Asthma	39	14	24	1	-	-	2	2	3	7	1	-	1	1	9	5	7
3. Other respiratory	112	53	59	4	1	2	2	7	9	28	3	1	1	3	14	10	27
I. Digestive diseases	317	198	118	2	1	2	24	66	41	63	1	1	2	9	25	22	57
1. Peptic ulcer	29	17	12	-	-	-	1	4	4	9	-	-	-	-	2	2	8
2. Cirrhosis of the liver	141	104	37	-	-	1	16	44	22	20	-	1	1	4	12	8	11
3. Appendicitis	2	1	1	-	1	-	-	-	-	-	-	-	-	-	-	-	-
4. Other digestive	145	76	69	2	1	1	6	18	15	34	1	-	2	4	11	12	39
J. Genito-urinary diseases	104	53	51	1	1	2	3	8	9	30	1	1	2	3	8	8	28
1. Nephritis and nephrosis	75	37	38	1	1	1	3	6	7	19	1	1	1	2	6	6	20
2. Benign prostatic hypertrophy	4	4	-	-	-	-	-	-	-	4	-	-	-	-	-	-	-
3. Other genito-urinary	25	11	13	-	-	1	1	1	2	8	-	-	1	-	2	2	8
K. Skin diseases	6	2	4	-	-	-	-	-	-	1	-	-	-	-	-	-	2

Males and Females columns are headed by age group (0-4, 5-14, 15-29, 30-44, 45-59, 60-69, 70+).

Annex Table 18g, continued. Deaths by age, sex and cause (thousands): Latin America and the Caribbean, 2020, pessimistic scenario

Cause	Total	Male	Female	Males							Females						
				0-4	5-14	15-29	30-44	45-59	60-69	70+	0-4	5-14	15-29	30-44	45-59	60-69	70+
L. Musculo-skeletal diseases	17	5	12	-	-	-	-	1	1	3	-	-	-	1	2	2	6
1. Rheumatoid arthritis	3	1	2	-	-	-	-	-	-	1	-	-	-	-	-	1	1
3. Other musculo-skeletal	13	4	9	-	-	-	-	1	1	2	-	-	-	1	2	1	4
M. Congenital anomalies	37	18	19	15	-	1	1	-	-	-	15	-	1	1	1	-	1
N. Oral conditions	-	-	-	-	-	-	-	-	-	-	-	-	-	-	-	-	-
III. Injuries	*635*	*476*	*159*	*15*	*28*	*135*	*132*	*89*	*34*	*43*	*12*	*14*	*40*	*30*	*22*	*13*	*28*
A. Unintentional injuries	405	288	117	12	23	65	71	57	24	35	9	12	24	19	17	11	26
1. Road traffic accidents	199	144	55	3	12	37	38	30	12	12	2	7	15	11	9	5	5
2. Poisonings	7	4	3	-	-	1	1	1	-	1	-	-	1	-	1	-	-
3. Falls	37	22	15	-	1	2	4	4	3	8	-	-	1	1	1	1	11
4. Fires	9	6	4	1	1	1	1	1	-	1	1	-	1	1	1	-	1
5. Drownings	33	27	7	2	4	8	6	4	1	1	1	2	2	1	1	-	-
6. Other unintentional	120	85	34	5	5	16	21	18	8	12	4	2	7	5	5	3	8
B. Intentional injuries	229	188	42	3	5	69	61	32	10	8	3	2	15	11	6	3	2
1. Self-inflicted injuries	41	29	12	-	-	7	8	7	3	4	-	-	4	3	2	1	1
2. Violence	164	144	20	1	3	57	50	24	6	4	1	-	8	6	3	1	1
3. War	25	14	10	2	1	5	4	1	1	-	2	1	4	3	1	1	-

Notes:
Causes responsible for no deaths have been omitted from this table.
A dash (-) symbol indicates fewer than 500 deaths.
*IA6 is Bacterial meningitis and meningococcaemia; IC3 is Hypertensive disorders of pregnancy; ID is Conditions arising during the perinatal period; IIE6 is Dementia and other degenerative and hereditary CNS disorders; IIH1 is Chronic obstructive pulmonary disease.

Annex Table 18h. Deaths by age, sex and cause (thousands): Middle Eastern Crescent, 2020, pessimistic scenario

Cause	Total	Male	Female	Males 0-4	5-14	15-29	30-44	45-59	60-69	70+	Females 0-4	5-14	15-29	30-44	45-59	60-69	70+
Population (millions)	*983*	*496*	*487*	*60*	*106*	*137*	*97*	*61*	*23*	*12*	*57*	*102*	*132*	*95*	*60*	*25*	*16*
All causes	*7 621*	*4 263*	*3 358*	*917*	*164*	*269*	*337*	*732*	*693*	*1 151*	*818*	*133*	*173*	*181*	*392*	*437*	*1 224*
I. Communicable, maternal, perinatal and nutritional conditions	*1 755*	*918*	*837*	*698*	*32*	*19*	*21*	*31*	*47*	*72*	*627*	*30*	*24*	*26*	*23*	*30*	*76*
A. Infectious and parasitic diseases	770	423	347	309	16	17	19	27	18	17	275	14	8	8	15	11	16
1. Tuberculosis	105	67	38	4	2	10	10	19	13	10	3	1	5	4	10	7	9
2. STDs excluding HIV	13	6	6	6	-	-	-	-	-	1	5	-	1	-	-	-	1
a. Syphilis	13	6	6	6	-	-	-	-	-	1	5	-	1	-	-	-	1
b. Chlamydia	-	-	-	-	-	-	-	-	-	-	-	-	-	-	-	-	-
c. Gonorrhoea	-	-	-	-	-	-	-	-	-	-	-	-	-	-	-	-	-
3. HIV	16	13	3	1	-	4	5	2	-	-	1	-	1	1	-	-	-
4. Diarrhoeal diseases	360	189	170	181	5	-	-	1	1	1	162	5	1	1	1	1	2
5. Childhood-cluster diseases	197	103	93	95	7	-	-	1	-	-	86	6	1	-	-	-	-
a. Pertussis	44	23	21	22	1	-	-	-	-	-	19	1	-	-	-	-	-
b. Poliomyelitis	3	2	1	2	1	-	-	-	-	-	1	-	-	-	-	-	-
c. Diphtheria	1	1	-	-	-	-	-	-	-	-	-	-	-	-	-	-	-
d. Measles	79	41	38	37	4	-	-	-	-	-	34	4	-	-	-	-	-
e. Tetanus	70	36	33	34	1	-	-	-	-	-	31	1	1	-	-	-	-
6. Bacterial meningitis*	17	9	8	4	-	-	1	1	1	1	4	-	-	1	1	1	1
7. Hepatitis B and hepatitis C	14	8	6	1	-	-	1	2	1	2	1	-	-	-	1	1	2
8. Malaria	5	3	2	1	1	1	-	-	-	-	1	1	-	-	-	-	-
9. Tropical-cluster diseases	3	2	1	-	1	-	1	1	-	-	-	1	-	1	-	-	-
a. Trypanosomiasis	-	-	-	-	-	-	-	-	-	-	-	-	-	-	-	-	-
b. Chagas disease	-	-	-	-	-	-	-	-	-	-	-	-	-	-	-	-	-
c. Schistosomiasis	2	1	1	-	-	1	-	1	-	-	-	-	1	-	1	-	-
d. Leishmaniasis	1	1	-	-	1	-	-	-	-	-	-	-	-	-	-	-	-
10. Leprosy	-	-	-	-	-	-	-	-	-	-	-	-	-	-	-	-	-
11. Dengue	-	-	-	-	-	-	-	-	-	-	-	-	-	-	-	-	-
12. Japanese encephalitis	-	-	-	-	-	-	-	-	-	-	-	-	-	-	-	-	-
13. Trachoma	-	-	-	-	-	-	-	-	-	-	-	-	-	-	-	-	-
14. Intestinal nematode infections	1	1	-	-	1	1	1	1	-	-	-	1	-	-	-	-	-
a. Ascariasis	-	-	-	-	-	-	-	-	-	-	-	-	-	-	-	-	-
b. Trichuriasis	-	-	-	-	-	-	-	-	-	-	-	-	-	-	-	-	-
c. Ancylostomiasis, necatoriasis	-	-	-	-	-	-	-	-	-	-	-	-	-	-	-	-	-
15. Other infectious and parasitic	39	21	18	15	1	1	1	1	1	2	13	1	1	1	1	1	1

Annex Table 18h, continued. Deaths by age, sex and cause (thousands): Middle Eastern Crescent, 2020, pessimistic scenario

				Males							Females						
Cause	Total	Male	Female	0-4	5-14	15-29	30-44	45-59	60-69	70+	0-4	5-14	15-29	30-44	45-59	60-69	70+
B. Respiratory infections	**525**	**272**	**253**	**173**	**13**	**2**	**1**	**3**	**28**	**52**	**154**	**14**	**2**	**2**	**5**	**19**	**57**
1. Lower respiratory infections	517	268	249	170	13	2	1	3	28	52	152	14	2	2	5	19	57
2. Upper respiratory infections	5	3	3	2						1	2						1
3. Otitis media	3	1	1	1							1						
C. Maternal conditions	**32**	**–**	**32**										**13**	**16**	**3**		
1. Maternal haemorrhage	8		8										3	4			
2. Maternal sepsis	5		5										2	3			
3. Hypertensive disorders*	5		5										2	3	1		
4. Obstructed labour	3		3										1	1	1		
5. Abortion	3		3										1	1	1		
6. Other maternal	8		8										3	4			
D. Perinatal conditions*	**346**	**181**	**165**	**181**							**165**						
E. Nutritional deficiencies	**83**	**42**	**40**	**35**	**3**			**1**	**1**	**2**	**32**	**3**	**1**	**1**	**1**		**3**
1. Protein-energy malnutrition	55	29	26	26				1	1	1	24		1	1	1		2
2. Iodine deficiency	3	1	1	1							1						
3. Vitamin A deficiency	16	8	8	6	2						6	2					
4. Iron-deficiency anaemia	9	4	5	2			1			1	1						1
II. Noncommunicable diseases	**4 989**	**2 769**	**2 220**	**153**	**70**	**63**	**173**	**630**	**620**	**1 060**	**129**	**69**	**61**	**99**	**342**	**390**	**1 131**
A. Malignant neoplasms	**638**	**396**	**242**	**4**	**12**	**11**	**36**	**137**	**102**	**93**	**4**	**10**	**10**	**26**	**69**	**61**	**61**
1. Mouth and oropharynx cancers	39	25	14			1	3	6	8	6				1	2	2	5
2. Oesophagus cancer	24	15	10				1	7	4	3					2	3	5
3. Stomach cancer	52	32	20			1	3	14	8	6			1	1	5	3	3
4. Colon and rectum cancers	31	15	16				2	4	5	4				1	2	6	7
5. Liver cancer	21	14	8			1	1	6	3	3				1	2	6	6
6. Pancreas cancer	12	7	5				1	3	2	1					1	2	2
7. Trachea, bronchus, lung cancers	177	151	27				11	59	39	40				2	10	8	6
8. Melanoma and other skin cancers	3	2	1					1	1								
9. Breast cancer	30	–	30										2	4	12	6	6
10. Cervix uteri cancer	19		19										1	2	8	4	4
11. Corpus uteri cancer	5		5												2	2	2
12. Ovary cancer	9		9											2	3	1	2
13. Prostate cancer	11	11	–					2	5	4							
14. Bladder cancer	24	19	5					7	6	5					1	1	2
15. Lymphomas, multiple myeloma	21	14	7				1	3	3	2			1	1	1	2	2
16. Leukaemia	27	14	13	1	3	1	3	2	2	2	1	3	1	2	1	2	2
17. Other cancers	132	78	55	3	6	3	8	24	18	15	2	5	3	8	14	12	11

Annex Table 18h, continued. Deaths by age, sex and cause (thousands): Middle Eastern Crescent, 2020, pessimistic scenario

Cause	Total	Male	Female	Males							Females						
				0-4	5-14	15-29	30-44	45-59	60-69	70+	0-4	5-14	15-29	30-44	45-59	60-69	70+
B. Other neoplasms	9	5	4	–	1	–	1	1	1	1	–	1	–	–	1	1	1
C. Diabetes mellitus	107	48	59	1	2	1	4	12	12	15	1	2	1	2	12	17	23
D. Endocrine disorders	23	12	11	4	1	1	1	2	1	2	4	2	1	1	1	1	1
E. Neuro-psychiatric conditions	91	49	43	9	7	6	5	6	5	11	7	7	4	3	4	4	13
2. Bipolar disorder	2	1	1	–	–	–	–	1	–	–	–	–	1	–	–	–	–
3. Schizophrenia	7	3	3	–	–	–	1	1	–	1	–	–	2	1	–	–	–
4. Epilepsy	12	7	5	1	1	2	1	1	–	1	1	1	2	1	–	–	–
5. Alcohol use	1	1	–	–	–	–	1	–	–	–	–	–	–	–	–	–	–
6. Dementia*	18	8	10	–	–	–	–	1	2	5	–	–	–	1	1	2	6
7. Parkinson disease	5	3	2	–	–	–	–	–	1	2	–	–	–	–	–	1	1
8. Multiple sclerosis	3	1	1	–	–	–	1	–	–	–	–	–	1	–	–	–	–
9. Drug use	2	2	–	–	–	1	1	–	–	–	–	–	–	–	–	–	–
13. Other neuro-psychiatric	42	22	19	8	5	2	1	2	1	2	6	5	2	1	1	1	2
F. Sense organ diseases	–	–	–	–	–	–	–	–	–	–	–	–	–	–	–	–	–
1. Glaucoma	–	–	–	–	–	–	–	–	–	–	–	–	–	–	–	–	–
2. Cataracts	–	–	–	–	–	–	–	–	–	–	–	–	–	–	–	–	–
G. Cardiovascular diseases	3 119	1 678	1 441	50	32	29	91	348	387	741	35	28	27	46	182	237	886
1. Rheumatic heart disease	36	18	18	–	3	5	6	3	1	–	–	3	5	3	3	1	–
2. Ischaemic heart disease	1 590	874	717	–	–	4	44	190	217	419	–	–	4	19	83	127	484
3. Cerebrovascular disease	524	255	269	3	6	4	11	51	61	118	2	5	2	6	35	46	173
4. Inflammatory heart diseases	135	76	60	9	6	5	9	18	10	18	8	5	5	6	11	6	20
5. Other cardiovascular	834	456	377	38	18	10	21	86	99	185	25	16	11	12	49	57	207
H. Respiratory diseases	480	281	199	18	5	3	9	51	60	134	15	8	5	6	32	36	97
1. COPD*	261	159	101	4	–	1	2	26	37	88	4	1	1	1	15	21	58
2. Asthma	32	18	15	–	1	1	2	4	4	8	–	1	–	1	3	3	7
3. Other respiratory	187	104	83	14	4	2	5	21	19	38	11	6	4	4	14	12	32
I. Digestive diseases	258	153	105	16	4	5	14	49	34	31	17	4	4	7	25	20	28
1. Peptic ulcer	13	9	4	–	–	–	1	3	2	2	–	–	–	–	1	1	2
2. Cirrhosis of the liver	92	55	38	–	–	1	5	21	14	12	–	–	1	3	11	9	12
3. Appendicitis	5	3	2	–	1	1	1	–	–	–	–	1	1	–	–	–	–
4. Other digestive	148	86	62	15	3	2	8	25	17	17	17	2	2	4	12	10	15
J. Genito-urinary diseases	151	89	62	3	3	5	10	22	17	29	3	3	5	6	14	11	19
1. Nephritis and nephrosis	62	35	27	2	2	2	4	7	6	12	2	2	3	3	5	4	8
2. Benign prostatic hypertrophy	3	3	–	–	–	–	–	–	1	2	–	–	–	–	–	–	–
3. Other genito-urinary	86	51	34	1	1	3	6	14	10	15	1	1	2	3	9	7	11
K. Skin diseases	3	1	2	–	–	–	–	–	–	–	–	–	–	–	–	–	1

Annex Table 18h, continued. Deaths by age, sex and cause (thousands): Middle Eastern Crescent, 2020, pessimistic scenario

Cause	Total	Male	Female	Males							Females						
				0-4	5-14	15-29	30-44	45-59	60-69	70+	0-4	5-14	15-29	30-44	45-59	60-69	70+
L. Musculo-skeletal diseases	**3**	**2**	**2**	-	-	-	-	-	-	-	-	-	-	-	-	-	-
1. Rheumatoid arthritis	-	-	-	-	-	-	-	-	-	-	-	-	-	-	-	-	-
3. Other musculo-skeletal	3	2	2	-	-	-	-	-	-	-	-	-	-	-	-	-	-
M. Congenital anomalies	**105**	**54**	**50**	46	3	2	1	1	1	-	42	3	2	1	2	1	1
N. Oral conditions	-	-	-	-	-	-	-	-	-	-	-	-	-	-	-	-	-
III. Injuries	*878*	*576*	*301*	*66*	*63*	*187*	*144*	*72*	*26*	*19*	*62*	*34*	*88*	*56*	*28*	*17*	*17*
A. Unintentional injuries	*376*	*270*	*106*	32	30	72	71	40	13	11	28	14	20	16	12	6	10
1. Road traffic accidents	153	119	34	4	13	39	36	18	5	4	3	7	7	7	5	2	3
2. Poisonings	24	16	8	2	1	2	5	4	1	1	2	-	2	1	1	1	1
3. Falls	21	15	6	2	2	3	3	3	1	2	2	1	2	1	1	1	2
4. Fires	25	11	14	3	1	2	2	1	1	-	3	1	5	2	1	-	1
5. Drownings	42	30	12	8	6	8	5	2	1	1	7	2	4	1	-	1	-
6. Other unintentional	111	79	32	14	7	18	19	12	5	4	11	3	4	4	3	2	4
B. Intentional injuries	*502*	*306*	*195*	33	33	115	73	31	13	8	34	21	67	40	16	10	7
1. Self-inflicted injuries	98	67	31	-	13	19	15	12	4	4	-	6	9	5	4	3	4
2. Violence	73	49	24	8	3	16	13	6	2	1	9	4	4	4	2	1	1
3. War	330	190	140	25	17	80	46	14	7	2	25	11	55	32	9	7	2

Notes:
Causes responsible for no deaths have been omitted from this table.
A dash (-) symbol indicates fewer than 500 deaths.
"IA6 is Bacterial meningitis and meningococcaemia; IC3 is Hypertensive disorders of pregnancy; ID is Conditions arising during the perinatal period; IIE6 is Dementia and other degenerative and hereditary CNS disorders; IIH1 is Chronic obstructive pulmonary disease.

Annex Table 18i. Deaths by age, sex and cause (thousands): World, 2020, pessimistic scenario

Cause	Total	Male	Female	Males 0-4	5-14	15-29	30-44	45-59	60-69	70+	Females 0-4	5-14	15-29	30-44	45-59	60-69	70+
Population (millions)	*7 666*	*3 819*	*3 848*	*362*	*665*	*949*	*790*	*625*	*253*	*174*	*347*	*639*	*917*	*775*	*638*	*288*	*244*
All causes	*78 144*	*43 254*	*34 890*	*5 429*	*1 042*	*2 439*	*3 480*	*8 340*	*8 128*	*14 396*	*4 597*	*852*	*1 579*	*1 884*	*4 371*	*5 103*	*16 504*
I. Communicable, maternal, perinatal and nutritional conditions	16 898	9 036	7 862	4 434	325	544	808	831	615	1 478	3 735	337	632	685	565	417	1 492
A. Infectious and parasitic diseases	10 535	5 869	4 666	2 451	231	521	780	776	431	678	2 032	234	496	534	502	279	589
1. Tuberculosis	3 275	1 897	1 378	55	36	224	292	550	308	433	52	45	216	202	372	187	304
2. STDs excluding HIV	192	90	101	63	-	-	1	3	4	19	55	-	6	7	4	5	25
a. Syphilis	179	90	89	63	-	-	1	3	4	19	55	-	1	1	3	5	25
b. Chlamydia	8	-	8	-	-	-	-	-	-	-	-	-	3	4	-	-	-
c. Gonorrhoea	4	-	4	-	-	-	-	-	-	-	-	-	2	2	-	-	-
3. HIV	1 755	1 024	731	156	22	243	414	132	37	19	146	22	225	268	50	13	7
4. Diarrhoeal diseases	2 204	1 183	1 020	988	46	8	12	16	28	85	802	47	10	13	18	24	107
5. Childhood-cluster diseases	1 486	795	691	698	64	5	10	7	4	7	599	61	5	7	7	3	8
a. Pertussis	262	141	121	133	8	-	-	-	-	-	113	8	-	-	-	-	-
b. Poliomyelitis	17	10	7	9	-	-	-	-	-	-	7	-	-	-	-	-	-
c. Diphtheria	6	3	3	3	-	-	-	-	-	-	3	-	-	-	-	-	-
d. Measles	839	450	389	403	47	-	-	-	-	-	345	43	-	-	-	-	-
e. Tetanus	362	191	171	150	9	5	10	7	4	7	132	10	5	7	7	3	8
6. Bacterial meningitis*	130	67	63	28	2	1	9	9	9	9	25	2	1	7	9	8	12
7. Hepatitis B and hepatitis C	94	54	40	5	2	2	5	13	8	19	3	2	2	3	5	8	18
8. Malaria	812	454	358	364	29	20	16	14	6	6	271	28	18	14	14	6	7
9. Tropical-cluster diseases	93	52	40	2	11	10	9	11	5	5	2	9	7	7	8	4	4
a. Trypanosomiasis	38	20	17	1	5	5	3	5	1	-	1	5	4	3	3	1	-
b. Chagas disease	23	11	12	-	-	-	1	4	3	3	-	-	-	2	4	3	3
c. Schistosomiasis	7	5	3	-	-	-	1	1	1	1	-	-	1	1	1	-	-
d. Leishmaniasis	25	16	9	1	6	4	3	-	-	-	1	3	2	1	-	-	-
10. Leprosy	3	2	1	-	-	-	-	-	1	-	-	-	-	1	-	-	-
11. Dengue	8	4	4	1	3	-	-	-	-	-	1	3	-	-	-	-	-
12. Japanese encephalitis	2	1	1	1	-	-	-	-	-	-	1	-	-	-	-	-	-
13. Trachoma	-	-	-	-	-	-	-	-	-	-	-	-	-	-	-	-	-
14. Intestinal nematode infections	11	6	6	-	4	-	-	-	1	1	-	3	-	-	-	1	1
a. Ascariasis	4	2	2	-	2	-	-	-	-	-	-	2	-	-	-	-	-
b. Trichuriasis	3	1	1	-	1	-	-	-	-	-	-	1	-	-	-	-	-
c. Ancylostomiasis, necatoriasis	4	2	2	-	-	-	-	-	1	1	-	-	-	-	-	1	1
15. Other infectious and parasitic	470	238	232	90	14	7	12	19	22	75	76	14	5	6	14	20	96

Annex Table 18i, continued. Deaths by age, sex and cause (thousands): World, 2020, pessimistic scenario

Cause	Total	Male	Female	Males							Females						
				0-4	5-14	15-29	30-44	45-59	60-69	70+	0-4	5-14	15-29	30-44	45-59	60-69	70+
B. Respiratory infections	3 977	2 056	1 922	969	79	19	24	48	173	744	805	80	20	19	43	127	828
1. Lower respiratory infections	3 921	2 026	1 895	951	78	19	23	47	171	737	789	79	19	18	43	126	820
2. Upper respiratory infections	39	20	19	10	1	-	-	-	2	7	8	1	-	-	-	1	8
3. Otitis media	18	9	8	8	1	-	-	-	-	-	7	1	-	-	-	-	-
C. Maternal conditions	253	-	253								-	7	110	126	10	-	-
1. Maternal haemorrhage	62		62									2	27	31	3		
2. Maternal sepsis	39		39									1	17	20	1		
3. Hypertensive disorders*	32		32									1	14	16	1		
4. Obstructed labour	20		20									-	9	10	1		
5. Abortion	34		34									1	15	17	1		
6. Other maternal	66		66									2	29	33	3		
D. Perinatal conditions*	1 623	864	759	863								759						
E. Nutritional deficiencies	510	248	262	150	15	4	4	8	11	56	139	15	6	6	10	11	75
1. Protein-energy malnutrition	308	155	153	111	2	1	1	3	6	30	104	3	1	1	3	5	37
2. Iodine deficiency	12	6	6	5	1	-	-	-	-	-	4	1	-	-	-	-	-
3. Vitamin A deficiency	69	36	33	26	10	1	-	-	-	-	23	9	-	-	-	-	-
4. Iron-deficiency anaemia	117	49	67	7	2	3	3	4	5	25	8	3	4	4	7	6	36
II. Noncommunicable diseases	53 039	28 839	24 200	571	287	361	1 458	6 609	7 131	12 422	516	258	305	761	3 393	4 438	14 528
A. Malignant neoplasms	12 504	7 563	4 941	29	74	95	502	2 424	2 062	2 378	32	54	90	304	1 249	1 247	1 966
1. Mouth and oropharynx cancers	630	417	213	1	1	7	34	134	115	126	1	1	5	13	52	63	77
2. Oesophagus cancer	831	569	262	-	-	3	22	198	172	174	-	-	3	5	63	88	104
3. Stomach cancer	1 624	1 072	552	-	-	6	42	362	314	348	-	-	5	24	119	150	253
4. Colon and rectum cancers	872	465	407	-	1	5	25	104	123	208	-	1	3	14	65	103	221
5. Liver cancer	1 204	896	307	1	2	14	116	405	202	156	1	2	4	20	90	84	108
6. Pancreas cancer	334	193	141	-	-	1	7	54	54	77	-	-	1	2	21	36	80
7. Trachea, bronchus, lung cancers	2 345	1 764	581	-	1	6	88	660	578	431	-	-	2	15	151	183	230
8. Melanoma and other skin cancers	82	43	39	-	-	1	4	13	9	16	-	-	1	3	8	9	19
9. Breast cancer	543	-	543								-	-	11	51	179	117	185
10. Cervix uteri cancer	413	-	413								-	-	11	37	170	89	106
11. Corpus uteri cancer	110	-	110								-	-	1	3	28	27	49
12. Ovary cancer	176	-	176								-	-	5	17	50	42	60
13. Prostate cancer	388	388	-	-	-	-	-	29	101	256							
14. Bladder cancer	264	200	64	-	-	-	1	40	57	97	1	-	1	2	9	16	37
15. Lymphomas, multiple myeloma	389	233	155	5	15	9	26	55	52	71	3	8	4	10	27	35	68
16. Leukaemia	365	203	162	8	21	14	33	45	32	51	10	15	11	21	29	27	49
17. Other cancers	1 935	1 119	816	14	33	27	99	325	254	368	17	24	23	67	188	179	319

Annex Table 18i, continued. Deaths by age, sex and cause (thousands): World, 2020, pessimistic scenario

Age-group columns 0-4 … 70+ appear first for **Males**, then for **Females**.

Cause	Total	Male	Female	M 0-4	M 5-14	M 15-29	M 30-44	M 45-59	M 60-69	M 70+	F 0-4	F 5-14	F 15-29	F 30-44	F 45-59	F 60-69	F 70+
B. Other neoplasms	**145**	**73**	**72**	3	5	3	6	14	14	28	3	4	3	4	11	13	34
C. Diabetes mellitus	**940**	**379**	**561**	5	7	4	21	76	93	172	5	7	5	11	77	137	319
D. Endocrine disorders	**208**	**92**	**117**	13	4	4	7	13	13	37	12	6	4	5	12	13	65
E. Neuro-psychiatric conditions	**998**	**500**	**498**	26	21	35	60	79	69	210	25	18	21	22	39	60	314
2. Bipolar disorder	25	7	18	-	-	2	-	-	1	4	-	-	1	2	-	-	15
3. Schizophrenia	78	38	39	-	-	2	6	7	6	17	-	-	1	2	5	6	26
4. Epilepsy	79	48	32	2	4	8	12	10	5	6	2	3	7	5	5	4	6
5. Alcohol use	79	64	11	-	-	2	16	26	11	9	-	-	1	2	2	3	3
6. Dementia*	337	129	208	2	-	-	3	10	19	92	4	-	-	2	9	22	170
7. Parkinson disease	99	52	47	-	-	-	-	1	7	44	-	-	-	-	-	5	42
8. Multiple sclerosis	34	14	20	-	-	-	4	5	3	3	-	-	-	3	7	5	5
9. Drug use	11	10	2	-	-	4	4	2	-	-	-	-	1	1	-	-	-
13. Other neuro-psychiatric	258	137	121	22	16	16	15	17	17	34	19	14	10	5	9	14	47
F. Sense organ diseases	**29**	**15**	**15**	1	-	-	-	4	5	4	1	-	-	-	3	5	5
1. Glaucoma	10	5	5	-	-	-	-	1	2	2	-	-	-	-	1	2	2
2. Cataracts	9	5	4	-	-	-	-	2	1	1	-	-	-	-	1	1	1
G. Cardiovascular diseases	**26 816**	**13 803**	**13 013**	131	92	121	537	2 723	3 377	6 822	98	85	99	264	1 303	2 077	9 086
1. Rheumatic heart disease	561	265	296	-	7	20	36	90	49	64	-	9	18	33	81	51	103
2. Ischaemic heart disease	11 891	6 257	5 633	16	-	12	198	1 239	1 592	3 215	6	-	8	83	483	918	4 136
3. Cerebrovascular disease	8 314	4 100	4 214	26	22	29	129	766	1 049	2 090	12	17	17	69	432	711	2 955
4. Inflammatory heart diseases	839	453	386	-	18	20	52	127	71	64	25	17	16	27	68	48	185
5. Other cardiovascular	5 212	2 727	2 484	89	46	41	122	501	616	1 314	55	42	40	52	239	349	1 707
H. Respiratory diseases	**6 335**	**3 506**	**2 829**	56	24	23	85	554	940	1 824	45	25	22	46	355	544	1 793
1. COPD*	4 744	2 637	2 107	14	4	5	29	388	752	1 445	14	4	3	17	229	423	1 416
2. Asthma	325	165	160	1	4	5	15	38	36	66	-	2	3	9	36	35	74
3. Other respiratory	1 266	705	561	41	17	13	41	128	152	314	30	18	15	20	90	86	302
I. Digestive diseases	**3 131**	**1 935**	**1 196**	37	21	37	184	608	432	617	37	22	28	66	241	225	576
1. Peptic ulcer	319	194	125	-	-	3	13	47	41	89	-	-	2	5	18	20	80
2. Cirrhosis of the liver	1 353	942	412	2	3	14	103	373	231	215	2	4	8	29	123	102	145
3. Appendicitis	55	33	22	1	6	8	9	4	2	2	1	5	3	5	3	2	2
4. Other digestive	1 404	767	637	34	12	12	58	184	157	311	34	13	13	28	96	102	350
J. Genito-urinary diseases	**1 128**	**593**	**534**	20	21	22	45	98	108	280	15	20	18	28	82	96	275
1. Nephritis and nephrosis	810	411	399	16	18	18	34	73	76	176	14	18	14	22	62	73	197
2. Benign prostatic hypertrophy	49	49	-	-	-	-	-	1	9	39	-	-	-	-	-	-	-
3. Other genito-urinary	268	133	135	3	3	4	10	25	24	64	2	2	4	6	20	23	78
K. Skin diseases	**65**	**30**	**34**	7	1	1	1	3	3	14	5	-	1	1	2	3	21

Annex Table 18i, continued. Deaths by age, sex and cause (thousands): World, 2020, pessimistic scenario

Cause	Total	Male	Female	Males							Females						
				0-4	5-14	15-29	30-44	45-59	60-69	70+	0-4	5-14	15-29	30-44	45-59	60-69	70+
L. Musculo-skeletal diseases	**151**	**54**	**97**	**1**	**1**	**1**	**2**	**6**	**12**	**32**	**1**	**1**	**3**	**4**	**10**	**12**	**67**
1. Rheumatoid arthritis	25	7	18	-	-	-	-	1	2	5	-	-	-	-	2	3	12
3. Other musculo-skeletal	125	46	79	1	1	1	2	5	10	27	1	1	3	4	8	10	54
M. Congenital anomalies	**586**	**296**	**289**	**243**	**16**	**14**	**9**	**8**	**3**	**5**	**237**	**16**	**11**	**6**	**9**	**4**	**6**
N. Oral conditions	**2**	**1**	**1**	-	-	-	-	-	-	-	-	-	-	-	-	-	-
III. Injuries	***8 207***	***5 379***	***2 828***	***424***	***430***	***1 534***	***1 215***	***899***	***382***	***495***	***346***	***257***	***642***	***438***	***414***	***247***	***483***
A. Unintentional injuries	**4 965**	**3 270**	**1 694**	**317**	**326**	**741**	**695**	**588**	**249**	**355**	**239**	**194**	**273**	**213**	**250**	**156**	**370**
1. Road traffic accidents	1 934	1 387	547	57	132	372	330	267	111	119	37	79	112	84	109	57	69
2. Poisonings	321	193	128	37	11	22	40	48	17	19	26	8	24	19	20	12	20
3. Falls	462	246	216	12	12	27	36	46	30	82	12	6	6	9	20	23	142
4. Fires	389	168	222	39	14	29	30	25	8	23	34	21	57	39	23	14	33
5. Drownings	559	373	186	83	92	73	51	36	15	24	55	41	21	15	18	11	26
6. Other unintentional	1 298	903	395	91	65	217	209	165	68	88	76	40	53	47	60	38	81
B. Intentional injuries	**3 242**	**2 108**	**1 133**	**107**	**104**	**793**	**519**	**312**	**133**	**140**	**107**	**63**	**369**	**226**	**164**	**91**	**114**
1. Self-inflicted injuries	1 200	696	503	-	25	152	156	167	86	112	-	12	144	92	104	58	93
2. Violence	1 027	821	206	28	27	383	224	108	30	22	30	16	56	41	35	15	14
3. War	1 015	591	425	79	53	258	140	37	18	7	77	35	170	93	25	18	7

Notes:
Causes responsible for no deaths have been omitted from this table.
A dash (-) symbol indicates fewer than 500 deaths.
*IA6 is Bacterial meningitis and meningococcaemia; IC3 is Hypertensive disorders of pregnancy; ID is Conditions arising during the perinatal period;
IIE6 is Dementia and other degenerative and hereditary CNS disorders; IIH1 is Chronic obstructive pulmonary disease.

Annex Table 19a. DALYs by age, sex and cause (thousands): Established Market Economies, 2020, pessimistic scenario

Cause	Total	Male	Female	Males 0-4	5-14	15-44	45-59	60+	Females 0-4	5-14	15-44	45-59	60+
Population (millions)	*890*	*434*	*456*	*29*	*57*	*161*	*85*	*102*	*27*	*55*	*156*	*87*	*131*
All causes	*109 929*	*62 296*	*47 633*	*2 269*	*1 241*	*19 945*	*15 168*	*23 673*	*1 842*	*950*	*12 846*	*9 591*	*22 404*
I. Communicable, maternal, perinatal and nutritional conditions	7 656	4 924	2 732	900	96	2 470	555	903	701	93	923	185	829
A. Infectious and parasitic diseases	4 303	3 245	1 058	143	32	2 391	478	201	115	33	658	88	165
1. Tuberculosis	96	69	27	–	–	9	16	44	–	–	3	5	19
2. STDs excluding HIV	247	17	230	–	–	15	1	1	–	2	223	2	2
a. Syphilis	4	3	2			1					1		
b. Chlamydia	212	9	203			9				3	199		
c. Gonorrhoea	27	5	22			5					22		
3. HIV	3 328	2 848	480	52	9	2 319	428	41	38	9	377	47	9
4. Diarrhoeal diseases	135	69	66	28	6	16	7	13	25	5	12	7	16
5. Childhood-cluster diseases	22	12	10	9	1	–	–	1	7	1	–	–	1
a. Pertussis	12	6	6	6					6				
b. Poliomyelitis	2	1	1					1					1
c. Diphtheria		1	1							1			
d. Measles	7	4	2	3	1				1	1			
e. Tetanus	1	–	1										
6. Bacterial meningitis*	108	59	50	38	6	6	4	5	32	6	3	3	4
7. Hepatitis B and hepatitis C	33	21	12	1	–	6	6	8	1	–	3	3	3
8. Malaria	1	1	–	–	–	–	–	–	–	–	–	–	–
9. Tropical-cluster diseases	1	1	–	–	–	–	–	–	–	–	–	–	–
a. Trypanosomiasis													
b. Chagas disease													
c. Schistosomiasis													
d. Leishmaniasis	1	1											
e. Lymphatic filariasis													
f. Onchocerciasis													
10. Leprosy													
11. Dengue													
12. Japanese encephalitis													
13. Trachoma													
14. Intestinal nematode infections													
a. Ascariasis													
b. Trichuriasis													
c. Ancylostomiasis and necatoriasis													

Annex Table 19a, continued. DALYs by age, sex and cause (thousands): Established Market Economies, 2020, pessimistic scenario

Cause	Total	Male	Female	Males 0-4	5-14	15-44	45-59	60+	Females 0-4	5-14	15-44	45-59	60+
B. Respiratory infections	**1 457**	**787**	**669**	**46**	**30**	**41**	**60**	**611**	**32**	**28**	**24**	**35**	**550**
1. Lower respiratory infections	1 368	741	626	35	8	36	57	605	24	8	20	33	542
2. Upper respiratory infections	38	20	18	5	2	4	2	6	3	1	4	2	8
3. Otitis media	51	26	25	6	20	–	–	–	5	19	–	–	–
C. Maternal conditions	**121**		**121**								**120**		
1. Maternal haemorrhage	7		7								7		
2. Maternal sepsis	12		12								12		
3. Hypertensive disorders of pregnancy	5		5								5		
4. Obstructed labour	86		86								86		
5. Abortion	4		4								4		
D. Perinatal conditions*	**1 186**	**670**	**516**	**669**	**1**				**515**				
E. Nutritional deficiencies	**590**	**222**	**368**	**41**	**34**	**38**	**18**	**91**	**39**	**32**	**121**	**62**	**115**
1. Protein-energy malnutrition	67	32	35	20	–	1	1	10	19	–	–	1	14
2. Iodine deficiency	–	–	–	–	–	–	–	–	–	–	–	–	–
3. Vitamin A deficiency	–	–	–	–	–	–	–	–	–	–	–	–	–
4. Iron-deficiency anaemia	517	187	330	21	33	37	16	80	19	32	119	61	99
II. Noncommunicable diseases	**91 343**	**49 805**	**41 537**	**1 124**	**746**	**12 499**	**13 442**	**21 995**	**966**	**619**	**10 223**	**8 803**	**20 927**
A. Malignant neoplasms	**18 785**	**11 050**	**7 735**	**29**	**83**	**1 023**	**3 900**	**6 014**	**26**	**59**	**901**	**2 382**	**4 366**
1. Mouth and oropharynx cancers	449	367	82			42	186	138			10	28	43
2. Oesophagus cancer	451	371	81			20	164	187			3	22	56
3. Stomach cancer	1 356	899	457			63	295	541			52	116	289
4. Colon and rectum cancers	2 089	1 168	921			70	355	743			54	224	642
5. Liver cancer	406	321	85		1	20	144	156		1	5	22	56
6. Pancreas cancer	760	448	312			27	158	263			14	79	220
7. Trachea, bronchus, lung cancers	4 345	3 029	1 317			238	1 414	1 376			76	457	784
8. Melanoma and other skin cancers	277	174	104			46	63	65			30	32	42
9. Breast cancer	1 538		1 538								254	613	671
10. Cervix uteri cancer	192		192								61	68	64
11. Corpus uteri cancer	211		211								19	72	120
12. Ovary cancer	416		416								48	160	208
13. Prostate cancer	854	854					83	767					
14. Bladder cancer	519	425	94			4	72	345			3	14	77
15. Lymphomas and multiple myeloma	817	491	327	2	9	106	153	221	1	3	50	79	192
16. Leukaemia	652	388	264	9	33	103	90	152	9	22	65	56	112
C. Diabetes mellitus	**2 536**	**1 179**	**1 358**	**2**	**3**	**182**	**377**	**615**	**2**	**4**	**135**	**319**	**898**
D. Endocrine disorders	**1 120**	**489**	**632**	**72**	**50**	**125**	**71**	**171**	**68**	**38**	**135**	**154**	**237**

Annex Table 19a, continued. DALYs by age, sex and cause (thousands): Established Market Economies, 2020, pessimistic scenario

Cause	Total	Male	Female	Males					Females				
				0-4	5-14	15-44	45-59	60+	0-4	5-14	15-44	45-59	60+
E. Neuro-psychiatric conditions	**24 891**	**12 726**	**12 166**	**108**	**312**	**8 278**	**1 871**	**2 157**	**93**	**264**	**6 655**	**1 848**	**3 306**
1. Unipolar major depression	6 566	2 297	4 269	-	-	1 602	491	204	-	-	2 922	903	445
2. Bipolar disorder	1 587	800	788	-	-	674	81	44	-	-	652	82	54
3. Schizophrenia	1 987	1 037	950	-	-	1 003	10	25	-	-	913	3	34
4. Epilepsy	405	222	183	6	41	109	43	23	6	43	69	33	31
5. Alcohol use	4 383	3 702	681	-	-	2 938	585	179	-	-	529	103	49
6. Dementia*	4 231	1 677	2 554	36	17	41	297	1 286	35	14	32	312	2 161
7. Parkinson disease	668	308	359	-	-	-	83	225	-	-	-	90	269
8. Multiple sclerosis	209	90	119	-	-	68	14	8	-	-	87	20	12
9. Drug use	1 359	1 029	331	4	91	887	42	9	6	31	283	14	3
10. Post-traumatic stress disorder	260	98	161	-	17	62	12	4	-	28	102	19	7
11. Obsessive-compulsive disorders	1 390	590	800	-	56	440	52	41	-	72	565	94	69
12. Panic disorder	665	221	444	-	19	146	55	1	-	19	310	88	27
F. Sense organ diseases	**148**	**68**	**80**	-	-	**3**	**27**	**38**	-	-	**2**	**28**	**50**
1. Glaucoma	100	45	55	-	-	2	22	21	-	-	1	24	31
2. Cataracts	43	21	22	-	-	1	4	16	-	-	1	3	18
G. Cardiovascular diseases	**22 756**	**13 721**	**9 036**	**54**	**25**	**1 102**	**3 802**	**8 738**	**42**	**17**	**510**	**999**	**7 469**
1. Rheumatic heart disease	172	71	102	-	-	11	24	35	-	-	10	24	67
2. Ischaemic heart disease	11 364	7 308	4 056	-	-	381	2 232	4 695	-	-	97	408	3 552
3. Cerebrovascular disease	6 104	3 203	2 901	9	6	305	768	2 116	6	4	219	373	2 300
4. Inflammatory heart diseases	720	459	260	11	6	128	156	159	12	4	58	44	143
H. Respiratory diseases	**5 975**	**3 223**	**2 752**	**74**	**126**	**538**	**766**	**1 719**	**42**	**94**	**491**	**684**	**1 442**
1. COPD*	3 162	1 849	1 313	3	1	98	440	1 307	1	1	54	327	930
2. Asthma	1 281	633	648	31	108	284	126	83	16	82	275	152	123
I. Digestive diseases	**5 355**	**3 158**	**2 197**	**34**	**15**	**525**	**1 281**	**1 302**	**26**	**13**	**352**	**657**	**1 150**
1. Peptic ulcer	313	196	117	-	1	33	59	103	1	-	18	25	73
2. Cirrhosis of the liver	1 961	1 410	551	1	1	230	713	466	1	1	89	234	227
3. Appendicitis	34	21	14	-	2	8	4	6	-	1	6	2	5
J. Genito-urinary diseases	**1 372**	**794**	**578**	**14**	**2**	**56**	**213**	**509**	**11**	**4**	**46**	**84**	**432**
1. Nephritis and nephrosis	534	284	249	11	1	32	46	195	9	3	13	27	198
2. Benign prostatic hypertrophy	304	304	-	-	-	-	129	176	-	-	-	-	-
L. Musculo-skeletal diseases	**4 916**	**1 668**	**3 248**	**2**	**3**	**360**	**890**	**415**	**1**	**10**	**709**	**1 387**	**1 141**
1. Rheumatoid arthritis	1 113	280	833	-	-	51	113	116	-	4	287	202	339
2. Osteoarthritis	3 349	1 269	2 079	-	-	283	746	241	-	-	323	1 105	651

Annex Table 19a, continued. DALYs by age, sex and cause (thousands): Established Market Economies, 2020, pessimistic scenario

Cause	Total	Male	Female	Males					Females				
				0-4	5-14	15-44	45-59	60+	0-4	5-14	15-44	45-59	60+
M. Congenital anomalies	1 506	806	700	708	25	50	12	11	627	23	28	11	12
N. Oral conditions	994	474	520	14	75	158	104	123	14	71	154	111	169
1. Dental caries	428	213	215	14	75	77	20	28	13	71	74	20	36
2. Periodontal disease	33	16	16	-	-	14	2	1	-	-	13	2	1
3. Edentulism	525	241	284	-	-	67	81	93	-	-	66	88	130
III. Injuries	10 930	7 566	3 364	245	400	4 976	1 171	775	176	238	1 700	603	648
A. Unintentional injuries	7 811	5 272	2 539	220	363	3 386	746	558	152	216	1 214	417	540
1. Road traffic accidents	3 937	2 698	1 239	60	174	2 092	247	124	45	119	830	149	97
2. Poisonings	230	161	69	3	3	122	24	10	2	2	43	13	8
3. Falls	1 325	716	608	35	62	305	145	170	23	31	146	147	261
4. Fires	219	129	90	18	27	49	19	16	14	27	25	11	13
5. Drownings	221	173	49	22	25	86	23	16	12	7	15	7	8
6. Other unintentional	1 879	1 395	484	81	72	733	288	222	55	30	155	90	153
B. Intentional injuries	3 119	2 294	825	25	37	1 590	425	217	24	22	486	186	107
1. Self-inflicted injuries	2 186	1 588	598	-	15	1 015	360	199	-	4	332	164	97
2. Violence	931	704	227	25	22	575	65	18	24	17	154	22	10
3. War	2	2	-	-	-	1	-	1	-	-	-	-	-

Notes:
A dash (-) symbol indicates fewer than 500 DALYs.
*IA6 is Bacterial meningitis and meningococcaemia; ID is Conditions arising during the perinatal period;
IIE6 is Dementia and other degenerative and hereditary CNS disorders; IIH1 is Chronic obstructive pulmonary disease.

Annex Table 19b. DALYs by age, sex and cause (thousands): Formerly Socialist Economies of Europe, 2020, pessimistic scenario

Cause	Total	Male	Female	Males					Females				
				0-4	5-14	15-44	45-59	60+	0-4	5-14	15-44	45-59	60+
Population (millions)	*361*	*170*	*191*	*12*	*25*	*75*	*29*	*29*	*12*	*24*	*74*	*33*	*48*
All causes	*68 546*	*41 954*	*26 592*	*1 948*	*900*	*14 432*	*12 926*	*11 748*	*1 545*	*603*	*8 017*	*5 460*	*10 967*
I. Communicable, maternal, perinatal and nutritional conditions	*3 247*	*1 571*	*1 676*	*893*	*83*	*216*	*126*	*253*	*678*	*80*	*550*	*63*	*306*
A. Infectious and parasitic diseases	1 062	519	543	197	26	156	77	63	169	27	264	23	60
1. Tuberculosis	189	161	28	1	-	68	59	33	1	1	8	7	11
2. STDs excluding HIV	241	35	206	4	1	29	1	-	4	3	198	1	1
a. Syphilis	2		1			1					1		
b. Chlamydia	186	13	172	1		12			1	2	167		
c. Gonorrhoea	50	18	32	2		15			2		29		
3. HIV	198	107	91	63	10	32	3	-	62	10	17	2	-
4. Diarrhoeal diseases	115	61	54	45	3	7	3	3	39	2	6	3	4
5. Childhood-cluster diseases	18	9	9	7		1			6	2			
a. Pertussis	10	5	6	5					5	1			
b. Poliomyelitis													
c. Diphtheria													
d. Measles	5	3	2	2					1	1			
e. Tetanus	1	1	1										
6. Bacterial meningitis*	113	65	48	41	4	9	5	7	32	3	5	3	6
7. Hepatitis B and hepatitis C	18	10	8	4	1	3	1	2	3	-	2	1	1
8. Malaria													
9. Tropical-cluster diseases													
a. Trypanosomiasis													
b. Chagas disease													
c. Schistosomiasis													
d. Leishmaniasis													
e. Lymphatic filariasis													
f. Onchocerciasis													
10. Leprosy													
11. Dengue													
12. Japanese encephalitis													
13. Trachoma													
14. Intestinal nematode infections	1		1								1		
a. Ascariasis													
b. Trichuriasis													
c. Ancylostomiasis and necatoriasis													

Annex Table 19b, continued. DALYs by age, sex and cause (thousands): Formerly Socialist Economies of Europe, 2020, pessimistic scenario

Cause	Total	Male	Female	Males 0-4	5-14	15-44	45-59	60+	Females 0-4	5-14	15-44	45-59	60+
B. Respiratory infections	827	444	383	175	22	42	42	163	133	20	18	14	198
1. Lower respiratory infections	791	425	365	169	13	40	41	162	128	12	16	13	196
2. Upper respiratory infections	13	7	7	2	–	2	1	1	2	–	2	1	2
3. Otitis media	23	12	11	4	8	–	–	–	3	8	–	–	–
C. Maternal conditions	209	–	209	–	–	–	–	–	–	–	209	–	–
1. Maternal haemorrhage	5		5								5		
2. Maternal sepsis	41		41								41		
3. Hypertensive disorders of pregnancy	4		4								4		
4. Obstructed labour	57		57								57		
5. Abortion	58		58								58		
D. Perinatal conditions*	799	470	329	470					329				
E. Nutritional deficiencies	350	138	212	51	35	18	7	28	47	33	59	26	48
1. Protein-energy malnutrition	59	29	30	26				3	24				5
2. Iodine deficiency	–												
3. Vitamin A deficiency	–												
4. Iron-deficiency anaemia	254	94	160	19	32	15	5	22	17	30	52	23	37
II. Noncommunicable diseases	53 995	31 817	22 178	707	367	8 309	11 357	11 076	596	298	6 028	4 922	10 333
A. Malignant neoplasms	10 625	7 342	3 283	31	67	973	3 608	2 663	27	41	594	1 127	1 495
1. Mouth and oropharynx cancers	399	365	34		1	57	232	76			7	11	15
2. Oesophagus cancer	198	180	18			18	115	47			2	6	10
3. Stomach cancer	1 561	1 149	411			128	622	399			56	129	226
4. Colon and rectum cancers	956	579	377	1		63	262	253			39	115	222
5. Liver cancer	280	195	86	1	1	20	98	75	1		8	25	52
6. Pancreas cancer	417	298	118			34	159	105			10	37	71
7. Trachea, bronchus, lung cancers	2 780	2 390	390		1	235	1 177	976		1	42	145	202
8. Melanoma and other skin cancers	139	86	53			26	37	23			18	14	20
9. Breast cancer	531	–	531								124	232	175
10. Cervix uteri cancer	194		194								58	67	69
11. Corpus uteri cancer	143		143								21	58	64
12. Ovary cancer	197		197								41	86	70
13. Prostate cancer	187	187				4	49	134					
14. Bladder cancer	241	208	34	1		8	86	113			3	8	22
15. Lymphomas and multiple myeloma	319	222	97	4	13	74	88	44	2	4	34	25	31
16. Leukaemia	352	227	125	10	26	68	73	50	9	16	39	28	34
C. Diabetes mellitus	609	258	351	–	1	64	86	106	1	1	49	89	211
D. Endocrine disorders	185	78	107	16	6	39	12	6	15	6	43	27	16

Annex Table 19b, continued. DALYs by age, sex and cause (thousands): Formerly Socialist Economies of Europe, 2020, pessimistic scenario

Cause	Total	Male	Female	Males					Females				
				0-4	5-14	15-44	45-59	60+	0-4	5-14	15-44	45-59	60+
E. Neuro-psychiatric conditions	**10 704**	**5 393**	**5 311**	**88**	**181**	**3 919**	**665**	**540**	**76**	**145**	**3 305**	**720**	**1 065**
1. Unipolar major depression	3 185	1 077	2 107	-	-	822	186	69	-	-	1 538	379	191
2. Bipolar disorder	844	412	432	-	-	358	34	20	-	-	352	37	42
3. Schizophrenia	844	438	406	-	-	423	8	7	-	-	394	3	9
4. Epilepsy	289	183	107	6	39	100	25	13	6	28	42	16	14
5. Alcohol use	1 747	1 538	209	-	-	1 280	200	58	-	-	182	16	11
6. Dementia*	1 176	408	768	16	8	18	87	278	15	7	16	110	620
7. Parkinson disease	159	62	97	-	-	-	19	43	-	-	-	24	72
8. Multiple sclerosis	112	48	65	-	-	36	7	5	-	-	47	9	9
9. Drug use	523	418	105	-	30	372	14	3	-	8	93	3	1
10. Post-traumatic stress disorder	116	43	73	2	7	29	4	1	3	12	49	7	2
11. Obsessive-compulsive disorders	647	270	377	-	25	214	19	13	-	32	281	37	27
12. Panic disorder	311	100	210	-	9	72	20	-	-	9	156	35	11
F. Sense organ diseases	**81**	**37**	**44**	-	-	**1**	**9**	**26**	-	-	**2**	**14**	**28**
1. Glaucoma	36	12	23	-	-	-	4	8	-	-	1	11	11
2. Cataracts	45	25	21	-	-	1	5	18	-	-	1	3	17
G. Cardiovascular diseases	**18 241**	**11 181**	**7 061**	**22**	**11**	**1 354**	**4 252**	**5 542**	**17**	**7**	**426**	**1 065**	**5 545**
1. Rheumatic heart disease	402	223	179	-	2	71	117	33	-	1	41	87	50
2. Ischaemic heart disease	9 210	6 094	3 116	3	-	669	2 601	2 824	2	-	105	439	2 572
3. Cerebrovascular disease	5 444	2 872	2 573	4	2	286	949	1 631	5	2	185	433	1 951
4. Inflammatory heart diseases	530	352	178	-	3	121	135	89	-	2	43	39	90
H. Respiratory diseases	**5 193**	**3 502**	**1 691**	**27**	**41**	**505**	**1 530**	**1 399**	**15**	**28**	**327**	**467**	**854**
1. COPD*	2 083	1 540	543	14	39	155	735	649	7	26	67	116	359
2. Asthma	620	334	286	-	-	143	83	54	-	-	131	67	56
I. Digestive diseases	**2 783**	**1 630**	**1 153**	**36**	**8**	**519**	**655**	**413**	**26**	**7**	**279**	**398**	**443**
1. Peptic ulcer	218	160	58	1	1	44	67	49	-	1	15	18	24
2. Cirrhosis of the liver	820	565	255	-	1	115	283	165	1	1	42	108	103
3. Appendicitis	15	9	6	-	-	4	2	2	-	-	3	1	2
J. Genito-urinary diseases	**878**	**456**	**422**	**5**	**5**	**121**	**151**	**174**	**4**	**6**	**111**	**149**	**152**
1. Nephritis and nephrosis	231	133	97	2	3	56	39	33	2	4	30	27	34
2. Benign prostatic hypertrophy	137	137	-	-	-	-	56	81	-	-	-	-	-
L. Musculo-skeletal diseases	**2 872**	**1 048**	**1 824**	**1**	**3**	**620**	**274**	**150**	**1**	**6**	**691**	**708**	**418**
1. Rheumatoid arthritis	523	124	399	-	-	67	31	26	-	3	216	106	75
2. Osteoarthritis	2 146	868	1 278	-	-	521	229	118	-	-	408	552	318

Annex Table 19b, continued. DALYs by age, sex and cause (thousands): Formerly Socialist Economies of Europe, 2020, pessimistic scenario

Cause	Total	Males	Females	Males					Females				
				0-4	5-14	15-44	45-59	60+	0-4	5-14	15-44	45-59	60+
M. Congenital anomalies	**929**	**502**	**427**	**455**	**17**	**25**	**4**	**1**	**391**	**16**	**14**	**4**	**1**
N. Oral conditions	**505**	**227**	**278**	**14**	**19**	**95**	**65**	**34**	**14**	**28**	**99**	**79**	**59**
1. Dental caries	246	113	133	14	19	45	21	14	14	28	44	23	24
2. Periodontal disease	17	7	10	-	-	5	1	1	-	-	8	1	1
3. Edentulism	241	107	134	-	-	45	43	18	-	-	47	54	34
III. Injuries	*11 305*	*8 567*	*2 738*	*348*	*450*	*5 908*	*1 443*	*418*	*271*	*225*	*1 439*	*474*	*329*
A. Unintentional injuries	**7 676**	**5 948**	**1 729**	**240**	**356**	**4 020**	**1 041**	**291**	**164**	**164**	**817**	**335**	**248**
1. Road traffic accidents	3 102	2 434	668	35	143	1 856	309	91	21	79	403	101	63
2. Poisonings	820	631	188	28	10	358	195	40	21	8	76	58	25
3. Falls	987	653	334	37	54	396	109	57	27	22	126	70	89
4. Fires	160	111	49	12	11	57	23	9	10	8	14	7	9
5. Drownings	492	417	75	22	56	272	54	13	10	21	29	9	6
6. Other unintentional	2 114	1 700	415	105	81	1 082	351	80	76	25	169	89	59
B. Intentional injuries	**3 629**	**2 619**	**1 010**	**108**	**94**	**1 888**	**401**	**127**	**106**	**62**	**622**	**139**	**81**
1. Self-inflicted injuries	1 661	1 323	338	-	17	899	302	104	-	4	184	90	60
2. Violence	850	652	198	9	9	538	79	17	7	8	134	35	15
3. War	1 117	644	474	99	67	451	20	6	100	50	303	14	6

Notes:
A dash (-) symbol indicates fewer than 500 DALYs.
*IA6 is Bacterial meningitis and meningococcaemia; ID is Conditions arising during the perinatal period;
IIE6 is Dementia and other degenerative and hereditary CNS disorders; IIH1 is Chronic obstructive pulmonary disease.

Annex Table 19c. DALYs by age, sex and cause (thousands): India, 2020, pessimistic scenario

Cause	Total	Male	Female	Males					Females				
				0-4	5-14	15-44	45-59	60+	0-4	5-14	15-44	45-59	60+
Population (millions)	*1 196*	*608*	*589*	*50*	*100*	*302*	*100*	*56*	*48*	*94*	*285*	*98*	*63*
All causes	*291 330*	*157 833*	*133 497*	*33 866*	*10 800*	*48 483*	*38 126*	*26 557*	*33 295*	*9 179*	*42 953*	*24 139*	*23 931*
I. Communicable, maternal, perinatal and nutritional conditions	*104 188*	*54 194*	*49 994*	*24 785*	*2 919*	*15 938*	*6 576*	*3 975*	*24 812*	*3 220*	*14 835*	*4 206*	*2 921*
A. Infectious and parasitic diseases	68 647	38 243	30 404	12 169	2 037	14 925	6 199	2 914	12 073	2 013	10 878	3 651	1 788
1. Tuberculosis	23 354	14 865	8 489	422	389	6 779	5 062	2 213	326	305	3 883	2 910	1 065
2. STDs excluding HIV	3 184	1 103	2 081	508	8	547	14	26	506	28	1 487	20	39
a. Syphilis	910	442	468	323	1	81	12	25	334	-	82	14	38
b. Chlamydia	1 331	213	1 118	45	3	164	1	-	42	20	1 051	4	1
c. Gonorrhoea	942	448	494	140	4	302	2	-	131	7	354	2	-
3. HIV	15 042	8 383	6 660	1 296	244	5 964	707	171	1 404	266	4 628	303	59
4. Diarrhoeal diseases	12 636	6 206	6 430	5 265	311	290	112	227	5 411	410	217	113	278
5. Childhood-cluster diseases	7 597	3 912	3 685	3 352	325	177	38	20	3 129	359	133	40	24
a. Pertussis	1 247	640	607	589	51	-	1	-	558	50	-	-	-
b. Poliomyelitis	563	331	232	322	1	7	1	-	227	1	3	-	-
c. Diphtheria	62	32	30	29	3	1	-	-	27	3	-	-	-
d. Measles	2 890	1 472	1 418	1 297	172	2	1	-	1 245	171	2	1	-
e. Tetanus	2 834	1 437	1 397	1 116	97	167	37	20	1 071	135	127	39	24
6. Bacterial meningitis*	679	357	322	235	9	69	27	18	220	8	46	27	22
7. Hepatitis B and hepatitis C	179	102	77	19	9	31	24	18	15	9	20	12	20
8. Malaria	483	263	219	63	65	100	24	11	54	68	65	21	11
9. Tropical-cluster diseases	1 285	905	380	49	262	533	53	8	26	123	147	74	10
a. Trypanosomiasis	-	-	-	-	-	-	-	-	-	-	-	-	-
b. Chagas disease	-	-	-	-	-	-	-	-	-	-	-	-	-
c. Schistosomiasis	-	-	-	-	-	-	-	-	-	-	-	-	-
d. Leishmaniasis	511	324	187	24	114	171	10	4	16	78	83	7	4
e. Lymphatic filariasis	774	581	193	24	148	361	43	4	10	45	64	67	7
f. Onchocerciasis	-	-	-	-	-	-	-	-	-	-	-	-	-
10. Leprosy	60	31	29	-	7	17	4	2	1	7	16	4	2
11. Dengue	152	71	82	17	50	2	1	-	20	59	2	1	-
12. Japanese encephalitis	33	17	16	10	5	2	-	-	10	5	1	-	-
13. Trachoma	22	6	16	-	-	1	2	3	-	-	2	5	9
14. Intestinal nematode infections	398	212	186	1	89	88	22	12	1	83	68	21	13
a. Ascariasis	83	43	40	1	42	2	1	-	1	39	2	1	-
b. Trichuriasis	54	28	26	-	28	-	-	-	-	26	-	-	-
c. Ancylostomiasis and necatoriasis	260	141	120	-	20	88	21	12	-	18	68	21	13

Annex Table 19c, continued. DALYs by age, sex and cause (thousands): India, 2020, pessimistic scenario

Cause	Total	Male	Female	Males 0-4	5-14	15-44	45-59	60+	Females 0-4	5-14	15-44	45-59	60+
B. Respiratory infections	**15 605**	**7 587**	**8 017**	**5 593**	**504**	**387**	**219**	**883**	**5 747**	**834**	**281**	**228**	**927**
1. Lower respiratory infections	15 184	7 383	7 801	5 457	460	377	216	874	5 600	786	273	224	917
2. Upper respiratory infections	167	82	85	54	6	10	3	10	55	9	7	4	10
3. Otitis media	254	122	132	82	39	1	–	–	92	38	1	–	–
C. Maternal conditions	**2 828**	**–**	**2 828**								**2 784**	**43**	
1. Maternal haemorrhage	325		325								316	10	
2. Maternal sepsis	479		479								473	6	
3. Hypertensive disorders of pregnancy	159		159								154	5	
4. Obstructed labour	571		571								568	3	
5. Abortion	609		609								603	6	
D. Perinatal conditions*	**11 238**	**5 635**	**5 603**	**5 635**					**5 603**				
E. Nutritional deficiencies	**5 871**	**2 728**	**3 143**	**1 388**	**378**	**626**	**158**	**178**	**1 389**	**373**	**891**	**284**	**205**
1. Protein-energy malnutrition	2 175	1 065	1 110	1 003	13	20	8	21	1 033	34	9	6	28
2. Iodine deficiency	155	81	74	71	7	3	–	–	65	7	2	–	–
3. Vitamin A deficiency	287	148	139	100	43	4	–	–	95	42	3	–	–
4. Iron-deficiency anaemia	3 254	1 435	1 819	214	315	599	150	156	196	291	877	278	177
II. Noncommunicable diseases	***140 664***	***76 689***	***63 975***	***5 248***	***1 669***	***20 133***	***27 917***	***21 722***	***5 231***	***1 666***	***19 665***	***17 348***	***20 066***
A. Malignant neoplasms	**16 595**	**9 220**	**7 375**	**126**	**205**	**2 000**	**4 695**	**2 193**	**71**	**100**	**1 923**	**3 461**	**1 821**
1. Mouth and oropharynx cancers	2 300	1 371	929	2	4	261	775	329	2	4	201	480	242
2. Oesophagus cancer	1 253	647	606			94	381	171			102	301	203
3. Stomach cancer	1 184	769	415		1	146	448	174			96	194	125
4. Colon and rectum cancers	543	299	245			94	131	73		1	47	108	89
5. Liver cancer	317	227	90	1	2	47	127	49	1	1	18	40	30
6. Pancreas cancer	187	115	72			22	66	27			16	30	25
7. Trachea, bronchus, lung cancers	3 451	2 988	462		1	476	1 676	836			71	231	159
8. Melanoma and other skin cancers	32	17	15			4	10	2			4	8	4
9. Breast cancer	1 035		1 035								335	498	202
10. Cervix uteri cancer	1 450		1 450								336	855	259
11. Corpus uteri cancer	76		76								8	40	28
12. Ovary cancer	327		327								127	115	83
13. Prostate cancer	156	156					45	107					
14. Bladder cancer	142	112	30			4	54	44			4	11	14
15. Lymphomas and multiple myeloma	554	384	170	21	37	155	129	43	4	7	52	55	51
16. Leukaemia	558	333	225	38	66	141	67	21	22	36	98	48	21
C. Diabetes mellitus	**2 715**	**1 313**	**1 402**	**63**	**89**	**303**	**491**	**368**	**65**	**85**	**215**	**488**	**549**
D. Endocrine disorders	**107**	**56**	**51**	**22**	**4**	**15**	**13**	**3**	**16**	**1**	**11**	**12**	**10**

Annex Table 19c, continued. DALYs by age, sex and cause (thousands): India, 2020, pessimistic scenario

Cause	Total	Male	Female	Males					Females				
				0-4	5-14	15-44	45-59	60+	0-4	5-14	15-44	45-59	60+
E. Neuro-psychiatric conditions	**30 059**	**13 582**	**16 478**	**394**	**357**	**10 119**	**1 723**	**989**	**500**	**427**	**12 135**	**2 069**	**1 346**
1. Unipolar major depression	13 071	4 698	8 372	-	-	3 807	736	156	-	-	6 750	1 307	316
2. Bipolar disorder	3 607	1 848	1 759	-	-	1 680	130	37	-	-	1 588	125	47
3. Schizophrenia	2 512	1 337	1 175	-	-	1 313	14	10	-	-	1 152	6	17
4. Epilepsy	870	502	368	35	75	305	58	30	41	109	170	19	29
5. Alcohol use	1 393	1 273	120	-	-	1 130	123	20	-	-	109	8	3
6. Dementia*	1 744	812	932	47	19	60	232	454	57	20	55	235	565
7. Parkinson disease	266	123	143	-	-	-	54	70	-	-	-	63	79
8. Multiple sclerosis	320	142	178	-	-	121	15	5	-	-	151	19	8
9. Drug use	112	100	11	-	5	90	4	1	-	1	10	-	-
10. Post-traumatic stress disorder	439	169	270	7	30	117	14	2	11	48	186	21	3
11. Obsessive-compulsive disorders	2 447	1 069	1 378	-	104	875	65	25	-	131	1 096	113	38
12. Panic disorder	1 167	379	788	-	4	304	71	-	-	36	626	110	15
F. Sense organ diseases	**6 543**	**3 498**	**3 045**	**5**	-	**215**	**1 936**	**1 341**	**3**	-	**144**	**1 361**	**1 536**
1. Glaucoma	1 173	657	517	-	-	52	480	126	-	-	19	346	151
2. Cataracts	5 367	2 839	2 528	3	-	164	1 456	1 215	3	-	125	1 014	1 385
G. Cardiovascular diseases	**46 215**	**27 275**	**18 940**	**517**	**210**	**3 284**	**10 983**	**12 281**	**440**	**283**	**1 880**	**5 040**	**11 298**
1. Rheumatic heart disease	2 312	1 139	1 173	1	24	484	511	119	1	31	488	503	150
2. Ischaemic heart disease	22 769	13 838	8 931	-	-	754	6 002	7 082	-	-	380	2 359	6 193
3. Cerebrovascular disease	8 404	4 716	3 688	100	37	430	1 686	2 463	86	41	319	801	2 441
4. Inflammatory heart diseases	2 612	1 533	1 079	95	49	534	590	265	96	70	311	337	265
H. Respiratory diseases	**16 160**	**9 313**	**6 848**	**394**	**379**	**1 544**	**3 987**	**3 008**	**332**	**283**	**1 389**	**2 675**	**2 169**
1. COPD*	6 956	4 365	2 591	42	27	504	2 105	1 688	42	29	361	1 174	986
2. Asthma	2 310	1 352	959	73	173	622	339	146	37	103	467	231	113
I. Digestive diseases	**7 673**	**5 160**	**2 512**	**145**	**71**	**1 605**	**2 545**	**794**	**155**	**65**	**824**	**995**	**474**
1. Peptic ulcer	1 180	784	396	2	4	278	352	148	3	7	149	152	85
2. Cirrhosis of the liver	3 809	2 784	1 026	27	14	767	1 494	483	35	32	293	457	209
3. Appendicitis	273	160	114	4	25	112	15	4	4	23	74	9	3
J. Genito-urinary diseases	**2 298**	**1 465**	**833**	**85**	**151**	**178**	**726**	**324**	**45**	**214**	**188**	**180**	**205**
1. Nephritis and nephrosis	1 562	776	786	67	145	163	215	186	41	213	176	164	191
2. Benign prostatic hypertrophy	631	631	-	-	-	-	500	131	-	-	-	-	-
L. Musculo-skeletal diseases	**2 643**	**1 027**	**1 617**	**2**	**5**	**357**	**498**	**165**	**2**	**5**	**508**	**743**	**359**
1. Rheumatoid arthritis	305	84	221	1	1	55	17	10	-	3	108	84	27
2. Osteoarthritis	2 309	924	1 384	-	-	296	476	152	-	-	397	657	330

Annex Table 19c, continued. DALYs by age, sex and cause (thousands): India, 2020, pessimistic scenario

Cause	Total	Males	Females	Males					Females				
				0-4	5-14	15-44	45-59	60+	0-4	5-14	15-44	45-59	60+
M. Congenital anomalies	7 550	3 710	3 840	3 414	111	147	28	9	3 529	130	126	39	16
N. Oral conditions	1 740	855	885	36	70	265	255	229	34	68	263	256	265
1. Dental caries	997	503	494	35	69	215	110	74	33	66	203	108	84
2. Periodontal disease	117	60	57	-	-	45	10	4	-	-	43	10	4
3. Edentulism	599	286	313	-	-	-	134	152	-	-	-	137	177
III. Injuries	*46 477*	*26 950*	*19 527*	*3 834*	*6 211*	*12 411*	*3 633*	*860*	*3 252*	*4 293*	*8 452*	*2 585*	*945*
A. Unintentional injuries	40 052	23 382	16 670	3 647	6 035	9 958	2 994	749	3 015	4 126	6 512	2 162	855
1. Road traffic accidents	10 775	7 740	3 035	531	1 296	4 540	1 101	272	157	974	1 120	562	223
2. Poisonings	1 058	482	576	138	65	217	49	12	96	45	261	162	12
3. Falls	8 117	4 844	3 274	826	2 650	957	313	97	947	1 067	733	422	105
4. Fires	5 566	1 634	3 932	352	281	749	215	37	304	805	2 452	254	117
5. Drownings	2 410	1 323	1 087	293	372	521	102	34	243	331	346	112	55
6. Other unintentional	12 126	7 360	4 766	1 506	1 371	2 973	1 213	297	1 268	903	1 601	650	344
B. Intentional injuries	6 425	3 568	2 857	187	176	2 454	640	111	237	167	1 940	423	90
1. Self-inflicted injuries	4 211	2 147	2 064	-	104	1 581	410	52	-	104	1 734	205	21
2. Violence	2 046	1 252	794	187	72	704	229	60	237	63	206	218	69
3. War	168	168	-	-	-	168	-	-	-	-	-	-	-

Notes:
A dash (-) symbol indicates fewer than 500 DALYs.
*IA6 is Bacterial meningitis and meningococcaemia; ID is Conditions arising during the perinatal period;
IIE6 is Dementia and other degenerative and hereditary CNS disorders; IIH1 is Chronic obstructive pulmonary disease.

Annex Table 19d. DALYs by age, sex and cause (thousands): China, 2020, pessimistic scenario

Cause	Total	Male	Female	Males					Females				
				0-4	5-14	15-44	45-59	60+	0-4	5-14	15-44	45-59	60+
Population (millions)	*1 447*	*727*	*721*	*56*	*101*	*316*	*161*	*93*	*53*	*96*	*302*	*159*	*110*
All causes	*257 121*	*146 350*	*110 772*	*12 681*	*3 934*	*38 689*	*50 244*	*40 801*	*12 906*	*3 040*	*31 610*	*29 622*	*33 593*
I. Communicable, maternal, perinatal and nutritional conditions	*20 332*	*10 113*	*10 218*	*5 185*	*742*	*1 491*	*1 129*	*1 567*	*5 564*	*737*	*1 459*	*937*	*1 521*
A. Infectious and parasitic diseases	6 879	3 730	3 148	976	388	664	800	902	969	379	448	542	810
1. Tuberculosis	2 253	1 370	884	34	7	226	503	599	36	24	144	306	373
2. STDs excluding HIV	52	12	39	1	-	9	1	1	1	1	36	-	1
a. Syphilis	4	2	2	-	-	-	-	1	-	-	-	-	1
b. Chlamydia	32	4	29	-	-	3	-	-	-	-	28	-	-
c. Gonorrhoea	15	6	9	1	-	5	-	-	1	-	8	-	-
3. HIV	182	99	83	16	3	66	12	3	11	2	62	6	-
4. Diarrhoeal diseases	1 370	662	708	305	43	127	66	122	372	40	91	66	138
5. Childhood-cluster diseases	768	416	353	370	28	12	4	2	320	25	5	2	1
a. Pertussis	264	139	125	126	13	-	-	-	113	13	-	-	-
b. Poliomyelitis	125	74	52	70	-	3	-	-	49	-	2	-	-
c. Diphtheria	2	1	1	1	-	-	-	-	1	-	-	-	-
d. Measles	174	91	83	79	9	2	1	1	71	9	1	1	-
e. Tetanus	202	110	92	94	5	7	2	1	86	3	2	1	1
6. Bacterial meningitis*	479	247	232	129	6	49	33	30	118	6	35	36	37
7. Hepatitis B and hepatitis C	271	180	92	22	3	52	70	32	17	3	13	17	41
8. Malaria	18	9	8	2	2	3	1	1	1	2	2	1	1
9. Tropical-cluster diseases	71	58	13	2	7	39	7	4	1	1	6	3	2
a. Trypanosomiasis													
b. Chagas disease													
c. Schistosomiasis	13	8	5	-	-	2	3	3	-	-	1	2	2
d. Leishmaniasis													
e. Lymphatic filariasis	58	50	8	2	6	36	4	1	-	1	5	1	-
f. Onchocerciasis													
10. Leprosy	2	1	1	1	-	-	-	-	-	-	-	-	-
11. Dengue	9	4	5	1	3	-	-	-	1	3	-	-	-
12. Japanese encephalitis	152	79	73	49	24	5	1	1	46	22	3	-	1
13. Trachoma	296	77	219	-	-	6	22	49	-	-	11	61	147
14. Intestinal nematode infections	537	275	262	4	247	15	5	4	4	237	12	5	4
a. Ascariasis	245	125	120	4	119	1	-	-	4	114	1	-	-
b. Trichuriasis	240	122	117	-	122	-	-	-	-	117	-	-	-
c. Ancylostomiasis and necatoriasis	52	27	25	-	6	14	5	3	-	5	11	5	4

Annex Table 19d, continued. DALYs by age, sex and cause (thousands): China, 2020, pessimistic scenario

Cause	Total	Male	Female	Males					Females				
				0-4	5-14	15-44	45-59	60+	0-4	5-14	15-44	45-59	60+
B. Respiratory infections	**4 934**	**2 369**	**2 566**	**1 742**	**96**	**53**	**63**	**414**	**1 959**	**98**	**46**	**43**	**419**
1. Lower respiratory infections	4 773	2 289	2 484	1 704	65	50	61	409	1 918	68	43	41	413
2. Upper respiratory infections	58	28	30	16	1	3	2	5	18	1	3	2	6
3. Otitis media	103	51	52	22	29	–	–	–	23	29	–	–	–
C. Maternal conditions	**534**		**534**								**505**	**30**	
1. Maternal haemorrhage	83		83								75	8	
2. Maternal sepsis	93		93								92	1	
3. Hypertensive disorders of pregnancy	19		19								17	2	
4. Obstructed labour	113		113								113	2	
5. Abortion	16		16								15	2	
D. Perinatal conditions*	**3 909**	**1 931**	**1 978**	**1 931**					**1 978**				
E. Nutritional deficiencies	**4 075**	**2 083**	**1 992**	**535**	**258**	**773**	**266**	**251**	**657**	**260**	**461**	**322**	**292**
1. Protein-energy malnutrition	735	317	417	287	1	2	3	24	391	1	2	2	22
2. Iodine deficiency	164	86	78	77	6	3	–	–	69	6	2	–	–
3. Vitamin A deficiency	109	57	52	41	14	2	–	–	37	13	1	–	–
4. Iron-deficiency anaemia	3 067	1 623	1 444	130	237	766	263	227	160	239	455	319	270
II. Noncommunicable diseases	**198 008**	**113 643**	**84 364**	**4 506**	**1 405**	**25 199**	**45 088**	**37 446**	**4 497**	**1 008**	**22 792**	**25 725**	**30 342**
A. Malignant neoplasms	**43 480**	**29 991**	**13 489**	**155**	**405**	**5 371**	**15 184**	**8 876**	**234**	**196**	**2 449**	**5 628**	**4 981**
1. Mouth and oropharynx cancers	1 267	921	346	6	9	313	395	198			99	151	95
2. Oesophagus cancer	4 658	3 419	1 239			324	1 736	1 359			51	474	714
3. Stomach cancer	8 487	5 986	2 501		9	489	3 172	2 316		8	388	955	1 150
4. Colon and rectum cancers	2 329	1 390	939		8	291	631	459		10	150	395	385
5. Liver cancer	9 785	7 777	2 007	6	25	2 070	4 228	1 448	8	23	365	936	675
6. Pancreas cancer	733	491	242			59	226	206	1		13	78	149
7. Trachea, bronchus, lung cancers	7 409	5 789	1 620	6	16	573	3 174	2 020			91	787	743
8. Melanoma and other skin cancers	30	19	11			4	8	6			2	4	5
9. Breast cancer	765		765								232	357	176
10. Cervix uteri cancer	570		570								102	281	188
11. Corpus uteri cancer	200		200								25	137	37
12. Ovary cancer	303		303						5	7	98	131	62
13. Prostate cancer	91	91				4	17	70					
14. Bladder cancer	419	343	76			27	118	197			4	19	53
15. Lymphomas and multiple myeloma	668	461	208		34	104	194	129			40	116	51
16. Leukaemia	2 214	1 241	973	87	203	521	338	92	108	101	436	222	106
C. Diabetes mellitus	**1 485**	**676**	**809**	**7**	**8**	**132**	**287**	**240**	**7**	**8**	**86**	**303**	**405**
D. Endocrine disorders	**527**	**165**	**362**	**17**	**8**	**46**	**57**	**36**	**118**	**18**	**116**	**48**	**62**

Annex Table 19d, continued. DALYs by age, sex and cause (thousands): China, 2020, pessimistic scenario

Cause	Total	Male	Female	Males 0-4	5-14	15-44	45-59	60+	Females 0-4	5-14	15-44	45-59	60+
E. Neuro-psychiatric conditions	**34 647**	**15 400**	**19 248**	**214**	**322**	**11 140**	**2 458**	**1 264**	**175**	**326**	**13 343**	**3 436**	**1 968**
1. Unipolar major depression	15 962	5 685	10 277	-	-	4 183	1 233	268	-	-	7 511	2 212	555
2. Bipolar disorder	4 184	2 128	2 056	-	-	1 853	215	59	-	-	1 767	213	76
3. Schizophrenia	2 718	1 463	1 255	15	55	1 425	18	20	14	59	1 210	25	20
4. Epilepsy	711	385	326	-	-	217	72	25	-	-	175	50	29
5. Alcohol use	1 706	1 583	123	-	-	1 363	194	26	-	-	110	11	2
6. Dementia*	2 813	1 242	1 572	58	22	61	369	732	56	18	56	393	1 048
7. Parkinson disease	200	95	106	-	-	-	44	51	-	-	-	44	62
8. Multiple sclerosis	374	162	212	-	13	129	25	8	-	1	162	35	14
9. Drug use	199	179	20	-	30	153	11	1	-	-	17	1	-
10. Post-traumatic stress disorder	484	185	299	7	-	122	22	3	12	49	197	34	6
11. Obsessive-compulsive disorders	2 711	1 168	1 543	-	106	916	105	41	-	134	1 161	183	65
12. Panic disorder	1 377	470	907	-	37	318	114	1	-	37	664	179	26
F. Sense organ diseases	**4 127**	**1 729**	**2 398**	**38**	-	**89**	**835**	**766**	**30**	**12**	**166**	**1 252**	**938**
1. Glaucoma	1 663	478	1 186	6	-	32	291	149	8	-	74	853	251
2. Cataracts	2 176	1 156	1 020	14	-	48	500	593	2	-	38	337	643
G. Cardiovascular diseases	**41 890**	**25 753**	**16 136**	**308**	**86**	**2 624**	**10 949**	**11 787**	**174**	**44**	**1 777**	**4 769**	**9 371**
1. Rheumatic heart disease	3 289	1 644	1 646	-	14	433	729	468	18	14	406	639	569
2. Ischaemic heart disease	11 902	7 396	4 507	72	37	650	3 172	3 574	45	13	349	1 209	2 949
3. Cerebrovascular disease	20 890	13 016	7 873	54	14	1 115	5 508	6 285	36	9	672	2 421	4 722
4. Inflammatory heart diseases	1 667	1 016	651	-	-	293	453	202	-	-	213	214	179
H. Respiratory diseases	**44 119**	**25 712**	**18 407**	**564**	**269**	**3 585**	**10 088**	**11 207**	**410**	**140**	**2 593**	**5 857**	**9 407**
1. COPD*	38 605	22 423	16 182	97	5	2 417	9 242	10 661	168	3	1 720	5 361	8 931
2. Asthma	3 588	2 114	1 474	119	243	943	601	208	56	123	739	391	165
I. Digestive diseases	**10 702**	**6 268**	**4 433**	**526**	**65**	**1 162**	**2 783**	**1 732**	**575**	**57**	**738**	**1 692**	**1 371**
1. Peptic ulcer	587	365	222	4	2	82	148	129	4	2	41	73	103
2. Cirrhosis of the liver	4 190	2 855	1 335	27	9	650	1 396	773	9	11	191	626	499
3. Appendicitis	210	122	88	2	22	76	16	6	2	19	53	10	4
J. Genito-urinary diseases	**3 096**	**2 066**	**1 030**	**66**	**44**	**413**	**1 132**	**411**	**64**	**30**	**268**	**315**	**353**
1. Nephritis and nephrosis	1 631	912	719	44	44	378	235	211	64	30	224	176	224
2. Benign prostatic hypertrophy	927	927	-	6	-	7	804	110	-	-	-	-	-
L. Musculo-skeletal diseases	**6 008**	**1 995**	**4 013**	-	**17**	**304**	**890**	**783**	**19**	**14**	**878**	**2 033**	**1 069**
1. Rheumatoid arthritis	1 183	365	818	-	-	87	213	65	-	6	183	428	201
2. Osteoarthritis	4 008	1 334	2 674	-	-	175	612	547	-	-	547	1 458	669

Annex Table 19d, continued. DALYs by age, sex and cause (thousands): China, 2020, pessimistic scenario

Cause	Total	Males	Females	Males					Females				
				0-4	5-14	15-44	45-59	60+	0-4	5-14	15-44	45-59	60+
M. Congenital anomalies	5 208	2 548	2 660	2 318	100	121	8	-	2 410	103	137	10	-
N. Oral conditions	1 484	709	776	175	36	66	218	214	166	36	83	225	265
1. Dental caries	640	325	316	173	35	45	51	20	165	33	43	50	24
2. Periodontal disease	39	20	19	-	-	16	3	1	-	-	15	3	1
3. Edentulism	768	357	411	-	-	-	164	192	-	-	-	171	240
III. Injuries	*38 782*	*22 593*	*16 189*	*2 991*	*1 786*	*12 000*	*4 028*	*1 788*	*2 845*	*1 295*	*7 359*	*2 960*	*1 730*
A. Unintentional injuries	27 093	17 463	9 630	2 816	1 645	8 777	3 006	1 220	2 524	1 160	3 032	1 787	1 127
1. Road traffic accidents	9 444	6 678	2 767	140	588	4 009	1 418	522	102	568	1 202	670	225
2. Poisonings	1 353	794	559	151	37	292	232	83	44	48	288	88	91
3. Falls	3 775	2 016	1 759	402	186	978	286	164	493	118	389	378	381
4. Fires	559	302	256	82	40	108	34	38	53	55	38	48	63
5. Drownings	2 966	1 853	1 113	680	448	542	114	69	539	207	199	81	87
6. Other unintentional	8 996	5 821	3 176	1 362	346	2 847	921	344	1 293	163	916	523	280
B. Intentional injuries	11 689	5 130	6 559	175	141	3 223	1 022	569	321	136	4 327	1 173	603
1. Self-inflicted injuries	9 917	4 067	5 850	-	94	2 509	927	537	-	70	4 107	1 105	568
2. Violence	1 746	1 037	709	175	47	689	95	31	321	66	220	68	35
3. War	26	26	-	-	-	26	-	-	-	-	-	-	-

Notes:
A dash (-) symbol indicates fewer than 500 DALYs.

*IA6 is Bacterial meningitis and meningococcaemia; ID is Conditions arising during the perinatal period;
IIE6 is Dementia and other degenerative and hereditary CNS disorders; IIH1 is Chronic obstructive pulmonary disease.

Annex Table 19e. DALYs by age, sex and cause (thousands): Other Asia and Islands, 2020, pessimistic scenario

Cause	Total	Male	Female	Males					Females				
				0-4	5-14	15-44	45-59	60+	0-4	5-14	15-44	45-59	60+
Population (millions)	*1 002*	*497*	*505*	*43*	*81*	*238*	*85*	*51*	*41*	*79*	*234*	*89*	*62*
All causes	**203 969**	**113 244**	**90 725**	**22 482**	**7 824**	**39 957**	**24 396**	**18 585**	**18 068**	**5 555**	**30 916**	**17 019**	**19 128**
I. Communicable, maternal, perinatal and nutritional conditions	*52 300*	*26 726*	*25 575*	*15 580*	*2 021*	*5 466*	*1 779*	*1 880*	*12 230*	*1 781*	*7 746*	*1 798*	*2 020*
A. Infectious and parasitic diseases	29 930	15 849	14 081	7 241	1 271	4 711	1 518	1 108	5 573	1 107	4 792	1 400	1 209
1. Tuberculosis	4 817	2 449	2 368	21	41	752	851	784	7	40	566	874	880
2. STDs excluding HIV	2 656	932	1 723	451	6	436	13	26	354	23	1 288	21	37
a. Syphilis	729	402	327	307	1	57	11	26	212	1	63	15	36
b. Chlamydia	1 123	165	958	33	2	129	1	-	33	17	904	4	-
c. Gonorrhoea	804	365	439	111	3	250	1	-	109	6	321	2	-
3. HIV	6 733	3 796	2 937	618	111	2 667	325	74	397	77	2 269	162	32
4. Diarrhoeal diseases	7 149	4 067	3 082	3 667	214	78	46	62	2 673	162	108	68	71
5. Childhood-cluster diseases	4 113	2 184	1 930	1 843	206	96	25	13	1 607	201	78	29	15
a. Pertussis	665	353	311	324	29	-	1	-	286	26	-	1	-
b. Poliomyelitis	211	123	88	116	-	6	-	-	82	-	4	-	-
c. Diphtheria	41	22	19	20	2	-	-	-	17	2	-	-	-
d. Measles	1 961	1 043	918	921	118	2	1	-	813	103	2	1	-
e. Tetanus	1 236	643	593	462	56	87	24	13	408	70	73	28	15
6. Bacterial meningitis*	508	265	243	152	8	54	30	21	137	8	42	33	22
7. Hepatitis B and hepatitis C	265	156	109	27	13	40	42	34	20	11	26	21	31
8. Malaria	1 280	694	586	111	193	287	75	28	99	168	205	84	31
9. Tropical-cluster diseases	349	241	108	6	38	150	41	7	4	12	51	35	6
a. Trypanosomiasis													
b. Chagas disease													
c. Schistosomiasis	10	6	4	-	-	2	2	2	-	-	1	2	2
d. Leishmaniasis	38	25	14	1	5	16	2	1	-	3	8	1	-
e. Lymphatic filariasis	300	211	90	5	32	131	37	5	4	8	42	32	4
f. Onchocerciasis													
10. Leprosy	31	16	15	-	4	6	4	2	3	3	6	2	1
11. Dengue	110	52	58	13	37	1	1	-	15	41	1	1	-
12. Japanese encephalitis	87	46	40	28	14	4	1	-	25	12	3	1	-
13. Trachoma	58	14	43	-	-	2	5	8	-	-	4	14	26
14. Intestinal nematode infections	831	428	403	4	311	81	21	11	4	294	70	22	14
a. Ascariasis	246	127	119	4	122	1	-	-	3	115	1	-	-
b. Trichuriasis	332	171	162	-	171	-	-	-	-	161	-	-	-
c. Ancylostomiasis and necatoriasis	253	131	123	-	18	80	20	11	-	18	69	22	14

Annex Table 19e, continued. DALYs by age, sex and cause (thousands): Other Asia and Islands, 2020, pessimistic scenario

Cause	Total	Male	Female	Males					Females				
				0-4	5-14	15-44	45-59	60+	0-4	5-14	15-44	45-59	60+
B. Respiratory infections	8 956	4 978	3 978	3 513	515	196	111	644	2 595	456	153	123	651
1. Lower respiratory infections	8 711	4 845	3 866	3 442	470	188	108	637	2 541	414	147	121	643
2. Upper respiratory infections	104	57	47	34	6	7	2	7	25	6	6	3	8
3. Otitis media	141	76	66	36	38	1	-	-	29	36	1	-	-
C. Maternal conditions	1 961		1 961								1 922	39	-
1. Maternal haemorrhage	191		191								183	9	
2. Maternal sepsis	344		344								338	6	
3. Hypertensive disorders of pregnancy	93		93								89	4	
4. Obstructed labour	438		438								436	3	
5. Abortion	375		375								370	5	
D. Perinatal conditions*	6 786	3 727	3 058	3 727					3 058				
E. Nutritional deficiencies	4 667	2 172	2 495	1 099	235	560	150	128	1 005	217	879	235	160
1. Protein-energy malnutrition	1 541	806	735	783	6	3	5	9	714	4	4	5	8
2. Iodine deficiency	87	45	42	39	4	2	-	-	37	4	2	-	-
3. Vitamin A deficiency	301	161	140	107	50	4	-	-	94	43	2	-	-
4. Iron-deficiency anaemia	2 738	1 160	1 578	171	175	551	144	119	160	166	871	230	151
II. Noncommunicable diseases	121 176	65 597	55 579	4 415	3 128	21 744	20 182	16 128	3 674	2 342	18 556	14 269	16 737
A. Malignant neoplasms	19 851	11 476	8 375	217	632	2 353	4 651	3 622	253	398	1 953	2 857	2 915
1. Mouth and oropharynx cancers	1 849	1 158	691	6	18	273	315	546	8	14	154	131	383
2. Oesophagus cancer	638	426	212			40	223	163			28	77	107
3. Stomach cancer	1 684	1 136	549	1	2	183	577	374		1	92	212	243
4. Colon and rectum cancers	1 070	569	501	2	6	135	151	275		4	90	118	286
5. Liver cancer	2 132	1 664	468	8	23	363	925	346	7	11	74	182	193
6. Pancreas cancer	259	167	92			29	75	63			7	35	47
7. Trachea, bronchus, lung cancers	3 068	2 375	693	3	7	354	1 281	731	1	4	52	292	341
8. Melanoma and other skin cancers	69	32	38		1	9	14	7			8	13	17
9. Breast cancer	929		929							3	280	433	211
10. Cervix uteri cancer	1 086		1 086							1	269	574	242
11. Corpus uteri cancer	112		112							2	15	52	43
12. Ovary cancer	364		364						10	15	157	113	69
13. Prostate cancer	267	267				5	59	200					
14. Bladder cancer	274	204	70			18	81	106		1	6	16	47
15. Lymphomas and multiple myeloma	735	467	268	28	79	154	93	113	16	24	68	45	115
16. Leukaemia	1 066	604	462	76	214	200	52	63	92	141	121	40	68
C. Diabetes mellitus	2 151	1 006	1 145	8	18	252	417	311	9	17	179	421	519
D. Endocrine disorders	496	223	273	94	31	37	34	26	76	17	57	58	66

Annex Table 19e, continued. DALYs by age, sex and cause (thousands): Other Asia and Islands, 2020, pessimistic scenario

Cause	Total	Male	Female	Males					Females				
				0-4	5-14	15-44	45-59	60+	0-4	5-14	15-44	45-59	60+
E. Neuro-psychiatric conditions	29 289	14 497	14 792	184	421	11 320	1 702	870	183	400	10 825	2 068	1 316
1. Unipolar major depression	10 815	3 773	7 042	-	-	3 005	626	143	-	-	5 545	1 189	308
2. Bipolar disorder	2 925	1 470	1 455	-	-	1 327	110	33	-	-	1 298	113	44
3. Schizophrenia	3 347	1 750	1 597	-	-	1 711	24	15	-	-	1 560	10	27
4. Epilepsy	870	491	379	14	102	270	81	25	15	111	183	45	25
5. Alcohol use	2 935	2 717	218	-	-	2 447	229	42	-	-	199	14	5
6. Dementia*	1 890	802	1 088	38	17	50	258	439	45	18	46	286	693
7. Parkinson disease	238	125	113	-	-	-	54	71	-	-	-	46	66
8. Multiple sclerosis	259	112	147	-	-	95	13	4	-	-	121	18	7
9. Drug use	1 357	1 223	134	-	61	1 091	60	10	-	7	119	7	1
10. Post-traumatic stress disorder	360	135	225	6	24	92	11	2	9	40	153	19	3
11. Obsessive-compulsive disorders	2 003	854	1 149	-	85	691	55	23	-	109	900	103	37
12. Panic disorder	990	330	660	-	30	240	60	-	-	30	514	100	15
F. Sense organ diseases	4 055	1 785	2 270	6	4	105	930	741	6	-	126	1 193	945
1. Glaucoma	1 281	374	907	-	-	20	257	96	-	-	61	673	172
2. Cataracts	2 757	1 400	1 357	-	-	82	672	644	-	-	64	519	771
G. Cardiovascular diseases	30 101	16 998	13 104	1 084	1 104	3 744	5 102	5 963	811	802	2 273	2 709	6 508
1. Rheumatic heart disease	245	116	130	-	6	32	32	46	-	8	35	31	56
2. Ischaemic heart disease	9 266	5 286	3 980	-	-	842	1 863	2 581	-	-	438	864	2 678
3. Cerebrovascular disease	8 484	4 599	3 885	135	221	876	1 472	1 894	105	151	515	921	2 192
4. Inflammatory heart diseases	2 593	1 527	1 065	212	246	572	340	158	191	185	338	179	173
H. Respiratory diseases	8 020	4 543	3 477	592	367	1 034	1 151	1 399	372	241	854	735	1 275
1. COPD*	3 023	1 813	1 210	59	20	303	595	836	40	16	179	297	678
2. Asthma	2 128	1 171	958	91	210	574	198	99	45	132	459	202	119
I. Digestive diseases	13 512	8 330	5 182	394	238	1 723	3 890	2 085	326	192	934	2 050	1 680
1. Peptic ulcer	625	405	220	3	6	103	158	134	3	5	48	64	100
2. Cirrhosis of the liver	4 460	3 361	1 099	23	23	812	1 801	701	16	23	195	499	366
3. Appendicitis	255	150	105	2	41	90	13	4	2	36	56	8	3
J. Genito-urinary diseases	2 769	1 557	1 211	57	132	280	736	353	38	97	249	326	502
1. Nephritis and nephrosis	1 720	828	892	41	113	235	208	231	38	84	183	219	367
2. Benign prostatic hypertrophy	496	496		-	-	-	449	47	-	-	-	-	-
L. Musculo-skeletal diseases	4 324	1 844	2 479	16	17	350	1 067	395	16	20	574	1 329	541
1. Rheumatoid arthritis	429	123	306	-	-	6	42	75	-	2	73	70	161
2. Osteoarthritis	3 503	1 584	1 919	-	-	315	987	282	-	-	429	1 197	294

Annex Table 19e, continued. DALYs by age, sex and cause (thousands): Other Asia and Islands, 2020, pessimistic scenario

Cause	Total	Males	Females	Males					Females				
				0-4	5-14	15-44	45-59	60+	0-4	5-14	15-44	45-59	60+
M. Congenital anomalies	3 486	1 837	1 649	1 659	72	79	20	7	1 501	69	49	21	10
N. Oral conditions	2 455	1 163	1 292	30	43	394	386	310	29	43	401	421	398
1. Dental caries	876	431	445	29	42	170	134	56	28	41	167	141	69
2. Periodontal disease	57	28	29	-	-	20	6	2	-	-	20	6	3
3. Edentulism	1 500	700	800	-	-	201	246	253	-	-	201	273	326
III. Injuries	30 493	20 922	9 571	2 487	2 676	12 746	2 435	578	2 163	1 432	4 613	952	411
A. Unintentional injuries	24 572	17 045	7 527	2 387	2 480	9 812	1 925	441	2 055	1 305	3 048	779	339
1. Road traffic accidents	7 432	5 274	2 158	471	753	3 286	597	167	433	418	931	255	122
2. Poisonings	1 176	618	558	61	65	358	102	33	56	71	341	58	33
3. Falls	4 089	2 709	1 380	627	405	1 353	271	53	485	198	514	142	41
4. Fires	454	241	213	52	57	106	20	7	76	67	53	10	7
5. Drownings	2 308	1 593	715	480	478	524	82	30	302	196	166	31	19
6. Other unintentional	9 113	6 610	2 503	697	723	4 186	853	151	704	355	1 044	284	116
B. Intentional injuries	5 921	3 877	2 044	100	196	2 934	510	137	108	127	1 565	173	72
1. Self-inflicted injuries	2 857	1 603	1 254	-	69	1 212	235	88	-	43	1 050	110	51
2. Violence	2 289	1 824	465	43	89	1 397	252	43	50	55	301	46	13
3. War	775	450	324	57	37	326	23	6	57	29	214	17	8

Notes:

A dash (-) symbol indicates fewer than 500 DALYs.

[a]IA6 is Bacterial meningitis and meningococcaemia; ID is Conditions arising during the perinatal period;
IIE6 is Dementia and other degenerative and hereditary CNS disorders; IIH1 is Chronic obstructive pulmonary disease.

Annex Table 19f. DALYs by age, sex and cause (thousands): Sub-Saharan Africa, 2020, pessimistic scenario

Cause	Total	Male	Female	Males					Females				
				0-4	5-14	15-44	45-59	60+	0-4	5-14	15-44	45-59	60+
Population (millions)	*1 120*	*555*	*565*	*85*	*140*	*255*	*49*	*26*	*82*	*137*	*260*	*54*	*31*
All causes	*422 751*	*233 605*	*189 147*	*98 585*	*23 057*	*83 207*	*17 302*	*11 453*	*80 636*	*19 371*	*60 018*	*15 852*	*13 270*
I. Communicable, maternal, perinatal and nutritional conditions	*221 955*	*113 951*	*108 003*	*83 200*	*8 382*	*17 527*	*3 121*	*1 721*	*67 257*	*8 262*	*27 510*	*2 954*	*2 021*
A. Infectious and parasitic diseases	*153 179*	*80 164*	*73 015*	*53 007*	*6 342*	*16 780*	*2 965*	*1 069*	*42 567*	*6 248*	*20 255*	*2 759*	*1 186*
1. Tuberculosis	*25 966*	*12 237*	*13 729*	*1 241*	*990*	*7 538*	*1 897*	*572*	*1 323*	*1 414*	*8 589*	*1 817*	*587*
2. STDs excluding HIV	**5 833**	**2 336**	**3 497**	**1 621**	**13**	**645**	**18**	**39**	**1 478**	**49**	**1 887**	**28**	**56**
a. Syphilis	2 726	1 420	1 306	1 250	2	115	16	38	1 096	2	133	21	55
b. Chlamydia	1 503	215	1 288	69	4	142	1	-	71	32	1 181	4	-
c. Gonorrhoea	1 604	701	902	303	8	389	2	-	311	16	573	3	-
3. HIV	*20 640*	*9 501*	*11 139*	*3 011*	*461*	*5 583*	*373*	*73*	*2 864*	*479*	*7 470*	*279*	*47*
4. Diarrhoeal diseases	*32 897*	*18 497*	*14 400*	*16 952*	*1 089*	*273*	*65*	*118*	*12 703*	*1 073*	*394*	*81*	*150*
5. Childhood-cluster diseases	**30 836**	**16 701**	**14 135**	**14 905**	**1 620**	**133**	**27**	**15**	**12 461**	**1 516**	**120**	**24**	**14**
a. Pertussis	5 674	3 084	2 590	2 850	234				2 378	212			
b. Poliomyelitis	619	364	256	356	2	6			250	1	4		
c. Diphtheria	65	35	30	32	3				26	3			
d. Measles	20 128	10 880	9 248	9 621	1 257	2			8 086	1 160	2		
e. Tetanus	4 349	2 338	2 012	2 047	124	125	26	15	1 721	140	114	23	14
6. Bacterial meningitis*	**993**	**520**	**472**	**432**	**14**	**49**	**17**	**9**	**381**	**13**	**48**	**18**	**13**
7. Hepatitis B and hepatitis C	**278**	**157**	**121**	**43**	**20**	**41**	**29**	**24**	**30**	**18**	**35**	**14**	**23**
8. Malaria	*27 277*	*15 256*	*12 021*	*13 472*	*893*	*738*	*116*	*37*	*10 283*	*850*	*713*	*125*	*50*
9. Tropical-cluster diseases	**4 487**	**2 890**	**1 597**	**101**	**895**	**1 470**	**329**	**94**	**107**	**505**	**693**	**229**	**63**
a. Trypanosomiasis	1 126	590	536	20	202	272	82	14	36	196	240	55	10
b. Chagas disease													
c. Schistosomiasis	1 013	633	381	27	217	311	52	25	17	136	178	33	16
d. Leishmaniasis	361	244	117	13	129	97	4		6	62	47	3	
e. Lymphatic filariasis	1 231	968	263	33	280	583	67	5	43	60	102	52	7
f. Onchocerciasis	756	456	300	8	67	206	125	50	6	51	127	86	30
10. Leprosy	**25**	**13**	**12**		**4**	**7**	**1**			**3**	**7**	**1**	
11. Dengue	**17**	**8**	**9**	**2**	**6**				**2**	**7**			
12. Japanese encephalitis													
13. Trachoma	*376*	*101*	*275*			**22**	*32*	*47*			*47*	*86*	*142*
14. Intestinal nematode infections	**411**	**212**	**199**	**2**	**99**	**90**	**14**	**7**	**1**	**95**	**79**	**15**	**8**
a. Ascariasis	77	40	38	2	38				1	36			
b. Trichuriasis	77	40	38		40					38			
c. Ancylostomiasis and necatoriasis	257	133	123		22	90	14	7		21	79	15	8

Annex Table 19f, continued. DALYs by age, sex and cause (thousands): Sub-Saharan Africa, 2020, pessimistic scenario

Cause	Total	Male	Female	Males					Females				
				0-4	5-14	15-44	45-59	60+	0-4	5-14	15-44	45-59	60+
B. Respiratory infections	**32 321**	**18 120**	**14 202**	**15 567**	**1 524**	**361**	**89**	**579**	**11 716**	**1 240**	**400**	**98**	**748**
1. Lower respiratory infections	31 601	17 721	13 880	15 271	1 439	351	87	573	11 490	1 163	391	96	740
2. Upper respiratory infections	334	187	147	154	18	8	2	6	115	15	8	2	8
3. Otitis media	387	212	175	143	68	2			110	62	2		
C. Maternal conditions	**6 649**		**6 649**								**6 361**	**6**	
1. Maternal haemorrhage	960		960								893	1	
2. Maternal sepsis	1 262		1 262								1 218	1	
3. Hypertensive disorders of pregnancy	475		475								442	1	
4. Obstructed labour	1 162		1 162								1 140		
5. Abortion	1 170		1 170								1 133	1	
D. Perinatal conditions*	**20 595**	**10 922**	**9 673**	**10 922**					**9 673**				
E. Nutritional deficiencies	**9 210**	**4 746**	**4 464**	**3 704**	**516**	**386**	**67**	**72**	**3 301**	**491**	**494**	**92**	**86**
1. Protein-energy malnutrition	5 696	3 001	2 695	2 924	30	19	9	20	2 602	30	32	8	22
2. Iodine deficiency	128	64	64	57	5	2			54	6	6	1	
3. Vitamin A deficiency	1 128	596	531	427	162	7			370	154	7		
4. Iron-deficiency anaemia	2 258	1 084	1 173	297	319	358	58	52	275	301	450	83	64
II. Noncommunicable diseases	***108 136***	***55 285***	***52 851***	***7 301***	***4 057***	***23 300***	***11 515***	***9 112***	***6 951***	***4 282***	***18 826***	***11 953***	***10 838***
A. Malignant neoplasms	**14 056**	**7 914**	**6 142**	**237**	**726**	**2 521**	**2 375**	**2 056**	**308**	**723**	**1 353**	**2 152**	**1 606**
1. Mouth and oropharynx cancers	645	393	252	2	6	123	88	174	10	28	55	46	114
2. Oesophagus cancer	665	505	159			115	257	134			26	65	68
3. Stomach cancer	915	551	364	1	3	128	250	169	1		61	189	114
4. Colon and rectum cancers	395	223	171	1	3	77	52	91	1		36	40	93
5. Liver cancer	2 061	1 614	447	5	19	817	568	205	7		128	171	121
6. Pancreas cancer	199	118	81			32	55	31			16	41	24
7. Trachea, bronchus, lung cancers	697	445	252		1	138	174	132		1	52	122	78
8. Melanoma and other skin cancers	214	96	119		1	21	46	28			13	49	55
9. Breast cancer	523		523								140	244	135
10. Cervix uteri cancer	955		955							3	214	465	274
11. Corpus uteri cancer	87		87								11	39	36
12. Ovary cancer	248		248								68	97	53
13. Prostate cancer	643	643				16	165	462					
14. Bladder cancer	363	240	123			47	93	99			26	49	47
15. Lymphomas and multiple myeloma	1 194	740	454	83	296	189	81	91	77	208	69	46	55
16. Leukaemia	398	182	217	15	52	67	17	31	34	93	36	28	26
C. Diabetes mellitus	**757**	**366**	**391**	**24**	**58**	**90**	**111**	**84**	**28**	**56**	**57**	**118**	**133**
D. Endocrine disorders	**1 633**	**817**	**817**	**347**	**48**	**212**	**152**	**58**	**218**	**90**	**172**	**176**	**161**

Annex Table 19f, continued. DALYs by age, sex and cause (thousands): Sub-Saharan Africa, 2020, pessimistic scenario

Cause	Total	Male	Female	Males 0-4	5-14	15-44	45-59	60+	Females 0-4	5-14	15-44	45-59	60+
E. Neuro-psychiatric conditions	**27 521**	**13 283**	**14 239**	**326**	**564**	**11 137**	**926**	**330**	**379**	**588**	**11 499**	**1 174**	**599**
1. Unipolar major depression	11 157	3 809	7 348	-	-	3 351	381	78	-	-	6 429	750	169
2. Bipolar disorder	3 209	1 584	1 625	-	-	1 499	67	18	-	-	1 527	74	23
3. Schizophrenia	1 093	568	525	-	-	560	5	3	-	-	518	3	5
4. Epilepsy	731	410	320	38	114	214	33	12	44	107	140	18	12
5. Alcohol use	4 277	3 463	814	-	-	3 257	182	24	-	-	765	37	12
6. Dementia*	748	240	508	28	13	27	59	114	75	35	51	68	279
7. Parkinson disease	111	58	53	-	-	-	27	31	-	-	-	24	29
8. Multiple sclerosis	245	105	140	-	-	96	7	2	-	-	125	11	4
9. Drug use	890	803	87	-	51	724	24	4	-	6	78	3	-
10. Post-traumatic stress disorder	432	160	272	11	42	99	7	1	18	70	171	12	2
11. Obsessive-compulsive disorders	2 208	932	1 276	-	146	742	32	12	-	191	1 004	62	19
12. Panic disorder	1 048	347	701	-	52	259	35	-	-	53	579	61	8
F. Sense organ diseases	**4 368**	**2 046**	**2 322**	**11**	**1**	**159**	**990**	**885**	**11**	**1**	**134**	**1 126**	**1 051**
1. Glaucoma	951	377	574	-	-	3	182	192	-	-	5	292	277
2. Cataracts	3 403	1 660	1 743	11	1	147	807	693	11	1	124	834	774
G. Cardiovascular diseases	**21 769**	**10 724**	**11 045**	**694**	**802**	**3 706**	**2 696**	**2 826**	**647**	**985**	**1 888**	**3 185**	**4 340**
1. Rheumatic heart disease	871	455	416	2	131	292	24	6	2	171	193	38	11
2. Ischaemic heart disease	5 067	2 518	2 549	-	-	745	836	937	-	-	279	834	1 245
3. Cerebrovascular disease	9 278	4 352	4 926	112	277	1 485	1 135	1 343	107	247	691	1 565	2 317
4. Inflammatory heart diseases	2 377	1 215	1 162	185	128	482	232	188	240	191	258	201	271
H. Respiratory diseases	**14 583**	**7 761**	**6 822**	**1 050**	**709**	**2 580**	**1 730**	**1 693**	**795**	**652**	**1 630**	**2 092**	**1 653**
1. COPD*	4 297	2 482	1 815	87	49	751	689	906	73	54	289	670	730
2. Asthma	2 445	1 235	1 210	132	340	589	102	72	81	283	581	174	91
I. Digestive diseases	**7 860**	**4 641**	**3 219**	**457**	**367**	**1 630**	**1 482**	**705**	**442**	**516**	**842**	**763**	**656**
1. Peptic ulcer	496	320	175	-	-	179	103	38	-	-	71	63	41
2. Cirrhosis of the liver	1 087	787	300	-	31	302	310	144	-	18	89	113	80
3. Appendicitis	488	304	184	7	114	168	13	3	7	104	60	10	3
J. Genito-urinary diseases	**3 752**	**2 272**	**1 480**	**433**	**447**	**500**	**658**	**233**	**318**	**347**	**287**	**306**	**221**
1. Nephritis and nephrosis	2 591	1 463	1 128	361	377	405	161	159	306	302	185	186	149
2. Benign prostatic hypertrophy	427	427	-	-	-	-	409	18	-	-	-	-	-
L. Musculo-skeletal diseases	**2 542**	**851**	**1 690**	-	-	**443**	**281**	**127**	-	**4**	**684**	**743**	**259**
1. Rheumatoid arthritis	212	59	153	-	-	38	16	6	-	4	94	42	13
2. Osteoarthritis	2 298	778	1 520	-	-	397	262	118	-	-	580	696	243

Annex Table 19f, continued. DALYs by age, sex and cause (thousands): Sub-Saharan Africa, 2020, pessimistic scenario

Cause	Total	Males	Females	Males					Females				
				0-4	5-14	15-44	45-59	60+	0-4	5-14	15-44	45-59	60+
M. Congenital anomalies	6 711	3 261	3 450	3 009	117	112	16	6	3 246	127	47	22	9
N. Oral conditions	848	407	441	84	100	117	26	80	82	103	127	29	100
1. Dental caries	593	296	297	82	97	85	23	8	79	95	87	25	10
2. Periodontal disease	66	32	33	-	-	30	3	-	-	-	30	3	-
3. Edentulism	161	71	90	-	-	-	-	71	-	-	-	-	90
III. Injuries	92 661	64 369	28 292	8 085	10 617	42 380	2 667	620	6 427	6 828	13 682	944	411
A. Unintentional injuries	51 640	35 853	15 787	5 943	8 470	19 382	1 658	398	4 456	5 527	5 033	520	251
1. Road traffic accidents	12 349	8 717	3 632	638	2 621	4 907	444	107	433	1 376	1 636	152	34
2. Poisonings	2 182	1 272	911	861	207	155	35	13	642	101	153	9	6
3. Falls	3 648	2 102	1 546	399	851	695	111	46	442	511	441	69	83
4. Fires	6 000	2 990	3 009	1 120	895	846	94	36	976	1 195	727	67	45
5. Drownings	5 012	3 661	1 351	958	1 687	925	70	21	494	651	182	16	7
6. Other unintentional	22 449	17 111	5 339	1 968	2 209	11 854	905	175	1 468	1 693	1 896	206	76
B. Intentional injuries	41 021	28 516	12 505	2 141	2 147	22 998	1 009	222	1 971	1 301	8 649	424	160
1. Self-inflicted injuries	1 132	906	226	-	103	736	52	14	-	-	207	18	2
2. Violence	15 718	13 599	2 119	275	662	12 026	541	95	136	273	1 558	117	34
3. War	24 170	14 011	10 160	1 866	1 381	10 236	416	112	1 835	1 028	6 884	289	123

Notes:
A dash (-) symbol indicates fewer than 500 DALYs.
*IA6 is Bacterial meningitis and meningococcaemia; ID is Conditions arising during the perinatal period;
IIE6 is Dementia and other degenerative and hereditary CNS disorders; IIH1 is Chronic obstructive pulmonary disease.

Annex Table 19g. DALYs by age, sex and cause (thousands): Latin America and the Caribbean, 2020, pessimistic scenario

Cause	Total	Male	Female	Males					Females				
				0-4	5-14	15-44	45-59	60+	0-4	5-14	15-44	45-59	60+
Population (millions)	667	331	336	28	54	156	55	37	27	52	155	57	44
All causes	128 606	72 131	56 475	10 948	4 268	31 540	14 246	11 129	8 553	3 127	21 071	12 501	11 222
I. Communicable, maternal, perinatal and nutritional conditions	25 672	14 278	11 395	7 624	777	4 401	782	693	5 772	812	3 614	556	641
A. Infectious and parasitic diseases	14 698	8 884	5 814	3 196	527	4 144	625	392	2 467	542	2 109	385	311
1. Tuberculosis	1 309	759	550	30	33	348	189	159	23	48	259	121	99
2. STDs excluding HIV	863	232	631	119	1	104	3	5	99	9	511	5	7
a. Syphilis	228	122	106	101	-	13	2	5	82	-	15	3	7
b. Chlamydia	429	40	389	4	-	34	-	-	4	7	377	1	-
c. Gonorrhoea	206	70	136	13	1	56	-	-	13	2	120	-	-
3. HIV	4 602	3 634	967	196	18	3 151	219	51	182	21	726	31	8
4. Diarrhoeal diseases	3 136	1 789	1 348	1 531	100	72	36	49	1 060	104	83	41	59
5. Childhood-cluster diseases	1 902	1 016	885	931	73	7	3	2	798	73	9	4	2
a. Pertussis	402	213	189	196	17	-	-	-	172	17	-	-	-
b. Poliomyelitis	119	69	49	67	-	2	-	-	48	-	1	-	-
c. Diphtheria	9	4	4	3	1	-	-	-	2	2	-	-	-
d. Measles	986	522	464	474	47	1	-	-	410	50	3	-	-
e. Tetanus	386	207	179	191	7	4	3	2	166	3	5	3	2
6. Bacterial meningitis*	331	168	163	93	6	36	18	15	84	6	35	20	19
7. Hepatitis B and hepatitis C	74	33	41	11	8	7	4	3	8	8	16	6	3
8. Malaria	271	137	133	23	30	63	15	6	20	32	57	17	7
9. Tropical-cluster diseases	588	307	281	5	12	180	72	37	4	8	158	75	36
a. Trypanosomiasis	497	250	246	1	1	150	64	34	1	5	142	69	34
b. Chagas disease	53	29	24	-	5	17	5	2	-	5	12	5	2
c. Schistosomiasis	30	22	8	4	5	11	1	-	2	3	3	-	-
d. Leishmaniasis	6	4	1	-	1	2	1	-	-	-	-	-	-
e. Lymphatic filariasis	2	1	1	-	1	1	1	-	-	-	-	-	-
f. Onchocerciasis													
10. Leprosy	21	11	10	-	2	4	2	2	-	2	4	2	1
11. Dengue													
12. Japanese encephalitis													
13. Trachoma													
14. Intestinal nematode infections	402	205	197	2	158	32	8	5	2	154	27	8	5
a. Ascariasis	132	66	65	2	64	-	-	-	2	63	-	-	-
b. Trichuriasis	170	86	84	-	86	-	-	-	-	84	-	-	-
c. Ancylostomiasis and necatoriasis	100	52	48	-	8	32	8	5	-	8	27	8	5

Annex Table 19g, continued. DALYs by age, sex and cause (thousands): Latin America and the Caribbean, 2020, pessimistic scenario

Cause	Total	Male	Female	Males					Females				
				0-4	5-14	15-44	45-59	60+	0-4	5-14	15-44	45-59	60+
B. Respiratory infections	**3 186**	**1 708**	**1 478**	**1 156**	**121**	**123**	**102**	**206**	**891**	**131**	**157**	**86**	**213**
1. Lower respiratory infections	3 074	1 650	1 424	1 136	93	118	100	204	875	103	151	84	210
2. Upper respiratory infections	41	22	19	12	2	4	2	3	8	2	4	2	3
3. Otitis media	70	35	35	8	27	-	-	-	7	26	1	-	-
C. Maternal conditions	**917**	**-**	**917**						**-**	**3**	**912**	**2**	**-**
1. Maternal haemorrhage	87		87							1	86	1	
2. Maternal sepsis	158		158								157		
3. Hypertensive disorders of pregnancy	54		54								53		
4. Obstructed labour	223		223								222		
5. Abortion	240		240							1	239	1	
D. Perinatal conditions*	**4 534**	**2 636**	**1 899**	**2 636**					**1 899**				
E. Nutritional deficiencies	**2 337**	**1 051**	**1 287**	**636**	**129**	**135**	**56**	**95**	**515**	**136**	**436**	**83**	**117**
1. Protein-energy malnutrition	1 039	561	477	454	19	19	20	49	351	25	25	18	58
2. Iodine deficiency	52	26	26	22	2	1	-	-	21	5	2	1	-
3. Vitamin A deficiency	100	52	48	38	13	2	-	-	33	14	1	-	-
4. Iron-deficiency anaemia	1 134	406	728	119	94	112	35	46	106	94	406	64	58
II. Noncommunicable diseases	***81 323***	***41 839***	***39 484***	***2 405***	***1 599***	***16 426***	***11 560***	***9 849***	***2 098***	***1 387***	***14 356***	***11 378***	***10 263***
A. Malignant neoplasms	**9 591**	**4 384**	**5 207**	**65**	**254**	**766**	**1 570**	**1 729**	**67**	**170**	**1 244**	**2 098**	**1 628**
1. Mouth and oropharynx cancers	347	257	90	-	2	49	129	77	-	1	15	35	40
2. Oesophagus cancer	236	169	66	-	-	14	85	70	-	-	5	24	38
3. Stomach cancer	868	535	333	-	-	70	212	254	-	-	46	116	171
4. Colon and rectum cancers	552	258	294	-	1	47	96	114	-	1	38	101	155
5. Liver cancer	125	64	61	-	2	12	25	25	-	1	7	21	31
6. Pancreas cancer	175	91	84	-	-	11	38	42	-	-	6	31	46
7. Trachea, bronchus, lung cancers	1 344	818	526	-	1	145	408	264	-	-	40	274	211
8. Melanoma and other skin cancers	90	42	47	-	1	15	16	10	-	1	15	18	13
9. Breast cancer	919	-	919						-	-	242	439	238
10. Cervix uteri cancer	784	-	784						-	-	259	363	161
11. Corpus uteri cancer	180	-	180						-	2	25	95	59
12. Ovary cancer	176	-	176						-	5	61	63	46
13. Prostate cancer	361	361	-	-	-	6	53	302					
14. Bladder cancer	184	139	45	-	-	11	46	81	-	-	4	13	27
15. Lymphomas and multiple myeloma	474	275	198	12	44	99	70	50	8	24	52	54	60
16. Leukaemia	425	238	187	21	76	85	31	26	19	55	55	30	29
C. Diabetes mellitus	**2 453**	**1 096**	**1 357**	**10**	**20**	**235**	**423**	**408**	**9**	**17**	**202**	**487**	**642**
D. Endocrine disorders	**1 532**	**735**	**796**	**265**	**63**	**197**	**113**	**98**	**212**	**52**	**215**	**161**	**156**

Annex Table 19g, continued. DALYs by age, sex and cause (thousands): Latin America and the Caribbean, 2020, pessimistic scenario

Cause	Total	Male	Female	Males 0-4	5-14	15-44	45-59	60+	Females 0-4	5-14	15-44	45-59	60+
E. Neuro-psychiatric conditions	23 719	13 308	10 411	199	440	10 369	1 557	743	179	407	7 668	1 294	863
1. Unipolar major depression	6 804	2 359	4 445	-	-	1 879	385	94	-	-	3 518	729	198
2. Bipolar disorder	1 827	913	914	-	-	824	67	22	-	-	818	69	26
3. Schizophrenia	1 905	992	913	-	-	963	18	12	-	-	893	7	13
4. Epilepsy	703	407	296	11	83	233	61	20	10	77	165	26	17
5. Alcohol use	6 016	5 532	484	-	-	4 666	678	188	-	-	440	32	12
6. Dementia*	1 344	556	788	38	22	33	138	325	38	18	34	189	508
7. Parkinson disease	85	46	39	-	-	-	19	26	-	-	-	16	23
8. Multiple sclerosis	176	75	101	-	-	63	9	3	-	-	83	13	5
9. Drug use	1 645	1 072	572	-	57	954	52	9	-	31	509	28	5
10. Post-traumatic stress disorder	238	89	149	4	16	60	7	1	6	27	101	12	2
11. Obsessive-compulsive disorders	1 272	539	732	-	55	435	34	16	-	70	574	64	25
12. Panic disorder	605	200	405	-	18	146	36	-	-	19	317	60	10
F. Sense organ diseases	1 369	625	744	20	4	29	172	400	13	6	29	210	484
1. Glaucoma	206	75	131	-	-	1	38	35	-	-	4	75	53
2. Cataracts	1 103	519	583	3	-	21	132	364	2	-	18	133	429
G. Cardiovascular diseases	16 498	8 995	7 502	138	100	1 580	3 260	3 918	100	74	1 322	2 421	3 585
1. Rheumatic heart disease	269	91	178	1	12	39	27	12	1	14	79	61	23
2. Ischaemic heart disease	6 853	3 904	2 948	-	-	512	1 542	1 850	-	-	350	980	1 618
3. Cerebrovascular disease	5 387	2 825	2 562	11	19	533	1 023	1 239	8	15	476	873	1 190
4. Inflammatory heart diseases	800	432	368	26	22	175	129	80	23	16	145	107	77
H. Respiratory diseases	7 786	3 439	4 347	459	210	921	843	1 005	315	178	1 004	1 718	1 132
1. COPD*	2 867	1 329	1 538	45	7	261	411	605	34	6	217	685	595
2. Asthma	1 678	756	922	50	130	401	107	68	32	109	331	315	136
I. Digestive diseases	6 377	3 858	2 519	140	79	1 094	1 705	840	108	63	767	880	701
1. Peptic ulcer	306	196	110	1	2	57	74	63	1	1	30	34	44
2. Cirrhosis of the liver	2 257	1 705	553	7	6	533	861	297	6	6	157	247	137
3. Appendicitis	58	34	24	1	8	20	3	2	-	6	14	2	1
J. Genito-urinary diseases	1 793	1 019	774	62	53	132	537	235	54	62	256	182	220
1. Nephritis and nephrosis	806	388	418	36	43	91	97	121	33	48	115	95	127
2. Benign prostatic hypertrophy	427	427	-	-	-	-	389	38	-	-	-	-	-
L. Musculo-skeletal diseases	5 953	2 317	3 636	6	21	716	1 237	336	4	29	1 192	1 744	666
1. Rheumatoid arthritis	1 019	221	798	-	6	104	85	33	-	6	463	236	93
2. Osteoarthritis	4 475	1 985	2 490	-	-	579	1 125	280	-	-	546	1 428	517

Annex Table 19q, continued. DALYs by age, sex and cause (thousands): Latin America and the Caribbean, 2020, pessimistic scenario

Cause	Total	Males	Females	Males					Females				
				0-4	5-14	15-44	45-59	60+	0-4	5-14	15-44	45-59	60+
M. Congenital anomalies	2 131	1 063	1 067	968	53	32	7	4	966	45	42	10	4
N. Oral conditions	1 371	680	691	36	246	267	52	79	35	238	265	55	98
1. Dental caries	1 122	566	556	35	245	260	17	8	34	237	258	18	10
2. Periodontal disease	39	19	20	-	-	5	9	4	-	-	5	10	5
3. Edentulism	199	90	109	-	-	-	24	66	-	-	-	27	82
III. Injuries	21 611	16 014	5 597	919	1 893	10 712	1 904	586	683	928	3 101	566	318
A. Unintentional injuries	15 063	10 755	4 308	809	1 686	6 395	1 395	469	585	822	2 153	466	283
1. Road traffic accidents	6 228	4 453	1 775	130	711	2 884	570	158	97	388	1 028	191	73
2. Poisonings	162	95	68	21	12	45	11	5	15	11	33	5	3
3. Falls	1 834	1 291	543	148	336	590	132	86	72	119	189	76	87
4. Fires	312	173	139	35	46	68	16	8	32	49	42	10	6
5. Drownings	906	714	192	72	153	418	57	14	46	58	75	9	4
6. Other unintentional	5 620	4 029	1 591	403	429	2 390	609	199	322	198	786	175	110
B. Intentional injuries	6 548	5 259	1 289	110	206	4 317	509	117	99	106	949	101	35
1. Self-inflicted injuries	934	619	315	-	17	453	107	42	-	14	250	38	14
2. Violence	4 695	4 107	588	43	142	3 479	375	67	32	57	442	44	13
3. War	919	533	386	67	47	385	27	7	67	35	257	19	8

Notes:
A dash (-) symbol indicates fewer than 500 DALYs.
*IA6 is Bacterial meningitis and meningococcaemia; ID is Conditions arising during the perinatal period;
IIE6 is Dementia and other degenerative and hereditary CNS disorders; IIH1 is Chronic obstructive pulmonary disease.

Annex Table 19h. DALYs by age, sex and cause (thousands): Middle Eastern Crescent, 2020, pessimistic scenario

Cause	Total	Male	Female	Males					Females				
				0-4	5-14	15-44	45-59	60+	0-4	5-14	15-44	45-59	60+
Population (millions)	*983*	*496*	*487*	*60*	*106*	*234*	*61*	*35*	*57*	*102*	*227*	*60*	*41*
All causes	*205 409*	*112 690*	*92 719*	*38 102*	*9 005*	*35 055*	*17 207*	*13 322*	*34 303*	*6 958*	*28 050*	*11 509*	*11 900*
I. Communicable, maternal, perinatal and nutritional conditions	*60 937*	*30 631*	*30 305*	*26 039*	*1 604*	*1 667*	*588*	*733*	*23 571*	*1 518*	*3 941*	*540*	*736*
A. Infectious and parasitic diseases	25 808	13 849	11 959	10 975	765	1 340	493	276	9 782	660	873	343	300
1. Tuberculosis	2 046	1 344	702	154	74	662	301	153	91	44	292	166	109
2. STDs excluding HIV	673	258	415	199	1	53	2	3	181	5	222	3	4
a. Syphilis	394	205	189	189	–	11	2	3	171	–	12	2	4
b. Chlamydia	197	24	173	3	–	20	–	–	3	4	166	–	–
c. Gonorrhoea	82	30	53	8	–	22	–	–	7	1	44	–	–
3. HIV	461	364	97	44	2	276	39	3	45	2	45	4	1
4. Diarrhoeal diseases	12 433	6 542	5 891	6 233	219	58	17	16	5 588	209	60	18	16
5. Childhood-cluster diseases	7 146	3 768	3 379	3 473	269	17	7	3	3 101	233	31	11	2
a. Pertussis	1 667	876	791	811	65	–	–	–	731	60	–	–	–
b. Poliomyelitis	405	238	167	232	1	4	–	–	164	1	3	–	–
c. Diphtheria	34	18	16	16	1	1	–	–	15	1	–	–	–
d. Measles	2 712	1 419	1 294	1 267	150	1	–	–	1 150	141	2	–	–
e. Tetanus	2 327	1 217	1 111	1 146	51	11	6	3	1 042	30	26	11	2
6. Bacterial meningitis*	588	309	278	223	11	44	19	13	204	10	32	19	14
7. Hepatitis B and hepatitis C	217	126	91	32	14	30	29	20	24	12	22	14	19
8. Malaria	269	144	126	33	49	47	10	4	30	45	36	10	5
9. Tropical-cluster diseases	208	133	75	19	44	52	13	5	12	25	28	7	3
a. Trypanosomiasis	–	–	–	–	–	–	–	–	–	–	–	–	–
b. Chagas disease	–	–	–	–	–	–	–	–	–	–	–	–	–
c. Schistosomiasis	111	72	39	2	17	37	11	5	1	7	22	6	2
d. Leishmaniasis	87	53	33	17	26	9	1	–	11	17	5	–	–
e. Lymphatic filariasis	10	7	3	–	–	5	1	1	–	–	1	1	1
f. Onchocerciasis	–	–	–	–	–	–	–	–	–	–	–	–	–
10. Leprosy	6	3	2	1	1	1	–	–	–	1	1	–	–
11. Dengue	–	–	–	–	–	–	–	–	–	–	–	–	–
12. Japanese encephalitis	–	–	–	–	–	–	–	–	–	–	–	–	–
13. Trachoma	285	78	207	–	–	14	26	38	–	–	28	68	110
14. Intestinal nematode infections	142	75	67	1	39	27	5	3	1	36	22	5	3
a. Ascariasis	65	34	31	1	32	1	–	–	1	30	–	–	–
b. Trichuriasis	1	–	–	–	–	–	–	–	–	–	–	–	–
c. Ancylostomiasis and necatoriasis	76	41	36	–	6	26	5	3	–	6	22	5	3

Annex Table 19h, continued. DALYs by age, sex and cause (thousands): Middle Eastern Crescent, 2020, pessimistic scenario

Cause	Total	Male	Female	Males					Females				
				0-4	5-14	15-44	45-59	60+	0-4	5-14	15-44	45-59	60+
B. Respiratory infections	**13 866**	**7 213**	**6 654**	**6 089**	**555**	**106**	**49**	**414**	**5 472**	**585**	**136**	**74**	**387**
1. Lower respiratory infections	13 509	7 026	6 482	5 969	501	100	48	409	5 364	534	130	72	382
2. Upper respiratory infections	147	76	71	59	6	5	1	5	53	7	5	2	4
3. Otitis media	211	110	101	62	48	-	-	-	56	45	1	-	-
C. Maternal conditions	**2 319**	**-**	**2 319**	**-**	**-**	**-**	**-**	**-**	**-**	**-**	**2 264**	**54**	**-**
1. Maternal haemorrhage	236	-	236	-	-	-	-	-	-	-	224	12	-
2. Maternal sepsis	490	-	490	-	-	-	-	-	-	-	482	8	-
3. Hypertensive disorders of pregnancy	152	-	152	-	-	-	-	-	-	-	144	8	-
4. Obstructed labour	635	-	635	-	-	-	-	-	-	-	631	4	-
5. Abortion	226	-	226	-	-	-	-	-	-	-	222	4	-
D. Perinatal conditions*	**13 161**	**6 826**	**6 335**	**6 826**					**6 335**				
E. Nutritional deficiencies	**5 782**	**2 744**	**3 038**	**2 149**	**284**	**222**	**46**	**43**	**1 981**	**271**	**668**	**69**	**49**
1. Protein-energy malnutrition	3 081	1 608	1 473	1 586	5	4	3	9	1 450	5	7	3	5
2. Iodine deficiency	206	105	102	92	9	3	-	-	85	9	6	1	-
3. Vitamin A deficiency	573	288	285	210	74	4	-	-	205	76	4	-	-
4. Iron-deficiency anaemia	1 922	744	1 179	261	197	210	42	34	241	181	651	65	40
II. Noncommunicable diseases	***109 679***	***59 428***	***50 251***	***8 662***	***3 886***	***19 520***	***15 121***	***12 239***	***7 604***	***3 496***	***17 916***	***10 341***	***10 895***
A. Malignant neoplasms	**9 042**	**5 417**	**3 625**	**141**	**468**	**1 336**	**2 162**	**1 311**	**134**	**400**	**1 079**	**1 151**	**861**
1. Mouth and oropharynx cancers	528	347	181	2	8	131	102	105	2	8	61	44	66
2. Oesophagus cancer	306	186	120	-	1	36	103	45	1	2	27	50	40
3. Stomach cancer	664	426	239	1	3	101	220	101	-	2	55	91	91
4. Colon and rectum cancers	377	201	176	1	2	72	60	67	1	5	45	38	87
5. Liver cancer	272	178	95	2	6	41	90	39	2	5	19	37	31
6. Pancreas cancer	145	93	52	-	-	23	49	21	-	-	8	24	20
7. Trachea, bronchus, lung cancers	2 070	1 746	323	2	8	316	919	502	2	7	53	155	107
8. Melanoma and other skin cancers	46	29	17	-	1	10	15	4	-	-	8	6	3
9. Breast cancer	473	-	473	-	-	-	-	-	1	3	187	200	82
10. Cervix uteri cancer	287	-	287	-	-	-	-	-	-	1	95	136	55
11. Corpus uteri cancer	62	-	62	-	-	-	-	-	-	1	12	29	21
12. Ovary cancer	150	-	150	-	-	-	-	-	2	8	68	50	20
13. Prostate cancer	102	102	-	-	-	6	33	61	-				
14. Bladder cancer	304	247	57	-	1	53	114	76	-	2	12	23	20
15. Lymphomas and multiple myeloma	399	273	126	16	68	114	42	31	11	38	40	15	22
16. Leukaemia	613	329	284	30	123	119	31	27	37	128	69	19	31
C. Diabetes mellitus	**2 286**	**1 146**	**1 140**	**44**	**69**	**323**	**434**	**276**	**42**	**66**	**237**	**410**	**385**
D. Endocrine disorders	**1 300**	**652**	**648**	**323**	**82**	**129**	**83**	**35**	**307**	**129**	**117**	**59**	**36**

Annex Table 19h, continued. DALYs by age, sex and cause (thousands): Middle Eastern Crescent, 2020, pessimistic scenario

Cause	Total	Male	Female	Males 0-4	5-14	15-44	45-59	60+	Females 0-4	5-14	15-44	45-59	60+
E. Neuro-psychiatric conditions	**25 409**	**12 132**	**13 277**	**750**	**756**	**9 294**	**942**	**390**	**599**	**657**	**10 288**	**1 206**	**527**
1. Unipolar major depression	9 880	3 501	6 379			2 957	446	97			5 379	802	198
2. Bipolar disorder	2 768	1 405	1 363			1 304	78	22			1 259	77	26
3. Schizophrenia	2 931	1 533	1 398		101	1 510	14	9		118	1 371	16	11
4. Epilepsy	633	342	291	42		158	30	11	34		110	21	8
5. Alcohol use	540	485	54			448	31	6			51	2	1
6. Dementia*	617	294	323	54	17	37	60	127	61	18	38	39	167
7. Parkinson disease	153	82	71				36	46				30	40
8. Multiple sclerosis	237	103	133			92	9	3			117	12	4
9. Drug use	1 881	1 690	191		103	1 510	66	11		12	171	7	1
10. Post-traumatic stress disorder	368	140	228	8	32	90	8	1	13	52	148	13	2
11. Obsessive-compulsive disorders	1 934	837	1 097		110	673	39	15		140	864	69	24
12. Panic disorder	888	302	586		37	224	41	-		37	475	64	9
F. Sense organ diseases	**2 397**	**1 208**	**1 189**	**4**	**1**	**66**	**587**	**551**	**5**	**1**	**55**	**537**	**591**
1. Glaucoma	275	104	171			2	70	33			4	122	45
2. Cataracts	2 103	1 095	1 008	3		60	515	517	3		47	413	545
G. Cardiovascular diseases	**33 330**	**19 334**	**13 996**	**1 777**	**1 230**	**3 840**	**5 996**	**6 492**	**1 242**	**1 090**	**2 500**	**3 245**	**5 919**
1. Rheumatic heart disease	1 032	505	527	2	109	338	48	9	2	128	328	56	13
2. Ischaemic heart disease	13 526	8 229	5 297			1 339	3 259	3 631			660	1 456	3 181
3. Cerebrovascular disease	5 297	2 875	2 422	94	213	594	910	1 064	63	171	339	668	1 181
4. Inflammatory heart diseases	2 820	1 609	1 211	340	230	540	324	174	293	188	374	200	155
H. Respiratory diseases	**11 783**	**6 488**	**5 295**	**1 329**	**542**	**1 368**	**1 486**	**1 764**	**1 034**	**489**	**1 129**	**1 394**	**1 250**
1. COPD*	3 645	1 982	1 663	142	31	340	431	1 037	130	56	283	584	611
2. Asthma	1 640	1 067	573	111	249	474	152	81	30	99	255	118	72
I. Digestive diseases	**8 301**	**4 695**	**3 606**	**1 185**	**239**	**1 053**	**1 538**	**680**	**1 324**	**191**	**678**	**880**	**533**
1. Peptic ulcer	249	176	73		4	69	71	32		2	29	26	16
2. Cirrhosis of the liver	1 438	858	581	13	29	206	411	199	9	65	118	230	158
3. Appendicitis	158	93	65	2	29	54	6	2	2	25	32	4	2
J. Genito-urinary diseases	**4 627**	**2 832**	**1 796**	**193**	**178**	**863**	**1 160**	**437**	**156**	**163**	**621**	**526**	**329**
1. Nephritis and nephrosis	1 073	554	520	81	91	179	109	93	70	116	172	88	73
2. Benign prostatic hypertrophy	487	487	-			1	447	38			-	-	-
L. Musculo-skeletal diseases	**1 988**	**863**	**1 125**	**18**	**12**	**443**	**291**	**100**	**14**	**9**	**417**	**459**	**226**
1. Rheumatoid arthritis	363	209	155			198	8	3		3	77	55	19
2. Osteoarthritis	1 461	579	882			217	271	91			299	386	197

Annex Table 19h, continued. DALYs by age, sex and cause (thousands): Middle Eastern Crescent, 2020, pessimistic scenario

Cause	Total	Males	Females	Males					Females				
				0-4	5-14	15-44	45-59	60+	0-4	5-14	15-44	45-59	60+
M. Congenital anomalies	**5 749**	**2 947**	**2 802**	**2 725**	**97**	**101**	**18**	**6**	**2 587**	**107**	**76**	**24**	**9**
N. Oral conditions	**2 923**	**1 447**	**1 476**	**125**	**167**	**614**	**374**	**166**	**119**	**162**	**610**	**386**	**199**
1. Dental caries	1 314	663	651	124	166	223	96	54	119	159	215	95	63
2. Periodontal disease	42	21	20	-	-	20	1	-	-	-	19	1	-
3. Edentulism	1 545	758	787	-	-	368	277	112	-	-	362	290	136
III. Injuries	***34 793***	***22 631***	***12 162***	***3 401***	***3 514***	***13 867***	***1 498***	***350***	***3 129***	***1 944***	***6 192***	***628***	***270***
A. Unintentional injuries	**17 124**	**12 021**	**5 103**	**2 152**	**2 171**	**6 559**	**936**	**202**	**1 862**	**1 036**	**1 756**	**314**	**135**
1. Road traffic accidents	5 183	4 036	1 146	152	684	2 812	326	63	131	354	533	94	35
2. Poisonings	604	385	219	85	25	201	63	12	79	20	88	23	9
3. Falls	2 432	1 571	861	457	477	539	80	18	395	200	202	47	17
4. Fires	1 065	473	592	144	132	165	26	6	149	138	275	21	10
5. Drownings	1 298	924	374	264	231	388	33	8	229	64	70	7	3
6. Other unintentional	6 542	4 632	1 910	1 051	622	2 454	410	95	879	261	588	122	61
B. Intentional injuries	**17 669**	**10 610**	**7 059**	**1 249**	**1 343**	**7 308**	**562**	**148**	**1 267**	**908**	**4 436**	**314**	**135**
1. Self-inflicted injuries	2 636	1 780	856	-	502	1 043	183	52	-	231	510	74	41
2. Violence	2 187	1 456	732	288	128	933	87	21	311	134	238	37	11
3. War	12 845	7 374	5 471	961	714	5 332	291	75	956	543	3 688	203	83

Notes:
A dash (-) symbol indicates fewer than 500 DALYs.
*IA6 is Bacterial meningitis and meningococcaemia; ID is Conditions arising during the perinatal period;
IIE6 is Dementia and other degenerative and hereditary CNS disorders; IIH1 is Chronic obstructive pulmonary disease.

Annex Table 19i. DALYs by age, sex and cause (thousands): World, 2020, pessimistic scenario

Cause	Total	Male	Female	Males 0-4	5-14	15-44	45-59	60+	Females 0-4	5-14	15-44	45-59	60+
Population (millions)	*7 666*	*3 819*	*3 848*	*362*	*665*	*1 739*	*625*	*427*	*347*	*639*	*1 692*	*638*	*532*
All causes	**1 687 661**	**940 102**	**747 559**	**220 883**	**61 029**	**311 308**	**189 615**	**157 267**	**191 148**	**48 783**	**235 481**	**125 691**	**146 455**
I. Communicable, maternal, perinatal and nutritional conditions	***496 286***	***256 388***	***239 898***	***164 206***	***16 624***	***49 177***	***14 655***	***11 725***	***140 585***	***16 502***	***60 578***	***11 239***	***10 994***
A. Infectious and parasitic diseases	**304 505**	**164 482**	**140 023**	**87 905**	**11 387**	**45 110**	**13 155**	**6 925**	**73 715**	**11 011**	**40 277**	**9 191**	**5 829**
1. Tuberculosis	60 032	33 255	26 777	1 902	1 535	16 383	8 879	4 556	1 807	1 875	13 744	6 206	3 144
2. STDs excluding HIV	13 747	4 925	8 822	2 904	30	1 837	52	102	2 623	120	5 853	79	147
a. Syphilis	4 997	2 596	2 400	2 171	3	279	43	100	1 895	4	306	55	141
b. Chlamydia	5 013	682	4 331	156	10	513	3	1	154	84	4 073	16	3
c. Gonorrhoea	3 731	1 644	2 086	578	17	1 044	5	1	574	33	1 472	7	1
3. HIV	51 187	28 733	22 454	5 296	858	20 058	2 105	416	5 003	866	15 594	833	158
4. Diarrhoeal diseases	69 872	37 894	31 978	34 026	1 984	922	353	609	27 871	2 005	971	398	733
5. Childhood-cluster diseases	52 403	28 017	24 386	24 891	2 522	443	105	56	21 429	2 410	375	111	61
a. Pertussis	9 943	5 317	4 626	4 908	409	–	–	–	4 247	379	16	2	–
b. Poliomyelitis	2 045	1 200	845	1 163	6	28	3	1	821	5	1	–	1
c. Diphtheria	214	113	101	100	11	2	–	–	89	11	1	–	–
d. Measles	28 864	15 434	13 430	13 664	1 755	11	3	1	11 779	1 636	11	3	1
e. Tetanus	11 337	5 953	5 385	5 056	341	402	99	54	4 494	380	346	106	59
6. Bacterial meningitis*	3 800	1 991	1 809	1 343	64	315	152	117	1 206	60	245	160	137
7. Hepatitis B and hepatitis C	1 335	785	551	160	67	211	207	141	118	62	138	88	145
8. Malaria	29 598	16 504	13 094	13 703	1 233	1 240	241	87	10 486	1 166	1 079	258	105
9. Tropical-cluster diseases	6 989	4 534	2 454	182	1 257	2 423	516	156	154	674	1 083	423	121
a. Trypanosomiasis	1 126	590	536	20	202	272	82	14	36	196	240	55	10
b. Chagas disease	497	250	246	1	1	150	64	34	1	–	142	69	34
c. Schistosomiasis	1 202	748	454	30	239	370	74	36	18	149	214	48	24
d. Leishmaniasis	1 028	668	360	59	280	305	18	6	36	162	145	12	5
e. Lymphatic filariasis	2 378	1 821	557	65	468	1 120	153	15	57	115	215	153	18
f. Onchocerciasis	758	457	301	8	67	206	125	50	6	51	128	86	30
10. Leprosy	145	76	70	2	18	36	12	6	5	16	35	10	4
11. Dengue	288	135	153	34	96	3	2	–	38	110	3	2	0
12. Japanese encephalitis	272	143	129	86	43	10	2	1	80	39	7	2	1
13. Trachoma	1 036	276	760	–	–	44	87	145	–	–	92	234	434
14. Intestinal nematode infections	2 722	1 407	1 315	14	944	333	75	41	14	898	279	76	48
a. Ascariasis	848	435	413	14	417	3	1	–	13	397	2	1	–
b. Trichuriasis	874	448	427	–	447	–	–	–	–	426	–	–	–
c. Ancylostomiasis and necatoriasis	998	524	474	–	80	330	74	41	–	76	275	75	48

Annex Table 19i, continued. DALYs by age, sex and cause (thousands): World, 2020, pessimistic scenario

Cause	Total	Male	Female	Males					Females				
				0-4	5-14	15-44	45-59	60+	0-4	5-14	15-44	45-59	60+
B. Respiratory infections	**81 152**	**43 205**	**37 947**	**33 881**	**3 367**	**1 309**	**733**	**3 915**	**28 545**	**3 392**	**1 216**	**700**	**4 093**
1. Lower respiratory infections	79 010	42 081	36 929	33 184	3 049	1 260	718	3 871	27 940	3 088	1 172	684	4 044
2. Upper respiratory infections	902	479	423	335	41	44	15	44	279	41	38	16	49
3. Otitis media	1 240	645	595	362	276	5	-	-	326	263	6	-	-
C. Maternal conditions	**15 539**		**15 539**							**287**	**15 077**	**175**	
1. Maternal haemorrhage	1 895		1 895							66	1 789	40	
2. Maternal sepsis	2 878		2 878							44	2 813	22	
3. Hypertensive disorders of pregnancy	961		961							33	908	20	
4. Obstructed labour	3 286		3 286							22	3 253	11	
5. Abortion	2 698		2 698							37	2 643	18	
D. Perinatal conditions*	**62 208**	**32 817**	**29 391**	**32 816**	**1**	**-**	**-**	**-**	**29 391**				
E. Nutritional deficiencies	**32 883**	**15 884**	**16 998**	**9 604**	**1 869**	**2 758**	**767**	**886**	**8 933**	**1 812**	**4 008**	**1 173**	**1 072**
1. Protein-energy malnutrition	14 392	7 420	6 973	7 083	73	69	50	145	6 584	99	79	42	167
2. Iodine deficiency	793	407	386	358	33	14	1	-	331	34	18	3	-
3. Vitamin A deficiency	2 497	1 302	1 195	923	357	22	-	-	834	342	19	-	-
4. Iron-deficiency anaemia	15 144	6 732	8 411	1 230	1 403	2 650	713	736	1 175	1 333	3 883	1 124	896
II. Noncommunicable diseases	*904 323*	*494 103*	*410 220*	*34 368*	*16 858*	*147 129*	*156 181*	*139 566*	*31 618*	*15 097*	*128 364*	*104 740*	*130 401*
A. Malignant neoplasms	**142 026**	**86 794**	**55 232**	**1 001**	**2 841**	**16 343**	**38 146**	**28 464**	**1 119**	**2 087**	**11 495**	**20 856**	**19 673**
1. Mouth and oropharynx cancers	7 784	5 180	2 604	19	49	1 249	2 221	1 643	23	57	602	926	997
2. Oesophagus cancer	8 404	5 903	2 502	-	1	661	3 064	2 176	1	2	244	1 019	1 236
3. Stomach cancer	16 719	11 451	5 269	3	17	1 308	5 795	4 327	1	11	846	2 002	2 410
4. Colon and rectum cancers	8 312	4 688	3 624	4	21	850	1 737	2 076	5	21	499	1 141	1 958
5. Liver cancer	15 379	12 040	3 338	25	78	3 391	6 204	2 342	26	62	625	1 434	1 191
6. Pancreas cancer	2 874	1 822	1 053	-	-	236	827	758	2	2	91	356	603
7. Trachea, bronchus, lung cancers	25 164	19 581	5 583	12	35	2 474	10 222	6 837	5	12	477	2 463	2 625
8. Melanoma and other skin cancers	898	493	404	1	4	134	209	146	1	9	97	144	159
9. Breast cancer	6 713		6 713							4	1 793	3 015	1 891
10. Cervix uteri cancer	5 518		5 518							3	1 394	2 808	1 312
11. Corpus uteri cancer	1 072		1 072							4	135	522	407
12. Ovary cancer	2 182		2 182						28	60	668	813	612
13. Prostate cancer	2 662	2 662		1	4	50	503	2 104					
14. Bladder cancer	2 446	1 918	529	2	6	184	664	1 060	2	3	62	154	308
15. Lymphomas and multiple myeloma	5 161	3 313	1 848	165	580	994	851	722	120	310	407	434	577
16. Leukaemia	6 280	3 542	2 738	286	793	1 304	698	461	329	592	917	471	428
C. Diabetes mellitus	**14 992**	**7 040**	**7 952**	**159**	**265**	**1 582**	**2 625**	**2 409**	**161**	**254**	**1 159**	**2 635**	**3 743**
D. Endocrine disorders	**6 899**	**3 214**	**3 685**	**1 156**	**292**	**798**	**535**	**433**	**1 029**	**350**	**864**	**696**	**744**

Annex Table 19i, continued. DALYs by age, sex and cause (thousands): World, 2020, pessimistic scenario

Cause	Total	Male	Female	Males					Females				
				0-4	5-14	15-44	45-59	60+	0-4	5-14	15-44	45-59	60+
E. Neuro-psychiatric conditions	**206 241**	**100 320**	**105 920**	**2 263**	**3 354**	**75 576**	**11 845**	**7 283**	**2 185**	**3 214**	**75 718**	**13 813**	**10 990**
1. Unipolar major depression	77 439	27 200	50 240	-	1	21 607	4 484	1 109	-	1	39 591	8 269	2 379
2. Bipolar disorder	20 952	10 559	10 392	-	-	9 519	784	255	-	-	9 261	792	338
3. Schizophrenia	17 338	9 118	8 220	-	-	8 908	110	101	-	-	8 012	73	135
4. Epilepsy	5 212	2 943	2 269	167	609	1 605	402	160	171	652	1 054	227	164
5. Alcohol use	22 997	20 294	2 703	-	-	17 528	2 223	542	-	-	2 385	223	96
6. Dementia*	14 562	6 030	8 532	314	135	325	1 500	3 756	383	148	327	1 632	6 042
7. Parkinson disease	1 880	900	980	-	-	-	336	562	-	-	1	338	640
8. Multiple sclerosis	1 932	837	1 095	-	-	699	98	39	-	-	893	138	63
9. Drug use	7 965	6 515	1 451	-	413	5 782	272	48	-	95	1 281	64	12
10. Post-traumatic stress disorder	2 697	1 019	1 678	48	199	671	85	15	79	325	1 108	138	28
11. Obsessive-compulsive disorders	14 613	6 260	8 353	-	688	4 984	402	185	-	880	6 446	725	302
12. Panic disorder	7 051	2 349	4 701	-	205	1 709	433	2	-	240	3 642	698	122
F. Sense organ diseases	**23 087**	**10 996**	**12 091**	**84**	**11**	**668**	**5 484**	**4 749**	**68**	**22**	**657**	**5 720**	**5 624**
1. Glaucoma	5 685	2 121	3 564	6	-	112	1 344	659	8	-	169	2 396	991
2. Cataracts	16 997	8 715	8 283	35	3	523	4 092	4 062	25	3	417	3 256	4 582
G. Cardiovascular diseases	**230 801**	**133 981**	**96 820**	**4 594**	**3 567**	**21 234**	**47 040**	**57 546**	**3 474**	**3 302**	**12 576**	**23 433**	**54 036**
1. Rheumatic heart disease	8 593	4 243	4 350	6	296	1 700	1 511	729	25	367	1 579	1 440	940
2. Ischaemic heart disease	89 958	54 572	35 385	-	-	5 892	21 508	27 173	191	-	2 658	8 548	23 988
3. Cerebrovascular disease	69 290	38 458	30 831	535	812	5 625	13 451	18 035	423	643	3 416	8 055	18 294
4. Inflammatory heart diseases	14 118	8 144	5 975	927	697	2 847	2 358	1 316	896	665	1 740	1 321	1 353
H. Respiratory diseases	**113 620**	**63 982**	**49 638**	**4 490**	**2 642**	**12 075**	**21 582**	**23 193**	**3 314**	**2 106**	**9 415**	**15 622**	**19 182**
1. COPD*	64 638	37 783	26 855	475	142	4 829	14 646	17 690	488	165	3 170	9 213	13 819
2. Asthma	15 691	8 660	7 031	620	1 491	4 031	1 707	811	304	957	3 237	1 651	882
I. Digestive diseases	**62 564**	**37 742**	**24 823**	**2 918**	**1 081**	**9 312**	**15 879**	**8 551**	**2 981**	**1 103**	**5 415**	**8 315**	**7 008**
1. Peptic ulcer	3 974	2 603	1 371	10	19	846	1 033	695	12	17	400	455	487
2. Cirrhosis of the liver	20 023	14 324	5 700	98	112	3 616	7 268	3 228	76	155	1 174	2 514	1 781
3. Appendicitis	1 492	892	600	18	241	532	72	29	18	215	297	47	23
J. Genito-urinary diseases	**20 584**	**12 461**	**8 123**	**917**	**1 012**	**2 542**	**5 313**	**2 677**	**690**	**924**	**2 027**	**2 068**	**2 414**
1. Nephritis and nephrosis	10 147	5 338	4 809	642	818	1 540	1 109	1 229	563	801	1 098	983	1 365
2. Benign prostatic hypertrophy	3 837	3 837	-	-	-	9	3 182	639	-	-	-	-	-
L. Musculo-skeletal diseases	**31 246**	**11 613**	**19 633**	**45**	**77**	**3 593**	**5 428**	**2 470**	**58**	**98**	**5 653**	**9 146**	**4 679**
1. Rheumatoid arthritis	5 148	1 466	3 682	1	2	606	524	334	-	30	1 502	1 222	927
2. Osteoarthritis	23 549	9 322	14 227	-	-	2 783	4 709	1 829	-	-	3 529	7 479	3 219

Annex Table 19i, continued. DALYs by age, sex and cause (thousands): World, 2020, pessimistic scenario

Cause	Total	Males	Females	Males					Females				
				0-4	5-14	15-44	45-59	60+	0-4	5-14	15-44	45-59	60+
M. Congenital anomalies	33 270	16 674	16 596	15 256	592	668	114	44	15 257	619	521	138	61
N. Oral conditions	12 321	5 963	6 358	514	757	1 975	1 479	1 236	492	749	2 002	1 562	1 553
1. Dental caries	6 218	3 111	3 107	507	749	1 120	472	262	485	730	1 091	482	319
2. Periodontal disease	409	203	206	-	-	154	35	15	-	-	153	36	17
3. Edentulism	5 538	2 609	2 929	-	-	681	970	958	-	-	676	1 039	1 214
III. Injuries	*287 051*	*189 611*	*97 440*	*22 309*	*27 546*	*115 001*	*18 778*	*5 976*	*18 946*	*17 183*	*46 539*	*9 712*	*5 060*
A. Unintentional injuries	191 032	127 738	63 294	18 214	23 207	68 289	13 701	4 328	14 813	14 356	23 567	6 780	3 778
1. Road traffic accidents	58 450	42 029	16 421	2 156	6 970	26 386	5 013	1 504	1 418	4 275	7 683	2 173	873
2. Poisonings	7 586	4 438	3 148	1 349	424	1 747	711	208	956	306	1 282	415	188
3. Falls	26 207	15 902	10 305	2 931	5 021	5 813	1 445	692	2 884	2 267	2 739	1 352	1 063
4. Fires	14 335	6 054	8 281	1 814	1 489	2 148	446	157	1 615	2 342	3 626	428	269
5. Drownings	15 614	10 659	4 956	2 791	3 451	3 676	535	206	1 875	1 536	1 081	273	190
6. Other unintentional	68 840	48 656	20 184	7 173	5 853	28 519	5 549	1 562	6 065	3 629	7 156	2 139	1 196
B. Intentional injuries	96 019	61 873	34 146	4 095	4 340	46 712	5 078	1 648	4 133	2 827	22 972	2 932	1 282
1. Self-inflicted injuries	25 536	14 034	11 502	-	922	9 447	2 578	1 088	-	469	8 374	1 805	854
2. Violence	30 461	24 631	5 830	1 045	1 172	20 340	1 722	352	1 118	673	3 251	586	201
3. War	40 022	23 207	16 815	3 050	2 246	16 925	778	209	3 014	1 685	11 347	541	228

Notes:

A dash (-) symbol indicates fewer than 500 DALYs.

*IA6 is Bacterial meningitis and meningococcaemia; ID is Conditions arising during the perinatal period;

IIE6 is Dementia and other degenerative and hereditary CNS disorders; IIH1 is Chronic obstructive pulmonary disease.

Annex Table 20a. Deaths by age, sex and cause (thousands): Established Market Economies, 2020, optimistic scenario

Cause	Total	Male	Female	Males 0-4	5-14	15-29	30-44	45-59	60-69	70+	Females 0-4	5-14	15-29	30-44	45-59	60-69	70+
Population (millions)	*911*	*444*	*466*	*29*	*58*	*85*	*77*	*87*	*51*	*58*	*28*	*55*	*81*	*75*	*87*	*56*	*84*
All causes	**8 119**	**4 365**	**3 753**	*22*	*7*	*85*	*115*	*521*	*744*	*2 871*	*16*	*5*	*25*	*53*	*187*	*332*	*3 136*
I. Communicable, maternal, perinatal and nutritional conditions	**446**	**235**	**211**	*10*	-	*5*	*17*	*9*	*9*	*185*	*7*	-	*1*	*2*	*2*	*5*	*193*
A. Infectious and parasitic diseases	**97**	**61**	**36**	*1*	-	*5*	*16*	*8*	*3*	*28*	*1*	-	*1*	*2*	*1*	*2*	*29*
1. Tuberculosis	**13**	**9**	**4**	-	-	-	-	-	1	7	-	-	-	-	-	-	4
2. STDs excluding HIV	1	-	-	-	-	-	-	-	-	-	-	-	-	-	-	-	-
a. Syphilis	-	-	-	-	-	-	-	-	-	-	-	-	-	-	-	-	-
b. Chlamydia	-	-	-	-	-	-	-	-	-	-	-	-	-	-	-	-	-
c. Gonorrhoea	-	-	-	-	-	-	-	-	-	-	-	-	-	-	-	-	-
3. HIV	**34**	**30**	**5**	-	-	5	16	7	1	1	-	-	1	2	1	-	1
4. Diarrhoeal diseases	**3**	**1**	**2**	-	-	-	-	-	-	1	-	-	-	-	-	-	1
5. Childhood-cluster diseases	-	-	-	-	-	-	-	-	-	-	-	-	-	-	-	-	-
a. Pertussis	-	-	-	-	-	-	-	-	-	-	-	-	-	-	-	-	-
b. Poliomyelitis	-	-	-	-	-	-	-	-	-	-	-	-	-	-	-	-	-
c. Diphtheria	-	-	-	-	-	-	-	-	-	-	-	-	-	-	-	-	-
d. Measles	-	-	-	-	-	-	-	-	-	-	-	-	-	-	-	-	-
e. Tetanus	-	-	-	-	-	-	-	-	-	-	-	-	-	-	-	-	-
6. Bacterial meningitis*	**2**	**1**	**1**	-	-	-	-	-	-	1	-	-	-	-	-	-	1
7. Hepatitis B and hepatitis C	**2**	**1**	**1**	-	-	-	-	-	-	1	-	-	-	-	-	-	1
8. Malaria	-	-	-	-	-	-	-	-	-	-	-	-	-	-	-	-	-
9. Tropical-cluster diseases	-	-	-	-	-	-	-	-	-	-	-	-	-	-	-	-	-
a. Trypanosomiasis	-	-	-	-	-	-	-	-	-	-	-	-	-	-	-	-	-
b. Chagas disease	-	-	-	-	-	-	-	-	-	-	-	-	-	-	-	-	-
c. Schistosomiasis	-	-	-	-	-	-	-	-	-	-	-	-	-	-	-	-	-
d. Leishmaniasis	-	-	-	-	-	-	-	-	-	-	-	-	-	-	-	-	-
10. Leprosy	-	-	-	-	-	-	-	-	-	-	-	-	-	-	-	-	-
11. Dengue	-	-	-	-	-	-	-	-	-	-	-	-	-	-	-	-	-
12. Japanese encephalitis	-	-	-	-	-	-	-	-	-	-	-	-	-	-	-	-	-
13. Trachoma	-	-	-	-	-	-	-	-	-	-	-	-	-	-	-	-	-
14. Intestinal nematode infections	-	-	-	-	-	-	-	-	-	-	-	-	-	-	-	-	-
a. Ascariasis	-	-	-	-	-	-	-	-	-	-	-	-	-	-	-	-	-
b. Trichuriasis	-	-	-	-	-	-	-	-	-	-	-	-	-	-	-	-	-
c. Ancylostomiasis, necatoriasis	-	-	-	-	-	-	-	-	-	-	-	-	-	-	-	-	-
15. Other infectious and parasitic	**42**	**19**	**23**	-	-	-	-	-	1	17	-	-	-	-	-	1	22

Annex Table 20a, continued. Deaths by age, sex and cause (thousands): Established Market Economies, 2020, optimistic scenario

Cause	Total	Male	Female	Males							Females						
				0-4	5-14	15-29	30-44	45-59	60-69	70+	0-4	5-14	15-29	30-44	45-59	60-69	70+
B. Respiratory infections	**314**	**157**	**157**	1	-	-	-	1	5	149	-	-	-	-	1	3	153
1. Lower respiratory infections	311	156	155	-	-	-	-	1	5	148	-	-	-	-	1	3	151
2. Upper respiratory infections	3	1	2	-	-	-	-	-	-	1	-	-	-	-	-	-	1
3. Otitis media	-	-	-	-	-	-	-	-	-	-	-	-	-	-	-	-	-
C. Maternal conditions																	
1. Maternal haemorrhage	-	-	-	-	-	-	-	-	-	-	-	-	-	-	-	-	-
2. Maternal sepsis	-	-	-	-	-	-	-	-	-	-	-	-	-	-	-	-	-
3. Hypertensive disorders*	-	-	-	-	-	-	-	-	-	-	-	-	-	-	-	-	-
4. Obstructed labour	-	-	-	-	-	-	-	-	-	-	-	-	-	-	-	-	-
5. Abortion	-	-	-	-	-	-	-	-	-	-	-	-	-	-	-	-	-
6. Other maternal	-	-	-	-	-	-	-	-	-	-	-	-	-	-	-	-	-
D. Perinatal conditions*	**14**	**8**	**6**	8	-	-	-	-	-	-	6	-	-	-	-	-	-
E. Nutritional deficiencies	**21**	**9**	**12**	-	-	-	-	-	-	8	-	-	-	-	-	-	12
1. Protein-energy malnutrition	7	2	4	-	-	-	-	-	-	2	-	-	-	-	-	-	4
2. Iodine deficiency	-	-	-	-	-	-	-	-	-	-	-	-	-	-	-	-	-
3. Vitamin A deficiency	-	-	-	-	-	-	-	-	-	-	-	-	-	-	-	-	-
4. Iron-deficiency anaemia	14	6	8	-	-	-	-	-	-	6	-	-	-	-	-	-	8
II. Noncommunicable diseases	***7 239***	***3 854***	***3 385***	7	2	14	59	466	707	2 595	6	2	6	32	162	308	2 868
A. Malignant neoplasms	**2 148**	**1 240**	**908**	-	2	5	25	211	297	700	-	1	3	20	112	181	590
1. Mouth and oropharynx cancers	38	29	8	-	-	-	1	9	8	12	-	-	-	-	1	2	5
2. Oesophagus cancer	51	40	11	-	-	-	1	8	11	20	-	-	-	-	-	2	8
3. Stomach cancer	172	109	63	-	-	-	2	14	23	70	-	-	-	1	5	9	48
4. Colon and rectum cancers	254	136	118	-	-	-	2	16	28	90	-	-	-	1	9	18	89
5. Liver cancer	43	32	11	-	-	-	1	7	10	14	-	-	-	-	1	3	7
6. Pancreas cancer	100	54	46	-	-	-	1	8	13	32	-	-	-	-	4	8	34
7. Trachea, bronchus, lung cancers	534	349	185	-	-	-	9	94	111	136	-	-	-	3	28	51	103
8. Melanoma and other skin cancers	24	15	10	-	-	-	1	3	3	7	-	-	-	1	-	1	6
9. Breast cancer	134	-	134	-	-	-	-	-	-	-	-	-	-	6	27	28	73
10. Cervix uteri cancer	14	-	14	-	-	-	-	-	-	-	-	-	-	1	3	3	7
11. Corpus uteri cancer	26	-	26	-	-	-	-	-	-	-	-	-	-	1	3	5	17
12. Ovary cancer	41	-	41	-	-	-	-	-	-	-	-	-	-	1	7	10	23
13. Prostate cancer	133	133	-	-	-	-	-	3	16	114	-	-	-	-	-	-	-
14. Bladder cancer	62	47	15	-	-	-	-	3	8	36	-	-	-	-	1	2	13
15. Lymphomas, multiple myeloma	90	50	40	-	-	1	2	7	11	29	-	-	1	1	4	7	28
16. Leukaemia	63	37	26	-	1	1	1	4	7	22	-	1	1	1	3	4	18
17. Other cancers	369	210	159	-	1	2	5	35	49	117	-	-	1	3	15	28	112

Annex Table 20a, continued. Deaths by age, sex and cause (thousands): Established Market Economies, 2020, optimistic scenario

Cause	Total	Male	Female	Males							Females						
				0-4	5-14	15-29	30-44	45-59	60-69	70+	0-4	5-14	15-29	30-44	45-59	60-69	70+
B. Other neoplasms	**37**	**17**	**20**	-	-	-	-	**2**	**2**	**12**	-	-	-	-	**1**	**1**	**17**
C. Diabetes mellitus	**169**	**60**	**109**	-	-	-	-	**4**	**8**	**46**	-	-	-	-	**2**	**7**	**100**
D. Endocrine disorders	**49**	**20**	**29**	-	-	-	**1**	**1**	**3**	**14**	-	-	-	-	**1**	**2**	**26**
E. Neuro-psychiatric conditions	**237**	**98**	**139**	**1**	-	**3**	**4**	**7**	**9**	**74**	-	-	**1**	**1**	**3**	**5**	**129**
2. Bipolar disorder	1	-	1	-	-	-	-	-	-	-	-	-	-	-	-	-	-
3. Schizophrenia	17	6	11	-	-	-	-	-	1	5	-	-	-	-	-	1	10
4. Epilepsy	5	3	2	-	-	-	1	1	-	1	-	-	-	-	-	1	1
5. Alcohol use	10	8	2	-	-	-	1	3	2	2	-	-	-	-	1	-	1
6. Dementia*	123	42	81	-	-	-	-	1	3	37	-	-	-	-	-	2	78
7. Parkinson disease	40	20	21	-	-	-	-	-	1	19	-	-	-	-	-	1	20
8. Multiple sclerosis	4	2	2	-	-	-	-	-	-	1	-	-	-	-	1	-	1
9. Drug use	2	2	-	-	-	1	1	1	-	-	-	-	-	-	-	-	-
13. Other neuro-psychiatric	36	16	20	1	-	1	1	1	2	10	-	-	1	-	1	1	17
F. Sense organ diseases				-	-	-	-	-	-	-	-	-	-	-	-	-	-
1. Glaucoma				-	-	-	-	-	-	-	-	-	-	-	-	-	-
2. Cataracts				-	-	-	-	-	-	-	-	-	-	-	-	-	-
G. Cardiovascular diseases	**3 597**	**1 871**	**1 726**	**1**	-	**3**	**20**	**189**	**313**	**1 346**	**1**	-	**1**	**5**	**20**	**72**	**1 627**
1. Rheumatic heart disease	19	7	12	-	-	-	-	1	2	4	-	-	-	-	1	1	10
2. Ischaemic heart disease	1 911	1 043	867	-	-	-	10	118	191	724	-	-	-	2	10	41	815
3. Cerebrovascular disease	899	414	485	-	-	1	4	30	52	328	-	-	-	2	6	16	461
4. Inflammatory heart diseases	68	38	30	-	-	1	2	8	5	23	-	-	-	-	-	1	27
5. Other cardiovascular	700	368	332	1	-	1	4	32	64	266	1	-	1	1	3	12	314
H. Respiratory diseases	**408**	**246**	**162**	-	-	**1**	**1**	**9**	**30**	**205**	-	-	-	**1**	**7**	**21**	**133**
1. COPD*	295	188	108	-	-	1	-	5	23	159	-	-	-	-	4	15	88
2. Asthma	24	11	13	-	-	-	-	1	2	7	-	-	-	-	1	2	9
3. Other respiratory	89	47	41	-	-	-	1	2	6	38	-	-	-	-	2	3	36
I. Digestive diseases	**374**	**213**	**161**	-	-	**1**	**7**	**39**	**38**	**128**	-	-	-	**3**	**14**	**14**	**129**
1. Peptic ulcer	42	24	18	-	-	-	-	2	3	19	-	-	-	-	1	1	17
2. Cirrhosis of the liver	128	89	39	-	-	-	5	28	23	33	-	-	-	2	9	7	20
3. Appendicitis	2	1	1	-	-	-	-	-	-	-	-	-	-	-	1	-	-
4. Other digestive	202	99	103	-	-	1	2	9	12	76	-	-	-	1	4	6	92
J. Genito-urinary diseases	**149**	**65**	**84**	-	-	-	**1**	**2**	**5**	**57**	-	-	-	-	**2**	**3**	**79**
1. Nephritis and nephrosis	96	43	53	-	-	-	-	2	4	37	-	-	-	-	2	2	50
2. Benign prostatic hypertrophy	5	5	-	-	-	-	-	-	1	4	-	-	-	-	-	-	-
3. Other genito-urinary	49	18	31	-	-	-	-	1	-	16	-	-	-	-	-	1	29
K. Skin diseases	**15**	**4**	**11**	-	-	-	-	-	-	**4**	-	-	-	-	-	-	**11**

Annex Table 20a, continued. Deaths by age, sex and cause (thousands): Established Market Economies, 2020, optimistic scenario

Cause	Total	Male	Female	Males							Females						
				0-4	5-14	15-29	30-44	45-59	60-69	70+	0-4	5-14	15-29	30-44	45-59	60-69	70+
L. Musculo-skeletal diseases	37	9	28	–	–	–	–	–	1	7	–	–	–	–	1	1	25
1. Rheumatoid arthritis	11	2	8	–	–	–	–	–	–	2	–	–	–	–	–	1	7
3. Other musculo-skeletal	26	7	19	–	–	–	–	–	1	6	–	–	–	–	1	1	18
M. Congenital anomalies	18	10	8	6	–	–	–	–	–	1	5	–	–	–	–	–	2
N. Oral conditions	–	–	–	–	–	–	–	–	–	–	–	–	–	–	–	–	–
III. Injuries	*434*	*277*	*157*	*3*	*4*	*66*	*39*	*46*	*28*	*91*	*3*	*3*	*18*	*18*	*23*	*19*	*74*
A. Unintentional injuries	259	151	108	3	3	41	15	18	12	60	2	2	11	11	12	11	59
1. Road traffic accidents	93	57	37	2	2	34	7	4	2	6	1	2	9	8	6	4	7
2. Poisonings	9	6	4	–	–	1	2	1	–	1	–	–	–	1	1	1	1
3. Falls	79	38	41	–	–	1	1	3	3	30	–	–	–	–	1	3	36
4. Fires	9	5	4	–	–	1	1	1	1	1	–	–	–	–	1	1	2
5. Drownings	10	7	3	–	–	1	1	1	1	2	–	–	1	–	–	–	2
6. Other unintentional	58	38	20	1	1	4	4	7	5	18	–	–	1	1	3	3	11
B. Intentional injuries	175	126	49	1	1	25	25	28	16	31	1	–	6	8	11	8	16
1. Self-inflicted injuries	143	103	41	–	–	16	18	24	15	30	–	–	4	6	10	7	14
2. Violence	31	23	8	1	–	9	6	4	1	2	1	–	2	2	1	1	1
3. War	–	–	–	–	–	–	–	–	–	–	–	–	–	–	–	–	–

Notes:

Causes responsible for no deaths have been omitted from this table.

A dash (–) symbol indicates fewer than 500 deaths.

*IA6 is Bacterial meningitis and meningococcaemia; IC3 is Hypertensive disorders of pregnancy; ID is Conditions arising during the perinatal period; IIE6 is Dementia and other degenerative and hereditary CNS disorders; IIH1 is Chronic obstructive pulmonary disease.

Annex Table 20b. Deaths by age, sex and cause (thousands): Formerly Socialist Economies of Europe, 2020, optimistic scenario

Cause	Total	Male	Female	Males							Females						
				0-4	5-14	15-29	30-44	45-59	60-69	70+	0-4	5-14	15-29	30-44	45-59	60-69	70+
Population (millions)	*366*	*172*	*194*	*12*	*25*	*37*	*38*	*30*	*17*	*13*	*12*	*24*	*36*	*39*	*33*	*24*	*27*
All causes	*4 708*	*2 634*	*2 073*	*26*	*9*	*77*	*144*	*578*	*585*	*1 215*	*20*	*5*	*25*	*43*	*135*	*240*	*1 605*
I. Communicable, maternal, perinatal and nutritional conditions	*124*	*56*	*68*	*10*	-	-	*1*	*3*	*3*	*39*	*7*	-	-	-	*1*	*2*	*58*
A. Infectious and parasitic diseases	**23**	**12**	**11**	**2**	-	-	**1**	**1**	**1**	**6**	**1**	-	-	-	-	-	**8**
1. Tuberculosis	**7**	**5**	**2**	-	-	-	-	**1**	**1**	**2**	-	-	-	-	-	-	**1**
2. STDs excluding HIV	-	-	-	-	-	-	-	-	-	-	-	-	-	-	-	-	-
a. Syphilis	-	-	-	-	-	-	-	-	-	-	-	-	-	-	-	-	-
b. Chlamydia	-	-	-	-	-	-	-	-	-	-	-	-	-	-	-	-	-
c. Gonorrhoea	-	-	-	-	-	-	-	-	-	-	-	-	-	-	-	-	-
3. HIV	**2**	**1**	**1**	**1**	-	-	-	-	-	-	**1**	-	-	-	-	-	-
4. Diarrhoeal diseases	**1**	**1**	**1**	**1**	-	-	-	-	-	-	**1**	-	-	-	-	-	-
5. Childhood-cluster diseases	-	-	-	-	-	-	-	-	-	-	-	-	-	-	-	-	-
a. Pertussis	-	-	-	-	-	-	-	-	-	-	-	-	-	-	-	-	-
b. Poliomyelitis	-	-	-	-	-	-	-	-	-	-	-	-	-	-	-	-	-
c. Diphtheria	-	-	-	-	-	-	-	-	-	-	-	-	-	-	-	-	-
d. Measles	-	-	-	-	-	-	-	-	-	-	-	-	-	-	-	-	-
e. Tetanus	-	-	-	-	-	-	-	-	-	-	-	-	-	-	-	-	-
6. Bacterial meningitis*	**2**	**1**	**1**	-	-	-	-	-	-	**1**	-	-	-	-	-	-	**1**
7. Hepatitis B and hepatitis C	**1**	**1**	-	-	-	-	-	-	-	-	-	-	-	-	-	-	-
8. Malaria	-	-	-	-	-	-	-	-	-	-	-	-	-	-	-	-	-
9. Tropical-cluster diseases	-	-	-	-	-	-	-	-	-	-	-	-	-	-	-	-	-
a. Trypanosomiasis	-	-	-	-	-	-	-	-	-	-	-	-	-	-	-	-	-
b. Chagas disease	-	-	-	-	-	-	-	-	-	-	-	-	-	-	-	-	-
c. Schistosomiasis	-	-	-	-	-	-	-	-	-	-	-	-	-	-	-	-	-
d. Leishmaniasis	-	-	-	-	-	-	-	-	-	-	-	-	-	-	-	-	-
10. Leprosy	-	-	-	-	-	-	-	-	-	-	-	-	-	-	-	-	-
11. Dengue	-	-	-	-	-	-	-	-	-	-	-	-	-	-	-	-	-
12. Japanese encephalitis	-	-	-	-	-	-	-	-	-	-	-	-	-	-	-	-	-
13. Trachoma	-	-	-	-	-	-	-	-	-	-	-	-	-	-	-	-	-
14. Intestinal nematode infections	-	-	-	-	-	-	-	-	-	-	-	-	-	-	-	-	-
a. Ascariasis	-	-	-	-	-	-	-	-	-	-	-	-	-	-	-	-	-
b. Trichuriasis	-	-	-	-	-	-	-	-	-	-	-	-	-	-	-	-	-
c. Ancylostomiasis, necatoriasis	-	-	-	-	-	-	-	-	-	-	-	-	-	-	-	-	-
15. Other infectious and parasitic	**10**	**3**	**7**	-	-	-	-	-	-	**3**	-	-	-	-	-	-	**6**

Annex Table 20b, continued. Deaths by age, sex and cause (thousands): Formerly Socialist Economies of Europe, 2020, optimistic scenario

				Males							Females						
Cause	Total	Male	Female	0-4	5-14	15-29	30-44	45-59	60-69	70+	0-4	5-14	15-29	30-44	45-59	60-69	70+
B. Respiratory infections	**85**	**37**	**49**	**2**	**-**	**-**	**-**	**-**	**2**	**31**	**2**	**-**	**-**	**-**	**-**	**1**	**45**
1. Lower respiratory infections	85	36	48	2	-	-	-	-	2	31	2	-	-	-	-	1	45
2. Upper respiratory infections	-	-	-	-	-	-	-	-	-	-	-	-	-	-	-	-	-
3. Otitis media	-	-	-	-	-	-	-	-	-	-	-	-	-	-	-	-	-
C. Maternal conditions	-	-	-	-	-	-	-	-	-	-	-	-	-	-	-	-	-
1. Maternal haemorrhage	-	-	-	-	-	-	-	-	-	-	-	-	-	-	-	-	-
2. Maternal sepsis	-	-	-	-	-	-	-	-	-	-	-	-	-	-	-	-	-
3. Hypertensive disorders*	-	-	-	-	-	-	-	-	-	-	-	-	-	-	-	-	-
4. Obstructed labour	-	-	-	-	-	-	-	-	-	-	-	-	-	-	-	-	-
5. Abortion	-	-	-	-	-	-	-	-	-	-	-	-	-	-	-	-	-
6. Other maternal	-	-	-	-	-	-	-	-	-	-	-	-	-	-	-	-	-
D. Perinatal conditions*	**9**	**6**	**3**	**6**	**-**	**-**	**-**	**-**	**-**	**-**	**3**	**-**	**-**	**-**	**-**	**-**	**-**
E. Nutritional deficiencies	**7**	**2**	**5**	**-**	**-**	**-**	**-**	**-**	**-**	**2**	**-**	**-**	**-**	**-**	**-**	**-**	**4**
1. Protein-energy malnutrition	2	1	1	-	-	-	-	-	-	-	-	-	-	-	-	-	1
2. Iodine deficiency	-	-	-	-	-	-	-	-	-	-	-	-	-	-	-	-	-
3. Vitamin A deficiency	-	-	-	-	-	-	-	-	-	-	-	-	-	-	-	-	-
4. Iron-deficiency anaemia	3	1	2	-	-	-	-	-	-	1	-	-	-	-	-	-	2
II. Noncommunicable diseases	***4 176***	***2 297***	***1 880***	***10***	***3***	***10***	***71***	***508***	***556***	***1 140***	***8***	***2***	***5***	***25***	***112***	***223***	***1 505***
A. Malignant neoplasms	**986**	**660**	**326**	**1**	**1**	**4**	**27**	**215**	**199**	**213**	**1**	**1**	**3**	**15**	**59**	**87**	**161**
1. Mouth and oropharynx cancers	28	25	3	-	-	-	2	13	6	4	-	-	-	-	-	1	2
2. Oesophagus cancer	17	14	3	-	-	-	1	7	4	3	-	-	-	-	-	1	2
3. Stomach cancer	149	101	48	-	-	-	4	36	28	34	-	-	-	2	7	12	28
4. Colon and rectum cancers	98	55	43	-	-	-	2	14	15	24	-	-	-	1	6	10	25
5. Liver cancer	30	19	11	-	-	-	1	6	6	6	-	-	-	-	1	3	6
6. Pancreas cancer	42	27	15	-	-	-	1	10	8	9	-	-	-	-	2	4	9
7. Trachea, bronchus, lung cancers	280	235	45	-	-	-	8	77	84	66	-	-	-	1	9	15	19
8. Melanoma and other skin cancers	12	7	5	-	-	-	1	2	1	3	-	-	-	-	1	1	3
9. Breast cancer	41	-	41	-	-	-	-	-	-	-	-	-	-	4	12	11	15
10. Cervix uteri cancer	16	-	16	-	-	-	-	-	-	-	-	-	-	2	3	4	6
11. Corpus uteri cancer	14	-	14	-	-	-	-	-	-	-	-	-	-	-	3	4	7
12. Ovary cancer	16	-	16	-	-	-	-	-	-	-	-	-	-	1	5	5	5
13. Prostate cancer	26	26	-	-	-	-	-	3	6	18	-	-	-	-	-	-	-
14. Bladder cancer	25	21	4	-	-	-	-	5	6	10	-	-	-	-	-	1	3
15. Lymphomas, multiple myeloma	22	15	7	-	-	1	2	5	4	3	-	-	-	1	1	2	3
16. Leukaemia	24	15	9	-	1	1	1	4	4	4	1	-	1	1	1	2	3
17. Other cancers	145	99	46	-	1	2	6	35	27	29	-	1	1	2	7	11	24

Annex Table 20b, continued.   Deaths by age, sex and cause (thousands): Formerly Socialist Economies of Europe, 2020, optimistic scenario

Cause	Total	Male	Female	Males							Females						
				0-4	5-14	15-29	30-44	45-59	60-69	70+	0-4	5-14	15-29	30-44	45-59	60-69	70+
B. Other neoplasms	**5**	**2**	**3**	-	-	-	-	-	-	**1**	-	-	-	-	**1**	**1**	**1**
C. Diabetes mellitus	**25**	**9**	**17**	-	-	-	-	**1**	**2**	**4**	-	-	-	-	**1**	**4**	**12**
D. Endocrine disorders	**2**	**1**	**1**	-	-	-	-	-	-	**1**	-	-	-	-	-	-	**1**
E. Neuro-psychiatric conditions	**61**	**24**	**37**	**1**	**1**	**1**	**2**	**4**	**3**	**13**	**1**	-	**1**	**1**	**1**	**3**	**30**
2. Bipolar disorder	7	1	5	-	-	-	-	-	-	1	-	-	-	1	-	-	5
3. Schizophrenia	4	2	2	-	-	-	1	-	-	1	-	-	-	-	-	-	2
4. Epilepsy	4	2	2	1	1	1	1	1	1	1	-	-	-	-	-	-	1
5. Alcohol use	5	4	1	-	-	-	1	1	1	1	-	-	-	-	-	-	-
6. Dementia*	19	5	14	-	-	-	-	-	1	4	-	-	-	-	-	1	13
7. Parkinson disease	8	3	5	-	-	-	-	-	-	2	-	-	-	-	-	-	5
8. Multiple sclerosis	3	1	2	-	-	-	-	-	-	1	-	-	-	-	-	-	1
9. Drug use	-	-	-	-	-	-	-	-	-	-	-	-	-	-	-	-	-
13. Other neuro-psychiatric	11	6	6	1	-	1	-	1	1	2	1	-	1	-	-	1	4
F. Sense organ diseases	**-**	**-**	**-**	-	-	-	-	-	-	-	-	-	-	-	-	-	-
1. Glaucoma	-	-	-	-	-	-	-	-	-	-	-	-	-	-	-	-	-
2. Cataracts	-	-	-	-	-	-	-	-	-	-	-	-	-	-	-	-	-
G. Cardiovascular diseases	**2 600**	**1 281**	**1 319**	-	-	**2**	**33**	**236**	**281**	**728**	-	-	**1**	**6**	**34**	**101**	**1 177**
1. Rheumatic heart disease	22	13	9	-	-	-	2	7	3	1	-	-	-	1	3	3	3
2. Ischaemic heart disease	1 309	679	630	-	-	1	19	144	148	367	-	-	-	2	15	48	565
3. Cerebrovascular disease	789	349	440	-	-	1	5	52	80	211	-	-	-	2	13	37	388
4. Inflammatory heart diseases	46	26	20	-	-	1	2	7	4	12	-	-	-	-	1	1	17
5. Other cardiovascular	434	215	219	-	-	-	5	26	46	137	-	-	-	1	2	13	203
H. Respiratory diseases	**321**	**216**	**105**	-	-	-	**2**	**27**	**47**	**139**	-	-	-	**1**	**6**	**14**	**83**
1. COPD*	165	111	54	-	-	-	1	13	24	73	-	-	-	1	2	7	44
2. Asthma	14	7	7	-	-	-	-	1	1	4	-	-	-	-	1	1	5
3. Other respiratory	142	98	44	-	-	1	1	13	21	62	-	-	-	-	3	6	34
I. Digestive diseases	**122**	**73**	**49**	-	-	-	**4**	**21**	**18**	**29**	-	-	-	**2**	**7**	**9**	**30**
1. Peptic ulcer	15	11	5	-	-	-	1	3	3	5	-	-	-	-	-	1	3
2. Cirrhosis of the liver	50	33	17	-	-	-	2	12	10	10	-	-	-	1	4	4	8
3. Appendicitis	1	-	-	-	-	-	-	-	-	-	-	-	-	-	-	-	-
4. Other digestive	56	29	27	-	-	-	2	6	6	14	-	-	-	1	3	4	19
J. Genito-urinary diseases	**35**	**20**	**15**	-	-	-	**1**	**3**	**3**	**13**	-	-	-	-	**2**	**3**	**9**
1. Nephritis and nephrosis	14	7	7	-	-	-	1	2	1	3	-	-	-	-	1	1	4
2. Benign prostatic hypertrophy	6	6	-	-	-	-	-	-	1	6	-	-	-	-	-	-	-
3. Other genito-urinary	15	7	8	-	-	-	-	1	1	4	-	-	-	-	1	2	5
K. Skin diseases	**1**	**1**	**1**	-	-	-	-	-	-	-	-	-	-	-	-	-	-

Annex Table 20b, continued. Deaths by age, sex and cause (thousands): Formerly Socialist Economies of Europe, 2020, optimistic scenario

Cause	Total	Male	Female	Males							Females						
				0-4	5-14	15-29	30-44	45-59	60-69	70+	0-4	5-14	15-29	30-44	45-59	60-69	70+
L. Musculo-skeletal diseases	3	1	2	-	-	-	-	-	-	-	-	-	-	-	-	1	1
1. Rheumatoid arthritis	1	-	-	-	-	-	-	-	-	-	-	-	-	-	-	1	1
3. Other musculo-skeletal	3	1	2	-	-	-	-	-	-	-	-	-	-	-	-	-	1
M. Congenital anomalies	14	8	6	7	-	-	-	-	-	-	6	-	-	-	-	-	-
N. Oral conditions	-	-	-	-	-	-	-	-	-	-	-	-	-	-	-	-	-
III. Injuries	407	281	126	6	6	67	72	67	26	36	5	4	20	18	22	16	42
A. Unintentional injuries	254	172	82	3	4	42	41	42	16	24	2	2	11	10	14	10	33
1. Road traffic accidents	113	79	35	1	2	31	18	14	5	7	1	1	9	6	6	4	8
2. Poisonings	38	27	11	-	-	2	8	11	3	2	-	-	1	2	4	2	2
3. Falls	35	17	18	-	-	1	2	3	2	8	-	-	-	-	1	1	15
4. Fires	7	4	3	-	-	-	1	1	-	1	-	-	-	-	-	-	2
5. Drownings	17	13	3	-	1	3	4	3	1	1	-	-	1	-	1	-	2
6. Other unintentional	44	32	12	1	1	5	8	9	3	4	1	-	1	1	3	2	4
B. Intentional injuries	153	109	44	3	2	25	31	26	10	12	3	1	8	8	8	6	10
1. Self-inflicted injuries	93	70	23	-	-	11	19	20	8	11	-	-	2	3	5	4	8
2. Violence	32	23	9	-	-	7	9	5	1	1	-	-	1	2	2	1	2
3. War	29	17	12	3	2	7	3	1	-	-	3	1	5	2	1	-	-

Notes:
Causes responsible for no deaths have been omitted from this table.
A dash (-) symbol indicates fewer than 500 deaths.
ᵃIA6 is Bacterial meningitis and meningococcaemia; IC3 is Hypertensive disorders of pregnancy; ID is Conditions arising during the perinatal period;
IIE6 is Dementia and other degenerative and hereditary CNS disorders; IIH1 is Chronic obstructive pulmonary disease.

Annex Table 20c. Deaths by age, sex and cause (thousands): India, 2020, optimistic scenario

Cause	Total	Male	Female	Males							Females						
				0-4	5-14	15-29	30-44	45-59	60-69	70+	0-4	5-14	15-29	30-44	45-59	60-69	70+
Population (millions)	*1 245*	*613*	*632*	*53*	*105*	*160*	*149*	*104*	*38*	*22*	*50*	*100*	*152*	*141*	*102*	*41*	*27*
All causes	**10 670**	**6 092**	**4 578**	**455**	**91**	**232**	**447**	**1 414**	**1 473**	**1 980**	**415**	**79**	**174**	**223**	**650**	**760**	**2 276**
I. Communicable, maternal, perinatal and nutritional conditions	*1 502*	*812*	*690*	*293*	*14*	*38*	*82*	*59*	*61*	*266*	*273*	*17*	*35*	*53*	*34*	*37*	*240*
A. Infectious and parasitic diseases	**937**	**534**	**403**	**148**	**10**	**36**	**80**	**55**	**40**	**165**	**138**	**11**	**31**	**48**	**29**	**21**	**126**
1. Tuberculosis	**263**	**176**	**88**	3	1	4	9	27	22	110	2	1	1	2	15	9	58
2. STDs excluding HIV	**19**	**8**	**10**	4	–	–	–	–	–	4	4	–	–	–	–	–	5
a. Syphilis	18	8	10	4	–	–	–	–	–	4	4	–	–	–	–	–	5
b. Chlamydia	–	–	–	–	–	–	–	–	–	–	–	–	–	–	–	–	–
c. Gonorrhoea	–	–	–	–	–	–	–	–	–	–	–	–	–	–	–	–	–
3. HIV	**261**	**152**	**109**	19	3	30	67	22	7	4	20	3	28	44	9	2	1
4. Diarrhoeal diseases	**206**	**102**	**104**	68	2	1	1	2	5	24	64	2	–	–	2	4	31
5. Childhood-cluster diseases	**88**	**47**	**41**	40	2	–	1	1	–	2	35	2	–	–	1	–	3
a. Pertussis	14	7	6	7	–	–	–	–	–	–	6	–	–	–	–	–	–
b. Poliomyelitis	2	1	1	1	–	–	–	–	–	–	1	–	–	–	–	–	–
c. Diphtheria	1	–	–	1	–	–	–	–	–	–	–	–	–	–	–	–	–
d. Measles	34	18	16	17	1	–	–	–	–	–	15	1	–	–	–	–	–
e. Tetanus	37	20	18	15	1	–	–	–	–	–	13	1	–	–	–	–	2
6. Bacterial meningitis*	**9**	**5**	**5**	2	–	–	–	–	1	1	2	–	–	–	–	1	1
7. Hepatitis B and hepatitis C	**6**	**3**	**3**	–	–	–	–	–	–	2	–	–	–	–	–	–	2
8. Malaria	**4**	**2**	**2**	1	–	–	–	–	–	1	1	–	–	–	–	–	1
9. Tropical-cluster diseases	**3**	**2**	**1**	–	1	–	–	–	–	–	–	–	–	–	–	–	–
a. Trypanosomiasis	–	–	–	–	–	–	–	–	–	–	–	–	–	–	–	–	–
b. Chagas disease	–	–	–	–	–	–	–	–	–	–	–	–	–	–	–	–	–
c. Schistosomiasis	–	–	–	–	–	–	–	–	–	–	–	–	–	–	–	–	–
d. Leishmaniasis	3	2	1	1	1	–	–	–	–	–	1	–	–	–	–	–	–
10. Leprosy	–	–	–	–	–	–	–	–	–	–	–	–	–	–	–	–	–
11. Dengue	**1**	**1**	–	–	–	–	–	–	–	–	–	–	–	–	–	–	–
12. Japanese encephalitis	–	–	–	–	–	–	–	–	–	–	–	–	–	–	–	–	–
13. Trachoma	–	–	–	–	–	–	–	–	–	–	–	–	–	–	–	–	–
14. Intestinal nematode infections	**1**	**1**	–	–	–	–	–	–	–	–	–	–	–	–	–	–	–
a. Ascariasis	–	–	–	–	–	–	–	–	–	–	–	–	–	–	–	–	–
b. Trichuriasis	–	–	–	–	–	–	–	–	–	–	–	–	–	–	–	–	–
c. Ancylostomiasis, necatoriasis	1	–	–	–	–	–	–	–	–	–	–	–	–	–	–	–	–
15. Other infectious and parasitic	**75**	**36**	**40**	11	1	–	1	2	4	17	10	1	–	–	1	3	23

Annex Table 20c, continued. Deaths by age, sex and cause (thousands): India, 2020, optimistic scenario

Cause	Total	Male	Female	Males 0-4	5-14	15-29	30-44	45-59	60-69	70+	Females 0-4	5-14	15-29	30-44	45-59	60-69	70+
B. Respiratory infections	397	197	201	71	3	1	2	4	20	95	67	6	1	1	4	15	107
1. Lower respiratory infections	391	194	198	69	3	1	2	4	20	94	65	6	1	1	4	15	106
2. Upper respiratory infections	4	2	2	1	-	-	-	-	-	1	1	-	1	-	-	-	1
3. Otitis media	2	1	1	1	-	-	-	-	-	-	1	-	-	-	-	-	-
C. Maternal conditions	8	-	8	-	-	-	-	-	-	-	-	-	3	4	1	-	-
1. Maternal haemorrhage	2	-	2	-	-	-	-	-	-	-	-	-	1	1	-	-	-
2. Maternal sepsis	1	-	1	-	-	-	-	-	-	-	-	-	-	1	-	-	-
3. Hypertensive disorders*	1	-	1	-	-	-	-	-	-	-	-	-	-	1	-	-	-
4. Obstructed labour	1	-	1	-	-	-	-	-	-	-	-	-	-	-	1	-	-
5. Abortion	1	-	1	-	-	-	-	-	-	-	-	-	1	-	-	-	-
6. Other maternal	2	-	2	-	-	-	-	-	-	-	-	-	1	1	-	-	-
D. Perinatal conditions*	128	67	62	67	-	-	-	-	-	-	62	-	-	-	-	-	-
E. Nutritional deficiencies	31	14	17	7	1	-	-	1	1	6	7	1	-	-	1	1	7
1. Protein-energy malnutrition	17	8	9	4	-	-	-	1	1	2	4	-	-	-	1	1	3
2. Iodine deficiency	1	-	1	-	-	-	-	-	-	-	-	1	-	-	-	-	-
3. Vitamin A deficiency	3	2	1	1	1	-	-	-	-	-	1	-	-	-	-	-	-
4. Iron-deficiency anaemia	10	5	6	2	-	-	-	-	-	3	2	-	-	-	-	-	4
II. Noncommunicable diseases	7 775	4 459	3 317	104	17	32	176	1 154	1 346	1 631	101	14	37	84	496	662	1 924
A. Malignant neoplasms	1 359	792	567	4	5	14	59	310	184	216	3	2	19	41	206	130	165
1. Mouth and oropharynx cancers	189	119	70	-	-	2	6	49	26	36	-	-	2	4	27	17	20
2. Oesophagus cancer	121	66	56	-	-	1	3	26	14	22	-	-	2	2	18	14	21
3. Stomach cancer	105	70	35	-	1	1	4	29	13	22	-	1	1	2	11	9	12
4. Colon and rectum cancers	49	26	22	-	-	1	3	8	5	9	-	-	1	1	6	6	9
5. Liver cancer	31	22	9	-	-	-	1	9	4	8	-	-	-	1	2	2	4
6. Pancreas cancer	18	11	7	-	-	-	-	5	2	4	-	-	-	-	2	2	3
7. Trachea, bronchus, lung cancers	290	249	41	-	-	1	18	112	83	35	-	-	1	2	15	13	10
8. Melanoma and other skin cancers	3	1	1	-	-	-	-	1	-	-	-	-	-	-	1	-	-
9. Breast cancer	72	-	72	-	-	-	-	-	-	-	-	-	3	7	30	15	17
10. Cervix uteri cancer	102	-	102	-	-	-	-	-	-	-	-	-	3	7	51	20	20
11. Corpus uteri cancer	8	-	8	-	-	-	-	-	-	-	-	-	-	1	2	2	3
12. Ovary cancer	25	-	25	-	-	-	-	-	-	-	-	-	1	3	7	6	7
13. Prostate cancer	29	29	-	-	-	-	-	3	5	21	-	-	-	-	-	-	-
14. Bladder cancer	17	13	4	-	-	-	-	3	3	7	-	-	-	-	1	1	2
15. Lymphomas, multiple myeloma	40	26	15	1	1	1	4	9	3	6	1	-	1	1	3	3	6
16. Leukaemia	29	17	11	1	2	1	4	5	2	3	1	1	1	2	3	2	2
17. Other cancers	232	142	89	2	2	5	15	52	23	43	1	1	4	9	27	20	28

Annex Table 20c, continued. Deaths by age, sex and cause (thousands): India, 2020, optimistic scenario

Cause	Total	Male	Female	Males 0-4	5-14	15-29	30-44	45-59	60-69	70+	Females 0-4	5-14	15-29	30-44	45-59	60-69	70+
B. Other neoplasms	4	2	1	-	-	-	1	-	-	-	-	-	-	-	-	-	-
C. Diabetes mellitus	107	44	63	2	1	1	3	10	11	17	2	1	1	1	9	18	31
D. Endocrine disorders	2	1	1	-	-	-	-	-	-	-	-	-	-	-	-	-	-
E. Neuro-psychiatric conditions	105	54	51	6	2	2	7	9	10	18	7	1	2	2	3	9	27
2. Bipolar disorder	3	1	2	-	-	-	-	1	1	1	-	-	-	-	-	1	2
3. Schizophrenia	5	2	3	-	-	1	-	1	1	1	-	-	1	-	-	1	2
4. Epilepsy	10	6	4	-	1	-	2	2	1	1	1	-	1	-	-	1	1
5. Alcohol use	5	4	-	-	-	1	2	2	1	-	-	-	-	-	-	-	-
6. Dementia*	27	11	16	-	-	-	-	1	2	7	-	-	-	-	1	2	12
7. Parkinson disease	8	4	3	-	-	-	-	-	1	3	-	-	-	-	1	1	2
8. Multiple sclerosis	3	1	2	-	-	-	-	1	-	-	-	-	-	-	1	-	-
9. Drug use	-	-	-	-	-	-	-	-	-	-	-	-	-	-	-	-	-
13. Other neuro-psychiatric	44	23	21	5	1	1	3	3	5	5	6	1	1	1	1	4	8
F. Sense organ diseases	-	-	-	-	-	-	-	-	-	-	-	-	-	-	-	-	-
1. Glaucoma	-	-	-	-	-	-	-	-	-	-	-	-	-	-	-	-	-
2. Cataracts	-	-	-	-	-	-	-	-	-	-	-	-	-	-	-	-	-
G. Cardiovascular diseases	4 977	2 827	2 150	14	2	7	75	650	957	1 121	9	3	6	24	194	425	1 489
1. Rheumatic heart disease	109	62	46	-	2	2	11	32	13	5	-	-	2	7	20	9	8
2. Ischaemic heart disease	2 703	1 552	1 151	-	-	-	23	354	549	626	-	-	-	7	92	234	817
3. Cerebrovascular disease	989	543	445	3	1	-	8	98	188	245	2	1	1	3	29	91	319
4. Inflammatory heart diseases	146	87	59	2	-	2	8	33	19	22	2	1	1	3	12	9	31
5. Other cardiovascular	1 031	582	449	9	1	2	25	133	189	224	5	1	2	3	41	82	314
H. Respiratory diseases	678	402	276	3	3	2	9	78	130	177	2	2	4	6	50	56	156
1. COPD*	392	241	152	1	-	-	2	40	81	116	1	-	1	1	23	32	94
2. Asthma	50	28	22	-	-	-	2	7	7	11	-	-	-	1	5	4	11
3. Other respiratory	236	134	103	2	2	1	5	31	42	49	2	2	3	4	22	19	52
I. Digestive diseases	288	205	83	1	1	4	18	85	39	58	1	1	3	6	24	14	34
1. Peptic ulcer	54	36	18	-	-	1	2	12	8	13	-	-	-	1	4	3	3
2. Cirrhosis of the liver	182	136	46	-	-	2	10	59	25	39	-	1	1	3	15	7	19
3. Appendicitis	6	3	2	-	-	1	1	1	-	-	-	-	-	1	-	-	-
4. Other digestive	47	30	17	1	-	1	4	13	5	6	1	-	1	2	5	3	6
J. Genito-urinary diseases	93	52	41	2	2	1	3	10	13	22	1	3	1	2	7	9	19
1. Nephritis and nephrosis	80	40	40	2	2	1	3	9	9	15	1	3	1	1	6	8	19
2. Benign prostatic hypertrophy	11	11	-	-	-	-	-	-	4	7	-	-	-	-	-	-	-
3. Other genito-urinary	2	1	1	-	-	-	-	1	-	-	-	-	-	-	-	-	-
K. Skin diseases	2	1	1	-	-	-	-	-	-	-	-	-	-	-	-	-	-

Annex Table 20c, continued. Deaths by age, sex and cause (thousands): India, 2020, optimistic scenario

Cause	Total	Male	Female	Males							Females						
				0-4	5-14	15-29	30-44	45-59	60-69	70+	0-4	5-14	15-29	30-44	45-59	60-69	70+
L. Musculo-skeletal diseases	2	1	1	-	-	-	-	-	-	-	-	-	-	-	-	-	1
1. Rheumatoid arthritis	2	1	1	-	-	-	-	-	-	-	-	-	-	-	-	-	1
3. Other musculo-skeletal	-	-	-	-	-	-	-	-	-	-	-	-	-	-	-	-	-
M. Congenital anomalies	158	77	81	70	1	2	2	1	1	1	74	2	1	1	2	1	1
N. Oral conditions	-	-	-	-	-	-	-	-	-	-	-	-	-	-	-	-	-
III. Injuries	1 393	821	571	58	60	162	189	201	67	83	42	47	102	86	120	62	112
A. Unintentional injuries	1 131	670	461	53	56	124	148	159	58	73	35	43	64	63	95	54	107
1. Road traffic accidents	606	415	191	15	37	100	94	100	35	35	4	29	26	26	46	25	35
2. Poisonings	29	15	14	4	1	2	6	3	1	1	2	1	3	3	3	-	1
3. Falls	64	37	27	3	3	2	6	9	5	10	3	1	1	2	4	4	13
4. Fires	133	41	92	7	1	5	10	10	3	4	6	3	24	20	14	8	18
5. Drownings	81	40	40	8	6	5	8	6	2	5	6	4	4	4	7	3	11
6. Other unintentional	219	123	96	17	8	10	26	30	12	19	14	5	7	8	18	14	29
B. Intentional injuries	261	151	110	5	5	38	42	42	9	11	6	4	38	24	25	7	6
1. Self-inflicted injuries	165	92	73	-	3	27	25	27	4	6	-	3	34	21	12	1	2
2. Violence	91	54	37	5	2	8	14	15	5	5	6	1	4	3	13	6	3
3. War	5	5	-	-	-	3	2	-	-	-	-	-	-	-	-	-	-

Notes:
Causes responsible for no deaths have been omitted from this table.
A dash (-) symbol indicates fewer than 500 deaths.
*IA6 is Bacterial meningitis and meningococcaemia; IC3 is Hypertensive disorders of pregnancy; ID is Conditions arising during the perinatal period; IIE6 is Dementia and other degenerative and hereditary CNS disorders; IIH1 is Chronic obstructive pulmonary disease.

Annex Table 20d. Deaths by age, sex and cause (thousands): China, 2020, optimistic scenario

Cause	Total	Male	Female	Males							Females						
				0-4	5-14	15-29	30-44	45-59	60-69	70+	0-4	5-14	15-29	30-44	45-59	60-69	70+
Population (millions)	*1 479*	*742*	*738*	*57*	*103*	*169*	*150*	*164*	*63*	*37*	*54*	*98*	*161*	*143*	*162*	*70*	*50*
All causes	**12 921**	**7 690**	**5 232**	**128**	**36**	**184**	**356**	**1 867**	**2 035**	**3 083**	**130**	**27**	**147**	**167**	**703**	**907**	**3 150**
I. Communicable, maternal, perinatal and nutritional conditions	*484*	*254*	*230*	*50*	*1*	*1*	*2*	*10*	*18*	*171*	*51*	*1*	*1*	*1*	*6*	*13*	*156*
A. Infectious and parasitic diseases	**212**	**120**	**92**	**9**	**1**	**1**	**2**	**9**	**14**	**84**	**8**	**1**	**-**	**-**	**5**	**9**	**68**
1. Tuberculosis	**126**	**78**	**48**	-	-	-	1	6	11	59	-	-	-	-	4	6	37
2. STDs excluding HIV	-	-	-	-	-	-	-	-	-	-	-	-	-	-	-	-	-
a. Syphilis	-	-	-	-	-	-	-	-	-	-	-	-	-	-	-	-	-
b. Chlamydia	-	-	-	-	-	-	-	-	-	-	-	-	-	-	-	-	-
c. Gonorrhoea	-	-	-	-	-	-	-	-	-	-	-	-	-	-	-	-	-
3. HIV	**2**	**1**	**1**	-	-	-	1	-	-	-	-	-	-	-	-	-	-
4. Diarrhoeal diseases	**39**	**18**	**21**	3	-	-	-	-	1	13	3	-	-	-	-	1	17
5. Childhood-cluster diseases	**7**	**4**	**3**	3	-	-	-	-	-	-	3	-	-	-	-	-	-
a. Pertussis	2	1	1	1	-	-	-	-	-	-	1	-	-	-	-	-	-
b. Poliomyelitis	-	-	-	-	-	-	-	-	-	-	-	-	-	-	-	-	-
c. Diphtheria	-	-	-	-	-	-	-	-	-	-	-	-	-	-	-	-	-
d. Measles	2	1	1	1	-	-	-	-	-	-	1	-	-	-	-	-	-
e. Tetanus	2	1	1	1	-	-	-	-	-	-	1	-	-	-	-	-	-
6. Bacterial meningitis*	**9**	**4**	**5**	1	-	-	-	-	1	2	1	-	-	-	-	1	2
7. Hepatitis B and hepatitis C	**11**	**6**	**5**	-	-	-	-	1	-	4	-	-	-	-	1	-	4
8. Malaria	-	-	-	-	-	-	-	-	-	-	-	-	-	-	-	-	-
9. Tropical-cluster diseases	**1**	-	-	-	-	-	-	-	-	-	-	-	-	-	-	-	-
a. Trypanosomiasis	-	-	-	-	-	-	-	-	-	-	-	-	-	-	-	-	-
b. Chagas disease	-	-	-	-	-	-	-	-	-	-	-	-	-	-	-	-	-
c. Schistosomiasis	1	-	-	-	-	-	-	-	-	-	-	-	-	-	-	-	-
d. Leishmaniasis	-	-	-	-	-	-	-	-	-	-	-	-	-	-	-	-	-
10. Leprosy	-	-	-	-	-	-	-	-	-	-	-	-	-	-	-	-	-
11. Dengue	-	-	-	-	-	-	-	-	-	-	-	-	-	-	-	-	-
12. Japanese encephalitis	-	-	-	-	-	-	-	-	-	-	-	-	-	-	-	-	-
13. Trachoma	-	-	-	-	-	-	-	-	-	-	-	-	-	-	-	-	-
14. Intestinal nematode infections	**1**	-	-	-	-	-	-	-	-	-	-	-	-	-	-	-	-
a. Ascariasis	-	-	-	-	-	-	-	-	-	-	-	-	-	-	-	-	-
b. Trichuriasis	-	-	-	-	-	-	-	-	-	-	-	-	-	-	-	-	-
c. Ancylostomiasis, necatoriasis	-	-	-	-	-	-	-	-	-	-	-	-	-	-	-	-	-
15. Other infectious and parasitic	**16**	**8**	**8**	-	-	-	-	1	1	6	-	-	-	-	1	1	7

Annex Table 20d, continued. Deaths by age, sex and cause (thousands): China, 2020, optimistic scenario

Cause	Total	Male	Female	Males 0-4	5-14	15-29	30-44	45-59	60-69	70+	Females 0-4	5-14	15-29	30-44	45-59	60-69	70+
B. Respiratory infections	**209**	**105**	**104**	**19**	–	–	–	**1**	**3**	**81**	**19**	–	–	–	**1**	**3**	**80**
1. Lower respiratory infections	206	103	103	18	–	–	–	1	3	80	19	–	–	–	1	3	80
2. Upper respiratory infections	2	1	1	–	–	–	–	–	–	1	–	–	–	–	–	–	1
3. Otitis media	–	–	–	–	–	–	–	–	–	–	–	–	–	–	–	–	–
C. Maternal conditions	**1**	–	**1**	–	–	–	–	–	–	–	–	–	**1**	–	–	–	–
1. Maternal haemorrhage	–	–	–	–	–	–	–	–	–	–	–	–	–	–	–	–	–
2. Maternal sepsis	–	–	–	–	–	–	–	–	–	–	–	–	–	–	–	–	–
3. Hypertensive disorders*	–	–	–	–	–	–	–	–	–	–	–	–	1	–	–	–	–
4. Obstructed labour	–	–	–	–	–	–	–	–	–	–	–	–	–	–	–	–	–
5. Abortion	–	–	–	–	–	–	–	–	–	–	–	–	–	–	–	–	–
6. Other maternal	–	–	–	–	–	–	–	–	–	–	–	–	–	–	–	–	–
D. Perinatal conditions*	**40**	**20**	**20**	**20**	–	–	–	–	–	–	**20**	–	–	–	–	–	–
E. Nutritional deficiencies	**22**	**9**	**13**	**2**	–	–	–	–	–	**6**	**4**	–	–	–	–	**1**	**8**
1. Protein-energy malnutrition	12	6	7	1	–	–	–	–	–	4	2	–	–	–	–	1	4
2. Iodine deficiency	1	1	–	–	–	–	–	–	–	–	–	–	–	–	–	–	–
3. Vitamin A deficiency	1	1	–	–	–	–	–	–	–	–	–	–	–	–	–	–	–
4. Iron-deficiency anaemia	8	3	5	–	–	–	–	–	–	2	1	–	–	–	–	–	4
II. Noncommunicable diseases	***10 977***	***6 691***	***4 286***	***40***	***12***	***44***	***233***	***1 699***	***1 917***	***2 745***	***43***	***7***	***23***	***92***	***550***	***802***	***2 768***
A. Malignant neoplasms	**3 518**	**2 386**	**1 132**	**3**	**8**	**22**	**152**	**888**	**746**	**566**	**5**	**4**	**12**	**57**	**300**	**334**	**420**
1. Mouth and oropharynx cancers	80	58	22	–	–	1	8	21	15	12	–	–	–	2	7	6	6
2. Oesophagus cancer	458	324	134	–	–	–	10	100	109	105	–	–	–	1	26	52	55
3. Stomach cancer	763	530	234	–	–	1	15	175	179	159	–	–	1	10	49	72	102
4. Colon and rectum cancers	189	111	78	–	–	2	7	34	32	37	–	–	1	4	20	23	31
5. Liver cancer	690	525	165	–	1	4	65	244	130	82	–	1	1	10	50	46	57
6. Pancreas cancer	76	49	28	–	–	–	1	13	16	18	–	–	–	–	4	10	13
7. Trachea, bronchus, lung cancers	691	517	174	–	–	1	19	209	199	87	–	–	–	3	48	56	66
8. Melanoma and other skin cancers	3	2	1	–	–	–	–	–	–	1	–	–	–	–	–	–	1
9. Breast cancer	51	–	51	–	–	–	–	–	–	–	–	–	–	7	18	11	15
10. Cervix uteri cancer	44	–	44	–	–	–	–	–	–	–	–	–	–	3	15	13	13
11. Corpus uteri cancer	13	–	13	–	–	–	–	–	–	–	–	–	–	1	7	3	3
12. Ovary cancer	19	–	19	–	–	–	–	–	–	–	–	–	–	2	7	4	5
13. Prostate cancer	12	12	–	–	–	–	–	1	5	6	–	–	–	–	–	–	–
14. Bladder cancer	45	36	9	–	–	–	–	6	14	15	–	–	–	1	–	3	5
15. Lymphomas, multiple myeloma	48	33	15	–	1	2	1	11	11	7	–	–	–	1	6	3	4
16. Leukaemia	99	55	44	2	4	6	10	19	7	7	2	2	5	7	12	7	9
17. Other cancers	237	135	102	1	2	4	14	54	28	32	2	1	2	8	30	25	34

Annex Table 20d, continued. Deaths by age, sex and cause (thousands): China, 2020, optimistic scenario

Cause	Total	Male	Female	Males							Females						
				0-4	5-14	15-29	30-44	45-59	60-69	70+	0-4	5-14	15-29	30-44	45-59	60-69	70+
B. Other neoplasms	16	8	8	1	-	1	1	2	2	2	1	-	-	-	1	2	3
C. Diabetes mellitus	60	23	37	-	-	-	1	5	6	10	-	-	-	-	5	10	22
D. Endocrine disorders	12	4	8	1	-	-	-	1	1	2	1	-	-	-	-	1	5
E. Neuro-psychiatric conditions	85	37	48	1	1	5	5	5	4	16	1	-	2	2	4	6	33
2. Bipolar disorder	3	1	3	-	-	1	-	-	-	-	-	-	-	2	-	-	2
3. Schizophrenia	11	7	4	-	-	1	2	1	1	3	-	-	1	1	1	1	2
4. Epilepsy	7	4	3	-	-	1	1	1	1	1	-	-	1	-	1	-	1
5. Alcohol use	3	3	-	-	-	1	1	1	-	-	-	-	-	-	-	-	-
6. Dementia*	34	10	23	-	-	-	-	-	1	7	-	-	-	-	1	2	19
7. Parkinson disease	7	3	4	-	-	-	-	-	-	3	-	-	-	-	-	-	4
8. Multiple sclerosis	4	2	2	-	-	-	-	-	-	1	-	-	-	-	-	-	1
9. Drug use	-	-	-	-	-	2	-	-	-	-	-	-	1	-	-	-	-
13. Other neuro-psychiatric	16	8	9	1	-	2	1	1	1	2	1	-	1	-	1	1	5
F. Sense organ diseases	16	8	8	-	-	-	-	2	2	3	-	-	-	-	2	3	3
1. Glaucoma	6	3	3	-	-	-	-	1	1	1	-	-	-	-	-	1	2
2. Cataracts	5	3	2	-	-	-	-	1	1	1	-	-	-	-	1	1	1
G. Cardiovascular diseases	4 431	2 633	1 799	4	1	7	47	583	729	1 261	3	-	4	17	125	241	1 409
1. Rheumatic heart disease	225	122	104	-	-	2	7	39	27	46	-	-	1	4	16	15	67
2. Ischaemic heart disease	1 346	776	570	-	-	1	15	164	207	389	-	-	1	5	31	73	460
3. Cerebrovascular disease	2 240	1 359	881	1	-	2	18	292	401	644	1	-	1	6	65	129	679
4. Inflammatory heart diseases	92	57	35	1	-	1	3	11	11	20	1	-	1	2	5	5	24
5. Other cardiovascular	528	318	210	3	-	-	3	67	83	162	1	-	-	1	8	20	179
H. Respiratory diseases	2 196	1 237	958	2	-	3	8	133	351	741	2	-	1	6	73	164	712
1. COPD*	2 074	1 168	906	1	-	1	6	123	335	702	1	-	1	5	67	157	675
2. Asthma	47	28	20	1	-	1	1	7	7	12	-	-	-	1	4	4	10
3. Other respiratory	75	42	33	1	-	1	1	3	8	27	-	-	-	-	1	3	27
I. Digestive diseases	427	248	179	2	-	1	13	69	63	99	2	-	1	5	32	29	109
1. Peptic ulcer	42	23	19	-	-	-	1	4	5	14	-	-	-	-	2	2	15
2. Cirrhosis of the liver	197	127	70	-	-	1	10	45	37	34	-	-	-	3	18	16	32
3. Appendicitis	4	2	2	-	-	-	-	1	-	-	-	-	-	-	-	-	-
4. Other digestive	184	95	89	2	-	-	2	20	20	51	2	-	1	2	12	11	61
J. Genito-urinary diseases	106	57	48	1	-	1	4	10	10	29	1	-	1	2	6	10	28
1. Nephritis and nephrosis	80	42	38	1	-	1	4	8	8	18	1	-	1	2	5	8	21
2. Benign prostatic hypertrophy	7	7	-	-	-	-	-	-	6	6	-	-	-	-	-	-	-
3. Other genito-urinary	19	9	11	-	-	-	1	1	2	5	-	-	-	-	1	2	7
K. Skin diseases	11	6	5	-	-	-	-	1	1	4	-	-	-	-	-	1	3

Annex Table 20d, continued. Deaths by age, sex and cause (thousands): China, 2020, optimistic scenario

Cause	Total	Male	Female	Males							Females						
				0-4	5-14	15-29	30-44	45-59	60-69	70+	0-4	5-14	15-29	30-44	45-59	60-69	70+
L. Musculo-skeletal diseases	**40**	**15**	**24**	–	–	–	–	1	3	11	–	–	–	–	1	2	20
1. Rheumatoid arthritis	2	1	1	–	–	–	–	–	–	1	–	–	–	–	–	–	1
3. Other musculo-skeletal	38	15	23	–	–	–	–	1	3	10	–	–	–	–	1	2	19
M. Congenital anomalies	**59**	**28**	**30**	25	1	2	–	–	–	–	27	1	1	–	–	–	–
N. Oral conditions	–	–	–	–	–	–	–	–	–	–	–	–	–	–	–	–	–
III. Injuries	***1 461***	***745***	***716***	*38*	*22*	*139*	*121*	*158*	*100*	*167*	*36*	*19*	*123*	*74*	*146*	*92*	*226*
A. Unintentional injuries	**855**	**456**	**399**	33	19	88	68	90	51	107	27	16	50	28	77	49	152
1. Road traffic accidents	379	230	149	4	10	65	44	49	26	32	3	12	41	18	40	17	19
2. Poisonings	69	35	33	2	–	2	4	11	4	12	1	1	3	3	6	6	14
3. Falls	120	37	83	1	–	2	2	5	6	21	2	–	–	1	8	11	61
4. Fires	35	15	20	1	–	1	1	1	1	10	1	–	–	–	3	2	13
5. Drownings	93	49	44	14	6	7	4	5	3	11	11	3	3	2	5	5	16
6. Other unintentional	159	90	69	12	2	12	13	19	11	21	11	1	3	3	15	7	29
B. Intentional injuries	**606**	**289**	**317**	4	4	51	54	68	49	60	8	3	73	46	69	43	73
1. Self-inflicted injuries	542	252	291	–	3	39	45	62	45	59	–	2	71	42	65	41	70
2. Violence	63	36	26	4	1	12	9	6	3	1	8	1	2	5	4	3	3
3. War	1	1	–	–	–	–	–	–	–	1	–	–	–	–	–	–	–

Notes:
Causes responsible for no deaths have been omitted from this table.
A dash (–) symbol indicates fewer than 500 deaths.
*IA6 is Bacterial meningitis and meningococcaemia; IC3 is Hypertensive disorders of pregnancy; ID is Conditions arising during the perinatal period; IIE6 is Dementia and other degenerative and hereditary CNS disorders; IIH1 is Chronic obstructive pulmonary disease.

Annex Table 20e. Deaths by age, sex and cause (thousands): Other Asia and Islands, 2020, optimistic scenario

Cause	Total	Male	Female	Males							Females						
				0-4	5-14	15-29	30-44	45-59	60-69	70+	0-4	5-14	15-29	30-44	45-59	60-69	70+
Population (millions)	1 029	511	518	44	84	125	118	87	33	20	42	81	121	116	91	39	28
All causes	7 382	4 220	3 161	305	81	187	369	869	854	1 555	227	51	102	172	388	500	1 721
I. Communicable, maternal, perinatal and nutritional conditions	931	493	438	199	11	17	36	30	40	158	140	9	18	29	26	28	188
A. Infectious and parasitic diseases	545	292	253	96	7	16	36	28	25	85	67	5	15	26	22	20	97
1. Tuberculosis	202	98	103	-	-	1	3	13	17	63	-	-	1	2	13	16	71
2. STDs excluding HIV	17	8	9	4	-	-	-	-	-	4	3	-	1	-	-	-	5
a. Syphilis	17	8	8	4	-	-	-	-	-	4	3	-	1	-	-	-	5
b. Chlamydia	-	-	-	-	-	-	-	-	-	-	-	-	-	-	-	-	-
c. Gonorrhoea	-	-	-	-	-	-	-	-	-	-	-	-	-	-	-	-	-
3. HIV	118	69	49	9	1	13	30	10	3	2	6	1	14	22	5	1	1
4. Diarrhoeal diseases	102	59	43	51	1	-	-	1	1	5	34	1	-	-	1	1	6
5. Childhood-cluster diseases	52	28	24	24	1	-	-	-	-	1	20	1	-	-	-	-	2
a. Pertussis	8	4	3	4	1	-	-	-	-	-	3	1	-	-	-	-	-
b. Poliomyelitis	1	-	-	-	-	-	-	-	-	-	-	-	-	-	-	-	-
c. Diphtheria	1	-	-	-	-	-	-	-	-	-	-	-	-	-	-	-	-
d. Measles	25	14	11	13	1	-	-	-	-	1	10	1	-	-	-	-	1
e. Tetanus	18	10	9	7	-	-	-	-	-	1	5	-	-	-	-	-	2
6. Bacterial meningitis*	8	4	4	1	-	-	-	1	1	1	1	-	-	-	1	-	1
7. Hepatitis B and hepatitis C	10	5	4	-	-	1	-	1	1	3	-	-	-	-	1	-	3
8. Malaria	15	8	7	1	1	1	1	1	1	1	1	1	1	1	1	1	2
9. Tropical-cluster diseases	1	1	-	-	-	-	-	-	-	-	-	-	-	-	-	-	-
a. Trypanosomiasis	-	-	-	-	-	-	-	-	-	-	-	-	-	-	-	-	-
b. Chagas disease	-	-	-	-	-	-	-	-	-	-	-	-	-	-	-	-	-
c. Schistosomiasis	-	-	-	-	-	-	-	-	-	-	-	-	-	-	-	-	-
d. Leishmaniasis	-	-	-	-	-	-	-	-	-	-	-	-	-	-	-	-	-
10. Leprosy	-	-	-	-	-	-	-	-	-	-	-	-	-	-	-	-	-
11. Dengue	1	1	-	-	-	-	-	-	-	-	-	-	-	-	-	-	-
12. Japanese encephalitis	-	-	-	-	-	-	-	-	-	-	-	-	-	-	-	-	-
13. Trachoma	-	-	-	-	-	-	-	-	-	-	-	-	-	-	-	-	-
14. Intestinal nematode infections	1	1	1	-	-	-	-	-	-	-	1	-	-	-	-	-	-
a. Ascariasis	-	-	-	-	-	-	-	-	-	-	-	-	-	-	-	-	-
b. Trichuriasis	-	-	-	-	-	-	-	-	-	-	-	-	-	-	-	-	-
c. Ancylostomiasis, necatoriasis	1	-	-	-	-	-	-	-	-	-	-	-	-	-	-	-	-
15. Other infectious and parasitic	19	10	9	4	-	-	-	1	1	4	3	-	-	-	-	-	5

Annex Table 20e, continued. Deaths by age, sex and cause (thousands): Other Asia and Islands, 2020, optimistic scenario

Cause	Total	Male	Female	Males							Females						
				0-4	5-14	15-29	30-44	45-59	60-69	70+	0-4	5-14	15-29	30-44	45-59	60-69	70+
B. Respiratory infections	271	139	132	47	4	1	1	2	15	70	32	3	1	1	2	7	86
1. Lower respiratory infections	268	138	130	46	4	1	1	2	15	69	31	3	-	1	2	7	85
2. Upper respiratory infections	3	1	1	-	-	-	-	-	-	1	-	-	-	-	-	-	1
3. Otitis media	1	-	-	-	-	-	-	-	-	-	-	-	-	-	1	-	-
C. Maternal conditions	5	-	5	-	-	-	-	-	-	-	-	-	2	3	1	-	-
1. Maternal haemorrhage	1	-	1	-	-	-	-	-	-	-	-	-	-	1	-	-	-
2. Maternal sepsis	1	-	1	-	-	-	-	-	-	-	-	-	-	-	-	-	-
3. Hypertensive disorders*	1	-	1	-	-	-	-	-	-	-	-	-	-	-	1	-	-
4. Obstructed labour	-	-	-	-	-	-	-	-	-	-	-	-	-	-	-	-	-
5. Abortion	1	-	1	-	-	-	-	-	-	-	-	-	1	-	-	-	-
6. Other maternal	1	-	1	-	-	-	-	-	-	-	-	-	-	1	-	-	-
D. Perinatal conditions*	85	49	36	49	-	-	-	-	-	-	36	-	-	-	-	-	-
E. Nutritional deficiencies	24	12	12	7	-	-	-	-	1	4	6	-	-	-	1	-	5
1. Protein-energy malnutrition	11	6	5	5	-	-	-	-	1	-	4	-	-	-	1	-	-
2. Iodine deficiency	-	-	-	-	-	-	-	-	-	-	-	-	-	-	-	-	-
3. Vitamin A deficiency	3	2	1	1	-	-	-	-	-	-	1	-	-	-	-	-	-
4. Iron-deficiency anaemia	9	4	5	-	-	-	-	-	-	3	-	-	-	-	-	-	4
II. Noncommunicable diseases	5 642	3 187	2 455	66	35	31	195	733	773	1 353	53	23	23	92	319	444	1 501
A. Malignant neoplasms	1 634	988	646	6	15	9	74	287	275	322	7	9	10	49	156	180	234
1. Mouth and oropharynx cancers	177	113	64	-	-	1	8	18	40	47	-	-	-	4	7	22	30
2. Oesophagus cancer	61	43	18	-	-	-	1	14	13	15	-	-	1	-	4	5	7
3. Stomach cancer	150	101	49	-	-	1	6	34	28	33	-	-	-	2	11	15	20
4. Colon and rectum cancers	105	57	48	-	-	1	4	9	20	23	-	-	-	2	6	17	23
5. Liver cancer	174	132	42	-	1	2	12	57	28	33	-	-	-	2	10	12	17
6. Pancreas cancer	26	16	9	-	-	-	1	5	5	6	-	-	-	-	2	3	4
7. Trachea, bronchus, lung cancers	293	222	72	-	-	-	13	85	56	67	-	-	1	-	18	25	27
8. Melanoma and other skin cancers	6	2	3	-	-	-	-	-	1	-	-	-	-	-	1	-	1
9. Breast cancer	62	-	62	-	-	-	-	-	-	-	-	-	1	7	23	13	17
10. Cervix uteri cancer	74	-	74	-	-	-	-	-	-	-	-	-	1	7	31	15	20
11. Corpus uteri cancer	10	-	10	-	-	-	-	-	-	-	-	-	-	-	3	3	4
12. Ovary cancer	22	-	22	-	-	-	-	-	-	-	-	-	1	4	6	4	6
13. Prostate cancer	36	36	-	-	-	-	-	3	15	17	-	-	-	-	-	-	-
14. Bladder cancer	30	22	8	-	-	-	-	5	8	9	-	-	-	-	1	3	4
15. Lymphomas, multiple myeloma	56	33	22	1	2	1	5	6	9	11	-	1	-	2	2	7	10
16. Leukaemia	50	28	22	2	3	1	6	3	5	6	3	3	1	3	2	4	6
17. Other cancers	303	182	121	2	6	2	18	49	49	54	3	4	3	13	28	31	39

Annex Table 20e, continued. Deaths by age, sex and cause (thousands): Other Asia and Islands, 2020, optimistic scenario

Cause	Total	Male	Female	Males							Females						
				0-4	5-14	15-29	30-44	45-59	60-69	70+	0-4	5-14	15-29	30-44	45-59	60-69	70+
B. Other neoplasms	**9**	**5**	**4**	-	-	-	1	1	1	1	-	-	-	-	1	1	2
C. Diabetes mellitus	**79**	**31**	**47**	-	-	-	2	7	8	13	-	-	-	1	6	13	27
D. Endocrine disorders	**9**	**4**	**6**	1	-	-	-	1	1	1	1	-	-	1	1	1	3
E. Neuro-psychiatric conditions	**82**	**42**	**40**	2	1	3	6	8	6	16	2	1	1	-	3	6	25
2. Bipolar disorder	3	1	2	-	-	1	-	-	-	-	-	-	1	1	-	-	-
3. Schizophrenia	8	4	4	-	-	1	1	1	1	-	-	-	1	1	1	-	1
4. Epilepsy	7	4	3	1	1	1	1	-	-	-	-	1	1	-	-	-	1
5. Alcohol use	6	5	1	-	-	-	1	2	1	1	-	-	-	-	1	-	-
6. Dementia*	28	11	17	-	-	-	-	1	2	8	-	-	-	-	1	2	14
7. Parkinson disease	6	4	3	-	-	-	-	-	1	3	-	-	-	-	-	1	2
8. Multiple sclerosis	2	1	1	-	-	-	-	1	-	-	-	-	-	-	1	-	-
9. Drug use	1	1	-	-	-	1	-	-	-	-	-	-	-	-	-	-	-
13. Other neuro-psychiatric	21	11	9	1	-	1	2	2	1	4	1	1	1	1	1	-	4
F. Sense organ diseases	-	-	-	-	-	-	-	-	-	-	-	-	-	-	-	-	-
1. Glaucoma	-	-	-	-	-	-	-	-	-	-	-	-	-	-	-	-	-
2. Cataracts	-	-	-	-	-	-	-	-	-	-	-	-	-	-	-	-	-
G. Cardiovascular diseases	**2 777**	**1 497**	**1 280**	23	12	13	80	287	353	729	15	8	7	28	94	167	961
1. Rheumatic heart disease	20	10	10	-	-	-	1	1	2	5	-	-	-	1	1	2	7
2. Ischaemic heart disease	1 090	585	505	-	-	-	25	101	145	313	-	-	-	8	30	68	399
3. Cerebrovascular disease	854	443	411	3	3	3	17	82	117	218	3	2	2	6	31	59	310
4. Inflammatory heart diseases	103	62	41	4	4	3	10	18	8	17	3	2	1	3	6	4	22
5. Other cardiovascular	710	397	312	16	7	7	27	85	80	175	9	4	4	9	27	35	223
H. Respiratory diseases	**368**	**211**	**157**	3	2	1	5	21	37	142	2	1	1	3	13	25	111
1. COPD*	218	130	89	-	-	-	1	11	23	94	-	-	-	1	6	14	67
2. Asthma	42	21	21	-	1	-	1	4	4	11	-	-	1	1	2	4	10
3. Other respiratory	108	60	47	3	1	1	2	6	10	38	1	1	1	1	3	6	34
I. Digestive diseases	**491**	**320**	**171**	2	2	2	22	110	81	101	2	1	1	7	34	36	88
1. Peptic ulcer	44	27	17	-	-	-	1	6	6	14	-	-	-	1	2	3	12
2. Cirrhosis of the liver	212	158	55	-	-	1	14	68	41	34	-	-	1	3	16	15	21
3. Appendicitis	5	3	2	-	1	1	-	1	-	-	-	-	1	-	1	-	-
4. Other digestive	229	132	97	2	1	1	7	36	34	53	2	1	1	4	16	19	56
J. Genito-urinary diseases	**123**	**53**	**69**	1	1	1	4	9	10	26	1	1	1	2	9	14	42
1. Nephritis and nephrosis	105	45	60	1	1	1	4	8	9	21	1	1	1	2	8	12	36
2. Benign prostatic hypertrophy	1	1	-	-	-	-	-	1	-	-	-	-	-	-	-	-	-
3. Other genito-urinary	16	7	9	-	-	-	-	1	1	4	-	-	-	-	1	2	6
K. Skin diseases	**3**	**1**	**1**	-	-	-	-	-	-	-	-	-	-	-	-	-	1

Annex Table 20e, continued. Deaths by age, sex and cause (thousands): Other Asia and Islands, 2020, optimistic scenario

Cause	Total	Male	Female	Males							Females						
				0-4	5-14	15-29	30-44	45-59	60-69	70+	0-4	5-14	15-29	30-44	45-59	60-69	70+
L. Musculo-skeletal diseases	11	4	7	–	–	–	–	1	1	1	–	–	–	–	1	1	5
1. Rheumatoid arthritis	1	–	1	–	–	–	–	–	–	–	–	–	–	–	–	–	1
3. Other musculo-skeletal	10	3	7	–	–	–	–	1	1	1	–	–	–	–	1	1	4
M. Congenital anomalies	56	30	26	26	1	1	1	1	–	–	22	1	1	1	1	–	–
N. Oral conditions	–	–	–	–	–	–	–	–	–	–	–	–	–	–	–	–	–
III. Injuries	*809*	*541*	*268*	*40*	*35*	*139*	*138*	*106*	*41*	*43*	*34*	*19*	*61*	*51*	*44*	*27*	*33*
A. Unintentional injuries	582	385	198	37	30	94	90	73	29	31	31	16	36	32	34	22	27
1. Road traffic accidents	289	191	98	13	16	60	44	32	13	13	12	10	22	17	17	11	10
2. Poisonings	42	22	20	1	1	4	5	6	3	2	1	1	5	4	4	3	3
3. Falls	43	30	13	3	1	4	8	8	3	4	2	–	1	1	3	2	3
4. Fires	10	6	4	1	–	1	1	1	–	1	1	–	1	–	1	–	1
5. Drownings	62	42	20	12	7	7	6	5	2	3	8	3	2	2	2	1	2
6. Other unintentional	136	94	42	7	5	19	26	21	7	7	7	2	5	7	8	5	7
B. Intentional injuries	227	156	71	3	5	44	48	33	11	12	3	3	25	19	10	5	6
1. Self-inflicted injuries	118	73	45	–	2	21	19	15	8	8	–	1	17	12	6	4	5
2. Violence	88	71	17	1	2	19	25	16	3	4	1	1	4	5	3	1	1
3. War	21	12	9	2	1	5	3	1	1	–	2	1	3	2	1	1	–

Notes:

Causes responsible for no deaths have been omitted from this table.

A dash (-) symbol indicates fewer than 500 deaths.

*IA6 is Bacterial meningitis and meningococcaemia; IC3 is Hypertensive disorders of pregnancy; ID is Conditions arising during the perinatal period; IIE6 is Dementia and other degenerative and hereditary CNS disorders; IIH1 is Chronic obstructive pulmonary disease.

Annex Table 20f. Deaths by age, sex and cause (thousands): Sub-Saharan Africa, 2020, optimistic scenario

Cause	Total	Male	Female	Males							Females						
				0-4	5-14	15-29	30-44	45-59	60-69	70+	0-4	5-14	15-29	30-44	45-59	60-69	70+
Population (millions)	1 178	584	595	91	152	170	94	50	17	10	87	148	170	100	56	20	13
All causes	9 846	5 601	4 244	1 543	317	888	696	679	553	926	1 181	226	430	328	507	424	1 148
I. Communicable, maternal, perinatal and nutritional conditions	3 421	1 823	1 597	1 236	72	131	114	94	50	126	928	75	176	142	86	49	142
A. Infectious and parasitic diseases	2 385	1 273	1 113	797	56	129	113	92	39	48	596	60	160	126	83	37	51
1. Tuberculosis	632	304	328	23	15	84	60	73	30	18	25	22	97	69	68	29	18
2. STDs excluding HIV	51	26	25	20	-	-	-	-	1	5	16	-	1	1	-	1	6
a. Syphilis	49	26	24	20	-	-	-	-	1	5	16	-	1	1	-	1	6
b. Chlamydia	1	-	1	-	-	-	-	-	-	-	-	-	-	-	-	-	-
c. Gonorrhoea	-	-	-	-	-	-	-	-	-	-	-	-	-	-	-	-	-
3. HIV	308	145	163	41	6	37	46	11	3	2	39	6	56	51	8	2	1
4. Diarrhoeal diseases	509	293	216	266	9	1	1	1	2	14	185	8	1	1	1	2	16
5. Childhood-cluster diseases	441	247	194	229	14	-	1	1	-	1	179	13	-	1	-	-	1
a. Pertussis	78	44	34	42	2	-	-	-	-	-	33	1	-	-	-	-	-
b. Poliomyelitis	3	2	1	2	-	-	-	-	-	-	1	-	-	-	-	-	-
c. Diphtheria	1	1	-	1	-	-	-	-	-	-	-	-	-	-	-	-	-
d. Measles	293	164	129	153	11	-	-	-	-	-	119	10	-	-	-	-	-
e. Tetanus	67	37	29	32	1	1	1	-	-	1	25	-	1	1	-	-	1
6. Bacterial meningitis*	13	7	6	5	-	-	-	-	-	-	4	-	-	-	-	-	-
7. Hepatitis B and hepatitis C	8	4	4	1	-	-	-	1	1	2	-	-	-	-	-	-	2
8. Malaria	363	212	152	193	7	4	2	2	1	2	135	7	3	2	2	1	2
9. Tropical-cluster diseases	15	9	6	-	3	2	2	2	1	1	-	2	1	1	1	-	1
a. Trypanosomiasis	12	7	5	-	2	1	2	2	1	1	-	2	1	1	1	-	-
b. Chagas disease	-	-	-	-	-	-	-	-	-	-	-	-	-	-	-	-	-
c. Schistosomiasis	1	1	-	-	-	-	-	-	-	-	-	-	-	-	-	-	-
d. Leishmaniasis	3	2	1	-	-	-	-	-	-	1	-	-	-	-	-	-	1
10. Leprosy	-	-	-	-	-	-	-	-	-	-	-	-	-	-	-	-	-
11. Dengue	-	-	-	-	-	-	-	-	-	-	-	-	-	-	-	-	-
12. Japanese encephalitis	-	-	-	-	-	-	-	-	-	-	-	-	-	-	-	-	-
13. Trachoma	-	-	-	-	-	-	-	-	-	-	-	-	-	-	-	-	-
14. Intestinal nematode infections	1	1	-	1	-	-	-	-	-	-	-	-	-	-	-	-	-
a. Ascariasis	-	-	-	-	-	-	-	-	-	-	-	-	-	-	-	-	-
b. Trichuriasis	-	-	-	-	-	-	-	-	-	-	-	-	-	-	-	-	-
c. Ancylostomiasis, necatoriasis	-	-	-	-	-	-	-	-	-	-	-	-	-	-	-	-	-
15. Other infectious and parasitic	44	25	19	18	2	1	1	1	1	3	13	2	-	-	1	1	3

Annex Table 20f, continued. Deaths by age, sex and cause (thousands): Sub-Saharan Africa, 2020, optimistic scenario

Cause	Total	Male	Female	Males							Females						
				0-4	5-14	15-29	30-44	45-59	60-69	70+	0-4	5-14	15-29	30-44	45-59	60-69	70+
B. Respiratory infections	**630**	**346**	**284**	**242**	**14**	**2**	**1**	**2**	**10**	**74**	**168**	**11**	**2**	**1**	**2**	**11**	**87**
1. Lower respiratory infections	620	341	279	237	14	2	1	2	10	74	165	11	2	1	2	11	86
2. Upper respiratory infections	6	3	3	2	-	-	-	-	-	1	2	-	-	-	-	-	1
3. Otitis media	4	2	1	2	-	-	-	-	-	-	1	-	-	-	-	-	-
C. Maternal conditions	**31**	**-**	**31**	-	-	-	-	-	-	-	-	-	**14**	**14**	-	-	-
1. Maternal haemorrhage	7	-	7	-	-	-	-	-	-	-	-	-	3	3	-	-	-
2. Maternal sepsis	5	-	5	-	-	-	-	-	-	-	-	-	2	2	-	-	-
3. Hypertensive disorders*	4	-	4	-	-	-	-	-	-	-	-	-	2	2	-	-	-
4. Obstructed labour	2	-	2	-	-	-	-	-	-	-	-	-	1	1	-	-	-
5. Abortion	4	-	4	-	-	-	-	-	-	-	-	-	2	2	-	-	-
6. Other maternal	8	-	8	-	-	-	-	-	-	-	-	-	4	4	-	-	-
D. Perinatal conditions*	**296**	**162**	**135**	**162**	-	-	-	-	-	-	**135**	-	-	-	-	-	-
E. Nutritional deficiencies	**79**	**43**	**36**	**36**	**2**	-	-	-	-	**4**	**29**	**2**	-	-	-	-	**4**
1. Protein-energy malnutrition	57	31	26	28	-	-	-	-	-	3	22	-	-	-	-	-	3
2. Iodine deficiency	1	-	-	-	-	-	-	-	-	-	-	-	-	-	-	-	-
3. Vitamin A deficiency	15	8	7	6	1	-	-	-	-	-	5	1	-	-	-	-	-
4. Iron-deficiency anaemia	6	3	3	1	-	-	-	-	-	1	1	-	-	-	-	-	1
II. Noncommunicable diseases	**4 065**	**2 100**	**1 965**	**117**	**54**	**58**	**230**	**437**	**449**	**756**	**110**	**51**	**33**	**76**	**374**	**350**	**971**
A. Malignant neoplasms	**1 100**	**647**	**453**	**9**	**21**	**20**	**77**	**159**	**157**	**204**	**13**	**19**	**12**	**33**	**129**	**106**	**141**
1. Mouth and oropharynx cancers	61	39	22	-	-	-	3	6	13	17	-	-	1	1	3	7	10
2. Oesophagus cancer	61	46	15	-	-	-	4	17	10	14	-	-	-	1	6	4	4
3. Stomach cancer	82	51	31	-	-	1	4	16	13	17	-	-	-	1	11	10	9
4. Colon and rectum cancers	39	22	17	-	-	-	2	4	7	9	-	-	-	1	2	6	8
5. Liver cancer	146	111	36	1	1	7	25	39	16	22	-	1	1	3	11	8	11
6. Pancreas cancer	18	11	7	-	-	-	1	4	2	3	-	-	-	-	2	2	3
7. Trachea, bronchus, lung cancers	58	38	20	-	-	1	5	11	10	11	-	-	-	2	6	6	5
8. Melanoma and other skin cancers	21	9	12	-	-	-	1	3	2	3	-	-	-	2	3	4	5
9. Breast cancer	40	-	40	-	-	-	-	-	-	-	-	-	1	3	15	9	12
10. Cervix uteri cancer	78	-	78	-	-	-	-	-	-	-	-	-	2	5	28	18	25
11. Corpus uteri cancer	9	-	9	-	-	-	-	-	-	-	-	-	-	-	2	3	4
12. Ovary cancer	17	-	17	-	-	-	-	-	-	-	-	-	1	2	6	4	5
13. Prostate cancer	92	92	-	-	-	-	-	11	35	47	-	-	-	-	-	-	-
14. Bladder cancer	36	25	11	-	-	-	1	6	7	10	-	-	-	-	3	3	5
15. Lymphomas, multiple myeloma	64	41	22	8	8	7	3	4	7	10	3	5	2	2	3	3	5
16. Leukaemia	23	12	11	1	2	1	-	3	2	3	1	2	-	1	2	2	2
17. Other cancers	255	150	105	5	10	6	23	35	33	38	3	9	4	10	28	21	26

Annex Table 20f, continued. Deaths by age, sex and cause (thousands): Sub-Saharan Africa, 2020, optimistic scenario

Cause	Total	Male	Female	Males							Females						
				0-4	5-14	15-29	30-44	45-59	60-69	70+	0-4	5-14	15-29	30-44	45-59	60-69	70+
B. Other neoplasms	11	5	5	–	1	–	1	1	1	1	1	1	–	–	1	1	1
C. Diabetes mellitus	28	12	17	1	1	–	1	2	3	4	1	1	–	–	2	5	7
D. Endocrine disorders	30	13	16	4	1	1	2	3	1	2	3	1	1	1	2	2	7
E. Neuro-psychiatric conditions	52	30	22	4	2	3	5	4	3	7	4	2	1	1	3	3	9
2. Bipolar disorder	1	1	1	–	–	–	–	–	–	–	–	–	–	–	–	–	1
3. Schizophrenia	2	1	1	–	–	–	–	–	1	–	–	–	–	–	–	1	–
4. Epilepsy	6	4	2	–	–	1	1	1	1	–	–	–	1	1	1	–	–
5. Alcohol use	5	4	1	–	–	1	1	1	1	1	–	–	–	–	1	1	–
6. Dementia*	12	5	7	–	–	–	–	–	1	3	–	–	–	–	–	1	4
7. Parkinson disease	3	2	1	–	–	–	–	–	–	1	–	–	–	–	–	–	1
8. Multiple sclerosis	2	1	1	–	–	–	–	1	1	–	–	–	1	1	1	–	–
9. Drug use	1	1	–	–	–	–	–	–	–	–	–	–	–	–	–	–	–
13. Other neuro-psychiatric	20	12	8	3	2	2	2	1	1	1	3	1	2	2	1	1	2
F. Sense organ diseases	–	–	–	–	–	–	–	–	–	–	–	–	–	–	–	–	–
1. Glaucoma	–	–	–	–	–	–	–	–	–	–	–	–	–	–	–	–	–
2. Cataracts	–	–	–	–	–	–	–	–	–	–	–	–	–	–	–	–	–
G. Cardiovascular diseases	1 792	815	977	24	11	17	88	167	183	324	17	12	9	28	155	161	595
1. Rheumatic heart disease	20	11	8	–	2	3	4	2	1	–	–	2	2	2	2	1	1
2. Ischaemic heart disease	496	236	260	–	4	1	24	49	60	103	5	4	2	6	39	48	161
3. Cerebrovascular disease	884	370	514	–	4	7	36	73	87	158	3	2	2	13	77	84	332
4. Inflammatory heart diseases	119	61	58	6	2	1	9	13	12	17	6	2	2	2	9	10	28
5. Other cardiovascular	274	137	137	14	4	4	15	31	24	45	3	4	3	5	28	19	74
H. Respiratory diseases	620	328	291	9	6	6	29	49	64	164	5	5	5	7	56	46	167
1. COPD*	342	184	157	2	1	1	7	25	40	108	1	1	1	1	26	27	100
2. Asthma	38	19	19	–	1	1	3	3	3	8	1	–	1	1	4	4	10
3. Other respiratory	240	125	115	7	4	4	19	22	21	48	4	4	3	4	26	16	57
I. Digestive diseases	204	132	72	3	3	5	18	41	28	34	3	5	2	4	14	16	28
1. Peptic ulcer	21	13	9	–	–	1	2	4	2	4	–	–	–	1	2	1	5
2. Cirrhosis of the liver	52	38	14	–	–	1	5	14	9	9	–	1	1	1	4	4	5
3. Appendicitis	9	6	3	–	1	1	2	1	–	–	–	1	1	–	1	–	–
4. Other digestive	122	76	46	3	2	2	10	22	16	22	2	3	2	2	8	11	18
J. Genito-urinary diseases	114	62	51	10	4	2	8	9	9	15	10	4	2	2	10	9	15
1. Nephritis and nephrosis	99	54	45	10	4	1	6	7	8	13	10	4	1	2	8	7	13
2. Benign prostatic hypertrophy	1	1	–	–	–	–	–	1	1	1	–	–	–	–	–	–	–
3. Other genito-urinary	14	7	6	1	1	–	1	1	2	1	–	–	2	–	2	1	2
K. Skin diseases	13	8	6	7	–	–	–	–	–	–	5	–	–	–	–	–	–

Annex Table 20f, continued. Deaths by age, sex and cause (thousands): Sub-Saharan Africa, 2020, optimistic scenario

Cause	Total	Male	Female	Males							Females						
				0-4	5-14	15-29	30-44	45-59	60-69	70+	0-4	5-14	15-29	30-44	45-59	60-69	70+
L. Musculo-skeletal diseases	1	1	–	–	–	–	–	–	–	–	–	–	–	–	–	–	–
1. Rheumatoid arthritis	–	–	–	–	–	–	–	–	–	–	–	–	–	–	–	–	–
3. Other musculo-skeletal	1																
M. Congenital anomalies	101	48	53	43	2	1	1	1	–	1	48	2	1	–	1	1	1
N. Oral conditions	–	–	–	–	–	–	–	–	–	–	–	–	–	–	–	–	–
III. Injuries	*2 360*	*1 678*	*682*	*190*	*191*	*698*	*351*	*148*	*55*	*44*	*144*	*99*	*220*	*111*	*47*	*25*	*36*
A. Unintentional injuries	**1 175**	**836**	**339**	**131**	**136**	**250**	**159**	**90**	**35**	**35**	**90**	**70**	**75**	**38**	**25**	**12**	**29**
1. Road traffic accidents	527	386	141	18	80	130	77	47	19	13	12	41	46	20	13	4	4
2. Poisonings	67	40	27	27	4	2	2	2	1	1	20	1	3	1	1	–	1
3. Falls	40	23	18	2	2	6	3	4	3	4	2	1	1	1	1	2	10
4. Fires	120	63	57	26	6	12	7	5	2	5	22	6	10	5	4	3	7
5. Drownings	127	94	33	31	30	17	8	5	2	2	15	10	3	2	1	–	1
6. Other unintentional	294	229	65	27	16	83	60	26	8	9	19	10	13	8	6	3	5
B. Intentional injuries	**1 185**	**842**	**343**	**60**	**55**	**448**	**192**	**58**	**20**	**9**	**54**	**30**	**145**	**73**	**22**	**13**	**6**
1. Self-inflicted injuries	39	32	7	–	3	15	8	3	1	1	–	–	4	1	1	–	–
2. Violence	512	441	71	8	17	268	101	35	9	5	4	7	32	16	7	3	2
3. War	634	368	266	52	35	165	83	20	10	4	50	23	109	56	14	10	4

Notes:
Causes responsible for no deaths have been omitted from this table.
A dash (-) symbol indicates fewer than 500 deaths.
*IA6 is Bacterial meningitis and meningococcaemia; IC3 is Hypertensive disorders of pregnancy; ID is Conditions arising during the perinatal period; IIE6 is Dementia and other degenerative and hereditary CNS disorders; IIH1 is Chronic obstructive pulmonary disease.

Annex Table 20g. Deaths by age, sex and cause (thousands): Latin America and the Caribbean, 2020, optimistic scenario

Cause	Total	Male	Female	Males 0-4	5-14	15-29	30-44	45-59	60-69	70+	Females 0-4	5-14	15-29	30-44	45-59	60-69	70+
Population (millions)	*681*	*338*	*344*	*29*	*56*	*84*	*75*	*56*	*22*	*16*	*28*	*54*	*82*	*75*	*59*	*25*	*22*
All causes	*4 491*	*2 507*	*1 984*	*138*	*37*	*173*	*230*	*454*	*448*	*1 026*	*101*	*24*	*72*	*106*	*293*	*290*	*1 099*
I. Communicable, maternal, perinatal and nutritional conditions	*424*	*246*	*178*	*98*	*3*	*24*	*23*	*15*	*14*	*69*	*66*	*3*	*8*	*8*	*8*	*10*	*75*
A. Infectious and parasitic diseases	**221**	**139**	**82**	42	2	24	23	12	10	27	30	2	7	6	6	6	26
1. Tuberculosis	**32**	**20**	**12**	1	–	1	1	3	4	9	1	–	1	1	2	3	6
2. STDs excluding HIV	**4**	**2**	**2**	1	–	–	–	–	–	1	1	–	–	–	–	–	1
a. Syphilis	4	2	2	1	–	–	–	–	–	1	1	–	–	–	–	–	1
b. Chlamydia	–	–	–	–	–	–	–	–	–	–	–	–	–	–	–	–	–
c. Gonorrhoea	–	–	–	–	–	–	–	–	–	–	–	–	–	–	–	–	–
3. HIV	**66**	**53**	**13**	2	–	22	20	6	2	1	2	–	5	4	1	1	–
4. Diarrhoeal diseases	**51**	**29**	**22**	21	–	–	–	1	1	6	13	–	–	–	1	1	7
5. Childhood-cluster diseases	**23**	**13**	**10**	12	2	–	–	–	–	–	10	2	–	–	–	–	–
a. Pertussis	4	2	2	2	–	–	–	–	–	–	2	–	–	–	–	–	–
b. Poliomyelitis	–	–	–	–	–	–	–	–	–	–	–	–	–	–	–	–	–
c. Diphtheria	–	–	–	–	–	–	–	–	–	–	–	–	–	–	–	–	–
d. Measles	13	7	6	7	–	–	–	–	–	–	5	1	–	–	–	–	–
e. Tetanus	6	3	3	3	–	–	–	–	–	–	2	–	–	–	–	–	–
6. Bacterial meningitis*	**5**	**3**	**3**	1	–	–	–	–	–	1	1	–	–	–	–	–	1
7. Hepatitis B and hepatitis C	**1**	**1**	**1**	–	–	–	–	–	–	1	–	–	–	–	–	–	1
8. Malaria	**3**	**2**	**1**	–	–	–	–	1	1	–	–	–	–	–	–	1	–
9. Tropical-cluster diseases	**10**	**5**	**5**	–	–	–	–	1	1	2	–	–	–	–	1	1	2
a. Trypanosomiasis	–	–	–	–	–	–	–	–	–	–	–	–	–	–	–	–	–
b. Chagas disease	9	5	5	–	–	–	–	1	1	2	–	–	–	–	1	1	2
c. Schistosomiasis	–	–	–	–	–	–	–	–	–	–	–	–	–	–	–	–	–
d. Leishmaniasis	–	–	–	–	–	–	–	–	–	–	–	–	–	–	–	–	–
10. Leprosy	–	–	–	–	–	–	–	–	–	–	–	–	–	–	–	–	–
11. Dengue	–	–	–	–	–	–	–	–	–	–	–	–	–	–	–	–	–
12. Japanese encephalitis	–	–	–	–	–	–	–	–	–	–	–	–	–	–	–	–	–
13. Trachoma	–	–	–	–	–	–	–	–	–	–	–	–	–	–	–	–	–
14. Intestinal nematode infections	**1**	**1**	**–**	–	–	–	–	–	–	–	–	–	–	–	–	–	–
a. Ascariasis	–	–	–	–	–	–	–	–	–	–	–	–	–	–	–	–	–
b. Trichuriasis	–	–	–	–	–	–	–	–	–	–	–	–	–	–	–	–	–
c. Ancylostomiasis, necatoriasis	–	–	–	–	–	–	–	–	–	–	–	–	–	–	–	–	–
15. Other infectious and parasitic	**24**	**12**	**12**	3	2	1	1	1	1	3	2	–	1	–	1	1	7

Annex Table 20g, continued. Deaths by age, sex and cause (thousands): Latin America and the Caribbean, 2020, optimistic scenario

Cause	Total	Male	Female	Males							Females						
				0-4	5-14	15-29	30-44	45-59	60-69	70+	0-4	5-14	15-29	30-44	45-59	60-69	70+
B. Respiratory infections	**105**	**54**	**51**	**16**	**1**	**-**	**1**	**2**	**3**	**31**	**10**	**1**	**1**	**1**	**2**	**2**	**34**
1. Lower respiratory infections	103	53	50	16	1	-	1	2	3	30	10	1	1	1	2	2	34
2. Upper respiratory infections	1	1	1	-	-	-	-	-	-	1	-	-	-	-	-	-	-
3. Otitis media	-	-	-	-	-	-	-	-	-	-	-	-	-	-	-	-	-
C. Maternal conditions	**2**		**2**										**1**	**1**			
1. Maternal haemorrhage	-	-	-	-	-	-	-	-	-	-	-	-	-	1	-	-	-
2. Maternal sepsis	-	-	-	-	-	-	-	-	-	-	-	-	-	-	-	-	-
3. Hypertensive disorders*	-	-	-	-	-	1	1	-	-	-	-	-	1	1	-	-	-
4. Obstructed labour	-	-	-	-	-	-	-	-	-	-	-	-	-	-	-	-	-
5. Abortion	-	-	-	-	-	-	-	-	-	-	-	-	-	-	-	-	-
6. Other maternal	-	-	-	-	-	-	-	-	-	-	-	-	-	-	-	-	-
D. Perinatal conditions*	**55**	**34**	**22**	**34**	-	-	-	-	-	-	**22**	-	-	-	-	-	-
E. Nutritional deficiencies	**41**	**19**	**21**	**6**	-	-	-	**1**	**1**	**11**	**4**	-	-	-	**1**	**1**	**14**
1. Protein-energy malnutrition	29	14	15	5	-	-	-	1	1	8	3	-	-	-	1	1	10
2. Iodine deficiency	-	-	-	-	-	-	-	-	-	-	-	-	-	-	-	-	-
3. Vitamin A deficiency	1	1	1	1	-	-	-	-	-	-	1	-	-	-	-	-	-
4. Iron-deficiency anaemia	10	4	6	1	-	-	-	-	-	3	1	-	-	-	-	1	4
II. Noncommunicable diseases	*3 441*	*1 811*	*1 630*	*27*	*11*	*12*	*88*	*358*	*403*	*911*	*24*	*8*	*15*	*66*	*260*	*266*	*991*
A. Malignant neoplasms	**840**	**429**	**411**	**2**	**6**	**4**	**22**	**94**	**110**	**193**	**2**	**4**	**6**	**32**	**112**	**99**	**156**
1. Mouth and oropharynx cancers	30	21	8	-	-	-	1	7	5	8	-	-	-	-	2	2	4
2. Oesophagus cancer	26	18	8	-	-	-	1	5	5	7	-	-	-	-	1	2	5
3. Stomach cancer	94	58	36	-	-	-	2	12	16	27	-	-	-	1	6	9	20
4. Colon and rectum cancers	56	26	30	-	-	-	1	5	7	13	-	-	-	2	5	8	15
5. Liver cancer	13	7	7	-	-	-	1	1	2	3	-	-	-	1	1	2	3
6. Pancreas cancer	20	10	10	-	-	-	1	2	3	4	-	-	-	-	1	3	6
7. Trachea, bronchus, lung cancers	126	75	51	-	-	-	5	27	21	22	-	-	-	1	17	16	16
8. Melanoma and other skin cancers	7	3	4	-	-	-	-	1	1	1	-	-	-	1	1	1	1
9. Breast cancer	65	-	65	-	-	-	-	-	-	-	-	-	1	6	23	14	21
10. Cervix uteri cancer	52	-	52	-	-	-	-	-	-	-	-	-	1	7	19	10	15
11. Corpus uteri cancer	15	-	15	-	-	-	-	-	-	-	-	-	-	-	5	4	6
12. Ovary cancer	12	-	12	-	-	-	-	-	-	-	-	-	-	1	3	3	4
13. Prostate cancer	56	56	-	-	-	-	-	3	17	36	-	-	-	-	-	-	-
14. Bladder cancer	22	16	5	-	-	-	-	2	5	9	-	-	-	-	1	1	3
15. Lymphomas, multiple myeloma	33	18	15	1	1	1	3	4	3	6	1	1	-	1	3	4	6
16. Leukaemia	22	12	10	1	2	2	2	2	2	1	1	2	-	1	1	2	3
17. Other cancers	191	109	82	1	3	1	5	21	23	54	2	2	2	10	22	18	28

Annex Table 20g, continued. Deaths by age, sex and cause (thousands): Latin America and the Caribbean, 2020, optimistic scenario

Cause	Total	Male	Female	Males 0-4	Males 5-14	Males 15-29	Males 30-44	Males 45-59	Males 60-69	Males 70+	Females 0-4	Females 5-14	Females 15-29	Females 30-44	Females 45-59	Females 60-69	Females 70+
B. Other neoplasms	10	5	5	-	-	-	-	1	1	2	-	-	-	-	1	1	3
C. Diabetes mellitus	124	46	78	-	-	-	2	9	11	23	-	-	-	1	10	17	50
D. Endocrine disorders	31	14	17	3	-	-	1	2	1	6	2	-	-	1	2	2	10
E. Neuro-psychiatric conditions	51	31	20	2	1	2	5	7	4	9	2	1	1	2	2	2	10
2. Bipolar disorder	-	1	1	-	-	-	-	-	-	1	-	-	-	-	-	-	1
3. Schizophrenia	5	3	3	-	-	-	-	1	1	1	-	-	-	-	1	1	1
4. Epilepsy	4	3	2	-	1	1	1	-	-	-	-	1	-	1	-	-	-
5. Alcohol use	12	11	1	-	-	-	3	4	2	2	-	-	-	-	1	-	-
6. Dementia*	11	5	6	-	-	-	-	1	1	3	-	-	-	-	-	1	5
7. Parkinson disease	3	2	2	-	-	-	-	-	-	2	-	-	-	-	-	-	2
8. Multiple sclerosis	2	1	1	-	-	-	-	-	-	-	-	-	-	1	-	-	-
9. Drug use	1	1	-	-	-	1	-	-	-	-	-	-	-	-	-	-	-
13. Other neuro-psychiatric	11	6	5	2	-	-	1	1	1	1	-	-	1	-	1	-	1
F. Sense organ diseases	1	-	-	-	-	-	-	-	-	-	-	-	-	-	-	-	-
1. Glaucoma	-	-	-	-	-	-	-	-	-	-	-	-	-	-	-	-	-
2. Cataracts	-	-	-	-	-	-	-	-	-	-	-	-	-	-	-	-	-
G. Cardiovascular diseases	1729	934	796	3	1	3	37	179	214	497	2	1	3	19	83	96	592
1. Rheumatic heart disease	11	4	6	-	-	1	-	1	1	1	-	-	-	1	3	-	2
2. Ischaemic heart disease	791	434	357	-	-	-	15	83	102	233	-	-	-	6	33	45	273
3. Cerebrovascular disease	547	290	257	-	-	1	12	57	67	154	-	-	-	7	30	32	186
4. Inflammatory heart diseases	43	24	19	1	-	-	3	7	4	10	2	-	-	2	3	2	12
5. Other cardiovascular	337	181	156	2	-	1	7	31	40	99	1	-	-	3	14	17	119
H. Respiratory diseases	310	153	156	2	1	1	4	14	26	106	1	-	2	4	28	29	92
1. COPD*	181	94	87	-	-	-	1	7	16	70	-	-	-	1	13	17	55
2. Asthma	33	13	21	1	-	-	1	2	2	7	-	-	-	1	5	4	10
3. Other respiratory	96	46	49	1	1	-	2	5	8	29	1	-	2	2	10	8	27
I. Digestive diseases	232	146	86	1	-	-	13	48	30	52	1	-	-	5	17	14	48
1. Peptic ulcer	22	13	9	-	-	-	-	3	3	7	-	-	-	-	1	1	7
2. Cirrhosis of the liver	100	75	25	-	-	-	9	32	16	17	-	-	-	2	8	5	9
3. Appendicitis	1	1	-	-	-	-	-	-	-	-	-	-	-	-	-	-	-
4. Other digestive	108	57	51	1	-	-	3	13	11	28	2	-	-	2	7	8	33
J. Genito-urinary diseases	69	34	34	1	-	-	2	5	5	21	1	-	-	1	4	5	22
1. Nephritis and nephrosis	49	24	25	1	-	-	2	4	4	13	1	-	-	1	3	4	16
2. Benign prostatic hypertrophy	3	3	-	-	-	-	-	-	-	3	-	-	-	-	-	-	-
3. Other genito-urinary	16	8	9	-	-	-	-	1	1	5	-	-	-	-	1	1	6
K. Skin diseases	4	2	3	-	-	-	-	-	-	2	-	-	-	-	-	-	2

Annex Table 20g, continued. Deaths by age, sex and cause (thousands): Latin America and the Caribbean, 2020, optimistic scenario

Cause	Total	Male	Female	Males							Females						
				0-4	5-14	15-29	30-44	45-59	60-69	70+	0-4	5-14	15-29	30-44	45-59	60-69	70+
L. Musculo-skeletal diseases	11	3	8	-	-	-	-	-	-	2	-	-	-	-	1	1	5
1. Rheumatoid arthritis	2	1	1	-	-	-	-	-	-	-	-	-	-	-	-	1	1
3. Other musculo-skeletal	8	3	6	-	-	-	-	-	-	1	-	-	-	-	1	-	3
M. Congenital anomalies	30	15	15	13	1	-	-	-	-	-	13	1	-	-	-	-	-
N. Oral conditions	-	-	-	-	-	-	-	-	-	-	-	-	-	-	-	-	-
III. Injuries	*627*	*450*	*177*	*14*	*23*	*136*	*119*	*81*	*31*	*46*	*11*	*13*	*48*	*33*	*25*	*14*	*33*
A. Unintentional injuries	393	259	134	11	18	66	57	49	21	38	8	10	33	21	19	11	31
1. Road traffic accidents	218	143	75	3	12	47	33	25	10	12	3	8	26	15	11	5	7
2. Poisonings	5	3	2	-	-	-	1	1	-	1	-	-	-	-	-	-	-
3. Falls	37	20	17	1	-	2	3	3	2	9	1	-	-	1	1	1	13
4. Fires	8	5	4	-	-	-	1	1	-	1	1	1	1	1	1	-	1
5. Drownings	25	20	5	2	2	5	5	3	1	1	1	1	1	-	-	-	-
6. Other unintentional	100	69	32	4	3	11	15	15	7	13	4	1	5	4	5	3	9
B. Intentional injuries	233	191	43	3	5	71	62	33	10	8	3	2	15	11	6	3	2
1. Self-inflicted injuries	42	30	12	-	-	7	8	7	4	4	-	-	4	3	2	1	1
2. Violence	167	146	20	1	3	58	50	24	6	4	1	1	8	6	3	1	1
3. War	25	15	11	2	1	5	4	1	1	-	2	1	4	3	1	1	-

Notes:
Causes responsible for no deaths have been omitted from this table.
A dash (-) symbol indicates fewer than 500 deaths.
*IA6 is Bacterial meningitis and meningococcaemia; IC3 is Hypertensive disorders of pregnancy; ID is Conditions arising during the perinatal period;
IIE6 is Dementia and other degenerative and hereditary CNS disorders; IIH1 is Chronic obstructive pulmonary disease.

Annex Table 20h. Deaths by age, sex and cause (thousands): Middle Eastern Crescent, 2020, optimistic scenario

Cause	Total	Male	Female	Males							Females						
				0-4	5-14	15-29	30-44	45-59	60-69	70+	0-4	5-14	15-29	30-44	45-59	60-69	70+
Population (millions)	*1 005*	*507*	*499*	*62*	*110*	*140*	*98*	*61*	*23*	*12*	*59*	*106*	*135*	*96*	*61*	*26*	*17*
All causes	**6 499**	**3 757**	**2 741**	**579**	**113**	**242**	**302**	**681**	**676**	**1 164**	**488**	**82**	**131**	**135**	**305**	**351**	**1 249**
I. Communicable, maternal, perinatal and nutritional conditions	***883***	***473***	***410***	***371***	***11***	***5***	***6***	***10***	***20***	***51***	***314***	***10***	***5***	***6***	***7***	***13***	***55***
A. Infectious and parasitic diseases	**370**	**206**	**164**	**163**	**5**	**5**	**5**	**9**	**7**	**12**	**136**	**4**	**2**	**2**	**5**	**4**	**12**
1. Tuberculosis	42	26	15	2	1	3	3	6	5	7	1	-	1	1	3	3	6
2. STDs excluding HIV	7	3	3	3	-	-	-	-	-	-	2	-	-	-	-	-	1
a. Syphilis	7	3	3	3	-	-	-	-	-	-	2	-	-	-	-	-	1
b. Chlamydia																	
c. Gonorrhoea																	
3. HIV	5	4	1	-	-	1	1	1	-	-	-	-	1	1	-	-	-
4. Diarrhoeal diseases	182	99	83	96	2	-	-	-	-	1	80	1	-	-	-	-	1
5. Childhood-cluster diseases	98	53	45	50	2	-	-	-	1	-	43	2	-	-	-	-	-
a. Pertussis	22	12	10	11	-	-	-	-	-	-	10	-	-	-	-	-	-
b. Poliomyelitis	2	1	1	1	-	-	-	-	-	-	1	-	-	-	-	-	-
c. Diphtheria																	
d. Measles	39	21	18	20	1	-	-	-	-	-	17	1	-	-	-	-	-
e. Tetanus	35	19	16	18	-	-	-	-	-	-	15	-	-	-	-	-	-
6. Bacterial meningitis*	8	4	4	2	-	-	-	-	-	1	2	-	-	-	-	-	1
7. Hepatitis B and hepatitis C	7	4	3	-	-	-	-	1	1	2	-	-	-	-	-	-	2
8. Malaria	2	1	1	-	-	-	-	-	-	-	-	-	-	-	-	-	-
9. Tropical-cluster diseases	1	1		-	-	-	-	-	-	-							
a. Trypanosomiasis																	
b. Chagas disease																	
c. Schistosomiasis	1	1		-	-	-	-	-	-	-							
d. Leishmaniasis	1	1		-	-	-	-	-	-	-							
10. Leprosy																	
11. Dengue																	
12. Japanese encephalitis																	
13. Trachoma																	
14. Intestinal nematode infections																	
a. Ascariasis																	
b. Trichuriasis																	
c. Ancylostomiasis, necatoriasis																	
15. Other infectious and parasitic	19	10	9	8	-	-	-	-	-	1	7	-	-	-	-	-	1

Annex Table 20h, continued. Deaths by age, sex and cause (thousands): Middle Eastern Crescent, 2020, optimistic scenario

Cause	Total	Male	Female	Males 0-4	5-14	15-29	30-44	45-59	60-69	70+	Females 0-4	5-14	15-29	30-44	45-59	60-69	70+
B. Respiratory infections	**281**	**148**	**133**	**91**	**5**	**1**	-	**1**	**12**	**37**	**77**	**5**	**1**	**1**	**2**	**8**	**41**
1. Lower respiratory infections	277	145	131	90	5	1	-	1	12	37	75	5	1	-	2	8	41
2. Upper respiratory infections	3	1	1	1	-	-	-	-	-	-	1	-	-	-	-	-	-
3. Otitis media	1	1	1	1	-	-	-	-	-	-	1	-	-	-	-	-	-
C. Maternal conditions	**7**	-	**7**	-	-	-	-	-	-	-	-	-	**3**	**3**	**1**	-	-
1. Maternal haemorrhage	2	-	2	-	-	-	-	-	-	-	-	-	1	1	1	-	-
2. Maternal sepsis	1	-	1	-	-	-	-	-	-	-	-	-	1	-	-	-	-
3. Hypertensive disorders*	1	-	1	-	-	-	-	-	-	-	-	-	-	1	-	-	-
4. Obstructed labour	1	-	1	-	-	-	-	-	-	-	-	-	1	-	-	-	-
5. Abortion	1	-	1	-	-	-	-	-	-	-	-	-	1	-	-	-	-
6. Other maternal	2	-	2	-	-	-	-	-	-	-	-	-	-	1	1	-	-
D. Perinatal conditions*	**184**	**98**	**85**	**98**	-	-	-	-	-	-	**85**	-	-	-	-	-	-
E. Nutritional deficiencies	**41**	**22**	**19**	**19**	**1**	-	-	-	-	**2**	**16**	**1**	-	-	-	-	**2**
1. Protein-energy malnutrition	29	15	13	14	-	-	-	-	-	1	12	-	-	-	-	-	1
2. Iodine deficiency	1	1	1	1	-	-	-	-	-	-	1	-	-	-	-	-	-
3. Vitamin A deficiency	7	4	3	3	1	-	-	-	-	-	3	-	-	-	-	-	-
4. Iron-deficiency anaemia	4	2	2	1	-	-	-	-	-	1	1	-	-	-	-	-	1
II. Noncommunicable diseases	**4 709**	**2 690**	**2 019**	**142**	**42**	**43**	**150**	**594**	**628**	**1 090**	**112**	**38**	**35**	**72**	**268**	**320**	**1 173**
A. Malignant neoplasms	**648**	**412**	**236**	**4**	**12**	**11**	**36**	**138**	**109**	**102**	**5**	**9**	**9**	**25**	**65**	**60**	**62**
1. Mouth and oropharynx cancers	40	27	13	-	-	1	3	6	9	7	-	-	-	1	2	4	5
2. Oesophagus cancer	25	16	9	-	-	-	1	7	4	3	-	-	-	1	3	3	3
3. Stomach cancer	53	33	20	-	-	1	3	14	9	7	-	-	1	1	5	6	5
4. Colon and rectum cancers	32	16	15	-	-	1	-	4	6	5	-	-	-	1	5	6	6
5. Liver cancer	22	14	8	-	2	-	1	4	4	3	-	1	-	-	2	2	2
6. Pancreas cancer	12	8	5	-	-	-	1	3	2	2	-	-	-	-	2	1	2
7. Trachea, bronchus, lung cancers	180	153	27	-	-	1	11	60	39	41	-	-	-	2	10	9	7
8. Melanoma and other skin cancers	3	2	1	-	-	-	-	1	1	-	-	-	-	-	1	-	-
9. Breast cancer	29	-	29	-	-	-	-	-	-	-	-	-	2	4	11	5	6
10. Cervix uteri cancer	19	-	19	-	-	-	-	-	-	-	-	-	1	2	8	4	4
11. Corpus uteri cancer	5	-	5	-	-	-	-	-	-	-	-	-	-	-	1	2	2
12. Ovary cancer	8	-	8	-	-	-	-	-	-	-	-	-	-	2	3	1	2
13. Prostate cancer	12	12	-	-	-	-	1	2	5	4	-	-	-	-	-	-	-
14. Bladder cancer	25	21	5	-	-	-	1	7	6	5	-	-	-	-	1	1	2
15. Lymphomas, multiple myeloma	21	14	7	-	1	1	1	3	3	2	-	-	-	1	1	1	2
16. Leukaemia	27	15	12	1	3	3	3	2	2	2	1	3	1	2	1	2	2
17. Other cancers	135	82	53	3	6	3	8	24	20	18	3	4	3	7	13	12	11

Annex Table 20h, continued. Deaths by age, sex and cause (thousands): Middle Eastern Crescent, 2020, optimistic scenario

Cause	Total	Male	Female	Males							Females						
				0-4	5-14	15-29	30-44	45-59	60-69	70+	0-4	5-14	15-29	30-44	45-59	60-69	70+
B. Other neoplasms	**6**	**3**	**3**	-	1	-	-	1	-	1	-	-	-	1	1	-	1
C. Diabetes mellitus	**75**	**33**	**42**	1	1	1	3	8	8	11	1	1	1	1	7	12	19
D. Endocrine disorders	**18**	**9**	**9**	4	1	-	1	1	1	1	4	1	1	-	1	1	1
E. Neuro-psychiatric conditions	**68**	**36**	**32**	8	4	3	3	4	4	8	8	4	2	2	3	3	10
2. Bipolar disorder	1	-	1	-	-	-	-	-	-	-	-	-	-	-	-	-	1
3. Schizophrenia	5	2	2	-	-	1	1	-	-	-	-	-	1	1	-	-	-
4. Epilepsy	8	5	3	1	1	1	1	1	-	-	-	1	-	1	1	-	-
5. Alcohol use	1	1	-	-	-	-	1	-	-	-	-	-	-	-	-	-	-
6. Dementia*	14	6	8	-	-	-	-	1	1	4	-	-	-	1	1	1	5
7. Parkinson disease	4	2	2	-	-	-	-	-	1	1	-	-	-	-	-	1	1
8. Multiple sclerosis	2	1	1	-	-	1	1	-	-	-	-	-	1	1	1	-	-
9. Drug use	2	2	-	-	-	1	1	-	-	-	-	-	-	-	-	-	-
13. Other neuro-psychiatric	32	18	15	9	3	1	1	1	1	1	7	3	1	1	1	-	2
F. Sense organ diseases				-	-	-	-	-	-	-	-	-	-	-	-	-	-
1. Glaucoma				-	-	-	-	-	-	-	-	-	-	-	-	-	-
2. Cataracts				-	-	-	-	-	-	-	-	-	-	-	-	-	-
G. Cardiovascular diseases	**2 994**	**1 675**	**1 319**	50	16	18	82	342	408	760	28	13	13	32	135	183	917
1. Rheumatic heart disease	25	14	11	-	1	3	5	3	1	-	-	1	2	3	2	1	1
2. Ischaemic heart disease	1 563	886	676	-	-	2	39	186	228	430	-	-	2	13	61	99	502
3. Cerebrovascular disease	506	255	250	3	3	3	10	51	65	121	2	2	1	4	27	35	179
4. Inflammatory heart diseases	118	70	47	9	3	3	8	18	10	18	6	2	2	4	8	4	21
5. Other cardiovascular	784	450	334	38	9	6	19	84	104	190	20	7	5	8	36	43	214
H. Respiratory diseases	**492**	**283**	**209**	12	4	3	8	44	57	156	8	5	4	5	30	36	121
1. COPD*	278	167	112	3	1	-	2	22	36	103	2	1	-	1	14	21	73
2. Asthma	34	18	16	-	-	-	2	3	3	9	-	-	1	1	3	3	8
3. Other respiratory	180	99	81	9	3	2	4	18	18	44	6	4	3	3	13	12	40
I. Digestive diseases	**194**	**119**	**75**	8	2	2	9	41	29	28	9	2	2	4	17	15	25
1. Peptic ulcer	10	7	3	-	-	-	1	3	2	2	-	-	-	-	1	1	1
2. Cirrhosis of the liver	73	45	28	-	-	1	3	17	12	11	-	1	1	2	8	7	11
3. Appendicitis	3	2	1	-	1	-	-	-	-	-	-	-	-	-	-	-	-
4. Other digestive	108	65	43	8	1	1	5	21	14	15	9	1	2	2	9	8	13
J. Genito-urinary diseases	**104**	**62**	**42**	3	2	3	7	14	11	21	3	2	3	3	9	8	15
1. Nephritis and nephrosis	43	24	19	2	1	1	2	5	4	9	2	1	-	1	4	3	6
2. Benign prostatic hypertrophy	2	2	-	-	-	-	-	-	-	2	-	-	-	-	-	-	-
3. Other genito-urinary	59	35	24	2	1	2	4	10	7	11	1	-	1	2	5	5	9
K. Skin diseases	**2**	**1**	**1**	-	-	-	-	-	-	-	-	-	-	-	-	-	-

Annex Table 20h, continued. Deaths by age, sex and cause (thousands): Middle Eastern Crescent, 2020, optimistic scenario

Cause	Total	Male	Female	Males							Females						
				0-4	5-14	15-29	30-44	45-59	60-69	70+	0-4	5-14	15-29	30-44	45-59	60-69	70+
L. Musculo-skeletal diseases	2	1	1	-	-	-	-	-	-	-	-	-	-	-	-	-	1
1. Rheumatoid arthritis	-	-	-	-	-	-	-	-	-	-	-	-	-	-	-	-	-
3. Other musculo-skeletal	2	1	1	-	-	-	-	-	-	-	-	-	-	-	-	-	1
M. Congenital anomalies	103	53	50	48	1	1	1	1	-	1	45	1	1	1	1	-	1
N. Oral conditions	-	-	-	-	-	-	-	-	-	-	-	-	-	-	-	-	-
III. Injuries	907	594	313	66	60	194	146	77	28	23	62	34	90	57	30	18	21
A. Unintentional injuries	395	282	113	32	26	77	73	45	15	15	27	13	21	17	14	7	14
1. Road traffic accidents	196	150	46	4	15	52	42	23	7	6	4	8	11	9	6	3	4
2. Poisonings	22	14	8	2	-	2	4	4	1	1	2	-	1	1	1	1	1
3. Falls	20	13	6	2	1	2	3	3	1	2	2	-	1	1	1	1	1
4. Fires	22	10	13	3	1	2	2	1	1	1	3	1	4	2	2	1	2
5. Drownings	36	25	10	8	4	6	5	2	1	1	7	1	1	1	-	-	-
6. Other unintentional	99	69	30	13	5	13	17	12	5	5	11	2	3	4	4	2	5
B. Intentional injuries	512	312	200	34	35	117	73	32	13	8	35	22	69	41	16	11	7
1. Self-inflicted injuries	100	68	31	-	14	19	15	12	4	4	-	6	9	5	4	3	4
2. Violence	75	50	25	9	3	16	13	6	2	1	9	4	4	4	2	1	1
3. War	337	194	143	26	17	82	46	14	7	2	25	12	56	32	9	7	2

Notes:
Causes responsible for no deaths have been omitted from this table.
A dash (-) symbol indicates fewer than 500 deaths.

*IA6 is Bacterial meningitis and meningococcaemia; IC3 is Hypertensive disorders of pregnancy; ID is Conditions arising during the perinatal period; IIE6 is Dementia and other degenerative and hereditary CNS disorders; IIH1 is Chronic obstructive pulmonary disease.

Annex Table 20i. Deaths by age, sex and cause (thousands): World, 2020, optimistic scenario

Cause	Total	Male	Female	Males							Females						
				0-4	5-14	15-29	30-44	45-59	60-69	70+	0-4	5-14	15-29	30-44	45-59	60-69	70+
Population (millions)	7 895	3 929	3 967	377	693	969	799	639	264	188	360	666	938	784	651	301	267
All causes	64 635	36 867	27 768	3 196	692	2 067	2 659	7 063	7 369	13 821	2 578	500	1 107	1 229	3 167	3 803	15 384
I. Communicable, maternal, perinatal and nutritional conditions	8 214	4 393	3 821	2 266	112	222	282	230	215	1 065	1 786	116	246	241	171	156	1 106
A. Infectious and parasitic diseases	4 791	2 636	2 154	1 257	80	215	274	213	140	456	977	83	216	211	152	101	415
1. Tuberculosis	1 317	716	601	30	17	94	77	131	91	277	29	24	101	75	106	66	201
2. STDs excluding HIV	99	49	50	32	-	-	-	1	2	14	26	-	1	1	1	2	19
a. Syphilis	96	49	47	32	-	-	-	1	1	14	26	-	-	1	1	2	18
b. Chlamydia	1	-	1	-	-	-	-	-	-	-	-	-	1	-	-	-	-
c. Gonorrhoea	1	-	1	-	-	-	-	-	-	-	-	-	1	-	-	-	-
3. HIV	795	455	341	73	11	108	181	57	17	9	68	11	105	125	23	6	3
4. Diarrhoeal diseases	1 093	601	492	504	14	2	3	4	10	63	380	13	2	2	5	9	81
5. Childhood-cluster diseases	709	392	318	360	20	1	2	2	1	5	288	18	1	1	2	1	6
a. Pertussis	128	71	57	68	3	-	-	-	-	-	55	2	-	-	-	-	-
b. Poliomyelitis	8	5	3	5	-	-	-	-	-	-	3	-	-	-	-	-	-
c. Diphtheria	3	2	1	2	-	-	-	-	-	-	1	-	-	-	-	-	-
d. Measles	406	225	181	210	15	-	-	-	-	-	168	13	-	-	-	-	-
e. Tetanus	165	90	75	75	3	1	2	2	1	5	62	3	1	1	2	1	6
6. Bacterial meningitis*	56	29	27	14	1	-	2	3	3	7	11	-	-	1	3	3	9
7. Hepatitis B and hepatitis C	45	25	20	2	-	1	1	4	3	14	2	-	-	-	2	3	13
8. Malaria	387	224	163	196	9	5	4	4	2	4	137	8	3	3	4	2	5
9. Tropical-cluster diseases	31	18	13	1	3	2	3	3	2	4	1	3	1	1	2	1	1
a. Trypanosomiasis	12	7	5	-	2	1	1	1	1	1	-	1	1	1	1	1	-
b. Chagas disease	9	4	5	-	-	-	1	2	1	-	-	-	-	-	1	1	2
c. Schistosomiasis	3	2	1	-	-	-	-	-	-	-	-	-	-	-	-	-	1
d. Leishmaniasis	7	5	2	1	2	1	1	-	-	-	1	1	-	-	-	-	-
10. Leprosy	1	1	-	-	-	-	-	-	-	-	-	-	-	-	-	-	-
11. Dengue	2	1	1	-	1	-	-	-	-	-	1	-	-	-	-	-	-
12. Japanese encephalitis	1	-	-	-	-	-	-	-	-	-	-	-	-	-	-	-	-
13. Trachoma	-	-	-	-	-	-	-	-	-	-	-	-	-	-	-	-	-
14. Intestinal nematode infections	4	2	2	1	1	-	-	-	-	-	1	1	-	-	-	-	-
a. Ascariasis	1	1	-	1	-	-	-	-	-	-	-	-	-	-	-	-	-
b. Trichuriasis	1	-	1	-	-	-	-	-	-	-	1	-	-	-	-	-	-
c. Ancylostomiasis, necatoriasis	2	1	1	-	1	-	-	-	-	-	-	1	-	-	-	-	-
15. Other infectious and parasitic	249	124	126	45	4	2	3	5	8	58	35	4	1	1	4	7	74

Annex Table 20i, continued. Deaths by age, sex and cause (thousands): World, 2020, optimistic scenario

Cause	Total	Male	Female	Males							Females						
				0-4	5-14	15-29	30-44	45-59	60-69	70+	0-4	5-14	15-29	30-44	45-59	60-69	70+
B. Respiratory infections	2 291	1 182	1 109	489	27	5	6	15	71	568	375	26	5	4	14	51	634
1. Lower respiratory infections	2 261	1 166	1 095	480	27	5	6	15	70	563	368	26	5	4	14	51	628
2. Upper respiratory infections	22	11	11	5	-	-	-	-	1	5	4	-	-	-	-	1	6
3. Otitis media	8	5	4	4	-	-	-	-	-	-	3	-	-	-	-	-	-
C. Maternal conditions	54		54										24	25	3		
1. Maternal haemorrhage	13		13										6	6	1		
2. Maternal sepsis	8		8										4	4			
3. Hypertensive disorders*	7		7										3	3			
4. Obstructed labour	4		4										2	2			
5. Abortion	7		7										3	3	1		
6. Other maternal	14		14										6	7			
D. Perinatal conditions*	812	444	368	444								368					
E. Nutritional deficiencies	266	131	135	76	4	1	1	2	4	42	65	4	1	1	3	4	57
1. Protein-energy malnutrition	164	83	80	57	1	-	-	1	2	22	49	1	-	1	1	2	28
2. Iodine deficiency	5	3	2	2	-	-	-	-	-	-	2	-	-	-	-	-	-
3. Vitamin A deficiency	30	16	14	13	3	-	-	-	-	-	11	3	-	-	-	-	-
4. Iron-deficiency anaemia	64	28	37	4	1	1	1	1	2	19	3	1	1	1	2	2	27
II. Noncommunicable diseases	48 023	27 087	20 936	513	178	245	1 201	5 949	6 779	12 222	457	146	178	539	2 540	3 375	13 701
A. Malignant neoplasms	12 231	7 553	4 678	29	69	89	472	2 302	2 077	2 515	36	48	75	273	1 140	1 177	1 930
1. Mouth and oropharynx cancers	642	431	211		1	6	32	128	121	142	1	1	4	12	49	62	81
2. Oesophagus cancer	819	566	253			3	20	183	170	190			2	5	57	83	107
3. Stomach cancer	1 570	1 053	517			6	38	331	308	369			4	21	105	139	248
4. Colon and rectum cancers	821	450	371			5	22	93	119	211			3	12	56	93	207
5. Liver cancer	1 149	861	289	1	2	14	106	369	199	171	1	1	3	17	79	78	109
6. Pancreas cancer	313	186	127			1	7	49	51	78			1	2	19	32	73
7. Trachea, bronchus, lung cancers	2 452	1 838	614			6	88	674	604	464			2	15	153	191	253
8. Melanoma and other skin cancers	78	41	37			1	3	12	9	16			1	2	8	8	18
9. Breast cancer	493		493										10	45	158	105	175
10. Cervix uteri cancer	399		399										9	34	159	87	110
11. Corpus uteri cancer	100		100											3	25	25	46
12. Ovary cancer	161		161									1	5	16	44	38	57
13. Prostate cancer	396	396					1	28	103	262							
14. Bladder cancer	262	201	61			1	5	38	57	100				1	8	15	35
15. Lymphomas, multiple myeloma	374	230	143	1	2	9	25	51	51	74	4	8	3	9	23	32	64
16. Leukaemia	337	192	146	7	18	13	30	41	31	51	9	13	9	18	26	24	46
17. Other cancers	1 866	1 109	757	14	31	25	94	305	254	386	18	22	19	61	170	166	301

Annex Table 20i, continued. Deaths by age, sex and cause (thousands): World, 2020, optimistic scenario

Cause	Total	Male	Female	Males							Females						
				0-4	5-14	15-29	30-44	45-59	60-69	70+	0-4	5-14	15-29	30-44	45-59	60-69	70+
B. Other neoplasms	**99**	**48**	**50**	**3**	**2**	**2**	**4**	**9**	**8**	**21**	**3**	**2**	**1**	**2**	**6**	**7**	**29**
C. Diabetes mellitus	**668**	**258**	**410**	**5**	**3**	**3**	**13**	**47**	**57**	**129**	**5**	**3**	**2**	**5**	**42**	**83**	**269**
D. Endocrine disorders	**154**	**66**	**88**	**13**	**2**	**3**	**5**	**8**	**8**	**27**	**12**	**3**	**2**	**2**	**7**	**8**	**54**
E. Neuro-psychiatric conditions	**741**	**352**	**390**	**26**	**12**	**22**	**38**	**49**	**42**	**163**	**26**	**10**	**11**	**11**	**22**	**37**	**274**
2. Bipolar disorder	20	5	15	-	-	1	-	1	-	3	-	-	-	1	1	-	13
3. Schizophrenia	56	26	30	-	-	1	4	5	3	13	-	-	-	1	3	4	22
4. Epilepsy	52	32	20	2	2	5	8	6	3	5	2	2	4	2	2	2	5
5. Alcohol use	48	41	7	-	-	1	10	16	7	7	-	-	-	1	2	2	2
6. Dementia*	267	95	172	2	1	1	2	6	11	72	3	-	1	2	4	13	149
7. Parkinson disease	79	39	40	-	-	-	-	1	4	35	-	-	-	-	1	3	36
8. Multiple sclerosis	22	9	13	-	-	-	2	3	2	2	-	-	-	1	4	3	5
9. Drug use	7	6	1	-	-	3	3	-	-	-	-	-	1	-	-	-	-
13. Other neuro-psychiatric	191	99	92	22	9	10	10	11	11	26	20	8	5	4	5	9	41
F. Sense organ diseases	**18**	**9**	**9**	**1**	**-**	**-**	**-**	**2**	**2**	**3**	**1**	**-**	**-**	**-**	**2**	**3**	**4**
1. Glaucoma	6	3	3	-	-	-	-	1	1	1	-	-	-	-	1	1	1
2. Cataracts	5	3	2	-	-	-	-	1	1	1	-	-	-	-	-	1	1
G. Cardiovascular diseases	**24 897**	**13 532**	**11 365**	**120**	**45**	**69**	**464**	**2 631**	**3 438**	**6 766**	**74**	**36**	**42**	**159**	**841**	**1 446**	**8 766**
1. Rheumatic heart disease	451	244	207	-	4	11	31	87	49	63	-	4	8	19	47	32	98
2. Ischaemic heart disease	11 208	6 191	5 017	-	-	7	170	1 200	1 630	3 185	-	-	3	49	311	656	3 992
3. Cerebrovascular disease	7 708	4 024	3 684	15	12	17	111	733	1 056	2 080	10	9	7	43	277	482	2 855
4. Inflammatory heart diseases	734	425	309	24	8	11	46	124	73	139	19	7	7	16	45	34	182
5. Other cardiovascular	4 797	2 648	2 149	81	21	23	106	488	631	1 299	40	17	17	32	160	242	1 641
H. Respiratory diseases	**5 392**	**3 077**	**2 315**	**32**	**16**	**18**	**66**	**375**	**742**	**1 829**	**20**	**15**	**17**	**33**	**263**	**392**	**1 575**
1. COPD*	3 946	2 282	1 664	8	3	4	20	247	577	1 425	6	3	2	11	156	290	1 196
2. Asthma	281	144	138	1	2	4	11	27	30	69	-	1	3	7	27	28	72
3. Other respiratory	1 164	651	513	24	11	10	34	102	135	336	14	11	12	16	80	75	306
I. Digestive diseases	**2 332**	**1 456**	**877**	**17**	**7**	**17**	**104**	**454**	**326**	**530**	**17**	**9**	**12**	**37**	**159**	**149**	**493**
1. Peptic ulcer	251	153	98	-	-	6	8	36	32	77	1	1	1	3	12	13	69
2. Cirrhosis of the liver	995	701	294	1	1	6	58	276	173	187	-	1	3	16	81	66	125
3. Appendicitis	30	18	11	-	2	4	5	3	2	2	-	2	2	3	2	1	1
4. Other digestive	1 056	583	473	16	4	6	34	139	120	265	16	5	6	16	64	68	297
J. Genito-urinary diseases	**792**	**407**	**385**	**21**	**11**	**13**	**29**	**62**	**67**	**203**	**17**	**10**	**9**	**13**	**47**	**60**	**229**
1. Nephritis and nephrosis	567	280	286	18	10	11	22	45	47	128	15	9	7	10	36	46	164
2. Benign prostatic hypertrophy	35	35	-	-	-	-	-	1	6	28	-	-	-	-	-	-	-
3. Other genito-urinary	191	92	99	3	-	2	7	16	15	47	2	1	2	3	12	14	65
K. Skin diseases	**52**	**24**	**28**	**8**	**-**	**-**	**1**	**2**	**2**	**10**	**6**	**-**	**1**	**-**	**1**	**2**	**18**

Annex Table 20i, continued. Deaths by age, sex and cause (thousands): World, 2020, optimistic scenario

Cause	Total	Male	Female	Males 0-4	5-14	15-29	30-44	45-59	60-69	70+	Females 0-4	5-14	15-29	30-44	45-59	60-69	70+
L. Musculo-skeletal diseases	**107**	**36**	**72**	1	1	1	1	3	7	23	1	-	1	2	5	7	56
1. Rheumatoid arthritis	18	5	13	-	-	1	-	-	1	3	-	-	-	-	1	2	10
3. Other musculo-skeletal	88	30	58	1	-	1	1	3	6	19	1	-	1	2	4	5	45
M. Congenital anomalies	**539**	**269**	**269**	237	8	8	6	5	2	3	240	8	5	3	5	3	5
N. Oral conditions	**1**	**-**	**1**	-	-	-	-	-	-	-	-	-	-	-	-	-	-
III. Injuries	***8 398***	***5 387***	***3 011***	*416*	*402*	*1 601*	*1 176*	*884*	*375*	*533*	*335*	*238*	*683*	*448*	*456*	*273*	*577*
A. Unintentional injuries	**5 045**	**3 211**	**1 834**	304	292	782	650	565	237	381	223	172	303	219	289	177	451
1. Road traffic accidents	2 421	1 651	770	59	175	520	359	295	118	124	38	110	191	119	145	73	94
2. Poisonings	281	162	119	37	6	15	30	39	14	21	26	4	16	15	20	13	24
3. Falls	439	215	224	11	7	19	28	39	25	87	10	3	4	7	20	25	155
4. Fires	346	149	197	40	9	21	24	22	8	26	34	11	39	29	24	15	45
5. Drownings	449	290	159	75	56	50	40	30	13	26	48	22	15	11	18	11	33
6. Other unintentional	1 110	744	366	82	39	157	169	141	59	97	67	22	38	38	62	40	100
B. Intentional injuries	**3 352**	**2 176**	**1 176**	112	110	818	526	318	138	152	112	66	380	229	167	96	126
1. Self-inflicted injuries	1 242	719	523	-	26	154	157	170	89	122	-	13	146	92	106	61	104
2. Violence	1 059	846	213	29	29	397	227	110	31	23	31	16	58	42	36	16	15
3. War	1 051	611	441	83	56	267	142	38	18	7	81	37	176	95	25	19	7

Notes:
Causes responsible for no deaths have been omitted from this table.
A dash (-) symbol indicates fewer than 500 deaths.
ªIA6 is Bacterial meningitis and meningococcaemia; IC3 is Hypertensive disorders of pregnancy; ID is Conditions arising during the perinatal period; IIE6 is Dementia and other degenerative and hereditary CNS disorders; IIH1 is Chronic obstructive pulmonary disease.

Annex Table 21a. DALYs by age, sex and cause (thousands): Established Market Economies, 2020, optimistic scenario

Cause	Total	Male	Female	Males					Females				
				0–4	5–14	15–44	45–59	60+	0–4	5–14	15–44	45–59	60+
Population (millions)	*911*	*444*	*466*	*29*	*58*	*162*	*87*	*108*	*28*	*55*	*156*	*87*	*140*
All causes	*89 847*	*51 213*	*38 634*	*1 193*	*841*	*16 212*	*12 392*	*20 576*	*980*	*706*	*10 993*	*7 463*	*18 492*
I. Communicable, maternal, perinatal and nutritional conditions	*3 329*	*1 961*	*1 369*	*433*	*36*	*671*	*160*	*661*	*323*	*35*	*309*	*68*	*634*
A. Infectious and parasitic diseases	1 390	963	427	57	10	643	131	122	45	11	232	26	113
1. Tuberculosis	52	37	15	-	-	2	5	29	-	-	1	2	13
2. STDs excluding HIV	133	10	124	-	-	8	-	1	-	-	119	1	2
a. Syphilis	2	1	1	-	-	-	-	1	-	-	-	-	-
b. Chlamydia	114	5	109	-	-	5	-	-	-	2	107	1	-
c. Gonorrhoea	15	3	12	-	-	3	-	-	-	-	12	-	-
3. HIV	889	761	128	14	2	620	114	11	10	2	101	12	2
4. Diarrhoeal diseases	61	31	30	13	2	4	2	9	11	2	2	2	12
5. Childhood-cluster diseases	10	6	4	4	-	-	-	1	3	-	-	-	1
a. Pertussis	6	3	3	3	-	-	-	-	3	-	-	-	-
b. Poliomyelitis	1	1	1	-	-	-	-	-	-	-	-	-	-
c. Diphtheria	-	-	-	-	-	-	-	-	-	-	-	-	-
d. Measles	3	2	1	1	-	-	-	-	1	-	-	-	-
e. Tetanus	1	-	-	-	-	-	-	-	-	-	-	-	-
6. Bacterial meningitis*	48	26	22	18	2	2	1	3	15	2	1	1	4
7. Hepatitis B and hepatitis C	14	9	5	-	-	2	2	5	-	-	1	1	3
8. Malaria	-	-	-	-	-	-	-	-	-	-	-	-	-
9. Tropical-cluster diseases	-	-	-	-	-	-	-	-	-	-	-	-	-
a. Trypanosomiasis	-	-	-	-	-	-	-	-	-	-	-	-	-
b. Chagas disease	-	-	-	-	-	-	-	-	-	-	-	-	-
c. Schistosomiasis	-	-	-	-	-	-	-	-	-	-	-	-	-
d. Leishmaniasis	-	-	-	-	-	-	-	-	-	-	-	-	-
e. Lymphatic filariasis	-	-	-	-	-	-	-	-	-	-	-	-	-
f. Onchocerciasis	-	-	-	-	-	-	-	-	-	-	-	-	-
10. Leprosy	-	-	-	-	-	-	-	-	-	-	-	-	-
11. Dengue	-	-	-	-	-	-	-	-	-	-	-	-	-
12. Japanese encephalitis	-	-	-	-	-	-	-	-	-	-	-	-	-
13. Trachoma	-	-	-	-	-	-	-	-	-	-	-	-	-
14. Intestinal nematode infections	-	-	-	-	-	-	-	-	-	-	-	-	-
a. Ascariasis	-	-	-	-	-	-	-	-	-	-	-	-	-
b. Trichuriasis	-	-	-	-	-	-	-	-	-	-	-	-	-
c. Ancylostomiasis and necatoriasis	-	-	-	-	-	-	-	-	-	-	-	-	-

Annex Table 21a, continued. DALYs by age, sex and cause (thousands): Established Market Economies, 2020, optimistic scenario

Cause	Total	Male	Female	Males					Females				
				0-4	5-14	15-44	45-59	60+	0-4	5-14	15-44	45-59	60+
B. Respiratory infections	**1 008**	**535**	**473**	**22**	**11**	**13**	**22**	**468**	**15**	**10**	**6**	**13**	**429**
1. Lower respiratory infections	969	515	454	17	3	11	21	463	11	3	5	12	423
2. Upper respiratory infections	20	10	10	2	1	1	1	5	1	-	1	1	-
3. Otitis media	20	10	9	3	7	-	-	-	2	7	-	-	6
C. Maternal conditions	**28**	**-**	**28**	-	-	-	-	-	-	-	**28**	-	-
1. Maternal haemorrhage	2	-	2	-	-	-	-	-	-	-	2	-	-
2. Maternal sepsis	3	-	3	-	-	-	-	-	-	-	3	-	-
3. Hypertensive disorders of pregnancy	1	-	1	-	-	-	-	-	-	-	1	-	-
4. Obstructed labour	20	-	20	-	-	-	-	-	-	-	20	-	-
5. Abortion	1	-	1	-	-	-	-	-	-	-	1	-	-
D. Perinatal conditions*	**576**	**332**	**244**	**331**	-	-	-	-	**244**	-	-	-	-
E. Nutritional deficiencies	**327**	**131**	**197**	**22**	**15**	**15**	**7**	**71**	**20**	**14**	**43**	**29**	**91**
1. Protein-energy malnutrition	38	18	20	10	-	-	-	7	9	-	-	-	11
2. Iodine deficiency	-	-	-	-	-	-	-	-	-	-	-	-	-
3. Vitamin A deficiency	-	-	-	-	-	-	-	-	-	-	-	-	-
4. Iron-deficiency anaemia	286	111	175	12	15	15	7	63	11	14	43	28	79
II. Noncommunicable diseases	**77 218**	**43 065**	**34 153**	**590**	**551**	**11 275**	**11 361**	**19 288**	**528**	**484**	**9 033**	**6 803**	**17 304**
A. Malignant neoplasms	**16 011**	**9 712**	**6 300**	**14**	**61**	**827**	**3 351**	**5 459**	**13**	**42**	**679**	**1 896**	**3 670**
1. Mouth and oropharynx cancers	355	292	63	-	-	31	143	118	-	-	7	21	34
2. Oesophagus cancer	364	301	63	-	-	14	126	161	-	-	3	16	44
3. Stomach cancer	1 102	744	358	-	-	46	227	471	-	-	38	86	233
4. Colon and rectum cancers	1 693	969	723	-	-	51	273	645	-	-	40	167	517
5. Liver cancer	323	258	65	-	-	15	111	131	-	-	4	16	44
6. Pancreas cancer	609	366	243	-	-	20	121	225	-	-	10	59	174
7. Trachea, bronchus, lung cancers	4 480	3 122	1 358	-	-	239	1 438	1 445	-	-	75	461	822
8. Melanoma and other skin cancers	217	138	79	-	-	34	48	56	-	-	22	24	34
9. Breast cancer	1 176	-	1 176	-	-	-	-	-	-	-	186	459	531
10. Cervix uteri cancer	145	-	145	-	-	-	-	-	-	-	44	50	50
11. Corpus uteri cancer	162	-	162	-	-	-	-	-	-	-	14	54	94
12. Ovary cancer	317	-	317	-	-	-	-	-	-	-	35	119	163
13. Prostate cancer	746	746	-	-	-	3	64	679	-	-	-	-	-
14. Bladder cancer	439	364	74	-	-	5	56	303	-	-	2	10	62
15. Lymphomas and multiple myeloma	647	396	251	1	7	81	118	189	1	2	37	59	152
16. Leukaemia	510	309	200	5	24	80	69	131	5	16	48	42	89
C. Diabetes mellitus	**1 660**	**768**	**892**	**1**	**1**	**117**	**223**	**425**	**1**	**2**	**62**	**149**	**677**
D. Endocrine disorders	**684**	**308**	**376**	**39**	**26**	**85**	**42**	**116**	**37**	**20**	**63**	**76**	**180**

Annex Table 21a, continued. DALYs by age, sex and cause (thousands): Established Market Economies, 2020, optimistic scenario

Cause	Total	Male	Female	Males					Females				
				0-4	5-14	15-44	45-59	60+	0-4	5-14	15-44	45-59	60+
E. Neuro-psychiatric conditions	**24 370**	**12 410**	**11 960**	**71**	**264**	**8 152**	**1 784**	**2 139**	**65**	**221**	**6 525**	**1 770**	**3 380**
1. Unipolar major depression	6 642	2 329	4 314	-	-	1 612	499	217	-	-	2 929	910	475
2. Bipolar disorder	1 600	808	793	-	-	679	83	46	-	-	654	82	57
3. Schizophrenia	1 975	1 030	945	-	-	1 006	6	18	-	-	915	2	28
4. Epilepsy	245	143	103	3	23	75	26	16	3	25	36	16	22
5. Alcohol use	4 344	3 676	668	-	-	2 938	564	175	-	-	525	95	48
6. Dementia*	4 296	1 680	2 616	31	14	35	288	1 312	30	12	28	303	2 243
7. Parkinson disease	661	299	362	-	-	-	83	216	-	-	-	90	272
8. Multiple sclerosis	183	80	103	-	-	65	10	5	-	-	83	12	7
9. Drug use	1 342	1 016	326	-	92	874	42	9	-	31	279	14	3
10. Post-traumatic stress disorder	262	99	162	4	17	63	12	4	6	28	102	19	7
11. Obsessive-compulsive disorders	1 404	597	807	-	57	443	53	44	-	72	566	95	74
12. Panic disorder	671	223	448	-	19	147	56	1	-	19	311	89	29
F. Sense organ diseases	**143**	**66**	**77**	**-**	**-**	**3**	**26**	**37**	**-**	**-**	**2**	**27**	**48**
1. Glaucoma	104	46	58	-	-	2	22	22	-	-	1	24	33
2. Cataracts	34	18	17	-	-	-	4	14	-	-	-	2	14
G. Cardiovascular diseases	**17 921**	**11 622**	**6 299**	**24**	**12**	**772**	**3 293**	**7 520**	**21**	**7**	**252**	**417**	**5 602**
1. Rheumatic heart disease	117	59	59	-	-	7	21	30	-	-	5	10	44
2. Ischaemic heart disease	9 119	6 239	2 880	5	3	273	1 924	4 042	4	2	47	166	2 667
3. Cerebrovascular disease	4 761	2 733	2 028	5	3	215	675	1 835	6	2	113	163	1 747
4. Inflammatory heart diseases	522	364	158	-	-	87	135	135	-	-	28	18	105
H. Respiratory diseases	**4 080**	**2 301**	**1 779**	**19**	**74**	**335**	**395**	**1 477**	**9**	**80**	**304**	**383**	**1 003**
1. COPD*	2 272	1 410	862	1	1	56	227	1 125	-	1	33	183	644
2. Asthma	801	388	414	8	63	182	65	69	3	70	170	85	84
I. Digestive diseases	**3 985**	**2 357**	**1 629**	**11**	**6**	**335**	**986**	**1 018**	**9**	**6**	**252**	**504**	**858**
1. Peptic ulcer	238	149	88	-	-	21	46	82	-	-	13	19	56
2. Cirrhosis of the liver	1 449	1 048	401	-	-	149	549	351	-	-	66	180	155
3. Appendicitis	23	14	9	1	1	5	3	5	1	1	4	2	3
J. Genito-urinary diseases	**1 056**	**644**	**413**	**8**	**1**	**36**	**181**	**418**	**6**	**2**	**21**	**41**	**342**
1. Nephritis and nephrosis	372	192	180	6	1	20	27	137	5	1	6	14	155
2. Benign prostatic hypertrophy	312	312	-	-	-	-	131	181	-	-	-	-	-
L. Musculo-skeletal diseases	**4 843**	**1 662**	**3 181**	**1**	**1**	**353**	**891**	**416**	**1**	**7**	**657**	**1 354**	**1 162**
1. Rheumatoid arthritis	1 126	284	842	-	-	51	114	120	-	4	288	200	350
2. Osteoarthritis	3 432	1 300	2 133	-	-	284	759	257	-	-	324	1 114	695

Annex Table 21a, continued. DALYs by age, sex and cause (thousands): Established Market Economies, 2020, optimistic scenario

Cause	Total	Male	Female	Males					Females				
				0-4	5-14	15-44	45-59	60+	0-4	5-14	15-44	45-59	60+
M. Congenital anomalies	**826**	**444**	**383**	**381**	**13**	**35**	**7**	**7**	**344**	**12**	**13**	**5**	**8**
N. Oral conditions	**1 018**	**486**	**533**	**14**	**75**	**159**	**105**	**131**	**14**	**72**	**155**	**112**	**180**
1. Dental caries	436	217	219	14	75	77	21	30	13	72	74	21	38
2. Periodontal disease	33	17	17	-	-	14	2	1	-	-	13	2	2
3. Edentulism	543	249	293	-	-	67	82	100	-	-	66	89	138
III. Injuries	***9 299***	***6 187***	***3 112***	***170***	***254***	***4 266***	***871***	***627***	***129***	***186***	***1 650***	***592***	***554***
A. Unintentional injuries	**6 142**	**3 863**	**2 278**	**144**	**217**	**2 666**	**439**	**397**	**105**	**164**	**1 163**	**404**	**442**
1. Road traffic accidents	3 315	2 155	1 160	61	109	1 852	91	42	46	97	819	134	64
2. Poisonings	166	104	62	2	1	77	16	8	1	1	39	13	8
3. Falls	1 022	492	530	18	35	192	101	145	13	21	132	149	215
4. Fires	153	82	71	9	15	31	14	13	8	18	23	11	11
5. Drownings	147	109	39	12	15	54	16	13	7	5	13	7	7
6. Other unintentional	1 337	921	416	42	41	461	201	176	31	21	138	91	136
B. Intentional injuries	**3 157**	**2 324**	**833**	**25**	**37**	**1 600**	**433**	**229**	**24**	**22**	**487**	**187**	**113**
1. Self-inflicted injuries	2 217	1 612	605	-	15	1 021	366	210	-	5	333	165	102
2. Violence	938	710	228	25	23	578	66	18	24	17	154	22	10
3. War	2	2	-	-	-	1	-	1	-	-	-	-	-

Notes:
A dash (-) symbol indicates fewer than 500 DALYs.
*IA6 is Bacterial meningitis and meningococcaemia; ID is Conditions arising during the perinatal period;
IIE6 is Dementia and other degenerative and hereditary CNS disorders; IIH1 is Chronic obstructive pulmonary disease.

Annex Table 21b. DALYs by age, sex and cause (thousands): Formerly Socialist Economies of Europe, 2020, optimistic scenario

Cause	Total	Male	Female	Males					Females				
				0-4	5-14	15-44	45-59	60+	0-4	5-14	15-44	45-59	60+
Population (millions)	366	172	194	12	25	76	30	30	12	24	75	33	51
All causes	60 348	37 670	22 678	1 281	652	12 919	11 573	11 245	1 026	446	7 027	4 451	9 728
I. Communicable, maternal, perinatal and nutritional conditions	1 510	745	765	437	30	69	42	167	312	29	186	24	215
A. Infectious and parasitic diseases	439	201	238	85	8	49	24	35	68	8	117	7	37
1. Tuberculosis	64	54	11	1	-	17	19	17	-	-	2	2	6
2. STDs excluding HIV	129	20	109	3	-	17	-	-	3	2	103	1	1
a. Syphilis	1	1	-	-	-	-	-	-	-	-	-	-	-
b. Chlamydia	99	8	91	1	-	7	-	-	1	-	87	-	-
c. Gonorrhoea	28	11	17	2	-	9	-	-	2	-	15	-	-
3. HIV	55	30	25	17	3	9	1	-	17	3	5	-	-
4. Diarrhoeal diseases	51	27	23	22	1	2	1	1	18	1	1	1	2
5. Childhood-cluster diseases	8	4	4	3	1	-	-	-	3	1	-	-	-
a. Pertussis	5	2	2	2	1	-	-	-	2	1	-	-	-
b. Poliomyelitis	-	-	-	-	-	-	-	-	-	-	-	-	-
c. Diphtheria	-	-	-	-	-	-	-	-	-	-	-	-	-
d. Measles	2	1	1	1	-	-	-	-	1	-	-	-	-
e. Tetanus	1	1	-	1	-	-	-	-	-	-	-	-	-
6. Bacterial meningitis*	50	29	21	20	1	2	2	4	15	1	1	1	3
7. Hepatitis B and hepatitis C	7	4	3	2	-	1	-	1	1	-	-	-	1
8. Malaria	-	-	-	-	-	-	-	-	-	-	-	-	-
9. Tropical-cluster diseases	-	-	-	-	-	-	-	-	-	-	-	-	-
a. Trypanosomiasis	-	-	-	-	-	-	-	-	-	-	-	-	-
b. Chagas disease	-	-	-	-	-	-	-	-	-	-	-	-	-
c. Schistosomiasis	-	-	-	-	-	-	-	-	-	-	-	-	-
d. Leishmaniasis	-	-	-	-	-	-	-	-	-	-	-	-	-
e. Lymphatic filariasis	-	-	-	-	-	-	-	-	-	-	-	-	-
f. Onchocerciasis	-	-	-	-	-	-	-	-	-	-	-	-	-
10. Leprosy	-	-	-	-	-	-	-	-	-	-	-	-	-
11. Dengue	-	-	-	-	-	-	-	-	-	-	-	-	-
12. Japanese encephalitis	-	-	-	-	-	-	-	-	-	-	-	-	-
13. Trachoma	-	-	-	-	-	-	-	-	-	-	-	-	-
14. Intestinal nematode infections	-	-	-	-	-	-	-	-	-	-	-	-	-
a. Ascariasis	-	-	-	-	-	-	-	-	-	-	-	-	-
b. Trichuriasis	-	-	-	-	-	-	-	-	-	-	-	-	-
c. Ancylostomiasis and necatoriasis	-	-	-	-	-	-	-	-	-	-	-	-	-

Annex Table 21b, continued. DALYs by age, sex and cause (thousands): Formerly Socialist Economies of Europe, 2020, optimistic scenario

Cause	Total	Male	Female	Males 0-4	5-14	15-44	45-59	60+	Females 0-4	5-14	15-44	45-59	60+
B. Respiratory infections	453	234	220	86	7	13	15	112	61	7	4	5	142
1. Lower respiratory infections	438	226	213	83	5	12	15	111	59	4	4	5	141
2. Upper respiratory infections	6	3	3	1	-	1	-	-	1	-	-	-	1
3. Otitis media	9	5	4	2	3	-	-	-	1	2	-	-	-
C. Maternal conditions	45		45								45		
1. Maternal haemorrhage	1		1								1		
2. Maternal sepsis	9		9								9		
3. Hypertensive disorders of pregnancy	1		1								1		
4. Obstructed labour	12		12								12		
5. Abortion	12		12								12		
D. Perinatal conditions*	398	239	159	239					159				
E. Nutritional deficiencies	175	71	103	27	15	7	3	20	24	14	19	11	35
1. Protein-energy malnutrition	30	15	15	13	-	-	-	2	11	-	-	-	4
2. Iodine deficiency	-	-	-										
3. Vitamin A deficiency	-	-	-										
4. Iron-deficiency anaemia	130	50	79	11	14	6	2	16	10	13	18	10	28
II. Noncommunicable diseases	*48 194*	*29 127*	*19 067*	*546*	*267*	*7 381*	*10 248*	*10 685*	*475*	*218*	*5 274*	*3 935*	*9 165*
A. Malignant neoplasms	10 065	7 102	2 962	25	58	897	3 433	2 690	23	33	513	992	1 401
1. Mouth and oropharynx cancers	370	340	30	-	-	51	213	75	-	-	6	10	14
2. Oesophagus cancer	184	168	16	-	-	16	106	47	-	-	2	5	9
3. Stomach cancer	1 453	1 085	368	-	-	115	572	397	-	-	48	111	209
4. Colon and rectum cancers	890	551	338	-	-	57	241	253	-	-	34	99	205
5. Liver cancer	261	184	77	1	1	18	90	75	1	-	7	21	48
6. Pancreas cancer	387	281	106	-	-	30	147	104	-	-	9	32	66
7. Trachea, bronchus, lung cancers	2 842	2 444	398	1	1	236	1 197	1 009	-	-	41	146	210
8. Melanoma and other skin cancers	127	80	47	-	-	23	34	23	-	-	16	12	19
9. Breast cancer	468		468						-	-	107	200	161
10. Cervix uteri cancer	171		171						-	-	50	57	63
11. Corpus uteri cancer	127		127						-	-	18	50	59
12. Ovary cancer	173		173						-	-	35	74	64
13. Prostate cancer	184	184	-	-	-	4	45	135					
14. Bladder cancer	230	200	30	1	-	7	79	113	-	-	2	7	21
15. Lymphomas and multiple myeloma	289	205	84	3	11	67	81	44	2	4	29	21	28
16. Leukaemia	318	209	109	8	22	61	67	50	7	13	33	24	31
C. Diabetes mellitus	390	169	221	-	-	41	55	72	1	1	23	48	148
D. Endocrine disorders	114	52	62	12	3	25	8	4	12	3	20	15	11

Annex Table 21b, continued. DALYs by age, sex and cause (thousands): Formerly Socialist Economies of Europe, 2020, optimistic scenario

Cause	Total	Male	Female	Males					Females				
				0-4	5-14	15-44	45-59	60+	0-4	5-14	15-44	45-59	60+
E. Neuro-psychiatric conditions	10 306	5 173	5 133	73	135	3 815	631	520	65	109	3 207	690	1 062
1. Unipolar major depression	3 211	1 087	2 123	-	-	826	190	71	-	-	1 542	382	199
2. Bipolar disorder	839	411	428	-	-	358	34	19	-	-	352	37	39
3. Schizophrenia	834	432	402	-	-	422	5	5	-	-	393	2	7
4. Epilepsy	179	117	62	5	22	65	16	9	5	15	22	9	10
5. Alcohol use	1 724	1 521	203	-	-	1 276	192	54	-	-	181	13	10
6. Dementia*	1 182	404	778	15	7	15	86	281	14	6	13	109	634
7. Parkinson disease	153	59	94	-	-	-	19	40	-	-	-	24	70
8. Multiple sclerosis	96	41	55	-	-	33	5	4	-	-	42	6	7
9. Drug use	526	421	105	-	31	373	14	3	-	8	93	3	1
10. Post-traumatic stress disorder	117	43	73	2	7	29	4	1	3	12	49	7	3
11. Obsessive-compulsive disorders	652	272	380	-	25	215	19	13	-	32	281	38	28
12. Panic disorder	313	101	212	-	9	72	20	-	-	9	156	36	11
F. Sense organ diseases	77	36	42	-	-	1	9	26	-	-	1	14	26
1. Glaucoma	37	13	24	-	-	-	4	8	-	-	1	11	12
2. Cataracts	41	23	17	-	-	1	5	18	-	-	1	2	14
G. Cardiovascular diseases	16 128	10 480	5 648	16	5	1 083	4 011	5 366	11	3	248	628	4 757
1. Rheumatic heart disease	308	199	109	-	1	55	110	32	-	-	23	51	35
2. Ischaemic heart disease	8 266	5 726	2 540	-	-	543	2 448	2 735	-	-	61	254	2 225
3. Cerebrovascular disease	4 749	2 715	2 035	3	1	228	901	1 582	2	1	111	262	1 659
4. Inflammatory heart diseases	438	311	127	3	1	93	127	86	3	1	24	22	77
H. Respiratory diseases	4 218	2 808	1 410	12	25	360	1 084	1 327	5	19	236	358	791
1. COPD*	1 719	1 247	472	-	-	110	521	616	-	-	48	89	335
2. Asthma	461	244	216	6	24	103	59	51	2	18	94	51	50
I. Digestive diseases	2 011	1 200	811	15	3	311	529	342	11	3	166	287	343
1. Peptic ulcer	162	121	42	-	-	26	54	40	-	-	9	13	19
2. Cirrhosis of the liver	616	435	181	-	-	70	229	136	-	-	25	78	77
3. Appendicitis	10	6	4	-	-	2	1	2	-	-	2	1	1
J. Genito-urinary diseases	587	337	250	4	3	78	117	136	3	3	53	85	106
1. Nephritis and nephrosis	144	87	57	2	2	36	25	22	2	2	14	15	24
2. Benign prostatic hypertrophy	129	129	-	-	-	-	56	73	-	-	-	-	-
L. Musculo-skeletal diseases	2 822	1 040	1 781	1	2	612	273	153	1	4	658	692	427
1. Rheumatoid arthritis	528	125	403	-	-	67	31	26	-	3	217	107	77
2. Osteoarthritis	2 178	879	1 299	-	-	524	233	122	-	-	409	557	332

Annex Table 21b, continued. DALYs by age, sex and cause (thousands): Formerly Socialist Economies of Europe, 2020, optimistic scenario

Cause	Total	Male	Female	Males					Females				
				0-4	5-14	15-44	45-59	60+	0-4	5-14	15-44	45-59	60+
M. Congenital anomalies	731	392	339	364	9	16	2	1	321	8	7	2	1
N. Oral conditions	512	231	282	14	19	95	66	35	14	28	99	79	61
1. Dental caries	249	115	135	14	19	45	21	15	14	28	44	24	25
2. Periodontal disease	17	8	10	-	-	5	1	2	-	-	8	1	1
3. Edentulism	245	108	137	-	-	46	44	19	-	-	47	55	35
III. Injuries	*10 644*	*7 798*	*2 846*	*298*	*354*	*5 469*	*1 283*	*393*	*238*	*198*	*1 567*	*493*	*349*
A. Unintentional injuries	6 985	5 156	1 828	189	260	3 571	875	261	131	136	944	353	265
1. Road traffic accidents	3 376	2 485	891	35	135	1 983	256	77	21	86	599	117	69
2. Poisonings	664	495	169	21	6	267	165	35	16	5	64	59	26
3. Falls	804	499	305	28	32	292	92	55	20	13	105	71	95
4. Fires	126	85	41	9	6	42	19	8	8	5	12	8	9
5. Drownings	364	305	59	16	33	197	46	12	7	12	24	9	6
6. Other unintentional	1 650	1 288	362	79	48	791	297	73	58	15	141	90	59
B. Intentional injuries	3 660	2 642	1 017	110	94	1 898	408	132	108	62	623	140	84
1. Self-inflicted injuries	1 679	1 337	342	-	18	904	308	108	-	4	185	91	63
2. Violence	856	657	199	9	9	541	81	17	7	8	134	35	15
3. War	1 124	648	476	101	68	453	20	6	101	51	304	14	7

Notes:
A dash (-) symbol indicates fewer than 500 DALYs.
*IA6 is Bacterial meningitis and meningococcaemia; ID is Conditions arising during the perinatal period;
IIE6 is Dementia and other degenerative and hereditary CNS disorders; IIH1 is Chronic obstructive pulmonary disease.

Annex Table 21c. DALYs by age, sex and cause (thousands): India, 2020, optimistic scenario

Cause	Total	Male	Female	Males 0-4	5-14	15-44	45-59	60+	Females 0-4	5-14	15-44	45-59	60+
Population (millions)	*1 245*	*632*	*613*	*53*	*105*	*309*	*104*	*60*	*50*	*100*	*293*	*102*	*69*
All causes	*214 319*	*121 113*	*93 206*	*19 988*	*6 695*	*35 949*	*32 336*	*26 144*	*18 724*	*5 147*	*29 165*	*18 392*	*21 777*
I. Communicable, maternal, perinatal and nutritional conditions	**35 694**	**18 508**	**17 186**	**10 990**	**785**	**4 099**	**1 011**	**1 622**	**10 335**	**867**	**3 870**	**692**	**1 423**
A. Infectious and parasitic diseases	**21 419**	**11 554**	**9 866**	**5 348**	**509**	**3 806**	**888**	**1 003**	**5 005**	**509**	**3 109**	**508**	**734**
1. Tuberculosis	**2 335**	**1 562**	**772**	**96**	**31**	**374**	**433**	**628**	**65**	**22**	**116**	**246**	**323**
2. STDs excluding HIV	**1 527**	**569**	**959**	**271**	**4**	**273**	**5**	**16**	**253**	**15**	**660**	**6**	**25**
a. Syphilis	400	200	200	142	-	38	3	16	137	-	35	4	24
b. Chlamydia	627	116	510	31	2	83	-	-	28	11	469	2	1
c. Gonorrhoea	501	253	248	97	2	152	1	-	88	4	155	1	-
3. HIV	**7 149**	**3 979**	**3 169**	**630**	**118**	**2 809**	**339**	**82**	**683**	**129**	**2 185**	**145**	**29**
4. Diarrhoeal diseases	**5 108**	**2 590**	**2 518**	**2 304**	**75**	**57**	**28**	**126**	**2 203**	**94**	**30**	**29**	**162**
5. Childhood-cluster diseases	**2 999**	**1 600**	**1 398**	**1 467**	**78**	**35**	**10**	**11**	**1 273**	**83**	**19**	**10**	**14**
a. Pertussis	508	270	238	258	12	-	-	-	227	11	-	-	-
b. Poliomyelitis	236	143	93	141	1	1	-	-	93	-	-	-	-
c. Diphtheria	25	13	12	12	1	-	-	-	11	-	-	-	-
d. Measles	1 156	610	546	568	41	-	-	-	507	39	-	-	-
e. Tetanus	1 073	564	508	488	23	33	9	11	436	31	18	10	13
6. Bacterial meningitis*	**248**	**133**	**115**	**103**	**2**	**13**	**7**	**8**	**89**	**2**	**6**	**7**	**10**
7. Hepatitis B and hepatitis C	**58**	**33**	**25**	**8**	**2**	**6**	**6**	**10**	**6**	**2**	**3**	**3**	**11**
8. Malaria	**133**	**75**	**59**	**27**	**16**	**20**	**6**	**6**	**22**	**16**	**9**	**5**	**7**
9. Tropical-cluster diseases	**302**	**214**	**88**	**21**	**65**	**109**	**14**	**4**	**11**	**29**	**22**	**20**	**6**
a. Trypanosomiasis	-	-	-	-	-	-	-	-	-	-	-	-	-
b. Chagas disease	-	-	-	-	-	-	-	-	-	-	-	-	-
c. Schistosomiasis	-	-	-	-	-	-	-	-	-	-	-	-	-
d. Leishmaniasis	118	77	40	11	28	34	2	2	7	18	12	2	2
e. Lymphatic filariasis	185	137	48	11	37	75	12	2	4	11	10	18	4
f. Onchocerciasis	-	-	-	-	-	-	-	-	-	-	-	-	-
10. Leprosy	**57**	**29**	**28**	**-**	**8**	**17**	**3**	**1**	**1**	**7**	**16**	**3**	**1**
11. Dengue	**43**	**20**	**22**	**8**	**12**	**-**	**-**	**-**	**8**	**14**	**-**	**-**	**-**
12. Japanese encephalitis	**11**	**6**	**5**	**4**	**1**	**-**	**-**	**-**	**4**	**1**	**-**	**-**	**-**
13. Trachoma	**9**	**2**	**7**	**-**	**-**	**-**	**1**	**2**	**-**	**-**	**-**	**1**	**5**
14. Intestinal nematode infections	**144**	**78**	**66**	**1**	**33**	**29**	**8**	**8**	**1**	**30**	**19**	**8**	**9**
a. Ascariasis	30	16	14	1	15	-	-	-	1	14	-	-	-
b. Trichuriasis	20	10	9	-	10	-	-	-	-	9	-	-	-
c. Ancylostomiasis and necatoriasis	95	52	42	-	8	29	8	8	-	7	19	8	9

Annex Table 21c, continued. DALYs by age, sex and cause (thousands): India, 2020, optimistic scenario

Cause	Total	Male	Female	Males 0-4	5-14	15-44	45-59	60+	Females 0-4	5-14	15-44	45-59	60+
B. Respiratory infections	**6 500**	**3 253**	**3 247**	**2 448**	**142**	**93**	**65**	**506**	**2 339**	**230**	**56**	**67**	**554**
1. Lower respiratory infections	6 337	3 172	3 165	2 388	129	91	64	500	2 279	217	55	66	548
2. Upper respiratory infections	67	34	33	23	2	2	1	5	22	3	1	1	6
3. Otitis media	96	47	48	36	11	-	-	-	38	11	-	-	-
C. Maternal conditions	**470**	**-**	**470**						**-**	**-**	**459**	**11**	**-**
1. Maternal haemorrhage	54	-	54								52	2	
2. Maternal sepsis	80	-	80								78	2	
3. Hypertensive disorders of pregnancy	27	-	27								25	1	
4. Obstructed labour	94	-	94								94	1	
5. Abortion	101	-	101								99	2	
D. Perinatal conditions*	**4 970**	**2 566**	**2 404**	**2 566**					**2 404**				
E. Nutritional deficiencies	**2 334**	**1 135**	**1 199**	**629**	**135**	**200**	**58**	**113**	**586**	**128**	**246**	**105**	**134**
1. Protein-energy malnutrition	907	460	448	439	3	4	2	12	420	8	1	2	17
2. Iodine deficiency	62	33	28	31	2	1	-	-	26	2	-	-	-
3. Vitamin A deficiency	104	55	49	44	10	1	-	-	38	10	-	-	-
4. Iron-deficiency anaemia	1 261	587	674	115	119	195	56	101	100	109	244	104	117
II. Noncommunicable diseases	***132 963***	***75 101***	***57 862***	***5 323***	***1 080***	***18 138***	***27 137***	***23 423***	***5 388***	***1 005***	***17 740***	***14 702***	***19 027***
A. Malignant neoplasms	**17 353**	**9 891**	**7 462**	**138**	**204**	**2 030**	**4 935**	**2 584**	**89**	**94**	**1 816**	**3 458**	**2 005**
1. Mouth and oropharynx cancers	2 435	1 495	940	3	4	264	818	406	3	4	189	478	267
2. Oesophagus cancer	1 330	710	621	-	-	96	403	211	-	-	96	300	225
3. Stomach cancer	1 259	838	422	-	1	148	473	216	-	-	90	193	138
4. Colon and rectum cancers	576	325	251	-	-	95	138	91	-	1	44	108	98
5. Liver cancer	339	247	93	1	2	47	135	61	1	1	17	40	34
6. Pancreas cancer	200	126	74	-	-	22	70	34	-	-	15	30	28
7. Trachea, bronchus, lung cancers	3 614	3 131	483	-	1	484	1 746	901	-	-	71	239	172
8. Melanoma and other skin cancers	33	18	16	-	-	4	10	3	-	-	4	8	4
9. Breast cancer	1 035	-	1 035								316	496	222
10. Cervix uteri cancer	1 452	-	1 452								316	852	284
11. Corpus uteri cancer	79	-	79								8	40	31
12. Ovary cancer	328	-	328								120	115	91
13. Prostate cancer	186	186	-			4	47	134					
14. Bladder cancer	158	126	32			13	58	55			4	11	16
15. Lymphomas and multiple myeloma	579	406	173	23	37	157	136	53	5	7	49	55	56
16. Leukaemia	573	347	226	42	66	143	70	26	27	34	93	47	24
C. Diabetes mellitus	**1 814**	**884**	**930**	**69**	**43**	**192**	**322**	**259**	**73**	**41**	**99**	**289**	**428**
D. Endocrine disorders	**84**	**45**	**40**	**23**	**2**	**9**	**8**	**2**	**18**	**1**	**5**	**8**	**8**

Annex Table 21c, continued. DALYs by age, sex and cause (thousands): India, 2020, optimistic scenario

Cause	Total	Male	Female	Males					Females				
				0-4	5-14	15-44	45-59	60+	0-4	5-14	15-44	45-59	60+
E. Neuro-psychiatric conditions	**29 972**	**13 376**	**16 595**	**425**	**274**	**10 072**	**1 654**	**951**	**559**	**349**	**12 244**	**2 097**	**1 347**
1. Unipolar major depression	13 466	4 832	8 634	-	-	3 897	766	169	-	-	6 941	1 353	341
2. Bipolar disorder	3 699	1 891	1 808	-	-	1 718	134	39	-	-	1 631	128	48
3. Schizophrenia	2 554	1 355	1 199	-	-	1 338	9	7	-	-	1 181	4	14
4. Epilepsy	555	330	225	37	40	194	38	21	46	58	87	12	22
5. Alcohol use	1 384	1 264	121	-	-	1 134	112	18	-	-	111	7	2
6. Dementia*	1 780	826	954	50	19	53	233	472	62	19	47	235	592
7. Parkinson disease	267	121	146	-	-	-	55	66	-	-	-	65	81
8. Multiple sclerosis	303	134	168	-	-	119	11	4	-	-	148	14	6
9. Drug use	112	101	11	-	5	90	4	1	-	1	10	-	-
10. Post-traumatic stress disorder	454	174	280	7	32	119	14	2	11	51	192	22	4
11. Obsessive-compulsive disorders	2 524	1 100	1 424	-	110	895	68	27	-	139	1 127	117	41
12. Panic disorder	1 202	389	813	-	4	311	74	-	-	38	644	114	17
F. Sense organ diseases	**6 346**	**3 591**	**2 755**	**5**	**-**	**184**	**1 943**	**1 459**	**3**	**-**	**107**	**1 181**	**1 464**
1. Glaucoma	1 230	689	541	-	-	53	500	136	-	-	20	358	163
2. Cataracts	5 114	2 900	2 214	4	-	131	1 443	1 322	3	-	87	823	1 301
G. Cardiovascular diseases	**44 276**	**28 757**	**15 519**	**486**	**89**	**2 725**	**11 584**	**13 873**	**326**	**107**	**1 030**	**3 579**	**10 478**
1. Rheumatic heart disease	1 820	1 064	756	1	10	379	539	135	1	11	265	355	124
2. Ischaemic heart disease	22 671	14 998	7 673	-	-	665	6 332	8 001	-	-	228	1 667	5 779
3. Cerebrovascular disease	8 149	5 039	3 110	96	19	370	1 776	2 777	69	19	183	583	2 256
4. Inflammatory heart diseases	2 186	1 446	740	88	20	415	622	300	70	25	163	238	243
H. Respiratory diseases	**13 541**	**7 826**	**5 715**	**234**	**233**	**1 212**	**3 235**	**2 912**	**152**	**149**	**1 094**	**2 268**	**2 051**
1. COPD*	6 032	3 784	2 248	25	17	395	1 707	1 639	19	15	284	995	935
2. Asthma	1 801	1 054	747	43	106	488	275	142	17	54	367	196	113
I. Digestive diseases	**5 064**	**3 561**	**1 503**	**63**	**22**	**820**	**1 963**	**694**	**68**	**23**	**387**	**641**	**385**
1. Peptic ulcer	785	543	242	1	1	140	271	130	1	2	70	98	70
2. Cirrhosis of the liver	2 611	1 980	630	12	4	390	1 152	422	15	11	138	294	172
3. Appendicitis	129	77	52	2	8	52	12	4	2	8	34	6	3
J. Genito-urinary diseases	**1 705**	**1 191**	**514**	**93**	**74**	**111**	**669**	**246**	**51**	**103**	**87**	**111**	**162**
1. Nephritis and nephrosis	998	516	483	73	71	102	141	130	46	102	82	101	152
2. Benign prostatic hypertrophy	631	631	-	-	-	-	520	111	-	-	-	-	-
L. Musculo-skeletal diseases	**2 733**	**1 059**	**1 675**	**3**	**2**	**362**	**516**	**175**	**2**	**4**	**519**	**763**	**386**
1. Rheumatoid arthritis	305	83	222	1	-	56	17	9	-	3	109	81	28
2. Osteoarthritis	2 409	964	1 445	-	-	303	496	165	-	-	408	680	357

Annex Table 21c, continued. DALYs by age, sex and cause (thousands): India, 2020, optimistic scenario

Cause	Total	Male	Female	Males					Females				
				0-4	5-14	15-44	45-59	60+	0-4	5-14	15-44	45-59	60+
M. Congenital anomalies	7 994	3 868	4 125	3 700	54	89	19	6	3 969	62	58	24	12
N. Oral conditions	1 821	895	926	37	74	270	265	248	36	71	267	265	287
1. Dental caries	1 041	525	516	36	73	221	115	80	35	70	209	112	91
2. Periodontal disease	121	61	59	-	-	47	11	4	-	-	44	11	5
3. Edentulism	637	304	333	-	-	-	140	165	-	-	-	141	191
III. Injuries	45 662	27 504	18 158	3 674	4 830	13 712	4 189	1 099	3 001	3 275	7 555	2 999	1 327
A. Unintentional injuries	39 020	23 823	15 197	3 478	4 644	11 199	3 522	979	2 752	3 098	5 555	2 561	1 230
1. Road traffic accidents	17 122	12 091	5 030	557	1 996	7 202	1 862	474	165	1 564	1 971	905	425
2. Poisonings	847	382	465	130	36	161	43	12	87	22	173	168	15
3. Falls	5 790	3 344	2 446	775	1 481	709	275	104	857	520	495	437	138
4. Fires	3 962	1 263	2 699	330	157	549	188	39	276	392	1 620	262	148
5. Drownings	1 785	986	800	275	208	377	90	37	220	161	230	116	72
6. Other unintentional	9 514	5 756	3 757	1 412	766	2 201	1 064	313	1 147	440	1 066	673	431
B. Intentional injuries	6 642	3 682	2 961	196	186	2 513	666	120	249	177	1 999	437	97
1. Self-inflicted injuries	4 345	2 213	2 132	-	110	1 620	427	56	-	110	1 787	212	22
2. Violence	2 125	1 296	829	196	76	720	239	64	249	67	212	226	75
3. War	173	173	-	-	-	173	-	-	-	-	-	-	-

Notes:
A dash (-) symbol indicates fewer than 500 DALYs.
*IA6 is Bacterial meningitis and meningococcaemia; ID is Conditions arising during the perinatal period;
IIE6 is Dementia and other degenerative and hereditary CNS disorders; IIH1 is Chronic obstructive pulmonary disease.

Annex Table 21d. DALYs by age, sex and cause (thousands): China, 2020, optimistic scenario

Cause	Total	Male	Female	Males 0-4	5-14	15-44	45-59	60+	Females 0-4	5-14	15-44	45-59	60+
Population (millions)	*1 479*	*742*	*738*	*57*	*103*	*319*	*164*	*99*	*54*	*98*	*304*	*162*	*120*
All causes	**201 701**	**116 722**	**84 979**	**6 943**	**2 335**	**31 452**	**39 756**	**36 236**	**7 036**	**1 973**	**27 145**	**21 792**	**27 033**
I. **Communicable, maternal, perinatal and nutritional conditions**	**7 669**	**3 898**	**3 771**	**2 085**	**219**	**374**	**286**	**934**	**2 068**	**212**	**277**	**251**	**962**
A. Infectious and parasitic diseases	**2 404**	**1 280**	**1 125**	**384**	**110**	**127**	**177**	**481**	**351**	**105**	**81**	**122**	**466**
1. Tuberculosis	**767**	**471**	**296**	**13**	**1**	**38**	**110**	**309**	**13**	**5**	**17**	**68**	**193**
2. STDs excluding HIV	**24**	**6**	**18**	1	-	4	-	1	1	-	16	-	1
a. Syphilis	2	1	1	-				1					1
b. Chlamydia	15	2	13			2					13		
c. Gonorrhoea	7	3	4			3					4		
3. HIV	**62**	**34**	**28**	5	1	22	4	1	4	1	21	2	-
4. Diarrhoeal diseases	**497**	**235**	**262**	**120**	**9**	**21**	**14**	**71**	**135**	**8**	**11**	**15**	**94**
5. Childhood-cluster diseases	**277**	**155**	**122**	**145**	**6**	**2**	**1**	**1**	**116**	**5**	**1**	-	-
a. Pertussis	95	52	43	50	3				41	2			
b. Poliomyelitis	46	28	18	28					18				
c. Diphtheria	1												
d. Measles	62	33	28	31	2				26	2			
e. Tetanus	73	40	32	37	1	1	1	1	31	1	-	-	-
6. Bacterial meningitis*	**153**	**80**	**72**	**51**	1	8	7	13	**43**	1	4	8	17
7. Hepatitis B and hepatitis C	**83**	**51**	**32**	9	1	9	15	17	6	1	1	4	20
8. Malaria	**4**	**2**	**2**	1	-	1	2	-	1	-	-	-	-
9. Tropical-cluster diseases	**16**	**13**	**3**	1	1	7	2	2	-	-	1	1	1
a. Trypanosomiasis													
b. Chagas disease													
c. Schistosomiasis	4	2	2				1	1					
d. Leishmaniasis													
e. Lymphatic filariasis	12	10	1			6	1	1			1		
f. Onchocerciasis													
10. Leprosy	**2**	**1**	**1**										
11. Dengue	**2**	**1**	**1**		1					1			
12. Japanese encephalitis	**47**	**25**	**22**	19	5	1	-	-	16	4	-	-	-
13. Trachoma	**149**	**37**	**112**	-	-	1	5	31	-	-	2	14	96
14. Intestinal nematode infections	**179**	**92**	**87**	2	81	4	2	2	2	77	3	2	3
a. Ascariasis	80	41	39	2	39				2	37			
b. Trichuriasis	79	41	39		41					38			
c. Ancylostomiasis and necatoriasis	19	10	9		2	4		2		2	3		3

Annex Table 21d, continued. DALYs by age, sex and cause (thousands): China, 2020, optimistic scenario

Cause	Total	Males						Females					
		Male	0-4	5-14	15-44	45-59	60+	Female	0-4	5-14	15-44	45-59	60+
B. Respiratory infections	**2 056**	**1 042**	685	23	11	16	279	**1 042**	708	23	8	11	291
1. Lower respiratory infections	2 002	987	670	16	10	16	276	1 015	693	16	7	11	288
2. Upper respiratory infections	23	11	6	-	1	-	4	12	7	-	-	-	4
3. Otitis media	31	16	9	7	-	-	-	15	8	7	-	-	-
C. Maternal conditions	**76**							**76**			69	7	-
1. Maternal haemorrhage	12							12			10	2	
2. Maternal sepsis	13							13			13		
3. Hypertensive disorders of pregnancy	3							3			2		
4. Obstructed labour	16							16			16		
5. Abortion	2							2			2		
D. Perinatal conditions*	**1 549**	**792**	792					**757**	757				
E. Nutritional deficiencies	**1 583**	**812**	225	86	236	92	173	**770**	252	84	119	111	205
1. Protein-energy malnutrition	286	129	113	-	-	1	15	157	141	-	-	-	14
2. Iodine deficiency	59	32	30	1	1	-	-	27	25	1	-	-	-
3. Vitamin A deficiency	36	19	16	3	-	-	-	16	14	3	-	-	-
4. Iron-deficiency anaemia	1 203	632	66	82	235	91	158	571	72	80	119	110	190
II. Noncommunicable diseases	*159 531*	*94 532*	*2 751*	*882*	*20 759*	*36 413*	*33 728*	*64 999*	*2 906*	*672*	*18 870*	*18 409*	*24 142*
A. Malignant neoplasms	**39 834**	**27 849**	102	314	4 661	13 823	8 948	**11 985**	165	150	1 938	4 948	4 785
1. Mouth and oropharynx cancers	1 117	821	4	7	267	348	195	296			77	130	89
2. Oesophagus cancer	4 270	3 157			276	1 530	1 351	1 114			39	406	668
3. Stomach cancer	7 739	5 524		6	417	2 797	2 304	2 216		6	306	818	1 086
4. Colon and rectum cancers	2 096	1 269		6	248	557	458	827		7	118	339	363
5. Liver cancer	8 689	6 940	4	19	1 764	3 727	1 426	1 748	5	17	290	802	634
6. Pancreas cancer	674	455			50	199	206	219			10	67	140
7. Trachea, bronchus, lung cancers	7 644	5 961		12	567	3 236	2 143	1 684			85	800	799
8. Melanoma and other skin cancers	27	17			4	7	6	10			2	4	4
9. Breast cancer	659							659			186	306	166
10. Cervix uteri cancer	497							497			81	240	176
11. Corpus uteri cancer	172							172			19	118	35
12. Ovary cancer	256							256		5	76	112	58
13. Prostate cancer	88	88				15	70						
14. Bladder cancer	393	324			23	104	196	69			3	16	50
15. Lymphomas and multiple myeloma	594	416		28	90	171	127	178			31	99	48
16. Leukaemia	1 841	1 055	58	158	448	298	91	787	77	79	341	190	100
C. Diabetes mellitus	**794**	**376**	5	4	73	153	141	**418**	5	3	33	133	243
D. Endocrine disorders	**301**	**94**	12	4	26	31	22	**207**	88	7	45	22	44

Annex Table 21d, continued. DALYs by age, sex and cause (thousands): China, 2020, optimistic scenario

Cause	Total	Male	Female	Males					Females				
				0-4	5-14	15-44	45-59	60+	0-4	5-14	15-44	45-59	60+
E. Neuro-psychiatric conditions	**33 934**	**14 988**	**18 945**	**170**	**262**	**10 863**	**2 406**	**1 287**	**147**	**283**	**13 107**	**3 381**	**2 028**
1. Unipolar major depression	16 170	5 759	10 411	-	-	4 214	1 257	288	-	-	7 561	2 247	603
2. Bipolar disorder	4 217	2 146	2 071	-	-	1 865	218	63	-	-	1 778	215	78
3. Schizophrenia	2 616	1 401	1 215	11	26	1 379	9	13	10	27	1 191	12	12
4. Epilepsy	373	218	155	-	-	128	38	15	-	-	76	23	18
5. Alcohol use	1 677	1 557	119	-	-	1 347	185	25	-	-	109	9	2
6. Dementia*	2 848	1 252	1 596	55	20	53	362	763	53	17	47	382	1 096
7. Parkinson disease	196	92	104	-	-	-	44	48	-	-	-	43	61
8. Multiple sclerosis	329	145	184	-	13	124	16	5	-	2	155	21	8
9. Drug use	197	177	20	-	31	151	11	2	-	50	17	1	-
10. Post-traumatic stress disorder	490	187	302	8	-	123	22	4	12	-	199	35	6
11. Obsessive-compulsive disorders	2 743	1 181	1 562	-	108	922	107	44	-	136	1 169	186	70
12. Panic disorder	1 392	475	917	-	38	321	116	1	-	38	669	182	29
F. Sense organ diseases	**3 645**	**1 542**	**2 103**	**31**	-	**72**	**737**	**702**	**26**	**9**	**143**	**1 129**	**796**
1. Glaucoma	1 671	470	1 201	4	-	29	288	149	6	-	75	859	262
2. Cataracts	1 727	990	737	10	-	35	412	533	1	-	22	216	498
G. Cardiovascular diseases	**33 802**	**23 407**	**10 395**	**153**	**29**	**1 804**	**10 001**	**11 420**	**86**	**13**	**735**	**2 230**	**7 330**
1. Rheumatic heart disease	2 270	1 389	881	-	4	272	662	451	8	4	160	289	420
2. Ischaemic heart disease	9 855	6 801	3 055	-	-	462	2 876	3 462	-	-	144	547	2 363
3. Cerebrovascular disease	17 148	12 010	5 137	41	14	795	5 063	6 097	26	5	299	1 167	3 640
4. Inflammatory heart diseases	1 161	822	339	25	4	186	412	194	17	2	83	97	140
H. Respiratory diseases	**27 252**	**16 241**	**11 011**	**146**	**129**	**1 974**	**5 326**	**8 665**	**87**	**80**	**1 434**	**3 118**	**6 292**
1. COPD*	24 260	14 461	9 798	25	3	1 316	4 880	8 238	36	1	938	2 854	5 970
2. Asthma	1 963	1 149	814	31	117	525	317	158	12	70	418	208	107
I. Digestive diseases	**6 137**	**3 645**	**2 492**	**152**	**18**	**543**	**1 736**	**1 197**	**177**	**16**	**347**	**1 011**	**941**
1. Peptic ulcer	362	223	138	1	1	38	92	91	1	1	19	43	74
2. Cirrhosis of the liver	2 505	1 713	793	8	3	311	870	521	3	3	93	374	320
3. Appendicitis	91	53	38	1	6	32	10	4	1	5	24	6	3
J. Genito-urinary diseases	**2 106**	**1 576**	**529**	**48**	**18**	**234**	**992**	**284**	**48**	**13**	**103**	**146**	**219**
1. Nephritis and nephrosis	882	514	368	32	18	215	125	124	48	13	86	82	139
2. Benign prostatic hypertrophy	931	931	-	4	-	4	817	106	-	-	-	-	-
L. Musculo-skeletal diseases	**5 810**	**1 928**	**3 883**	-	**7**	**288**	**875**	**758**	**14**	**9**	**790**	**1 983**	**1 086**
1. Rheumatoid arthritis	1 209	371	838	-	-	87	216	68	-	6	183	433	216
2. Osteoarthritis	4 146	1 387	2 759	-	-	176	624	587	-	-	551	1 481	727

Annex Table 21d, continued. DALYs by age, sex and cause (thousands): China, 2020, optimistic scenario

Cause	Total	Male	Female	Males					Females				
				0-4	5-14	15-44	45-59	60+	0-4	5-14	15-44	45-59	60+
M. Congenital anomalies	**3 695**	**1 786**	**1 909**	**1 669**	**42**	**71**	**4**	**-**	**1 808**	**43**	**53**	**5**	**-**
N. Oral conditions	**1 535**	**732**	**803**	**178**	**37**	**66**	**222**	**229**	**169**	**36**	**80**	**229**	**288**
1. Dental caries	654	331	323	177	36	45	52	22	168	34	43	51	26
2. Periodontal disease	39	20	19	-	-	16	3	1	-	-	15	3	1
3. Edentulism	809	374	435	-	-	-	168	206	-	-	-	174	261
III. Injuries	*34 502*	*18 292*	*16 209*	*2 107*	*1 234*	*10 319*	*3 057*	*1 575*	*2 062*	*1 089*	*7 998*	*3 132*	*1 928*
A. Unintentional injuries	**22 616**	**13 074**	**9 542**	**1 929**	**1 091**	**7 072**	**2 015**	**967**	**1 735**	**951**	**3 640**	**1 940**	**1 276**
1. Road traffic accidents	10 614	6 359	4 254	143	566	4 360	926	366	104	661	2 438	804	247
2. Poisonings	949	517	432	101	18	168	159	71	29	24	187	89	102
3. Falls	2 730	1 258	1 473	268	92	557	196	144	332	58	261	384	438
4. Fires	407	199	208	54	20	62	23	39	36	27	25	49	72
5. Drownings	1 891	1 120	772	453	223	304	79	60	363	102	126	82	99
6. Other unintentional	6 024	3 621	2 403	909	172	1 621	633	286	871	80	602	532	319
B. Intentional injuries	**11 886**	**5 218**	**6 668**	**178**	**144**	**3 246**	**1 042**	**608**	**328**	**138**	**4 358**	**1 192**	**652**
1. Self-inflicted injuries	10 088	4 142	5 946	-	95	2 527	945	575	-	71	4 137	1 123	615
2. Violence	1 772	1 050	722	178	48	694	96	33	328	67	221	69	38
3. War	26	26	-	-	-	26	-	-	-	-	-	-	-

Notes:
A dash (-) symbol indicates fewer than 500 DALYs.
*IA6 is Bacterial meningitis and meningococcaemia; ID is Conditions arising during the perinatal period;
IIE6 is Dementia and other degenerative and hereditary CNS disorders; IIH1 is Chronic obstructive pulmonary disease.

Annex Table 21e. DALYs by age, sex and cause (thousands): Other Asia and Islands, 2020, optimistic scenario

Cause	Total	Male	Female	Males					Females				
				0-4	5-14	15-44	45-59	60+	0-4	5-14	15-44	45-59	60+
Population (millions)	*1 029*	*511*	*518*	*44*	*84*	*242*	*87*	*53*	*42*	*81*	*237*	*91*	*66*
All causes	*155 242*	*88 685*	*66 557*	*13 149*	*4 541*	*32 835*	*20 786*	*17 375*	*10 334*	*3 007*	*23 265*	*13 125*	*16 827*
I. Communicable, maternal, perinatal and nutritional conditions	*22 214*	*11 858*	*10 356*	*7 530*	*644*	*2 089*	*578*	*1 017*	*5 527*	*554*	*2 515*	*557*	*1 203*
A. Infectious and parasitic diseases	*12 606*	*6 792*	*5 814*	*3 485*	*402*	*1 846*	*486*	*573*	*2 511*	*341*	*1 870*	*419*	*673*
1. Tuberculosis	**1 641**	**822**	**819**	**10**	**11**	**164**	**232**	**405**	**3**	**10**	**90**	**237**	**479**
2. STDs excluding HIV	1 318	497	821	250	4	224	4	16	193	12	585	7	24
a. Syphilis	343	193	150	147	-	28	3	15	94	-	28	4	23
b. Chlamydia	539	92	447	24	1	67	1	-	23	9	413	2	-
c. Gonorrhoea	435	211	224	79	2	129	1	-	76	3	144	1	-
3. HIV	**3 199**	**1 802**	**1 397**	**301**	**54**	**1 256**	**156**	**36**	**193**	**37**	**1 074**	**77**	**15**
4. Diarrhoeal diseases	**3 157**	**1 861**	**1 297**	**1 743**	**56**	**17**	**13**	**31**	**1 178**	**40**	**17**	**18**	**43**
5. Childhood-cluster diseases	1 753	965	788	876	54	21	7	7	708	50	12	8	9
a. Pertussis	294	162	132	154	8	-	-	-	126	6	-	-	-
b. Poliomyelitis	94	57	37	55	-	1	-	-	36	-	1	-	-
c. Diphtheria	18	10	8	9	-	-	-	-	8	-	-	-	-
d. Measles	855	470	385	438	31	-	-	-	358	26	-	-	-
e. Tetanus	492	267	225	220	15	19	7	7	180	17	12	8	9
6. Bacterial meningitis*	**193**	**104**	**89**	**72**	**2**	**12**	**8**	**10**	**60**	**2**	**7**	**9**	**11**
7. Hepatitis B and hepatitis C	**94**	**54**	**39**	**13**	**3**	**9**	**11**	**18**	**9**	**3**	**4**	**6**	**18**
8. Malaria	**356**	**200**	**156**	**53**	**51**	**63**	**20**	**13**	**44**	**42**	**33**	**23**	**16**
9. Tropical-cluster diseases	90	63	27	3	10	34	12	4	2	3	9	10	3
a. Trypanosomiasis	-	-	-	-	-	-	-	-	-	-	-	-	-
b. Chagas disease	-	-	-	-	-	-	-	-	-	-	-	-	-
c. Schistosomiasis	3	2	2	-	-	-	1	1	-	-	-	-	-
d. Leishmaniasis	9	6	3	-	1	4	1	1	-	1	1	-	1
e. Lymphatic filariasis	77	55	23	3	9	30	11	3	2	2	7	9	2
f. Onchocerciasis	-	-	-	-	-	-	-	-	-	-	-	-	-
10. Leprosy	**24**	**12**	**12**	-	**3**	**6**	**2**	**1**	**2**	**3**	**6**	**2**	-
11. Dengue	**34**	**17**	**17**	**6**	**10**	-	-	-	**6**	**10**	-	-	-
12. Japanese encephalitis	**33**	**18**	**15**	**13**	**4**	**1**	-	-	**11**	**3**	-	-	-
13. Trachoma	**27**	**6**	**21**	-	-	-	**1**	**4**	-	-	**1**	**4**	**16**
14. Intestinal nematode infections	317	166	152	2	120	28	8	7	2	111	21	8	10
a. Ascariasis	93	49	45	2	46	-	-	-	2	43	-	-	-
b. Trichuriasis	128	67	61	-	66	-	-	-	-	61	-	-	-
c. Ancylostomiasis and necatoriasis	96	50	46	-	8	28	8	7	-	7	20	8	10

Annex Table 21e, continued. DALYs by age, sex and cause (thousands): Other Asia and Islands, 2020, optimistic scenario

Cause	Total	Male	Female	Males 0-4	5-14	15-44	45-59	60+	Females 0-4	5-14	15-44	45-59	60+
B. Respiratory infections	**4 048**	**2 277**	**1 771**	**1 670**	**156**	**52**	**35**	**364**	**1 144**	**135**	**34**	**39**	**420**
1. Lower respiratory infections	3 951	2 223	1 728	1 637	143	50	34	360	1 120	123	32	38	415
2. Upper respiratory infections	45	25	20	16	2	2	1	4	11	2	1	1	5
3. Otitis media	53	29	24	17	12	-	-	-	13	11	-	-	-
C. Maternal conditions	**365**		**365**								**354**	**11**	
1. Maternal haemorrhage	36		36								34	2	
2. Maternal sepsis	64		64								62	2	
3. Hypertensive disorders of pregnancy	18		18								16	1	
4. Obstructed labour	81		81								80	1	
5. Abortion	69		69								68	1	
D. Perinatal conditions*	**3 249**	**1 836**	**1 413**	**1 836**					**1 413**				
E. Nutritional deficiencies	**1 946**	**953**	**993**	**539**	**86**	**192**	**57**	**80**	**459**	**78**	**257**	**89**	**110**
1. Protein-energy malnutrition	704	381	323	372	1	1	1	5	315	1	1	1	5
2. Iodine deficiency	37	20	17	18	1	-	-	-	16	1	-	-	-
3. Vitamin A deficiency	118	65	53	51	13	1	-	-	42	11	1	-	-
4. Iron-deficiency anaemia	1 087	488	600	97	70	190	55	75	86	65	256	88	105
II. Noncommunicable diseases	***105 155***	***58 230***	***46 925***	***3 388***	***1 867***	***19 228***	***17 971***	***15 777***	***2 860***	***1 327***	***16 058***	***11 532***	***15 148***
A. Malignant neoplasms	**19 159**	**11 353**	**7 806**	**196**	**564**	**2 237**	**4 506**	**3 850**	**250**	**335**	**1 714**	**2 617**	**2 890**
1. Mouth and oropharynx cancers	1 808	1 159	650	5	16	256	299	582	8	12	135	119	376
2. Oesophagus cancer	622	423	199			37	212	173			25	70	105
3. Stomach cancer	1 632	1 120	513	1	2	172	547	399	-	1	81	192	239
4. Colon and rectum cancers	1 044	570	473	2	5	127	143	293	3	4	79	107	281
5. Liver cancer	2 051	1 615	436	7	20	342	877	369	7	9	65	164	190
6. Pancreas cancer	252	166	86			28	72	67	1	-	6	32	46
7. Trachea, bronchus, lung cancers	3 158	2 440	717	2	7	356	1 307	768	3	4	50	299	362
8. Melanoma and other skin cancers	66	31	35		1	9	13	8			7	12	16
9. Breast cancer	849		849						2	3	245	393	207
10. Cervix uteri cancer	992		992							1	235	518	238
11. Corpus uteri cancer	104		104								13	47	42
12. Ovary cancer	330		330						10	13	137	102	68
13. Prostate cancer	276	276				4	56	213					
14. Bladder cancer	273	206	67	1	2	17	76	113			5	15	46
15. Lymphomas and multiple myeloma	702	453	249	26	73	145	89	121	16	20	60	41	113
16. Leukaemia	987	565	422	69	191	188	49	67	91	121	107	36	67
C. Diabetes mellitus	**1 297**	**623**	**674**	**8**	**9**	**153**	**253**	**201**	**8**	**8**	**79**	**223**	**356**
D. Endocrine disorders	**345**	**161**	**184**	**86**	**15**	**22**	**21**	**17**	**72**	**8**	**25**	**32**	**47**

Annex Table 21e, continued. DALYs by age, sex and cause (thousands): Other Asia and Islands, 2020, optimistic scenario

Cause	Total	Male	Female	Males 0-4	5-14	15-44	45-59	60+	Females 0-4	5-14	15-44	45-59	60+
E. Neuro-psychiatric conditions	28 753	14 161	14 592	173	333	11 219	1 602	836	176	310	10 783	2 011	1 312
1. Unipolar major depression	11 018	3 844	7 175	-	-	3 055	639	150	-	-	5 632	1 215	328
2. Bipolar disorder	2 968	1 492	1 477	-	-	1 347	111	33	-	-	1 317	115	44
3. Schizophrenia	3 362	1 756	1 606	-	-	1 731	14	10	-	-	1 581	5	20
4. Epilepsy	503	299	204	12	54	167	49	16	14	57	91	25	17
5. Alcohol use	2 926	2 710	216	-	-	2 464	208	38	-	-	200	11	4
6. Dementia*	1 883	792	1 091	38	16	44	253	441	45	17	40	281	708
7. Parkinson disease	232	121	111	-	-	-	54	66	-	-	-	47	65
8. Multiple sclerosis	240	104	136	-	-	92	9	3	-	-	119	12	5
9. Drug use	1 360	1 226	134	-	64	1 091	61	11	-	7	118	7	1
10. Post-traumatic stress disorder	368	138	230	6	25	94	12	2	10	41	155	20	4
11. Obsessive-compulsive disorders	2 043	871	1 172	-	88	703	57	24	-	113	914	105	39
12. Panic disorder	1 009	336	672	-	31	244	61	-	-	31	522	103	16
F. Sense organ diseases	3 747	1 692	2 055	5	3	86	862	735	5	-	104	1 074	872
1. Glaucoma	1 318	385	934	-	-	21	262	101	-	-	62	688	184
2. Cataracts	2 413	1 297	1 116	1	-	62	599	634	3	-	42	385	687
G. Cardiovascular diseases	24 643	15 144	9 499	816	474	2 864	4 868	6 121	531	300	1 166	1 685	5 817
1. Rheumatic heart disease	192	103	89	-	2	24	31	47	-	3	18	19	49
2. Ischaemic heart disease	8 320	5 130	3 190	-	-	707	1 773	2 650	-	-	244	530	2 417
3. Cerebrovascular disease	7 215	4 257	2 957	109	112	679	1 413	1 945	77	69	282	588	1 942
4. Inflammatory heart diseases	1 781	1 162	619	157	101	418	324	162	123	66	167	110	154
H. Respiratory diseases	5 993	3 374	2 619	260	216	719	820	1 359	129	145	589	552	1 203
1. COPD*	2 495	1 486	1 009	26	12	209	424	815	14	10	123	223	639
2. Asthma	1 469	797	671	40	124	399	141	94	16	79	317	152	108
I. Digestive diseases	8 996	5 686	3 310	164	78	924	2 870	1 650	139	69	480	1 343	1 278
1. Peptic ulcer	431	283	148	-	2	55	117	107	-	2	24	42	79
2. Cirrhosis of the liver	3 047	2 334	712	10	7	440	1 329	548	7	8	103	327	268
3. Appendicitis	119	71	48	1	13	44	10	3	1	13	27	6	2
J. Genito-urinary diseases	1 891	1 165	727	52	64	169	632	247	36	45	110	181	354
1. Nephritis and nephrosis	1 047	510	537	37	55	143	126	150	36	39	81	122	259
2. Benign prostatic hypertrophy	507	507	-	-	-	-	458	48	-	-	-	-	-
L. Musculo-skeletal diseases	4 276	1 838	2 438	14	8	343	1 073	399	15	10	541	1 327	545
1. Rheumatoid arthritis	440	126	315	-	-	6	42	78	-	2	74	70	169
2. Osteoarthritis	3 596	1 625	1 971	-	-	320	1 008	297	-	-	435	1 223	313

Annex Table 21e, continued. DALYs by age, sex and cause (thousands): Other Asia and Islands, 2020, optimistic scenario

Cause	Total	Male	Female	Males					Females				
				0-4	5-14	15-44	45-59	60+	0-4	5-14	15-44	45-59	60+
M. Congenital anomalies	**3 103**	**1 615**	**1 488**	**1 516**	**35**	**48**	**12**	**4**	**1 416**	**32**	**22**	**12**	**7**
N. Oral conditions	**2 529**	**1 196**	**1 333**	**31**	**45**	**400**	**394**	**327**	**30**	**44**	**406**	**430**	**424**
1. Dental caries	900	442	458	30	44	173	136	59	29	42	169	144	73
2. Periodontal disease	58	29	29	–	–	20	6	2	–	–	20	6	3
3. Edentulism	1 552	722	831	–	–	204	251	266	–	–	204	279	347
III. Injuries	*27 873*	*18 597*	*9 275*	*2 231*	*2 029*	*11 518*	*2 237*	*581*	*1 947*	*1 126*	*4 691*	*1 036*	*476*
A. Unintentional injuries	**21 831**	**14 641**	**7 190**	**2 128**	**1 826**	**8 534**	**1 717**	**437**	**1 836**	**994**	**3 100**	**859**	**399**
1. Road traffic accidents	8 926	5 980	2 947	486	827	3 901	588	177	446	513	1 510	323	155
2. Poisonings	895	460	435	52	37	253	87	31	48	39	252	59	37
3. Falls	3 127	2 023	1 103	537	234	971	231	51	415	108	388	145	47
4. Fires	335	176	159	44	33	75	17	7	65	36	40	10	8
5. Drownings	1 695	1 152	543	411	277	366	69	29	258	107	124	32	22
6. Other unintentional	6 852	4 849	2 003	597	418	2 967	725	142	603	193	787	290	131
B. Intentional injuries	**6 042**	**3 956**	**2 086**	**103**	**204**	**2 985**	**521**	**144**	**111**	**131**	**1 591**	**176**	**76**
1. Self-inflicted injuries	2 916	1 636	1 279	–	72	1 233	240	92	–	44	1 068	113	54
2. Violence	2 335	1 859	475	45	93	1 420	257	45	52	57	305	47	14
3. War	792	460	332	58	39	332	24	7	59	30	218	17	8

Notes:
A dash (-) symbol indicates fewer than 500 DALYs.
*IA6 is Bacterial meningitis and meningococcaemia; ID is Conditions arising during the perinatal period;
IIE6 is Dementia and other degenerative and hereditary CNS disorders; IIH1 is Chronic obstructive pulmonary disease.

Annex Table 21f. DALYs by age, sex and cause (thousands): Sub-Saharan Africa, 2020, optimistic scenario

Cause	Total	Male	Female	Males 0-4	5-14	15-44	45-59	60+	Females 0-4	5-14	15-44	45-59	60+
Population (millions)	1 178	584	595	91	152	264	50	26	87	148	271	56	33
All causes	311 759	180 254	131 504	62 091	16 389	74 091	16 094	11 590	48 959	12 014	43 754	13 814	12 963
I. Communicable, maternal, perinatal and nutritional conditions	112 225	59 760	52 465	45 058	3 304	8 715	1 634	1 048	34 376	3 310	11 947	1 568	1 264
A. Infectious and parasitic diseases	78 415	41 752	36 664	28 572	2 518	8 451	1 574	637	21 668	2 567	10 209	1 491	728
1. Tuberculosis	16 440	7 723	8 717	806	651	4 736	1 174	356	856	923	5 419	1 143	375
2. STDs excluding HIV	3 155	1 342	1 813	952	8	352	7	24	831	28	909	10	35
a. Syphilis	1 426	765	661	676	1	59	5	24	556	1	62	7	35
b. Chlamydia	777	132	645	51	2	78	-	-	51	18	574	2	-
c. Gonorrhoea	952	445	507	224	5	215	1	-	224	9	273	1	-
3. HIV	9 436	4 342	5 094	1 402	215	2 520	172	34	1 334	222	3 388	128	22
4. Diarrhoeal diseases	16 627	9 667	6 960	9 139	363	74	21	70	6 419	343	79	26	93
5. Childhood-cluster diseases	15 450	8 628	6 821	8 036	539	36	9	8	6 296	485	24	8	8
a. Pertussis	2 884	1 615	1 269	1 537	78	-	-	-	1 202	68	-	-	-
b. Poliomyelitis	322	194	128	192	1	2	-	-	126	1	1	-	-
c. Diphtheria	32	18	14	18	1	1	-	-	13	-	-	-	-
d. Measles	10 063	5 606	4 457	5 187	419	1	-	-	4 086	371	-	-	-
e. Tetanus	2 148	1 196	953	1 103	41	34	9	8	870	45	23	8	8
6. Bacterial meningitis*	479	260	218	233	5	13	5	5	192	4	10	6	6
7. Hepatitis B and hepatitis C	109	63	46	23	7	11	9	13	15	6	7	5	13
8. Malaria	13 494	7 817	5 678	7 263	297	201	37	18	5 196	272	145	41	25
9. Tropical-cluster diseases	1 414	932	482	55	305	409	108	55	54	164	150	76	37
a. Trypanosomiasis	338	186	152	11	67	74	26	7	18	63	49	18	4
b. Chagas disease	-	-	-										
c. Schistosomiasis	322	208	114	15	75	87	17	14	9	45	40	11	10
d. Leishmaniasis	112	79	33	7	43	27	1	-	3	20	10	1	-
e. Lymphatic filariasis	389	303	86	18	97	163	22	3	22	20	23	17	4
f. Onchocerciasis	253	157	96	4	23	58	41	31	3	17	29	29	19
10. Leprosy	22	11	11	-	4	6	1	-	-	4	6	1	-
11. Dengue	6	3	3	1	2	-	-	-	1	2	-	-	-
12. Japanese encephalitis	-												
13. Trachoma	173	45	127	-	-	6	10	29	-	-	11	29	88
14. Intestinal nematode infections	172	91	81	1	44	35	6	5	1	41	11	7	6
a. Ascariasis	33	17	16	1	16	-	-	-	1	15	-	-	-
b. Trichuriasis	34	17	16	-	17	-	-	-	-	16	-	-	-
c. Ancylostomiasis and necatoriasis	105	56	48	-	10	35	6	5	-	9	27	7	6

Annex Table 21f, continued. DALYs by age, sex and cause (thousands): Sub-Saharan Africa, 2020, optimistic scenario

Cause	Total	Male	Female	Males 0-4	5-14	15-44	45-59	60+	Females 0-4	5-14	15-44	45-59	60+
B. Respiratory infections	**16 483**	**9 480**	**7 003**	**8 392**	**576**	**116**	**32**	**364**	**5 920**	**460**	**109**	**36**	**477**
1. Lower respiratory infections	16 133	9 281	6 852	8 233	544	113	32	360	5 806	432	107	35	472
2. Upper respiratory infections	168	96	71	83	7	2	1	4	58	5	2	1	5
3. Otitis media	183	103	80	77	26	1	-	-	56	23	1	-	-
C. Maternal conditions	**1 563**		**1 563**						-	**90**	**1 471**	**2**	-
1. Maternal haemorrhage	228		228							21	207		
2. Maternal sepsis	296		296							14	282		
3. Hypertensive disorders of pregnancy	113		113							10	102		
4. Obstructed labour	271		271							7	264		
5. Abortion	274		274							12	262		
D. Perinatal conditions*	**11 172**	**6 075**	**5 097**	**6 075**					**5 097**				
E. Nutritional deficiencies	**4 591**	**2 453**	**2 138**	**2 019**	**210**	**148**	**28**	**48**	**1 690**	**193**	**158**	**38**	**58**
1. Protein-energy malnutrition	2 955	1 607	1 348	1 576	10	5	3	13	1 315	10	7	2	14
2. Iodine deficiency	63	33	30	31	2	-	-	-	27	2	1	-	-
3. Vitamin A deficiency	524	286	238	230	54	2	-	-	187	49	2	-	-
4. Iron-deficiency anaemia	1 049	527	523	182	144	140	25	35	161	132	149	36	44
II. Noncommunicable diseases	*104 845*	*54 235*	*50 609*	*8 256*	*2 956*	*21 901*	*11 364*	*9 757*	*7 749*	*2 838*	*17 640*	*11 192*	*11 190*
A. Malignant neoplasms	**15 057**	**8 631**	**6 426**	**307**	**791**	**2 682**	**2 513**	**2 338**	**462**	**719**	**1 367**	**2 153**	**1 725**
1. Mouth and oropharynx cancers	698	432	266	2	7	131	94	199	15	28	55	45	122
2. Oesophagus cancer	712	547	165			123	272	152			27	65	73
3. Stomach cancer	971	599	372	1	3	137	266	193			61	188	123
4. Colon and rectum cancers	424	245	179	1	3	82	55	104	1	1	36	40	100
5. Liver cancer	2 197	1 737	460	7	20	872	602	235	11	19	129	171	131
6. Pancreas cancer	211	128	83			34	59	35			16	41	25
7. Trachea, bronchus, lung cancers	717	456	261		1	142	178	135		1	53	126	82
8. Melanoma and other skin cancers	227	104	123		1	22	49	32		1	13	49	59
9. Breast cancer	534	-	534							3	141	244	146
10. Cervix uteri cancer	978		978							1	216	464	295
11. Corpus uteri cancer	90		90						1		11	39	39
12. Ovary cancer	257		257						13	22	68	97	57
13. Prostate cancer	721	721	-			17	175	529					
14. Bladder cancer	390	263	127			50	98	113			27	49	51
15. Lymphomas and multiple myeloma	1 311	820	491	106	323	201	86	104	110	206	70	46	59
16. Leukaemia	437	201	236	19	57	71	18	35	50	93	37	28	28
C. Diabetes mellitus	**549**	**265**	**284**	**29**	**33**	**62**	**79**	**62**	**35**	**31**	**30**	**79**	**110**
D. Endocrine disorders	**1 414**	**744**	**670**	**425**	**28**	**141**	**108**	**42**	**272**	**50**	**92**	**121**	**135**

Annex Table 21f, continued. DALYs by age, sex and cause (thousands): Sub-Saharan Africa, 2020, optimistic scenario

Cause	Total	Male	Female	Males					Females				
				0-4	5-14	15-44	45-59	60+	0-4	5-14	15-44	45-59	60+
E. Neuro-psychiatric conditions	**27 999**	**13 397**	**14 602**	**394**	**490**	**11 304**	**897**	**311**	**461**	**520**	**11 834**	**1 180**	**608**
1. Unipolar major depression	11 579	3 938	7 641			3 470	388	80			6 685	778	178
2. Bipolar disorder	3 326	1 637	1 688			1 551	68	18			1 588	77	24
3. Schizophrenia	1 125	582	543			576	4	2			538	2	4
4. Epilepsy	520	296	224	47	71	145	23	9	56	64	82	12	10
5. Alcohol use	4 393	3 557	837			3 359	176	21			792	33	11
6. Dementia*	755	233	522	31	12	23	57	110	84	35	50	66	287
7. Parkinson disease	109	56	53				27	29				24	28
8. Multiple sclerosis	244	104	140			96	6	2			128	9	3
9. Drug use	912	822	90		55	740	24	4		6	81	3	
10. Post-traumatic stress disorder	454	168	286	12	45	102	7	1	19	75	178	12	2
11. Obsessive-compulsive disorders	2 306	971	1 335		158	768	33	12		206	1 044	65	20
12. Panic disorder	1 092	361	731		56	269	36			57	602	63	8
F. Sense organ diseases	**4 354**	**2 092**	**2 262**	**12**	**1**	**138**	**994**	**947**	**12**	**1**	**104**	**1 060**	**1 085**
1. Glaucoma	986	386	600			3	186	197			6	303	291
2. Cataracts	3 356	1 698	1 658	12	1	127	808	749	12	1	94	757	793
G. Cardiovascular diseases	**19 672**	**10 398**	**9 274**	**861**	**440**	**3 184**	**2 809**	**3 105**	**591**	**468**	**1 225**	**2 697**	**4 293**
1. Rheumatic heart disease	552	320	232	2	67	218	25	7	2	77	111	32	10
2. Ischaemic heart disease	4 900	2 591	2 308			689	872	1 030			205	701	1 230
3. Cerebrovascular disease	8 592	4 240	4 352	134	168	1 284	1 181	1 473	102	135	479	1 336	2 300
4. Inflammatory heart diseases	2 052	1 166	886	230	66	420	242	208	218	86	151	169	262
H. Respiratory diseases	**14 083**	**7 375**	**6 708**	**891**	**526**	**2 388**	**1 688**	**1 881**	**511**	**394**	**1 471**	**2 281**	**2 051**
1. COPD*	4 475	2 496	1 979	74	36	703	672	1 011	47	32	262	730	908
2. Asthma	2 131	1 081	1 049	112	253	537	100	80	52	171	525	190	112
I. Digestive diseases	**5 385**	**3 333**	**2 052**	**268**	**143**	**954**	**1 307**	**660**	**255**	**229**	**441**	**550**	**576**
1. Peptic ulcer	354	232	122			105	91	35		8	38	46	38
2. Cirrhosis of the liver	805	599	207		12	179	273	134		8	48	81	70
3. Appendicitis	244	154	90	4	44	91	12	3	4	46	30	7	2
J. Genito-urinary diseases	**3 033**	**1 894**	**1 139**	**530**	**260**	**336**	**595**	**174**	**398**	**193**	**154**	**211**	**182**
1. Nephritis and nephrosis	2 062	1 160	902	441	219	270	115	115	383	168	99	128	123
2. Benign prostatic hypertrophy	435	435					418	17					
L. Musculo-skeletal diseases	**2 622**	**871**	**1 751**			**456**	**286**	**130**		**4**	**707**	**769**	**271**
1. Rheumatoid arthritis	219	60	158			39	15	6		4	98	43	13
2. Osteoarthritis	2 382	801	1 582			411	268	122			603	722	256

Annex Table 21f, continued. DALYs by age, sex and cause (thousands): Sub-Saharan Africa, 2020, optimistic scenario

Cause	Total	Male	Female	Males					Females				
				0-4	5-14	15-44	45-59	60+	0-4	5-14	15-44	45-59	60+
M. Congenital anomalies	8 019	3 837	4 182	3 680	68	73	12	4	4 064	70	26	15	7
N. Oral conditions	890	427	462	91	107	121	27	82	87	109	131	30	106
1. Dental caries	629	314	315	88	105	88	24	9	85	103	90	26	11
2. Periodontal disease	68	34	35	-	-	31	3	-	-	-	31	3	-
3. Edentulism	167	73	94	-	-	-	-	73	-	-	-	-	94
III. Injuries	*94 689*	*66 259*	*28 430*	*8 776*	*10 128*	*43 475*	*3 095*	*785*	*6 834*	*5 866*	*14 166*	*1 055*	*508*
A. Unintentional injuries	51 800	36 493	15 307	6 481	7 804	19 585	2 066	557	4 730	4 465	5 157	615	340
1. Road traffic accidents	18 501	13 189	5 312	684	3 970	7 470	835	232	463	2 089	2 464	234	62
2. Poisonings	2 136	1 260	876	941	136	132	36	15	682	58	120	9	8
3. Falls	3 035	1 735	1 299	436	558	578	112	52	469	292	353	72	112
4. Fires	5 071	2 652	2 419	1 224	587	706	95	41	1 035	684	574	70	56
5. Drownings	4 079	3 012	1 067	1 047	1 106	765	71	24	524	373	144	17	9
6. Other unintentional	18 978	14 645	4 334	2 150	1 448	9 935	917	195	1 557	969	1 501	214	93
B. Intentional injuries	42 889	29 766	13 123	2 295	2 325	23 890	1 029	227	2 104	1 401	9 010	440	168
1. Self-inflicted injuries	1 180	944	236	-	112	764	53	15	-	-	215	19	2
2. Violence	16 383	14 163	2 220	295	718	12 501	552	98	145	294	1 623	122	36
3. War	25 326	14 660	10 667	2 000	1 495	10 625	424	115	1 959	1 108	7 171	300	130

Notes:
A dash (-) symbol indicates fewer than 500 DALYs.
*IA6 is Bacterial meningitis and meningococcaemia; ID is Conditions arising during the perinatal period;
IIE6 is Dementia and other degenerative and hereditary CNS disorders; IIH1 is Chronic obstructive pulmonary disease.

Annex Table 21g. DALYs by age, sex and cause (thousands): Latin America and the Caribbean, 2020, optimistic scenario

Cause	Total	Male	Female	Males					Females				
				0-4	5-14	15-44	45-59	60+	0-4	5-14	15-44	45-59	60+
Population (millions)	*681*	*338*	*344*	*29*	*56*	*158*	*56*	*39*	*28*	*54*	*157*	*59*	*47*
All causes	*100 830*	*57 989*	*42 842*	*6 298*	*2 826*	*26 483*	*12 096*	*10 285*	*4 849*	*1 992*	*16 601*	*9 684*	*9 716*
I. Communicable, maternal, perinatal and nutritional conditions	*10 622*	*6 201*	*4 421*	*3 702*	*250*	*1 617*	*252*	*380*	*2 616*	*253*	*1 013*	*167*	*372*
A. Infectious and parasitic diseases	5 848	3 629	2 219	1 525	167	1 542	203	193	1 097	166	682	111	162
1. Tuberculosis	371	227	144	14	9	78	52	75	10	12	42	33	47
2. STDs excluding HIV	416	119	297	61	1	53	1	3	49	5	238	2	4
a. Syphilis	106	59	48	49	-	6	-	3	37	-	6	1	4
b. Chlamydia	205	21	183	3	-	18	-	-	3	4	176	1	-
c. Gonorrhoea	105	39	66	9	-	29	-	-	9	1	56	-	-
3. HIV	1 876	1 481	395	81	8	1 282	90	21	75	9	295	12	3
4. Diarrhoeal diseases	1 374	816	558	734	27	16	10	29	472	27	13	11	35
5. Childhood-cluster diseases	847	470	377	447	20	2	1	1	355	19	1	1	1
a. Pertussis	180	99	81	94	5	-	-	-	76	4	-	-	-
b. Poliomyelitis	54	33	22	32	-	-	-	-	21	-	-	-	-
c. Diphtheria	3	2	1	1	-	-	-	-	1	1	-	-	-
d. Measles	436	240	196	227	13	-	1	-	183	13	1	-	-
e. Tetanus	174	96	77	92	2	1	-	-	74	1	-	1	-
6. Bacterial meningitis*	125	66	58	45	2	8	5	7	37	2	6	5	9
7. Hepatitis B and hepatitis C	23	12	11	5	2	2	1	2	4	2	3	2	2
8. Malaria	75	40	34	11	8	14	4	3	9	8	9	5	3
9. Tropical-cluster diseases	155	85	69	3	3	41	20	18	2	2	28	21	17
a. Trypanosomiasis	130	70	60	-	-	34	18	17	-	-	25	19	16
b. Chagas disease	14	8	6	-	1	4	1	1	-	1	2	1	1
c. Schistosomiasis	9	7	2	2	1	2	-	-	-	1	2	-	-
d. Leishmaniasis	2	1	-	-	-	1	-	-	1	-	-	-	-
e. Lymphatic filariasis	1	-	-	-	-	-	-	-	-	-	-	-	-
f. Onchocerciasis	-	-	-	-	-	-	-	-	-	-	-	-	-
10. Leprosy	17	9	8	-	2	4	1	1	-	2	4	1	1
11. Dengue	-	-	-	-	-	-	-	-	-	-	-	-	-
12. Japanese encephalitis	-	-	-	-	-	-	-	-	-	-	-	-	-
13. Trachoma	-	-	-	-	-	-	-	-	-	-	-	-	-
14. Intestinal nematode infections	155	80	75	1	62	11	3	3	1	59	8	3	4
a. Ascariasis	51	26	25	1	25	-	-	-	1	23	-	-	-
b. Trichuriasis	66	34	32	-	34	-	-	-	-	32	-	-	-
c. Ancylostomiasis and necatoriasis	38	20	18	-	3	11	3	3	-	3	8	3	4

Annex Table 21g, continued. DALYs by age, sex and cause (thousands): Latin America and the Caribbean, 2020, optimistic scenario

Cause	Total	Male	Female	Males					Females				
				0-4	5-14	15-44	45-59	60+	0-4	5-14	15-44	45-59	60+
B. Respiratory infections	**1 418**	**784**	**634**	**554**	**38**	**33**	**32**	**127**	**396**	**40**	**35**	**27**	**136**
1. Lower respiratory infections	1 377	762	615	545	29	32	31	125	389	32	34	26	134
2. Upper respiratory infections	17	10	7	6	1	1	1	2	4	1	1	1	2
3. Otitis media	24	12	12	4	8	-	-	-	3	8	1	-	-
C. Maternal conditions	**174**		**174**							**1**	**173**	**1**	
1. Maternal haemorrhage	16		16								16		
2. Maternal sepsis	30		30								30		
3. Hypertensive disorders of pregnancy	10		10								10		
4. Obstructed labour	42		42								42		
5. Abortion	46		46								45		
D. Perinatal conditions*	**2 193**	**1 308**	**884**	**1 308**						**884**			
E. Nutritional deficiencies	**989**	**480**	**509**	**314**	**45**	**42**	**18**	**59**	**239**	**45**	**123**	**28**	**74**
1. Protein-energy malnutrition	472	263	209	218	5	4	5	30	156	7	4	5	37
2. Iodine deficiency	22	12	11	11	1				9	1			
3. Vitamin A deficiency	40	22	18	18	3				15	4			
4. Iron-deficiency anaemia	449	181	268	67	36	37	12	29	57	34	118	23	37
II. Noncommunicable diseases	***69 804***	***37 232***	***32 572***	***1 789***	***1 095***	***14 858***	***10 146***	***9 344***	***1 626***	***949***	***12 105***	***8 905***	***8 987***
A. Malignant neoplasms	**8 981**	**4 268**	**4 713**	**55**	**218**	**714**	**1 493**	**1 789**	**62**	**138**	**1 065**	**1 883**	**1 564**
1. Mouth and oropharynx cancers	327	245	82		1	45	119	79			12	30	37
2. Oesophagus cancer	225	164	61			13	79	72			4	21	36
3. Stomach cancer	826	522	303			64	196	262			39	102	162
4. Colon and rectum cancers	519	251	269			43	89	118			33	89	147
5. Liver cancer	117	61	55		2	11	23	26		1	6	19	30
6. Pancreas cancer	165	88	77			10	35	43			5	27	44
7. Trachea, bronchus, lung cancers	1 379	837	542		1	145	416	275			39	280	222
8. Melanoma and other skin cancers	82	40	42			14	15	11		1	13	16	13
9. Breast cancer	818		818								206	387	225
10. Cervix uteri cancer	692		692								221	319	152
11. Corpus uteri cancer	161		161								22	84	56
12. Ovary cancer	156		156						2	4	52	55	44
13. Prostate cancer	367	367					49	312					
14. Bladder cancer	179	137	41			6	43	84			3	12	26
15. Lymphomas and multiple myeloma	433	257	176	10	39	91	65	52	8	20	44	47	57
16. Leukaemia	380	216	163	18	65	78	28	27	17	45	47	26	27
C. Diabetes mellitus	**1 454**	**670**	**785**	**8**	**10**	**141**	**252**	**259**	**8**	**8**	**88**	**253**	**427**
D. Endocrine disorders	**1 011**	**507**	**504**	**229**	**30**	**118**	**67**	**63**	**189**	**24**	**94**	**88**	**109**

Annex Table 21g, continued. DALYs by age, sex and cause (thousands): Latin America and the Caribbean, 2020, optimistic scenario

Cause	Total	Male	Female	Males					Females				
				0-4	5-14	15-44	45-59	60+	0-4	5-14	15-44	45-59	60+
E. Neuro-psychiatric conditions	**23 080**	**12 964**	**10 116**	**176**	**307**	**10 278**	**1 477**	**726**	**164**	**285**	**7 522**	**1 267**	**879**
1. Unipolar major depression	6 906	2 394	4 511	-	-	1 903	392	99	-	-	3 557	745	210
2. Bipolar disorder	1 846	924	923			834	68	22			826	70	27
3. Schizophrenia	1 902	988	914			970	10	8			901	4	9
4. Epilepsy	398	244	154	9	43	143	36	12	9	39	81	14	11
5. Alcohol use	5 973	5 498	475			4 669	647	183			436	27	11
6. Dementia*	1 345	548	797	36	16	29	135	332	37	14	28	189	529
7. Parkinson disease	82	44	39				19	24				16	22
8. Multiple sclerosis	162	70	92			62	6	2			80	9	3
9. Drug use	1 640	1 071	569	-	59	950	52	9	-	31	504	28	5
10. Post-traumatic stress disorder	242	91	151	4	17	61	8	1	6	27	103	13	2
11. Obsessive-compulsive disorders	1 291	548	743	-	56	440	35	16	-	72	580	65	26
12. Panic disorder	614	203	411	-	19	147	37		-	19	320	61	10
F. Sense organ diseases	**1 218**	**582**	**637**	**19**	**4**	**23**	**154**	**383**	**13**	**5**	**22**	**173**	**423**
1. Glaucoma	213	77	136	-		1	39	37	2		4	76	56
2. Cataracts	950	476	474	2		16	113	345	2		11	95	366
G. Cardiovascular diseases	**13 616**	**8 333**	**5 283**	**97**	**42**	**1 253**	**3 041**	**3 900**	**63**	**27**	**686**	**1 447**	**3 060**
1. Rheumatic heart disease	169	71	97	1	5	29	25	12	1	5	39	36	17
2. Ischaemic heart disease	5 844	3 692	2 153			416	1 434	1 842			183	577	1 393
3. Cerebrovascular disease	4 460	2 643	1 818	9	9	428	961	1 235	6	7	261	536	1 008
4. Inflammatory heart diseases	580	360	220	18	9	134	120	80	14	6	72	63	66
H. Respiratory diseases	**5 584**	**2 452**	**3 132**	**184**	**121**	**614**	**578**	**954**	**100**	**110**	**668**	**1 246**	**1 007**
1. COPD*	2 240	1 054	1 186	18	4	173	282	577	11	4	144	497	531
2. Asthma	1 142	498	644	20	75	267	73	63	10	67	219	228	119
I. Digestive diseases	**4 130**	**2 563**	**1 566**	**57**	**26**	**586**	**1 245**	**650**	**45**	**22**	**396**	**581**	**522**
1. Peptic ulcer	207	134	72	-	1	30	54	49	-	1	15	23	33
2. Cirrhosis of the liver	1 498	1 149	349	3	2	289	629	227	2	2	84	163	98
3. Appendicitis	28	17	12	-	3	10	3	2	-	2	7	1	1
J. Genito-urinary diseases	**1 241**	**802**	**439**	**54**	**25**	**79**	**484**	**160**	**48**	**28**	**112**	**99**	**152**
1. Nephritis and nephrosis	481	241	240	31	20	55	58	77	29	22	50	52	87
2. Benign prostatic hypertrophy	429	429	-				396	33					
L. Musculo-skeletal diseases	**5 856**	**2 315**	**3 541**	**6**	**10**	**711**	**1 249**	**339**	**4**	**16**	**1 099**	**1 742**	**680**
1. Rheumatoid arthritis	1 031	223	808	-	-	105	86	33	-	6	467	239	96
2. Osteoarthritis	4 581	2 025	2 556			587	1 146	292			552	1 459	545

Annex Table 21q, continued. DALYs by age, sex and cause (thousands): Latin America and the Caribbean, 2020, optimistic scenario

Cause	Total	Male	Female	Males					Females				
				0-4	5-14	15-44	45-59	60+	0-4	5-14	15-44	45-59	60+
M. Congenital anomalies	1 797	887	910	837	25	19	4	2	863	20	18	5	3
N. Oral conditions	1 401	694	707	37	253	270	52	82	36	244	268	56	103
1. Dental caries	1 144	577	566	36	252	263	18	8	35	242	261	18	10
2. Periodontal disease	40	19	21	-	-	5	10	4	-	-	5	10	5
3. Edentulism	208	94	114	-	-	-	25	69	-	-	-	27	87
III. Injuries	20 404	14 555	5 849	807	1 481	10 008	1 698	561	607	790	3 483	612	357
A. Unintentional injuries	13 758	9 216	4 541	694	1 269	5 635	1 180	440	506	682	2 523	509	320
1. Road traffic accidents	7 152	4 638	2 514	133	707	3 171	486	141	99	441	1 663	228	82
2. Poisonings	123	70	53	17	7	32	10	4	13	6	25	5	4
3. Falls	1 380	928	451	122	194	416	111	86	60	66	147	77	101
4. Fires	228	125	103	29	26	48	14	8	27	27	32	11	7
5. Drownings	638	498	140	59	88	289	48	13	39	32	56	9	4
6. Other unintentional	4 238	2 957	1 280	333	247	1 678	512	188	269	110	600	179	123
B. Intentional injuries	6 646	5 338	1 308	113	212	4 373	519	122	101	108	960	103	37
1. Self-inflicted injuries	949	629	320	-	18	459	109	44	-	14	253	39	14
2. Violence	4 764	4 167	597	44	146	3 525	382	70	33	58	447	45	14
3. War	934	542	392	69	48	390	28	8	68	36	260	19	8

Notes:
A dash (-) symbol indicates fewer than 500 DALYs.
*IA6 is Bacterial meningitis and meningococcaemia; ID is Conditions arising during the perinatal period;
IIE6 is Dementia and other degenerative and hereditary CNS disorders; IIH1 is Chronic obstructive pulmonary disease.

Annex Table 21h. DALYs by age, sex and cause (thousands): Middle Eastern Crescent, 2020, optimistic scenario

Cause	Total	Male	Female	Males					Females				
				0–4	5–14	15–44	45–59	60+	0–4	5–14	15–44	45–59	60+
Population (millions)	*1 005*	*507*	*499*	*62*	*110*	*238*	*61*	*36*	*59*	*106*	*230*	*61*	*42*
All causes	**161 582**	**92 300**	**69 282**	**25 059**	**6 261**	**31 992**	**15 852**	**13 135**	**21 460**	**4 462**	**22 922**	**9 435**	**11 005**
I. Communicable, maternal, perinatal and nutritional conditions	***29 491***	***15 525***	***13 967***	***13 875***	***563***	***504***	***195***	***387***	***11 840***	***514***	***1 010***	***182***	***420***
A. Infectious and parasitic diseases	**12 284**	**6 712**	**5 571**	**5 788**	**248**	**384**	**158**	**135**	**4 847**	**204**	**248**	**110**	**162**
1. Tuberculosis	673	451	222	81	23	178	96	72	45	13	57	52	54
2. STDs excluding HIV	350	140	210	108	–	29	1	2	92	3	111	1	3
a. Syphilis	202	108	94	100	–	6	1	2	85	–	6	1	3
b. Chlamydia	102	14	88	2	–	11	–	–	2	2	83	–	–
c. Gonorrhoea	46	18	28	6	–	12	–	–	5	1	22	–	–
3. HIV	131	103	27	13	1	78	11	1	13	1	13	1	–
4. Diarrhoeal diseases	6 252	3 390	2 862	3 292	69	15	6	8	2 773	63	12	6	9
5. Childhood-cluster diseases	3 546	1 927	1 619	1 834	85	5	2	1	1 539	70	6	4	1
a. Pertussis	830	449	381	428	21	1	–	–	362	18	–	–	–
b. Poliomyelitis	206	124	82	122	–	1	–	–	81	–	–	–	–
c. Diphtheria	17	9	8	9	–	–	–	–	7	–	–	–	–
d. Measles	1 331	717	614	669	48	–	–	–	571	42	–	–	–
e. Tetanus	1 163	627	535	605	16	3	2	1	517	9	5	3	1
6. Bacterial meningitis*	268	145	123	118	3	12	6	6	101	3	6	6	7
7. Hepatitis B and hepatitis C	84	49	35	17	4	8	9	11	12	4	4	4	10
8. Malaria	92	51	41	17	16	13	3	2	15	13	7	3	2
9. Tropical-cluster diseases	69	46	24	10	14	14	4	3	6	8	6	2	2
a. Trypanosomiasis	–	–	–	–	–	–	–	–	–	–	–	–	–
b. Chagas disease	–	–	–	–	–	–	–	–	–	–	–	–	–
c. Schistosomiasis	34	23	11	1	6	10	4	2	–	2	5	2	1
d. Leishmaniasis	32	20	12	9	9	3	–	–	5	5	1	–	–
e. Lymphatic filariasis	3	2	1	–	–	1	–	–	–	–	1	–	–
f. Onchocerciasis	–	–	–	–	–	–	–	–	–	–	–	–	–
10. Leprosy	5	3	2	–	1	1	–	–	–	1	1	–	–
11. Dengue	–	–	–	–	–	–	–	–	–	–	–	–	–
12. Japanese encephalitis	–	–	–	–	–	–	–	–	–	–	–	–	–
13. Trachoma	126	33	93	–	–	4	9	20	–	–	6	23	64
14. Intestinal nematode infections	60	32	27	1	17	11	2	2	1	15	7	2	2
a. Ascariasis	28	15	13	1	14	–	–	–	1	12	–	–	–
b. Trichuriasis	–	–	–	–	–	–	–	–	–	–	–	–	–
c. Ancylostomiasis and necatoriasis	31	17	14	–	3	11	2	2	–	3	7	2	2

Annex Table 21h, continued. DALYs by age, sex and cause (thousands): Middle Eastern Crescent, 2020, optimistic scenario

Cause	Total	Male	Female	Males					Females				
				0-4	5-14	15-44	45-59	60+	0-4	5-14	15-44	45-59	60+
B. Respiratory infections	6 900	3 693	3 207	3 216	199	34	18	226	2 715	203	36	26	227
1. Lower respiratory infections	6 735	3 605	3 131	3 152	180	32	17	224	2 661	186	34	26	224
2. Upper respiratory infections	71	38	33	31	2	2	-	3	26	2	1	1	3
3. Otitis media	93	50	43	33	17	-	-	-	28	15	-	-	-
C. Maternal conditions	522	-	522	-	-	-	-	-	-	-	505	17	-
1. Maternal haemorrhage	54	-	54	-	-	-	-	-	-	-	50	4	-
2. Maternal sepsis	110	-	110	-	-	-	-	-	-	-	107	2	-
3. Hypertensive disorders of pregnancy	35	-	35	-	-	-	-	-	-	-	32	2	-
4. Obstructed labour	142	-	142	-	-	-	-	-	-	-	141	1	-
5. Abortion	51	-	51	-	-	-	-	-	-	-	49	1	-
D. Perinatal conditions*	6 990	3 716	3 274	3 716	-	-	-	-	3 274	-	-	-	-
E. Nutritional deficiencies	2 796	1 404	1 392	1 156	116	86	19	26	1 004	106	222	29	31
1. Protein-energy malnutrition	1 575	847	728	838	2	1	1	5	719	3	1	1	5
2. Iodine deficiency	99	52	47	49	3	-	-	-	42	3	-	-	-
3. Vitamin A deficiency	261	135	125	111	23	1	-	-	102	23	1	-	-
4. Iron-deficiency anaemia	861	369	492	159	88	83	18	21	140	79	219	28	26
II. Noncommunicable diseases	97 425	54 268	43 157	7 801	2 549	17 479	14 075	12 363	6 506	2 155	15 629	8 586	10 281
A. Malignant neoplasms	8 990	5 521	3 468	152	455	1 336	2 170	1 408	164	361	1 006	1 077	861
1. Mouth and oropharynx cancers	530	358	172	2	8	131	101	116	3	7	57	40	65
2. Oesophagus cancer	304	191	114	-	2	36	103	50	1	2	25	46	40
3. Stomach cancer	663	436	227	1	-	101	219	111	1	-	51	84	91
4. Colon and rectum cancers	377	208	169	1	1	72	60	74	2	4	42	35	86
5. Liver cancer	272	182	90	2	6	41	90	43	2	5	18	34	31
6. Pancreas cancer	145	96	49	-	-	23	49	23	-	-	7	22	20
7. Trachea, bronchus, lung cancers	2 097	1 768	329	2	7	318	928	512	2	6	52	157	111
8. Melanoma and other skin cancers	46	30	16	-	1	10	15	4	-	-	7	6	3
9. Breast cancer	444	-	444	-	-	-	-	-	-	-	173	185	82
10. Cervix uteri cancer	270	-	270	-	-	-	-	-	-	1	89	126	54
11. Corpus uteri cancer	59	-	59	-	-	-	-	-	-	-	11	27	21
12. Ovary cancer	141	-	141	-	-	-	-	-	3	8	64	46	20
13. Prostate cancer	109	109	-	-	-	6	33	68	-	-	-	-	-
14. Bladder cancer	309	255	54	1	3	53	114	84	-	1	11	21	20
15. Lymphomas and multiple myeloma	397	276	120	17	67	115	42	35	13	34	37	14	22
16. Leukaemia	606	331	275	32	120	119	31	30	45	117	65	18	31
C. Diabetes mellitus	1 505	774	731	46	37	211	290	191	45	34	118	250	284
D. Endocrine disorders	1 061	542	519	337	44	82	55	24	329	67	59	37	27

Annex Table 21h, continued. DALYs by age, sex and cause (thousands): Middle Eastern Crescent, 2020, optimistic scenario

Cause	Total	Male	Female	Males					Females				
				0-4	5-14	15-44	45-59	60+	0-4	5-14	15-44	45-59	60+
E. Neuro-psychiatric conditions	**24 907**	**11 834**	**13 074**	**781**	**573**	**9 219**	**898**	**363**	**640**	**491**	**10 245**	**1 181**	**518**
1. Unipolar major depression	10 036	3 549	6 487			2 998	451	100			5 466	815	206
2. Bipolar disorder	2 805	1 422	1 383			1 321	79	22			1 279	78	26
3. Schizophrenia	2 949	1 542	1 406			1 527	9	6			1 388	10	8
4. Epilepsy	415	232	182	44	58	102	20	8	36	66	61	13	6
5. Alcohol use	540	486	55			451	29	6			51	2	1
6. Dementia*	594	282	312	55	16	33	56	121	64	17	34	35	163
7. Parkinson disease	148	78	70				36	43				30	39
8. Multiple sclerosis	227	99	127				6	2				9	3
9. Drug use	1 885	1 693	192		107	1 510	66	11		12	171	7	1
10. Post-traumatic stress disorder	376	143	234	8	33	92	8	1	13	54	151	13	2
11. Obsessive-compulsive disorders	1 970	851	1 118		114	682	40	16		146	878	70	25
12. Panic disorder	904	307	596		38	227	41			39	483	66	10
F. Sense organ diseases	**2 229**	**1 178**	**1 051**	**3**		**54**	**559**	**561**	**4**	**1**	**39**	**450**	**557**
1. Glaucoma	280	106	175			2	71	33			4	124	47
2. Cataracts	1 931	1 064	867	3		48	486	527	2		31	324	509
G. Cardiovascular diseases	**29 000**	**18 165**	**10 835**	**1 770**	**630**	**3 111**	**5 890**	**6 764**	**989**	**486**	**1 471**	**2 405**	**5 485**
1. Rheumatic heart disease	649	360	290	2	54	248	47	10	1	55	181	42	11
2. Ischaemic heart disease	12 598	8 142	4 456			1 160	3 199	3 783			418	1 073	2 965
3. Cerebrovascular disease	4 665	2 709	1 956	95	125	486	896	1 107	54	90	214	506	1 093
4. Inflammatory heart diseases	2 183	1 367	816	339	114	414	318	182	233	81	213	148	142
H. Respiratory diseases	**9 945**	**5 484**	**4 461**	**853**	**368**	**1 123**	**1 285**	**1 855**	**516**	**307**	**910**	**1 325**	**1 403**
1. COPD*	3 431	1 861	1 570	91	21	281	372	1 095	65	35	228	555	688
2. Asthma	1 321	847	474	71	169	390	131	85	15	62	205	112	79
I. Digestive diseases	**5 386**	**3 195**	**2 191**	**621**	**90**	**602**	**1 288**	**592**	**698**	**80**	**358**	**622**	**433**
1. Peptic ulcer	176	129	47		1	39	60	28		1	16	18	13
2. Cirrhosis of the liver	1 039	653	386	7	11	119	344	173	5	28	63	163	128
3. Appendicitis	80	48	32	1	11	29	5	2	1	11	16	3	1
J. Genito-urinary diseases	**3 230**	**2 091**	**1 139**	**201**	**95**	**558**	**928**	**309**	**167**	**84**	**311**	**332**	**245**
1. Nephritis and nephrosis	717	385	331	84	48	115	73	64	75	60	86	56	54
2. Benign prostatic hypertrophy	487	487	-			1	451	35					-
L. Musculo-skeletal diseases	**1 968**	**853**	**1 115**	**18**	**6**	**438**	**290**	**100**	**15**	**6**	**403**	**459**	**232**
1. Rheumatoid arthritis	368	211	157			200	8	3		3	78	56	20
2. Osteoarthritis	1 488	587	901			220	274	93			304	392	205

Annex Table 21h, continued. DALYs by age, sex and cause (thousands): Middle Eastern Crescent, 2020, optimistic scenario

Cause	Total	Male	Female	Males					Females				
				0-4	5-14	15-44	45-59	60+	0-4	5-14	15-44	45-59	60+
M. Congenital anomalies	5 858	2 971	2 887	2 839	52	64	12	4	2 773	55	38	15	6
N. Oral conditions	2 980	1 473	1 507	129	173	623	378	170	123	167	618	392	207
1. Dental caries	1 347	678	668	128	172	226	97	55	122	165	219	97	65
2. Periodontal disease	42	21	21	-	-	20	1	-	-	-	19	1	-
3. Edentulism	1 571	768	803	-	-	373	280	114	-	-	368	294	141
III. Injuries	*34 666*	*22 508*	*12 158*	*3 382*	*3 149*	*14 009*	*1 583*	*385*	*3 113*	*1 792*	*6 282*	*667*	*304*
A. Unintentional injuries	16 624	11 688	4 936	2 095	1 756	6 589	1 015	234	1 806	850	1 768	348	164
1. Road traffic accidents	6 586	5 052	1 534	157	820	3 557	428	90	135	452	773	124	49
2. Poisonings	529	336	193	82	16	166	60	12	77	12	72	23	10
3. Falls	2 009	1 277	732	443	300	439	76	19	381	116	166	48	20
4. Fires	865	387	478	139	83	133	25	7	144	80	221	21	12
5. Drownings	1 076	750	326	256	145	309	32	8	222	37	56	7	3
6. Other unintentional	5 560	3 887	1 673	1 018	391	1 986	394	98	848	152	480	124	69
B. Intentional injuries	18 042	10 819	7 222	1 288	1 393	7 420	568	151	1 307	943	4 514	319	140
1. Self-inflicted injuries	2 694	1 817	877	-	520	1 059	185	53	-	240	519	76	43
2. Violence	2 236	1 484	752	297	132	946	88	21	321	139	242	38	12
3. War	13 112	7 518	5 594	991	740	5 415	294	77	986	563	3 753	206	86

Notes:
A dash (-) symbol indicates fewer than 500 DALYs.
*IA6 is Bacterial meningitis and meningococcaemia; ID is Conditions arising during the perinatal period;
IIE6 is Dementia and other degenerative and hereditary CNS disorders; IIH1 is Chronic obstructive pulmonary disease.

Annex Table 21i. DALYs by age, sex and cause (thousands): World, 2020, optimistic scenario

Cause	Total	Male	Female	Males					Females				
				0-4	5-14	15-44	45-59	60+	0-4	5-14	15-44	45-59	60+
Population (millions)	*7 895*	*3 929*	*3 967*	*377*	*693*	*1 768*	*639*	*452*	*360*	*666*	*1 722*	*651*	*568*
All causes	*1 295 628*	*745 946*	*549 682*	*136 002*	*40 539*	*261 933*	*160 885*	*146 587*	*113 368*	*29 746*	*180 870*	*98 156*	*127 541*
I. Communicable, maternal, perinatal and nutritional conditions	*222 754*	*118 455*	*104 299*	*84 111*	*5 831*	*18 138*	*4 157*	*6 217*	*67 397*	*5 774*	*21 128*	*3 507*	*6 493*
A. Infectious and parasitic diseases	134 807	72 883	61 924	45 244	3 970	16 848	3 641	3 180	35 593	3 912	16 548	2 795	3 076
1. Tuberculosis	22 343	11 347	10 995	1 022	726	5 587	2 121	1 891	994	986	5 744	1 783	1 489
2. STDs excluding HIV	7 053	2 703	4 350	1 645	17	960	18	62	1 422	66	2 741	28	93
a. Syphilis	2 483	1 328	1 155	1 115	2	137	13	61	910	2	137	17	89
b. Chlamydia	2 477	390	2 087	112	6	270	1	1	108	47	1 922	8	2
c. Gonorrhoea	2 090	984	1 106	418	10	552	3	1	404	18	680	3	1
3. HIV	22 797	12 533	10 264	2 464	401	8 596	887	186	2 329	404	7 080	379	72
4. Diarrhoeal diseases	33 127	18 618	14 510	17 368	601	206	95	347	13 207	578	166	108	450
5. Childhood-cluster diseases	24 889	13 755	11 134	12 813	783	100	29	30	10 294	712	63	31	34
a. Pertussis	4 801	2 652	2 150	2 526	126	–	1	–	2 039	111	–	–	–
b. Poliomyelitis	960	579	381	570	–	6	1	–	376	3	3	1	–
c. Diphtheria	97	53	44	49	3	–	1	–	41	3	–	1	–
d. Measles	13 908	7 680	6 228	7 122	554	2	1	–	5 731	494	2	1	–
e. Tetanus	5 123	2 792	2 332	2 545	99	90	28	29	2 107	103	58	30	33
6. Bacterial meningitis*	1 562	843	719	659	18	69	41	55	552	16	40	43	66
7. Hepatitis B and hepatitis C	473	275	197	78	20	46	55	76	54	17	24	24	79
8. Malaria	14 154	8 184	5 970	7 372	388	311	71	42	5 285	352	203	77	53
9. Tropical-cluster diseases	2 046	1 353	694	93	400	615	159	86	75	207	216	129	67
a. Trypanosomiasis	338	186	152	11	67	74	26	7	18	63	49	18	4
b. Chagas disease	130	70	60	–	–	34	18	17	–	–	25	19	16
c. Schistosomiasis	378	243	135	16	82	102	24	20	9	49	47	15	14
d. Leishmaniasis	280	189	91	29	82	70	5	3	16	45	25	3	3
e. Lymphatic filariasis	667	508	159	32	145	277	46	9	28	34	42	45	11
f. Onchocerciasis	253	157	96	4	23	58	41	31	3	17	29	29	19
10. Leprosy	126	64	62	2	18	34	8	3	3	17	33	8	2
11. Dengue	85	41	44	15	24	1	–	–	16	27	–	1	–
12. Japanese encephalitis	91	49	42	37	10	2	1	1	31	9	1	1	–
13. Trachoma	484	124	360	–	–	12	26	86	–	–	19	70	270
14. Intestinal nematode infections	1 027	540	487	8	357	119	29	27	7	332	85	30	33
a. Ascariasis	315	164	152	8	154	1	–	–	7	144	1	–	–
b. Trichuriasis	327	169	158	–	169	–	–	–	–	157	–	–	–
c. Ancylostomiasis and necatoriasis	384	207	177	–	34	118	29	27	–	31	84	30	32

Annex Table 21i, continued. DALYs by age, sex and cause (thousands): World, 2020, optimistic scenario

Cause	Total	Male	Female	Males 0-4	Males 5-14	Males 15-44	Males 45-59	Males 60+	Females 0-4	Females 5-14	Females 15-44	Females 45-59	Females 60+
B. Respiratory infections	**38 867**	**21 270**	**17 597**	**17 073**	**1 153**	**364**	**234**	**2 447**	**13 299**	**1 109**	**289**	**223**	**2 677**
1. Lower respiratory infections	37 943	20 771	17 172	16 724	1 048	350	229	2 419	13 019	1 012	279	218	2 645
2. Upper respiratory infections	417	227	190	169	14	12	5	27	130	13	9	5	32
3. Otitis media	507	272	235	180	91	2	–	–	149	84	1	–	–
C. Maternal conditions	**3 243**		**3 243**							**92**	**3 104**	**48**	
1. Maternal haemorrhage	403		403							21	371	11	
2. Maternal sepsis	603		603							14	583	6	
3. Hypertensive disorders of pregnancy	207		207							11	190	6	
4. Obstructed labour	678		678							7	668	3	
5. Abortion	556		556							12	540	5	
D. Perinatal conditions*	**31 097**	**16 863**	**14 234**	**16 863**					**14 234**				
E. Nutritional deficiencies	**14 740**	**7 439**	**7 301**	**4 932**	**708**	**926**	**283**	**590**	**4 273**	**661**	**1 188**	**441**	**739**
1. Protein-energy malnutrition	6 966	3 718	3 248	3 578	21	16	14	89	3 087	27	14	12	108
2. Iodine deficiency	342	182	159	170	9	1	–	–	146	9	3	1	–
3. Vitamin A deficiency	1 082	583	499	470	107	5	–	–	397	99	3	–	–
4. Iron-deficiency anaemia	6 327	2 945	3 382	709	569	901	268	498	638	526	1 165	427	625
II. Noncommunicable diseases	***795 135***	***445 790***	***349 344***	***30 445***	***11 249***	***131 018***	***138 714***	***134 364***	***28 039***	***9 648***	***112 349***	***84 063***	***115 245***
A. Malignant neoplasms	**135 450**	**84 328**	**51 122**	**989**	**2 666**	**15 383**	**36 223**	**29 066**	**1 227**	**1 872**	**10 097**	**19 024**	**18 902**
1. Mouth and oropharynx cancers	7 641	5 142	2 498	16	44	1 176	2 136	1 769	29	53	539	873	1 004
2. Oesophagus cancer	8 012	5 660	2 352	–	1	611	2 830	2 217	1	2	219	929	1 201
3. Stomach cancer	15 645	10 866	4 780	3	15	1 199	5 297	4 352	1	8	714	1 774	2 282
4. Colon and rectum cancers	7 618	4 389	3 229	4	18	776	1 555	2 036	6	17	424	983	1 798
5. Liver cancer	14 249	11 224	3 025	23	71	3 109	5 654	2 367	27	53	535	1 267	1 141
6. Pancreas cancer	2 643	1 706	937	–	–	216	752	738	2	2	79	310	544
7. Trachea, bronchus, lung cancers	25 931	20 159	5 772	10	29	2 485	10 446	7 189	6	11	467	2 508	2 780
8. Melanoma and other skin cancers	825	457	368	1	3	119	192	142	1	2	82	129	152
9. Breast cancer	5 983		5 983						5	8	1 560	2 669	1 741
10. Cervix uteri cancer	5 197		5 197						2	3	1 252	2 627	1 313
11. Corpus uteri cancer	955		955						2	4	115	457	376
12. Ovary cancer	1 957		1 957						31	54	587	719	566
13. Prostate cancer	2 677	2 677	–	–	–	48	484	2 140					
14. Bladder cancer	2 369	1 875	495	1	4	179	628	1 060	2	3	58	141	291
15. Lymphomas and multiple myeloma	4 952	3 230	1 722	186	585	946	788	725	155	293	356	382	536
16. Leukaemia	5 650	3 233	2 418	251	704	1 190	631	457	320	518	770	412	397
C. Diabetes mellitus	**9 463**	**4 528**	**4 935**	**166**	**137**	**989**	**1 627**	**1 609**	**175**	**128**	**534**	**1 425**	**2 673**
D. Endocrine disorders	**5 014**	**2 453**	**2 561**	**1 163**	**151**	**508**	**340**	**290**	**1 019**	**179**	**403**	**400**	**560**

Annex Table 21i, continued. DALYs by age, sex and cause (thousands): World, 2020, optimistic scenario

Cause	Total	Male	Female	Males 0-4	5-14	15-44	45-59	60+	Females 0-4	5-14	15-44	45-59	60+
E. Neuro-psychiatric conditions	**203 320**	**98 303**	**105 018**	**2 262**	**2 638**	**74 921**	**11 348**	**7 134**	**2 276**	**2 568**	**75 466**	**13 576**	**11 132**
1. Unipolar major depression	79 028	27 732	51 296	-	-	21 976	4 583	1 173	-	1	40 313	8 444	2 539
2. Bipolar disorder	21 300	10 730	10 570			9 673	795	261			9 424	802	343
3. Schizophrenia	17 317	9 086	8 230			8 950	67	69			8 088	40	103
4. Epilepsy	3 188	1 879	1 309	170	338	1 019	246	106	181	352	535	125	116
5. Alcohol use	22 962	20 269	2 693			17 637	2 113	519			2 406	199	89
6. Dementia*	14 683	6 018	8 665	311	119	285	1 471	3 832	389	137	288	1 600	6 252
7. Parkinson disease	1 848	870	979			1	337	531	1		1	339	638
8. Multiple sclerosis	1 783	778	1 005			682	69	26			871	92	42
9. Drug use	7 974	6 527	1 447		425	5 779	273	49		97	1 274	64	12
10. Post-traumatic stress disorder	2 762	1 044	1 719	50	208	683	87	16	82	339	1 128	141	30
11. Obsessive-compulsive disorders	14 933	6 392	8 541		717	5 068	411	196		917	6 562	740	322
12. Panic disorder	7 196	2 396	4 800		214	1 738	442	2		250	3 708	713	130
F. Sense organ diseases	**21 760**	**10 779**	**10 981**	**76**	**8**	**561**	**5 284**	**4 850**	**64**	**16**	**522**	**5 108**	**5 271**
1. Glaucoma	5 839	2 171	3 668	4		110	1 372	684	6		172	2 443	1 047
2. Cataracts	15 566	8 466	7 100	32	2	421	3 870	4 142	24	2	288	2 604	4 182
G. Cardiovascular diseases	**199 058**	**126 306**	**72 752**	**4 222**	**1 722**	**16 796**	**45 497**	**58 069**	**2 617**	**1 410**	**6 813**	**15 088**	**46 823**
1. Rheumatic heart disease	6 077	3 565	2 513	6	143	1 231	1 460	724	14	155	801	834	709
2. Ischaemic heart disease	81 574	53 319	28 255			4 916	20 857	27 546	173		1 530	5 514	21 037
3. Cerebrovascular disease	59 739	36 346	23 393	492	451	4 487	12 866	18 051	338	327	1 941	5 142	15 645
4. Inflammatory heart diseases	10 903	6 999	3 904	867	319	2 167	2 299	1 348	683	268	900	864	1 188
H. Respiratory diseases	**84 695**	**47 862**	**36 834**	**2 600**	**1 694**	**8 725**	**14 411**	**20 431**	**1 510**	**1 284**	**6 707**	**11 532**	**15 801**
1. COPD*	46 924	27 798	19 126	260	94	3 244	9 084	15 116	191	99	2 060	6 126	10 649
2. Asthma	11 088	6 058	5 030	331	931	2 891	1 161	744	128	592	2 315	1 223	772
I. Digestive diseases	**41 093**	**25 540**	**15 553**	**1 351**	**387**	**5 075**	**11 924**	**6 803**	**1 402**	**448**	**2 827**	**5 540**	**5 337**
1. Peptic ulcer	2 714	1 814	900	4	6	455	785	564	5	6	205	302	382
2. Cirrhosis of the liver	13 571	9 912	3 659	39	40	1 946	5 375	2 512	33	60	620	1 660	1 286
3. Appendicitis	724	439	285	8	86	266	55	23	9	86	143	31	17
J. Genito-urinary diseases	**14 850**	**9 700**	**5 149**	**989**	**539**	**1 601**	**4 597**	**1 974**	**758**	**471**	**952**	**1 206**	**1 763**
1. Nephritis and nephrosis	6 702	3 605	3 097	705	434	956	690	820	624	408	505	569	992
2. Benign prostatic hypertrophy	3 861	3 861	-	5		5	3 246	605					
L. Musculo-skeletal diseases	**30 930**	**11 565**	**19 365**	**43**	**37**	**3 563**	**5 452**	**2 470**	**52**	**63**	**5 373**	**9 088**	**4 789**
1. Rheumatoid arthritis	5 226	1 484	3 743	1	1	611	530	342	-	31	1 513	1 229	969
2. Osteoarthritis	24 213	9 568	14 645			2 826	4 808	1 934			3 586	7 629	3 430

Annex Table 21i, continued. DALYs by age, sex and cause (thousands): World, 2020, optimistic scenario

Cause	Total	Male	Female	Males					Females				
				0-4	5-14	15-44	45-59	60+	0-4	5-14	15-44	45-59	60+
M. Congenital anomalies	32 022	15 800	16 222	14 985	297	416	73	30	15 556	304	·236	82	44
N. Oral conditions	12 687	6 135	6 552	532	783	2 004	1 510	1 306	508	770	2 025	1 593	1 655
1. Dental caries	6 399	3 199	3 199	525	777	1 139	483	277	501	756	1 110	493	340
2. Periodontal disease	419	208	211	-	-	157	36	15	-	-	156	37	18
3. Edentulism	5 731	2 692	3 039	-	-	691	989	1 012	-	-	686	1 059	1 295
III. Injuries	277 739	181 701	96 038	21 445	23 460	112 776	18 014	6 006	17 932	14 324	47 393	10 586	5 804
A. Unintentional injuries	178 774	117 955	60 820	17 137	18 865	64 852	12 828	4 272	13 601	11 341	23 851	7 591	4 437
1. Road traffic accidents	75 592	51 950	23 642	2 256	9 129	33 495	5 472	1 598	1 478	5 903	12 237	2 870	1 154
2. Poisonings	6 309	3 624	2 685	1 346	258	1 255	576	189	953	166	932	425	209
3. Falls	19 896	11 556	8 339	2 627	2 926	4 153	1 194	657	2 548	1 195	2 047	1 383	1 167
4. Fires	11 147	4 968	6 179	1 839	928	1 646	395	161	1 598	1 269	2 547	441	324
5. Drownings	11 676	7 931	3 745	2 529	2 094	2 662	450	196	1 640	829	773	280	223
6. Other unintentional	54 154	37 925	16 229	6 540	3 531	21 641	4 742	1 471	5 384	1 979	5 315	2 191	1 360
B. Intentional injuries	98 965	63 746	35 218	4 308	4 595	47 924	5 186	1 734	4 332	2 983	23 542	2 995	1 367
1. Self-inflicted injuries	26 067	14 331	11 736	-	960	9 585	2 634	1 152	-	488	8 497	1 837	915
2. Violence	31 408	25 387	6 022	1 089	1 244	20 925	1 761	368	1 159	708	3 338	602	214
3. War	41 489	24 028	17 461	3 219	2 391	17 414	791	214	3 173	1 787	11 706	556	238

Notes:
A dash (-) symbol indicates fewer than 500 DALYs.
*IA6 is Bacterial meningitis and meningococcaemia; ID is Conditions arising during the perinatal period;
IIE6 is Dementia and other degenerative and hereditary CNS disorders; IIH1 is Chronic obstructive pulmonary disease.

INDEX